HYPERTENSION PRIMER
THIRD EDITION

This book was developed with an educational grant from
AstraZeneca Pharmaceuticals

HYPERTENSION PRIMER
THIRD EDITION

The Essentials of High Blood Pressure

Senior Editors
Joseph L. Izzo, Jr, MD, and Henry R. Black, MD

Section Editors
Theodore L. Goodfriend, MD; James R. Sowers, MD; Alan B. Weder, MD; Lawrence J. Appel, MD, MPH; Donald G. Vidt, MD; Sheldon G. Sheps, MD; Domenic A. Sica, MD

From the Council on High Blood Pressure Research
American Heart Association

Editor: Ruth Weinberg
Managing Editor: Jennifer Kullgren
Production Editor: Lucinda Myers Ewing, Silverchair Science + Communications
Marketing Manager: Sara Bodison
Purchasing Manager, Clinical and Healthcare: Jennifer Jett
Compositor: Silverchair Science + Communications
Printer: Victor Graphics, Inc.

© 2003 American Heart Association

Dallas, Texas

Format, design, and index © 2003
Lippincott Williams & Wilkins
530 Walnut Street
Philadelphia, PA 19106 USA
LWW.com

Printed in the USA

Cataloging-in-Publication data is on file with the Library of Congress.
ISBN: 0-7817-4509-8

Care has been taken to confirm the accuracy of the information presented and to describe generally accepted practices. However, the authors, editors, and publisher are not responsible for errors or omissions or for any consequences from application of the information in this book and make no warranty, expressed or implied, with respect to the currency, completeness, or accuracy of the contents of the publication. Application of this information in a particular situation remains the professional responsibility of the practitioner.

The authors, editors, and publisher have exerted every effort to ensure that drug selection and dosage set forth in this text are in accordance with current recommendations and practice at the time of publication. However, in view of ongoing research, changes in government regulations, and the constant flow of information relating to drug therapy and drug reactions, the reader is urged to check the package insert for each drug for any change in indications and dosage and for added warnings and precautions. This is particularly important when the recommended agent is a new or infrequently employed drug.

Some drugs and medical devices presented in this publication have Food and Drug Administration (FDA) clearance for limited use in restricted research settings. It is the responsibility of the health care provider to ascertain the FDA status of each drug or device planned for use in their clinical practice.

03 04 05 06
1 2 3 4 5 6 7 8 9 10

Preface

We are delighted to bring you the *Hypertension Primer, Third Edition*, a decade after the *First Edition* was launched. Given the breadth and depth of information available in the continuously expanding field of hypertension, our *Primer* remains a "small introductory book" on the subject. Nonetheless, previous readers will immediately note a substantial expansion in scope and substance. In addition, the *Third Edition* is fundamentally different from its predecessors in that it has been formatted to appear as an electronic version as well as in print form. Thus, one of our remaining goals for this unique hypertext system has been realized. In the *Third Edition*, many areas have been expanded, including genetics, molecular and cellular mechanisms, population medicine, and, perhaps most important, clinical management. The clinical section has received the greatest additional attention, especially the chapters on individual drugs and specific management issues.

The basic format of the *Primer* remains the same: short, state-of-the-art chapters written by widely acknowledged experts, each of which provides a unique synthesis of information on a single aspect of the broader whole. This format has been very popular with readers, because it allows them to quickly and easily find the answers to specific questions. Although each chapter is written so that it can stand alone, it is best viewed in the context of several larger themes. This need is met by the inclusion of the "See Alsos" in each chapter that link the reader to important related information in basic science, population science, or clinical management. Other hypertext linkages will be possible as the electronic version is further developed.

The *Primer* is the fruit of the labor of many scholar-contributors who represent the Council for High Blood Pressure Research (CHBPR) of the American Heart Association. Each has achieved a substantial personal reputation for specific expertise in our field, and it is the desire to illuminate and disseminate their individual wisdom that has been the rationale for the *Hypertension Primer* project. We owe a very large debt of gratitude to each of the 220 scholars who wrote our 174 chapters. Each has distilled the essence of an individual topic into a pithy summary for medical specialists, primary care clinicians, trainees, and other health professionals. *Primer* contributors and members of the CHBPR can take pride that the royalties from the book have been returned to the CHBPR for support of recurring educational programs, such as the Hypertension Summer School for promising research scholars.

The *Primer* would not have been possible without the skilled editors and staff who have guided the process. The section editors provided the initial review and editing of the original submissions. In the Basic Science area, Drs. Theodore Goodfriend and James Sowers have been with us on all three editions, whereas Dr. Alan Weder has joined us on the *Third Edition*. To oversee the Population Science area, we were fortunate to attract Dr. Lawrence Appel. In the Clinical Management area, Drs. Domenic Sica, Sheldon Sheps, and Donald Vidt returned by popular demand. We thank all of them for their superb counsel and dedication. In addition, the administrative staff performed superbly. We are particularly indebted to Julie Kostyo, who has again kept us all together in her role as Project Manager, and to Norma Sandoval.

We are grateful to AstraZeneca Pharmaceuticals for their continued educational grant support for the *Hypertension Primer* project. We would like to recognize specifically Tammi Gaskins, David Snow, and Robert Lamb for their ongoing support of this critical publication.

On a more solemn note, we mourn the passing of four of our colleagues and contributors from the *Second Edition*: Donald J. Reis, MD; David H. P. Streeten, MB, DPhil, FRCP, FACP; Jay M. Sullivan, MD; and Roger R. Williams, MD. We can only hope that these outstanding physician-scientists would approve of our continuing efforts and the contributions of those of us who remain.

Finally, to you, our readers, we hope that this edition provides enough useful and up-to-date information on hypertension that you will join with us in studying the condition and working for its control in our patients. Hypertension remains the most common reason Americans visit a physician. In 2003, the publication of the *Hypertension Primer, Third Edition* and the Seventh Report of the Seventh Joint National Committee on the Prevention, Detection, Evaluation and Treatment of High Blood Pressure (JNC VII) should provide an improved knowledge base and clearer guidance to accomplish the task.

Joseph L. Izzo, Jr, MD
Henry R. Black, MD

Contents

Contributing Authors

Greti Aguilera, MD
Chief, Section on Endocrine Physiology
Developmental Endocrinology Branch
National Institute of Child Health and Human Development
National Institutes of Health
Bethesda, Maryland

Suhail Ahmad, MD
Acting Section Chief, Department of Nephrology
Medical Director, Department of Dialysis/Apheresis
University of Washington School of Medicine
Medical Director
Scribner Kidney Center
Lake City Kidney Center
Seattle, Washington

Michael H. Alderman, MD
Professor, Departments of Medicine and Epidemiology and Social Medicine
Albert Einstein College of Medicine of Yeshiva University
Bronx, New York

Sharon Anderson, MD
Professor, Department of Medicine
Division of Nephrology and Hypertension
Oregon Health & Science University School of Medicine
Portland, Oregon

Lawrence J. Appel, MD, MPH
Professor of Medicine, Epidemiology, and International Health
Center for Human Nutrition
Department of Medicine
Johns Hopkins Hospital
Baltimore, Maryland

Donna K. Arnett, MSPH, PhD
Associate Professor, Department of Epidemiology
University of Minnesota Medical School—Twin Cities
Minneapolis, Minnesota

Kenneth M. Baker, MD
Professor and Director, Division of Molecular Cardiology
Mayborn Chair in Cardiovascular Research
The Texas A&M University System Health Science Center College of Medicine
College Station, Texas

George L. Bakris, MD
Professor of Preventive and Internal Medicine
Department of Preventive Medicine
Rush-Presbyterian–St. Luke's Medical Center
Chicago, Illinois

Tamas Balla, MD, PhD
Senior Investigator, Endocrinology and Reproduction Research Branch
National Institute of Child Health and Human Development
National Institutes of Health
Bethesda, Maryland

Jan N. Basile, MD
Associate Professor of Medicine
Department of Primary Care
Ralph H. Johnson VA Medical Center
Medical University of South Carolina College of Medicine
Charleston, South Carolina

Gary L. Baumbach, MD
Professor of Medicine
Department of Pathology
University of Iowa Hospitals and Clinics
Iowa City, Iowa

William H. Beierwaltes, PhD
Professor, Department of Medicine
Hypertension and Vascular Research Division
Henry Ford Hospital
Detroit, Michigan

Kathleen H. Berecek, PhD
Professor, Departments of Physiology and Biophysics
University of Alabama at Birmingham
Birmingham, Alabama

Bradford C. Berk, MD, PhD
Chair, Department of Medicine
Director, Center for Cardiovascular Research
Paul N. Yu Professor of Cardiology
Department of Cardiology
University of Rochester School of Medicine and Dentistry
Rochester, New York

Henry R. Black, MD
Associate Vice President for Research
Associate Dean for Research
Rush Medical College
Charles J. and Margaret Roberts Professor and Chair, Department of Preventive Medicine
Professor, Internal Medicine
Rush-Presbyterian–St. Luke's Medical Center
Chicago, Illinois

Mordecai P. Blaustein, MD
Professor and Chair, Department of Physiology
University of Maryland School of Medicine
Baltimore, Maryland

George W. Booz, PhD
Assistant Professor, Department of Molecular Cardiology
The Texas A&M University System Health Science Center College of Medicine
College Station, Texas

Emmanuel L. Bravo, MD
Consultant/Staff
Department of Nephrology/Hypertension
Cleveland Clinic Foundation
Cleveland, Ohio

Robert D. Brown, Jr, MD, MPH
Associate Professor, Department of Neurology
Mayo Medical School
Chair, Division of Cerebrovascular Diseases
Mayo Clinic
Rochester, Minnesota

David A. Calhoun, MD
Associate Professor of Medicine
Vascular Biology and Hypertension Program
University of Alabama School of Medicine
Birmingham, Alabama

Vito M. Campese, MD
Professor of Medicine
Department of Internal Medicine and Nephrology
Keck School of Medicine of the University of Southern California
Los Angeles, California

Vincent J. Canzanello, MD
Associate Professor of Medicine
Mayo Medical School
Division of Hypertension and Internal Medicine
Mayo Clinic
Rochester, Minnesota

Robert M. Carey, MD
David A. Harrison III Professor of Medical Science
Department of Medicine
University of Virginia School of Medicine
Charlottesville, Virginia

Oscar A. Carretero, MD
Division Head, Hypertension and Vascular Research Division
Professor of Medicine
Case Western Reserve University
Henry Ford Health System
Detroit, Michigan

Kevin J. Catt, MD, PhD
Endocrinology and Reproduction Research Branch
National Institute of Child Health and Human Development
National Institutes of Health
Bethesda, Maryland

Mark W. Chapleau, PhD
Associate Professor of Medicine
Department of Internal Medicine
University of Iowa Roy J. and Lucille A. Carver School of Medicine
Research Health Science Specialist
Veterans Affairs Medical Center
Iowa City, Iowa

Mark C. Chappell, PhD
Associate Professor, Hypertension and Vascular Disease Center
Wake Forest University School of Medicine
Winston-Salem, North Carolina

Kanchan A. Chitaley, PhD
Postdoctoral Fellow, Department of Physiology
University of Michigan Medical School
Ann Arbor, Michigan

George T. Cicila, PhD
Associate Professor, Departments of Physiology and Molecular Medicine
Medical College of Ohio
Toledo, Ohio

Jay N. Cohn, MD
Professor, Department of Medicine
Cardiovascular Division
University of Minnesota Medical School
Minneapolis, Minnesota

Thomas G. Coleman, PhD
Professor Emeritus, Department of Physiology and Biophysics
University of Mississippi School of Medicine
Jackson, Mississippi

Richard S. Cooper, MD
Professor and Chair, Department of Preventive Medicine and
    Epidemiology
Loyola University Chicago Stritch School of Medicine
Maywood, Illinois

Allen W. Cowley, Jr, PhD
Professor and Chair, Department of Physiology
Medical College of Wisconsin
Milwaukee, Wisconsin

Carlos J. Crespo, PhD, MS
Associate Professor, Department of Social and Preventive Medicine
State University of New York at Buffalo
Buffalo, New York

Michael D. Cressman, DO
Senior Medical Director, Cardiovascular Therapeutic Area
AstraZeneca Pharmaceuticals
Wilmington, Delaware

Michael H. Criqui, MD, MPH
Professor and Vice Chair, Department of Family and
    Preventive Medicine
University of California, San Diego, School of Medicine
La Jolla, California

William C. Cushman, MD
Professor of Preventive Medicine and Medicine
Preventive Medicine Section
Veterans Affairs Medical Center
Memphis, Tennessee

Jeffrey A. Cutler, MD, MPH
Senior Scientific Advisor
Division of Epidemiology and Clinical Applications
National Heart, Lung, and Blood Institute
Bethesda, Maryland

Robert C. Davidson, MD
Department of Medicine and Nephrology
University of Washington School of Medicine
Seattle, WA

Prakash C. Deedwania, MD
Professor of Medicine
Department of Cardiology
University of California, San Francisco, School of Medicine
Fresno, California

Julie O. Denenberg, MA
Staff Research Associate II
Department of Family and Preventive Medicine
University of California, San Diego, School of Medicine
La Jolla, California

Richard B. Devereux, MD
Professor, Department of Medicine
Weill Medical College of Cornell University
New York, New York

Donald J. DiPette, MD
Professor, Department of Medicine
Texas A&M University Health Science Center College of Medicine
College Station, Texas
Scott and White Memorial Hospital and Clinic
Temple, Texas

Robert G. Dluhy, MD
Professor of Medicine
Division of Endocrinology, Diabetes, and Hypertension
Harvard Medical School
Brigham and Women's Hospital
Boston, Massachusetts

Mark E. Dunlap, MD
Associate Professor, Department of Medicine, Physiology, and Biophysics
Case Western Reserve University
Director of Cardiovascular Research
Louis Stokes Cleveland VA Medical Center
Cleveland, Ohio

Brent M. Egan, MD
Professor of Medicine and Pharmacology
Medical University of South Carolina College of Medicine
Charleston, South Carolina

Graeme F. Eisenhofer, PhD
Staff Scientist, Clinical Neurocardiology Section
National Institute of Neurological Disorders and Stroke
National Institutes of Health
Bethesda, Maryland

Paul Elliott, PhD, FRCP, FFPHM, FMedSci
Professor of Epidemiology and Public Health Medicine
Department of Epidemiology and Public Health
Division of Primary Care and Population Health Sciences Faculty of Medicine
Imperial College of Science, Technology, and Medicine
London, United Kingdom

William J. Elliott, MD, PhD
Professor of Preventive Medicine, Internal Medicine, and Pharmacology
Department of Preventive Medicine
Rush Medical College of Rush University
Rush-Presbyterian–St. Luke's Medical Center
Chicago, Illinois

Murray Epstein, MD, FACP
Professor, Department of Medicine
University of Miami School of Medicine
Miami, Florida

Ervin G. Erdös, MD
Professor, Department of Pharmacology
University of Illinois College of Medicine
Chicago, Illinois

Bonita E. Falkner, MD
Professor of Medicine and Pediatrics
Department of Nephrology
Jefferson Medical College of Thomas Jefferson University
Philadelphia, Pennsylvania

Ross D. Feldman, MD
R. W. Gunton Professor of Therapeutics
Departments of Medicine and Physiology and Pharmacology
University of Western Ontario
Faculty of Medicine and Dentistry
London, Ontario, Canada

Andrew Fenves, MD, FACP
Dallas Nephrology Associates
Baylor University Medical Center
University of Texas Southwestern Medical Center at Dallas
Dallas, Texas

Keith C. Ferdinand, MD
Professor of Clinical Pharmacology
Director, Heartbeats Life Center
Xavier University
New Orleans, Louisiana

Carlos M. Ferrario, MD
Professor and Director
Hypertension and Vascular Disease Center
Wake Forest University School of Medicine
Winston-Salem, North Carolina

John M. Flack, MD, MPH
Professor of Medicine
Department of Internal Medicine
Wayne State University School of Medicine
Detroit, Michigan

Robert N. Frank, MD
The Robert S. Jampel Professor of Ophthalmology
Professor of Anatomy and Cell Biology
Department of Opthalmology
Kresge Eye Institute
Wayne State University School of Medicine
Detroit, Michigan

Stanley S. Franklin, MD, FACP, FACC
Clinical Professor, Department of Medicine
University of California, Irvine, College of Medicine
Irvine, California

William H. Frishman, MD
Professor and Chairman, Department of Medicine
New York Medical College
Westchester Medical Center
Valhalla, New York

Edward D. Frohlich, MD
Alton Ochsner Distinguished Scientist
Ochsner Clinic Foundation
New Orleans, Louisiana

Arnost Fronek, MD, PhD
Professor of Surgery and Bioengineering
Department of Surgery
University of California, San Diego, School of Medicine
La Jolla, California

Curt D. Furberg, MD, PhD
Professor, Department of Public Health Sciences
Wake Forest University School of Medicine
Winston-Salem, North Carolina

Mario R. Garcia Palmieri, MD
University of Puerto Rico
Rio Pedras, Puerto Rico

James C. Garrison, PhD
Chair and Professor, Department of Pharmacology
University of Virginia School of Medicine
Charlottesville, Virginia

Benjamin Gavish, PhD
Intercure, Ltd.
Northern Industrial Area Lod, Israel

Haralambos Gavras, MD
Professor of Medicine
Medicine/Hypertension Section
Boston University School of Medicine
Boston, Massachusetts

Ray W. Gifford, Jr, MD, MS
Professor of Medicine
Department of Nephrology and Hypertension
Cleveland Clinic Foundation
Cleveland, Ohio

Thomas D. Giles, MD
Professor of Medicine
Department of Cardiology
Louisiana State University School of Medicine in New Orleans
New Orleans, Louisiana

David S. Goldstein, MD, PhD
Chief, Clinical Neurocardiology Section
National Institute of Neurological Disorders and Stroke
National Institutes of Health
Bethesda, Maryland

Mary K. Goldstein, MD, MS
Associate Professor, Department of Medicine
Stanford University School of Medicine
Veterans Administration Palo Alto Health Care System
Palo Alto, California

Celso E. Gomez-Sanchez, MD
Professor and Director of Endocrinology
Department of Medicine
University of Mississippi School of Medicine
Jackson, Mississippi

Theodore L. Goodfriend, MD
Professor of Medicine
Associate Chief of Staff for Research
University of Wisconsin Medical School
Madison, Wisconsin

Alan H. Gradman, MD
Professor, Department of Medicine
Temple University School of Medicine
Philadelphia, Pennsylvania
Chief, Division of Cardiovascular Diseases
Western Pennsylvania Hospital
Pittsburgh, Pennsylvania

John W. Graves, MD
Assistant Professor of Medicine
Divisions of Hypertension and Nephrology
Mayo Medical School
Mayo Clinic
Rochester, Minnesota

Suzanne G. Greenberg, PhD
Assistant Professor, Obstetrics and Gynecology
University of Cincinnati College of Medicine
Cincinnati, Ohio

Andrew S. Greene, PhD
Professor, Department of Physiology
Medical College of Wisconsin
Milwaukee, Wisconsin

Roger J. Grekin, MD
Professor, Department of Internal Medicine
University of Michigan Medical School
Veterans Administration Ann Arbor Healthcare System
Ann Arbor, Michigan

Kathy K. Griendling, PhD
Professor, Department of Medicine
Emory University School of Medicine
Atlanta, Georgia

Carlene M. Grim, MSN, SpDN
Shared Care Research and Education Consulting, Inc.
Milwaukee, Wisconsin

Clarence E. Grim, MS, MD
Professor of Medicine and Epidemiology
Department of Medicine
Medical College of Wisconsin
Milwaukee, Wisconsin

Richard H. Grimm, Jr, MD, PhD
Professor of Epidemiology and Cardiology
Department of Medicine
Division of Epidemiology
University of Minnesota Medical School—Twin Cities
Hennepin County Medical Center
Minneapolis, Minnesota

Ehud Grossman, MD
Professor, Department of Internal Medicine
Sackler Faculty of Medicine
Tel Aviv University
Head, Department of Internal Medicine
Sheba Medical Center
Tel Aviv, Israel

Rajeev Gupta, MD, FACC
Professor and Consultant, Department of Medicine
Mahatma Gandhi Institute of Medical Sciences
Monilek Hospital and Research Centre
Jaipur, India

Steven M. Haffner, MD
Professor, Department of Medicine
Division of Clinical Epidemiology
University of Texas Medical School at San Antonio
University of Texas Health Science Center
San Antonio, Texas

Julian P. J. Halcox, MA, MRCP
National Heart, Lung, and Blood Institute
National Institutes of Health
Rockville, Maryland

John E. Hall, PhD
Professor and Chair, Department of Physiology and Biophysics
University of Mississippi School of Medicine
University of Mississippi Medical Center
Jackson, Mississippi

John M. Hamlyn, PhD
Professor, Department of Physiology
University of Maryland School of Medicine
Baltimore, Maryland

David G. Harrison, MD
Professor, Department of Medicine
Division of Cardiology
Emory University School of Medicine
Atlanta, Georgia

William G. Haynes, MD
Associate Professor, Department of Internal Medicine
University of Iowa Roy J. and Lucille A. Carver College of
   Medicine
Iowa City, Iowa

Donald D. Heistad, MD
Professor of Internal Medicine
Department of Internal Medicine
University of Iowa Roy J. and Lucille A. Carver College of Medicine
Iowa City, Iowa

Linda A. Hershey, MD, PhD
Professor, Department of Neurology
State University of New York at Buffalo
VA WNY Healthcare System
Buffalo, New York

Carrie L. Hildebrant, MA
University of Minnesota Medical School—Twin Cities
Minneapolis, Minnesota

Martha N. Hill, RN, PhD
Dean and Professor, School of Nursing
Johns Hopkins University
Baltimore, Maryland

Brian B. Hoffman, MD
Professor, Department of Medicine
Stanford University School of Medicine
VA Palo Alto Healthcare System
Palo Alto, California

Norman K. Hollenberg, MD, PhD
Professor of Medicine
Departments of Radiology and Medicine
Harvard Medical School
Brigham and Women's Hospital
Boston, Massachusetts

Willa Hsueh, MD
Chief, Division of Endocrinology, Diabetes, and Hypertension
University of California, Los Angeles, School of Medicine
Los Angeles, California

Steven C. Hunt, PhD
Professor of Medicine
Departments of Cardiovascular Genetics and Internal Medicine
University of Utah School of Medicine
Salt Lake City, Utah

David J. Hyman, MD, MPH
Associate Professor, Departments of Medicine and Family and
   Community Medicine
Baylor College of Medicine
Ben Taub Hospital
Houston, Texas

Joseph L. Izzo, Jr, MD
Professor of Medicine and Pharmacology & Toxicology
Head, Division of Clinical Pharmacology
Department of Medicine
State University of New York at Buffalo
Buffalo, New York

Daniel W. Jones, MD
Associate Vice Chancellor for Health Affairs
Executive Associate Dean, School of Medicine
Herbert G. Langford Professor of Medicine
University of Mississippi School of Medicine
University of Mississippi Medical Center
Jackson, Mississippi

Stevo Julius, MD, ScD
Professor of Medicine and Physiology
Fredrick G. H. Huetwell Professor of Hypertension
Department of Internal Medicine
Division of Hypertension
University of Michigan Medical School
University of Michigan Health Systems
Ann Arbor, Michigan

William B. Kannel, MD, MPH
Professor of Medicine
Department of Epidemiology
Boston University School of Medicine
Senior Investigator
Framingham Heart Study
Boston, Massachusetts

Norman M. Kaplan, MD
Clinical Professor of Medicine
Department of Internal Medicine
University of Texas Southwestern Medical Center at Dallas Southwestern
   Medical School
Dallas, Texas

Tomas J. Kara, MD
Department of Medicine
Divisions of Cardiovascular Disease and Hypertension
Mayo Clinic and Mayo Foundation
Rochester, Minnesota

Sharon L. R. Kardia, PhD
Assistant Professor, Department of Epidemiology
University of Michigan Medical School
Ann Arbor, Michigan

Mofid N. Khalil-Ibrahim, MD, PhD
Department of Internal Medicine
Millard Fillmore Hospital
Buffalo, New York

Michael J. Klag, MD, MPH
Professor, Department of Medicine
The Johns Hopkins Medical Institutions
Baltimore, Maryland

Jyothsna Kodali, MD
Fellow, Department of Hypertension
Case Western Reserve University
University Hospitals of Cleveland
Cleveland, Ohio

John B. Kostis, MD
John C. Detwiler Professor of Cardiology
Professor of Medicine and Pharmacology
Chair, Department of Medicine
UMDNJ—Robert Wood Johnson Medical School
New Brunswick, New Jersey

Jane Morley Kotchen, MD, MPH
Professor, Department of Epidemiology
Health Policy Institute
Medical College of Wisconsin
Milwaukee, Wisconsin

Theodore A. Kotchen, MD
Professor of Medicine and Epidemiology
Associate Dean for Clinical Research
Department of Medicine
Medical College of Wisconsin
Milwaukee, Wisconsin

Lawrence R. Krakoff, MD
Professor of Medicine
Mount Sinai School of Medicine of New York University
New York, New York
Chief of Medicine
Englewood Hospital and Medical Center
Englewood, New Jersey

Daniel T. Lackland, PhD
Professor, Department of Biometry and Epidemiology
Medical University of South Carolina College of Medicine
Charleston, South Carolina

Edward G. Lakatta, MD
Director, Laboratory of Cardiovascular Science
National Institute on Aging
National Institutes of Health
Baltimore, Maryland

Lewis Landsberg, MD
Vice President for Medical Affairs
Dean and Professor of Medicine
Northwestern University, The Feinberg School of Medicine
Chicago, Illinois

Robert D. Langer, MD, MPH
Professor, Department of Family and Preventive Medicine
University of California, San Diego, School of Medicine
La Jolla, California

Farhana Latif, MD
Fellow, Department of Cardiology
Albert Einstein College of Medicine of Yeshiva University
Montefiore Medical Center
Bronx, New York

William J. Lawton, MD
Associate Professor, Department of Internal Medicine
University of Iowa Roy J. and Lucille A. Carver College of Medicine
Iowa City, Iowa

Thierry H. Le Jemtel, MD
Professor, Department of Medicine
Albert Einstein College of Medicine of Yeshiva University
Bronx, New York

Daniel Levy, MD
Director, Framingham Heart Study
National Heart, Lung, and Blood Institute
Framingham, Massachusetts

Marshall D. Lindheimer, MD
Emeritus Professor, Departments of Obstetrics and Gynecology and Medicine
University of Chicago Hospitals and Clinics
Chicago, Illinois

William M. Manger, MD, PhD
Professor of Clinical Medicine
Department of Medicine
New York University Medical Center
New York, New York

Barry J. Materson, MD, MBA
Professor of Medicine
University of Miami School of Medicine
Miami, Florida

Samy I. McFarlane, MD
Associate Professor, Department of Medicine
Division of Endocrinology, Diabetes and Hypertension
State University of New York–Downstate Medical Center and Kings
    County Hospital Center
Brooklyn, New York

John C. McGiff, MD
Professor and Chairman, Department of Pharmacology
New York Medical College
Valhalla, New York

Irene Meissner, MD, FRCPC
Associate Professor, Department of Neurology
Mayo Medical School
Mayo Clinic
Rochester, Minnesota

Franz H. Messerli, MD, FACC
Department of Internal Medicine
Section on Hypertensive Diseases
Ochsner Clinic Foundation
New Orleans, Louisiana

Mieczyslaw Michalkiewicz, DVM, PhD
Associate Professor, Department of Physiology
Medical College of Wisconsin
Milwaukee, Wisconsin

Edgar R. Miller III, MD, PhD
Assistant Professor of Medicine and Epidemiology
Department of Medicine
Johns Hopkins University School of Medicine
Baltimore, Maryland

Nancy Houston Miller, RN
Associate Director, Stanford Cardiac Rehabilitation Program
Departments of Medicine and Cardiovascular Medicine
Stanford University School of Medicine
Palo Alto, California

Brett M. Mitchell, PhD
Postdoctoral Fellow, Department of Physiology
Medical College of Georgia School of Medicine
Augusta, Georgia

Gary F. Mitchell, MD
Cardiovascular Engineering Inc.
Holliston, Massachusetts

Michael A. Moore, MD
Clinical Professor of Medicine and Nephrology
Hypertension and Vascular Center
Nephrology Division
Wake Forest University School of Medicine
Winston-Salem, North Carolina

Barbara J. Morgan, PhD
Associate Professor, Department of Orthopedics and Rehabilitation
University of Wisconsin Medical School
Madison, Wisconsin

Marvin Moser, MD
Clinical Professor of Medicine
Yale University School of Medicine
New Haven, Connecticut

Jerry L. Nadler, MD
Professor of Medicine
Department of Internal Medicine
Division of Endocrinology and Metabolism
University of Virginia School of Medicine
Charlottesville, Virginia

Joseph V. Nally, Jr, MD
Staff Nephrologist and Director of Nephrology Fellowship
Departments of Nephrology and Hypertension
Cleveland Clinic Foundation
Cleveland, Ohio

Alberto Nasjletti, MD
Professor, Department of Pharmacology
New York Medical College
Valhalla, New York

Samar A. Nasser, MS, PA-C
Physician Assistant, Department of Internal Medicine
University Health Center and Detroit Receiving Hospital
Detroit, Michigan

L. Gabriel Navar, PhD
Professor and Chair, Department of Physiology
Tulane University School of Medicine
New Orleans, Louisiana

Carrie A. Northcott, MS
Graduate Fellow, Department of Pharmacology and Toxicology
Michigan State University College of Human Medicine
East Lansing, Michigan

Jeffrey W. Olin, DO
Professor of Medicine
Mount Sinai School of Medicine of New York University
Director of Vascular Medicine
Zena and Michael A. Wiener Cardiovascular Institute
New York, New York

Suzanne Oparil, MD
Professor of Medicine, Physiology, and Biophysics
Director, Vascular Biology and Hypertension Program
University of Alabama School of Medicine
Birmingham, Alabama

Jeffrey L. Osborn, PhD
Professor, Department of Biology
Trinity College
Hartford, Connecticut

Vasilios Papademetriou, MD
Professor, Department of Medicine
Georgetown University School of Medicine
Washington, D.C.

Gianfranco Parati, MD, FAHA, FESC
Professor of Medicine
Department of Clinical Medicine, Prevention and Applied Technologies
University of Milano-Bicocca
S. Luca Hospital, Istituto Auxologico Italiano
Milano, Italy

Valory N. Pavlik, PhD, MPH
Assistant Professor, Department of Family and Community Medicine
Baylor College of Medicine
Houston, Texas

M. Ian Phillips, PhD, DSc
Professor of Medicine and Physiology
Associate Vice President for Research
Departments of Medicine and Physiology
University of Florida College of Medicine
Gainesville, Florida

Stephen J. Phillips, MBBS, FRCPC
Associate Professor, Department of Medicine
Dalhousie University Faculty of Medicine
Queen Elizabeth II Health Sciences Centre
Halifax, Nova Scotia, Canada

Xavier Pi-Sunyer, MD, MPH
Professor, Department of Medicine
Director, Division of Endocrinology
Columbia University College of Physicians and Surgeons
St. Luke's-Roosevelt Hospital Center
New York, New York

Thomas G. Pickering, MD, PhD
Professor, Department of Medicine
Mount Sinai School of Medicine of New York University
New York, New York

David W. Ploth, MD
Arthur V. Williams Professor, Department of Medicine
Director, Division of Nephrology
Medical University of South Carolina College of Medicine
Charleston, South Carolina

Jorge Plutzky, MD
Assistant Professor
Harvard Medical School
Department of Vascular Medicine
Brigham and Women's Hospital
Boston, Massachusetts

James L. Pool, MD
Professor of Medicine and Pharmacology
Baylor College of Medicine
Methodist Hospital
Houston, Texas

J. Howard Pratt, MD
Professor, Department of Medicine
Indiana University School of Medicine
Indianapolis, Indiana

[illegible]
Professor, Department of Pharmacology
University of California, San Diego, School of Medicine
La Jolla, California

L. Michael Prisant, MD
Professor of Medicine
Departments of Hypertension and Clinical Pharmacology
Medical College of Georgia School of Medicine
Augusta, Georgia

Bruce M. Psaty, MD, PhD
Professor of Medicine, Epidemiology, and Health Services
Cardiovascular Health Research Unit
University of Washington School of Medicine
Seattle, Washington

Patrick Pullicino, MD, PhD
Professor, Department of Neurology and Neurosciences
UMDNJ—New Jersey Medical School
Newark, New Jersey

Arshed A. Quyyumi, MD, FACC, FRCP
Professor of Medicine
Department of Cardiology
Emory University School of Medicine
Emory University Hospital
Atlanta, Georgia

Mahboob Rahman, MD, MS
Assistant Professor, Department of Medicine
Case Western Reserve University
University Hospitals of Cleveland
Louis Stokes Cleveland Veterans Affairs Medical Center
Cleveland, Ohio

C. Venkata S. Ram, MD, FACC, MACP
Texas Blood Pressure Institute
University of Texas Southwestern Medical Center
Dallas Nephrology Associates
Dallas, Texas

Lawrence M. Resnick, MD
Professor of Medicine
Department of Cardiovascular Pathophysiology
Weill Medical College of Cornell University
Hypertension Center
New York Presbyterian Hospital
New York, New York

Nour-Eddine Rhaleb, PhD
Senior Staff Scientist, Departments of Internal Medicine and
    Hypertension and Vascular Research
Henry Ford Hospital
Detroit, Michigan

David Robertson, MD
Professor of Medicine, Pharmacology, and Neurology
Vanderbilt University School of Medicine
Nashville, Tennessee

Edward J. Roccella, PhD, MPH
Coordinator, National High Blood Pressure Education Program
Office of Prevention, Education, and Control
National Heart, Lung, and Blood Institute
National Institutes of Health
Bethesda, Maryland

Albert P. Rocchini, MD
Professor, Department of Pediatrics
University of Michigan Medical School
Ann Arbor, Michigan

Richard J. Roman, PhD
Professor, Department of Physiology
Medical College of Wisconsin
Milwaukee, Wisconsin

Clive Rosendorff, MD, PhD, FRCP
Professor of Medicine and Associate Chair
Mount Sinai School of Medicine of New York University
New York, New York
Chief of Medicine
Bronx VA Medical Center
Bronx, New York

Frank M. Sacks, MD
Professor of Cardiovascular Disease Prevention
Department of Nutrition
Harvard School of Public Health
Boston, Massachusetts

Willis K. Samson, PhD
Professor, Department of Pharmacology and Physiology
Saint Louis University School of Medicine
Saint Louis, Missouri

Ernesto L. Schiffrin, MD, PhD, FRCPC
Professor of Medicine
Director, CIHR Multidisciplinary Hypertension Group
Clinical Research Institute of Montreal
Montreal, Quebec, Canada

Nicholas J. Schork, PhD
Professor of Psychiatry
University of California, San Diego
La Jolla, California

Ellen W. Seely, MD
Associate Professor, Department of Medicine
Harvard Medical School
Endocrine-Hypertension Division
Brigham and Women's Hospital
Boston, Massachusetts

Yoram Shenker, MD
Associate Professor of Medicine
Department of Internal Medicine
University of Wisconsin Medical School
William S. Middleton Veterans Administration Hospital
Madison, Wisconsin

Alexander M. M. Shepherd, MD, PhD
Professor, Department of Medicine and Pharmacology
University of Texas Health Science Center
San Antonio, Texas

Sheldon G. Sheps, MD
Emeritus Professor, Department of Medicine
Division of Hypertension
Mayo Medical School
Mayo Clinic
Rochester, Minnesota

Clarence Shub, MD
Professor of Medicine
Department of Cardiology
Mayo Medical School
Mayo Clinic
Rochester, Minnesota

Domenic A. Sica, MD
Professor of Medicine and Pharmacology
Chair, Section of Clinical Pharmacology and Hypertension
Department of Medicine
Virginia Commonwealth University School of Medicine
Medical College of Virginia Hospitals
Richmond, Virginia

Denise G. Simons-Morton, MD, PhD
Director, Clinical Applications and Prevention Program
Division of Epidemiology and Clinical Applications
National Heart, Lung, and Blood Institute
National Institutes of Health
Bethesda, Maryland

Alan R. Sinaiko, MD
Professor, Department of Pediatrics
University of Minnesota Medical School—Twin Cities
Minneapolis, Minnesota

Randal A. Skidgel, PhD
Professor, Department of Pharmacology
University of Illinois College of Medicine
Chicago, Illinois

Ellen Smit, PhD
Assistant Professor, Department of Social and
    Preventive Medicine
University of Buffalo, State University of New York School
    of Medicine and Biomedical Sciences
Buffalo, New York

Caren G. Solomon, MD, MPH
Assistant Professor, Department of Medicine
Harvard Medical School
Brigham and Women's Hospital
Boston, Massachusetts

Virend K. Somers, MD, PhD
Professor, Department of Medicine
Divisions of Cardiovascular Disease and Hypertension
Mayo Clinic and Mayo Foundation
Rochester, Minnesota

James R. Sowers, MD
Professor of Medicine, Cell Biology, and Biochemistry
Department of Medicine
State University of New York, Downstate Medical Center
    College of Medicine
Brooklyn, New York

J. David Spence, MD, MBA
Professor of Clinical Neurological Sciences, Internal Medicine, and
    Physiology and Pharmacology
Department of Clinical Neurological Science
University of Western Ontario Faculty of Medicine and Dentistry
London, Ontario, Canada

Jeremiah Stamler, MD
Professor Emeritus, Department of Preventive Medicine
Northwestern University, The Feinberg School of Medicine
Chicago, Illinois

Helmut O. Steinberg, MD
Associate Professor, Department of Medicine
Indiana University School of Medicine
Indianapolis, Indiana

Naftali Stern, MD
Professor of Medicine
Institute of Endocrinology, Metabolism, and Hypertension
Sackler Faculty of Medicine
Tel Aviv University
Tel Aviv–Sourasky Medical Center
Tel Aviv, Israel

Sandra J. Taler, MD
Assistant Professor of Medicine
Department of Hypertension
Mayo Medical School
Mayo Clinic
Rochester, Minnesota

William T. Talman, MD
Professor, Department of Neurology
University of Iowa Roy J. and Lucille A. Carver College of Medicine
Iowa City, Iowa

Addison A. Taylor, MD, PhD
Professor of Medicine and Pharmacology
Chief, Section of Hypertension and Clinical Pharmacology
Associate Dean of Clinical Research
Baylor College of Medicine
Houston, Texas

Meghan M. Taylor, PhD
Fellow, Department of Pharmacology and Physiology
Saint Louis University School of Medicine
Saint Louis, Missouri

Stephen C. Textor, MD
Professor, Department of Medicine
Divisions of Hypertension and Nephrology
Mayo Medical School
Mayo Clinic
Rochester, Minnesota

Thomas J. Thom, BA
Statistician
National Heart, Lung, and Blood Institute
National Institutes of Health
Bethesda, Maryland

Rhian M. Touyz, MD, PhD
Associate Professor of Medicine
Department of Experimental Hypertension
Clinical Research Institute of Montreal
Montreal, Quebec, Canada

Raymond R. Townsend, MD
Professor, Department of Medicine
University of Pennsylvania School of Medicine
Philadelphia, Pennsylvania

David J. Triggle, PhD, DSc (Hon)
University Professor
School of Pharmacy
State University of New York at Buffalo
Buffalo, New York

Michael Tuck, MD

Paul M. Vanhoutte, MD, PhD
Professor of Medicine, Pharmacology, and Physiology
Service de Pharmacologie
Université Paris VI
Morainvilliers, France

Douglas E. Vaughan, MD
Professor of Medicine and Pharmacology
Department of Cardiovascular Medicine
Vanderbilt University School of Medicine
Nashville, Tennessee

Donald G. Vidt, MD
Professor of Medicine
Department of Nephrology and Hypertension
Ohio State University College of Medicine and Public Health
Cleveland Clinic Foundation
Cleveland, Ohio

Ralph E. Watson, MD, FACP
Assistant Professor, Department of Medicine
Director, Hypertension Clinic
Michigan State University College of Human Medicine
East Lansing, Michigan

Stephanie W. Watts, PhD
Assistant Professor, Department of Pharmacology and Toxicology
Michigan State University College of Human Medicine
East Lansing, Michigan

R. Clinton Webb, PhD
Robert B. Greenblatt Professor and Chair, Department of Physiology
Medical College of Georgia School of Medicine
Augusta, Georgia

Michael A. Weber, MD
Professor and Associate Dean, Department of Medicine
State University of New York, Downstate Medical Center College of Medicine
New York, New York

Alan B. Weder, MD
Department of Internal Medicine
Division of Hypertension and Hyperlipidemia
University of Michigan Medical School
Ann Arbor, Michigan

Myron H. Weinberger, MD
Professor, Department of Medicine
Indiana University School of Medicine
Indianapolis, Indiana

Matthew R. Weir, MD
Professor and Director, Department of Medicine
Division of Nephrology
University of Maryland School of Medicine
Baltimore, Maryland

Paul K. Whelton, MD, MS
Professor, Departments of Epidemiology and Medicine
Tulane University School of Medicine
Tulane University Health Sciences Center
New Orleans, Louisiana

William B. White, MD
Professor of Medicine
Division Chief, Section of Hypertension and
    Clinical Pharmacology
University of Connecticut School of Medicine
Farmington, Connecticut

Michael F. Wilson, MD
Professor, Departments of Medicine and Nuclear Medicine
Kaleida Health
Buffalo, New York

Peter W. F. Wilson, MD
Professor, Department of Medicine
Boston University School of Medicine
Boston, Massachusetts

Philip A. Wolf, MD
Professor, Department of Neurology
Boston University School of Medicine
Boston, Massachusetts

Nathan D. Wong, PhD, MPH
Associate Professor
Director, Heart Disease Prevention Program
Division of Cardiology
University of California, Irvine, College of Medicine
Irvine, California

Jackson T. Wright, Jr, MD, PhD
Professor, Department of Medicine
Case Western Reserve University
University Hospitals of Cleveland
Cleveland, Ohio

J. Michael Wyss, PhD
Professor, Departments of Cell Biology and Medicine
University of Alabama School of Medicine
Birmingham, Alabama

William F. Young, Jr, MD, MSc
Professor of Medicine
Division of Endocrinology and Metabolism
Mayo Medical School
Mayo Clinic
Rochester, Minnesota

Jason X.-J. Yuan, MD, PhD
Associate Professor, Department of Medicine
University of California, San Diego, School of Medicine
San Diego, California

Part A. BASIC SCIENCE

Section 1. *Vasoactive Substances*

Chapter A1

Adrenergic and Dopaminergic Receptors and Actions

Kathleen H. Berecek, PhD; Robert M. Carey, MD

KEY POINTS

- There are 9 different adrenergic receptor subtypes in 3 main classes, $\alpha_{1A,B,D}$, $\alpha_{2A,B,C}$, and $\beta_{1,2,3}$, and 5 dopaminergic receptor subtypes in 2 main classes, D_1-like and D_2-like.

- Adrenergic and dopaminergic receptors are coupled to G proteins and activate cells through alterations in intracellular calcium, cyclic nucleotides, inositol phosphates, and protein phosphorylation.

- Receptor desensitization and downregulation reduce responses of cells to continuous exposure to catecholamines.

- Alterations in adrenergic and dopaminergic receptors and their functions may play a role in hypertension, cardiac ischemia, congestive heart failure, nocturnal asthma, and obesity.

See also Chapters A2, A28–A30, A33, A41, A42, A51, C140, and C141

ADRENERGIC RECEPTORS

Norepinephrine (NE) and epinephrine are endogenous catecholamines released by the postganglionic sympathetic nerve terminals and the adrenal gland that interact with cell surface receptor molecules in many diverse target organs. This interaction begins a cascade of membrane and intracellular events (see Chapters A28–A32) that culminate in altered cellular activity. Endogenous catecholamines are involved in regulation of virtually every organ system (**Table A1.1**), and drugs targeting adrenergic receptors (ARs) are among the most widely used therapeutic agents in clinical medicine. Activation of ARs increases heart rate and strength of cardiac contraction and causes cardiac and vascular hypertrophy, bronchodilation, vasoconstriction, sedation, and analgesia. Inhibition of AR results in vasodilation, decreased heart rate, and strength of contraction and relaxation of prostate smooth muscle. Each of these actions is important in treating diseases such as hypertension, congestive heart failure, and angina, as well as benign prostatic hypertrophy, acute and chronic pain, and asthma.

Adrenergic Receptor Subtype Classification

Classically, ARs were divided into 2 principal types: α and β. Synthetic compounds that specifically stimulate or inhibit adrenergic targets enabled further differentiation of AR into subtypes of α_1, α_2, β_1, and β_2. Recent pharmacologic and molecular cloning studies have identified several additional subtypes leading to the current division of 9 AR subtypes in 3 families: $\alpha_{1A,B,D}$, $\alpha_{2A,B,C}$, and $\beta_{1,2,3}$.

Signal Transduction Mechanisms

ARs are members of a large superfamily of receptors that mediate their activities through interaction with 1 of a series of guanosine nucleotide-binding regulatory proteins (G proteins). This process is critical in linking the effect of the first messenger on the receptor to the activity of the membrane-bound enzyme system that produces the second messenger. The G proteins to which AR are linked are heterotrimeric proteins with α, β, and γ subunits; each subunit is part of a family consisting of multiple members. Each type of AR preferentially couples to a different major subfamily of G_α proteins: α_1-AR to $G_{q\alpha}$, α_2-AR to $G_{i\alpha}$, and β-AR to $G_{s\alpha}$. Each of the G_α proteins can be linked to ion channels, numerous effector molecules, or both, although most target cells have preferred linkages. Thus, α_1-ARs are preferentially linked by G_q to activation of phospholipases, especially phospholipase C, and, in some tissues, to activation of Ca^{2+} channels, Na^+-H^+ and Na^+-Ca^+ exchangers and activation or inhibition of K^+ channels.

Table A1.1. Tissue Distribution, Responses, and Pharmacology of Adrenergic Receptor Subtypes

| RECEPTOR | PHYSIOLOGY | | PHARMACOLOGY | |
	TISSUE	RESPONSE	AGONISTS	ANTAGONISTS
$\alpha_{1A,B,C}$	Smooth muscle: vascular, iris, radial ureter, pilomotor, uterus, sphincters (gut, bladder)	Contraction	Methoxamine Phenylephrine	Prazosin Terazosin Doxazosin
	Smooth muscle (gut)	Relaxation		Corynanthine
	Heart	Positive inotrope ($\beta_1$xry) cell growth, hypertrophy		Phentolamine
	Salivary gland	Secretion		Phenoxybenzamine
	Adipose tissue	Glycogenolysis		
	Sweat glands	Secretion		
	Kidney (proximal tubule)	Gluconeogenesis, Na^+ reabsorption		
$\alpha_{2A,B,C,D}$	Presynaptic autoreceptor on sympathetic nerve endings	Inhibition of norepinephrine release	Guanfacine Clonidine	Yohimbine Piperoxan
	Platelets	Aggregation, granule release	α-Methyl-NE	Rauwolscine
	Endocrine pancreas	Inhibition of insulin release	Tramazoline	Phentolamine
	Adipose tissue	Inhibition of lipolysis	Xylazine	Phenoxybenzamine
	Vascular smooth tissue	Contraction	Guanadrel	
	Kidney	Inhibition of renin release (?)	Oxymetazoline	
β_1	Heart	Positive inotropic effect, positive chronotropic effect, cell growth, hypertrophy	Isoproterenol Prenaterol	Propranolol Betaxolol
	Adipose tissue	Lipolysis	Dobutamine	Atenolol
	Kidney	Renin release		Practolol Metoprolol
β_2	Liver	Glycogenolysis, gluconeogenesis	Isoproterenol	Propanolol
	Skeletal muscle	Glycogenolysis, lactate release	Terbutaline	Butoxamine
	Smooth muscle: bronchi, uterus, gut, vascular (skeletal muscle), detrusor	Relaxation	Salbutamol Rimiterol Albuterol	High concentration of β_1-antagonists
	Endocrine pancreas	Insulin secretion (?)		
	Salivary gland	Amylase secretion		
β_3	Adipose tissue	Lipolysis	BRL 37344	
	Striated muscle	Thermogenesis		

NE, norepinephrine.

Receptors of the α_2 subtype are linked by G_i to inhibition of adenylyl cyclase and, in some tissues, to regulation of K^+ and calcium Ca^{2+} channels. β-ARs are linked by G_s to activation of adenylyl cyclase and Ca^{2+} channels in some tissues.

Each of these linkages leads to changes in intracellular concentrations of second messengers such as adenosine 3',5'-cyclic monophosphate, Ca^{2+}, diacylglycerol, and 1,4,5-trisphosphate that regulate the phosphorylated states of cellular proteins by modifying the activity of a variety of protein kinases.

Structural Features

All G protein–coupled receptors share many features, such as extracellular amino terminals with sites for N-linked glycosylation, 7 α-helical domains that span the plasma membrane, and intracellular carboxy terminals containing amino acid sequences that are probable sites of phosphorylation by 1 or more protein kinases. Through various interactions with ion channels and second messengers, different AR subtypes enable NE and epinephrine to have a broad range of physiological actions (see Chapters A28, A29, A30).

Physiology and Pharmacology

AR subtypes, their tissue distributions, and the responses that they mediate are shown in Table A1.1. Also included in Table A1.1 are the pharmacologic agents that stimulate or inhibit various receptor subtypes. As shown in this table, individual AR subtypes are not restricted to a single cell. Moreover, most tissues contain more than one subtype. The response of a cell depends on the concentration of NE and epinephrine in the tissue, the subtypes and kinetics of the receptors on the cell, and the second messenger system(s) altered by occupancy of the receptors. ARs can be characterized by their physiology and pharmacology. The endogenous catecholamines NE and epinephrine are agonists for all AR subtypes, although with varying affinity.

α_1-Adrenergic receptors. α_1-ARs are located on postsynaptic cells in smooth muscle, heart, vas deferens, and brain. The α_1-AR subtypes are stimulated by the agonists methoxamine and phenylephrine and inhibited by antagonists such as prazosin, phentolamine, and corynanthine.

α_2-Adrenergic receptors. Many α_2-ARs are autoreceptors localized on the presynaptic membrane of postganglionic nerve terminals that synthesize NE. When activated by catecholamines, α_2-ARs act as negative feedback controllers, inhibiting further NE release. Activation of brain α_2-ARs by endogenous NE or by synthetic α_2-AR agonists such as clonidine, guanfacine, or α-methyl NE (formed from α-methyldopa) reduces systemic sympathetic outflow. Conversely, blockade of the α_2-AR with agents such as yohimbine or rauwolscine facilitates

additional release of NE from sympathetic nerve terminals. α_2-ARs are also located postsynaptically, where they cause mild vasoconstriction. Chronically, the presynaptic effects of α_2-AR stimulants (to limit catecholamine release and sympathetic outflow) are more powerful than the postsynaptic α_2-AR–mediated vasoconstrictor effects.

β_1-Adrenergic receptor. Activation of β_1-AR stimulates the rate and strength of cardiac contraction, lipolysis in fat cells, and renin release from the kidneys. This receptor is stimulated by isoproterenol, dobutamine, and prenaterol and is inhibited by β_1-AR blockers such as propranolol, metoprolol, or atenolol. The order of potency for stimulation of β_1-AR by catecholamines is isoproterenol > epinephrine = NE.

β_2-Adrenergic receptor. The β_2-AR relaxes smooth muscle cells in bronchi, blood vessels, uterus, gut, and bladder. This receptor is stimulated by isoproterenol, terbutaline, albuterol, salbutamol, and rimiterol and is inhibited by IPS 339 and ICI 118,551. For the β_2-AR, the order of potency is isoproterenol > epinephrine > NE.

Control of Adrenergic Receptors

Desensitization and downregulation. After stimulation, α- and β-ARs exhibit decreased response to further stimulation. In other words, they can be rapidly desensitized and downregulated after prolonged exposure to their agonist. One cascade that decreases β-adrenergic responses includes phosphorylation of agonist-occupied receptors, uncoupling of the receptors from G proteins, and internalization of receptors from the membrane into the cytoplasm. Immediately after agonist presentation, β-AR kinase catalyzes phosphorylation of consensus sequences near the carboxy terminus (cytoplasmic domain) of the receptor. Subsequent events, including G proteins, cause internalization of the receptor, after which the receptor can be degraded or reinserted into the plasma membrane.

In addition to desensitization and downregulation induced by the agonist itself (homologous desensitization), β-ARs display heterologous desensitization. In this case, β-ARs become less responsive to agonists after stimulation of the same cell by a nonadrenergic adenylyl cyclase activator, such as another neurotransmitter. This phenomenon is associated with adenosine 3',5'-cyclic monophosphate activation of protein kinases and subsequent phosphorylation and desensitization of the β-ARs.

Control mechanisms. Long-term regulation of β-ARs occurs principally at the gene level. Stimulation of β-ARs modifies the transcription rate and the steady-state level of β-AR messenger RNA. Adenosine 3',5'-cyclic monophosphate-responsive elements in the promoter region of the gene, as well as exposure of cells to several humoral agents (i.e., glucocorticoids and thyroid hormone), modify the expression of β-ARs. Regulation of α-ARs has been less completely examined. α-ARs appear to be subject to dynamic regulation by a variety of mechanisms including phosphorylation, protein–protein interactions, and protein trafficking and transcription, which produce homologous and heterologous desensitization. The mechanism of desensitization appears to involve both phosphorylation of the agonist-occupied receptor and uncoupling of the phosphorylated receptor from G protein by β-arrestins.

Clinical Impact

Alterations in AR structure and function may play a role in numerous disease states such as hypertension, cardiac ischemia, cardiac and vascular hypertrophy, hypothyroidism, diabetes, morbid obesity, and asthma. Increased expression of AR in myocardial ischemia and hypertension and decreased expression of β-AR in congestive heart failure have been reported as well as genetic polymorphisms in β_2-AR in patients with asthma and β_3-AR in patients with morbid obesity. Identification and characterization of AR subtypes may lead to the development of new therapeutic agents that are highly selective, more effective, and have fewer side effects than agents currently available.

DOPAMINERGIC RECEPTORS

Dopamine (DA) is an endogenous catecholamine that serves as a precursor of NE and epinephrine and as a neurotransmitter in its own right. DA is released by postganglionic sympathetic neurons and dopaminergic neurons and is also synthesized by nonchromaffin tissues such as proximal renal tubule cells and gastrointestinal epithelium. The vast majority of circulating DA derives from kidney. DA modulates a variety of physiological functions, including behavior, movement, nerve conduction, hormone synthesis and release, ion transport, vascular tone, and blood pressure.

General Characteristics

Peripheral dopaminergic receptors (DRs) have been divided into 2 major types: D_1-like and D_2-like (**Table A1.2**). Molecular studies have revealed 5 major subtypes (D_1 through D_5). D_1-like receptors include D_1 and D_5. D_2-like receptors include D_2, D_3, and D_4 receptors. DRs contain the 7 transmembrane domains that characterize the other G protein–coupled receptors. The D_1-like receptors have no introns and are encoded by a single exon, whereas the D_2-like family is encoded by a mosaic of exons and contains introns within its protein-coding regions. Therefore, it is likely that the D_1- and D_2-like receptors derive from 2 different gene families.

Signal Transduction Mechanisms

D_1-like and D_2-like receptors induce 2 different types of signal transduction. One of these, the adenylyl cyclase pathway, is obligatory for all cell systems. D_1-like receptors are associated with stimulation and D_2-like receptors with inhibition of adenylyl cyclase. The other pathways are different in different cells. These other pathways include activation of calcium or potassium channels and stimulation of phosphoinositide hydrolysis.

Distribution and Function

In peripheral tissues, DRs are distributed in the sympathetic nervous system, the pituitary gland, the cardiovascular system, kidney, and adrenal cortex. Molecular studies suggest that the peripheral D_1- and D_2-like receptors are identical to those in the central nervous system. D_1-like DRs are located postsynaptically in the heart (atrial and ventricular myocardium and coronary vessels), arterial blood vessels (vascular smooth muscle cells), adrenal cortex (zona glomerulosa), and

Table A1.2. **Classification of Dopamine Receptors**

GROUP	PHARMACOLOGIC CLASS				
	D₁-LIKE GROUP		D₂-LIKE GROUP		
G protein coupling	Gs		Gi/Go		
Signal transduction	+AC	+AC	−AC		
	+PLC		+K⁺channel		
			−Ca²⁺ channel		
Group selective agonists	Fenoldopam[a]		Bromocriptine[b]		
Group selective antagonists	SCH 23390 and 39166[b]		YM-09151[b]		
	SKF 83566[a]				
Molecular biologic subclass	D₁	D₅	D₂	D₃	D₄
Subclass-selective agonists	None	None	091356A	PD128907	PD168077
				Tramipexole	(+)N-propyl-norapomorphine
				Quinelorane	
Subclass-selective antagonists	None	None	L-741,6626	Nafadotride	U-101958
				U-99, 194A21	L-745,870
			Raclopride	(+)AJ76	L-741,742
				(+)S14297	NGD-94

+, stimulatory; −, inhibitory; AC, adenylyl cyclase; PLC, phospholipase C.
[a]Selective for D₁-like dopamine receptor but cannot distinguish D₁ from D₅.
[b]Selective for D₂-like dopamine receptor but cannot distinguish subtypes.

kidney (proximal tubule, thick ascending loop of Henle, cortical collecting duct, and vascular smooth muscle).

D₁-like renal effects and natriuresis. Stimulation of D₁-like receptors by fenoldopam, a selective D₁-like DR agonist, leads to vasodilation (renal and systemic), diuresis, natriuresis, and a decrease in systemic blood pressure without postural hypotension or increased plasma renin activity. DA-induced natriuresis is caused by an increase in renal blood flow and a decrease in renal tubule sodium reabsorption. In proximal tubule cells, inhibition of sodium transport from the tubule lumen is mediated by stimulation of adenylyl cyclase, increased protein kinase A activity, and inhibition of Na⁺/K⁺ antiport activity at the brush border membrane. In the medullary thick ascending loop of Henle, DA acts through D₁-like receptors to increase cyclic adenosine monophosphate–dependent protein kinase, which phosphorylates a protein, DARPP-32 (DA-related phosphoprotein), which phosphorylates basolateral membrane Na⁺/K⁺ adenosine triphosphatase, causing inactivation of this enzyme. D₁ receptor–selective antagonists include SCH-23390, SCH-39166, and SKF-83566.

DA synthesized in and released from renal proximal tubule cells is thought to act as a paracrine substance (cell-to-cell mediator) stimulating D₁-like DR on these cells to inhibit sodium reabsorption in tonic fashion. A defect in proximal tubule D₁ receptor–G protein complex recycling is present in spontaneously hypertensive rats and in human essential hypertension. It is now thought that G protein–coupled receptor kinase 4 hyperphosphorylates the D₁ receptor in the proximal renal tubule cell of humans with essential hypertension. This defect promotes renal sodium reabsorption and may contribute to the development of hypertension.

D₂-like effects. D₂-like DRs in the periphery are distributed presynaptically and postsynaptically in the sympathetic nervous system. Presynaptic D₂-like DRs inhibit NE release from sympathetic neurons. Postsynaptic and nonneuronal D₂-like DRs are present in the endothelial and adventitial layers of blood vessels, on pituitary lactotrophs (where they inhibit prolactin secretion

in response to DA), and in the adrenal zona glomerulosa (where they inhibit aldosterone secretion). D₃ receptors, 1 of the D₂-like DR group, have been identified in the glomeruli, proximal tubules, and blood vessels of the kidney, and a novel D₂-like receptor (the D₂ₖ receptor) has been described in inner medullary collecting duct cells. The functions of the D₃ and D₂ₖ receptors are unknown. However, knockout of the D₃ receptor in mice leads to angiotensin-dependent hypertension associated with increased renin secretion.

Aside from inhibition of NE, prolactin, and aldosterone secretion, the physiologic role of peripheral D₂-like DRs is not established, and it is unclear whether these receptors have a role in the pathophysiology of cardiovascular disease. Bromocriptine and domperidone are selective agonists at D₂-like receptors. New, relatively specific agonists for the D₃ receptor include PD 128907, quinelorane, and pramipexole.

SUGGESTED READING

1. Michelotti GA, Price DT, Schwinn DA. α₁-Adrenergic receptor regulation: basic science and clinical implications. *Pharmacol Ther.* 2000;88:281–309.
2. Naga Prasad SV, Nienaber J, Rockman HA. β-adrenergic axis and heart disease. *Trends Genet.* 2001;17:544–549.
3. Singh K, Xiao L, Remondino A, et al. Adrenergic regulation of cardiac myocyte apoptosis. *J Cell Physiol.* 2001;189:257–265.
4. Higashida H, Yokoyama S, Hoshi N, et al. Signal transduction from bradykinin, angiotensin, adrenergic and muscarinic receptors to effector enzymes, including ADP-ribosyl cyclase. *Biol Chem.* 2001;382:23–30.
5. Garcia-Sainz JA, Prado JV, del Carmen Medina L. α₁-Adrenoceptors: function and phosphorylation. *Eur J Pharmacol.* 2000;389:1–12.
6. Buscher R, Hermann V, Insel PA. Human adrenoceptors polymorphisms: evolving recognition and clinical significance. *Trends Pharmacol Sci.* 1999;20:94–99.
7. Eckhardt AD, Koch WJ. Transgenic studies of cardiac adrenergic receptor regulation. *J Pharmacol Exp Ther.* 2001;299:1–5.
8. Carey RM. Renal dopamine system: paracrine regulator of sodium homeostasis and blood pressure. *Hypertension.* 2001;38:298–302.
9. Jose PA, Eisner GM, Felder RA. Role of dopamine receptors in the kidney in the regulation of blood pressure. *Curr Opin Nephrol Hypertens.* 2002;11:87–92.
10. Felder RA, et al. G-protein coupled receptor kinase 4 gene variants in human essential hypertension. *Proc Natl Acad Sci U S A.* 2002;99:3872–3877.

Catecholamine Synthesis, Release, Reuptake, and Metabolism

David S. Goldstein, MD, PhD; Graeme F. Eisenhofer, PhD

KEY POINTS

- The endogenous catecholamines, norepinephrine (noradrenaline), epinephrine (adrenaline), and dopamine are the chemical effectors of the sympathetic nervous system, adrenomedullary hormonal system, and the DOPA-dopamine autocrine/paracrine system.

- The main determinants of the amount of norepinephrine available at its receptors are the sympathetic nerve traffic and the degree of catecholamine reuptake via the cell membrane norepinephrine transporter (Uptake 1).

- Catecholamines are metabolized by multiple enzymes; plasma levels and urinary excretion rates of catecholamine metabolites represent different physiologic pools.

See also Chapters A1, A51, C148, and C169

The 3 endogenous catecholamines in humans, norepinephrine (noradrenaline), epinephrine (adrenaline), and dopamine, act as the chemical effectors of the sympathetic nervous system, adrenomedullary hormonal system, and DOPA-dopamine autocrine/paracrine system. All 3 systems play important roles in tonic and phasic cardiovascular regulation.

Catecholamine Synthesis

The enzymatic rate-limiting step in catecholamine synthesis is conversion of tyrosine to the catechol amino acid, DOPA, which is catalyzed by tyrosine hydroxylase. This step, which follows uptake of tyrosine into the cell, requires tetrahydrobiopterin as a cofactor. A variety of cell types outside the central nervous system, including sympathetic neurons, adrenomedullary cells, and gastrointestinal parenchymal cells, express tyrosine hydroxylase (**Figure A2.1**).

Many tissues express aromatic-L-amino-acid decarboxylase, which catalyzes conversion of DOPA to dopamine, using pyridoxal phosphate as cofactor. Alpha-methyldopa and carbidopa inhibit this enzyme. In the kidneys, the main source of dopamine is uptake and decarboxylation of DOPA by tubular cells.

After translocation of dopamine into vesicles that contain dopamine-β-hydroxylase, dopamine undergoes hydroxylation to form norepinephrine, with ascorbic acid as cofactor. In tissues that synthesize epinephrine, the final synthetic step involves the action of phenylethanolamine *N*-methyltransferase, a cytoplasmic enzyme, which transfers a methyl group from *S*-adenosylmethionine to norepinephrine, forming epinephrine.

Catecholamine Release

Release of norepinephrine from sympathetic nerve endings and epinephrine from adrenomedullary cells occurs by exocytosis, in which vesicles containing the catecholamines fuse with the cell membrane, porate, and discharge their contents into the extracellular fluid. Exocytosis is triggered by depolarization of the cell membrane and entry of ionized calcium into the terminal. Nicotine potently stimulates ganglionic transmission and adrenomedullary secretion, whereas angiotensin II evokes adrenomedullary secretion by binding to specific stimulatory receptors on adrenomedullary cells. Norepinephrine release can also occur nonexocytotically in response to drugs that displace vesicular norepinephrine (the most well known is tyramine) and in the setting of anoxic ischemia (**Figure A2.2**).

Receptors on presynaptic membranes of postganglionic sympathetic nerves modulate the amount of norepinephrine released by electrical excitation of the sympathetic nerve fiber. In humans, norepinephrine can feedback-inhibit its own release via presynaptic α_2-adrenoceptors. α_2-adrenoceptor agonists such as clonidine act on these inhibitory receptors, causing decreased release of norepinephrine from sympathetic nerves. In contrast, circulating epinephrine augments norepinephrine release by stimulating β_2-adrenoceptors on sympathetic nerve terminals.

Catecholamine Reuptake

Neuronal reuptake (Uptake 1) via the cell membrane norepinephrine transporter is the main means of inactivation of norepinephrine released from sympathetic nerves. Tricyclic antidepressants and cocaine potently inhibit Uptake 1. Most of the norepinephrine taken up into the terminals is translocated into storage vesicles via the vesicular monoamine transporter. Reserpine inhibits this vesicular translocation, leading to norepinephrine depletion.

Nonneuronal catecholamine uptake (Uptake 2) is mediated by extraneuronal cell membrane transporters. Subsequent intracellular metabolism after Uptake 2 is the main means of inactivation of circulating catecholamines.

Catecholamine Metabolism

Catecholamines in cells undergo a complex metabolic fate, dependent on the actions of multiple enzymes, including

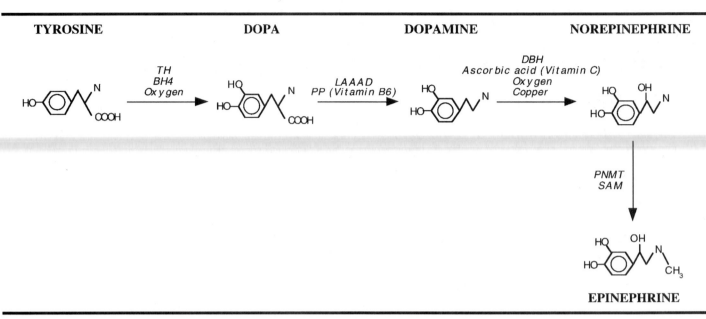

Figure A2.1. Enzymatic steps in catecholamine biosynthesis.

monoamine oxidase, aldose reductase, aldehyde reductase, aldehyde dehydrogenase (AD), alcohol dehydrogenase, catechol O-methyltransferase (COMT), and monoamine-preferring phenolsulfotransferase (PST) **(Figure A2.3)**.

Human plasma normally contains 6 unconjugated catechols—DOPA, dopamine, norepinephrine, epinephrine, dihydroxyphenylglycol (DHPG), and dihydroxyphenylacetic acid (DOPAC)—and 2 unconjugated metanephrines (MNs), normetanephrine (NMN) and MN. Because of the different sources of these compounds in sympathetic nerves, the adrenal

medulla, and nonchromaffin cells, and the different enzymes and sites of enzymatic reactions leading to their formation, plasma levels of catechols and MNs have distinctly different meanings in terms of functions and dysfunctions of catecholamine systems.

Norepinephrine and epinephrine metabolism. Under resting conditions, the main determinant of the loss of norepinephrine from a tissue is net leakage from storage vesicles into the axoplasm, a process that is independent of sympa-

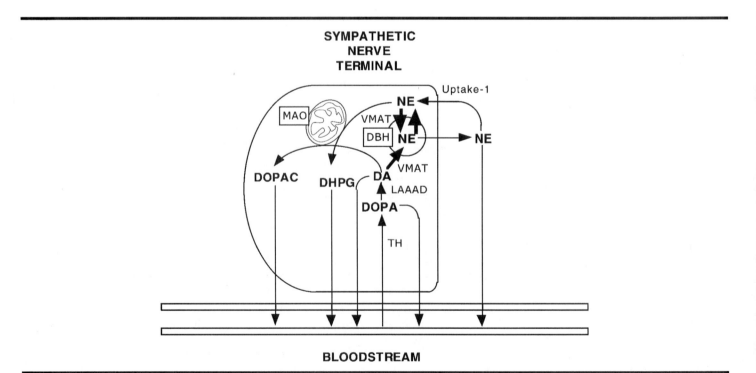

Figure A2.2. Sources of catechols in sympathetic nerve terminals and the circulation. DA, dopamine; DBH, dopamine β-hydroxylase; DHPG, dihydroxyphenylglycol; DOPA, 3,4-dihydroxyphenylalanine; MAO, monoamine oxidase; NE, norepinephrine; VMAT, vesicular monoamine transporter.

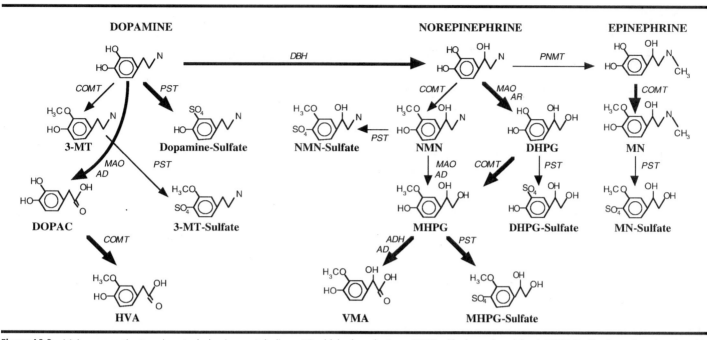

Figure A2.3. Main enzymatic steps in catecholamine metabolism. AR, aldehyde reductase; DHPG, dihydroxyphenylglycol; DOPAC, dihydroxyphenylacetic acid; HVA, homovanillic acid; MN, metanephrine; 3-MT, 3-methoxytyramine; NMN, normetanephrine; MHPG, methoxyhydroxyphenylglycol; VMA, vanillylmandelic acid.

thetic nerve traffic. Some of the norepinephrine in the axoplasm is metabolized to an aldehyde intermediate by monoamine oxidase A in the mitochondrial outer membrane. Subsequently, the aldehyde is converted by aldehyde reductase to DHPG, the main neuronal metabolite of norepinephrine. During sympathetic stimulation, released norepinephrine is also taken back up into the axoplasm via Uptake 1, providing a second source of DHPG. Most of the DHPG produced in sympathetically innervated organs eventually undergoes conversion by COMT within the organ to methoxyhydroxyphenylglycol (MHPG). In the liver, MHPG is converted by alcohol dehydrogenase and AD to vanillylmandelic acid, and in mesenteric organs, MHPG is converted to MHPG-sulfate by monoamine-preferring PST. Thus, the main end products of norepinephrine metabolism are vanillylmandelic acid, MHPG, and MHPG-sulfate.

Adrenomedullary cells also express COMT, which catalyzes conversion of norepinephrine to NMN and conversion of epinephrine to MN. Plasma levels of NMN arise partly from extraneuronal uptake of norepinephrine released from sympathetic nerves and partly from leakage of norepinephrine from storage vesicles into the cytoplasm of adrenomedullary cells. More than 90% of plasma MN is derived from epinephrine leaking from storage vesicles in adrenomedullary cells. Ongoing leakage and intracellular O-methylation help explain the extraordinary sensitivity of plasma unconjugated MNs (NMN and MN) for diagnosing pheochromocytoma.

Dopamine metabolism. Dopamine in neuronal and non-neuronal cells is metabolized by monoamine oxidase to form dihydroxyphenylacetaldehyde, which is rapidly metabolized further by AD to form DOPAC. DOPAC in turn is O-methylated via COMT to form homovanillic acid, the main end product of dopamine metabolism. Dopamine in non-neuronal cells is also extensively sulfoconjugated by monoamine-preferring PST to form dopamine sulfate. Another major end product of dopamine metabolism is 3-methoxytyramine sulfate, formed from the actions of COMT and monoamine-preferring PST on dopamine.

SUGGESTED READING

1. Goldstein DS. *The Autonomic Nervous System in Health and Disease.* New York, NY: Marcel Dekker, Inc.; 2001.
2. Cooper JR, Roth R, Bloom FE. *Biochemical Basis of Neuropharmacology.* New York, NY: Oxford University Press; 1996.
3. Eisenhofer G. Understanding catecholamine metabolism as a guide to the biochemical diagnosis of pheochromocytoma. *Rev Endo Metab Dis.* 2001; 2:297–311.
4. Kopin IJ. Catecholamine metabolism: basic aspects and clinical significance. *Pharmacol Rev.* 1985;37:333–364.
5. Lenders JW, Pacak K, Walther MM, et al. Biochemical diagnosis of pheochromocytoma: which test is best? *JAMA.* 2002;287:1427–1434.
6. Goldstein DS, Eisenhofer G, Stull R, et al. Plasma dihydroxyphenylglycol and the intraneuronal disposition of norepinephrine in humans. *J Clin Invest.* 1988;81: 213–220.
7. Kagedal B, Goldstein DS. Catecholamines and their metabolites. *J Chromatog.* 1988;429:177–233.

Angiotensins: Actions and Receptors

Theodore L. Goodfriend, MD

KEY POINTS

- Angiotensin II, by activating receptors of the AT_1 subtype, stimulates aldosterone secretion, constricts blood vessels, amplifies sympathetic nervous outflow, increases renal sodium retention, and promotes cell growth in the cardiovascular system.

- Angiotensin II effects are amplified or reduced by other autacoids, such as nitric oxide, eicosanoids, and growth factors, whose production is stimulated by angiotensin II.

- A second subtype of angiotensin receptor, AT_2, affects growth and development, mediates vasodilation in the adult kidney, and opposes AT_1-mediated actions of angiotensin II.

- Other angiotensin peptides are formed in humans and are postulated to have actions distinct from those of angiotensin II.

See also Chapters A4–A8, A14, A28, A29, A31, A33, A41, A48, A61, A63, A65, C144, and C145

General Characteristics

The multiple properties of angiotensin II (Ang II) itself, the contrasting effects of its 2 receptor subtypes, and the secondary effects of the many other substances released in response to Ang II make it difficult to simply characterize Ang II as a benefactor or culprit in cardiovascular homeostasis or disease.

Angiotensin peptides. Angiotensins are peptide hormones produced by a series of proteolytic reactions starting with the cleavage of angiotensinogen by renin. Some are identified by Roman numerals (e.g., Ang II), and all can be denoted by the use of arabic numbers referring to their amino acid sequence starting with the N-terminal aspartic acid of Ang I. (See Chapter A7). Ang I (Ang 1–10) has no known biologic role aside from serving as the precursor of Ang II and III; it is the major substrate of angiotensin converting enzyme (ACE). The peptide with the greatest cardiovascular potency is Ang II (Ang 1–8). Angiotensin III (Ang 2–8) is more lipid-soluble than Ang II and is found in relatively high concentrations in the brain and cerebrospinal fluid. Ang IV (Ang 2–8) and Ang 1–7 are both found in human blood.

Receptor subtypes. There are 2 well-characterized receptors for Ang II, denoted as AT_1 and AT_2, the subscript numbers of which should not be confused with the Roman numerals or amino acid numerals that are used to name the peptides themselves. Both receptor subtypes have strong affinity for Ang II and virtually none for Ang I. There is no specific receptor for Ang III (Ang 2–8) but the AT_2 subtype has higher affinity for that peptide than the AT_1 subtype has. Specific binding sites for Ang IV have been described, but these may be proteolytic enzymes, not signal-transducing receptors in cell membranes. There are no classic receptors known that have specificity for the other small fragments of Ang II.

AT_1 receptors, the subtype that mediates most of the classic effects of Ang II, are blocked by angiotensin receptor blockers (ARBs). The gene for AT_1 is located on human chromosome 3; the gene for AT_2 is located on the X chromosome. Both subtypes are typical of receptors that have 7 membrane-spanning sequences, but they share only 34% of their amino acid sequences.

Cellular Mechanisms of Angiotensin II Effects

AT_1 receptor mechanisms

Signal transduction. When Ang II binds to AT_1 receptors in the cell membrane, the G proteins associated with the intracellular loops of the receptor dissociate and activate phospholipase C, which cleaves phosphoinositides to form inositol trisphosphate and diacylglycerol (DAG) (see Chapters A29, A30, and A32). The G proteins associated with AT_1 receptors are primarily of the $G_{q/11}$ class. Inositol trisphosphate triggers release of calcium from intracellular stores. Activated AT_1 receptors also open calcium channels in the cell membrane. Calcium and DAG stimulate protein kinase C, which phosphorylates various intracellular proteins, the specific proteins varying with the target cell. It is the phosphoproteins that effect changes in function initiated by Ang II, such as contraction in vascular smooth muscle and aldosterone synthesis in the adrenal cortex. In addition to phospholipase C, Ang II stimulates 2 other phospholipases, A_2 and D. Phospholipase A_2 cleaves arachidonic acid from phospholipids and thereby provides substrate for enzymes that form eicosanoids. Phospholipase D cleaves phosphatidyl choline, a more abundant source of DAG than phosphatidyl inositol. Activation of phospholipase D helps prolong stimulation of targets by Ang II after phosphatidyl inositol is depleted. Ang II also stimulates the membrane Na^+/H^+ exchanger, leading to slight intracellular alkalinization. These events all occur outside the cell nucleus.

Gene transcription and protein synthesis. Binding of Ang II to membrane AT_1 receptors also initiates a series of events that

Table A3.1. Angiotensin Targets and Actions

TARGET ORGAN OR CELL	ACTION (STIMULATORY, MEDIATED BY THE AT$_1$ RECEPTOR SUBTYPE UNLESS INDICATED)
Vascular smooth muscle	Vasoconstriction, hypertrophy, hyperplasia
Vascular endothelium	Prostaglandin, nitric oxide, endothelin and type-1 plasminogen activator inhibitor production
Vascular connective tissue	Extracellular matrix synthesis
Myocardium	Strength of contraction, hypertrophy
Platelets	Aggregation by catecholamines
Monocytes	Adhesion to vessel wall
Bone marrow	Erythropoiesis
Adrenal glomerulosa	Aldosterone secretion
Adrenal medulla	Catecholamine release
Adrenal fasciculata	Cortisol secretion
Posterior pituitary	Antidiuretic hormone release
Kidney	Embryogenesis (AT$_1$ and AT$_2$), efferent vasoconstriction
Juxtaglomerular cells	Inhibit renin release
Mesangial cells	Contraction
Proximal tubule	Sodium reabsorption
Sympathetic neurons	Norepinephrine release
Brain	Pressor center activation, baroreceptor blunting, antidiuretic hormone synthesis, thirst, prostaglandin release (angiotensin 1–7)
Intestine	Salt and water absorption (AT$_2$)
Liver	Glycogenolysis, angiotensinogen synthesis

affect gene transcription and protein synthesis. These involve several cascades of protein phosphorylation, each of which includes several protein kinases (see Chapter A30). It is difficult to identify a protein kinase that is *not* activated in the course of events after Ang II binding to AT$_1$ and ending with increased gene transcription. Among the kinases close to the AT$_1$ receptor are those of the Src, JAK, and STAT families. At the other end of the cascades are kinases of the MAPK, MEK, and ERK families that alter proteins, such as nuclear factor κB, that interact with response elements regulating gene transcription. Responses to Ang II are also mediated by cyclic nucleotides. In the liver, activation of AT$_1$ inhibits adenylate cyclase and reduces levels of cyclic adenosine monophosphate. In other cells, activation of AT$_2$ stimulates formation of cyclic adenosine monophosphate and cyclic guanosine monophosphate.

Receptor downregulation. Binding of Ang II to AT$_1$ receptors leads to internalization of the hormone-receptor complex, part of the rapid downregulation or desensitization that is common to most G protein–linked receptor systems (see Chapter A29). This does not occur when antagonists like the ARBs bind to AT$_1$. The AT$_2$ receptor subtype is not internalized or acutely downregulated by Ang II or drugs.

AT$_2$ receptor mechanisms. Binding of Ang II to AT$_2$ receptors activates phosphatases that remove phosphate groups added to proteins by protein kinases. The G protein associated with AT$_2$ receptors is a member of the G$_i$ class, commonly associated with receptors that inhibit various intracellular signaling mechanisms. By stimulating dephosphorylation of proteins, AT$_2$ antagonizes the growth-promoting effects of Ang II mediated by AT$_1$ receptors. In the kidney, AT$_2$ receptors stimulate formation of bradykinin and nitric oxide that dilate blood vessels. Another inhibitory mechanism mediated by AT$_2$ is hyperpolarization of cell membranes by opening potassium channels.

Regulation of receptor density and responsiveness. The number of angiotensin receptors available for activation by Ang II depends on synthesis of the receptors themselves as well as the acute internalization process of the hormone-receptor complex. Synthesis of AT$_1$ receptors is increased by insulin, glucocorticoids, and epidermal growth factor. Synthesis of AT$_2$ receptors is increased by tissue injury and is elevated in the myocardium of failing hearts. Density of both subtypes in the myometrium varies during pregnancy and after parturition. In essential hypertension of animals and humans, virtually all of the pressor and growth-stimulating aspects of Ang II action are increased, from elevation of intracellular calcium to production of amplifying autacoids. So far, it has not been possible to identify 1 element of the signaling cascade that is responsible for this hyperreactivity.

Physiologic Effects of Ang II

Short-term actions mediated by AT$_1$ receptors
Cardiovascular homeostasis. The best-established biologic effects of Ang II are listed in **Table A3.1**, and some are depicted in **Figure A3.1**. Most of the rapid actions constitute a concerted response that supports the circulation when hemorrhage or dehydration depletes plasma volume. These actions include vasoconstriction, which reduces the capacity of the vascular tree, and aldosterone secretion, tubular sodium retention, and release of antidiuretic hormone, which conserve intravascular fluid volume. Most other rapid homeostatic actions of Ang II can be viewed as adjuncts to circulatory rescue: increased sympathetic nervous activity, increased thirst, intestinal fluid absorption, platelet agglutination, and increased cardiac contractility. In the absence of volume contraction, the rapid actions of Ang II can elevate blood pressure above baseline. This is particularly noticeable in renovascular hypertension, in which angiotensin formation is increased despite a normal plasma volume.

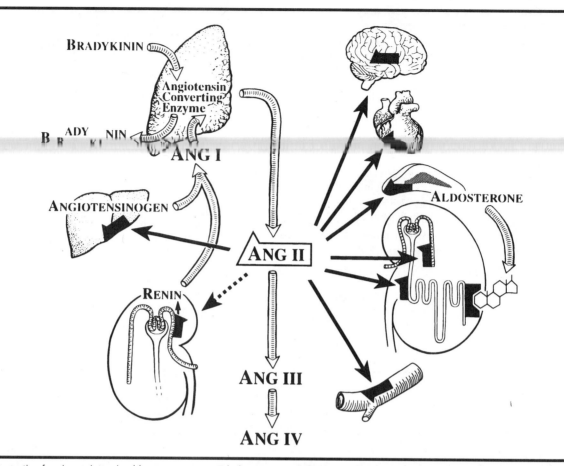

Figure A3.1. Schematic of renin-angiotensin-aldosterone system. Tubular arrows on left show pathway of formation of angiotensin (Ang) II and degradation of bradykinin by enzymes in blood and lung. Arrows in center show cascade of proteolytic cleavages that form smaller congeners of Ang II. Solid arrows indicate stimulatory actions of Ang II, and dashed arrow shows its principal inhibitory action: to reduce renin release. Solid symbols at end of arrows indicate angiotensin receptors. Except for brain, which has 2 subtypes, all receptors in this figure are the AT$_1$ subtype. Not shown are the formation and actions of Ang (1–7), and the synthesis of angiotensin within tissues independent of the blood-borne renin-angiotensin-aldosterone system.

Central nervous system. Angiotensin receptors of both subtypes are found in many regions of the brain. Some sites are in circum-ventricular organs, which lack the usual blood–brain barrier and can be activated by angiotensins in the circulation. Other sites are behind the blood–brain barrier and are probably activated by angiotensins formed from substrate and enzymes resident in the brain itself. Ang II and III in the brain increase release of antidiuretic hormone, stimulate thirst, and increase blood pressure by effects on hypothalamic and brain stem neurons. There is experimental evidence for effects of angiotensin peptides on memory and other cortical functions, but the relevance of these animal findings to humans is not established.

Feedback Interactions. Some actions of Ang II serve as afferent limbs of negative and positive feedback loops. Ang II directly inhibits release of renin by the juxtaglomerular cells (a negative feedback effect), and stimulates release of angiotensinogen by the liver (a positive feedback effect).

Long-term actions mediated by AT$_1$ receptors

Cell growth and organ hypertrophy. Administration of sub-pressor doses of Ang II to animals for days or weeks causes trophic changes in the heart and blood vessels, including sensitization of vessels to other constrictors, hypertrophy of myocardial and vascular contractile cells, and deposition of collagen and other macromolecules of the extracellular matrix. These effects are mediated by the AT$_1$ receptor subtype. Drugs that block the formation of Ang II (ACE-inhibitors) or block its action at AT$_1$ receptors (ARBs) can retard or reverse left ventricular hypertrophy and other structural manifestations of human hypertension.

Inflammation and remodeling. Ang II stimulates migration of monocytes, and when cellular and extracellular effects are viewed together, they represent many features of inflammation, causing some to regard Ang II and the AT$_1$ receptor as proinflammatory. The structural changes induced by prolonged elevations of Ang II also resemble the cardiovascular changes, called *remodeling,* seen in human hypertension and atherosclerosis.

Embryogenesis. One of the most important slow effects of Ang II is on the fetus. Experiments with ACE-inhibitors, ARBs and gene deletion in animals, and experience with ACE-inhibitors and ARBs in humans clearly show that Ang II is essential for normal embryogenesis. The organ whose development suffers most from loss of angiotensin action is the kidney, but a variety of other abnormalities have been observed in animals and humans when the renin-angiotensin axis is perturbed during fetal life.

Erythropoietic effects. Ang II acts with erythropoietin to increase red cell production. This action is evident in some patients whose hematocrit drops when they are treated with drugs that block angiotensin formation or action. The erythropoietic effect of Ang II is mediated by the AT$_1$ receptor subtype.

Other actions. There are receptors for Ang II in places where the function of the peptide is obscure. For example, the urinary bladder contains AT_1 receptors, and the rat bladder contracts when exposed to Ang II *in vitro*, but there is no known relevance of this effect in humans. Tissues of the male and female reproductive tract display angiotensin receptors, but the roles of the peptide in the function of the ovary, uterus, placenta, and testis are unknown. Similar mystery shrouds the function of Ang II receptors in adipocytes, synovium, skin, peripheral nerves, anterior pituitary, pancreas, and immune system.

Actions mediated by AT_2 receptors

Fetal development. AT_2 is the predominant subtype in fetal mammals. It is important in development of the kidney. Because they mediate vasodilation, not vasoconstriction, AT_2 receptors probably protect the fetus from ischemia that might result from any maternal angiotensin that crossed the placenta. In normal adult mammals, the AT_2 subtype is found almost exclusively in some regions of the brain, the uterus, the adrenal medulla, and the kidney, but in much smaller amounts than in the fetus.

Vasodilation. Activation of AT_2 receptors by Ang II initiate a vasodilatory cascade that begins with release of bradykinin, followed by production of nitric oxide and generation of intracellular cyclic guanosine monophosphate. In addition, AT_2 receptors mediate release of prostaglandins from tissues in which the receptor is present and activated by Ang II, especially the kidney. AT_2 receptors mediate inhibition of cell growth, an action directly opposite to those mediated by the AT_1 subtype. In fact, almost all of the actions mediated by AT_2 receptors are opposite to those mediated by AT_1. Because ARBs interfere with feedback inhibition of renin release, they cause increased plasma levels of Ang II, but they leave the AT_2 receptor open to the peptide. Therefore, activation of AT_2 subtypes may mediate some of the antihypertensive properties of these drugs.

Apoptosis and natriuresis. There is evidence that Ang II, when it binds to AT_2, induces apoptosis. In the kidney, AT_2 receptors promote natriuresis, again opposite to the renal effects of Ang II mediated by AT_1.

Other actions. Levels of AT_2 receptors in the adult heart are lower than those of AT_1, but they rise dramatically after myocardial infarction, as they do after injury in other tissues. The function of these receptors in injured tissue is unknown, but they may prevent vasoconstriction that might otherwise be mediated by Ang II acting through AT_1.

Modulation of Angiotensin II Actions

The acute and chronic effects of Ang II are increased or decreased by other autacoids released in response to the peptide.

Amplifiers and negative modulators. Aldosterone, catecholamines, and antidiuretic hormone are increased by Ang II; these hormones participate in the concerted actions to protect or expand circulating blood volume and maintain blood pressure. Aldosterone also amplifies the action of Ang II to release plasminogen activator inhibitor from endothelium and to stimulate fibrosis in the heart and blood vessels. Ang II stimulates release of endothelin and thromboxane from endothelium, and both of those autacoids contribute to vasoconstriction.

The slower actions of Ang II to stimulate growth, fibrosis, and "inflammation" in the cardiovascular system are amplified by growth factors such as platelet-derived growth factor, epidermal growth factor, insulin-like growth factor, basic fibroblast growth factor, and transforming growth factor β. By contrast, the vasodilators nitric oxide and prostacyclin released from blood vessels under the influence of Ang II protect the kidney and other vital organs from excessive vasoconstriction.

Oxidative stress. Along with the steroid aldosterone, thromboxane, catecholamines, growth factors, and peptides such as endothelin, Ang II exerts its pressor and hypertrophic effects on the cardiovascular system by increasing oxidative stress (see Chapters A19 and A65). Through the AT_1 receptor subtype, Ang II stimulates formation of reactive oxygen species such as peroxide and superoxide, which can damage cell membrane lipids, structural proteins, and nucleic acids and can combine with nitric oxide. Oxidative stress can stimulate vascular smooth muscle contraction and cell growth on the one hand, and impair endothelial cell integrity and function on the other.

Biologic Effects of Other Angiotensins

Ang 1–7 is a weak agonist that binds with low affinity to the AT_1 receptor, so the net effect of large amounts of that peptide is to inhibit Ang II action at that receptor. In addition, Ang 1–7 induces formation of nitric oxide and vasodilator prostaglandins and retards vascular smooth muscle growth by a mechanism that does not involve the AT_1 receptor. Levels of Ang 1–7 are increased during therapy with ACE-inhibitors. Angiotensin IV (Ang 2–8) has effects on the brain that suggest a role in memory. It also stimulates the release of plasminogen activator inhibitor from endothelial cells (see Chapters A6, A7, A23).

SUGGESTED READING

1. Goodfriend TL, Elliott ME, Catt KJ. Angiotensin receptors and their antagonists. *N Engl J Med.* 1996;334:1649–1654.
2. Goodfriend TL. Angiotensin receptors: history and mysteries. *Am J Hypertens.* 2000;13:442–449.
3. deGasparo M, Catt KJ, Inagami T, et al. International union of pharmacology. XXIII. The angiotensin II receptors. *Pharmacol Rev.* 2000;52:415–472.
4. Touyz RM, Schiffrin EL. Signal transduction mechanisms mediating the physiological and pathophysiological actions of angiotensin II in vascular smooth muscle cells. *Pharmacol Rev.* 2000;52:639–672.
5. Carey RM, Wang ZQ, Siragy HM. Role of the angiotensin type 2 (AT_2) receptor in the regulation of blood pressure and renal function. *Hypertension.* 2000;35:155–163.

Chapter A4

Angiotensinogen

Morton P. Printz, PhD

KEY POINTS

- Angiotensin peptides arise from angiotensinogen.

- There are multiple angiotensinogen systems.

- Plasma angiotensinogen correlates with arterial pressure in animals.

- Angiotensinogen gene polymorphisms are associated with hypertension in some ethnic populations.

See also Chapters A3, A5–A8, A41, A46, A75, A76, A78, and C148

Biochemistry

Angiotensinogen (AGT) is the only known precursor protein (prohormone) for the family of angiotensin (Ang) peptides, including Angs I, II, III (des-Asp^1-Ang II), IV (des-Asp^1-Arg^2-Ang II), and "1–7" (des-Phe^8-Ang II). AGT and renin are rate determinants for the formation of active Ang II in the circulation. AGT was originally known as *renin substrate*. After a single amide bond scission by renin, the inactive decapeptide Ang I is released, leaving behind in the circulation 98% of the original protein, des-Ang I-AGT. Prepro-AGT is processed and glycosylated in a species- and tissue-dependent manner, and post-translational processing and postsecretional glycolytic activity result in a mixture of electrophoretically distinguishable forms. Initial studies indicated that the carbohydrate adducts had minor but distinguishable effects on the kinetics of renin-AGT interaction; these effects have been confirmed in recent studies seeking a functional effect of the M235T polymorphic variant of human AGT. However, the exact role of the carbohydrate on *in vivo* functioning of AGT remains unclear.

Evidence for Multiple Angiotensinogen/Angiotensin Systems

Although attention focused for years on plasma AGT, we now know that there are at least 4 independent AGT systems: (a) systemic, (b) brain, (c) sex glands and fetoplacental, and (d) other tissue and organs. The first is the systemic system localized to the circulation. Here, AGT is synthesized by hepatocytes and immediately released into the circulation with no storage in the liver. The brain AGT system (and first "tissue" system) stems from the finding that cerebrospinal fluid (CSF) and brain AGT was not of hepatic (i.e., blood) origin but was synthesized directly within the central nervous system (CNS). The third AGT system is localized within sex glands of both genders and has a major role during pregnancy in functioning of the fetoplacental unit and in fetal development. The fourth system is a collection of other tissues and organs, all of which have been shown to express AGT messenger RNA (mRNA) and in which, in most cases, AGT formation is regulated in a manner independent of the systemic, brain, or uterine systems. These tissue AGT systems have local influences on organ function but, in the absence of a functioning systemic system, can exert systemic effects. Among the tissues in which local AGT is formed are the kidney, adrenal, cardiac, vascular, pulmonary, eye, and adipose. Within these tissues, a variety of cell types are implicated, namely cardiac myocytes, cardiac and pulmonary interstitial fibroblasts, endothelial and vascular smooth muscle cells, adipocytes, and renal tubular epithelial cells.

Control of Angiotensinogen Release

Systemic system. Early studies established the hepatocyte as the source of systemic (i.e., plasma) AGT. The protein is constitutively expressed as a preproprotein, processed and secreted into the venous outflow so as to maintain a steady-state plasma concentration of AGT. Because AGT is a protein substrate for the enzyme renin, it would be expected that plasma renin activity would be rate limiting; however, renin's Michaelis constant for AGT approximates AGT's steady-state plasma concentration so that the rate of Ang I release becomes a function of both renin and plasma AGT. There are excessively high amounts of plasma AGT due to steroid overstimulation of hepatocyte synthesis and secretion.

Plasma levels of AGT reflect control at several sites: constitutive expression, transcriptional regulation, mRNA lifetime, and protein half-life within the circulation. Among the many molecules found to exert transcriptional regulation are Ang II, estrogens, thyroid hormone, cytokines, and glucocorticoid. The hepatocyte Ang II AT$_1$ receptor subtype enhances synthesis and secretion of AGT and thereby exerts positive feedback regulation. AT1 signaling is multifactorial, with 1 pathway involving coupling to nuclear factor-κB, and a second related to enhanced mRNA lifetime (attributed to stimulated formation of a cytosolic protein that binds to 3' nontranslated sequence). The third mechanism regulating plasma AGT is its half-life in the circulation; the reaction half-time of intact AGT has been reported to vary between 6 and 20 hours, depending on species. Within the circulation, both intact AGT and des-Ang I-AGT are present, but the fate and importance of des-Ang I-AGT remain unknown.

Brain–central nervous system. Ang II is present in CSF in a high concentration (almost 2% of total protein), which is unusual for a neuronal source. Recent studies have demonstrated that rat brain AGT is produced both by glia and neurons in an approximate 2:1 to 3:1 ratio. It is likely that neuronal AGT is the source of nerve terminal Ang II, whereas glia export large amounts of AGT into CSF for a function not yet elucidated. It is unknown whether a brain renin or another protease is responsible for processing AGT to Ang I/II. The electrophoretic characteristics of CSF AGT also differ from the systemic protein.

Brain AGT formation is evident throughout fetal development and appears to correlate with developmental maturation of the CNS, starting initially with glial expression in and around the hypothalamus and radiating outward into cortices and brain parenchyma. Subsequently, AGT is found within neurons. AGT distribution correlates with expression of the Ang AT_2 receptor subtype implying that during development, AGT is processed to Ang peptides, which then bind to AT_2 receptors. Fetal expression of AGT is area-specific and highest in the hindbrain and spinal cord, whereas, in adult animals, expression is greater in hypothalamic and medullary brain nuclei. In transgenic rats, the level of AGT expression within the brain correlates with the density of Ang receptors at sites within, but not outside of, the blood–brain barrier. The autonomic nervous system ganglia also express AGT mRNA; thus, AGT is formed both within the CNS and the autonomic nervous system.

Brain AGT is regulated by hormones, steroids, and cytokines and, like hepatic AGT, is dependent on a basal level of thyroid hormone secretion. Hypothyroidism results in lowered hepatic and brain AGT, whereas hyperthyroidism, which greatly enhances hepatic synthesis, fails to stimulate overall brain synthesis. Glial AGT formation is reduced by adrenalectomy and, concomitantly, glucocorticoid has been shown to enhance AGT formation predominantly via the type II receptor.

Fetoplacental system. AGT and other components of the Ang system are present in the fetus and pregnant uterus throughout gestation. Estrogens and androgens affect AGT synthesis. During pregnancy, a high-molecular-weight form of human systemic AGT was identified and shown to increase in pregnancy-induced hypertension. However, the ratio of high- to normal-molecular-weight forms appears to reflect events within the fetoplacental unit, rather than an etiologic factor in the development of hypertension. The origins of this form of AGT and its function, if any, await further study.

Adipose system. Adipose tissue is a significant source of AGT, and studies performed in the late 1990s indicate that AGT mRNA expression increases more in adipose tissue of males with obesity than males who are not obese. Body weight correlated independently and positively with adipose AGT mRNA expression (adjusted for age and height), and adipose AGT expression also correlated with abdominal fat distribution in obesity. In a transgenic mouse with the AGT gene knocked out [i.e., AGT

(–/–)] and made transgenic with a rat AGT gene restricted to adipose tissue expression, rat AGT was found in the circulation (indicating export) and the normally *hypo*tensive AGT null mice were made *normo*tensive. However, when wild-type mice (AGT +/+) also had the rat transgene inserted, there was both systemic and adipose AGT expression with greatly increased plasma AGT and hypertension. Of interest was the finding that transgenic adipose expression in the AGT (–/–) mice also rescued the animals from developmental abnormalities of the kidney, normally found with total ablation of the AGT gene. This illustrates systemic effects of a local tissue AGT system.

Role of Angiotensinogen in Hypertension

The early demonstration of the link between oral contraceptive hypertension and systemic AGT was the forerunner of more recent evidence implicating AGT in potentially all forms of systemic arterial hypertension. In AGT null mice and in transgenic rats in which AGT formation is compromised through the use of antisense, systemic arterial pressure is directly related to the absence or functioning of the AGT gene. In mice in which integral numbers of functioning AGT genes are inserted, systemic arterial pressure is increased in proportion to the number of genes inserted. This would imply a direct connection between the AGT gene and level of systemic arterial pressure, indicating that blood pressure is a function of the reaction between renin and systemic AGT.

High levels of AGT are found in the spontaneously hypertensive rat (SHR) brain when compared to age-matched normotensive Wistar-Kyoto rats. However, these differences vary with age and tend to normalize when hypertension is fully expressed. Studies have documented greater AGT formation in selected brain areas in the SHR. In contrast, plasma (i.e., systemic) AGT is not different between SHR and Wistar-Kyoto rats at 6 weeks of age but is increased after 14 weeks. Thus, increased brain AGT in SHR parallels the development phase of hypertension. When brain AGT expression is inhibited in SHR, blood pressure is lowered, and conversely, in both transgenic rats and engineered mice, heightened arterial pressure and hypertension are coincident with increased expression of brain AGT.

Genetics of Angiotensinogen and Hypertension

Molecular aspects. The AGT gene has been cloned, the genomic sequence determined, and its chromosomal location determined. Only 1 copy of the gene is present in human and other mammalian genomes. The human AGT gene consists of 5 exons, 4 introns, and nontranslated-5' and -3' termini. Exon 1 encodes the 5'-nontranslated sequence of the mRNA whereas the signal peptide and the coding region for Ang I are encoded by exon 2. The other 3 exons contain the balance of information for the protein as well as the 3'-nontranslated region. In humans AGT is located on chromosome 1, in mice on chromosome 8, and in the rat on chromosome 17.

Genetic studies. Classic genetic efforts to demonstrate involvement of the AGT gene in genetic hypertension of humans and rodents have met with mixed success. Blood pressure quantitative trait loci found from studies of genetic hypertensive rodent models have not identified the AGT gene as a major gene determining the level of arterial pressure. Although genetically engineered mice implicate the AGT gene as an important part of blood pressure regulation, they have not established a definitive link with essential hypertension. Furthermore, few studies have addressed the role of genetic background on altered AGT gene function in murine and transgenic rat models. Human genetic studies in unique families did identify a quantitative trait loci near the human AGT gene and subsequent linkage, and sequence analysis implicated the T174M and M235T diallelic polymorphisms within the coding sequence as potentially contributory to essential hypertension. Since these findings, many association and linkage studies have examined the contribution to essential hypertension of these (and other) single nucleotide polymorphisms (SNPs) in different subsets of patients and normals and to other cardiovascular traits.

Ethnic populations. The association of AGT with hypertension has been confirmed in many ethnic-based studies, but not in all. The M235T polymorphism has received greatest attention and was found to be in linkage disequilibrium with an A(–6)G polymorphism in the 5'-promoter sequence. The M235T SNP was shown to be a determinant of plasma AGT concentration; however, except for oral contraceptive–induced hypertension, plasma AGT levels do not correlate tightly with level of blood pressure. There are many potential SNPs that could comprise a hypertension haplotype. In one study, a 14.4-kilobase genomic region spanning the AGT gene was

sequenced and 44 SNPs identified. Six major haplotypes were identified in a comparison of Caucasian and Japanese subjects and accounted for most of the genetic variation in this region. However, the 2 ethnic populations exhibited substantial differences in haplotype frequency, with Caucasians exhibiting a higher frequency of M235-associated haplotypes.

SUGGESTED READING

1. Bremer AA, Jamaluddin M, Han Y, et al. Angiotensin II induces gene transcription through cell-type-dependent effects on the nuclear factor-kappaB (NF-kappaB) transcription factor. *Mol Cell Biochem*. 2000;212:155–169.
2. Corvol P, Soubrier F, Jeunemaitre X. Molecular genetics of the renin-angiotensin-aldosterone system in human hypertension. *Pathol Biol (Paris)*. 1997;45:229–239.
3. Ding Y, Stec DE, Sigmund CD. Genetic evidence that lethality in angiotensinogen-deficient mice is due to loss of systemic but not renal angiotensinogen. *J Biol Chem*. 2001;276:7431–7436.
4. Kim HS, Lee G, John SW, et al. Molecular phenotyping for analyzing subtle genetic effects in mice: application to an angiotensinogen gene titration. *Proc Natl Acad Sci U S A*. 2002;99:4602–4607.
5. Lalouel JM, Rohrwasser A, Terreros D, et al. Angiotensinogen in essential hypertension: from genetics to nephrology. *J Am Soc Nephrol*. 2001;12:606–615.
6. Nakajima T, Jorde LB, Ishigami T, et al. Nucleotide diversity and haplotype structure of the human angiotensinogen gene in two populations. *Am J Hum Genet*. 2002;70:108–123.
7. Smithies O, Kim HS, Takahashi N, Edgell MH. Importance of quantitative genetic variations in the etiology of hypertension. *Kidney Int*. 2000;58:2265–2280.

Chapter A5

Renin Synthesis and Secretion

William H. Beierwaltes, PhD

KEY POINTS

- *Renin* is the rate-limiting enzyme in the formation of the vasoconstrictor angiotensin II.

- Renal juxtaglomerular cells are the site of renin synthesis, storage, and release, initiated by formation of first preprorenin, then inactive prorenin, which is deposited in storage granules and cleaved to form the active enzyme.

- Active renin is secreted in response to 4 regulatory mechanisms: the renal baroreceptor, the macula densa, β_1-receptor stimulation by renal nerves, and humoral factors.

See also Chapters A3, A4, A6–A8, A37, A48, A49, and C148

Renin Synthesis in Juxtaglomerular Cells

Renin catalyzes the rate-limiting step in a cascade that forms angiotensin II (Ang II) and its congeners (**Figure A5.1**). Renin is an aspartyl proteolytic enzyme whose substrate is angiotensinogen, a 60,000-d peptide formed within the liver and released into the general circulation. The target bond of renin action is located between leucine in position 10 and valine in position 11, between the body of the angiotensinogen molecule and its

amino-terminal decapeptide. The decapeptide released from the substrate is angiotensin I, which in turn is changed by angiotensin converting enzyme into the potent vasoactive hormone Ang II. Because renin catalyzes the critical rate-limiting step in the formation of Ang II, renin activity is generally used as an index of the endogenous formation of Ang II and reflects the importance of the signals that control renin synthesis and release.

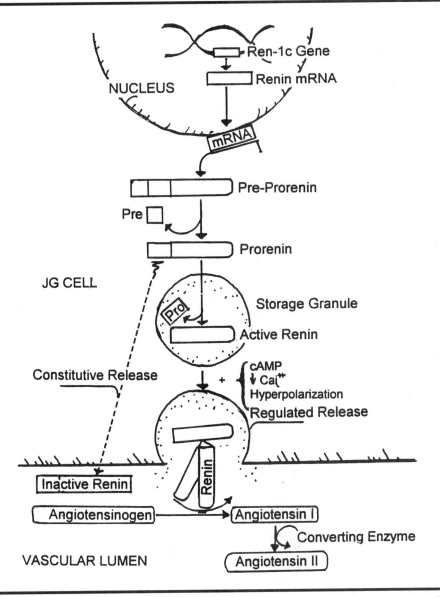

Figure A5.1. Cascade of renin synthesis, activation, and release in juxtaglomerular cell in afferent arteriole, leading to enzymatic formation of angiotensin II. cAMP, cyclic adenosine monophosphate; mRNA, messenger RNA.

The Ren-1ᶜ gene is responsible for renin messenger RNA formation, which then initiates synthesis of an enzymatically inactive preprorenin by renin messenger RNA. This intermediate form is transported into the rough endoplasmic reticulum. The 23–amino acid "pre" sequence is cleaved, leaving prorenin, which is also an inactive form of the enzyme (47,000 d); in turn, prorenin is passed through the Golgi apparatus, glycosylated, and deposited in lysosomal granules. There the carboxyl-terminal 43-amino-acid "pro" sequence is cleaved to form the enzymatically active form of renin (40,000 d). It is thought that cleavage and activation within the granules are initiated by the enzyme cathepsin B. Once the pro sequence is removed, unmasking the active aspartyl residues of the molecule, secretion or release of active renin occurs in response to various regulatory stimuli.

Renin-storing granules migrate to the cellular surface, where exocytosis causes the active enzyme to be released into the vascular lumen and possibly into the renal interstitium. There is constant basal (or constitutive) release of active renin into the circulation, accounting for basal plasma renin activity and circulating levels of angiotensin II, as well as various stimuli (discussed in the sections Renal Baroreceptors, Macula Densa, Renal Nerves, and Humoral Factors) that increase renin secretion in response to various physiologic or pathophysiologic conditions.

Release of inactive prorenin and its presence in the circulation, which under basal conditions is 2-fold to 5-fold greater than circulating active renin, are not regulated by acute control mechanisms and may only reflect synthesis. Any other significance of circulating prorenin is unknown. When active renin secretion is stimulated, circulating inactive renin tends to be diminished, presumably as more prorenin is channeled into storage granules or activated. Extrarenal activation of inactive renin remains controversial and unresolved.

Sources of Renin

Juxtaglomerular cells. Juxtaglomerular (JG) cells are the locus for renin synthesis, storage, and release. Renal renin is synthesized, stored, and released by the JG cells, which have been hypothesized to be derived from vascular smooth muscle, although it is now thought that the 2 cell types may be derived from a similar progenitor. They are located in the medial layer of the vascular wall near the terminus of the afferent arteriole, where they abut the glomerulus and macula densa. They are highly specialized epithelioid cells containing myofilaments, some mitochondria, and renin-containing granules, as well as gap junctions and myoendothelial junctions coupling them to other JG cells and smooth muscle and endothelial cells.

Renin in other tissues. In most mammals, the kidney is the primary source of synthesis and secretion of active renin, although prorenin has been found in a number of extrarenal sources, including the adrenal, pituitary, and submandibular glands. These extrarenal ("tissue") renin-angiotensin systems are discussed in Chapter A8.

Physiologic Regulation of Renin Release

Overall role of salt balance. Chronic sodium deprivation results in a unique metaplastic transformation or "recruitment" of non-JG afferent arteriolar cells upstream, which become renin-expressing as renin secretion and plasma renin activity increase under these conditions. Renin gene expression is mediated by hormones through hormone-response elements for androgens and thyroxine. Sodium restriction also leads to renin expression in the JG cell, as do chronic increases in cyclic adenosine monophosphate (cAMP), whereas angiotensin has been proposed as a negative (feedback) regulator of renin gene expression.

Modulatory mechanisms. Release of active renin is regulated by 4 factors: (a) the renal baroreceptor, (b) macula densa, (c) renal nerves, and (d) various humoral factors.

Renal baroreceptors. An intrarenal vascular stretch receptor in the afferent arteriole stimulates renin secretion in response to reduced renal perfusion pressure and attenuates it as renal perfusion is elevated. The renal baroreceptor is perhaps the most powerful regulator of renin release, and its chronic stimulation contributes to the hyperreninemic phase of renovascular hypertension, resulting in an increase in renin synthesis and release.

Macula densa. A modified plaque of sensory cells (macula densa) located in the distal tubule of the nephron at the end of the loop of Henle lies adjacent to the afferent arteriole, JG cells, and extraglomerular mesangium. All of these components make up the JG apparatus, which sends a feedback signal when the macula densa senses a decrease in distal tubular salt delivery. This signal initiates a series of steps that ultimately stimulates renin secretion. Although the specific nature of the feedback signal remains a topic of considerable interest, adenosine is most often implicated, although many other factors, including prostaglandin E_2 and nitric oxide, may be involved. Cyclooxygenase-2 and the neuronal isoform of nitric oxide synthase are localized to the macula densa cells and respond to signals that stimulate the macula densa pathway for renin regulation. The macula densa mechanism is most likely a chronic adaptive system for regulating renin rather than an acute mediator.

Renal nerves. JG cells are directly innervated by sympathetic nerves. Direct stimulation of the renal nerves increases renin release from the JG cells through a β_1-adrenergic–mediated mechanism. The renal nerves are stimulated via a pathway that involves cardiac mechanoreceptors, aortocarotid pressoreceptors, chemoreceptors, and vagal afferent fibers. Several central neural reflex pathways mediate stimulation of efferent sympathetic renal nerve traffic and subsequent stimulation of renin secretion. Renal nerve–mediated renin secretion constitutes an acute pathway by which rapid activation of the renin-angiotensin system is provoked by such stimuli as stress and posture.

Humoral factors. Although the 3 pathways discussed in the sections Renal Baroreceptors, Macula Densa, and Renal Nerves are the classic regulators of renin release, a series of humoral factors has also been implicated. The primary stimulatory intracellular "second messenger" for renin release is the cyclic nucleotide cAMP, which is probably the second messenger for stimulation by β-adrenergic nerves and prostaglandins. Humoral agents such as prostacyclin, endothelium-derived hyperpolarizing factor, and nitric oxide may hyperpolarize vascular smooth muscle cells and JG cells, leading to decreased influx of calcium across cell membranes. Integration of these humoral mechanisms into the more classic pathways of renin stimulation and the precise mechanisms of constitutive regulation of renin secretion remain the focus of considerable investigation.

Inhibitors of renin release

Intracellular calcium. Unlike most secretory responses (except parathyroid follicular cells that release parathyroid hormone), renin release is inhibited, not stimulated, by increased intracellular calcium. This occurs via a calmodulin-mediated process. Thus, there is an inverse relationship between intracellular calcium concentration and renin release. Electric depolarization of the JG cell permits calcium entry and inhibits renin release. Conversely, hyperpolarization leads to decreased JG cell calcium and increased renin release. Among the depolarizing, inhibitory humoral factors are vasoconstrictors such as angiotensin, α-adrenergic agonists, thromboxane (or the endoperoxide prostaglandin H_2), adenosine A_1 agonists, and endothelin.

Cyclic nucleotides. The cyclic nucleotide guanosine monophosphate (cGMP) may also act as an inhibitory second messenger. It is hypothesized that cGMP can inhibit renin secretion directly, acting through G-kinase II. Factors that stimulate guanylate cyclase, such as atrial natriuretic factor and nitric oxide, inhibit renin release. It is also possible that some of these inhibitory hormones stimulate phospholipase C, leading to release of intracellular calcium from sequestered stores that would also inhibit renin release. However, cGMP can also diminish the catabolism of renin-stimulating cAMP by selectively inhibiting phosphodiesterase-3, thereby indirectly stimulating renin.

SUGGESTED READING

1. Bader M, Ganten D. Regulation of renin: new evidence from cultured cells and genetically modified mice. *J Mol Med.* 2000;78:130–139.
2. Hsueh WA, Baxter JD. Human prorenin. *Hypertension.* 1991;17:469–477.
3. Keeton TK, Campbell WB. The pharmacologic alteration of renin release. *Pharmacol Rev.* 1980;32:81–227.

4. Kurtz A, Wagner C. Role of nitric oxide in the control of renin secretion. *Am J Physiol Renal Physiol.* 1998;275:F849–F862.

5. Kurtz A, Wagner C. Cellular control of renin secretion. *J Exp Biol.* 1999;202:219–225.

6. Navar LG, Inscho EW, Majid SA, et al. Paracrine regulation of the renal microcirculation. *Physiol Rev.* 1996;76:425–536.

7. Sigmund CD, Gross KW. Structure, expression, and regulation of the murine renin genes. *Hypertension.* 1991;18:446–457.

Chapter A6

Angiotensin I–Converting Enzyme and Neprilysin (Neutral Endopeptidase)

Randal A. Skidgel, PhD; Ervin G. Erdös, MD

KEY POINTS

- Angiotensin-converting enzyme hydrolyzes inactive angiotensin I to the active pressor angiotensin II and inactivates the vasodilator bradykinin.

- Angiotensin-converting enzyme is found on endothelial cells, especially in the lung, retina, and brain. It is also present on the microvillar structures in the choroid plexus, proximal tubules of the kidney, placenta, intestine, and testes.

- Neprilysin cleaves a variety of peptides. Among them are angiotensin I, bradykinin, enkephalins, substance P, and the atrial natriuretic peptide.

- Neprilysin is widely distributed in the body in kidney, brain, and male genital tract. Neprilysin is a marker of the malignant cells in acute lymphoblastic leukemia.

See also Chapters A3–A5, A7, A8, A14–A16, A23, C144, and C148

ANGIOTENSIN I–CONVERTING ENZYME

Activity

Angiotensin-converting enzyme (ACE) converts the inactive decapeptide angiotensin (Ang) I to the active octapeptide Ang II by releasing the C-terminal histidyl-leucine dipeptide. The enzyme is not specific for Ang, because it cleaves a variety of other peptides, including bradykinin luteinizing hormone-releasing hormone, enkephalins, and substance P. On the basis of enzyme kinetics, ACE is a better "kininase" than "converting enzyme" or "enkephalinase" because of the very low K_m of bradykinin. Thus, ACE activates the vasoconstrictor Ang, whereas it inactivates the vasodilator bradykinin (**Figure A6.1**). ACE inhibitors interfere with both reactions, prolonging the half-life of bradykinin while inhibiting the formation of Ang II. Some of the beneficial cardiac actions of ACE inhibitor therapy are attributed to potentiating and prolonging the effect of bradykinin. ACE is a metalloenzyme that always requires zinc as cofactor and also needs chloride ions to cleave most substrates; Ang I conversion is absolutely chloride dependent, whereas bradykinin hydrolysis is less affected.

Molecular Aspects

General properties. Human ACE has a molecular weight of 150,000 to 180,000 d, of which 146,000 d is protein and the balance is carbohydrate. The majority of ACE is membrane-bound and is present on the plasma membrane of various cell types (**Figure A6.2**). ACE is inserted into the membrane by a short hydrophobic region near the C-terminus. Proteolytic cleavage near the C-terminus results in the release of ACE from the plasma membrane. This is carried out *in vivo* by a zinc-dependent metalloprotease that may be a member of the ADAM (*a d*isintegrin *and m*etalloprotease) family that also is the α-secretase that cleaves the amyloid precursor protein from the membrane. As a result of this proteolytic release, ACE can be detected in many body fluids (Figure A6.2).

Structure. The primary structure of ACE, first determined by cloning and sequencing its complementary DNA from a human endothelial cell library, unexpectedly revealed the presence of 2 putative active centers (Figure A6.2) located within 2 highly homologous domains, which probably evolved through gene duplication. This is further supported by the fact that testicular ACE contains only 1 of these domains and, therefore, may represent the ancestral, nonduplicated form of the enzyme. Endothelial ACE contains 2 zinc ions and 2 inhibitor binding sites per molecule, also indicating the presence of 2 functional active sites. The K_m values for the classic substrates (Ang I or bradykinin) do not differ much between the active centers on the N- and C-domains, but the turnover number of the C-domain is higher *in vitro*. Some other physiologic peptide substrates are preferentially cleaved by the N-domain active site such as the hemoregulatory tetrapeptide, acetyl-Ser-Asp-Lys-Pro, Ang 1–7, and luteinizing hormone-releasing hormone. These rates of dissociation of inhibitors from the active centers in the 2 domains differ, so the duration of their inhibition also differs.

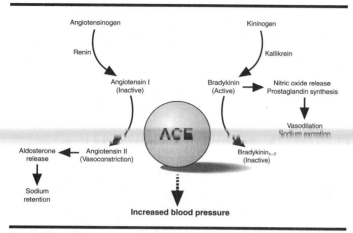

Figure A6.1. The role of angiotensin I–converting enzyme (ACE) in the metabolism of vasoactive peptides. ACE can contribute to the elevation of blood pressure by converting the inactive peptide angiotensin I to the active vasoconstrictor angiotensin II and by inactivating the vasodilator bradykinin. By blocking vasoconstriction and promoting sodium excretion, ACE inhibitors can lower blood pressure. (Modified with permission from Skidgel RA, Erdös EG. Biochemistry of angiotensin I converting enzyme. In: Robertson JIS, Nichols MG, eds. *The Renin Angiotensin System.* London: Gower Medical Publishing; 1993.)

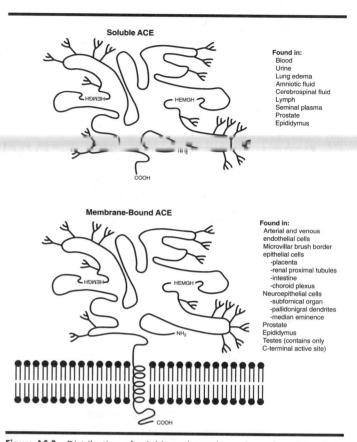

Figure A6.2. Distribution of soluble and membrane-bound angiotensin I–converting enzyme (ACE). ACE is widely distributed in tissues, cells, and body fluids. Membrane-bound ACE, shown in schematic, is attached to the lipid bilayer by a C-terminal hydrophobic anchor peptide, whereas soluble ACE lacks this portion of the molecule due to proteolytic cleavage. Most of the physiologic functions of ACE are attributed to the membrane-bound form. The His-Glu-Met-Gly-His (HEMGH) sequence represents the zinc-binding motif in the 2 active-site domains of ACE, and branched structures denote potential glycosylation sites.

Distribution

In vascular beds, ACE is bound to the plasma membrane of endothelial cells where it cleaves circulating peptides such as Ang I or bradykinin. Vessels of the lung, retina, and brain are especially rich in ACE. Some epithelial cells in humans have a higher concentration of ACE than do endothelial cells; the human kidney contains 5 to 6 times more ACE per wet weight than the lung; the proximal tubular brush border is a major site of kidney ACE. Other microvillar structures of epithelial linings in the small intestine, choroid plexus, and placenta are also very rich in ACE. ACE is concentrated in some regions of the brain besides the choroid plexus, such as the subfornical organ, area postrema, substantia nigra, and locus caeruleus.

Genetic Variation

Studies on the structure of the human ACE gene revealed an insertion (I)/deletion (D) polymorphism in a noncoding region, corresponding to the presence or absence of a 287-base pair sequence in intron 16. Individuals homozygous for the insertion polymorphism (II) have lower levels of ACE in plasma than do those with the DD genotype. The correlation of this polymorphism with cardiovascular and renal diseases has been the subject of many studies. Some investigations suggest an association of the D allele with an increased risk for hypertension, myocardial infarction, or diabetic nephropathy, and the I allele has been associated with enhanced endurance performance in athletes.

NEPRILYSIN (NEUTRAL ENDOPEPTIDASE)

Neprilysin (NEP) was found first in the kidney proximal tubules as neutral endopeptidase 24.11, then as enkephalinase in brain, and subsequently as common acute lymphoblastic leukemia antigen (CALLA of CD10) in lymphocytes.

Actions

NEP cleaves bradykinin, enkephalin, and the chemotactic peptide fMet-Leu-Phe at the same peptide bonds as ACE, and NEP cleaves numerous other vaso- and neuropeptides at different sites. In general, NEP hydrolyzes peptide substrates at the amino end of hydrophobic amino acids, such as phenylalanine. In contrast to ACE, NEP does not release Ang II from Ang I, but cleaves it to a hepta- and tripeptide, thereby liberating another active derivative, Ang 1–7 (see Chapter A7). Of the many peptides found to be cleaved by NEP, bradykinin, endothelin, substance P, and the atrial natriuretic peptide hormone are of interest. Substance P is released from sensory nerve granules in connection with painful stimuli. The concept that inhibition of the atrial natriuretic peptide and bradykinin breakdown by NEP would be beneficial in patients with hypertension or congestive heart failure led to the development of dual action ACE and NEP (or "vasopeptidase") inhibitors (see Chapter A15).

Structure

Human NEP is a type II integral membrane glycoprotein of 742 residues, inserted into the cell membrane near its N-terminus. It contains a short N-terminal cytoplasmic domain followed by a hydrophobic transmembrane sequence and a large extracellular domain. A single active center is present in the extracellular domain that contains the canonic HEXXH motif in which the glutamic acid serves as an important catalytic residue, and the 2 histidines (and a glutamic acid 60 residues downstream) act as the zinc coordinating ligands. NEP belongs to a family of related proteins termed the *M13* peptidase family that notably includes the endothelin converting enzyme. The structure of the extracellular domain of NEP was determined by x-ray crystallography and revealed the presence of 2 separate α-helical lobes. The larger N-terminal region contains all the required active site residues and resembles the structure of the related bacterial protease thermolysin. The smaller C-terminal region is not present in thermolysin and may function to restrict access of substrate to the active sites, explaining the well-known preference of NEP to cleave smaller peptides. The structure of NEP is stabilized by the presence of 6 disulfide bonds. Although not related in overall sequence, the active site residues and catalytic mechanisms used by ACE and NEP are very similar, helping guide the development of effective NEP and combined ACE/NEP inhibitors.

Distribution

ACE and NEP are highly concentrated in some of the same tissues—for example, in the microvilli of brush borders (e.g., proximal tubules) and in the male genital tract. ACE and NEP distribution differs in other organs and cell types. Vascular endothelial cells express more ACE, whereas epithelial cells and fibroblasts are richer in NEP. In leukocytes, NEP is involved in chemotactic peptide metabolism, and in the brain and the lungs, in enkephalin and substance P inactivation. Substance P can contract pulmonary smooth muscle.

SUGGESTED READING

1. Bralet J, Schwartz JC. Vasopeptidase inhibitors: an emerging class of cardiovascular drugs. *Trends Pharmacol Sci.* 2001;22:106–109.
2. Corvol P, Williams TA. Peptidyl-dipeptidase A/angiotensin I-converting enzyme. In: Barrett AJ, Rawlings ND, Woessner JF, eds. *Handbook of Proteolytic Enzymes.* San Diego, CA: Academic Press; 1998:1066–1076.
3. Erdös EG, Skidgel RA. Neutral endopeptidase 24.11 (enkephalinase) and related regulators of peptide hormones. *FASEB J.* 1989;3:145–151.
4. Erdös EG, Skidgel RA. Metabolism of bradykinin by peptidases in health and disease. In: Farmer SG, ed. *The Kinin System. Handbook of Immunopharmacology.* London, UK: Academic Press; 1997:112–141.
5. Gafford JT, Skidgel RA, Erdös EG, Hersh LB. Human kidney "enkephalinase," a neutral metalloendopeptidase that cleaves active peptides. *Biochemistry.* 1983;22:3265–3271.
6. Hooper NM, Turner AJ. Protein processing mechanisms: from angiotensinconverting enzyme to Alzheimer's disease. *Biochem Soc Trans.* 2000;28:441–446.
7. Linz W, Wiemer G, Gohlke P, et al. Contribution of kinins to the cardiovascular actions of angiotensin-converting enzyme inhibitors. *Pharmacol Rev.* 1995;47:25–49.
8. Soubrier F, Wei L, Hubert C, et al. Molecular biology of the angiotensin I-converting enzyme: II. Structure-function. Gene polymorphism and clinical implications. *J Hypertens.* 1993;11:599–604.
9. Turner AJ. Neprilysin. In: Barrett AJ, Rawlings ND, Woessner JF, eds. *Handbook of Proteolytic Enzymes.* San Diego, CA: Academic Press; 1998:1080–1085.
10. Woods DR, Humphries SE, Montgomery HE. The ACE I/D polymorphism and human physical performance. *Trends Endocrinol Metab.* 2000;11:416–420.

Chapter A7

Angiotensin Formation and Degradation

Carlos M. Ferrario, MD; Mark C. Chappell, PhD

KEY POINTS

- A family of angiotensins is derived from angiotensin I through the action of converting enzymes, chymase, aminopeptidases, and tissue endopeptidases.

- Angiotensin (1–7), a competitive inhibitor of angiotensin II, is increased during angiotensin-converting enzyme inhibition and angiotensin II receptor blockade, and may have vasodepressor and antigrowth functions.

- Chymases (angiotensin convertases) and angiotensin-converting enzyme 2 are resistant to angiotensin-converting enzyme inhibitors and degrade angiotensin I and angiotensin II to other effectors of the renin-angiotensin system, such as angiotensin (1–9) and angiotensin (1–7).

- Blockade of angiotensin-converting enzyme initially reduces angiotensin II levels; angiotensin II levels may increase during chronic therapy, probably because of tissue chymases.

See also Chapters A3–A6, A8, A23, C144, and C148

In mammalian systems, the concentration of a peptide hormone such as angiotensin (Ang) II at its receptor is controlled by numerous factors, including those that influence its synthesis, secretion, and removal. Major mechanisms by which peptides are removed include enzymatic degradation by peptidases, hemodynamic factors, and endocytosis of the ligand-receptor complex.

Metabolic Pathways

Figure A7.1 illustrates the enzymatic pathways leading to the production and metabolism of the active angiotensins.

Angiotensin-converting enzyme and tissue endopeptidases. Ang I, the prohormone decapeptide, is cleaved into the octapeptide Ang II primarily by angiotensin-converting

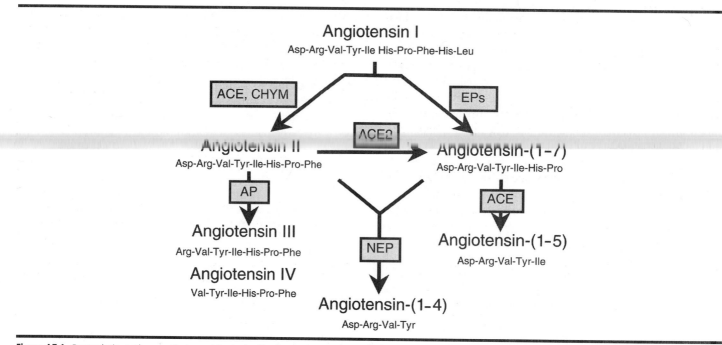

Figure A7.1. Proteolytic pathways that contribute to the formation and metabolism of products derived from angiotensin I. ACE, angiotensin-converting enzyme; NEP, neprilysin.

enzyme (ACE) and into the heptapeptide Ang (1–7) by tissue endopeptidases (EPs). One form of chymase (CHYM, angiotensin convertase) has been implicated in an alternative pathway for the production of Ang II.

Multiple EPs can form Ang (1–7) from Ang I, including prolyl EP (EC 3.4.21.26), neprilysin (NEP) (EC 3.4.24.11), thimet oligopeptidase (EC 3.4.24.15), and endothelin-converting enzyme (EC 3.4.24.23). NEP can also cleave Ang II and Ang (1–7) into the inactive fragment Ang (1–4).

Angiotensin-converting enzyme 2. A homolog of ACE, termed *ACE2*, has been identified, primarily in kidney and heart. In contrast to ACE, ACE2 exhibits a very high specificity for Ang II and directly generates Ang (1–7) (**Table A7.1**). This enzyme may constitute an important regulatory step to reduce Ang II and increase Ang (1–7).

Aminopeptidases. Aminopeptidases constitute another route for angiotensin metabolism. Glutamyl aminopeptidase (EC 3.4.11.7) cleaves Ang II to Ang III [Ang (2–8)], and arginyl aminopeptidase (EC 3.4.11.6) cleaves Ang III to Ang IV [Ang (3–8)].

Endocytosis. Another determinant of the duration of action of angiotensin peptides is endocytosis. AT_1 receptors are the primary mediators of intracellular transport of Ang II, but the internalization of the ligand-receptor complex may also be influenced by the AT_2-receptor subtype.

Function of Alternative Pathways

The possibility of forming 2 different active angiotensin peptides [Ang II and Ang (1–7)] from a common substrate, Ang I, could allow cells to regulate selective production of one or the other product. Further processing of these 2 active peptides into smaller fragments may add another level of specificity to the signaling process. The role of ACE, ACE2, and NEP in regulating the balance between constriction (Ang II) and dilation [Ang (1–7) and bradykinin] in peripheral tissues may be important in the regulation of blood pressure and the structural changes associated with hypertension.

Angiotensin Metabolic Changes during Angiotensin-Converting Enzyme Inhibition

Incomplete angiotensin-converting enzyme inhibition. Inhibition of ACE initially increases the concentration of Ang I and decreases Ang II and aldosterone. However, plasma levels of Ang II may not remain fully suppressed during chronic ACE inhibition, even though blood pressure remains controlled ("ACE escape"). Furthermore, ACE inhibition causes increases in renin and circulating Ang I, which may exceed the inhibitory capacity of the ACE inhibitors in plasma or tissues. Dissociation of the therapeutic effects of ACE inhibitors and the levels of plasma Ang II may indicate incomplete blockade of ACE.

Angiotensin (1–7). Chronic inhibition of ACE also raises the plasma concentration of Ang (1–7) in both humans and animals. Ang (1–7) is an endogenous competitive inhibitor of

Table A7.1. Substrate Properties of Human Angiotensin-Converting Enzyme 2

SUBSTRATE	MICHAELIS CONSTANT (µMOL/L)	K_{CAT}/K_M (MMOL/L^{-1} SEC^{-1})	BOND
Angiotensin II	2.0	1,800	Pro-Phe
Angiotensin I	6.9	4.9	His-Leu
Apelin-13	6.8	2,000	Pro-Phe
Casomorphin	31	220	Pro-Ile
Dynorphin A	5.5	2,900	Leu-Lys
[des-Arg^9]-Bradykinin	290	220	Pro-Phe
Neurotensin	300	190	Pro-Arg

native Ang II; blockade of Ang (1–7) activity or synthesis reduces the antihypertensive effects of ACE inhibition. Ang (1–7) can be degraded to the inactive product Ang (1–5) by ACE with K_{cat}/K_m Ang (1–7) comparable to that of bradykinin; therefore, ACE inhibitors have 2 actions that can increase levels of Ang (1–7). New findings using the mixed or combined ACE-NEP inhibitor omapatrilat reveal augmented renal excretion of Ang (1–7) in humans and animals. Elevated levels of Ang (1–7) may contribute to the diuretic and blood pressure–lowering actions of this class of ACE-NEP inhibitors.

Chymases. One form of mast cell chymase expressed in hypertension provides another route for the formation of Ang II during ACE-inhibitor therapy. The relative importance of alternative pathways in counteracting the antihypertensive effects of ACE inhibitors is the subject of continuing debate.

SUGGESTED READING

1. Albiston AL, McDowall SG, Matsacos D, et al. Evidence that the angiotensin IV (AT(4)) receptor is the enzyme insulin-regulated aminopeptidase. *J Biol Chem.* 2001;276:48623–48626.
2. Chappell MC, Allred AJ, Ferrario CM. Pathways of angiotensin-(1–7) metabolism in the kidney. *Nephrol Dial Transplant.* 2001;16:I22–I26.
3. Ferrario CM, Chappell MC, Tallant EA, et al. Counterregulatory actions of angiotensin-(1–7). *Hypertension.* 1997;30:535–541.
4. Ferrario CM, Smith RD, Brosnihan KB, et al. Effects of omapatrilat on the renin angiotensin system in salt sensitive hypertension. *Am J Hypertens.* 2002;15:557–564.
5. Guo C, Ju H, Leung D, et al. A novel vascular smooth muscle chymase is upregulated in hypertensive rats. *J Clin Invest.* 2001;107:703–715.
6. Iyer SN, Chappell MC, Averill DB, et al. Vasodepressor actions of angiotensin-(1–7) unmasked during combined treatment with lisinopril and losartan. *Hypertension.* 1998;31:699–705.
7. Luque M, Martin P, Martell N, et al. Effects of captopril related to increased levels of prostacyclin and angiotensin-(1–7) in essential hypertension. *J Hypertens.* 1996;14:799–805.
8. Tipnis SR, Hooper NM, Hyde R, et al. A human homolog of angiotensin-converting enzyme. Cloning and functional expression as a captopril-insensitive carboxypeptidase. *J Biol Chem.* 2000;275:33238–33243.
9. Urata H, Nishimura H, Ganten D. Chymase-dependent angiotensin II forming system in humans. *Am J Hypertens.* 1996;9:277–284.
10. Vickers C, Hales P, Kaushik V, et al. Hydrolysis of biological peptides by human angiotensin-converting enzyme-related carboxypeptidase. *J Biol Chem.* 2002;277:14838–14843.

Chapter A8

Tissue Renin-Angiotensin Systems

M. Ian Phillips, PhD, DSc

KEY POINTS

- Many tissues and organs can synthesize angiotensin II independent of the classic blood-borne renin-angiotensin system.

- Brain and testes contain significant amounts of angiotensin II despite the barriers that separate these tissues from the blood.

- Locally formed angiotensins can act as growth factors, neurotransmitters, and smooth muscle constrictors.

- Tissue angiotensin II is a target for antihypertensive and antihypertrophic effects of drugs.

See also Chapters A3–A7, A24, A63, A66, and C144

Renal juxtaglomerular cells are not the only source of renin in the body, and angiotensin II (Ang II) can be synthesized locally in many tissues, including the brain, pituitary, aorta, arteries, heart, ventricles, adrenal glands, kidneys, adipocytes, leukocytes, ovaries, testes, uterus, spleen, and skin (**Table A8.1**). Ang II levels (pg/g) are much higher in tissue than in plasma (pg/mL), so there must be local production of Ang II either intracellularly, extracellularly, or by intercellular activity. Collectively, these additional enzyme systems are referred to as *tissue renin-angiotensin systems.*

Brain

Renin-angiotensin system components. Except for specialized periventricular areas such as the area postrema, where there are fenestrated capillaries (i.e., no blood–brain barrier), the brain is separated from the blood-borne Ang II. However, central nervous system Ang II concentrations are not determined by circulating Ang II and do not correlate. Therefore, Ang II in the brain must come from local synthesis.

Angiotensinogen (AGT) messenger RNA (mRNA) is abundant in glial cells and is also expressed in some neurons. Renin mRNA is present in brain but in very low concentrations. Angiotensin-converting enzyme (ACE) is widely distributed in the brain, and, because ACE is an ectoenzyme, the brain synthesis of Ang II from Ang I must be predominantly extracellular or transcellular between glia and neurons.

The highest concentrations of Ang II in the brain is found in the hypothalamus and brain stem, with lesser amounts in the spinal cord, cerebellum, cortex, and amygdala. The levels vary

Table A8.1. Angiotensin II Concentration in Different Tissues[a]

TISSUE	PG ANGIOTENSIN II/G
Brain (hypothalamus)	200 ± 20
Aorta	85 ± 22
Mesenteric artery	184 ± 10
Kidney	142 ± 6
Left ventricle	54 ± 6
Right ventricle	68 ± 6
Adrenal (cortex)	3,320 ± 281
Brown fat	440 ± 5
White fat	52 ± 7
Ovary	259 ± 92
Uterus	147 ± 12
Spleen	2,134 ± 1,330
Plasma (human)	30 ± 10[a]

Note: Plasma is pg/mL.
[a]Picograms angiotensin II per g (± standard error) of tissue.

with physiologic conditions and gender. For example, females have lower hypothalamic Ang II than males at the beginning of the estrus cycle, but these concentrations rise severalfold after the surge of leuteinizing hormone at estrus.

Ang II injected directly into the brain causes drinking behavior, increased blood pressure, vasopressin release, and sodium appetite. The blood pressure response to Ang II results from combined effects of vasopressin release, sympathetic nervous system activation, and inhibition of baroreflexes.

Angiotensin II receptors. There are several types of Ang II receptors in the brain. Type 1 (AT_1) receptors are clustered on the hypothalamic neurons and in the nucleus of the tractus solitarius. AT_2 receptors are found in the thalamus, locus caeruleus, and the inferior olivary nucleus. AT_1 and AT_2 receptors are generally found on cells that synthesize catecholamines and are believed to modulate sympathetic neurotransmission. Ang IV receptors are found in the hippocampus, which is important in memory functions. Ang (1–7) receptors are found on vasopressin-forming neurons.

Brain AT_1 receptors are increased in genetically hypertensive rats. Inhibiting brain AT_1 receptors reduces blood pressure by sensitizing baroreflexes and by directly reducing central sympathetic outflow.

Pituitary

Ang II levels per gram of tissue are higher in the anterior pituitary than in the brain. Renin mRNA is present in the anterior and intermediate lobes but not in the posterior lobe. Ang II is concentrated in the gonadotrophs of the anterior pituitary and is colocalized with renin mRNA in the cells that produce luteinizing hormone. Ang II also inhibits prolactin release from lactotrophs. Thus, pituitary Ang II may modulate increased estrogen production in women, and testosterone production in men.

Blood Vessels

All the cellular and molecular components needed for the formation of Ang II are present in endothelial cells and vascular smooth muscle cells of blood vessels. However, much of the AGT mRNA is expressed in the adventitia and in the fatty tissue surrounding blood vessels. Vascular Ang II persists after bilateral nephrectomy (with dialysis) although plasma renin is undetectable, proving that local tissue synthesis exists.

Endothelial ACE controls activation of Ang II and degradation of bradykinin. Therefore, synthesis of vascular Ang II probably is intercellular, independent of the circulating renin-Ang system (RAS). Vascular Ang II plays a critical role in the development of atherosclerosis and inflammation. ACE accumulates in human plaque on inflammatory cells, leading to unstable plaque and myocardial infarction.

Heart

All the components of the RAS have also been demonstrated in cardiac tissue, and Ang II is synthesized in the heart. Cardiomyocytes also take up renin from plasma, which locally cleaves cardiac AGT to form Ang I. Conversion of Ang I to Ang II in the heart probably occurs extracellularly because of the location of ACE in the extracellular space. Most cardiac Ang II, however, is the result of cardiac chymase activity. Ang II itself is taken up into myocytes and fibroblasts. The atria contain higher levels of AGT than the ventricles, and the ventricles contain higher levels of renin than the atria. Ang AT_1 receptors are distributed in the valves and the myocardium and on coronary arteries. Cardiac RAS activity is increased by glucocorticoids, estrogen, thyroid hormone, and high-sodium diet, all of which increase AGT mRNA. Pressure overload on the heart is associated with a rise in ACE content and AGT mRNA. Cardiac ACE and Ang II are generally considered to be major causative factors in left ventricular hypertrophy and cardiac fibrosis, independent of blood pressure.

Adrenal Glands

The adrenal glands contain the highest levels of tissue Ang II that have been measured (Table A8.1). The majority of adrenal Ang II is localized within the zona glomerulosa and zona fasciculata of the cortex, where it stimulates aldosterone and corticosteroid synthesis. Cellular levels of renin in the rat adrenal cortex are independent of plasma renin levels. The adrenal medulla contains high levels of AT_2 receptors and is a major source of epinephrine and norepinephrine, which increase vasoconstriction and cardiac output. Aldosterone also stimulates growth of fibrotic tissue in the heart.

Kidney

In addition to the classic role of releasing renin into the circulation, the kidney contains all of the elements for local production of Ang. ACE is present in mesangial cells and tubular epithelial cells. Ang II is found in the proximal tubule cells and mesangial cells. Intrarenal Ang II constricts afferent and efferent arterioles and directly increases sodium reabsorption from the tubules. In addition, Ang II is a renal growth promoter. Excessive amounts of renal Ang II contribute to increased glomerular capillary pressure, nephrosclerosis, and renal failure. Therefore, ACE inhibitors are used to slow the progression of end-stage renal disease.

Testes

Because the testes have a blood–tissue barrier, circulating renin, angiotensinogen, and Ang II would not be expected to accumulate in testicular cells. Nevertheless, Ang I, II, and III have been measured in testes. AT_1 receptors are found on Leydig cells, which produce sperm, and in sperm tails. The testis has a unique form of ACE that is found in the luminal wall of the epididymis. Its role is not clear, but testicular Ang II may have a growth-regulating role in spermatogenesis.

Ovaries

There is a high rate of production of renin and its precursor, prorenin, in human ovarian cells. All the components of the RAS have been demonstrated in human ovarian follicular fluid. Ang receptors are also present in the ovaries, exclusively in follicular granulosa cells. Granulosa and theca cells, which secrete estrogen, contain renin and Ang. In contrast to the testes, the ovary secretes large amounts of prorenin and renin. Prorenin is secreted continuously by the ovary during pregnancy, and its presence implies a function for the ovarian RAS in normal pregnancy.

Adipose Tissue

Ang II is abundant in fat cells. The major source of AGT mRNA in blood vessels is the adipose tissue surrounding them. In obesity, fatty tissue is more highly vascularized. Therefore, it is possible that locally formed Ang II from adipocytes causes local and systemic vasoconstriction, altering local and systemic blood flow characteristics and perhaps increasing blood pressure. Although difficult to prove, this concept could explain why reducing weight also reduces high blood pressure.

Skin

Ang II and AGT mRNA are expressed in animal and human skin fibroblasts. The local concentration of Ang II is greatly elevated after injury, although plasma levels are unchanged. For this reason, it has been suggested that Ang II contributes to wound healing, perhaps by stimulating release of growth factors, such as transforming growth factor β, and promoting vascular smooth muscle cell growth.

Overview

Tissue RAS systems produce Ang II independent of the blood-borne system and control local blood flow. Ang II stimulates contraction in all smooth muscle contractile cells, such as vascular smooth muscle, kidney mesangial cells, cardiomyocytes, uterine wall cells, and sperm tails. In these and many other cells, Ang II also stimulates growth factor secretion and contributes to modeling and repair. Ang II may be formed in tissue by the enzymatic activity of renin or by nonrenin proteases such as tonin, chymase, and cathepsins. Because ACE is an ectoenzyme, Ang I can be formed in 1 cell and converted to Ang II extracellularly to be taken up into another cell. Ang II synthesized in 1 cell can have a paracrine action on a neighboring cell. Controlling tissue Ang II is clinically important because excess tissue Ang II contributes to atherosclerosis, thrombosis, ventricular hypertrophy, renal failure, stenosis, and high blood pressure. Tissue Ang II is a target for therapy to control hypertension and prevent target organ damage.

SUGGESTED READING

1. Bernstein KE. Molecular analysis of the renin-angiotensin system. *Semin Nephrol.* 1992;12(6):524–530.
2. Dostal DE, Baker KM. Evidence for a role of an intracardiac renin-angiotensin system in normal and failing hearts. *Trends Cardiovasc Med.* 1993;3:67–74.
3. Dzau VJ, Burt DW, Pratt RE. Molecular biology of the renin-angiotensin system. *Am J Physiol.* 1988;255:F563–F573.
4. Ghazi N, Grove KL, Wright JW, et al. Variations in angiotensin-II release from the rat brain during the estrous cycle. *Endocrinology.* 1994;135(5):1945–1950.
5. Kimura B, Sumners C, Phillips MI. Changes in skin angiotensin II receptors in rats during wound healing. *Biochem Biophys Res Commun.* 1992;187(2):1083–1090.
6. Navar LG, Harrison-Bernard LM, Nishiyama A, Kobori H. Regulation of intra-renal angiotensin II in hypertension. *Hypertension.* 2002;39(2):316–322.
7. Phillips MI. Functions of brain angiotensin. *Annu Rev Physiol.* 1987;49:413–435.
8. Phillips MI, Speakman EA, Kimura B. Levels of angiotensin and molecular biology of the tissue renin-angiotensin systems. *Regul Pept.* 1992;43:1–20.
9. Phillips MI, Kagiyama S. Angiotensin II as a pro-inflammatory mediator. *Curr Opin Investig Drugs.* 2002;3:569–577.
10. Trolliet MR, Phillips MI. The effect of chronic bilateral nephrectomy on plasma and brain angiotensin. *J Hypertens.* 1992;10:29–36.

Chapter A9

Mineralocorticoid Receptors

J. Howard Pratt, MD

KEY POINTS

- Binding of aldosterone to the mineralocorticoid receptor in kidney and other epithelia initiates gene transcription that increases the number of sodium channels and the transport of sodium.

- In epithelial cells, mineralocorticoid receptor binding is limited primarily to aldosterone (not the more available glucocorticoids) because the adjacent enzyme 11β-hydroxysteroid dehydrogenase-2 locally inactivates cortisol.

- Mineralocorticoid receptor–mediated responses to aldosterone and cortisol in cardiovascular and renal tissues may cause necrosis and fibrosis.

- Nongenomic mineralocorticoid receptor–mediated responses such as contraction or membrane calcium entry do not require gene transcription.

See also Chapters A3, A7, A8, A10, A50, A77, C140, and C170

The mineralocorticoid receptor (MR) is a member of a large family of nuclear receptors that includes the glucocorticoid receptor, the androgen receptor, the estrogen receptor, and the peroxisomal proliferation-activated receptor.

Aldosterone-Mediated Sodium Reabsorption

Aldosterone, the principal mineralocorticoid, diffuses freely across the outer cell membrane, reaching the cytoplasm where it binds to the MR. MR is expressed in epithelial cells in distal nephron, ducts of salivary and sweat glands, and colon. Nonepithelial sites include cardiac myocytes and certain areas in brain. The binding of aldosterone to MR initiates a cascade of events that leads to the renal reabsorption of sodium and excretion of potassium.

Aldosterone increases sodium reabsorption by amiloride-sensitive epithelial sodium channels (ENaC) on the apical surface of the principal cells of the renal cortical collecting duct. The reabsorbed sodium reaches the extracellular compartment through the action of Na^+/K^+ adenosine triphosphatase at the basolateral surface. Here there is exchange of potassium for sodium, with potassium traversing the cell, reaching the lumen at the apical surface. The movements of sodium and potassium in opposite directions maintain electroneutrality (**Figure A9.1**).

The mechanism whereby aldosterone increases ENaC function is indirect. The "activated" receptor (MR coupled to its ligand) functions within the nucleus as a transcription factor, increasing expression of the protein Sgk (serum and glucocorticoid-regulated kinase). The latter phosphorylates Nedd4-2, a ubiquitin ligase that normally binds to ENaC, targeting it for internalization and disposal. The phosphorylation step renders Nedd4-2 ineffective, ENaCs are retained at the cell surface, and sodium reabsorption is sustained (**Figure A9.2**).

Mineralocorticoid Receptor Specificity

Epithelial tissues: role of 11β-hydroxysteroid dehydrogenase type 2. The relative binding affinities of aldosterone and cortisol for MR are nearly identical but cortisol's ambient concentrations are several orders of magnitude higher than those of aldosterone. Thus, it would be expected that the actions of cortisol would predominate. In epithelial tissues such as renal distal tubule cells, however, the MR is protected from "overexposure" to cortisol by the enzyme 11β-hydroxysteroid dehydrogenase type 2 (11βHSD2), which converts cortisol to cortisone, the latter having no affinity for MR (Figure A9.1).

Nonepithelial tissues. In nonepithelial tissues, such as brain and heart, there is an absence of 11βHSD2 and cortisol is thought to be the predominant ligand regulating transcription.

Modulation of Mineralocorticoid Receptor Effects

Once aldosterone or cortisol binds to MR, other factors may influence the final transcriptional response, such as the coactivators and corepressors that have been better characterized for other nuclear receptors. These influences may arise in part from hormones and growth factors binding to cell surface receptors. It has also been suggested that at least for some targets of aldosterone, differential modification of transcription is determined by whether it is aldosterone or cortisol that binds to MR, possibly by affecting the folding and overall conformation of the receptor.

Nongenomic Actions of Aldosterone

It has been known from very early experiments that aldosterone administered to an animal increases vascular resistance within minutes, too rapidly for mediation by an increase in sodium reabsorption or an increase in gene expression (hence, the term *nongenomic*). It has since been shown repeatedly that

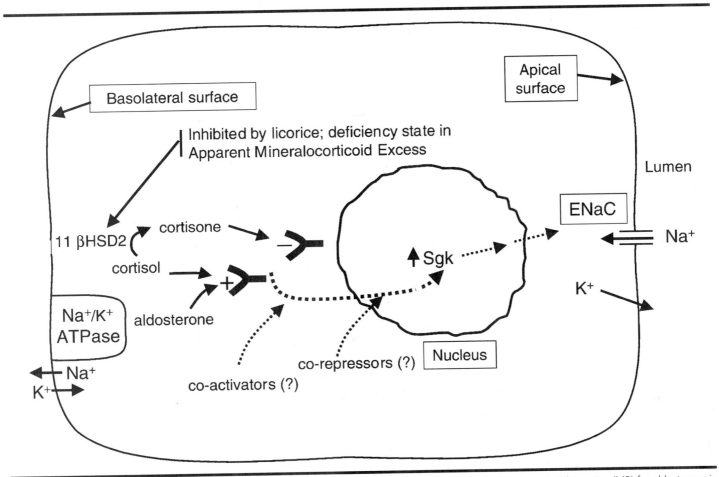

Figure A9.1. Aldosterone-mediated sodium reabsorption in the cortical collecting duct. The specificity of mineralocorticoid receptor (MR) for aldosterone is maintained by 11β-hydroxysteroid dehydrogenase type 2 (11βHSD2), which converts cortisol, a ligand with MR binding affinity equal to aldosterone, to cortisone, which has no affinity for MR. Activated MR's transcriptional capacities may be modified by other influences, such as coactivators and corepressors. Serum and glucocorticoid regulated kinase (Sgk) is an aldosterone-induced protein whose actions lead to retention of the epithelial sodium channel (ENaC) at the apical surface. ATPase, adenosine triphosphatase.

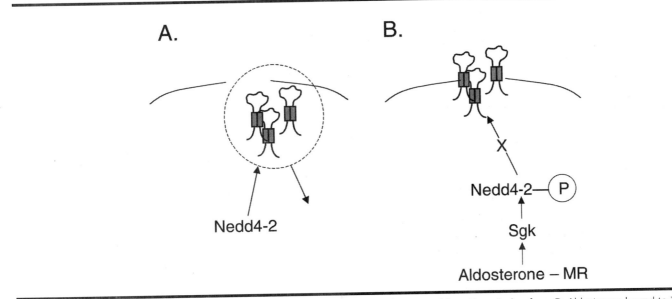

Figure A9.2. **A:** Nedd4-2, a ubiquitin ligase, normally targets the sodium channel for removal from the apical surface. **B:** Aldosterone bound to its receptor increases transcription of serum and glucocorticoid-regulated kinase (Sgk), a protein that phosphorylates Nedd4-2, rendering it ineffective. The net effect is an increase in the number of sodium channels retained at the cell surface and sustained sodium reabsorption. MR, mineralocorticoid receptor; P, indicates phosphorylation of Nedd4-2.

aldosterone can acutely increase calcium mobilization in peripheral mononuclear leukocytes and vascular smooth muscle cells. Such responses are unaffected by actinomycin D or cycloheximide (inhibitors of transcription and protein synthesis, respectively), again consistent with nonnuclear receptor mediation. Additionally, the acute effects of aldosterone are not prevented by coadministration of an MR antagonist (either canrenone or spironolactone), and responses are exaggerated in the MR knockout mouse. The nongenomic effects of aldosterone might contribute to some clinically important effects of an excess of aldosterone on nonepithelial tissues such as heart, effects not blocked by MR antagonists.

Mineralocorticoid Receptor and Hypertension

Molecular variation in mineralocorticoid receptor and hypertension. Molecular mutations in MR have now been recognized in conditions characterized by either extreme of sodium retention. In pseudohypoaldosteronism type 1, where there can be a life-threatening natriuresis early in life, loss of function molecular variations in MR have been identified. Recently, an activating mutation (S810L) in MR in a 15-year-old boy who presented with hypertension. In studies of the extended family, some of the female carriers of the mutation were identified as having had severe hypertension during pregnancy, a result of MR activation by progesterone, which normally binds to MR to inhibit aldosterone's actions (as does spironolactone). There are potentially numerous other modifications in MR that could alter function less severely but affect risk for hypertension. To date, however, there has been no demonstration of linkage of MR variants to essential hypertension.

Syndromes of altered 11β-hydroxysteroid dehydrogenase type-2 activity. Sodium retention and the potential for blood pressure elevation occurs if there is a loss of 11βHSD2 activity, as occurs with chronic ingestion of licorice (glycyrrhizinic acid) or with the genetically determined enzyme deficiency state known as *apparent mineralocorticoid excess* (see Chapters A10 and A77). It has been suggested that lesser degrees of 11βHSD2 activity may contribute to risk for common forms of hypertension.

Treatment of hypertension with mineralocorticoid receptor antagonists. Spironolactone, the only currently available MR antagonist, is enjoying a resurgence in use in essential hypertension and is the preferred drug for the medical management of primary aldosteronism. MR antagonists may be particularly useful in low-renin forms of hypertension, even in cases in which aldosterone levels are not increased.

Mineralocorticoid receptor and cardiac fibrosis. Aldosterone has important effects on nonepithelial targets. It has been known for some time that angiotensin II administered chronically to animals produces a series of injurious responses,

including necrosis and fibrosis in the kidney and the heart. Angiotensin-converting enzyme inhibitors and AT_1 receptor blockers ameliorate these effects, but MR antagonists also curtail the response, consistent with a direct role of aldosterone or cortisol. Indeed, aldosterone may mediate many of the adverse effects previously ascribed to angiotensin II. Autonomous hypersecretion of aldosterone in primary aldosteronism can result in left ventricular hypertrophy to a degree that is apparently disproportional to the degree of blood pressure elevation. On the other hand, the increase in aldosterone levels that accompanies a diet restricted in sodium apparently does not result in fibrosis.

Aldosterone antagonism and heart failure. Compelling evidence that aldosterone can have adverse cardiac effects has emerged from a trial in severe heart failure known as the Randomized Aldactone Evaluation Study (RALES). Patients with New York Heart Association class IV heart failure receiving a loop diuretic and an angiotensin-converting enzyme inhibitor were assigned to receive in addition either a small dose of spironolactone (25 mg) or placebo. Over a period of 24 months, there was a 30% reduction in risk of death among patients in the spironolactone group from either progressive heart failure or sudden death. The investigators speculated that the MR antagonist reduced sodium retention and myocardial fibrosis as well as prevented losses of potassium. Whether the effect of spironolactone was solely as an antagonist of aldosterone is unclear, because spironolactone may have its own agonist effects with induction of cardioprotective proteins.

SUGGESTED READING

1. Chen SY, Bhargava A, Mastroberardino L, et al. Epithelial sodium channel regulated by aldosterone-induced protein Sgk. *Proc Natl Acad Sci U S A*. 1999;96(5):2514–2519.
2. Delyani JA, Rocha R, Cook CS, et al. Eplerenone: a selective aldosterone receptor antagonist (SARA). *Cardiovasc Drug Rev*. 2001;19(3):185–200.
3. Geller DS, Farhi A, Pinkerton N, et al. Activating mineralocorticoid receptor mutation in hypertension exacerbated by pregnancy [see comments]. *Science*. 2000;289(5476):119–123.
4. Geller DS, Rodriguez-Soriano J, Boado AV, et al. Mutations in the mineralocorticoid receptor gene cause autosomal dominant pseudohypoaldosteronism type I. *Nat Genet*. 1998;19:279–281.
5. Mune T, Rogerson FM, Nikkila H, et al. Human hypertension caused by mutations in the kidney isozyme of 11 beta-hydroxysteroid dehydrogenase. *Nat Genet*. 1995;10(4):394–399.
6. Pitt B, Zannad F, Remme WJ, et al. The effect of spironolactone on morbidity and mortality in patients with severe heart failure. *N Engl J Med*. 1999;341:709–717.
7. Pratt JH, Eckert GJ, Newman S, Ambrosius WT. Blood pressure responses to small doses of amiloride and spironolactone in normotensive subjects. *Hypertension*. 2001;38(5):1124–1129.
8. Shigematsu Y, Hamada M, Okayama H, et al. Left ventricular hypertrophy precedes other target-organ damage in primary aldosteronism. *Hypertension*. 1997;29(3):723–727.
9. Wehling M. Specific, nongenomic actions of steroid hormones. *Annu Rev Physiol*. 1997;59:365–393.
10. Young WF, Jr. Primary aldosteronism. A common and curable form of hypertension. *Cardiol Rev*. 1999;7:207–214.

Adrenal Steroid Synthesis and Regulation

Celso E. Gomez-Sanchez, MD

KEY POINTS

- The adrenal cortex synthesizes aldosterone in the zona glomerulosa and cortisol in the zona fasciculata.

- Aldosterone is regulated primarily by angiotensin II and potassium.

- The adrenal cortex also synthesizes weaker sodium-retaining steroids, including deoxycorticosterone, 18-oxycortisol, 18-hydroxydeoxycorticosterone, and 19-nordeoxycorticosterone, which can be clinically significant in patients with adrenal adenomas or other syndromes of mineralocorticoid excess.

- Metabolism of cortisol in mineralocorticoid target organs determines that the mineralocorticoid receptor selectively responds to aldosterone.

See also Chapters A9, A50, and C170

Adrenal Cortex

The adrenal cortex contains 3 (or 2, depending on the species) distinct areas involved in adrenal steroid biosynthesis, each of which play different physiologic or pathophysiologic roles. The outer portion of the adrenal, zona glomerulosa, is the site of synthesis of aldosterone, the most important mineralocorticoid hormone. The next layer, or zona fasciculata (fasciculata-reticularis in some species), is the site of synthesis of cortisol (in species that express the cytochrome P-450 17α-hydroxylase, as in the human) or corticosterone (most rodents), the most important glucocorticoids.

The innermost layer of the cortex, the reticularis, is the site of synthesis of adrenal androgens. A progenitor area where cells are generated exists between the zona glomerulosa and fasciculata.

Regulation of Steroid Biosynthesis

Adrenocorticotropic hormone (ACTH) administration results within minutes in the release of cortisol and aldosterone, and ACTH is needed chronically for the trophic regulation and the maintenance of steroidogenic capacity of the zona fasciculata. The acute effects of ACTH are mediated by a cyclic adenosine monophosphate–mediated process resulting in the rapid mobilization of cholesterol for steroidogenesis via a labile protein (i.e., steroidogenic acute regulatory protein). ACTH also stimulates aldosterone secretion acutely, but continued ACTH stimulation does not result in a sustained response. Chronic aldosterone regulation is primarily under the control of angiotensin II and extracellular fluid potassium. Changes in vascular volume or sodium ingestion affect aldosterone secretion by altering levels of angiotensin II.

Synthetic Pathways

Most of the steroidogenic enzymes for the synthesis of cortisol and aldosterone from cholesterol are the same (**Figure A10.1**), but regulation of the enzymes and terminal reactions differ for each steroid.

Initial steps. Cholesterol is the fundamental building block for steroid synthesis; most cholesterol used by the adrenal for steroid synthesis is transported to the gland by HDL and LDL from the plasma. After deposition in intracellular lipid droplets, cholesterol is transported into the mitochondria by an incompletely understood mechanism that involves the steroidogenic acute regulatory protein and peripheral benzodiazepine receptor. In the inner mitochondrial membrane, the cytochrome P-450 side-chain cleavage enzyme performs successive hydroxylations of cholesterol, eliminating a portion of the side chain, to generate pregnenolone.

17-Hydroxylation. In the zona fasciculata, pregnenolone is hydroxylated to 17α-hydroxy pregnenolone by microsomal cytochrome P-450 17α-hydroxylase. Pregnenolone in the zona glomerulosa and 17α-hydroxypregnenolone in the zona fasciculata are then oxidized and isomerized by the microsomal enzyme 3β-ol dehydrogenase 4-5 isomerase to generate progesterone and 17α-hydroxyprogesterone, which are then hydroxylated by microsomal cytochrome P-450 21-hydroxylase to deoxycorticosterone (DOC) and 11-deoxycortisol.

11-Hydroxylation. DOC and 11-deoxycortisol then diffuse into the mitochondria of the zona glomerulosa and zona fasciculata, respectively, where they are transformed by 2 similar enzymes. In humans, 2 cytochrome P-450–11β-hydroxylases have been described: the 11β-hydroxylase in the fasciculata and aldosterone synthase in the glomerulosa; their genes are located on chromosome 8q24.3, separated by approximately 40 kilobases (kb). They have 9 exons spread over 7 kb of DNA and a sequence homology of 95% in the coding region and 90% in the introns.

Aldosterone synthase. The cytochrome P-450 aldosterone synthase on the inner mitochondrial membrane catalyzes 3 successive hydroxylations, binding DOC and converting it into corticosterone (11-hydroxylation), corticosterone to 18-hydroxycorticosterone (18-OH-B), and 18-OH-B to a germinal diol that spontaneously dehydrates to form aldosterone. This enzyme is a relatively inefficient partial processing enzyme

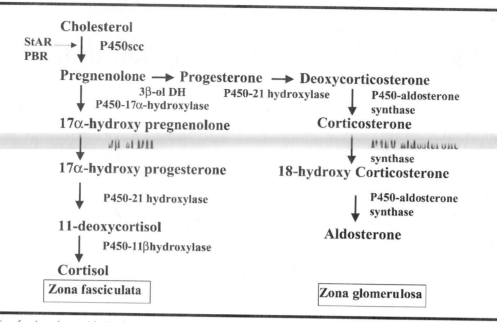

Figure A10.1. Biosynthesis of adrenal steroids in the human zona fasciculata and glomerulosa. DH, dehydrogenase; PBR, peripheral benzodiazepine receptor; StAR, steroidogenic acute regulatory protein.

from which a significant portion of the products of each enzymatic hydroxylation is released from the enzyme and secreted. As a consequence, the zona glomerulosa secretes significantly greater quantities of corticosterone and 18-OH-B than aldosterone. The free metabolites are less efficient substrates, especially 18-OH-B, which adopts a stable hemiacetal form and is a very poor substrate for the enzyme.

Cortisol synthesis. In the zona fasciculata, 11-deoxycortisol is also passively transferred into the mitochondria and hydroxylated by the cytochrome P-450 11β-hydroxylase to cortisol. Not all of the pregnenolone is hydroxylated to 17α-hydroxy pregnenolone in the human zona fasciculata; as in the zona glomerulosa, the remaining pregnenolone is successively hydroxylated to form DOC and corticosterone. Because the mass of fasciculata tissue is far larger than that of the glomerulosa, most of the DOC and corticosterone in plasma comes from the zona fasciculata.

Other Mineralocorticoids

Aldosterone is the most important mineralocorticoid, but other adrenal corticosteroids also have variable mineralocorticoid activity, including DOC, 18-oxocortisol, 19-nordeoxycorticosterone (19-norDOC), and 18-hydroxydeoxycorticosterone (18-OH-DOC). The 11β-hydroxylase has the ability, but to a lesser degree, to hydroxylate DOC or 11-deoxycortisol in other positions of the steroid molecule including the 18 position to generate 18-OH-DOC and the 19 position to generate 19-OH-DOC. The degree of alternative hydroxylations for this enzyme depends on the species.

Deoxycorticosterone. Increased production of DOC occurs in individuals with 11β-hydroxylase deficiency or in adrenal tumors having incomplete expression of this enzyme.

18-Hydroxydeoxycorticosterone. In the rat, approximately 25% of DOC is transformed into 18-OH-DOC. Although it has

weak mineralocorticoid properties, 18-OH-DOC is produced in large enough amounts to participate in the development of hypertension in the Dahl salt-sensitive rat. In this animal, a high-salt diet suppresses aldosterone, but not corticosterone or 18-OH-DOC (a side product of the 11β-hydroxylase) production. The human 11β-hydroxylase synthesizes a much smaller proportion of 18-OH-DOC, but there are cases of mineralocorticoid hypertension in which increased secretion of 18-OH-DOC has been demonstrated. However, no clear explanation of the biosynthetic pathway used is known.

19-Nordeoxycorticosterone and 19-noraldosterone. The steroid 19-norDOC, a potent mineralocorticoid, was initially identified in the urine of rats undergoing adrenal regeneration. 19-Hydroxylation of DOC by the 11β-hydroxylase occurs in small quantities and the product is further processed, probably by successive hydroxylations, to form 19-oxoDOC and 19-oicDOC. 19-NorDOC is formed extraadrenally, probably in the kidney, by the decarboxylation of the adrenal precursor 19-oicDOC. 19-NorDOC has been found to be elevated in the urine of some rat models of genetic hypertension and in very rare cases of hypertension associated with an adrenal adenomas. Another 19-nor steroid, 19-noraldosterone, a mineralocorticoid with similar potency to that of aldosterone, also has been shown to be excreted in excessive amounts in patients with primary aldosteronism. The biosynthetic pathway for the formation of this steroid is unknown, but the excretion is significantly lower than that of aldosterone.

Syndromes with Abnormal Steroid Synthesis

In aldosterone-producing adenomas and in glucocorticoid-suppressible aldosteronism (also known as *glucocorticoid-remediable aldosteronism*, or *GRA*), 11-deoxycortisol can be metabolized by aldosterone synthase to generate the aldosterone analogues 18-hydroxycortisol and 18-oxocortisol. In both cases, 11-deoxycortisol becomes available as a substrate for aldosterone synthase. Some adenomas express the 17α-hydroxylase and aldosterone synthase. In GRA there is a gene duplication resulting from the crossover of the genes CYP11B1 (11β-hydroxylase) and CYP11B2 (aldosterone synthase) with the formation of an additional gene that has sequences for the promoter region and first exons (2–4) of the 11β-hydroxylase followed by most of the coding region from the aldosterone synthase gene. This results in an enzyme expressed in the zona fasciculata and regulated by ACTH with the ability to synthesize aldosterone from DOC or 18-hydroxycortisol and 18-oxocortisol from 11-deoxycortisol. 18-Oxocortisol has approximately 2% of the mineralocorticoid activity of aldosterone and produces hypertension when infused in rats or sheep. Large amounts of 18-oxocortisol is also formed in GRA and seems to play a role in the pathogenesis of hypertension.

Extraadrenal Synthesis

Steroid transformations occur outside steroid-producing glands. Testosterone action is mediated to a significant degree by its peripheral conversion to estradiol, a reaction catalyzed by the aromatase enzyme, and also by conversion to 5α-dihydrotestosterone by the 5α-reductases. In addition, *de novo* synthesis of pregnenolone, progesterone, DOC, and reduced derivatives occurs in the brain to form neurosteroids. Corticosterone and aldosterone can be formed in vascular tissue, heart, and brain via the same steroidogenic enzymes present in the adrenal, which are also expressed in small amounts in these tissues. It is likely that corticosterone and aldosterone formed in vascular, heart, and brain tissue play a paracrine or autocrine role, because their contribution to circulating steroid levels is negligible, aldosterone and corticosterone levels become unmeasurable in plasma after adrenalectomy. The synthesis of these steroids in the heart may be altered in congestive heart failure, and the steroids may affect catecholamine synthetic enzymes in the brain and medulla.

Target Cell Metabolism and Receptor Specificity

The mineralocorticoid receptor exhibits similar affinity for aldosterone, corticosterone, and cortisol. Under normal conditions, corticosterone and cortisol are secreted and circulate in 100- to 1,000-fold greater quantities than aldosterone (see Chapter A9). Yet, aldosterone is able to successfully compete for its receptor in mineralocorticoid target cells such as those of the kidney tubule because specificity of the mineralocorticoid receptor for aldosterone depends on the coexpression in many target cells of enzymes that metabolize cortisol or corticosterone into inactive compounds such as cortisone or 11-dehydrocorticosterone. Two such specificity-conferring enzymes have been characterized (**Figure A10.2**). 11β-Hydroxysteroid dehydrogenase-1 is an NADP⁺-dependent, low affinity, bidirectional enzyme with preferential reduction of cortisone to cortisol. The 11β-hydroxysteroid dehydrogenase-2 is an NAD⁺-dependent, high affinity, unidirectional enzyme which, when expressed in the same cell as the mineralocorticoid receptor, protects the

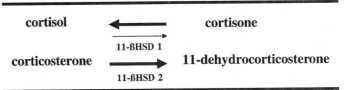

Figure A10.2. Regulation of the formation of cortisol and cortisone in peripheral tissues by the 11β-hydroxysteroid dehydrogenase (11-βHSD) enzymes.

receptor from binding by more abundant glucocorticoids. Congenital or acquired (by ingestion of licorice or derivatives) deficiency of the 11β-hydroxysteroid dehydrogenase-2 enzyme results in the syndrome of apparent mineralocorticoid excess. In these cases, cortisol is able to reach the receptor and produce transactivation.

Hepatic and Renal Metabolism of Adrenal Steroids

In the human, aldosterone is metabolized in the liver and kidney. In the liver, the principal metabolite (~30–40%) is 3α,5β-tetrahydroaldosterone, which is excreted in the urine as a 3-glucuronide, and, in the kidney, aldosterone is conjugated at the 18-position to form aldosterone-18-oxo-glucuronide (~5–10%). This renal metabolite is acid sensitive and generates aldosterone when incubated at pH 1. It is the most commonly measured urinary metabolite used in the diagnosis of alterations of aldosterone secretion.

Further metabolism of the glucocorticoids occurs primarily in the liver, where cortisol is reduced at the 3 and the 5 position of the steroid molecule to form tetrahydrocortisol (5β reduction) and allotetrahydrocortisol (5α reduction). Cortisone is similarly reduced at the 3 and 5 positions of the steroid molecule to form tetrahydrocortisone. These metabolites are excreted in the urine as glucuronide conjugates. The measurement of the ratio of tetrahydrocortisol plus allotetrahydrocortisol over tetrahydrocortisone is used for estimation of the *in vivo* 11β-hydroxysteroid dehydrogenase-2 activity.

SUGGESTED READING

1. Auchus RJ, Miller WL. The principles, pathways and enzymes of human steroidogenesis. In DeGroot LJ, Jameson JL, eds. *Endocrinology*. 4th ed. Philadelphia, PA: Saunders; 2001:1616–1631.
2. Farman N, Rafestin-Oblin ME. Multiple aspects of mineralocorticoid selectivity. *Am J Physiol Renal Physiol*. 2001;280(2):F181–F192.
3. Melby JC, Griffing GT, Gomez-Sanchez CE. 19-Nor-deoxycorticosterone (19-nor-DOC) in genetic and experimental hypertension in rats and in human hypertension. In: Biglieri EG, Melby JC, eds. *Endocrine Hypertension*. New York, NY: Raven Press Ltd; 1990:183–194.
4. Stocco DM. StAR protein and the regulation of steroid hormone biosynthesis. *Annu Rev Physiol*. 2001;63:193–213.
5. White PC. Inherited forms of mineralocorticoid hypertension. *Hypertension*. 1996;28:927–936.
6. White PC, Mune T, Agarwal AK. 11-Beta-hydroxysteroid dehydrogenase and the syndrome of apparent mineralocorticoid excess. *Endocr Rev*. 1997;18:135–156.

Leptin and Other Adipocyte Hormones

William G. Haynes, MD

KEY POINTS

- Leptin is an adipocyte hormone that acts in the central nervous system to decrease appetite and may function as the negative feedback signal that maintains stable adipose tissue mass.

- Leptin increases sympathetic nerve activity to thermogenic and cardiovascular tissues, including skeletal muscle, adrenal gland, and kidney, resulting in increased energy expenditure and elevated arterial pressure.

- Leptin expression and plasma leptin concentrations are elevated in obesity; abnormalities in leptin generation or resistance to the actions of leptin may contribute to the sympathetic, cardiovascular, and renal changes associated with obesity.

- Other adipocyte-derived hormones, such as adiponectin and resistin, have undetermined physiologic and pathologic roles.

See also Chapters A13, A34, A42, A44, A45, B97 , and C162

Adipose tissue was formerly considered almost exclusively as a passive tissue depot for storage of energy-dense triglycerides. It is now realized that adipocyte-derived hormones affect food intake, thermogenesis, and lipid and glucose metabolism. These hormones include leptin, tumor necrosis factor-α (TNF-α), angiotensinogen, adiponectin, and resistin. Leptin causes sympathetic, renal, and metabolic effects that may contribute to altered cardiovascular regulation in obesity. The roles of other adipocyte-derived hormones are as yet uncertain.

LEPTIN

Leptin is a 167-amino acid protein expressed and secreted exclusively from adipocytes. Leptin circulates in blood at low levels (5–15 ng/mL) in lean subjects, with approximately 50% as the free form.

Regulation of Fat Cell Mass

Body fat stores need to be regulated to maintain energy reserves and to prevent excessive changes in body weight. A central tenet of the "lipostat hypothesis" is that a negative feedback signal from adipose tissue to the central nervous system exists. Parabiosis experiments demonstrated that obesity in *ob* mice was due to lack of a circulating factor that acted to decrease body weight, whereas obesity in *db* mice was due to insensitivity to this same substance. Positional cloning has identified the mutated gene responsible for obesity in the *ob* mouse strain, named *leptin* from the Greek *leptos* for "thin" **(Figure A11.1)**.

Leptin Regulation

Leptin expression and plasma leptin concentrations are proportional to adipose tissue mass in genetic models of obesity other than experimentally induced obesity. Decreases in adipose tissue mass in obesity cause decreases in leptin concentrations.

Food intake, insulin, and corticosteroids increase leptin expression, whereas cold temperature and catecholamines decrease leptin expression. Sympathetic blockade increases leptin expression and plasma leptin levels, suggesting that endogenous sympathetic activity physiologically suppresses leptin expression and secretion. Leptin is too large to readily penetrate the blood–brain barrier by passive diffusion. Entry of leptin into cerebrospinal fluid appears to occur via a saturable specific transport mechanism that mediates binding and endocytosis of leptin by brain capillaries.

Receptors

The full leptin receptor (Ob-Rb) is a protein containing a single transmembrane domain with similarities to the class I cytokine receptors. It possesses 2 peptide motifs in a long intracellular C-terminal tail that interact with specific kinases to promote transcription through the signal transducers and activators of transcription (STAT) pathway and activation of PI3 kinase. The gene for the leptin receptor appears to encode for at least 6 alternatively spliced variants of the receptor. The Ob-Rb form encodes for the full receptor, including a long intracellular tail. Ob-Ra, Rc, and Rd with premature terminations and short intracellular tails may act to transport leptin across the blood–brain barrier. Messenger RNA (mRNA) for the leptin receptor is expressed in the hypothalamus and choroid plexus. The Ob-Re form lacks the transmembrane domain and may therefore be secreted as a soluble receptor, perhaps contributing to binding and inactivation of circulating leptin. Leptin receptor mRNA is expressed in adipose tissue, heart, kidney, liver, spleen, pancreatic islets, and testis, although the presence of the full-length receptor splice variant (Ob-Rb) has not been demonstrated in all these tissues. Full-length leptin receptor mRNA and protein has been demonstrated in vascular endothelial cells. Leptin appears to exert its effects on body fat stores through a number of hypothalamic mediators. These include neuropeptide Y (NPY), which acts to increase body fat and is

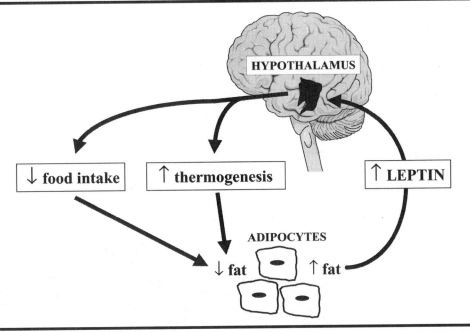

Figure A11.1. Leptin is a protein produced exclusively by adipocytes. Increases in adipose cell mass and insulin stimulate leptin expression and secretion. Leptin then circulates to cross the blood–brain barrier by a receptor-mediated saturable process. Leptin binds to leptin receptors in the hypothalamus, where it suppresses appetite and increases thermogenesis. Together, these actions decrease adipose cell mass. Therefore, leptin forms the afferent signaling component of a negative feedback loop that maintains stable body fat stores. ↑, increased; ↓, decreased.

suppressed by leptin and melanocortins and corticotropin-releasing factor (CRF), which act to decrease body fat stores and are stimulated by leptin.

Leptin and the Sympathetic Nervous System

Systemic and intracerebroventricular administration of leptin increases directly measured sympathetic nerve activity (SNA) to thermogenic brown adipose tissue. Quite low doses of leptin increase SNA to kidney, hindlimb, and adrenal gland.

Central effects. Full-length leptin receptors are abundantly expressed in the hypothalamus, especially in the arcuate nucleus, with neurons projecting to other hypothalamic areas, particularly the paraventricular nucleus, which modulates sympathetic outflow. Leptin does not cause sympathoactivation in obese Zucker rats, known to possess a mutation in the gene for the leptin receptor. These and other data suggest that the sympathetic effects of circulating leptin occur secondary to its passage across the blood–brain barrier, with subsequent binding to full-length leptin receptors expressed in the arcuate nucleus of the hypothalamus.

Neuropeptide modulation. Several hypothalamic neuropeptides that may mediate the effects of leptin on SNA, including α-melanocyte stimulating hormone, CRF, and NPY. In the neural melanocortin system, α-melanocyte–stimulating hormone is derived from proopiomelanocortin and acts on melanocortin-4 receptors to decrease appetite and weight. Leptin is known to stimulate proopiomelanocortin expression in the arcuate nucleus. Leptin appears to increase renal and hindlimb SNA through activation of a hypothalamic melanocortin system acting on melanocortin-4 receptors (**Figure A11.2**). Hypothalamic expression of mRNA for CRF is upregulated by leptin, which appears to increase sympa-

thetic activation of a hypothalamic CRF system. Leptin also downregulates hypothalamic NPY expression.

Nonsympathetic Actions of Leptin

High doses of leptin increase endothelial generation of nitric oxide in isolated blood vessels. It is possible that an endothelium-dependent vasorelaxant effect of leptin may constitute a counterregulatory mechanism opposing vasoconstrictor and pressor effects of leptin mediated via sympathoexcitation (Figure A11.2). With opposing increases in sympathetic activity and endothelial nitric oxide, leptin effects are similar in nature to the cardiovascular actions of insulin.

Leptin may also promote angiogenesis, though the mechanism and physiologic significance are unknown. The kidney has been shown to express mRNA for the full-length Ob-Rb leptin receptor, suggesting that leptin may exert functional effects in this organ. Indeed, human leptin acts directly to cause natriuresis and diuresis. Leptin inhibits glucose-mediated insulin secretion but appears to increase insulin-mediated glucose uptake, even in the absence of changes in food intake and adiposity. Finally, leptin receptors have been demonstrated on platelets, and physiologic concentrations of leptin appear to promote platelet aggregation.

Leptin and Hypertension

Given the multiple cardiovascular actions of leptin (Figure A11.2), its overall effect on arterial pressure depends crucially on the balance among these actions. Several studies have suggested that chronic hyperleptinemia can increase arterial pressure. The pressor effect of leptin is accompanied by increases in renal vascular resistance and heart rate, consistent with sympathetic activation. Sympathetic blockade prevents this pressor

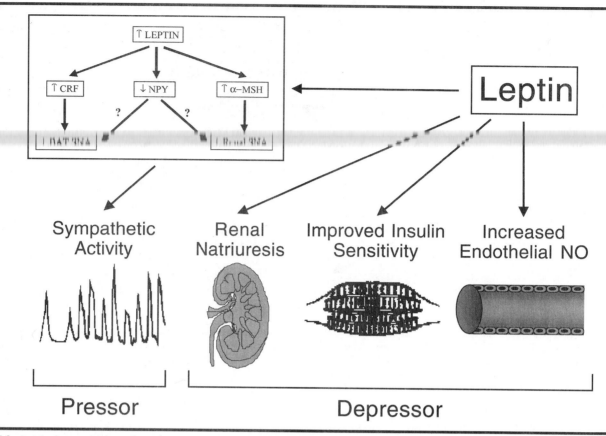

Figure A11.2. Leptin has multiple actions that may increase (sympathoactivation) or decrease arterial pressure (natriuresis, insulin sensitization, and vasodilatation). The inset panel shows proposed mechanisms for sympathoactivation. Increases in renal sympathetic nerve activity (SNA) caused by leptin appear to be mediated by increased α-melanocyte stimulating hormone (α-MSH), whereas increases in brown adipose tissue (BAT) SNA appear to be mediated by corticotropin-releasing factor (CRF). The role of neuropeptide Y (NPY) remains unclear. ↑, increased; ↓, decreased; NO, nitric oxide.

effect. Leptin does not produce natriuresis despite an increase in arterial pressure.

Mean arterial pressure is significantly lower in obese *ob* leptin-deficient mice than in their lean controls. The rare human cases of complete leptin deficiency also tend to have normal or low arterial pressure despite severe obesity, with attenuated pressor responses to sympathetic stimuli. These data support the concept that leptin may contribute importantly to the physiologic maintenance of arterial pressure.

Leptin Resistance and Obesity

Most obese humans have high circulating leptin concentrations. Obese subjects with normal leptin concentrations may be more likely to gain weight subsequently. However, for most obese humans, inadequate leptin production does not appear to underlie obesity. Circulating hyperleptinemia suggests that leptin resistance may contribute to obesity. Several mechanisms have been suggested to explain the phenomenon of leptin resistance, such as decreased transport of leptin across the blood–brain barrier, a defect in the leptin receptor, or impaired downstream signaling in the hypothalamus. In addition to multiple mechanisms of leptin resistance, there is emerging evidence that leptin resistance may be selective and spare some actions of leptin.

In monogenic and polygenic murine models, there is resistance to the metabolic effects of leptin (anorexia and weight loss) but preservation of its sympathoexcitatory and pressor effects. In support of the persistence of sympathetic action of leptin in obesity is

the finding that plasma leptin concentration correlates significantly with muscle SNA in obese subjects. Relative preservation of leptin-induced sympathoactivation might then contribute to obesity-related sodium chloride retention, hypertension, vascular and myocardial hypertrophy, and cardiac arrhythmias.

OTHER ADIPOCYTE-DERIVED HORMONES

Adipocytes secrete several other hormones that act in peripheral tissues to influence energy expenditure, metabolism of lipids and glucose, and cardiovascular function. These substances include inflammatory cytokines such as TNF-α and interleukin-6. Adipocyte secretion of these and other cytokines may be linked to the finding that markers of a systemic inflammatory state, such as C-reactive protein, are elevated in obesity. Angiotensinogen is expressed in most adipose tissues (visceral > subcutaneous), and there is increasing evidence that angiotensin-converting enzyme and the angiotensin AT_1 receptor are also expressed in adipocytes. Although renin gene expression has not been shown, other enzymes with angiotensinogen cleaving activity appear to be present in adipocytes.

Resistin

Resistin is a 114–amino acid protein that circulates as a homodimer of 2 peptides. Resistin gene expression is upregulated during adipocyte development and downregulated by peroxisomal proliferation-activated receptor-gamma agonists, such as the thiazolidinediones. Resistin inhibits insulin-stimulated glucose uptake, and blockade of resistin by antibodies improves insulin sensitivity in obese mice, suggesting that resistin may contribute to insulin resistance. Early studies in humans show increased adipose tissue expression of resistin in visceral adipose tissue. Genetic studies have failed to find an association between polymorphisms in the resistin gene and obesity or insulin resistance in humans. Nonetheless, resistin may be a potentially valuable therapeutic target for drug development.

Adiponectin

Adiponectin has opposite regulation and actions to resistin. Although adiponectin is exclusively secreted from adipose tissue, adiponectin levels are significantly decreased in obese and diabetic subjects, and this decrease may be at least partially genetically determined. Production of adiponectin is upregulated by peroxisomal proliferation-activated receptor-gamma agonists. Like leptin, adiponectin gene expression is downregulated with sympathetic activation.

The actions of adiponectin include increased expression of energy dissipation and fatty-acid combustion pathways, resulting in reduction of triglyceride stores and normalization of insulin resistance. These insulin-sensitizing effects of adiponectin appear to be synergistic with those of leptin. In addition to its metabolic actions, adiponectin has antiinflammatory effects. Adiponectin prevents TNF-α–induced adhesion of monocytes to endothelial cells, and expression of vascular cell adhesion molecule-1 and endothelial-leukocyte adhesion molecule-1 (E-selectin). Intriguingly, adiponectin levels are suppressed in atherosclerotic patients compared to weight-matched controls, suggesting potential involvement of this hormone in vascular disease.

SUGGESTED READING

1. Ahima RS, Flier JS. Adipose tissue as an endocrine organ. *Trends Endocrinol Metab.* 2000;11:327–333.
2. Correia ML, Haynes WG, Rahmouni K, et al. The concept of selective leptin resistance: evidence from agouti yellow obese mice. *Diabetes.* 2002;51:439–442.
3. Haynes WG, Morgan DA, Walsh SA, et al. Receptor-mediated regional sympathetic nerve activation by leptin. *J Clin Invest.* 1997;100:270–278.
4. Lembo G, Vecchione C, Fratta L, et al. Leptin induces direct vasodilation through distinct endothelial mechanisms. *Diabetes.* 2000;49:293–297.
5. Ouchi N, Kihara S, Arita Y, et al. Novel mediator for endothelial adhesion molecules: adipocyte-derived plasma protein adiponectin. *Circulation.* 1999;100:2473–2476.
6. Shek EW, Brands MW, Hall JE. Chronic leptin infusion increases arterial pressure. *Hypertension.* 1998;31:409–414.
7. Sivitz WI, Walsh SA, Morgan DA, et al. *Endocrinology.* 1997;138:3395–3401.
8. Steppan CM, Bailey ST, Bhat S, et al. The hormone resistin links obesity to diabetes. *Nature.* 2001;409:307–312.
9. Yamamuchi T, Kamon J, Waki H, et al. The fat-derived hormone adiponectin reverses insulin resistance associated with both lipoatrophy and obesity. *Nat Med.* 2001;7:887–888.
10. Zhang Y, Proenca R, Maffei M, et al. Positional cloning of the mouse *obese* gene and its human homologue. *Nature.* 1994;372:425–432.

Chapter A12

Endothelin

Ernesto L. Schiffrin, MD, PhD, FRCPC

KEY POINTS

- Endothelin-1 is a potent 21-amino acid vasoconstrictor peptide produced by the endothelium.
- Endothelin-1 may be overexpressed in blood vessels in salt-sensitive and severe forms of hypertension in experimental animals and in humans.
- Orally active endothelin receptor antagonists have been effective in some forms of experimental hypertension and heart failure and have been approved for treatment of primary pulmonary hypertension.

See also Chapters A3, A16, A19, A24, A28, A29, A31, A33, A41, A50, A63, A64, A66, and A67

Three endothelins (ETs) have been recognized in mammals (ET-1, ET-2, and ET-3) **(Figure A12.1)**. These 21–amino acid peptides were originally identified as products of vascular endothelial cells but are now known to be produced in different organs. They are important regulators of cardiovascular and noncardiovascular functions, including activity on smooth muscle tone, digestive tract function, endocrine glands, renal and genitourinary system, and the nervous system.

Synthesis and Release

Endothelial cells cleave proendothelin (183 residues) from the 203-residue preproendothelin and subsequently convert it to big ET (39 amino acids) via the action of ET-converting enzyme, a neutral metalloendopeptidase that is inhibited by phosphoramidon but not thiorphan. ET-converting enzyme may cleave big ET to active 21-residue ET inside or outside endothelial cells.

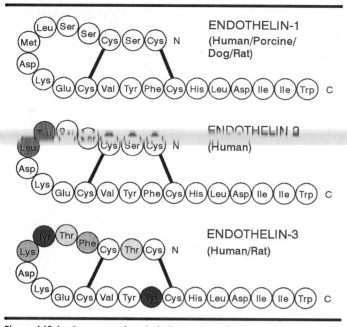

Figure A12.1. Structure of endothelin-1, -2, and -3. N and C are the N-terminal and C-terminal ends, respectively.

The main ET secreted by endothelium is ET-1, which is released in response to stimulation by pressure, low shear stress (high shear inhibits ET-1 production), angiotensin II, vasopressin, catecholamines, and transforming growth factor β. ET-1 produced by endothelial cells is mainly secreted abluminally. Plasma ET results from spillover from the vascular wall or may be secreted by the pituitary. Plasma concentrations of immunoreactive ET probably do not reliably reflect tissue production, particularly by endothelium of blood vessels, of ET-1.

Endothelin Receptors

ET receptors (ET$_A$ and ET$_B$) are 7-transmembrane domain receptors with less than 70% sequence homology. ET$_A$ and ET$_B$ are encoded by genes located in different chromosomes. They are G protein–coupled receptors signaling through activation of phospholipase C, intracellular calcium mobilization, protein kinase C activation, stimulation of the Na$^+$/H$^+$ antiporter, and intracellular alkalinization. Extracellular calcium influx in smooth muscle cells of some vascular beds and phospholipase D and phospholipase A$_2$ activation and stimulation of nonreceptor tyrosine kinases are other pathways that participate in intracellular signaling of ET receptors.

Endothelial ET-1 acts on ET$_A$ and ET$_B$ receptors to induce contraction, proliferation, and cell hypertrophy (**Figure A12.2**). ET-1 may also act on endothelial ET$_B$ receptors, inducing release of nitric oxide and prostacyclin, which explains ET-1's bifunctional constrictor and relaxant properties. It is unknown which effect is more important, although this probably varies according to the vascular bed. Mitogen-activated protein kinase stimulation of genes such as c-*jun*, c-*myc*, and c-*fos* may participate in the mitogenic and hypertrophic effects of ETs, whereas promotion of apoptosis may counterbalance ET-induced growth.

Functional Effects

Vascular effects. ET activation causes hypertrophy in small arteries (Figure A12.2) and promotes vascular fibrosis. In stroke-prone spontaneously hypertensive rats (SHRs) and in rats infused with angiotensin II (a known stimulant of ET-1 production) or aldosterone, vascular ET-1 expression is increased, and chronic administration of ET antagonists lowers blood pressure and reduces small artery hypertrophic remodeling. Effects on blood vessels and heart are probably exerted in a

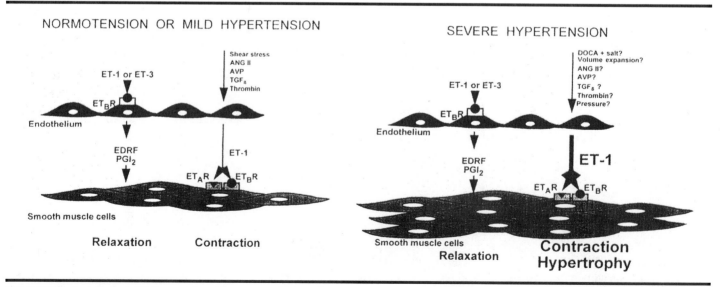

Figure A12.2. Endothelin-1 (ET-1) may play either a vasorelaxant role or a vasoconstrictor role in different vascular beds in normotension and in mild hypertension (left-hand side of figure). In moderate to severe hypertension, enhanced expression of ET-1 produces a predominant vasoconstrictor effect associated with enhanced growth, resulting in a contribution to elevated blood pressure. Growth of the vascular wall is accentuated and contributes to further elevate blood pressure and to complications of hypertension. ANG, angiotensin; AVP, arginine vasopressin; DOCA, deoxycorticosterone acetate; EDRF, endothelium-derived relaxing factor; ET$_A$R, ET$_A$ receptor; ET$_B$R, ET$_B$ receptor; PGI$_2$, prostaglandin I; TGF$_β$, transforming growth factor β.

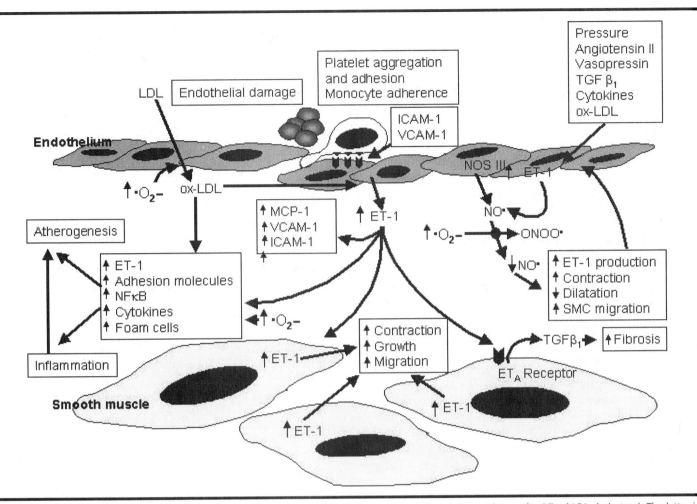

Figure A12.3. Endothelin-1 (ET-1) production is enhanced in part as a result of endothelial damage, hypertension, and oxidized LDL cholesterol. The latter is enhanced by increased oxidative stress. Smooth muscle cell (SMC) growth and migration are stimulated. Foam cells are formed, and inflammatory mediators (NFκB), adhesion molecules like intercellular adhesion module-1 (ICAM-1) and vascular cell adhesion molecule-1 (VCAM-1), and chemokines such as monocyte chemoattractant protein (MCP-1), are upregulated. Macrophages produce cytokines, and an inflammatory reaction is triggered, in large measure resulting from endothelial dysfunction. All these processes contribute to progression of vascular disease and atherosclerosis. LDL, low-density lipoprotein; NOS III, nitric oxide synthase III; oxLDL, oxidized low-density lipoprotein; TGFβ$_1$, transforming growth factor β$_1$.

paracrine or even autocrine fashion, by locally released ET acting on ET receptors in the immediate vicinity.

Smooth muscle cell growth and migration are stimulated by ET-1, which also may contribute to foam cell formation via stimulation of inflammatory mediators (e.g., NFκB), adhesion molecules (e.g., intercellular adhesion module-1 and vascular cell adhesion molecule-1), and chemokines (e.g., monocyte chemoattractant protein-1). Macrophages produce cytokines in response to ET-1, and the ensuing inflammatory reaction is a consequence of endothelial dysfunction. In the aorta and conduit arteries, ET-1 production is enhanced in part as a result of endothelial damage, hypertension, oxidized low-density lipoprotein cholesterol, and increased oxidative stress. All these processes contribute to progression of vascular disease and atherosclerosis (**Figure A12.3**).

Cardiac effects. In the coronary circulation, the virtual absence of endothelial ET$_B$ receptors suggests that ETs act only as coronary vasoconstrictors. ETs have positive chronotropic and inotropic effects on cardiac muscle and may induce cell hypertrophy. ET$_A$ receptors are present in cardiomyocytes and

fibroblasts, and ET-1 mediates the extensive cardiac fibrosis and microvascular remodeling that is found in deoxycorticosterone acetate (DOCA) -salt– and aldosterone-infused rats.

Renal effects. In the kidney, ET receptors are mainly present in blood vessels and mesangial cells. Although these are predominantly of the ET$_A$ subtype, renal ET$_B$ receptors may have pathophysiological significance, particularly in the distal tubules in which they stimulate sodium excretion.

Developmental effects. The role of the ET system in development has been emphasized by gene disruption experiments: Inactivation of the ET-1 or the ET$_A$ receptor genes in mice results in branchial arch abnormalities, inducing malformations of the mandibula, upper airway, and aortic arch (resembling the Pierre Robin syndrome), with hypoxia and hypercapnia. Surprisingly for a vasoconstrictor system, this is associated with elevation of blood pressure. This paradoxical result may be explained by the bifunctional constrictor (via ET$_A$ and ET$_B$ smooth muscle receptors) and relaxant effects of ETs (via ET$_B$ endothelial receptors, which stimulate the release of endothelial-derived nitric oxide, and prostacyclin) as shown in Figure A12.2. The slight blood pressure elevation found in this syndrome may result from hypoxia and hypercapnia, acting through sympathetic activation.

The inactivation of the ET-3 or the ET_B-receptor genes results in pigmentary abnormalities and in aganglionic megacolon, underlining the role of ET-3 and the ET_B receptor in migration of neural crest cells (melanocytes and neurons of the myenteric plexus). In humans, mutations in the ET_B receptor gene have been discovered in some of the familial and sporadic forms of Hirschsprung's disease. These results show that ET-1 is the main ligand of the ET_A receptor, whereas ET-3 is the main endogenous ligand of the ET_B receptor.

Endothelin System in Animal Models

Variation in endothelin activation. In many hypertensive models, plasma ET is normal. The ET system seems to be activated in severe forms of hypertension and in low-renin, salt-sensitive models. Other hypertensive models, including 1-kidney Goldblatt hypertensive rats, cyclosporine-induced hypertensive rats, and fructose-fed hypertensive rats, may also exhibit an ET-dependent component.

Salt-sensitive hypertension in rats. The ET system is activated in salt-dependent models of hypertension, such as the DOCA-salt hypertensive rat, the DOCA–salt-treated SHR, and the Dahl salt-sensitive rat. In all of these models, ET-1 is overexpressed in the endothelium, and blood pressure responds to ET receptor antagonists. In these models, severe hypertrophic remodeling of small arteries regresses with ET antagonist treatment.

Renovascular and spontaneous hypertension in rats. Two-kidney one clip (Goldblatt) renovascular hypertensive rats and SHRs without deoxycorticosterone or salt do not have an activated ET system. In these models, there is eutrophic rather than hypertrophic remodeling of small arteries.

Human Hypertension

The role of ETs in the pathophysiology of hypertension is still unclear. Figure A12.2 summarizes our current view of the potential implication of ET-1 in blood pressure elevation and vascular hypertrophy in moderate to severe hypertension. In humans, ET plasma levels are usually normal. Using *in situ* hybridization radioautography, the expression of the ET-1 gene has been shown to be enhanced in small arteries from gluteal subcutaneous biopsies in hypertensive patients.

Endothelin blockade. In healthy subjects, the acute intravenous administration of a mixed ET receptor antagonist results in minimal lowering of blood pressure. In hypertensive patients, endothelial dysfunction was shown to improve acutely with nonselective ET blockade (by combined infusion of BQ-123, an ET_A blocker, and BQ-788, an ET_B blocker). In mild essential hypertension, 1 study showed a moderate blood pressure–lowering effect after 4 weeks of oral administration of the combined ET_A/ET_B receptor antagonist bosentan.

Syndromes of endothelin activation. Certain populations of hypertensive subjects may exhibit chronic activation of the ET system. In blacks, hypertension is often severe, and salt sensitivity is a pathophysiologic characteristic. Severity of blood pressure elevation and salt sensitivity may be common denominators for activation of the vascular ET system in humans and experimental animals. Other forms of hypertension in which ETs may be involved in humans include rare cases of hemangioendotheliomas that produce ET, chronic renal failure, erythropoietin- and cyclosporine-induced hypertension, pheochromocytoma, and pregnancy-induced hypertension.

Primary Pulmonary Hypertension

ET antagonism has been shown to improve outcomes in primary pulmonary hypertension, and bosentan has been approved by the U.S. Food and Drug Administration for this indication.

SUGGESTED READING

1. Barton M, D'Uscio LV, Shaw S, et al. ET_A receptor blockade prevents increased tissue endothelin-1, vascular hypertrophy, and endothelial dysfunction in salt-sensitive hypertension. *Hypertension.* 1998;31:499–504.
2. Cardillo C, Kilcoyne CM, Waclawiw M, et al. Role of endothelin in the increased vascular tone of patients with essential hypertension. *Hypertension.* 1999;33:753–758.
3. Cardillo C, Campia U, Kilcoyne CM, et al. Improved endothelium-dependent vasodilation after blockade of endothelin receptors in patients with essential hypertension. *Circulation.* 2002;105:452–456.
4. Haynes WG, Ferro CJ, O'Kane KPJ, et al. Systemic endothelin receptor blockade decreases peripheral vascular resistance and blood pressure in humans. *Circulation.* 1996;93:1860–1870.
5. Krum H, Viskoper RJ, Lacourcière Y, et al. Bosentan Hypertension Investigators. The effect of an endothelin-receptor antagonist, bosentan, on blood pressure in patients with essential hypertension. *N Engl J Med.* 1998;338:784–790.
6. Lüscher TF, Oemar BS, Boulanger CM, Hahn AWA. Molecular and cellular biology of endothelin and its receptors—part I and II. *J Hypertens.* 1993;11:7–11;121–126.
7. Rubin LJ, Badesch DB, Barst RJ, et al. for the Bosentan Randomized Trial of Endothelin Antagonist Therapy Study Group. Bosentan therapy for pulmonary arterial hypertension. *N Engl J Med.* 2002;46:896–903.
8. Sakai S, Miyauchi T, Kobayashi M, et al. Inhibition of myocardial endothelin pathway improves long-term survival in heart failure. *Nature.* 1996;384:353–355.
9. Schiffrin EL. Endothelin: potential role in hypertension and vascular hypertrophy. *Hypertension.* 1995;25:1135–1143.
10. Schiffrin EL. Role of endothelin-1 in hypertension. *Hypertension.* 1999;34[part 2]:876–881.

Vasopressin and Neuropeptide Y

Allen W. Cowley, Jr, PhD; Mieczyslaw Michalkiewicz, DVM, PhD

KEY POINTS

- Vasopressin is a potent vasoconstrictor as well as a stimulus to water retention; it plays a significant role in normalizing blood pressure during conditions of acute hypotension.

- Vasopressin's long-term effect on blood pressure depends on water intake and counterregulatory mechanisms, but elevated levels of vasopressin may contribute to hypertension in a subset of human subjects.

- Neuropeptide Y accentuates the vasoconstrictor effects of sympathetic nerves and pressor hormones; its role in short- and long-term regulation of blood pressure remains to be established.

See also Chapters A2, A30, A33, A34, A37, A51, and C148

VASOPRESSIN

Physiologic regulation. Arginine vasopressin (AVP), also known as *antidiuretic hormone*, is a nonapeptide released from the posterior pituitary gland in response to (a) reduced cardiopulmonary blood volume, (b) decreased arterial blood pressure, or (c) increased plasma osmolality. Stimulation of AVP release is elicited by sudden decreases in cardiac stretch during cardiac mechanoreceptor "unloading" and aortic and carotid baroreflex stimulation. AVP release is also mediated directly by receptors in the hypothalamus, which sense osmotic changes of <1%. An increase from normal concentrations of 3 pg/mL plasma AVP to only 9 pg/mL reduces renal medullary blood flow and exerts powerful antidiuretic effects by increasing water permeability of the renal collecting ducts. These effects make AVP the major determinant of the rate of renal water excretion.

Under normal physiologic conditions, osmolality is the principal signal modulating AVP release. During hypovolemia or other conditions that reduce cardiac "preload," however, the hypovolemic stimulus can easily override the effect of the osmotic feedback loop so that AVP can be released despite significant hyponatremia. Very high concentrations of plasma AVP (20–400 pg/mL) can be attained during volume depletion and hypotension.

Vasopressin Receptors

AVP interacts with at least 2 types of receptors: V_{1a} and V_2.

V_{1a} receptors. The V_{1a} receptor gene is expressed in blood vessels from a wide variety of organs, including the kidneys. V_{1a} receptor–mediated vasoconstrictor responses of blood vessels and the glycogenolytic response of hepatocytes are linked to membrane phosphatidylinositol turnover, phospholipase C stimulation, and increased cytosolic free Ca^{2+}. V_{1a} receptors in distal segments of the mammalian nephron also promote prostaglandin E_2 generation.

V_2 receptors. The most important response to V_2 receptor stimulation is adenylyl cyclase–coupled stimulation of increased water permeability of the luminal membrane of the medullary and cortical collecting tubules. V_2 receptors in cells of the ascending limb of the loop of Henle also stimulate Na^+-K^+-Cl^- co-transport at this site. Vasodilation is observed in some parts of the systemic circulation (such as skeletal muscle) in response to selective vasopressin V_2 agonists, but V_2 receptor messenger RNA and proteins have not been found in blood vessels. Vasodilation after V_2 stimulation may be mediated through the release of paracrine hormones from the interstitial or parenchymal cells surrounding the vessels.

Physiologic Effects

AVP circulates normally at very low concentrations, ranging from 1 to 3 pg/mL (10 to 12 mol/L), and AVP is one of the most potent vasoactive peptides circulating in the blood. Concentrations that are well within the physiologic range (10–20 pg/mL) can produce significant renal vasoconstriction and blunt the pressure-diuresis-natriuresis relationship.

Blood pressure effects. Constrictive effects of AVP on skin, kidneys, and splanchnic and coronary beds are offset by vasodilation in skeletal muscle, contributing to variable effects on systemic blood pressure. AVP enhances the sympathoinhibitory influence of the arterial baroreflex and the central nervous system, which further buffers this powerful vasoconstrictor substance. As a result of these forces, only slight elevations of arterial pressure are normally observed with elevations of plasma AVP, which allows the antidiuretic action of AVP to occur without the offsetting effects of pressure-induced diuresis. In the absence of autonomic reflex mechanisms, the pressor activity of vasopressin is increased 9,000-fold.

Hypertension in animal models. AVP is elevated in many forms of experimental hypertension, but its contribution to the elevated pressure in these models is not entirely clear. AVP is a potent vasoconstrictor and can play an important role in blood pressure normalization after rapid hemorrhage. As shown in dogs, AVP release can bring about a rapid 70% compensation of arterial pressure in the absence of the autonomic reflexes and renin release.

Despite the vasoconstrictor and fluid-retaining effects of AVP, chronic administration of the endogenous peptide does not result in sustained hypertension in rats, dogs, or humans. Yet, chronic administration of a selective V_1 agonist intravenously or into the medullary interstitial space of the rat lowers blood flow to the renal medulla and produces sustained hypertension. The difference between the pressor action of the selective agonist and that of AVP itself is probably accounted for by the lack of depressor V_2 effect.

Several studies have now demonstrated that AVP-stimulated nitric oxide (NO) release from the renal medulla is mediated by V_2 receptors. Sustained increases of medullary interstitial NO have been found by microdialysis in response to chronic elevations of plasma AVP. However, it has also been shown that V_2 receptors are downregulated after dehydration when plasma AVP is elevated. This downregulation of V_2 receptors with sustained elevations of AVP could contribute to the so-called AVP escape mechanism and is consistent with the failure of AVP to cause a sustained elevation of blood volume and arterial pressure.

Recently, it was found that Dahl salt-sensitive rats exhibit lower medullary levels of NO synthase activity, messenger RNA, and protein and that in this strain of rats, chronic intravenous administration of very small amounts of AVP does result in sustained hypertension. It has been demonstrated that stimulation of NO release with AVP is necessary to prevent sustained hypertension with AVP infusion.

Human hypertension. The contribution of AVP to the maintenance of arterial hypertension in humans remains unclear. Plasma AVP levels are significantly elevated (5–20 pg/mL) in nearly 30% of male hypertensive patients and are directly correlated with systolic and diastolic blood pressure in men. By contrast, as few as 7% of female hypertensive subjects exhibit elevated plasma AVP. It is unknown whether changes in AVP concentrations in essential hypertension are primary or secondary. Plasma AVP levels can be higher (>20 pg/mL) in the malignant phase of hypertension or in congestive heart failure. AVP elevations of this magnitude could contribute to chronic redistribution of cardiac output and influence regional blood flow, body fluid volume status, and autonomic reflex mechanisms. Plasma AVP levels are higher in blacks than in whites, and selective vasopressin V_1 receptor inhibition was shown to lower mean arterial pressure in blacks (28 mm Hg) but not in whites.

The plasma AVP levels usually found in hypertensive humans are lower than those needed to produce pressor responses in normal subjects. However, sustained plasma levels of 10 to 20 pg/mL could result in fluid retention, volume expansion, and a rise of arterial pressure. The extent to which this occurs depends on the level of daily water intake. If hypertension does occur, as observed with chronic intravenous infusion of AVP with a fixed water intake, significant elevations of pressure are sustained for only 1 to 2 weeks because of the phenomenon known as *vasopressin escape*. Escape from the fluid-retaining effects of AVP results from pressure-induced diuresis similar to that observed in

patients with the syndrome of inappropriate antidiuretic hormone. It is possible that some human subjects resemble the genetically inbred Dahl S rat and fail to produce sufficient renal NO in response to AVP, thereby enabling small elevations of this peptide to contribute to the chronic hypertensive state.

NEUROPEPTIDE Y

Neuropeptide Y (NPY) is a 36-amino acid peptide that has been implicated in numerous physiologic processes, including thirst, appetite, blood pressure modulation, and energy metabolism. It is one of the most abundant peptides of the mammalian nervous systems.

Neurohumoral Effects

In the central nervous system, the peptide is expressed in the cluster of neurons involved in cardiovascular regulation, including the hypothalamus, the ventrolateral medulla, the nucleus tractus solitarii, the locus caeruleus, and the sympathetic lateral column of the spinal cord. In the peripheral nervous system, NPY is found mainly in sympathetic ganglia and sympathetic fibers innervating blood vessels, small arteries, heart, and kidney. A striking feature of this peptide is its close coexistence with norepinephrine in central and peripheral adrenergic neurons. It is released from noradrenergic nerve terminals, particularly during high-frequency prolonged stimulation.

Neuropeptide Receptors

Of the 5 proposed NPY receptor subtypes, Y_1 and Y_2 are believed to be the most relevant for control of vascular tone.

Y_1 receptors. Y_1 receptors are postsynaptic, coupled to the inhibition of adenylate cyclase, and act to increase intracellular calcium. Stimulation of Y_1 receptors results in direct vasoconstriction or potentiation of the vasoconstrictor effects of norepinephrine, angiotensin, or serotonin in some vessels. Small resistance vessels of the coronary, splanchnic, or cerebral vascular beds are particularly sensitive to NPY.

Y_2 receptors. Y_2 receptors are predominantly presynaptic, and they decrease intracellular calcium by inhibiting N-type calcium channels in nerve terminals. NPY receptors at presynaptic sites in the central nervous system, vasculature, heart, and kidney mediate inhibition of neurotransmitter release, including norepinephrine and glutamate. NPY is colocalized with vasopressin in magnocellular neurons of the hypothalamus and potentiates vasopressin release from the neuronal lobe of the rat pituitary gland.

Actions

Blood pressure effects. Exogenous NPY elicits a hypertensive or hypotensive effect depending on the site of administration. Injection of NPY into discrete areas of the central nervous system (such as the third ventricle, the paraventricular nucleus, the nucleus tractus solitarius, or ventrolateral medulla) causes potent blood pressure lowering and heart rate reduction. These sympatholytic effects are also associated with reduced sympathetic firing to the kidney and reduced norepinephrine release. On the other hand, acute administration of NPY into the systemic circulation effectively increases blood pressure in a pattern similar to an

α_2 agonist. Systemic or central administration of NPY also increases the sensitivity of the aortic baroreceptor reflex in the rat. Recently, NPY involvement in neurogenic angiogenesis in skeletal muscle ischemia and development has been demonstrated.

Renal effects. In contrast to the antidiuretic effects of most vasoconstrictor neurotransmitters and hormones, NPY enhances diuresis and natriuresis *in vivo* in anesthetized animals. NPY has been reported to reduce renin release, elevate plasma atrial natriuretic peptide, and directly modify sodium- and potassium-activated adenosine triphosphatase activity on renal proximal tubules.

Hypertension

Elevated plasma NPY levels have been found in conditions of intense and prolonged sympathetic activation, including stress, exercise, hemorrhage, or myocardial infarction. NPY release is also enhanced in some animal models of hypertension and in a subset of patients with essential hypertension, including hypertensive children and adolescents. In the brain of the spontaneously hypertensive rat (SHR), a reduced NPY content has been observed. The sympatholytic and blood pressure–reducing effects of central NPY administration is diminished in SHR.

Selective Y_1-receptor blockade failed to change blood pressure or heart rate in normal or SHRs; however, blockade of Y_1 receptor attenuates stress-induced vasoconstriction. The NPY or NPY Y_1-receptor gene deletion in mice does not affect blood pressure significantly, but transgenic NPY overexpression under natural promoter in rats is associated with a sym-patholytic effect and a hypotensive phenotype with a reduced blood pressure response to stress. The NPY locus cosegregates with high blood pressure in the SHR, and NPY gene polymorphism is associated with increased blood pressure and accelerated atherosclerotic progression in humans.

SUGGESTED READING

1. Cowley AW Jr, Liard JF. Cardiovascular actions of vasopressin. In: Gash DM, Boer GJ, eds. *Vasopressin: Principles and Properties.* New York, NY: Plenum Press; 1987:389–433.
2. Cowley AW Jr, Roman RJ. Role of the kidney in hypertension. *JAMA.* 1996;275:1581–1589.
3. Bakris G, Bursztzen M, Gavras I, et al. Role of vasopressin in essential hypertension: racial differences. *J Hypertens.* 1997;15:545–550.
4. Crofton JT, Ota M, Shore L. Role of vasopressin, the renin-angiotensin system and sex in Dahl salt-sensitive hypertension. *J Hypertens.* 1993;11:1031–1038.
5. Szentivanyi M Jr, Park F, Maeda CY, Cowley AW Jr. Nitric oxide in the renal medulla protects from vasopressin-induced hypertension. *Hypertension.* 2000;35:740–745.
6. Yuan B, Cowley AW Jr. Evidence that reduced renal medullary nitric oxide synthase activity of Dahl S rats enables small elevations of arginine vasopressin to produce sustained hypertension. *Hypertension.* 2001;37:524–528.
7. Michel MC, Rascher W. Neuropeptide Y: a possible role in hypertension. *J Hypertens.* 1995;13:385–395.
8. Zukowska-Grojec Z, Karwatowska-Prokopczuk E, Rose W, et al. Neuropeptide Y: a novel angiogenic factor from the sympathetic nerves and endothelium. *Circ Res.* 1998;83:187–195.
9. Michalkiewicz M, Michalkiewicz T, Kreulen D, McDougall S. Increased vascular responses in neuropeptide Y transgenic rats. *Am J Phys.* 2001;281:R417–R426.
10. Thorsell A, Michalkiewicz M, et al. Behavioral insensitivity to restraint stress, absent fear suppression of behavior and impaired spatial learning in neuropeptide Y transgenic rats. *Proc Natl Acad Sci.* 2000; 97:12852–12857.

Chapter A14

Kinins

Oscar A. Carretero, MD; Nour-Eddine Rhaleb, PhD

KEY POINTS

- Kinins are potent vasodilators cleaved from kininogens by kallikreins.

- Kinins stimulate release of nitric oxide, prostaglandins, and other mediators.

- Kinin formation increases with stimulation of secretory activity in some glands and with inflammation in some cases.

- Kinins are both natriuretic and diuretic, and they mediate part of the cardioprotective effect of angiotensin-converting enzyme inhibitors.

See also Chapters A6, A7, A16, A20, A24, A29, A33, A63, A66, A67, and C144

Kinins are vasodepressor autacoids that play an important role in the regulation of cardiovascular and renal function. In mammals, the main kinins are bradykinin and lysyl-bradykinin (kallidin). They are released from substrates known as *kininogens* by enzymes known as *kininogenases* (**Figure A14.1**). The main kininogenases are plasma and tissue (glandular) kal-likrein. These are separate enzymes that differ in function and are encoded by different genes.

Kallikrein-Kinin Bioregulation

There are 2 main kininogens, *high-molecular-weight kininogen* and *low-molecular-weight kininogen*. Both are synthesized

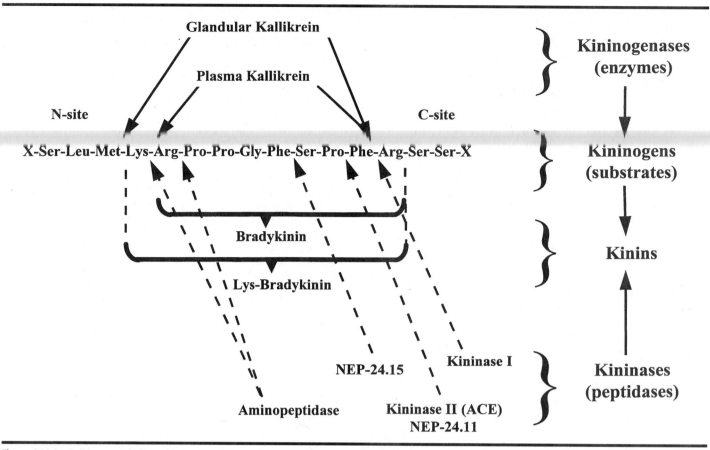

Figure A14.1. Solid arrows indicate kininogen cleavage by the main kininogenases, glandular and plasma kallikrein. Broken arrows indicate sites of kinin cleavage by kininases [kininase I, kininase II (ACE [angiotensin-converting enzyme]), neutral endopeptidases (NEP) 24.11 and 24.15, and aminopeptidases].

in the liver and are found in very high concentrations in plasma. They are encoded by a single gene, but their messenger RNA is generated by different splicing of the gene transcript. Plasma kallikrein releases kinins only from high-molecular-weight kininogen. All kininogens also inhibit thiol proteases, such as cathepsin M and H and calpains.

Kinins are destroyed by enzymes known as *kininases*, which are located mainly in the endothelial cells of the capillaries of the lungs and other tissues. The best-known kininases are angiotensin-converting enzyme (ACE, also known as *kininase II*), neutral endopeptidases 24.11 and 24.15, aminopeptidases, and carboxypeptidase N (known as *kininase I*) (Figure A14.1). However, even after inhibition of most of these enzymes, the half-life of kinins *in vivo* is less than 15 seconds, suggesting that other peptidases are also important in the metabolism of these peptides.

Receptors

Kinins act mainly as local autocrine and paracrine hormones via 2 different receptors: B_1 and B_2. B_1 receptors are selectively activated by des-Arg[9]-bradykinin and des-Arg[10]-kallidin, whereas B_2 receptors are activated by bradykinin or kallidin. B_1 receptors are expressed primarily during administration of lipopolysaccharides (such as endotoxin) and in inflammation. Nevertheless, in the absence of B_2 receptors, as in B_2-receptor knockout mice, B_1 receptors can be upregulated and assume some of the hemodynamic properties of B_2 recep-

tors. In wild-type animals and humans, most of the known physiologic effects of kinins are mediated by B_2 receptors. They belong to a family of peptide hormone receptors with 7 membrane-spanning regions linked to G proteins.

Functions

In some organs, kinins appear to play an important role in the regulation of blood flow to meet metabolic demands. In the submandibular salivary glands, kallikrein secretion and vasoconstriction are increased by sympathetic nerve stimulation. After stimulation, vasodilatation is mediated by kinins and is greatly magnified by blocking kinin hydrolysis with ACE inhibitors. Because other glands of the gastrointestinal tract contain kallikrein, it is possible that after a meal, kallikrein is secreted and kinins mediate part of the resultant vasodilatation. Similarly, eccrine (sweat) glands contain a kallikrein-like enzyme, and it is possible that kinins also participate in the regulation of sweat formation as well as the skin vasodilatation observed during sweating. Kinins may also mediate part of the vasodilatation and edema observed during inflammation. Kininogenase, low-molecular-weight and high-molecular-weight kininogens, and neutral endopeptidase 24.11 are present in leukocytes. Kinins can also stimulate release of cytokines such as interleukin-1 from monocytes. Prostaglandins, nitric oxide, endothelium-derived hyperpolarizing factor, and tissue plasminogen activator mediate some of the effects of kinins.

Renal Kallikrein-Kinin System

Renal kallikrein is located in the connecting cells of the tubules, and kinin receptors are present in the collecting duct. Kinins play an important role in the regulation of renal microcirculation and water and sodium excretion. The natriuretic and diuretic effects of kinins are mediated in part by prostaglandin E_2. *In vitro*, stimulation of the release of nitric oxide from endothelial cells by bradykinin or acetylcholine increases cyclic guanosine monophosphate and inhibits sodium transport by cortical collecting duct cells. *In vivo*, bradykinin causes natriuresis and diuresis without affecting the glomerular filtration rate. The diuretic and natriuretic effects of neutral endopeptidase 24.11 inhibitors are due in part to blockade of kinin and atrial natriuretic factor (ANF) hydrolysis of endogenous natriuretic peptides. These 2 peptides act in synergy to inhibit water and sodium transport in the nephron, so that blocking either peptide suppresses the natriuretic and diuretic effects of endopeptidase inhibitors.

Relationship to Hypertension

Decreased activity of the kallikrein-kinin system may play a role in hypertension. Low urinary kallikrein excretion in children is one of the major genetic markers associated with a family history of essential hypertension, and children with high urinary kallikrein excretion have less probability of a genetic background of hypertension. Urinary kallikrein excretion is decreased in various models of genetic hypertension. A restriction fragment-length polymorphism for the kallikrein gene family in spontaneously hypertensive rats has been linked to high blood pressure. Urinary and arterial tissue kallikrein are also decreased in renovascular hypertension. Mice with the bradykinin B_2 receptor deleted by homologous recombination (gene knockout) develop hypertension when fed a high-sodium diet. Thus, low kinin activity may be involved in the development and maintenance of salt-sensitive hypertension. In mineralocorticoid hypertension, circulating kinins and urinary kallikrein excretion are increased, but hypertension is not worsened in mice lacking B_2 receptors or kininogen-deficient rats.

Role of Kinins in the Antihypertensive Effect of Angiotensin-Converting Enzyme Inhibitors

Increased tissue kinin concentrations and potentiation of their effect may be involved in the therapeutic effect of ACE inhibitors. This hypothesis is supported by the following facts:

1. ACE is one of the main peptidases that hydrolyze kinins.
2. Tissue and urinary kinins increase after treatment with ACE inhibitors, possibly promoting vasodilatation and increased sodium and water excretion.
3. Inhibition of the kallikrein-kinin system with a kinin antagonist partially blocks the acute, but not the chronic, hypotensive effects of ACE inhibitors.
4. In kininogen- or kinin-deficient Brown Norway rats with experimental renovascular hypertension, the acute antihypertensive effect of ACE inhibitors is significantly reduced in both magnitude and duration.

Role of Kinins in the Therapeutic Effect of Angiotensin-Converting Enzyme Inhibitors

Components of the kallikrein-kinin system, especially tissue kallikrein, are present in the heart, arteries, and veins. Kinins are also found in the venous effluent of isolated perfused hearts, and their release is rapidly increased during ischemia and after administration of ACE inhibitors. Repeated brief periods of ischemia render the myocardium more resistant to injury from subsequent prolonged ischemia, a phenomenon called *ischemic preconditioning*.

ACE inhibitors reverse cardiac remodeling and improve function in heart failure due to myocardial infarction. In rats with heart failure, the benefit of ACE inhibitors is reversed by a kinin antagonist, suggesting that kinins have a cardioprotective effect. Moreover, the myocardial protection afforded by preconditioning or ACE inhibition is greatly attenuated in mice lacking B_2 receptors and kinin-deficient rats subjected to myocardial infarction, suggesting that kinins play a key role in preconditioning or ACE therapy.

Thrombosis

The bradykinin cascade interacts with the hemostatic system in several ways. Plasma kallikrein, high-molecular-weight kininogen, and Hageman factor are involved in the intrinsic pathway of blood clotting and in fibrinolysis. Kinins induce formation of nitric oxide and prostaglandin I_2, which inhibit platelet aggregation. Kinins are also potent stimulators of the release of tissue plasminogen activator and may promote fibrinolysis. These effects may help explain some of the beneficial properties of ACE inhibitors in patients with heart disease.

SUGGESTED READING

1. Bhoola KD, Figueroa CD, Worthy K. Bioregulation of kinins: kallikreins, kininogens, and kininases. *Pharmacol Rev*. 1992;44:1–80.
2. Carretero OA, Scicli AG. The kallikrein-kinin system. In: Fozzard HA, et al., eds. *The Heart and Cardiovascular System. Scientific Foundations*, Vol. 2. New York, NY: Raven Press, 1991;1851–1874.
3. Liu Y-H, Yang X-P, Mehta D, et al. Role of kinins in chronic heart failure and in the therapeutic effect of ACE inhibitors in kininogen-deficient rats. *Am J Physiol Heart Circ Physiol*. 2000;278:H507–H514.
4. Liu Y-H, Yang X-P, Sharov VG, et al. Effects of angiotensin-converting enzyme inhibitors and angiotensin II type 1 receptor antagonists in rats with heart failure. Role of kinins and angiotensin II type 2 receptors. *J Clin Invest*. 1997;99:1926–1935.
5. Margolius HS. Tissue kallikreins and kinins: regulation and roles in hypertensive and diabetic diseases. *Annu Rev Pharmacol Toxicol*. 1989;29:343–364.
6. Milia AF, Gross V, Plehm R, et al. Normal blood pressure and renal function in mice lacking the bradykinin B_2 receptor. *Hypertension*. 2001;37:1473–1479.
7. Nasjletti A, Malik KU. The renal kallikrein-kinin and prostaglandin systems interaction. *Annu Rev Physiol*. 1981;43:597–609.
8. Rhaleb N-E, Peng H, Alfie M, et al. Effect of ACE inhibitor on DOCA-salt- and aortic coarctation-induced hypertension in mice. Do kinin B_2 receptors play a role? *Hypertension*. 1999;33:329–334.
9. Rhaleb N-E, Yang X-P, Nanba M, et al. Effect of chronic blockade of the kallikrein-kinin system on the development of hypertension in rats. *Hypertension*. 2001;37:121–128.
10. Yang X-P, Liu Y-H, Scicli GM, et al. Role of kinins in the cardioprotective effect of preconditioning. Study of myocardial ischemia/reperfusion injury in B_2 kinin receptor knockout mice and kininogen-deficient rats. *Hypertension*. 1997;30:737–740.

Endogenous Natriuretic Peptides

Yoram Shenker, MD

KEY POINTS

- Atrial natriuretic peptide and brain natriuretic peptide are released from myocardium when it is stretched; C-type natriuretic peptide is released from endothelium.

- Atrial natriuretic peptide and brain natriuretic peptide enhance sodium excretion by a direct effect on the kidney; they also inhibit sympathetic nervous outflow, renin release, and aldosterone secretion.

- Natriuretic peptides relax vascular smooth muscle by 2 receptor-mediated mechanisms that generate cyclic guanosine monophosphate; a third type of receptor helps clear the peptides from the circulation.

- Measurement of brain natriuretic peptide plasma levels is useful in diagnosis and follow-up of congestive heart failure; synthetic atrial natriuretic peptide and brain natriuretic peptide are efficacious in the treatment of acute heart failure.

See also Chapters A5, A6, A16, A24, A29, A33, A37, A62, C121, and C156

The heart serves as an endocrine organ by synthesizing and releasing 2 hormones that affect cardiorenal homeostasis: atrial natriuretic peptide (ANP) and BNP, originally called *brain natriuretic peptide*. The actions of ANP (**Table A15.1**) include natriuresis, inhibition of the renin-angiotensin-aldosterone system (RAAS), modulation of the sympathetic nervous outflow, selective increases in capillary permeability, arterial vasodilation, and inhibition of vascular smooth muscle cell proliferation.

Synthesis

Atrial natriuretic peptide. The ANP prohormone contains 126 amino acids and is cleaved in cardiac tissue into 2 fragments; the C-terminal 28–amino acid peptide (proANP 99–126) is the biologically active circulating hormone. The sequence proANP 95–126, known as *urodilatin*, has been isolated from human urine and may arise by alternative processing of proANP in the kidney.

Brain natriuretic peptide. BNP complements ANP and exerts similar biologic actions (Table A15.1). BNP has a different amino acid sequence but is structurally related to ANP. It is synthesized and stored in atrial cardiomyocytes and cells of the central nervous system. BNP normally circulates at lower concentrations than ANP, but in patients with hypertension and congestive heart failure, it may circulate at levels that exceed those of ANP.

C-type natriuretic peptide. The third member of this family of peptides, C-type natriuretic peptide (CNP), is a product of endothelial cells and is not of cardiac origin. CNP is a potent vasoactive peptide (Table A15.1) that dilates veins and arteries. In addition, CNP is antimitogenic. Unlike ANP and BNP, CNP is only minimally natriuretic and does not inhibit the RAAS.

CNP probably functions in a paracrine manner, acting locally on vascular smooth muscle cells, whereas ANP and BNP function as circulating hormones.

Control of Secretion

ANP is normally synthesized in atrial myocytes and is released from the heart in response to atrial stretch during such conditions as intravascular volume expansion and atrial pressure overload. The increase in circulating ANP and BNP in chronic cardiovascular disease states follows recruitment of ventricular myocardium to synthesize peptides. This underscores the importance of the ventricle and the atrium as endocrine organs. Besides changes in atrial and ventricular wall tension, several vasoconstrictors including norepinephrine, endothelin-1, and angiotensin II stimulate ANP and BNP transcription and secretion. Cytokines such as interleukin-1β and tumor necrosis factor-α are also strong stimuli, particularly of BNP secretion. Secretion of BNP is very prompt in response to all these stimuli, suggesting that this peptide is an acute-phase reactant released in response to acute tissue injury.

Receptors

There are 3 different natriuretic peptide receptors (NPRs). Two of these, NPR-A and NPR-B, are guanylyl cyclases with identical extracellular domains. The C-terminal intracellular sequences of these 2 receptors are guanylyl cyclase catalytic domains. ANP and BNP bind to the A-receptor, whereas CNP binds exclusively to the B-receptor. This binding results in intracellular formation of cyclic guanosine monophosphate, a classic second messenger of vasodilators. The NPR-A receptor is highly expressed in vascular endothelial cells and in renal epithelial cells, whereas the NPR-B receptor is highly expressed in vascular smooth muscle cells.

Table A15.1. Biologic Actions of the Natriuretic Peptides

Atrial natriuretic peptide and brain natriuretic peptide
  Natriuresis
  Arterial vasodilation
  Inhibition of the renin-angiotensin-aldosterone system
  Inhibition of sympathetic nervous function
  Inhibition of endothelin
  Inhibition of vasopressin and adrenocorticotropic hormone
  Increase in capillary permeability
  Anti-mitogenesis
  Inhibition of cardiac fibroblasts
C-type natriuretic peptide
  Venous and arterial vasodilation
  Inhibition of endothelin
  Antimitogenesis
  Minimal natriuresis

The NPR-C receptor is homologous to the other natriuretic peptide receptors in its extracellular domain but lacks any intracellular domain or guanylyl cyclase activity. NPR-C may act as a "clearance" receptor that removes natriuretic peptides from the circulation.

Metabolism

Several tissues are involved in the metabolism of natriuretic peptides, including lungs, liver, and kidneys. In addition to clearance through binding to the NPR-C receptor, another degradative mechanism is inactivation by neutral endopeptidase (NEP), a widely distributed metallopeptidase. NEP inhibition increases levels of ANP and BNP to a similar extent, accounting for approximately half of the turnover of these peptides.

Physiologic Significance

The natriuretic peptides can be viewed as a "mirror image" of the RAAS. ANP and BNP are secreted in response to volume expansion and pressure overload in the heart. Not only do they inhibit renin and aldosterone release, but they also oppose the actions of angiotensin II and aldosterone through their effects on vascular contractility and cell growth and renal sodium reabsorption.

Administration of NPR-A and NPR-B receptor-antagonists impairs the natriuretic response to an acute intravenous volume load in rats. Mice that lack the ANP gene have higher blood pressure than controls, but they are able to cope with a sustained increase in dietary sodium. Altered structure of the ANP gene has been identified as a likely causative factor for stroke occurrence in the stroke-prone spontaneously hypertensive rats. These results suggest that ANP and BNP contribute to blood pressure regulation, but are not essential for chronic sodium and water homeostasis.

Clinical Significance

ANP and BNP are elevated in long-standing hypertension and congestive heart failure, but their levels appear inappropriately low for the degree of myocyte stretch caused by the chronic pressure and volume overload. Thus, these disease states may represent relative natriuretic peptide deficiency states. CNP is present in human plasma, but its role in cardiovascular disease states remains undefined.

Chronic heart failure diagnosis and management. Raised levels of ANP or BNP are good indicators of failing cardiac function and can serve as markers for titration of heart failure medications. The use of BNP levels in diagnosis and management of congestive heart failure is becoming routine in many U.S. medical centers. There are also early indications that plasma levels of ANP or other fragments of proANP may predict mortality in elderly patients.

Therapeutic uses. Therapeutic strategies are emerging that amplify the biologic actions of ANP and BNP. The effects of these peptides are limited by their removal by the NPR-C and their degradation by NEP. NRP-C receptor blockade and NEP inhibition potentiate the biologic actions of endogenous ANP and BNP, and these inhibitors have shown therapeutic use in the treatment of experimental hypertension and congestive heart failure. NEP inhibition has been combined with angiotensin-converting enzyme (ACE) inhibition in a series of new antihypertensive agents of which omapatrilat is the best studied. ACE-NEP inhibitors reduce blood pressure in patients with isolated systolic hypertension and are effective in high-renin and low-renin forms of hypertension. Omapatrilat has been found to cause more angioedema than ACE inhibitors, presumably because of the greater potentiation of bradykinin and its metabolites by the added NEP inhibition.

BNP and ANP infusions have been used in the treatment of acute heart failure. ANP is primarily used in Japan and BNP (nesiritide) in the United States. Infusion of these agents leads to a decrease in pulmonary capillary wedge pressure and systemic vascular resistance, improving cardiac function by reducing preload and afterload. Diuresis and natriuresis are markedly increased, but the other actions of the natriuretic peptides prevent activation of the RAAS despite vasodilatation and diuresis, which usually activate the RAAS.

SUGGESTED READING

1. Brunner-La Rocca HP, Kiowski W, Ramsay D, Sütsch G. Therapeutic benefits of increasing natriuretic peptide levels. *Cardiovasc Res.* 2001;51:510–520.
2. Levin ER, Gardner DG, Samson WK. Natriuretic peptides. *N Engl J Med.* 1998;339:321–328.
3. Maisel A. B-Type natriuretic peptide in the diagnosis and management of congestive heart failure. *Cardiol Clin.* 2001;19:557–571.
4. Nathisuwan S, Talbert RL. A review of vasopeptidase inhibitors: a new modality in the treatment of hypertension and chronic heart failure. *Pharmacotherapy.* 2002;22:27–42.
5. Rubattu S, Volpe M. The atrial natriuretic peptide: a changing view. *J Hypertens.* 2001;19:1923–1931.
6. Sagnella GA. Atrial natriuretic peptide mimetics and vasopeptidase inhibitors. *Cardiovasc Res.* 2001;51:416–428.
7. Villarreal D, Freeman RH, Reams GP. Natriuretic peptides and salt sensitivity: endocrine cardiorenal integration in heart failure. *Congest Heart Fail.* 2002;8:29–36.
8. Yoshimura M, Yasue H, Ogawa H. Pathophysiological significance and clinical application of ANP and BNP in patients with heart failure. *Can J Physiol Pharmacol.* 2001;79:730–735.

Vascular Nitric Oxide

Paul M. Vanhoutte, MD, PhD

KEY POINTS

- Endothelial cells contain the constitutive form of nitric oxide synthase, which produces moderate amounts of nitric oxide by metabolizing L-arginine.

- Endothelium-derived nitric oxide inhibits contraction and proliferation of the underlying vascular smooth muscle, adhesion of blood cells and platelets, and platelet aggregation.

- Release of nitric oxide can be augmented acutely by increases in blood flow velocity and shear stress and by a variety of hormones, autacoids, and by-products associated with blood coagulation; nitric oxide release can be modulated chronically by exercise, hormones, and diet.

- Endothelial production of nitric oxide decreases with age and in many vascular diseases, including hypertension.

See also Chapters A14, A15, A19, A29, A33, A45, A63, and A65–A67

Nitric oxide (NO) is a freely diffusible gas that can act as an intracellular and intercellular messenger molecule. The half-life of NO under physiologic conditions is only a few seconds, as NO is avidly scavenged by superoxide anions and heme-containing molecules, especially hemoglobin. NO contributes to many physiologic responses within and outside of the cardiovascular system. If produced in large amounts, it can facilitate apoptosis and cause cell death. In the cardiovascular system, the main source of NO is the endothelial cells, although certain nerves, blood cells, and even vascular smooth muscle cells can produce the mediator. Endothelial cells produce moderate amounts of NO, which act mainly on the vascular wall and the platelets, but NO also can contribute to the regulation of cardiac contractility.

Nitric Oxide Synthesis

In 1980, Furchgott and Zawadzki discovered that endothelial cells relaxed isolated aortic rings in response to acetylcholine. The labile, diffusible substance mediating endothelium-dependent relaxation was identified a few years later as NO. NO is formed from the guanidine-nitrogen terminal of L-arginine by an enzyme called *NO synthase* (NOS), of which there are 3 isoforms: NOS I, II, and III, more commonly referred to as *neuronal* (nNOS), *inducible* (iNOS), and *endothelial* (eNOS), respectively. The enzyme present in endothelial cells (the III isoform) is constitutively active, calmodulin-dependent, regulated by the intracellular Ca^{2+}-concentration, and requires reduced nicotinamide adenine dinucleotide phosphate and tetrahydrobiopterin as cofactors. eNOS can be inhibited competitively by L-arginine analogs, such as N^G-mono-methyl-L-arginine, which have permitted the exploration of the role of NO *in vivo*. A circulating, endogenous inhibitor of NOS also exists and has been identified as asymmetric dimethylarginine.

Endothelial Nitric Oxide Release

The activity of eNOS and the subsequent release of NO is modulated acutely by a number of physical and humoral stimuli.

Among physical stimuli, shear stress exerted by blood flow is one of the main factors affecting moment-to-moment changes in the local release of endothelium-derived NO. Several neurohumoral mediators augment the release of NO by activating specific endothelial receptors (**Figure A16.1**). The endogenous substances involved include circulating hormones such as catecholamines (stimulating α_2-adrenoceptors), vasopressin and oxytocin (V_1-receptors), endothelin-1 (ET_B-receptors), possibly angiotensin II (AT_2-receptors), serotonin ($5HT_{1D}$-receptors), adenine nucleotides (P_{2Y}-receptors), thrombin, histamine, and bradykinin (B_2-receptors). The endothelial cell membrane receptors for these different endogenous substances are coupled to the activation of eNOS by different G proteins. For example, α_2-adrenoceptors, $5HT_{1D}$-receptors, thrombin-receptors, and ET_B-receptors are coupled to pertussis toxin–sensitive G_i proteins, whereas B_2-receptors and P_{2Y} receptors couple with pertussis toxin–insensitive G_q proteins (**Figure A16.2**).

Cellular Effects of Nitric Oxide

Direct actions and cyclic guanosine monophosphate stimulation. The NO produced by eNOS acts on the endothelial cells themselves and also diffuses away in luminal and abluminal directions. In the endothelial cells, NO inhibits the production of endothelin-1, the oxidation of low-density lipoproteins to oxidized low-density lipoproteins, the expression of adhesion molecules, and, thus, the adhesion to the endothelium of platelets and white cells. At the interface with the blood, NO cannot penetrate deep into the blood stream because it is avidly scavenged by oxyhemoglobin. However, it acts in strong synergy with prostacyclin to inhibit platelet aggregation and also blocks release of vasoconstrictor substances such as serotonin and thromboxane A_2 and growth factors such as platelet-derived growth factor. In the underlying vascular smooth muscle, endothelium-derived NO inhibits the contractile process and proliferation of these cells (Figure A16.2).

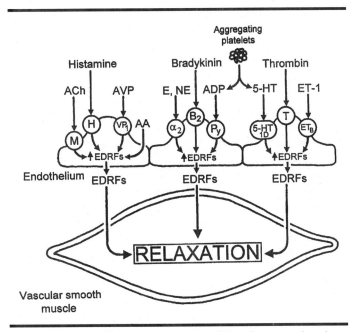

Figure A16.1. Some of the neurohumoral mediators that cause the release of endothelium-derived relaxing factors (EDRF), mainly nitric oxide through activation of specific endothelial receptors (*circles*). α, alpha-adrenergic receptor; AA, arachidonic acid; ACh, acetylcholine; ADP, adenosine diphosphate; AVP, arginine vasopressin; B, kinin receptor; E, epinephrine; ET, endothelin, endothelin receptor; H, histaminergic receptor; 5-HT, serotonin (5-hydroxytryptamine), serotoninergic receptor; M, muscarinic receptor; NE, norepinephrine; P, purinergic receptor; T, thrombin receptor; VP, vasopressinergic receptor. [From Vanhoutte PM. Endothelial dysfunction and inhibition of converting enzyme. *Eur Heart J.* 1998;19(suppl 1):J7–J15, with permission.]

Most of the cellular actions of NO (and of exogenous NO-donors such as nitrovasodilators) are explained by the activation of the cytosolic enzyme soluble guanylate cyclase, which catalyzes the formation of cyclic guanosine monophosphate (GMP) from guanosine triphosphate. The increased level of cyclic GMP activates protein kinase G, which in turn phosphorylates a number of proteins involved in the relaxation of vascular smooth muscle, the proliferative process, the expression of adhesion molecules, and the aggregation of platelets, among other actions. Vascular smooth muscle tone is dependent on the cyclic GMP–mediated effects of NO that contribute to endothelium-dependent relaxation, including (a) stimulation of sodium-potassium adenosine triphosphatase and opening of adenosine triphosphate-dependent potassium channels leading to cell membrane hyperpolarization; (b) inhibition of Ca^{2+}-channels, stimulation of plasma membrane–associated calcium adenosine triphosphatase and reduction of calcium release from the sarcoplasmic reticulum, leading to a reduced intracellular Ca^{2+} concentration; (c) inhibition of phospholipase C and thus decreased production of stimulatory phosphoinositides; and (d) phosphorylation of proteins accelerating the relaxation process and inhibition of Rho-kinase, with reduced interaction of the contractile proteins. In addition, NO can directly open certain Ca^{2+}-dependent K^+-channels, thus accelerating potassium efflux and causing hyperpolarization.

Indirect actions. Apart from the direct effects of NO on vascular smooth muscle cells described in the section Direct Actions and Cyclic Guanosine Monophosphate Stimulation, indirect actions of the endothelial media contribute to its vasodilator potential. These include the following: (a) inhibi-

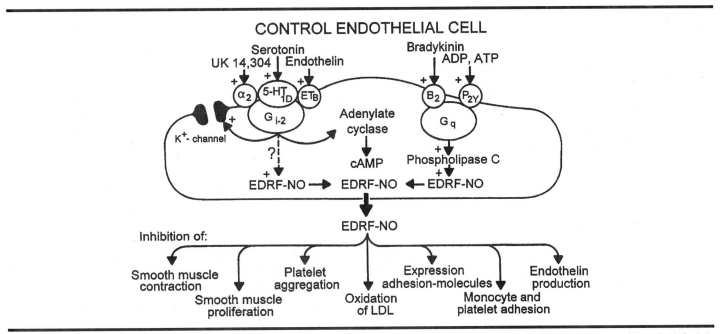

Figure A16.2. Signal transduction processes in endothelial cells. Activation of the cell causes the release of endothelin-derived relaxing factor (EDRF) nitric oxide (NO), which has important protective effects in the vascular wall. α, alpha-adrenergic receptor; 5-HT, serotonin receptor; ADP, adenosine diphosphate; ATP, adenosine triphosphate; B, bradykinin receptor; cAMP, cyclic adenosine monophosphate; ET, endothelin receptor; G, coupling proteins; LDL, low-density lipoproteins; NO, nitric oxide; P, purinoceptor; UK, urokinase. [From PM Vanhoutte. Endothelial dysfunction and atherosclerosis. *Eur Heart J.* 1997;18(suppl E):E19–E29, with permission.]

tion of phosphodiesterase II–mediated breakdown of cyclic adenosine monophosphate, thus leading to potentiation of the inhibitory response to prostacyclin and β-adrenergic agonists; (b) inhibition of renin release and thus of the production of angiotensin II; (c) inhibition of the production of endothelin; and (d) scavenging of superoxide anions and other radicals that promote endothelium-dependent vasoconstriction. These indirect actions all help to explain the vasoconstrictor responses observed *in vivo* with inhibitors of NOS.

Vascular Physiologic Effects

Flow-mediated dilation. The increase in NO release with increasing shear stress underlies flow-dependent vasodilatation in the intact organism and probably is the single most important local regulatory factor modulating the activity of eNOS. The action of catecholamines and vasopressin on endothelial cells in certain vascular beds (e.g., coronary and cerebral circulations) reinforces the preferential distribution of blood flow to those tissues. The release of NO evoked by angiotensin II and endothelin-1 may curtail exaggerated vasoconstriction evoked by these 2 peptides.

Wheal and flare reactions. The stimulation of eNOS by histamine and substance P explains the local vasodilatation and local reddening of the skin during allergic reactions and axon reflexes.

Bradykinin and angiotensin-converting enzyme inhibition. The local production of bradykinin and its effect via B_2-receptors not only sustains the secretion of exocrine glands but also contributes to flow-mediated dilation, which activates the local kinin-generating system in animal and human blood vessels. The potentiation of the effects of endogenously produced bradykinin partly explains the vasodilator and vascular protective effects of angiotensin-converting enzyme inhibitors, particularly in patients with low rennin levels.

Coagulation and vascular occlusion. The endothelial response to thrombin and platelet products is crucial to the protective role played by the normal endothelium against unwanted coagulation. Local platelet aggregation, resulting in the release of serotonin and adenosine diphosphate; local activation of the coagulation cascade; and the production of thrombin cause a massive local NO response, with diffusion of NO toward the underlying smooth muscle. The resulting vasodilatation helps to eliminate "microaggregates," whereas the release of NO toward the lumen, in synergy with prostacyclin, inhibits platelet adhesion and aggregation and eliminates the imminent danger of vascular occlusion.

Other Endothelium-Derived Mediators

In addition to NO, endothelial cells can release other vasodilators: endothelium-derived relaxing factors, prostacyclin, endothelium-derived hyperpolarizing factors, endothelium-derived contracting factors, superoxide anions, endoperoxides, isoprostanes, thromboxane A_2, endothelin-1, and other substances.

Chronic Endothelial Nitric Oxide Synthase Modulation and Disease

The expression of the messenger RNA of eNOS and the activity of the enzyme are upregulated chronically by regular increases in blood flow such as occurs with exercise training, estrogen therapy, and certain components of the diet (e.g., ω_3-unsaturated fatty acid in fish or polyphenols in red wine). The production of NO by the blood vessel wall is reduced with smoking, cholesterol-rich diets, and aging (after menopause in women).

The regenerated endothelial cells that reline the arterial intima after spontaneous desquamation or traumatic disruption (e.g., angioplasty) exhibit a selective loss of their G_i protein–mediated responses (Figure A16.2), which sets the stage for atherosclerosis. Hypertension, diabetes, atherosclerosis, and other chronic disorders associated with increases in oxidative stress are characteristically accompanied by a progressive reduction in endothelium-dependent release of NO. Augmented production of asymmetric dimethylarginine may also contribute to the endothelial dysfunction seen in vascular diseases. Reduced NO release also exacerbates the impact of endothelium-derived contracting factors.

Nonendothelial Nitric Oxide and Inducible Nitric Oxide Synthase Induction

Exposure of vascular smooth muscle cells *in vitro* or *in vivo* to certain inflammatory mediators, including interleukin-1B, tumor necrosis factor-α, endotoxin, or lipopolysaccharide, leads to the induction of another isoform of NO synthase, iNOS (NOS II). The induction of iNOS and the resulting massive production of large amounts of NO explain the vascular paralysis characteristic of septic shock. Whether this paralysis is harmful because of the resulting fall in arterial blood pressure or whether it constitutes a defense mechanism against exaggerated vasoconstriction and tissue damage is still a matter of debate.

Neural Nitric Oxide and Neuronal Nitric Oxide Synthase

Certain blood vessels, particularly in the brain and in corpora cavernosa, are endowed with nitroxidergic nerves containing the third isoform of the enzyme, nNOS (NOS I) that release NO on stimulation. In the brain, nerve-released NO may contribute, together with endothelium-derived NO, to optimal autoregulation, as well as to the prevention of cerebral vasospasm. In the corpora cavernosa, nerve-released NO may contribute to the erectile process.

SUGGESTED READING

1. Ferro CJ, Webb DJ. Endothelial dysfunction and hypertension. *Drugs.* 1997;53(suppl.1):30–41.
2. Furchgott RF, Vanhoutte PM. Endothelium-derived relaxing and contracting factors. *FASEB J.* 1989;3:2007–2017.
3. Ignarro L, Murad F. *Nitric Oxide: Biochemistry, Molecular Biology, and Therapeutic Implications. Advances in Pharmacology.* New York, NY: Academic Press; 1995.
4. Lüscher TF, Vanhoutte PM. *The Endothelium: Modulator of Cardiovascular Function.* Boca Raton, FL: CRC Press; 1990.
5. Moncada S, Palmer RMJ, Higgs EA. Nitric oxide: physiology, pathophysiology and pharmacology. *Pharmacol Rev.* 1991;43:109.
6. Schini-Kerth VB, Vanhoutte PM. Nitric oxide synthases in vascular cells. *Exp Physiol.* 1995;80:885–905.
7. Vane JR. The endothelium: maestro for the blood circulation. *Philos Trans Royal Soc London B Biol Sci.* 1994;343:225–246.
8. Vanhoutte PM. Say NO to ET. *J Auton Nerv Syst.* 2000;81:271–277.
9. Vanhoutte PM. Endothelial dysfunction and vascular disease. In: Panza JA, Cannon RO III, eds. *Endothelium, Nitric Oxide and Atherosclerosis. From Basic Mechanisms to Clinical Implications.* Armonk, NY: Futura Publishing; 1999:79–95.
10. Vanhoutte PM. Endothelial dysfunction in hypertension. *J Hypertens.* 1996;14:S83–S93.

Chapter A17

Acetylcholine, γ-Aminobutyric Acid, Serotonin, Adenosine, and Endogenous Ouabain

Roger J. Grekin, MD; John M. Hamlyn, PhD

KEY POINTS

- Acetylcholine dilates blood vessels via muscarinic receptors in vascular smooth muscle and in the central nervous system, and slows the heart and constricts blood vessels via nicotinic receptors in autonomic ganglia.

- Serotonin vasodilates through central and peripheral 5-hydroxytryptamine$_1$ receptors, and vasoconstricts via 5-hydroxytryptamine$_2$ receptors.

- Adenosine is a direct vasodilator, whereas γ-aminobutyric acid has tonic central depressor effects.

- Endogenous ouabain, a steroidal glycoside of probable adrenocortical origin, inhibits sodium- and potassium-activated adenosine triphosphatase and may increase central sympathetic outflow; plasma ouabain is increased in some patients with essential hypertension.

See also Chapters A27, A33, A34, and C148

ACETYLCHOLINE

Synthesis and Actions

Acetylcholine (ACh), a neurotransmitter with widespread cardiovascular and noncardiovascular actions, is synthesized in nerve terminals. Active uptake of choline is followed by acetylation, with subsequent storage in vesicles. ACh is released into synapses in response to electric stimulation and is rapidly degraded by acetylcholinesterase, an enzyme that is present in large amounts in neural tissue. ACh serves as the primary neurotransmitter for (a) postganglionic parasympathetic neurons; (b) sympathetic and parasympathetic ganglion cells and the adrenal medulla, which is innervated by preganglionic autonomic fibers; (c) motor end-plates in skeletal muscle; and (d) some neurons within the central nervous system.

Muscarinic effects. Postganglionic parasympathetic effects are mediated by muscarinic receptors. Cardiovascular effects mediated by muscarinic receptors include vasodilation and negative chronotropic and inotropic effects. Five functional subtypes of muscarinic receptors have been identified: M_2 receptors mediate the cardiac and coronary artery effects of ACh and M_3 receptors mediate endothelium-dependent vascular responses. M_1 and M_3 receptors also mediate direct smooth muscle vasoconstrictive effects, which are blocked by atropine. The vasodilatory effects of ACh are mediated through endothelial M_3 receptors, which results in endothelial release of nitric oxide. ACh also stimulates release of prostacyclin and endothelium-derived hyperpolarizing factor, which contributes to vasodilation of arterial smooth muscle. To date, there is no evidence that either neurally derived or circulating ACh is a significant regulator of vascular tone *in vivo*, and administration of atropine has minimal effects on systemic vascular resistance. Tonic vagal release of ACh is a predominant regulator of heart rate, particularly in young, healthy individuals;

atropine administration often increases heart rate by 30 to 40 beats per minute.

Nicotinic effects. Autonomic ganglionic neurotransmission is mediated by nicotinic cholinergic receptors. Ganglionic blocking agents result in inhibition of sympathetic and parasympathetic postganglionic neurons. Inhibition of adrenergic tone results in arterial and venous vasodilation with increased flow and decreased venous return. Postural hypotension is a particularly prominent response. Two ganglionic blockers, trimethaphan and mecamylamine, have been used as antihypertensive agents in the past. Because vagal effects usually predominate in the regulation of heart rate, ganglionic blockers commonly cause tachycardia.

Central Effects

Cholinergic neurotransmission in the central nervous system (CNS) has been implicated in the regulation of blood pressure. The most important of sites of action appear to be the rostral ventrolateral medulla (RVLM) (see Chapter A34) and several areas within the hypothalamus. Administration of muscarinic antagonists into the cerebrospinal fluid or directly into the hypothalamus or RVLM decreases blood pressure in most experimental forms of hypertension. Control animals are relatively unresponsive to muscarinic antagonists, suggesting that central cholinergic neurons are not important in normal blood pressure regulation but may play a role in the development of hypertension.

SEROTONIN

Synthesis and Metabolism

Serotonin, or 5-hydroxytryptamine (5-HT) (**Figure A17.1**), is synthesized in a 2-step process involving hydroxylation of tryptophan to 5-hydroxytryptophan followed by decarboxyla-

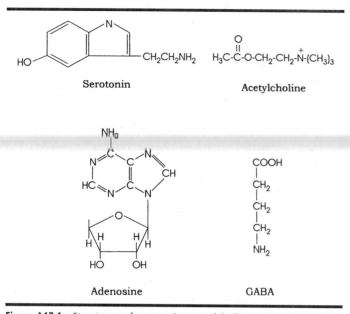

Figure A17.1. Structures of serotonin, acetylcholine, adenosine, and γ-aminobutyric acid (GABA).

tion. Serotonin is present in the enterochromaffin cells of the gastrointestinal tract, in the central and peripheral nervous systems, and in platelets. Within neural cells, serotonin is stored in granular vesicles similar to those of catecholamines. *De novo* synthesis occurs only in the enterochromaffin cells and the nervous system. Serotonin released from enterochromaffin cells is metabolized almost entirely in liver. The remainder of intestinal and neurally derived serotonin is taken up by high-affinity uptake systems in platelets and nerves. As a result, circulating concentrations of serotonin are extremely low.

Cardiovascular Effects

Serotonin may have either vasoconstricting or vasodilating effects, depending on the state of endothelial function and the specific vessel site. Different receptor subtypes mediate the different vasoactive actions of serotonin. Vasodilation is mediated through 5-HT$_{1A}$ receptors within the endothelium. Activation of these receptors results in release of nitric oxide, prostacyclin, and endothelium-derived hyperpolarizing factors. Vasoconstrictive effects are mediated through smooth muscle 5-HT$_2$ receptors. Serotonin-induced vasoconstriction is enhanced in hypertensive states, perhaps partly owing to endothelial damage and loss of vasodilating effects. In deoxycorticosterone acetate–salt hypertension, there is a switch from 5-HT$_{2A}$ to 5-HT$_{2B}$ receptors in vascular smooth muscle that results in marked enhancement of the vasoconstrictor effects of serotonin. Treatment of deoxycorticosterone acetate–salt rats with a 5HT$_{2B}$ receptor antagonist decreases blood pressure in animals with severe hypertension.

Central Effects

Serotonin effects within the CNS are also dimorphic. Central administration of serotonin may increase or decrease blood pressure. Activation of 5HT$_{1A}$ receptors in the RVLM results in a decrease in sympathetic outflow sand blood pressure. Renal sympathetic activity is particularly responsive to stimulation of cen-

tral 5HT$_{1A}$ receptors. Activation of 5HT$_2$ receptors in the RVLM causes increased renal and splanchnic sympathetic activity, vasoconstriction, and an increase in blood pressure. Hypothalamic serotonin levels are increased in spontaneously hypertensive rats during the development of hypertension and central administration of 5,6-dihydroxytryptamine.

ADENOSINE

Synthesis and Metabolism

Adenosine is a nucleotide composed of adenine and d-ribose. When combined with phosphate, energy-storing mono-, di-, and triphosphate forms (AMP, ADP, and ATP) are synthesized. Adenosine itself is distributed throughout all body tissues and is formed by breakdown of adenine nucleotides and by hydrolysis of *S*-adenosylmethionine and *S*-adenosylhomocysteine. Adenosine production is increased during periods of tissue ischemia, and through its powerful local vasodilatory actions, it probably serves to ameliorate the effects of ischemia. Adenosine is rapidly metabolized with a half-life of 1 to 7 seconds. Plasma levels are in the range of 1.5×10^{-7} mol/L in healthy individuals.

Receptors and Actions

Four types of adenosine receptors have been characterized. Cardiac effects are mediated mainly by A$_1$ receptors, which inhibit adenylate cyclase and activate K$^+$ channels. Adenosine suppresses sinus node automaticity and atrioventricular nodal conduction and decreases inotropy. A$_{2A}$ and A$_{2B}$ receptors stimulate adenylate cyclase and cause vasodilation. Adenosine has direct vasodilatory effects in coronary and systemic vascular beds and causes hypotension in anesthetized individuals. Adenosine administration has minor effects on blood pressure in conscious individuals but results in decreased vagal tone and reflex activation of the sympathetic nervous system. Adenosine is commonly used in the treatment of supraventricular tachycardias and as a test agent for coronary artery disease. By inducing coronary vasodilation, it produces a "steal" effect, revealing areas of coronary ischemia.

γ-AMINOBUTYRIC ACID

γ-Aminobutyric acid (GABA) is an inhibitory amino acid neurotransmitter distributed throughout the CNS. Tonic release of GABA by neurons in the posterior hypothalamus and ventral medulla plays a role in blood pressure homeostasis. Administration of GABA$_A$ agonists into these brain regions decreases blood pressure, and GABA$_A$ antagonists increase blood pressure. GABA$_B$ receptors in the anterior hypothalamus mediate increases in blood pressure. Spontaneously hypertensive rats have decreased GABA content and decreased GABA$_A$ receptors in the posterior hypothalamus and demonstrate no response to hypothalamic injection of GABA antagonists, suggesting that these animals may have a deficiency in tonic GABA-ergic input.

ENDOGENOUS OUABAIN

Endogenous "ouabain" (EO) is a mammalian steroidal counterpart to the plant glycoside ouabain (**Figure A17.2**). Pos-

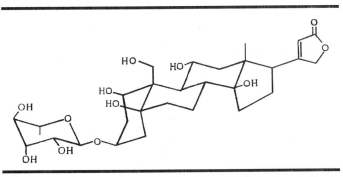

Figure A17.2. Structure of ouabain. The A/B and C/D rings are both *cis*-fused. A 5-member lactone ring is attached at C_{17} in the β-orientation. The deoxy-L-sugar rhamnose is linked to C_3. The steroid nucleus of ouabain is heavily oxygenated (positions 1, 3, 5, 14, and 19). In endogenous ouabain, the position and/or orientation of one or more of the steroidal oxygen atoms may differ.

sible structural differences between the mammalian- and plant-derived compounds are under investigation. Human EO is a high-affinity, reversible, and specific inhibitor of sodium- and potassium-activated adenosine triphosphatase with inotropic and vasopressor activity.

Synthesis

Circulating EO appears to arise from slow secretion by cells in the adrenal zona glomerulosa, which can be stimulated by adrenocorticotropic hormone and angiotensin II. Conserved binding sites with high affinity for EO exist on each of the 4 sodium pump isoforms. In addition, a new ouabain receptor has been described in the adrenal cortex, brain, and kidney. The adrenocortical source, specific receptors, and regulation of EO suggest it is part of a new mammalian hormone system.

Actions

The physiologic role and pathologic significance of EO are linked with the augmentation of cellular responses to stimulation, especially in key neuronal circuits involved in long-term arterial pressure and electrolyte homeostasis. In the rat, sustained plasma levels of ouabain ranging from 1 to 5 nmol/L have a slow pressor effect, leading to sustained hypertension. The severity of the hypertension is dose-dependent, resembles human essential hypertension, and is influenced by genetic factors and renal function. Clinical studies show that ~30% to 45% of whites with essential hypertension and hypertensive individuals with certain adrenocortical tumors have elevated circulating levels of EO that correlate with blood pressure. Elevated plasma EO has also been linked with cardiac cell growth *in vitro* and *in vivo* and may be a factor in the pathogenesis of congestive heart failure. These and related observations suggest that EO exerts multiple, significant, and chronic effects on cardiovascular function.

SUGGESTED READING

1. Walch L, Brink C, Norel X. The muscarinic receptor subtypes in human blood vessels. *Therapie.* 2001;56:223–226.
2. Ckuba T. Cholinergic mechanism and blood pressure regulation in the central nervous system. *Brain Res Bull.* 1998;46:475–481.
3. DeWardner HE. The hypothalamus and hypertension. *Physiol Rev.* 2001;71:1599–1658.
4. Chalmers J, Arnolda L, Llewellyn-Smith I, et al. Central neurons and neurotransmitters in the control of blood pressure. *Clin Exp Pharmacol Physiol.* 1994;21:819–829.
5. Hindle AT. Recent developments in the physiology and pharmacology of 5-hydroxytryptamine. *Br J Anaesth.* 1994;73:395–407.
6. Ramage AG. Central cardiovascular regulation and 5-hydroxytryptamine receptors. *Brain Res Bull.* 2001;56:425–439.
7. Pelleg A, Porter RS. The pharmacology of adenosine. *Pharmacotherapy.* 1990;10:157–174.
8. Blaustein MP. The physiological effects of endogenous ouabain: control of cell responsiveness. *Am J Physiol.* 1993;264:C1367–C1387.
9. Schoner W. Endogenous cardiotonic steroids. *Cell Mol Biol. (Noisy-le-grand.)* 2001;47(2):273–280.

Chapter A18

Adrenomedullin-Derived Peptides and Calcitonin Gene–Related Peptide

Meghan M. Taylor, PhD; Willis K. Samson, PhD

KEY POINTS

- Adrenomedullin exerts potent hypotensive actions via increased vascular nitric oxide production and via direct diuretic and natriuretic actions on the kidney; adrenomedullin and proadrenomedullin N-20 terminal peptide also inhibit aldosterone secretion.

- Proadrenomedullin N-20 terminal peptide is derived from the same prohormone as adrenomedullin, and it exerts its vasodilatory effects via presynaptic inhibition of vascular sympathetic terminals.

- Calcitonin gene–related peptide shares structural homology with adrenomedullin and exerts many similar actions, especially vasodilation; calcitonin gene–related peptide may be the major transmitter in vasodilatory nerves innervating resistance vessels.

- Adrenomedullin and calcitonin gene–related peptide receptors share a common receptor moiety, but specificity is directed by the type of associated receptor activity modifying protein: receptor activity modifying protein-1 for calcitonin gene–related peptide specificity, receptor activity modifying protein-2 for adrenomedullin specificity.

See also Chapters A10, A16, A28, A29, and A33

ADRENOMEDULLIN AND N-20 TERMINAL PEPTIDE (PROADRENOMEDULLIN N-20 TERMINAL PEPTIDE)

Synthesis and Cellular Effects

The 52–amino acid adrenomedullin (AM) and the 20–amino acid proadrenomedullin N-20 terminal peptide (PAMP) are products of the same gene and are produced by posttranslational processing of a larger preprohormone. The AM gene is expressed primarily in the vasculature and also in brain and kidney. Adrenomedullin exerts its potent hypotensive action via activation of nitric oxide synthase in endothelial cells. PAMP, on the other hand, does not activate nitric oxide synthase but activates potassium channels and exerts presynaptic inhibition of sympathetic nerves innervating blood vessels. Thus, the AM gene encodes at least 2 peptides with shared biologic activity but unique mechanisms of action.

Adrenomedullin and Calcitonin Gene–Related Peptide Receptors

AM is structurally similar to calcitonin gene–related peptide (CGRP), but exerts its effects via at least 1 unique G protein–linked AM receptor that activates adenylate cyclase and phospholipase C. The AM receptor has been identified as having 2 parts: the calcitonin receptor–like receptor (CRLR) and the associated receptor activity modifying protein-2. CGRP also binds CRLR, but only when the CRLR receptor is associated with receptor activity modifying protein-1. CGRP cannot bind to the AM receptor, and many of the actions of AM are not reproduced by CGRP. Two additional putative AM receptors have been identified, RDC1 and L1. The receptor for PAMP has not yet been identified.

Adrenomedullin Physiology

Potentially important extravascular actions of 1 or both peptides (AM or PAMP) have been reported (**Figure A18.1**). AM acts in a variety of sites to compensate for increased plasma volume by decreasing venous return, increasing urine volume, decreasing aldosterone, and decreasing fluid and salt intake. The venodilatory or "volume-unloading" effects of AM may be balanced by its sympathostimulatory and positive inotropic cardiac actions, which act to maintain adequate cardiac output. AM also has been demonstrated to exert antimitogenic effects in vascular tissue and kidney; however, these actions of AM remain controversial as they have not yet been demonstrated in a physiologic setting. Furthermore, AM has been demonstrated to be promitogenic in cancer tissue. Of all its effects, only the role of AM in salt appetite and thirst has been demonstrated to be unequivocally physiologically relevant.

Central nervous system and adrenal effects. AM and PAMP have been shown to act within the brain to stimulate sympathetic function. PAMP can inhibit nicotine-stimulated catecholamine release. In the pituitary gland, AM and PAMP inhibit adrenocorticotropin secretion. AM can inhibit water drinking and salt appetite by direct effects on the brain. The ability of AM to increase cerebral blood flow may protect against cerebral hypoperfusion. In the adrenal gland, AM and PAMP inhibit angiotensin II and potassium-stimulated aldosterone secretion, with PAMP being more potent.

Cardiac effects. Recently, direct positive inotropic and chronotropic effects of AM have been demonstrated.

Vascular effects. Shear stress elevates vascular production of AM, as do proinflammatory cytokines (e.g., tumor necrosis

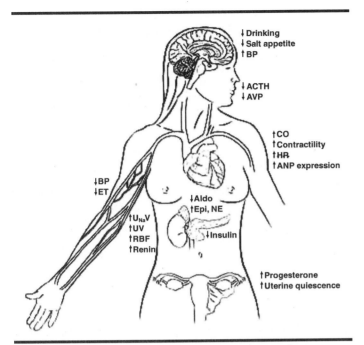

Figure A18.1. Pharmacologic actions of adrenomedullin. ↓, decreased; ↑, increased; ACTH, adrenocorticotropin; Aldo, aldosterone; ANP, atrial natriuretic peptide; AVP, arginine vasopressin; BP, blood pressure; CO, cardiac output; Epi, epinephrine; ET, endothelin; HR, heart rate; NE, norepinephrine; RBF, renal blood flow; $U_{Na}V$, urinary sodium excretion; UV, urine volume. (Reproduced from Jougasaki M, Burnett JC Jr. Adrenomedullin: potential in physiology and pathophysiology. *Life Sci.* 2000;66:855–872.)

factor, interleukin-1), leading to the hypothesis that the hypotension of sepsis is owing, at least in part, to excessive AM in the vasculature. (Excessive nitric oxide production via inducible nitric oxide synthase also occurs in sepsis; see Chapter A16.) Plasma AM levels not only correlate with the hypotension of sepsis but also predict survival rate.

Renal effects. AM increases renal blood flow even in the face of reductions in arterial pressure, has tubular effects to stimulate sodium excretion and prevent water reabsorption, and can directly stimulate renin secretion. Tubular effects of AM probably reflect physiologic actions of peptide produced within the kidney and AM that is not circulating. Renal effects of PAMP have not been reported. AM's ability to maintain renal blood flow even in the face of severe hypotension is thought to protect against cardiovascular collapse and renal failure.

Genetic Studies

Recently, 3 independent groups have attempted embryonic compromise of AM production. Unfortunately, the knock-out is embryonically lethal, with hypoxia caused by a ring of constriction in the umbilical vein. Heterozygotes can survive with half the normal levels of circulating AM, but heterozygotes are hypertensive and less able to heal after vascular injury. A surprising finding has been that the heterozygotes become obese as they age and develop type 2 diabetes mellitus.

Human Studies

Kinetics and dynamics. Adrenomedullin circulates in low (pg/mL) levels in normal humans. The presence of an AM binding protein has been demonstrated in human plasma and has been identified as *complement factor H*. The metabolic clearance rate of AM is 27.4 mL/kg per minute. In humans, AM has a plasma half-life of 22 minutes and a volume of distribution of approximately 900 mL/kg. Infusion of low doses of AM (2 and 8 ng/kg per minute) into healthy volunteers results in significant reductions in mean arterial pressure with no activation of the sympathetic nervous system, alteration in renin secretion, or change in renal function. Thus, the vascular actions of AM may have a lower threshold than do the extravascular effects.

Adrenomedullin in human diseases. Elevations of circulating AM levels have been reported in hypertension complicated by renal failure, heart failure, liver disease with ascites, acute asthma, and septic shock. High circulating AM levels may be caused by the disease state itself or by compensatory mechanisms activated by the disease.

CALCITONIN GENE–RELATED PEPTIDE

CGRP is an alternative product of calcitonin gene expression. Similar to AM, CGRP is a potent hypotensive agent whose receptor specificity is dependent on a specific receptor activity-modifying protein 1.

Distribution and Actions

There appear to be reciprocal inhibitory effects of CGRP and norepinephrine in the peripheral vascular beds. CGRP is found predominantly in peripheral and central nervous system neurons, often colocalized with acetylcholine. It is now believed that CGRP is the primary active neurotransmitter in nonadrenergic noncholinergic vasodilatory neurons innervating resistance vessels in the mesentery circulation. CGRP exerts positive inotropic effects on the heart via a calcium-dependent effect.

Calcitonin Gene–Related Peptide in Hypertension

CGRP knockout mice are hypertensive, suggesting a role for the peptide in the long-term regulation of peripheral resistance and blood pressure. Also, there appears to be a deficiency in CGRP release in spontaneously hypertensive animal models (i.e., spontaneously hypertensive rat). This deficiency may owe to the inhibitory effect of angiotensin II on the nonadrenergic noncholinergic neurons because angiotensin-converting enzyme inhibitors enhance CGRP release in the spontaneously hypertensive rat in response to perivascular nerve stimulation.

Other Clinical Conditions

Central and peripheral levels of CGRP are elevated in a variety of pathologic states, and there are potential therapeutic uses of CGRP in migraine and Raynaud's phenomenon.

SUGGESTED READING

1. Hinson JP, Kapas S, Smith DM. Adrenomedullin, a multifunctional regulatory peptide. *Endocr Rev.* 2000;21:138–167.

2. Jougasaki M, Burnett JC Jr. Adrenomedullin: potential in physiology and pathophysiology. *Life Sci.* 2000;66:855–872.
3. Kawasaki H. Regulation of vascular function by perivascular calcitonin gene–related peptide-containing nerves. *Jpn J Pharmacol.* 2002;8:39–43.
4. Lainchbury JG, Troughton RW, Lewis LK, et al. Hemodynamic, hormonal, and renal effects of short-term adrenomedullin infusion in healthy volunteers. *J Clin Endocrinol Metab.* 2000;85:1016–1020.
5. Nakamura M, Yoshida H, Makita S, et al. Potent and long-lasting vasodilatory effects of adrenomedullin in humans: comparisons between normal subjects and patients with chronic heart failure. *Circulation.* 1997;95:1214–1221.
6. Sextin PM, Albiston A, Morfis M, Tilakaratne N. Receptor activity modifying proteins. *Cell Signal.* 2001;13:73–83.
7. Taylor MM, Shimosawa T, Samson WK. Endocrine and metabolic actions of adrenomedullin. *Endocrinologist.* 2001;11:171–177.

Chapter A19

Reactive Oxygen Species and Mediators of Oxidative Stress

Rhian M. Touyz, MD, PhD

KEY POINTS

- The major reactive oxygen species in cardiovascular biology are superoxide, hydroxyl, hydrogen peroxide, nitric oxide, and peroxynitrite.

- Many enzyme systems generate superoxide in the vasculature, but nonphagocytic nicotinamide adenine dinucleotide phosphate oxidase is the most important; nicotinamide adenine dinucleotide phosphate oxidase enzyme is regulated by growth factors, cytokines, physical forces, and vasoactive agents.

- Superoxide and hydrogen peroxide are signal transduction intermediates that activate signaling cascades and reduction-oxidation–sensitive transcription factors important in regulating vascular smooth muscle cell growth, endothelial function, inflammatory responses, and extracellular matrix deposition.

- Oxidative stress, a consequence of an increase in formation of reactive oxygen species or a decrease in antioxidant reserve, contributes to hypertensive vascular damage.

See also Chapters A3, A16, A33, A65–A67, and C154

Metabolism of Biologically Important Reactive Oxygen Species

Reactive oxygen species (ROS), also termed *oxygen-derived species* or *oxidants*, are produced as intermediates in reduction-oxidation (redox) reactions leading from O_2 to H_2O. ROS are reactive chemical entities comprising 2 major groups: free radicals [e.g., superoxide ($\cdot O_2^-$), hydroxyl (OH·), nitric oxide (NO·)], and nonradical derivatives of O_2 (e.g., H_2O_2, ONOO$^-$) **(Table A19.1)**. A free radical is any species capable of independent existence (thus the term *free*) that contains 1 or more unpaired electron. The unpaired electron imparts high reactivity and renders the radical unstable. Nonradical derivatives are less reactive and more stable with a longer half-life than free radicals. When oxygen accepts electrons to its orbitals, it is "reduced" and functions as a strong oxidizing agent. The sequential univalent reduction of O_2 is

$$O_2 \xrightarrow{e^-} \cdot O_2^- \xrightarrow{e^-} H_2O_2 \xrightarrow{e^-} OH \cdot \xrightarrow{e^-} H_2O + O_2$$

Superoxide radical. Superoxide is produced by the 1-electron reduction of O_2 by enzymatic catalysis or by electron leaks from electron transfer reactions: $O_2 \rightarrow \cdot O_2^-$. In biologic fluids, $\cdot O_2^-$ is short-lived owing to its rapid reduction to H_2O_2 by superoxide dismutase (SOD). Superoxide can act as an oxidizing agent, in which it is reduced to H_2O_2, or as a reducing agent, in which it donates its extra electron to NO· to form ONOO$^-$. Nitric oxide reacts with $\cdot O_2^-$ at near diffusion-limited rates and is therefore one of the few biomolecules able to "outcompete" SOD for $\cdot O_2^-$. Hence, in most biologic systems, unless NO· levels are very high, production of $\cdot O_2^-$ usually results in H_2O_2 formation.

Hydrogen peroxide. Of the many ROS generated in vascular cells, H_2O_2 seems to be particularly important because it is relatively stable and uncharged. Hydrogen peroxide is lipid soluble, easily diffusible within and between cells, and is stable under physiologic conditions. H_2O_2 is only a weak oxidizing and reducing agent and is generally poorly reactive. In the presence of myeloperoxidase and chloride ion, H_2O_2 forms hypochlorous acid, followed by the formation of other nonradical oxidants, such as singlet oxygen ($^1O_2$). Hypochlorous acid is highly reactive and able to damage biomolecules, both directly and by decomposing to form chlorine. H_2O_2 is also a precursor of OH·. The main source of H_2O_2 in vascular tissue is the dismutation of $\cdot O_2^-$: $2 \cdot O_2^- + 2H^+ \rightarrow H_2O_2 + O_2$. This reaction can be spontaneous or it can be catalyzed by SOD. The SOD-catalyzed dismutation is favored when the concentra-

Table A19.1. Biologically Important Reactive Oxygen Species

Free radicals (species with an unpaired electron)

$\cdot O_2^-$	Superoxide anion radical
$OH\cdot$	Hydroxyl radical
$ROO\cdot$	Lipid peroxide
$RO_2\cdot$	Peroxyl
$NO\cdot$	Nitric oxide

Nonradicals

H_2O_2	Hydrogen peroxide
$HOCl$	Hypochlorous acid
$ONOO^-$	Peroxynitrite
O_3	Ozone
$^1O_2$	Singlet oxygen

tion of $\cdot O_2^-$ is low and when the concentration of SOD is high, which occurs normally. Three mammalian SOD isoforms are known: copper/zinc SOD (SOD1), mitochondrial SOD (Mn SOD, SOD2), and extracellular SOD (SOD3).

Hydroxyl radical. Hydroxyl radical is generated by 2 major reactions from H_2O_2: the Fenton reaction, in which H_2O_2 decomposes by accepting an electron from a reduced metal ($Fe^{2+} + H_2O_2 \rightarrow Fe^{3+} + OH\cdot + OH^-$), and the Haber-Weiss reaction, in which $OH\cdot$ is generated by the interaction of $\cdot O_2^-$ and H_2O_2 ($\cdot O_2^- + H_2O_2 \rightarrow O_2 + H_2O + OH\cdot$). Hydroxyl radical is highly reactive, and unlike $\cdot O_2^-$ and H_2O_2, which travel some distance from their site of generation, $OH\cdot$ induces local damage where it is formed.

Peroxynitrite. Peroxynitrite is a potent oxidant formed from the reaction between $\cdot O_2^-$ and $NO\cdot$ in a 1:1 stoichiometry: $NO\cdot + \cdot O_2^- \rightarrow ONOO^-$. A major regulator of $ONOO^-$ formation is the concentration of $NO\cdot$. When the level of $NO\cdot$ increases and overcomes dismutation by SOD (e.g., during ischemia, reperfusion, or both), $ONOO^-$ is produced. This reaction is biologically significant because $NO\cdot$ and $\cdot O_2^-$ can antagonize each other's biologic actions and because $ONOO^-$ is a powerful oxidizing species. The toxic effect of $ONOO^-$ and its protonated form, peroxynitrous acid, derives from its oxidation of zinc fingers, protein thiols, and membrane lipids. Intermediates are formed from the heterolytic cleavage of $ONOO^-$ to $OH\cdot$ and nitronium ion (NO_2^+), catalyzed by the transition metal of SOD and myeloperoxidase. Nitration of protein tyrosine residues produces 3-nitrotyrosine, which is often used as an assay for $ONOO^-$ in tissue and blood.

Vascular Reactive Oxygen Species Generation and Nicotinamide Adenine Dinucleotide Phosphate Activity

General features. Superoxide anion, H_2O_2, $OH\cdot$, and $ONOO^-$ are all produced to varying degrees in the vasculature. These oxygen derivatives, which are tightly regulated under physiologic conditions, act as second messengers to control vascular function and structure. In the vessel wall, virtually all types of cells produce $\cdot O_2^-$ and H_2O_2. Cellular production of ROS occurs via enzymatic and nonenzymatic processes (**Figure A19.1**). In addition to mitochondrial sources of ROS, $\cdot O_2^-$ is generated by xanthine

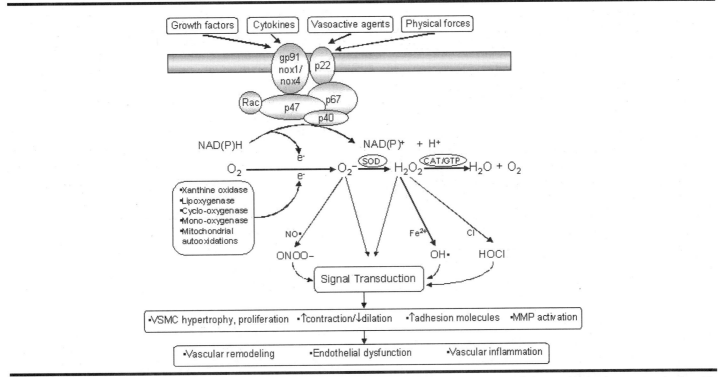

Figure A19.1. Generation of reactive oxygen species in vascular cells. The major source of $\cdot O_2^-$ in vascular cells is a multisubunit enzyme, nicotinamide adenine dinucleotide phosphate (NADPH) oxidase. Other enzymes also contribute to $\cdot O_2^-$ formation in vascular tissue, but their role is minor. $\cdot O_2^-$ is dismutated by superoxide dismutase (SOD) to form H_2O_2, which is converted by catalase (CAT) or glutathione peroxidase (GTP) to H_2O. Reactive oxygen species activate many signaling pathways, which regulate vascular function. Increased production of reactive oxygen species leads to increased vascular smooth muscle cell (VSMC) growth, altered vasomotor tone, and inflammatory responses, which contribute to vascular remodeling and endothelial dysfunction, characteristic features of hypertensive vascular damage. ↓, decreased; ↑, increased; MMP, matrix metalloproteinase.

oxidase, cyclooxygenase, lipoxygenase, nitric oxide synthase, heme oxygenases, hemoproteins (heme and hematin), peroxidases, and nicotinamide adenine dinucleotide phosphate (NADPH) oxidase.

Nicotinamide adenine dinucleotide phosphate activity.

Nonphagocytic NADPH oxidase, the primary physiologic enzymatic source of ROS in vascular tissue, is a multisubunit enzyme that catalyzes $\cdot O_2^-$ production by the 1-electron reduction of O_2 using NADPH as the electron donor. $2O_2 + NADPH \rightarrow 2O_2^- + NADP^+ + H^+$. The prototypical NADPH oxidase is that found in neutrophils and has 5 subunits: p40phox ("phox" stands for *pha*gocyte *ox*idase), p47phox, p67phox, p22phox, and gp91phox (Figure A19.1). In unstimulated cells, p40phox, p47phox, and p67phox exist in the cytosol, whereas p22phox and gp91phox are in the membrane, where they occur as a heterodimeric flavoprotein, cytochrome b558. On stimulation, p47phox becomes phosphorylated, and the cytosolic subunits form a complex that translocates to the membrane, where it associates with cytochrome b558 to assemble the active oxidase, which transfers electrons from the substrate to O_2 forming $\cdot O_2^-$. Activation also requires participation of Rac 2 (or Rac 1) and Rap 1A. In fibroblasts and endothelial cells, all phox subunits have been detected, whereas in vascular smooth muscle cells (VSMCs) only p22phox and p47phox have been definitively demonstrated in animal models. Whether a similar situation exists in human VSMCs awaits clarification. Because gp91phox is essential for NADPH oxidase activity, the possibility exists that there are gp91phox isoforms that are active in VSMCs. Homologues of gp91phox, nox-1 (for *no*n-phagocytic *ox*idase), and nox-4 have recently been cloned from rat aortic smooth muscle cells, and appear to be important in $\cdot O_2^-$ production in these cells.

Control of nicotinamide adenine dinucleotide phosphate activity.

How the NADPH subunits interact in vascular cells and how they generate $\cdot O_2^-$ is not fully known, but vascular NADPH oxidase is responsive to several growth factors (platelet-derived growth factor, epidermal growth factor, and transforming growth factor β), cytokines (tumor necrosis factor-α, interleukin-1, and platelet aggregation factor), mechanical forces (cyclic stretch, laminar and oscillatory shear stress) and vasoactive agents [serotonin, thrombin, bradykinin, endothelin, and angiotensin II (Ang II)]. Ang II is a major regulator of vascular NADPH oxidase. It activates NADPH oxidase via AT_1 receptors through stimulation of signaling pathways involving Src p21^{Ras}, PLD, and PLA$_2$. Ang II also influences gene expression of some NADPH oxidase subunits.

Antioxidant Defenses

Antioxidants are defined as substances that, when present at low concentrations relative to an oxidizable substrate, significantly delay or prevent oxidation of that substrate. Living organisms have evolved a number of antioxidant defenses to maintain their survival against oxidative stress (**Table A19.2**). These mechanisms are different in the intracellular and extracellular compartments and comprise enzymatic and nonenzymatic types.

Cellular mechanisms.

The major intracellular enzymatic antioxidants are SOD, catalase, and glutathione peroxidase. SOD catalyzes the dismutation of $\cdot O_2^-$ into H_2O_2 and O_2. H_2O_2 is destroyed

Table A19.2. Antioxidant Defense Mechanisms

Enzymatic defense enzymes	
Superoxide dismutase (SOD)	$2 \cdot O_2^- + 2H^+ \xrightarrow{SOD} H_2O_2 + O_2\cdot$
Catalase (CAT)	$2H_2O_2 \xrightarrow{CAT} O_2 + H_2O$
Glutathione peroxidase (GTP)	$2GSH + H_2O_2 \xrightarrow{GTP} GSSG + 2H_2O$
	$2GSH + ROOH \xrightarrow{GTP} GSSG + ROH + 2H_2O$
Nonenzymatic scavengers	
Vitamins—A, β-carotene, C (ascorbic acid), E (α-tocopherol)	
Transferrin, lactoferrin	
Ceruloplasmin	
Urate	
Bilirubin	
Albumin	
Cysteine	
Flavonoids	
Sulfhydryl group	

GSH, reduced glutathione; GSSG, oxidized glutathione; R, lipid chain.

by catalase and glutathione peroxidase to form H_2O and O_2. Catalase is important when H_2O_2 concentration is high. Glutathione peroxidase uses reduced glutathione to convert H_2O_2 to H_2O, and, in the process, glutathione is oxidized. This enzyme is important when H_2O_2 concentration is low. Glutathione peroxidase is the major enzyme protecting the cell membrane against lipid peroxidation, because reduced glutathione donates protons to the membrane lipids, maintaining them in a reduced state. Because of its extremely high reactivity, there are no specific scavengers of $OH\cdot$. However, numerous nonspecific antioxidants, such as α-tocopherol (vitamin E) and ascorbic acid (vitamin C), scavenge $OH\cdot$ as well as other radicals. Low antioxidant bioavailability promotes cellular oxidative stress.

Clinical studies.

Considerable attention has been paid to the potential clinical value of antioxidant scavengers. Clinical trials to date, however, are extremely disappointing. Vitamin E has been shown to be ineffective in reducing the incidence of ischemic cardiac events. Recent work suggests that the poor response to scavengers may be related to the low doses of scavengers that deliver insufficient amounts of active compound to the sites where they are needed at the appropriate moment (see Chapter A62).

SUGGESTED READING

1. Babior BM. NADPH oxidase: an update. *Blood.* 1999;93(5):1464–1476.
2. Berk BC. Redox signals that regulate the vascular response to injury. *Thromb Haemost.* 1999;82(2):810–817.
3. Droge W. Free radicals in the physiological control of cell function. *Physiol Rev.* 2001;82:47–95.
4. Fridovich I. Superoxide anion radical, superoxide dismutases, and related matters. *J Biol Chem.* 1997;272:18515–18517.
5. Griendling KK, Sorescu D, Lassegue B, Ushio-Fukai M. Modulation of protein kinase activity and gene expression by reactive oxygen species and their role in vascular physiology and pathophysiology. *Arterioscler Thromb Vasc Biol.* 2000;20:2175–2183.
6. Halliwell B, Gutteridge JMC. *Free Radicals in Biology and Medicine.* 3rd ed. New York, NY: Oxford University Press; 2000.
7. McIntyre M, Bohr DF, Dominiczak AF. Endothelial function in hypertension. The role of superoxide anion. *Hypertension.* 1999;34:539–545.
8. Thannickal VJ, Fanburg BL. Reactive oxygen species in cell signaling. *Am J Physiol.* 2000;279:L1005–L1028.
9. Touyz RM. Oxidative stress and vascular damage in hypertension. *Curr Hypertens Rep.* 2000;2:98–105.

Prostaglandins and P450 Metabolites

Alberto Nasjletti, MD; John C. McGiff, MD

KEY POINTS

- Prostaglandins and other eicosanoids are produced from arachidonic acid by the action of tissue cyclooxygenases, cytochromes, and lipoxygenases.

- Prostacyclin (prostaglandin I_2) and prostaglandin E_2 are vasodilators that counteract the pressor effects of norepinephrine and angiotensin II and stimulate diuresis and natriuresis.

- Thromboxane A_2, prostaglandin H_2, and prostaglandin F_2 are vasoconstrictors that blunt renal salt excretion.

- 20-Hydroxyeicosatetraenoic produced by cytochrome P450 4A enzymes has vasoconstrictor activity and exhibits complex effects on salt and water excretion.

See also Chapters A3, A14, A21, A24, A33, A35, A37, and C150

Arachidonic acid (AA) is liberated from tissue phospholipids by hormone-regulated phospholipases (**Figure A20.1**). Once free, AA is processed by cyclooxygenases (COXs), cytochrome (CYP) P450 oxygenases, or lipoxygenases to form an abundance of eicosanoids capable of affecting vascular and renal functions.

CYCLOOXYGENASE-DERIVED EICOSANOIDS

Synthesis

The constitutive form of cyclooxygenase, COX-1, is expressed in most tissues, including blood vessels, kidney, and platelets. The inducible form, COX-2, is usually undetectable but can be expressed in response to cytokines and growth factors. COXs catalyze the metabolism of AA to the endoperoxide prostaglandin H_2 (PGH_2), which subsequently is converted to thromboxane A_2 (TxA_2) by thromboxane synthase, to prostaglandin I_2 (PGI_2, or prostacyclin) by prostacyclin synthase, or to prostaglandins E_2 (PGE_2), D_2, or $F_2\alpha$ by specific isomerases (Figure A20.1).

Vasodilator Prostaglandins

The prostaglandins PGE_2 and PGI_2 dilate resistance blood vessels, reduce release of norepinephrine from sympathetic nerves, attenuate the vasoconstrictor responses to angiotensin II and other constrictor hormones, and facilitate renal excretion of salt and water.

The vasodilatory action of PGE_2 is linked to activation of EP_2 and EP_4 receptors. Mice lacking EP_2 receptors develop hypertension when placed on a high salt diet, implying that the actions of PGE_2 on this receptor serve an antihypertensive function. Inhibition of COX augments vascular resistance, increases vascular responsiveness to angiotensin II and other constrictor hormones, increases antidiuretic responsiveness to vasopressin, and blunts the pressure-natriuresis response.

Collectively, these observations support the concept that PGE_2 and PGI_2 serve as counterregulatory influences to pressor mechanisms mediated by the renin-angiotensin system, the sympathetic nervous system, and vasopressin. Conversely, PGE_2 and PGI_2 stimulate renin secretion, and COX inhibitors reduce plasma renin activity.

Vasoconstrictor Eicosanoids

TxA_2 and its immediate precursor, PGH_2, stimulate contraction of vascular smooth muscle directly via activation of shared receptors and indirectly by enhancing sympathetic nervous activity. In the kidney, activation of TxA_2/PGH_2 receptors produces renal vasoconstriction and salt and water retention. PGH_2 may mediate endothelium-dependent vasoconstriction.

Long-term systemic infusion of a synthetic agonist for TxA_2/PGH_2 receptors produces sustained elevation of blood pressure (BP), part of which is attributable to activation of central pressor mechanisms. Treatment with inhibitors of thromboxane synthase lowers BP in high renin models of experimental hypertension in rats.

Blood Pressure Responses to Cyclooxygenase Inhibition

BP can increase, decrease, or remain unaffected during treatment with COX inhibitors. This variability in BP response is not unexpected, because COX-derived eicosanoids subserve vasodilatory and vasoconstrictive functions. In general, COX inhibitors have little effect on BP in normal subjects but are likely to increase BP in patients with salt-sensitive hypertension. On the other hand, COX inhibitors can decrease BP in normotensive and hypertensive conditions in which the renin-angiotensin system is stimulated, presumably by disrupting prostanoid-mediated renin secretion and vasoconstrictor mechanisms. The net BP response to inhibition of COX thus seems to reflect the sum of alterations in BP regulatory mechanisms having a prostaglandin component.

CYTOCHROME P450–DERIVED EICOSANOIDS

The wide distribution of the CYP monooxygenases in the vasculature and transporting epithelia and the diverse circulatory and renal effects of CYP-derived AA products suggest their possible participation in BP regulation.

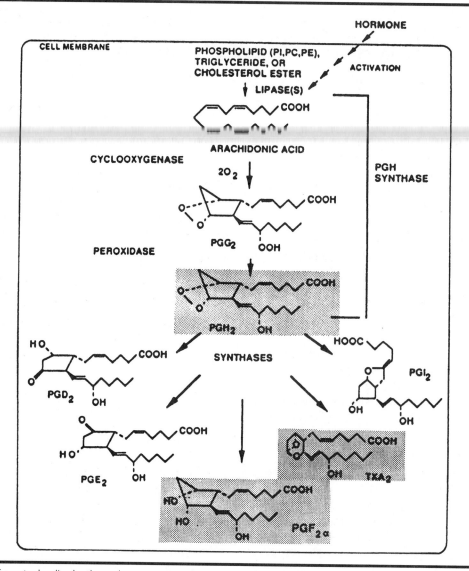

Figure A20.1. Formation of prostaglandins by the cyclooxygenase pathway. Shading indicates prostanoids that are prohypertensive. PGD$_2$, prostaglandin D$_2$; PGE$_2$, prostaglandin E; PGF$_{2\alpha}$, prostaglandin F$_{2\alpha}$; PGG$_2$, prostaglandin G$_2$; PGH$_2$, prostaglandin H$_2$; PGI$_2$, prostaglandin I$_2$; TXA$_2$, thromboxane A$_2$. (Reproduced from Smith WL. Prostanoid biosynthesis and mechanisms of action. *Am J Physiol.* 1992;263:F181–F191, with permission.)

Synthesis

CYP catalyzes transformation of AA by 3 types of oxidative reactions.

Epoxidation. Epoxidation of AA forms 4 epoxyeicosatrienoic acids (EETs) (**Figure A20.2**), characterized by the position of the epoxide oxygen (5,6-, 8,9-, 11,12-, or 14,15-EET), which are readily degraded by epoxide hydrolases (Figure A20.2). The 5,6- and 11,12-EETs are the most important, having the greatest vascular smooth muscle relaxing activity. The 5,6-EET can be further metabolized by COX to a bioactive product (Figure A20.2). Endothelial cells manufacture EETs, which stimulate calcium-activated potassium channels in vascular smooth muscle, producing hyperpolarization and vasodilation. Endothelium-derived EETs mediate the nitric oxide–independent action of bradykinin and other vasodilators and attenuate the vasoconstrictor action of angiotensin II.

Dietary salt loading upregulates EET production in the kidney. EETs subserve antihypertensive functions, because inhibitors of EET synthesis increase BP and vasoconstrictor responsiveness to pressor hormones. Interference with the degradation of EETs lowers BP and vasoconstrictor responsiveness.

Allylic oxidation. Allylic oxidation of AA forms hydroxyeicosatetraenoic acids (HETEs), one of which, 12(R)-HETE, is a potent inhibitor of sodium- and potassium-activated adenosine triphosphatase and exists in high levels in the vasculature in response to ischemic insults.

Hydroxylation. ω-Hydroxylation of AA by CYP oxygenases of the 4A family yields 20-HETE (Figure A20.2), which exhibits several properties that may affect BP. For example, 20-HETE inhibits the activity of calcium-activated potassium channels in vascular smooth muscle, which promotes accumulation of calcium in the cytosol, and leads to vasoconstriction. This action of 20-HETE is central to its ability to sensitize the vasculature to vasoconstrictor hormones and other constrictor stimuli.

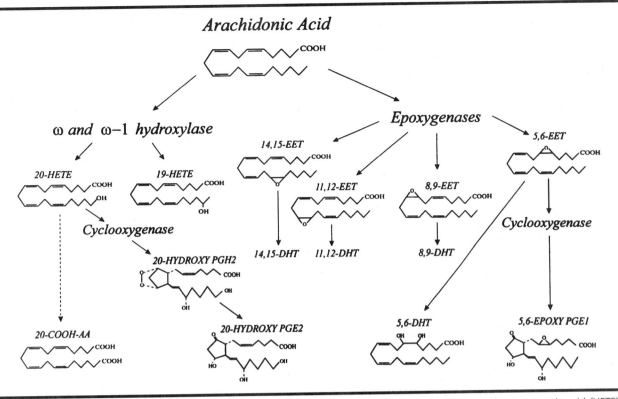

Figure A20.2. Pathways of arachidonic acid (AA) metabolism catalyzed by cytochrome P450 enzymes. 20-Hydroxyeicosatetraenoic acid (HETE) and 5,6-epoxyeicosatrienoic acid (EET) can be metabolized via cyclooxygenase to 5,6-EET and 20-COOH-AA prostaglandin analogs as shown. DHT, dihydroxyeicosatrienoic acid; PGH2, prostaglandin H_2; PGE1, prostaglandin E_1; PGE2, prostaglandin E_2.

20-Hydroxyeicosatetraenoic Acid

Regulation and effects. 20-HETE contributes to the mechanisms underlying preglomerular renal vasoconstriction in response to elevation of renal perfusion pressure and activation of the tubuloglomerular feedback mechanism. 20-HETE also inhibits sodium reabsorption in the proximal tubule and in the medullary thick ascending limb of the loop (mTAL) of Henle, which are actions attributable to inhibition of sodium- and potassium-activated adenosine triphosphatase and of the Na^+-K^+-$2Cl^-$ cotransporter, respectively. Accordingly, 20-HETE produced by arterial vessels may mediate prohypertensive functions by fostering vasoconstriction at renal and extrarenal sites. Conversely, 20-HETE produced by renal tubular structures may mediate antihypertensive functions by promoting sodium excretion. Another product of AA metabolism by CYP, 19-HETE, also may contribute to BP regulation, as it was shown to antagonize the vascular actions of 20-HETE.

Cytochrome P450 isoform regulation. The multiplicity of CYPs metabolizing AA is complicated further by the diversity of mechanisms by which the isoforms are regulated. The rat renal CYP 4A isoforms (4A1, 2, 3, and 8), which generate 20-HETE, may act in antihypertensive or prohypertensive mechanisms, based on differential distribution of the 4A isoforms among tubular segments and vasculature of the kidney. 20-HETE constricts preglomerular arterioles and also modulates ion movement in the mTAL, each site presumably served by a different ω-hydroxylase isoform that is subject to different regulatory factors.

Renal effects. Increased Cl^- transport in the mTAL is critical to BP elevation in the Dahl salt-sensitive rat and is attributable to deficient production of 20-HETE, which reduces the activity of the Na^+-K^+-$2Cl^-$ cotransporter responsible for Cl^- reabsorption. In agreement with this concept, induction of CYP4A ω-hydroxylase with clofibrate normalizes BP in the Dahl salt-sensitive rat. Conversely, in the spontaneously hypertensive rat, 20-HETE production at renal and vascular sites is increased and may contribute to the hypertension. For example, 20-HETE produced in preglomerular vessels may elevate BP by promoting renal vasoconstriction, which reduces glomerular filtration rate and facilitates salt and water reabsorption by decreasing renal interstitial pressure. Supporting this idea, BP in spontaneously hypertensive rats was decreased by interventions that decrease 20-HETE synthesis. 20-HETE also acts as a second messenger for the renal tubular and vascular actions of endothelins. The dependence of the renal functional effects of endothelins on generation of 20-HETE was shown in the deoxycorticosterone acetate/salt-induced hypertension model in rats. The appearance of severe renal injury and rapid elevation of BP coincided with increased production of endothelins and 20-HETE. The pressor response and proteinuria were markedly attenuated by inhibition of CYP450 metabolism of arachidonic acid.

SUGGESTED READING

1. Breyer MD, Jacobson HR, Breyer RM. Functional and molecular aspects of renal prostaglandin receptors. *J Am Soc Nephrol.* 1996;7:8–17.
2. Keen HL, Brands MW, Smith MJ Jr, et al. Thromboxane is required for full expression of angiotensin hypertension in rats. *Hypertension.* 1997;29:310–314.

3. Makita K, Takahashi K, Karara A, et al. Experimental and/or genetically controlled alterations of the renal microsomal cytochrome P450 epoxygenase induce hypertension in rats fed a high salt diet. *J Clin Invest.* 1994;94:2414–2420.
4. Nasjletti A. Arthur C. Corcoran Memorial Lecture: The role of eicosanoids in angiotensin-dependent hypertension. *Hypertension.* 1997;31:194–200.
5. Omata K, Abraham NG, Schwartzman ML. Renal cytochrome P450-arachidonic acid metabolism: localization and hormonal regulation in SHR. *Am J Physiol.* 1992;262:F591–F599.
6. Oyekan AO, McGiff JC. Cytochrome P-450-derived eicosanoids participate in the renal functional effects of ET-1 in the anesthetized rat. *Am J Physiol.* 1998;274:R52–R61.
7. Quilley J, Bell-Quilley CP, McGiff, JC. *Hypertension: Pathophysiology, Diagnosis, and Management.* New York, NY: Raven Press Ltd; 1995.
8. Roman RJ. P-450 metabolites of arachidonic acid in the control of cardiovascular function. *Physiol Rev.* 2002;82:131–186.
9. Sacerdoti D, Escalante B, Abraham NG, et al. Treatment with tin prevents the development of hypertension in spontaneously hypertensive rats. *Science.* 1989;243:388–390.

Chapter A21

Lipoxygenase Products

Jerry L. Nadler, MD

KEY POINTS

- Three lipoxygenase enzymes oxidize arachidonic acid to short-lived, potent autacoids such as hydroxyeicosatetraenoic acids.
- Hydroperoxy and hydroxyl radicals can be added to arachidonic acid at position 5, 12, or 15; 5-position derivatives can be metabolized further to leukotrienes.
- Lipoxygenase-derived eicosanoids may affect endothelial function, vascular smooth muscle contraction and growth, renin release, aldosterone secretion, and oxidation of low-density lipoproteins.
- Gene deletion studies in rodents suggest that 12 and 15 lipoxygenases play an important role in atherosclerosis development and response to vascular injury.

See also Chapters A19, A20, A33, A35, A37, A65–67, and C150

Eicosanoid Synthesis

Free arachidonic acid is released from membrane phospholipids by a variety of phospholipases after stimulation by cells, growth factors, vasoactive peptides, or inflammatory mediators. Arachidonic acid is then oxidized (**Figure A21.1**) by cyclooxygenase (COX) and cytochrome P450 pathways, as described in Chapter A20. Lipoxygenase enzymes, a group of nonheme iron-containing oxidases, are named for their ability to insert molecular oxygen at the 5-, 12-, or 15-carbon positions of arachidonic acid.

Cellular and Inflammatory Effects

There are several possible mechanisms by which the lipoxygenase products can produce their biologic effects, including increased intracellular free calcium levels and activation of protein kinase C. Arachidonic acid–derived products of the 12-lipoxygenase pathway have been shown to activate mitogen-activated protein kinase, stress-activated kinases, and inflammation-related transcription factors, suggesting a role in cell proliferation and inflammation. Additional results indicate that products of the 12-lipoxygenase pathway can increase monocyte binding to human aortic endothelial cells.

Table A21.1 lists examples of potential biologic effects of the 12- and 15-lipoxygenase products of arachidonic acid. The 15-

lipoxygenase enzyme is found in macrophage-rich atherosclerotic areas in the human blood vessel wall, raising speculation about a role in atherogenesis. Angiotensin II has been shown to increase 12-lipoxygenase products and to activate transcription of the 12-lipoxygenase gene in human adrenal glomerulosa and cultured human aortic smooth muscle.

Cyclooxygenase Inhibition

Antiinflammatory agents block various steps in the arachidonic acid cascades. Glucocorticoids inhibit phospholipases and reduce the release of arachidonic acid. Aspirin, a nonselective COX inhibitor, and selective nonsteroidal COX-2 antiinflammatory agents directly block COX enzymes. Currently, no inhibitors of the 12- or 15-lipoxygenase enzymes are available for clinical use.

Leukotriene Slow-Reacting Substance of Anaphylaxis Synthesis

The 5-lipoxygenase pathway converts arachidonic acid to 5-hydroperoxyeicosatetraenoic acid (5-HPETE, Figure A21.1). Another intermediate product of this pathway is leukotriene A_4 (LTA_4). LTA_4 hydrolase converts LTA_4 to LTB_4, a potent chemoattractant substance that causes polymorphonuclear cells to bind to vessel walls and may play a role in vascular pathology.

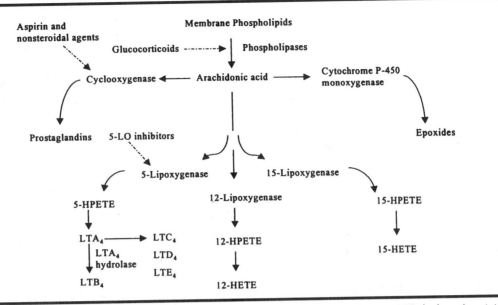

Figure A21.1. Pathways of arachidonic acid metabolism. Broken line illustrates possible areas for inhibition. HETE, hydroxyeicosatetraenoic acid; HPETE, hydroperoxyeicosatetraenoic acid; LO, lipoxygenase; LTA_4, leukotriene A_4; LTB_4, leukotriene B_4; LTC_4, leukotriene C_4; LTD_4, leukotriene D_4; LTE_4, leukotriene E_4.

Alternatively, LTA_4 can be converted to LTC_4, LTD_4, or LTE_4. These 3 leukotrienes together, formerly known as the *slow-reacting substance of anaphylaxis*, are potent vasoconstrictors in several vascular beds that also cause increased microvascular permeability.

Leukotrienes are synthesized primarily by mast cells, eosinophils, neutrophils, and macrophages. 5-Lipoxygenase is present in endothelium and can convert arachidonic acid to 5-hydroxyeicosatetraenoic acids (HETEs). Vascular endothelium and smooth muscle cells themselves have little capacity to produce leukotrienes, but they may convert intermediate products to leukotrienes under certain conditions.

Lipoxygenase Inhibition

A 5-lipoxygenase inhibitor, zileuton (Zyflo) and 2 leukotriene receptor antagonists, zafirlukast (Accolate) and montelukast (Singulair), have become clinically available for asthma control in recent years.

Lipoxins

Novel eicosanoids called *lipoxins* can be generated by transcellular metabolism of arachidonic acid between 5-lipoxygenase and either 12- or 15-lipoxygenase or aspirin-exposed COX-2.

The lipoxins generally have antiinflammatory actions and some actually can reduce endothelial cell migration and angiogenesis.

Endoperoxides and Hydroxyeicosatetraenoic Acids

The biologic role of products of the 12- and 15-lipoxygenase pathways has become clear only over the past several years. Both enzyme systems produce unstable endoperoxides or hydroperoxyeicosatetraenoic acids, which are subsequently converted to a variety of products, including more stable HETEs (Figure A21.1). 12- and 15-HETE production has been shown in vascular tissues, including cultured vascular smooth muscle cells, endothelial cells, aorta, and coronary arteries. These vascular cells have the capacity to incorporate HETEs into cell lipids and to produce additional metabolites. 12-HETE is a major product of platelets, adrenal glomerulosa cells, and certain sites within the renal cortex, including mesangial cells and the glomerulus. Stimulation of monocytes by interleukin-4 also produces 15-HETE. Growth factors such as angiotensin II and platelet-derived growth factor can increase 12-lipoxygenase expression and activity.

Lipoxygenase Activity and Atherosclerosis

When 12- and 15-lipoxygenase–deficient mice are cross-bred to apolipoprotein E–deficient or low-density lipoprotein–receptor-deficient mice, the proatherogenic role of the leukocyte type of 12-lipoxygenase is demonstrated, because these knock-out mice are protected from atherosclerosis development. In the rat carotid balloon angioplasty model, delivery of a 12-lipoxygenase ribozyme ("molecular scissors") markedly reduces the vascular injury response. Finally, in a diabetic porcine model of accelerated atherosclerosis, increased 12-lipoxygenase expression tracks directly with increased lesion formation.

Table A21.1. Potential Roles of the 12- and 15-Lipoxygenase Pathways in Cardiovascular Disorders

Inhibition of renin release (particularly 12-lipoxygenase pathway)
Mediation of angiotensin II action on blood vessels and adrenal glomerulosa (particularly 12-lipoxygenase pathway)
Inhibition of prostacyclin synthesis
Direct vasoconstriction of certain vascular beds
Growth-promoting effect on vascular smooth muscle cells
Oxidative modification of low-density lipoprotein
Promotion of monocyte binding to human endothelium
Progression of atherosclerosis

SUGGESTED READING

1. Folcik V, Nivar-Aristy R, Krajewskih L, Cathcart M. Lipoxygenase contributes to the oxidation of lipids in human atherosclerotic plaques. *J Clin Invest*. 1995;96:504–510.
2. Kim JA, Gu JL, Natarajan R, et al. A leukocyte-type of 12-lipoxygenase is expressed in human vascular and mononuclear cells: evidence for upregulation by angiotensin II. *Arterioscler Thromb Vasc Biol*. 1995;15:942–948.
3. Funk C. Prostaglandins and leukotrienes. *Adv Eicosanoid Biol Sci*. 2001;294:1871–1875.
4. Natarajan R, Gu JL, Nadler J, et al. Elevated glucose and angiotensin II increase 12-lipoxygenase activity and expression in porcine aortic smooth muscle cells. *Proc Natl Acad Sci U S A*. 1993;90:4947–4951.
5. Rao GN, Alexander RW, Runge MS. Linoleic acid and its metabolites, hydroperoxyoctadecadienoic acids, stimulate c-fos, c-jun, and c-myc mRNA expression, mitogen-activated protein kinase activation and growth in rat aortic smooth muscle cells. *J Clin Invest*. 1995;96:842–847.
6. Funk C, Cyrus T. 12/15 Lipoxygenase, oxidative modification of LDL and atherogenesis. *Trends Cardiovasc Med*. 2001;11:116–124.
7. Levy B, Clish C, Schmidt B, et al. Lipid mediator class switching during acute inflammation: signals in resolution. *Nat Immunol*. 2001;2:612–618.
8. Fang X, Kaduce TL, Spector AA. 13-(S)-hydroxyoctadecadienoic acid (13-HODE) incorporation and conversion to novel products by endothelial cells. *J Lipid Res*. 1999;40:699–707.
9. Gu JL, Pei H, Thomas L, Nadler J, et al. Ribozyme-mediated inhibition of rat leukocyte-type 12 lipoxygenase prevents intimal hyperplasia in balloon-injured rat carotid arteries. *Circulation*. 2001;103:1446–1452.
10. Natarajan R, Gerrity RG, Gu JL, et al. Role of 12-lipoxygenase and oxidant stress in hyperglycaemia-induced acceleration of atherosclerosis in a diabetic pig model. *Diabetologia*. 2002;45:125–133.

Chapter A22

Peroxisome Proliferator–Activated Receptors

Jorge Plutzky, MD

KEY POINTS

- There are three known classes of peroxisome proliferator–activated receptors: α, δ, and γ, each of which dimerizes with a retinoic acid receptor (retinoic X receptor) to regulate gene transcription.

- The putative endogenous ligands for proliferator-activated receptors include fatty acids and their oxidized derivatives. Synthetic peroxisome proliferator-activated receptor ligands include thiazolidinediones (peroxisome proliferator-activated receptor-γ) and fibrates (peroxisome proliferator-activated receptor-α). Genes activated by proliferator-activated receptors affect lipid metabolism, insulin sensitivity, and possibly inflammation.

- Proliferator-activated receptor activators may affect the vasculature directly by binding to proliferator-activated receptors in the arterial wall or inflammatory cells in atherosclerotic plaques.

See also Chapters A45, A66, A67, and C149

Peroxisomes are cellular organelles in which various molecules, including long-chain fatty acids, are oxidized. Fibric acid derivatives (e.g., gemfibrozil) increase the size and number of peroxisomes in rodents and are therefore called *peroxisome proliferators*. Similar peroxisome proliferation has not been seen in humans. Fibrates bind to a nuclear receptor through which they affect lipids—for example, increasing transcription of the apolipoprotein A-I component of high-density lipoprotein (HDL) or regulating by acid oxidation. Peroxisome proliferator–activated receptors (PPARs) were the subject of intense study in the 1990s, first for their role in metabolism, and, more recently, because of the implication that PPAR activation may influence vascular biology and atherosclerosis. PPAR ligands already in widespread therapeutic use include fibrates for dyslipidemia and thiazolidinediones (TZDs) as insulin-sensitizing antidiabetic agents.

Peroxisome Proliferator-Activated Receptor Subtypes and Gene Expression

PPARs are ligand-activated transcription factors that include PPAR-α, PPAR-γ, and PPAR-δ subtypes. Like other nuclear receptors such as the estrogen receptor and thyroid hormone receptor, PPARs contain both ligand binding domains and DNA binding domains (**Figure A22.1**). Divergence of amino acid sequences is greatest around the ligand binding domains, where receptor specificity is determined. During ligand binding, PPARs form a heterodimeric complex with another nuclear receptor, retinoic X receptor, which is activated by its own ligand (9-*cis* retinoic acid). This heterodimeric complex binds to defined PPAR-response elements in the promoters of specific target genes. In this way, PPAR ligands regulate gene expression.

Peroxisome Proliferator-Activated Receptor-α

Role in fatty acid metabolism. Many lines of evidence establish that PPAR-α, which is more widely expressed (heart, liver, kidney) than PPAR-γ, is a central regulator of fatty acid and lipid metabolism (**Table A22.1**). PPAR-α target genes are involved in the conversion of fatty acids to acyl coenzyme A derivatives, peroxisome β oxidation, and apolipoprotein expression (A-I, A-II, and C-III). Synthetic fibrates (gemfibrozil and fenofibrate), used clinically to lower triglycerides and raise HDL, are PPAR-α agonists. PPAR-α–deficient mice lack gross

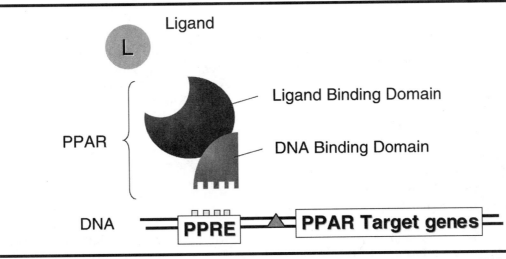

Figure A22.1. Schematic drawing of the peroxisome proliferator–activated receptors (PPARs) nuclear hormone receptor. PPARs are ligand-activated nuclear receptors that, on binding with cognate ligands, act as transcription factors controlling gene expression through interaction between their DNA binding domains and PPAR response elements. This occurs as part of a heterodimeric complex with retinoic X receptor nuclear hormone receptor (not shown). PPRE, PPAR-response elements.

phenotypic abnormalities, but they demonstrate increased total cholesterol and mildly increased total HDL levels, the latter owing to decreased HDL metabolism.

Vascular and antiinflammatory effects. PPAR-α expression in vascular cells as well as inflammatory cells, such as macrophages or lymphocytes, is now well established. In vascular smooth muscle cells (VSMCs), PPAR-α activators inhibit interleukin (IL)-1–dependent production of IL-6 and prostaglandins, as well as expression of cyclooxygenase-2. Aortic explants of PPAR-α–deficient mice demonstrate prolonged inflammatory responses and increased IL-6 production. PPAR-α agonists also inhibit expression of tissue factor, a major pro-coagulant that contributes to plaque formation. In endothelial cells, PPAR-α activators limit cytokine-induced vascular cell adhesion molecule-1 expression as well as monocyte adhesion. The site of activity is probably at the vascular cell adhesion molecule-1 promoter, through inhibition of NFκB, a common theme for PPAR-α target gene regulation.

Fibrate effects. Fibrates in clinical use decrease triglycerides and raise HDL. The beneficial effects of fibrates in recent cardiovascular trials (VA-HIT) in patients with relatively low low-

density lipoprotein raise the possibility that the beneficial results seen with such drugs stem, in part, from PPAR-α activation. Vascular benefits could also be mediated by the effect on lipoprotein.

Peroxisome Proliferator-Activated Receptor-γ

Role in adipogenesis. PPAR-γ, a key mediator in metabolic syndromes such as diabetes and obesity, was first identified as a part of a transcriptional complex necessary for adipocyte differentiation (Table A22.1). Overexpression of PPAR-γ in fibroblasts leads those cells to differentiate toward an adipocyte-like phenotype. There is high expression of PPAR-γ in adipose tissue. Homozygous PPAR-γ–deficient animals die *in utero* due to various abnormalities that include cardiac malformations and absent white fat. PPAR-γ also influences lipid metabolism, with target genes such as hydroxymethylglutaryl coenzyme A synthetase and apolipoprotein A-I.

Endogenous peroxisome proliferator-activated receptor ligands. Naturally occurring PPAR ligands probably exist, but their identity is uncertain. Oxidized linoleic acid, in the form of 9- or 13- hydroxy octadecadienoic acid, activates PPAR-γ and

Table A22.1. Synthetic Peroxisome Proliferator-Activated Receptor (PPAR) Ligands and Selected Examples of PPAR-Regulated Target Genes in Metabolic and Vascular Settings

NUCLEAR RECEPTOR	SYNTHETIC LIGANDS	METABOLIC TARGETS	VASCULAR TARGETS
PPAR-γ	Thiazolidinediones: pioglitazone (Actos), rosiglitazone (Avandia)	GLUT 4 (+) AP2 (+) CD36 (+)	Matrix metalloproteinase-9 (−) Selected cytokines (−) Selected chemokines (−) Adhesion molecules (−)
PPAR-α	Fibrates: gemfibrozil (Lopid), fenofibrate (Tricor)	Fatty acid β oxidation (+) Apolipoprotein A-I (+) Lipoprotein lipase (+)	Tissue factor (−)

+, gene induced; −, gene repressed.

may also have some PPAR-α activity. Similarly, the prostaglandin metabolite 15-deoxy-Δ12,14-prostaglandin J$_2$ (15d-PGJ$_2$) may be a PPAR-γ agonist.

Peroxisome proliferator-activated receptor-γ role in atherogenesis. PPAR-γ is expressed in lymphocytes, macrophages, VSMCs, and endothelial cells, in which there is evidence for PPAR-γ regulation of relevant target genes, including matrix metalloproteinases, enzymes implicated in plaque rupture, and various inflammatory targets. PPAR-γ activation appears to repress cytokine-induced chemokines (chemoattractant cytokines) in vascular endothelium and colonic epithelium, the latter suggesting a potential role for PPAR agonists in inflammatory bowel disease. PPAR-γ activation also inhibits monocyte production of cytokines, production of matrix metalloproteinases, and VSMC cell cycle progression. The significance of PPAR-γ induced expression of the oxidized low-density lipoprotein receptor (CD36) and remains unclear. Some macrophage effects may be offset by increases in cholesterol efflux through induction of adenosine triphosphate binding cassette protein-1 (ABC1).

Genetic studies. A dominant negative mutation in PPAR-γ, reported in at least 2 human kindreds, has been associated with severe insulin resistance, diabetes, and hypertension. A PPAR-γ mutation was seen in association with severe obesity in a subset of German patients, and another group has found that a single nucleotide polymorphism in PPAR-γ was linked to decreased risk of diabetes.

Thiazolidinediones. TZDs, as synthetic PPAR-γ ligands, were identified through chemical screening, with the subsequent realization that these agents sensitize patients to insulin by activating PPAR-γ. Drugs currently available in this class include pioglitazone (Actos) and rosiglitazone (Avandia). Troglitazone (Rezulin), a TZD with an α-tocopherol side chain, was withdrawn from the market because of sporadic liver damage. Perhaps the most instructive aspect of TZDs was to show that PPAR-γ represents an important player in insulin resistance/diabetes and atherosclerosis. In 4 different mouse models of atherosclerosis, various PPAR-γ agonists have reduced the severity of atherosclerotic lesions. Most recently, rosiglitazone has been shown in a large clinical trial to reduce myocardial ischemic events.

Additional clinical effects of thiazolidinediones. One prominent unexpected observation has been that TZDs modestly lower blood pressure. The mechanism for this has not been established but may include repression of angiotensin effects. Edema has also been seen among diabetic patients, with unknown significance and mechanism. Interestingly, the ligand-binding domain of PPAR-γ, as suggested by its crystal structure, is exceptionally large. This provides a structural basis through which unique TZD and non-TZD ligands may activate PPAR-γ in distinct ways, perhaps exerting different therapeutic and side-effect profiles.

Peroxisome Proliferator-Activated Receptor-δ

Although PPAR-γ and PPAR-α have received most of the attention over the past 5 years, PPAR-δ is an intriguing molecule with potential relevance to metabolic and vascular issues, as well as a potential therapeutic target. The ubiquitous expression of PPAR-δ in essentially all tissues suggests a fundamental role in homeostasis and cellular function. Like other PPAR relatives, PPAR-δ appears activated to some extent by fatty acids. Prostacyclin may be another endogenous agonist. Early studies with PPAR-δ agents have revealed marked increases in HDL, although liver toxicity poses a potential problem.

Unresolved Issues and Future Prospects

The rapid advance in understanding PPARs has brought with it some confusion, probably owing to the multilevel actions of PPAR agonists. Because some putative PPAR agonist responses can occur in the absence of the presumed target PPAR, the issue of nonspecific as well as nontranscriptional effects must be considered. The complex and overlapping antidiabetic and hypolipidemic effects of these agents also make dissection of primary effects difficult. Newer agents are also under development, including a dual PPAR-α and PPAR-γ agonist, which could potentially lower triglycerides, raise HDL, increase insulin sensitivity, and lower glucose. Although the complexity of these issues is challenging, they also suggest potential new ways for understanding and intervening in the cardiovascular dysmetabolic (insulin resistance) syndrome.

SUGGESTED READING

1. Altshuler D, Hirschhorn JN, Klannemark M, et al. The common PPAR-gamma Pro12Ala polymorphism is associated with decreased risk of type 2 diabetes. *Nat Genet.* 2000;26:76–80.
2. Barroso I, Gurnell M, Crowley VE, et al. Dominant negative mutations in human PPARgamma associated with severe insulin resistance, diabetes mellitus and hypertension [see comments]. *Nature.* 1999;402:880–883.
3. Bishop-Bailey D. Peroxisome proliferator-activated receptors in the cardiovascular system. *Br J Pharmacol.* 2000;129:823–834.
4. Henry RR. Thiazolidinediones. *Endocrinol Metab Clin North Am.* 1997;26:553–573.
5. Li AC, Brown KK, Silvestre MJ, et al. Peroxisome proliferator-activated receptor gamma ligands inhibit development of atherosclerosis in LDL receptor-deficient mice. *J Clin Invest.* 2000;106:523–531.
6. Marx N, Libby P, Plutzky J. Peroxisome proliferator-activated receptors (PPARs) and their role in the vessel wall: possible mediators of cardiovascular risk? *J Cardiovasc Risk.* 2001;8:203–210.
7. Parulkar AA, Pendergrass ML, Granda-Ayala R, et al. Nonhypoglycemic effects of thiazolidinediones. *Ann Intern Med.* 2001;134:61–71.
8. Plutzky J. Peroxisome proliferator-activated receptors in vascular biology and atherosclerosis: emerging insights for evolving paradigms. *Curr Atheroscler Rep.* 2000;2:327–335.
9. Schoonjans K, Auwerx J. Thiazolidinediones: an update. *Lancet.* 2000;355:1008–1010.
10. Wilson TM, Brown PJ, Sternbach DD, Henke BR. The PPARs: from orphan receptors to drug discovery. *J Med Chem.* 2000;43:527–550.

Plasminogen Activation and Fibrinolytic Balance

Douglas E. Vaughan, MD

KEY POINTS

- The plasminogen activator/plasmin (i.e., fibrinolytic) system serves as one of the endogenous defense mechanisms against intra-vascular thrombosis.

- Fibrinolytic activity is highly dependent on the balance between tissue-type plasminogen activator and plasminogen activator inhibitor-1.

- Angiotensin and aldosterone play important roles in regulating vascular plasminogen activator inhibitor-1 production, whereas bradykinin is a potent stimulus of vascular tissue-type plasminogen activation release.

- Angiotensin-converting enzyme plays a role in regulating vascular fibrinolytic balance.

See also Chapters A3, A6, A14, A16, A63, A66, A67, and C144

Fibrinolytic System

Plasminogen activators. The plasminogen activator/plasmin (i.e., fibrinolytic) system serves as an endogenous defense mechanism against intravascular thrombosis. As such, it complements the effects of protein anticoagulants such as proteins C and S and antithrombin III, and the short-acting, endothelial-derived platelet inhibitors nitric oxide (NO) and prostacyclin. The activity of the fibrinolytic system is ultimately dependent on the generation of the protease plasmin, which is produced from the inactive precursor plasminogen by the action of plasminogen activators (PAs). In mammals, 2 PAs have been identified: tissue-type plasminogen activator (t-PA) and urokinase-type plasminogen activator. Although both of these activators are synthesized in the endothelium, t-PA is felt to be the primary PA in blood.

Plasmin activator-inhibitor balance. Normally, there is an abundant supply of plasminogen in plasma that is available for activation and conversion to plasmin. However, little if any plasmin is produced, because t-PA circulates in trace concentrations in plasma and because t-PA is inhibited by very specific and rapidly acting plasminogen activator inhibitors (PAIs) that are also present in plasma. This balance prevents spontaneous hemorrhage or unwanted thrombosis.

Physiology and Regulation of Plasminogen Activator Inhibitor-1

The most important inhibitor of t-PA in the blood is plasminogen activator inhibitor-1 (PAI-1).

Genetic control. The gene for PAI-1 is located on human chromosome number 7, spans approximately 12 kilobases, and is composed of 9 introns and 8 exons. A variety of regulatory elements have been identified in the PAI-1 gene, including AP-1 sites; a glucocorticoid response element, which also mediates the aldosterone response; a very-low-density lipoprotein response site; and two Sp1 sites that appear to mediate glucose responsiveness. Recent studies have localized an angiotensin-responsive region that conforms with a putative JAK/STAT response element between the glucocorticoid response element and the second Sp1 site (**Figure A23.1**).

Plasminogen activator inhibitor-1 synthesis and metabolism in plasma. Plasma PAI-1 is derived from several sources, including the vascular endothelium, adipose tissue, and the liver. Platelets store large quantities of PAI-1 that are secreted after platelet aggregation. Several different fates are possible for PAI-1 after it is synthesized and secreted. Under normal conditions, PAI-1 concentrations exceed t-PA on a stoichiometric basis. The majority of PAI-1 circulates briefly in plasma and is removed via a hepatic clearance mechanism. Because the circulating half-life of PAI-1 is approximately 5 minutes, only a fraction of the secreted, active PAI-1 has the opportunity to react with plasma t-PA and form inert covalent complexes. There appears to be no endogenous mechanism for recycling PA–PAI-1 complexes, which are cleared through the low-density lipoprotein–related receptor and the very-low-density lipoprotein receptor. Active PAI-1 in plasma can also bind to vitronectin, which stabilizes PAI-1 in the active conformation.

Extracellular sterilization. PAI-1 also is present in the extracellular matrix of blood vessels, where it also associates with vitronectin. Tissue PAI-1 is derived from adjacent endothelium, vascular smooth muscle cells, and monocytes in areas of inflammation. The relative abundance of vitronectin in the subendothelial matrix provides a mechanism for preserving PAI-1 activity, and it is likely that vitronectin-bound PAI-1 represents the physiologically relevant form of the inhibitor in the extracellular matrix. PAI-1 bound to vitronectin has been shown to block the engagement of specific integrin receptors and thus impair cellular migration.

Endothelial production. A number of agents have been found to stimulate endothelial PAI-1 production. PAI-1 is classified as an acute phase reactant, and inflammatory cytokines such as interleukin-1 and tumor necrosis factor-α can induce

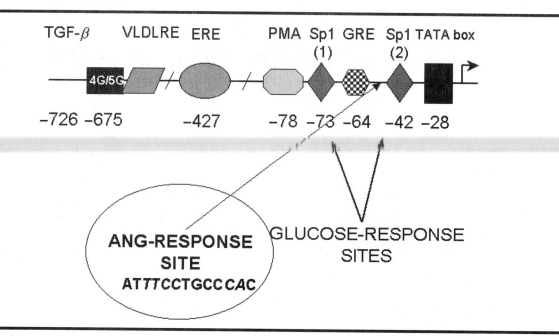

Figure A23.1. Schematic representation of the promoter region of plasminogen activator inhibitor-1. ANG, angiotensin; ERE, estrogen response element; GRE, glucocorticoid response element; PMA, phorbol myristate acetate; TGF-β, transforming growth factor β; VLDLRE, very-low-density lipoprotein response element.

PAI-1 production. These same factors promote vascular inflammation and atherosclerosis. Growth factors and hormones also regulate PAI-1 production, including transforming growth factor β (TGFβ), epidermal growth factor, thrombin, and insulin. Angiotensin II (Ang II) and Ang IV induce dose- and time-dependent increases in PAI-1 messenger RNA expression in vascular tissue *in vitro* and *in vivo*. Aldosterone interacts with Ang II to increase PAI-1 expression in vascular smooth muscle and endothelial cells.

Diurnal variation. There is a well-recognized circadian variation in plasma PAI-1, and this fluctuation in PAI-1 activity is responsible for the diurnal variation in net fibrinolytic activity. PAI-1 levels peak in the early morning and correspond with a nadir in net fibrinolytic activity, whereas the afternoon fall in plasma PAI-1 facilitates a peak in endogenous fibrinolysis. These diurnal fluctuations may have important clinical consequences, as the morning peak in PAI-1 corresponds with the circadian peak in the incidence of acute myocardial infarctions (MIs). The basic mechanisms that are responsible for this diurnal regulation of PAI-1 are poorly understood, although it has been reported that transcription factors involved in peripheral circadian gene expression regulate PAI-1 promoter activity *in vitro*. Activation of the renin-angiotensin system prolongs and exaggerates the morning peak in PAI-1. Furthermore, in salt-depleted, healthy human subjects and in hypertensive subjects treated with hydrochlorothiazide, there is a strong and statistically significant correlation between serum aldosterone and plasma PAI-1 levels that is abolished by spironolactone.

Plasminogen Activator Inhibitor-1 in Disease States

PAI-1 is readily detectable in plasma samples, and mean PAI-1 antigen levels in healthy adults are 15 to 30 ng/mL.

Hypertension. PAI-1 appears to play a role in hypertension and its sequelae. Plasma PAI-1 levels correlate with systolic blood pressure in healthy middle-aged men and women. Older populations tend to have higher PAI-1 levels, and mean PAI-1 antigen levels of 50 to 60 ng/mL are not uncommon in middle-aged male subjects.

Perivascular fibrosis and arteriosclerosis. Long-term inhibition of nitric oxide synthase (NOS) is known to induce hypertension and perivascular fibrosis in experimental animals and has been more recently shown to induce expression of PAI-1 in vascular tissues. NOS inhibition also induces vascular PAI-1 accumulation. Coronary perivascular fibrosis in PAI-1–deficient mice is significantly attenuated compared to controls during long-term NOS inhibition, suggesting that PAI-1 deficiency protects against the structural vascular changes that accompany hypertension. Direct inhibition of vascular PAI-1 activity may thus provide a new therapeutic strategy for the prevention of arterial stiffening and arteriosclerotic cardiovascular disease.

Atherogenesis. Aside from the role PAI-1 plays in thrombosis, the fibrinolytic system also plays an important role in vascular and tissue housekeeping. Several groups have reported excess PAI-1 in atherosclerotic plaques in humans, a finding that is exaggerated in type 2 diabetics. Impairment of the plasmin/plasminogen activator system appears to play an important role in the progression of atherosclerotic lesions. Local plasmin generation in the vessel wall is required for the activation of several matrix metalloproteinases, for the conversion of latent TGFβ to its active form, and for the dismantling of cholesterol aggregates. In a diseased vessel wall in which PAI-1 is overproduced, local plasmin production falls. Consequently, remodeling capacity is reduced due to decreased matrix metalloproteinase activation, smooth muscle cell proliferation is

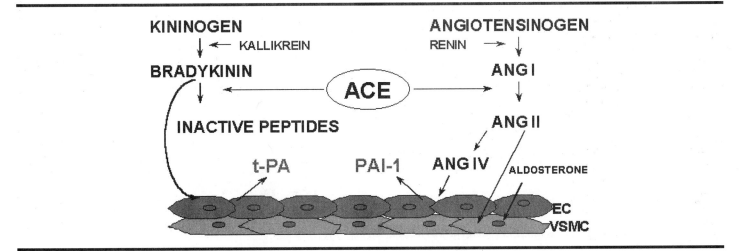

Figure A23.2. The dual functional roles of angiotensin-converting enzyme (ACE) and the strategic location of ACE in regulating vascular fibrinolytic balance. ANG, angiotensin; EC, endothelial cell; PA, plasminogen activators; PAI, plasminogen activator inhibitor; VSMC, vascular smooth muscle cell.

increased owing to decreased TGFβ activation, and cholesterol efflux may be impaired.

Increased PAI-1 in atherosclerotic plaques may augment the cellular content of vascular lesions, because PAI-1 retards smooth muscle cell migration by inhibiting the binding of vitronectin to the integrin $\alpha_v\beta_3$. It has been reported that plasminogen deficiency accelerates the development of atherosclerosis in ApoE-deficient (ApoE$^{-/-}$) mice, whereas PAI-1–deficient mice crossed into an ApoE$^{-/-}$ background appear to be partially protected against the development of atherosclerosis. Taken together, experimental data make it evident that plasmin plays a multifaceted housekeeping role in the vessel wall, and that fibrinolytic activity likely retards the progression of atherosclerotic lesions.

Acute myocardial infarction. It has been suggested that t-PA and urokinase-type plasminogen activator, in conjunction with thrombomodulin, serve as the critical endogenous defenders against thrombosis in the coronary circulation. If this hypothesis is correct, then an excess of PAI-1 would be expected to increase the risk of coronary thrombosis. There is substantial experimental and epidemiologic evidence that PAI-1 contributes to the development of ischemic cardiovascular disease. PAI-1 excess has been identified in youthful survivors that go on to develop recurrent MI, and a large prospective, nested case-control study identified a strong association between elevated plasma levels of PAI-1 antigen and activity with increased risk of MI, independent of other conventional risk factors.

Renin-Angiotensin-Aldosterone System Interactions

A substantial body of evidence supports the hypothesis that activation of the renin-angiotensin-aldosterone system (RAAS) promotes the development of atherosclerosis and ischemic cardiovascular disease independent of its effects of blood pressure, and angiotensin-converting enzyme (ACE) inhibitors ameliorate these diseases. For example, recent experiments demonstrate remarkable acceleration in the development of atherosclerosis in ApoE$^{-/-}$ mice that receive chronic infusions of Ang II.

Angiotensin-converting enzyme regulation of fibrinolysis. As illustrated in **Figure A23.2**, ACE is strategically located to play a crucial role in regulating the interaction between the RAAS and fibrinolysis. In addition to catalyzing the activation of Ang II, ACE catalyzes the rapid degradation of bradykinin. ACE inhibitors potentiate the hemodynamic effects of bradykinin, and bradykinin is one of the most potent stimuli for the release of t-PA in humans. Although systemic infusion of bradykinin induces a moderate (4-fold) increase in plasma t-PA levels, local infusions of bradykinin into humans stimulate the acute release of t-PA, yielding a >50-fold increase across the vascular bed, through a B_2-receptor–dependent, prostacyclin- and NO-independent mechanism.

Clinical studies. There is a growing body of clinical evidence that therapeutic interruption of the RAAS impacts vascular fibrinolytic balance. In the Healing and Early Afterload Reducing Therapy (HEART) study, ACE inhibition reduced plasma PAI-1 levels by >40% during the recovery phase after acute MI. Other studies confirm the effects of ACE inhibition on plasma fibrinolytic balance in healthy normotensive subjects, in postmenopausal women, and in hypertensives with insulin resistance.

SUGGESTED READING

1. Brown NJ, Agirbasli MA, Williams GH, et al. Effect of activation and inhibition of the renin-angiotensin system on plasma PAI-1. *Hypertension.* 1998;32:965–971.
2. Brown NJ, Kim KS, Chen YQ, et al. Synergistic effect of adrenal steroids and angiotensin II on plasminogen activator inhibitor-1 production. *J Clin Endocrinol Metabol.* 2000;85:336–344.
3. Kaikita K, Fogo AB, Ma L, et al. Plasminogen activator inhibitor-1 deficiency prevents hypertension and vascular fibrosis in response to long-term hypertension and vascular fibrosis in response to long-term nitric oxide synthase inhibition. *Circulation.* 2001;104:839–844.
4. Kerins DM, Hao Q, Vaughan DE. Angiotensin induction of PAI-1 expression in endothelial cells is mediated by the hexapeptide angiotensin IV. *J Clin Invest.* 1995;96:2515–2520.
5. Rosenberg RD, Aird WC. Vascular-bed-specific hemostasis and hypercoagulable states. *N Engl J Med.* 1999;340:1555–1564.

6. Sawathiparnich P. Spironolactone abolishes the relationship between aldosterone and plasminogen activator inhibitor-1 in humans. *J Clin Endocrinol Metab*. 2002;87:448–452.

7. Thogersen AM, Jansson JH, Boman K, et al. High plasminogen activator inhibitor and tissue plasminogen activator levels in plasma precede a first acute myocardial infarction in both men and women: evidence for the fibrinolytic system as an independent primary risk factor. *Circulation*. 1998;98:2241–2247.

8. Vaughan DE. Plasminogen activator inhibitor-1: a common denominator in cardiovascular disease. *J Invest Med*. 1998;46:370–376.

9. Vaughan DE, Rouleau J-L, Ridker PM, et al. Effects of ramipril on plasma fibrinolytic balance in patients with acute anterior myocardial infarction. *Circulation*. 1997;96:442–447.

10. Weiss D, Kools JJ, Taylor WR. Angiotensin II-induced hypertension accelerates the development of atherosclerosis in apoE-deficient mice. *Circulation*. 2001;103:448–454.

Chapter A24

Vasoactive Growth Factors and Adhesion Molecules

Carrie A. Northcott, MS; Stephanie W. Watts, PhD; Willa Hsueh, MD

KEY POINTS

- Classic peptide growth factors that promote cell growth (such as epidermal growth factor or platelet-derived growth factor) also tend to cause constriction, whereas growth factors that are antiproliferative (such as insulin-like growth factor, fibroblast growth factor, or vascular endothelial growth factor) tend to be vasodilatory.

- Signal transduction stimulated by growth factors and other vasoactive substances occurs by G protein–dependent and G protein–independent pathways and by transactivation, a process by which diverse agonists can stimulate tyrosine kinase activity via the same heptahelic receptor.

- Families of adhesion molecules include immunoglobulin-like cell adhesion molecules, integrins, selectins, and cadherins that are regulated by cytokines, growth factors, and shear stress. Adhesion molecules contribute to the inflammatory and prethrombotic process at the vessel wall.

- Integrins regulate remodeling and fibrosis in heart and vascular tissue, as well as inflammation and thrombosis.

See also Chapters A29, A32, A33, A59, A61, A63, A66, and A67

VASOACTIVE GROWTH FACTORS

Cellular Effects

Growth factors are peptides that interact with receptors that traverse the plasma membrane, typically 1 time. Epidermal growth factor (EGF) interacts with 1 of its monomeric receptors (ErbB1, ErbB3, ErbB4) to cause dimerization of these receptors or dimerization with ErbB2, an EGF receptor for which no known ligand has been defined. Dimerization of stimulated monomers results in activation of a tyrosine kinase on the cytoplasmic C-terminal end of the receptor. Activated tyrosine kinase phosphorylates tyrosine residues with src-homology 2 domains of its activated partner. Tyrosine-phosphorylated src-homology 2 domains are sites of protein-protein interaction that allows for scaffolding of proteins (Grb 2, Sos), which enables signal transduction pathways to proceed. The extracellular signal-regulated kinase (Erk) mitogen-activated protein kinase (MAPK) pathway depends on such a sequence of events. The end result of activation of the Erk MAPK pathway is translocation of MAPK to the nucleus, in which MAPK proteins phosphorylate and alter activation of transcription factors involved in growth. Thus, pathways such as the Erk MAPK pathway are "growth pathways" and substances that activate the pathway are "growth factors."

Receptor Effects

G protein–coupled receptor effects. G protein–coupled receptors interact with heterotrimeric G proteins (α, β, γ) to transduce an external signal to an internal event. Once activated, both the α and β/γ subunits of the G protein stimulate effector molecules, including phospholipases, adenylate cyclases, and ion channels, leading to biologic response such as smooth muscle contraction. For example, activation of the endothelin receptor in arterial smooth muscle results in activation of phospholipase C $\beta 1$ through the G protein Gq. Phospholipase C hydrolyzes phosphatidylinositol in the plasma membrane to release diacylglycerol and inositol (1,4,5) trisphosphate. Diacylglycerol activates classic forms of protein kinase C, and inositol (1,4,5) trisphosphate releases calcium from intracellular stores located in the sarcoplasmic reticulum.

Linked vasoactive and growth effects and transactivation. Classic heptahelic receptor agonists have previously been thought to work solely through stimulation of G proteins. It is now clear that many heptahelic receptors are also linked to growth pathways similar to those stimulated by growth factor receptors. A diverse group of agonists can activate the Erk-MAPK pathway by 1 mechanism dependent on G protein activation and 1 independent of G protein stimulation. Several different agonists can activate the tyrosine kinase intrinsic to the EGF receptor

Table A24.1. Heptahelic Receptor Agonists, Contractility, and Growth

SUBSTANCE	ARTERY/CELL	CONTRACTILE EFFECT	GROWTH EFFECT ON ARTERIAL SMOOTH MUSCLE
Adrenomedullin	Rat mesangial cells	Relaxation	–
Angiotensin II (via AT_1 receptor)	Multiple	Contraction	+
Atrial natriuretic peptide	Multiple	Relaxation	–
Bradykinin	Multiple	Relaxation/contraction	–
Endothelin-1 (via ET_A receptor)	Multiple	Contraction	+
Norepinephrine	Multiple	Contraction	+
Serotonin	Multiple	Contraction	+
Thrombin	Multiple	Contraction/relaxation	+
Vasoactive intestinal polypeptide	Smooth muscle cells	Relaxation	–

–, decrease; +, increase.

ErbB1 in a process called *transactivation*, which defines the complicated and no longer separate signal transduction of heptahelic and growth factor receptors. In vascular smooth muscle, angiotensin II, endothelin-1, thrombin, and arachidonic acid or eicosanoid derivatives can activate the epidermal growth factor receptor, affecting signaling and growth. Thus, epidermal growth factor receptor transactivation can occur independent of EGF. Transactivation by heptahelic receptors has also been described for the platelet-derived growth factor receptor as well, but the role of transactivation in smooth muscle contraction is still unclear. In **Table A24.1**, a small number of these studies is listed, and general trends have emerged. Agonists of heptahelic receptors that constrict arterial smooth muscle also typically stimulate smooth muscle cell growth. Conversely, agonists that relax smooth muscle tend to inhibit growth. Exceptions to this trend include insulin (**Table A24.2**), which causes endothelium-dependent relaxation and smooth muscle cell proliferation.

Vascular Responses

Platelet-derived growth factor causes a potent, concentration-dependent contraction of isolated rat aorta. Other classic growth factors have also been shown to modify arterial tone (Table A24.2). One mechanism by which growth factors modulate smooth muscle tone is through modulation of the activity of caldesmon, a substrate of Erk MAPK. In its unphosphorylated state, caldesmon inhibits the actinomyosin adenosine triphosphatase necessary for contraction. When phosphorylated by Erk MAPK, this inhibition is lifted and contraction proceeds. Growth factors also activate L-type calcium channels, although the mechanism by which this occurs is not well understood.

Blood Pressure Regulation

The role of growth factors in direct blood pressure regulation is probably minimal because their plasma levels are low. For example, the level of plasma EGF in humans is estimated at 30 pM. However, plasma levels of growth factors are not an accurate measure of artery exposure. The plasma membrane and extracellular matrix proteins are reservoirs for growth factors, from which they are released by proteases. Thus, acute and locally high concentrations of growth factors can occur at the arterial wall and exert both growth and contractile effects. In these ways, growth factors may indirectly affect chronic blood pressure levels.

ADHESION MOLECULES

Adhesion allows cells to adhere to each other or to molecules in the extracellular matrix (ECM). The process of adhesion is necessary for a variety of cell functions, including differentiation, growth, migration, and response of the cell to its external milieu. Four types of cell adhesion molecules have been described.

Table A24.2. Classic Growth Factors, Contractility, and Growth

SUBSTANCE	VESSEL	CONTRACTILE EFFECT	GROWTH EFFECT ON ARTERIAL SMOOTH MUSCLE
Basic fibroblast growth factor	Coronary arterioles	Relaxation, endothelium-dependent	+
Epidermal growth factor	Rabbit aorta	Contraction	+
	Rat aorta	Contraction	+
Insulin	Coronary artery	Relaxation (complex)	+ (complex)
Insulin-like growth factor-I	Coronary artery	Relaxation	+
Platelet-derived growth factor	Rat aorta	Contraction	+
	Rat mesangial cells	Contraction	+
Vascular endothelial growth factor	Coronary postcapillary venular endothelial cells	Relaxation	
	Rat aorta	Relaxation	
	Cavernous smooth muscle cells		+
	Multiple		– growth, + migration

–, decrease; +, increase.

Immunoglobulin-Like Cell Adhesion Molecules

Immunoglobulin-like cell adhesion molecules (ICAMs) include ICAM-1 (CD54), ICAM-2 (CD102), ICAM-3 (CD 50), ICAM-4 (Landsteiner-Wiener red cell), neural cell adhesion molecule (ICAM-5 or telencephalin), vascular cell adhesion molecule (VCAM), and platelet/endothelial cell adhesion molecule (PECAM). ICAMs are transmembrane glycoproteins that contain immunoglobulin-like domains. They play an important role in the adhesion and spreading of circulating leukocytes to endothelium in areas of tissue damage; these processes then allow for transendothelial migration of white cells via intercellular junctions between endothelial cells.

Roles in atherogenesis. The ICAM family and selectins play a key role in immune and inflammatory responses; this role is of particular importance in the development of the atherosclerotic plaque (see Chapter A67). The ICAMs found on endothelial cells, monocytes and macrophages, lymphocytes, and vascular smooth muscle cells contribute to the vascular injury response. They are induced by cytokines, such as tumor necrosis factor-α and interleukins; growth factors, such as endothelin and angiotensin II; shear stress; oxidized low-density lipoprotein; and thrombin. One of the earliest changes in the endothelium in the atherosclerotic process is the attachment of leukocytes owing to increased expression of ICAM-1 and VCAM-1, which can adhere in a ligand-receptor fashion to receptors on appropriately activated monocytes or T-lymphocytes. PECAM can lead to platelet adhesion if the endothelium is activated appropriately. Increased amounts of ICAM-1, VCAM-1, PECAM, and E-selectin have been found in human atherosclerotic plaques. ICAM-1 can be shed from the vasculature into the circulation in a soluble form. Increased soluble ICAM-1 has been associated with increased risk of myocardial infarction; inhibitors of ICAM-1 and VCAM-1 are under development. Whether attenuation of the inflammatory response by reduction of ICAM/VCAM function can affect atherosclerosis remains to be determined.

Integrins

Integrins are transmembrane receptors composed of α- and β-subunit heterodimers that consist of a large extracellular domain, a transmembrane region, and a relatively short cytoplasmic domain. There are at least 15 α- and 8 β-subunits described; the combinations of α- and β-subunits form at least 20 integrins, which are classified into subfamilies based on their structurally distinct β-chains. The extracellular domain binds to proteins in the ECM, such as fibronectin, collagen, vitronectin, osteopontin (OPN), and others, whereas the cytoplasmic domains interact with cytoskeletal proteins and intracellular signaling molecules. Integrins have a unique role, transmitting information from the external environment of the cell that then influences structural changes and signaling pathways within the cell, regulating cell activity.

Roles in cardiovascular disease. Integrins are intimately involved in a variety of cell activities that underlie atherosclerosis, cardiac and vascular remodeling, angiogenesis, and other cardiovascular processes. The engagement of integrins by certain ECM proteins initiates the localization of cytoskeletal proteins into focal adhesions, which are areas of tight association between the plasma membrane and the ECM. Focal adhesions represent the colocalization of cytoskeletal proteins such as talin and α-actinin, focal adhesion kinase (FAK), integrins, growth factor receptors, and other signaling molecules. In general, this colocalization is dependent on the integrin β-cytoplasmic domain, which is highly conserved between species and for each of the β-subtypes. Signaling molecules such as c-*src*, FAK, phosphatidylinositol 3-kinase, phospholipase C, MAPK, MEK, JNK, Ras, Raf, and others are associated with focal adhesions. The colocalization of all these molecules is likely an important means of facilitating their interactions. Activation of integrins can induce protooncogene expression and regulate the production of cell cycle proteins. Integrins may also affect the apoptotic process. The tyrosine kinase FAK is phosphorylated in various cells when the cells are attached to fibronectin, laminin, vitronectin, collagen, and other ECM proteins. FAK appears to be an important regulator of the movement of cells, because cells that are deficient in FAK have reduced motility *in vitro*, whereas overexpression of FAK is associated with increased motility. Integrins contribute to vascular smooth muscle cell (VSMC) growth and migration; inhibition of certain integrins on these cells can inhibit intimal hyperplasia and restenosis, which are dependent on these actions of VSMC. Atherosclerosis also involves migration and proliferation of VSMC; whether inhibition of integrins that regulates these processes impacts on atherosclerosis is unknown. Endothelial cell migration related to angiogenesis is highly integrin mediated; antibodies inhibiting $\alpha_v\beta_3$ integrins inhibit angiogenesis associated with certain cancers and may inhibit cancer growth and metastasis. Because of their effects on cell attachment to the ECM and influence on ECM production, integrins may also play a key role in the fibrotic response of the myocardium and vasculature, and thus, contribute to remodeling processes in these tissues.

Selectins

Selectins occur as P, E, and L forms and are expressed by leukocytes and endothelial cells. Selectins mediate loose contacts between leukocytes and endothelial cells that allow the "rolling" of leukocytes over the endothelium.

Cadherins

Cadherins are cell surface glycoproteins that confer calcium-dependent intercellular adhesion. They represent diverse families of adhesion proteins with multiple structural differences, although all have extracellular calcium binding domains, a transmembrane domain, and an intracellular domain that allows them to interact with cytoskeletal and signaling molecules. Their role in cardiovascular disease is less well described compared to the other classes of adhesion molecules, but they are known to be important in cardiac and vascular development and possibly in mechanical signal transduction in endothelial cells.

Osteopontin and Structural Protein Interactions

Increasing attention is being paid to the interaction of structural proteins as adhesion molecules. One of the best studied is OPN, which is a secreted, acidic phosphoprotein that plays an important role in cell adhesion. OPN participates in multiple pathologic processes in the cardiovascular system. OPN binds to extracellular matrix proteins such as collagens and fibronectin and contains an arginine-glycine-aspartate motif that facilitates its binding to a variety of integrins, including $\alpha_v\beta$, $\alpha_v\beta_3$, $\alpha_v\beta_5$, and others. Angiotensin II and other growth factors stimulate OPN expression in cardiovascular and renal tissues. Genetic knock-out of OPN in mice has shed light on its important role in cardiovascular disease; after myocardial infarction, OPN$^{-/-}$ have greater ventricular dilation and decreased function than their wild type (WT) counterparts. After angiotensin II infusion associated with hypertension, OPN$^{-/-}$ have less cardiac enlargement and less interstitial fibrosis than WT, suggesting that OPN contributes to the fibrotic process in the heart and may be necessary for healing after necrosis but may promote extensive fibrosis in a nonnecrotic model. OPN also plays a role in the inflammatory process. In a renal hydronephrosis model, OPN$^{-/-}$ have less macrophage infiltration into the kidney compared to WT. Knock-out of OPN in atherosclerosis-prone apolipoprotein E–deficient mice rescues the animal from atherosclerosis, an effect that is mediated primarily through OPN in monocytes. It is thus possible that OPN can emerge as a therapeutic target in cardiovascular remodeling and inflammation.

SUGGESTED READING

1. Ashizawa N, Graf K, Do Y, et al. Osteopontin is produced by rat cardiac fibroblasts and mediates AII-induced DNA synthesis and collagen gel contraction. *J Clin Invest.* 1996;98:2218–2227.
2. Berk BC. Vascular smooth muscle growth: autocrine growth mechanisms. *Physiol Rev.* 2001;81:999–1030.
3. Davis MJ, Gordon JL, Gearing AHJ, et al. The expression of the adhesion molecules ICAM-1, VCAM-1, PECAM, and E-selection in human atherosclerosis. *J Pathol.* 1993;171:223–229.
4. G Protein Function (movie). http://entochem.tamu.edu/Teaching/G-protein/Gproteinmovie.html. Accessed December 2, 2002.
5. G Proteins. http://gpcr.org. Accessed December 2, 2002.
6. Giachelli CM, Schwartz SM, Liaw L. Molecular and cellular biology of osteopontin. *Trends Cardiovasc Med.* 1995;5:88–95.
7. Growth Factors. http://www.growth-factor.net/. Accessed September 30, 2002.
8. Hsueh WA, Law RE, Do YS. Integrins, adhesion and cardiac remodeling. *Hypertension.* 1998;31:176–180.
9. Hollenberg MD. Tyrosine kinase pathways and the regulation of smooth muscle contractility. *Trends Pharmacol Sci.* 1994;15:108–114.
10. Marinissen MJ, Gutkind JS. G-protein coupled receptors and signaling networks: emerging paradigms. *Trends Pharmacol Sci.* 2001;22:368–376.
11. Meredith J, Winitxz S, McArthur LJ, et al. The regulation of growth and intracellular signaling by integrins. *Endocr Rev.* 1996;17:207.
12. Ridker PM, Hennekens CH, Roitman-Johnson B, et al. Plasma concentration of soluble intercellular adhesion molecule 1 and risks of future myocardial infarction in apparently healthy men. *Lancet.* 1998;351:88–92.
13. Signal Transduction. http://stke.sciencemag.org; http://vlib.org/science/Cell_Biology/signal_transduction.shtml; http://biocarta.com. Accessed December 2, 2002.

Section 2. *Ion Transport and Signal Transduction*

Chapter A25

Intracellular pH and Cell Volume

Bradford C. Berk, MD, PhD

KEY POINTS

- Anion and cation transporters and exchangers regulate intracellular pH and cell volume.

- Na$^+$-H$^+$ exchange is increased in most hypertensive humans and some animal models.

- Enzymes that regulate Na$^+$-H$^+$ exchange are candidate pathophysiologic genes for essential hypertension.

- Increased Na$^+$-H$^+$ exchange can cause cell swelling, sensitivity to pressors, and cell hypertrophy.

See also Chapters A24, A26, A27, A33, A47, A63, A75, and A76

Cells maintain a homeostatic balance that requires regulation of volume and intracellular pH (pH$_i$) around "set points." Both pH$_i$ and cell volume are regulated by ion transport systems that include the HCO$_3^-$-Cl$^-$ exchangers and the Na$^+$-H$^+$ exchangers.

REGULATION OF INTRACELLULAR PH

Vascular smooth muscle cells (VSMCs) maintain vessel tone by altering their contractile state and maintain vessel structure by altering their growth state. pH$_i$ plays a critical role in both functions. Regulation of pH$_i$ is due to "buffering" and transport of H$^+$ (or OH$^-$) across membranes. Intracellular buffering is complex and includes physicochemical buffering by the interaction of H$^+$ with cellular proteins, compartmentalization, and metabolic consumption.

Ion Transport Mechanisms

Three ion transport mechanisms participate in pH$_i$ homeostasis: (a) Na$^+$-H$^+$ exchange, (b) Na$^+$-dependent HCO$_3^-$-Cl$^-$ exchange, and (c) cation-independent HCO$_3^-$-Cl$^-$ exchange (**Figure A25.1**).

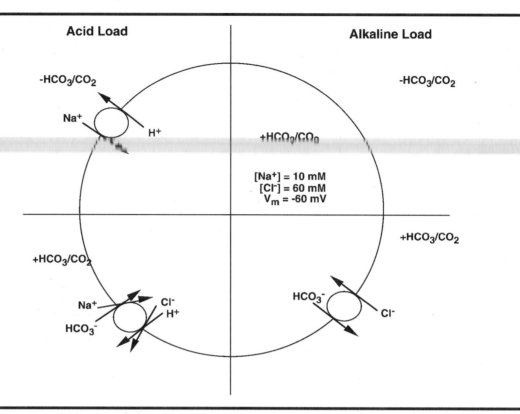

Figure A25.1. Regulation of intracellular pH. Shown are pH regulatory ion transport mechanisms in response to an acid load **(left)** or an alkaline load **(right)**. Nature of transport is also influenced by bicarbonate **(bottom)** or absence of bicarbonate **(top)**. There is no regulatory ion transport process for alkaline loads in absence of bicarbonate, and cell relies on intracellular generation of protons.

Na$^+$-H$^+$ exchange. Na$^+$-H$^+$ exchange is an electroneutral transport process that under physiologic conditions exchanges 1 intracellular H$^+$ for 1 extracellular Na$^+$. The Na$^+$-H$^+$ exchanger participates in multiple cellular functions, including regulation of pH$_i$ and transport of salt and water. It is now known that Na$^+$-H$^+$ exchange is mediated by a family of at least 6 related Na$^+$-H$^+$ exchanger gene products (NHE-1 through NHE-6). These have unique tissue distributions and sensitivities to inhibition by pharmacologic agents. The NHE-1 isoform appears to be ubiquitous and is dominant in VSMCs. The primary function of NHE-1 is to regulate pH$_i$, as evidenced by the pH$_i$ dependence of the rate of transport. Basal NHE-1 activity maintains normal VSMC pH$_i$ at 0.3 to 0.5 pH units above the Donnan equilibrium for H$^+$. Rapid increases in Na$^+$-H$^+$ exchange activity occur on exposure to growth factors and vasoconstrictors. This stimulation is characterized by a change in affinity for intracellular H$^+$ and extracellular Na$^+$. At normal pH$_i$ (7.4), the Na$^+$-H$^+$ exchanger is inactive, but it is greatly stimulated when the cell is acidified, indicating the existence of an intracellular H$^+$ sensor. The sensitivity of this intracellular site can be shifted to more acid pH$_i$ by depletion of adenosine triphosphate or to more alkaline pH$_i$ by growth factor stimulation or cell shrinkage. The efficiency of Na$^+$-H$^+$ exchange in restoring pH$_i$ of an acid-loaded cell is inversely proportional to the buffering power (β); only a few exchanges are required to induce a large pH recovery when β is low.

Na$^+$-dependent HCO$_3^-$-Cl$^-$ exchange. In the absence of CO$_2$-HCO$_3^-$, as might occur with decreased blood flow, the Na$^+$-H$^+$ exchanger is the dominant pH$_i$ regulator. In the presence of CO$_2$-HCO$_3^-$, the Na$^+$-dependent HCO$_3^-$-Cl$^-$ exchanger is dominant. This transporter normally exchanges extracellular Na$^+$ and HCO$_3^-$ for intracellular Cl$^-$ (and probably H$^+$), with stoichiometry for Na$^+$/Cl$^-$/acid-base equivalents of 1:1:2. It can be distinguished from Na$^+$-H$^+$ exchange by its sensitivity to stilbene derivatives and resistance to amiloride.

Cation-independent HCO$_3^-$-Cl$^-$ exchange. The cation-independent HCO$_3^-$-Cl$^-$ exchanger transports anions across the cell membrane with a stoichiometry of 1:1 and is electroneutral. Like Na$^+$-H$^+$ exchange, HCO$_3^-$-Cl$^-$ exchange has been shown to be mediated by a multigene family of transporters (AE1 through AE3). At normal intracellular Cl$^-$ and HCO$_3^-$ concentrations, net transport of the exchanger would be 1 intracellular HCO$_3^-$ for 1 extracellular Cl$^-$, producing intracellular acidification. Thus, as shown in Figure A25.1, HCO$_3^-$-Cl$^-$ exchange lowers pH$_i$ in alkaline-loaded cells. There is no alkaline pH$_i$ regulatory mechanism in the absence of HCO$_3^-$-CO$_2$ except for transporters that normally extrude H$^+$ working in reverse.

REGULATION OF CELL VOLUME

Cells regulate their volume by unloading excess water if swollen or by taking on water if shrunken. Usually, cell volume is corrected by altering the number of osmotically active particles in the cytoplasm, thereby causing obligate water movement. The volume-sensing mechanisms are unknown, but possibilities include changes in cytoplasmic electrolyte concentrations (e.g., protons and membrane potential), changes in cell shape (e.g., cytoskeleton-membrane interactions), or alterations in kinases that regulate shape (such as Rho kinase and myosin light-chain

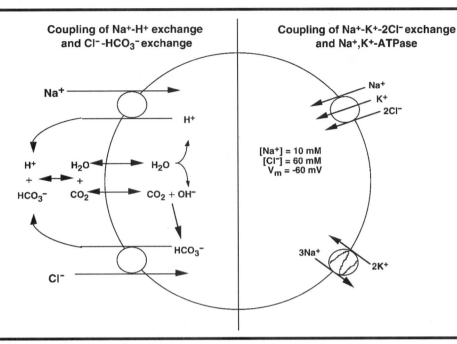

Figure A25.2. Coupling of several exchangers and sodium pump to regulate cell volume. Change in pH may regulate cell volume, and, conversely, changes in cell volume may alter intracellular pH as discussed in text. Na^+, K^+-ATPase, sodium- and potassium-activated adenosine triphosphatase.

kinase). Volume regulation is particularly important in VSMCs, because they undergo rapid transient volume changes during contraction and slower sustained volume changes during hypertrophy.

Role of Ion Pumps

Two mechanisms have been described that regulate volume in VSMCs: (a) Na^+-H^+ exchange and Cl^--HCO_3^- exchange–coupled transport and (b) Na^+-K^+-$2Cl^-$ cotransport and sodium- and potassium-activated adenosine triphosphatase–coupled transport (**Figure A25.2**). Na^+-H^+ and Cl^--HCO_3^- are functionally coupled with pH_i, because H^+ regulates Na^+-H^+ exchange and also determines the concentration of HCO_3^-. As an example of the link between pH_i and volume, consider the situation after sudden intracellular acidification. Because the β is not infinitely large, a finite amount of time is required for Na^+-H^+ exchange to restore pH_i to the basal level. The time required is dependent on the β and the rate of Na^+-H^+ exchange. Cell volume changes because Na^+-H^+ exchange is activated, resulting in an increased influx of Na^+ and water. H^+ ions are generated by intracellular metabolism "fueling" the exchange. If Cl^--HCO_3^- exchange is also present, the initial rate of pH recovery is faster, because intracellular Cl^- is exchanged for extracellular HCO_3^-, which raises pH_i. Although the loss of intracellular Cl^- initially causes a decrease in cell volume, this is followed by coupled Na^+-H^+ and Cl^--HCO_3^- exchange.

The result of this coupling is the inward movement of Na^+ by Na^+-H^+ exchange and of Cl^- by Cl^--HCO_3^- exchange. The H^+ and HCO_3^- transported out of the cell in exchange for Na^+ and Cl^- are converted into H_2O and CO_2, increasing cell volume (Figure A25.2). Key to this increase in cell volume are the facts that H^+ is generated from cell metabolism (and hence "created" *de novo*) and the Na^+-K^+-$2Cl^-$ cotransporter can mediate a net influx of Cl^- with increases in Na^+ and K^+. The changes in Na^+ activate sodium- and potassium-activated

adenosine triphosphatase, which works to maintain transcellular gradients for Na^+ and K^+. The net result is obligate inward movement of water and cell volume increase.

VASCULAR SMOOTH MUSCLE FUNCTION AND HYPERTENSION

Functional Aspects

The abnormalities of vessel tone and growth seen in hypertension may be, in part, the result of changes in the regulation of cell volume and pH_i. The Na^+-H^+ exchanger may play a pathogenic role in hypertension (**Figure A25.3**) by modifying pH_i and altering

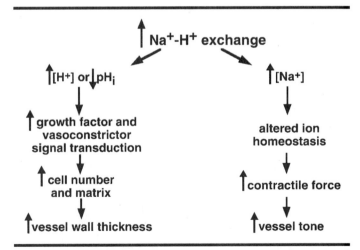

Figure A25.3. Effect of Na^+-H^+ exchange on vascular smooth muscle cell growth and tone. Increased activity leads to alterations in concentrations of H^+ and Na^+ that secondarily modulate signal transduction and contractile force. Chronic changes mediated by these alterations may lead to fixed structural abnormalities, such as medial hypertrophy and smooth muscle hyperplasia. pH_i, intracellular pH.

signal transduction pathways by which vasoactive agents regulate vascular tone and VSMC growth. The effect of increased Na^+-H^+ exchange on VSMC growth would most likely be an enhanced sensitivity to mitogens. Increased activity of the Na^+-H^+ exchanger could lead to increased vascular tone by 2 mechanisms. First, increased Na^+ entry would activate Na^+-Ca^{2+} exchange, leading to increased intracellular calcium. This phenomenon is important in conditions of ischemia and reperfusion such as occur with myocardial infarction, stroke, and microvascular occlusion. Second, increased pH_i would enhance the calcium sensitivity of the contractile apparatus, leading to an increase in contractility for a given intracellular calcium concentration. Owing to the activation of the Na^+-H^+ exchanger by hyperplastic and hypertrophic agents, it has been proposed that abnormal function of this protein may be involved in the pathophysiology of hypertension. Evidence for dysfunction of the Na^+-H^+ exchanger in hypertension includes observations that its activity is increased in skeletal muscle, VSMCs, lymphocytes, platelets from spontaneously hypertensive rats, and platelets from hypertensive patients.

Genetic Aspects

A large number of studies suggests that increased NHE-1 activity is prevalent in hypertension. Alterations in Na^+-H^+ exchange in hypertension could occur by (a) mutation in the gene, (b) increased expression of the gene product, and (c) altered posttranslational regulation of existing exchangers.

By RFLP analysis, there is no linkage between the human Na^+-H^+ exchanger gene and essential hypertension. There also does not appear to be any alteration in NHE-1 messenger RNA or protein expression in the spontaneously hypertensive rat. However, there is clearly an increase in both NHE-1 phosphorylation and cell growth in cells derived from the hypertensive rats and human hypertensive patients. These findings support the simple concept that increased activity of an NHE-1 kinase (or decreased activity of an NHE-1 phosphatase) is responsible for increased basal activity of the exchanger in tissues of hypertensive persons and animals.

Alternatively, an NHE-1 regulatory protein whose activity is modulated by phosphorylation may be altered in hypertension. Studies with mutated or deleted NHE-1 proteins indicate that modulation of NHE-1 by phosphorylation shifts the pH range over which the "pH_i sensor" of the exchanger regulates ion exchange. Thus, the primary alteration in Na^+-H^+ exchange in VSMCs in hypertension is likely to involve a change in phosphorylation of an NHE-1 regulatory protein or NHE-1 itself. Recent work has identified several NHE-1 kinases [p90RSK, ERK1/2, p160ROCK (a RhoA-activated kinase), and Nck interacting kinase] as well as several NHE-1 binding proteins (calcineurin B homologous protein, 14-3-3β, heat shock protein 70, ezrin, radixin, and moesin) that may play a role in gene expression.

SUGGESTED READING

1. Berk BC. Regulation of the Na^+/H^+ exchanger in vascular smooth muscle. In: Fliegel L, Austin RG. *The Na^+/H^+ Exchanger*. Austin, TX: Landes Co.; 1996:47–67.
2. Berk BC, Vallega G, Muslin AJ, et al. Spontaneously hypertensive rat vascular smooth muscle cells in culture exhibit increased growth and Na^+/H^+ exchange. *J Clin Invest.* 1989;83:822–829.
3. Chamberlin ME, Strange K. Anisosmotic cell volume regulation: a comparative view. *Am J Physiol.* 1989;257:C159–C173.
4. Lifton RP, Hunt SC, Williams RR, et al. Exclusion of the Na^+-H^+ antiporter as a candidate gene in human essential hypertension. *Hypertension.* 1991;17:8–14.
5. Orlov SN, Tremblay J, Hamet P. Cell volume in vascular smooth muscle is regulated by bumetanide-sensitive ion transport. *Am J Physiol.* 1996;270:C1388–C1397.
6. Orlowski J, Grinstein S. Na^+/H^+ exchangers of mammalian cells. *J Biol Chem.* 1997;272:22373–22376.
7. Rosskopf D, Dusing R, Siffert W. Membrane sodium-proton exchange and primary hypertension. *Hypertension.* 1993;21:607–617.
8. Siczkowski M, Davies JE, Ng LL. Na^+-H^+ exchanger isoform 1 phosphorylation in normal Wistar-Kyoto and spontaneously hypertensive rats. *Circ Res.* 1995;76:825–831.
9. Wakabayashi S, Fafournoux P, Sardet C, Pouyssegur J. The Na^+/H^+ antiporter cytoplasmic domain mediates growth factor signals and controls "H^+-sensing." *Proc Natl Acad Sci U S A.* 1992;89:2424–2428.

Chapter A26

Cellular Potassium Transport

Jason X.-J. Yuan, MD, PhD; Mordecai P. Blaustein, MD

KEY POINTS

- High intracellular K^+ concentration in vascular smooth muscle cells is maintained by the Na^+,K^+ pump (Na^+,K^+-ATPase).

- The activity of K^+ channels governs membrane potential in vascular smooth muscle cells and is a major determinant of cytosolic free Ca^{2+} concentration and vascular tone.

- Multiple types of K^+ channels are expressed in vascular smooth muscle cells: voltage-gated, Ca^{2+}-activated, and adenosine triphosphate–sensitive K^+ channels.

- Endothelium-derived relaxing factors regulate vascular tone by affecting K^+ channel activity.

- Dysfunction of K^+ channels in vascular smooth muscle cells is associated with membrane depolarization, increased Ca^{2+} concentration, and arterial hypertension.

See also Chapters A25, A27, A33, A47, and C148

Na^+,K^+-ATPase and K^+ Influx

Potassium ions are transported into virtually all mammalian cells against their electrochemical gradient. The mechanism responsible for this active transport is the ouabain-sensitive Na^+,K^+ pump (Na^+,K^+-ATPase; see Chapter 22) that expels 3 Na^+ ions in exchange for 2 entering K^+ ions. Hydrolysis of the terminal high-energy phosphate bond of adenosine triphosphate (ATP) provides sufficient energy so that the Na^+,K^+ pump can concentrate K^+ approximately 20-fold in cells and thus can extrude Na^+ against approximately a 20-fold concentration gradient. This transport is electrogenic because 1 net positive charge is extruded during each cycle. The resulting current flow usually adds approximately 1 to 2 mV to the resting membrane potential determined from ion gradients and permeabilities. The Na^+,K^+ pump compensates for the loss of K^+ through the various types of K^+-permeable channels.

K^+ Channels and K^+ Currents

The membrane potential (E_m) in vascular smooth muscle cells (VSMCs) is a function of the Na^+, K^+, and Cl^- concentration gradients across the plasma membrane and the relative ion permeabilities (P) as given by

$$E_m = 58 \log [(P_{Na}[Na^+]_{out} + P_K[K^+]_{out} + P_{Cl}[Cl^-]_{cyt})/(P_{Na}[Na^+]_{cyt} + P_K[K^+]_{cyt} + P_{Cl}[Cl^-]_{out})]$$

where *out* and *cyt* refer to the extracellular (out) and cytosolic (cyt) ion concentrations. In resting VSMCs, membrane potential is controlled primarily by K^+ permeability and gradient, because $P_K \gg P_{Cl} > P_{Na}$. K^+ permeability is directly related to the whole-cell K^+ current ($I_K = NiP_o$, where N is the number of membrane K^+ channels, i is the single-channel current, and P_o is the open-state probability of a K^+ channel). When K^+ chan-

nels close, P_K and I_K decrease and cell membrane potential becomes less negative (i.e., the membrane depolarizes).

At least 4 types of K^+ currents have been described in VSMCs: voltage-gated K^+ currents [$I_{K(V)}$], Ca^{2+}-activated K^+ currents [$I_{K(Ca)}$], ATP-sensitive K^+ currents [$I_{K(ATP)}$], and inward rectifier K^+ currents [$I_{K(IR)}$]. These currents are carried by 3 corresponding K^+ channels: voltage-gated channels (K_V), Ca^{2+}-activated channels (K_{Ca}), and inward rectifier channels (K_{IR}). Voltage-gated and Ca^{2+}-activated channels are composed of 2 structurally distinct types of subunits: large pore-forming α subunits, and small cytoplasmic β subunits. The kinetics and gating of the K^+ channels encoded by certain α subunits can be dramatically affected by their associated β subunits. Different K^+ channel subunits (α and β) can coassociate *in vivo* to yield a large number of functionally distinct K^+ channels.

Voltage-gated K^+ channels. Voltage-gated K^+ (K_V) channels of VSMCs carry a rapidly inactivating A-type current, a slowly inactivating delayed rectifier current, and a noninactivating delayed rectifier current. These are activated in the voltage range of resting E_m in VSMCs; the unitary conductance is 5 to 65 picoSiemens (pS). 4-Aminopyridine (4-AP) is a potent blocker of K_V channels. Functionally, the noninactivating or slowly inactivating delayed rectifier K_V channels are the major determinants of resting E_m and, thus, intracellular Ca^{2+} concentration ($[Ca^{2+}]_{cyt}$) and tonic tension in VSMCs. Inhibition of K_V channels (e.g., by 4-AP or hypoxia in pulmonary VSMCs) depolarizes the cells, induces Ca^{2+}-dependent action potentials, raises $[Ca^{2+}]_{cyt}$, and causes vasoconstriction. In contrast, activation of K_V channels by agents like nitric oxide hyperpolarizes VSMCs, closes voltage-gated Ca^{2+} channels, and causes vasodilation.

Native K_V channels are homomultimers or heteromultimers composed of 4 identical or similar α subunits and perhaps 4 β subunits. The α subunit consists of 6 transmembrane domains

(S1 through S6), a pore-forming region (H5, located in the loop between the S5 and S6 domains), and cytoplasmic N- and C-termini. Segment S4 is the voltage sensor. There are at least 13 subfamilies of K_V channel α subunits (K_V1 through K_V11, K_VLQT, and *eag*). Four (K_V5, K_V6, K_V8, and K_V9) are electrically silent modulatory α subunits, whereas the remainder are functional α subunits. There are three subfamilies of β subunits: $K_V\beta1$ through $K_V\beta3$.

Ca²⁺-activated K⁺ channels. Ca²⁺-activated K⁺ (K_{Ca}) channels are the major Ca²⁺-regulated channels. By opening when Ca²⁺ enters cells, K_{Ca} channels may contribute to negative-feedback regulation of membrane potential and vascular tone. There are 3 types of K_{Ca} channels: small-conductance (4 to 14 pS; SK channels), intermediate-conductance (100 to 200 pS; IK channels), and large-conductance (200 to 285 pS; BK or maxi-K channels). Apamin blocks SK channels but negligibly affects BK and IK channels. BK channels are very sensitive to charybdotoxin (from scorpion venom) and tetraethylammonium. Voltage and Ca²⁺ gating for K_{Ca} channels are synergistic; therefore, K_{Ca} channels play a critical role in coupling changes in $[Ca^{2+}]_{cyt}$ to changes in E_m. K_{Ca} channels are half-maximally activated between +12 and +30 mV, and most are closed in VSMCs under resting conditions, where E_m = –60 to –40 mV and $[Ca^{2+}]_{cyt}$ = 50 to 100 nmol/L. Toxins that inhibit K_{Ca} channels enhance evoked membrane depolarization and elevation of $[Ca^{2+}]_{cyt}$ in stimulated VSMCs. Normally, K_{Ca} channels control E_m and vascular tone by negative-feedback regulation of the degree of membrane depolarization caused by myogenic factors and vasoactive substances.

The α subunit of the BK channel is encoded by the slowpoke gene (*Slo*), first identified in *Drosophila*. The channel protein shares extensive homology with the K_V channels of the Shaker (K_V1) subfamily. In 1996, the small-conductance, apamin-sensitive K_{Ca} channel was also cloned; it has a membrane topology similar to those of K_V and BK channels. The β1 subunit of the BK channel tunes the Ca²⁺ sensitivity and voltage dependence of the channel. Deletion of the gene that encodes this subunit reduces the Ca²⁺ sensitivity of BK channels at given membrane potentials.

Inward rectifier K⁺ channels. Rectifiers conduct current in 1 direction only. K_{IR} channels conduct inward K⁺ current but little outward current. K_{IR} channels are blocked by intracellular Mg²⁺ and Cs⁺ and external Ba²⁺. K_{IR} channels in VSMCs set the resting E_m, prevent membrane hyperpolarization by the electrogenic Na⁺, K⁺-ATPase, mediate K⁺-induced vasodilation, and minimize loss of cell K⁺. In contrast to K_V and K_{Ca} channels, K_{IR} channels contain only 2 transmembrane domains (M1 and M2). Heteromultimeric combinations of different K_{IR} channel subunits form distinct K⁺ channels; for example, the acetylcholine-sensitive, G protein–gated K⁺ channel (I_{KACh}) is a heteromultimer composed of 2 distinct types of K_{IR} subunits, $K_{IR}3.1$ and $K_{IR}3.4$.

Adenosine triphosphate–sensitive K⁺ channels. Adenosine triphosphate–sensitive K⁺ (K_{ATP}) channels are inhibited by intracellular ATP and activated by adenosine diphosphate (ADP). They fall into 2 categories: low-conductance (10 to 50 pS) and large-conductance (=130 pS) K_{ATP} channels. Electrophysiologic studies demonstrate that $I_{K(ATP)}$ is voltage independent. Sulfonylureas, such as glibenclamide, are selective blockers of K_{ATP} channels. In coronary and cerebral arteries,

metabolic regulation of basal tone and blood flow involves modulation of K_{ATP} channels. During hypoxia or ischemia, ATP falls and ADP rises. This activates K_{ATP} channels, hyperpolarizes VSMCs, and contributes to vasodilation. K_{ATP} channels are heteromultimers: 4 $K_{IR}6.2$ (pore-forming) subunits and 4 SUR1 subunits are required to form a K_{ATP} channel. $K_{IR}6.2$ also serves as the ATP sensor, whereas SUR1 confers sensitivity to sulfonylureas, channel openers like diazoxide, and ADP.

Role of K⁺ Channels in Regulating Membrane Potential, Ca²⁺ Concentration, and Vascular Tone

Owing to the voltage dependence of sarcolemmal voltage-gated Ca²⁺ channels, E_m plays an important role in regulating intracellular Ca²⁺ in VSMCs. Closure or inactivation of K⁺ channels lowers E_m (depolarizes), which increases $[Ca^{2+}]_{cyt}$ by opening voltage-gated Ca²⁺ channels. This influx of Ca²⁺ causes vasoconstriction. In contrast, opening or activation of K⁺ channels hyperpolarizes VSMCs, closes voltage-gated Ca²⁺ channels, and causes vasodilation. Many vasodilators activate K⁺ channels, including β-adrenergic agonists, muscarinic agonists, and nitroglycerin. Endothelium-derived relaxing factors (e.g., nitric oxide and prostacyclin) open K_V and K_{Ca} channels in pulmonary and systemic vessels. Antihypertensive drugs such as diazoxide and cromakalim also open K_{ATP} channels.

Ca²⁺ entry through voltage-gated Ca²⁺ channels raises $[Ca^{2+}]_{cyt}$. This activates Ca²⁺- and ryanodine-sensitive sarcoplasmic reticulum (SR) Ca²⁺-release channels. The coordinated opening of clusters of these SR channels produces "Ca²⁺ sparks," which contribute to the global elevation of $[Ca^{2+}]_{cyt}$ and VSMC contraction. Ca²⁺ sparks that occur in regions of SR adjacent to the plasma membrane may activate nearby BK channels or Ca²⁺-activated Cl⁻ channels. Opening the latter depolarizes VSMC and thereby exerts positive feedback on the rise in $[Ca^{2+}]_{cyt}$. Opening of BK channels, however, hyperpolarizes VSMC and exerts a potent negative feedback effect on the $[Ca^{2+}]_{cyt}$ elevation and contraction. Thus, SR Ca²⁺ release contributes to positive and negative feedback regulation of vascular smooth muscle contraction.

Dysfunctional K⁺ Channels and Hypertension

Defective K⁺ channels have been implicated in some types of essential hypertension and pulmonary hypertension. In systemic (renal and mesenteric) VSMCs from spontaneously hypertensive rats, voltage-activated and cromakalim-activated K⁺ channels are significantly decreased compared with those in normotensive rats. In pulmonary VSMCs from patients with primary pulmonary hypertension, voltage-activated K⁺ current is significantly attenuated compared with that in control cells. Hypoxia and the anorexic agent fenfluramine can cause pulmonary hypertension. In pulmonary VSMCs, both hypoxia and fenfluramine reduce the 4-AP–sensitive K⁺ current, depolarize E_m, and increase cytoplasmic Ca²⁺. These observations fit the view that dysfunctional K⁺ channels in pulmonary and systemic VSMCs may play an etiologic role in the development of pulmonary and systemic arterial hypertension.

SUGGESTED READING

1. Brenner R, Perez GJ, Bonev AD, et al. Vasoregulation by the β1 subunit of the calcium-activated potassium channel. *Nature.* 2000;407:870–876.

2. Carl A, Lee HK, Sanders KM. Regulation of ion channels in smooth muscles by calcium. *Am J Physiol.* 1996;271:C9–C34.

3. Cook NS. The pharmacology of potassium channels and their therapeutic potential. *Trends Pharmacol Sci.* 1988;9:21–28.

4. Jaggar JH, Porter VA, Lederer WJ, Nelson MT. Calcium sparks in smooth muscle. *Am J Physiol Cell Physiol.* 2000;278:C235–C256.

5. Nelson MT, Patlak JB, Worley JF, Standen N. Calcium channels, potassium channels, and voltage dependence of arterial smooth muscle tone. *Am J Physiol.* 1990;259:C3–C18.

6. Nelson MT, Quayle JM. Physiological roles and properties of potassium channels in arterial smooth muscle. *Am J Physiol.* 1995;268:C799–C822.

7. Yuan X-J. Voltage-gated K^+ currents regulate resting membrane potential and $[Ca^{2+}]_i$ in pulmonary arterial myocytes. *Circ Res.* 1995;77:370–378.

8. Yuan X-J, Tod ML, Rubin LJ, Blaustein MP. NO hyperpolarizes pulmonary artery smooth muscle cells and decreases the intracellular Ca^{2+} concentration by activating voltage-gated K^+ channels. *Proc Natl Acad Sci U S A.* 1996;93:10489–10494.

Chapter A27

Calcium Transport and Calmodulin

David J. Triggle, PhD, DSc (Hon.)

KEY POINTS

- Intracellular calcium is a critical determinant of the stimulus-response paradigm, including excitation-contraction and stimulus-secretion coupling, gene activation, and cell death.

- Calcium is stored in intracellular pools, including the endoplasmic or sarcoplasmic reticulum and mitochondria, from which it is transiently released through the action of various pumps and channels that actively regulate intracellular calcium.

- Calmodulin, a Ca^{2+}-binding protein that is the most important transducer of intracellular Ca^{2+} signals, functions in diverse ways through protein kinases, ion channels, protein phosphatases such as calcineurin, and nitric oxide synthase.

- Calmodulin acts in a temporally and spatially heterogeneous manner that parallels the heterogeneous activation and distribution of Ca^{2+}; its expression is encoded by a family of nonallelic genes and is highly conserved across species.

- Movement of Ca^{2+} into cells occurs via 6 types of voltage-gated Ca^{2+} channels, 2 of which (T- and L-types) are of particular cardiovascular significance, and through ligand-gated ion channels.

See also Chapters A25, A26, A28, A32, A33, A47, and C146

Intracellular Calcium

Calcium is a cation of critical significance to cellular control mechanisms, serving as a ubiquitous second messenger and, in excitable cells, a current-carrying species. Both roles serve to link events at the plasma membrane with cellular responses, including muscle contraction, hormone and neurotransmitter release, gene activation, fertilization, and cell death and destruction. Calcium is thus both a physiologic and a pathologic cation—one that brings us into, and takes us out of, this world.

Calcium Gradients and Calcium Sparks

During excitation, intracellular Ca^{2+} concentration rises either by Ca^{2+} entry through the plasma membrane via voltage- or ligand-gated ion channels, or by release from intracellular stores. Ca^{2+} sensors that control the activities of pumps, enzymes, and other targets detect these increased Ca^{2+} levels and control processes that restore the physiologically low levels of intracellular Ca^{2+}.

In resting states, there is an extremely high Ca^{2+} gradient; free ionized intracellular Ca^{2+} is maintained at very low levels ($< 5 \times 10^{-8}$ mol/L) despite plasma concentrations in the milli-

molar range. Plasma levels are themselves tightly regulated through a triumvirate of hormones: vitamin D, parathyroid, and calcitonin. During stimulation, intracellular Ca^{2+} concentration can rise up to 200-fold, to approximately 10^{-5} mol/L. These elevated concentrations are coupled to cellular responses through a homologous group of Ca^{2+} binding proteins, including the ubiquitous calmodulin, which serve as intracellular Ca^{2+} sensors.

Changes in intracellular Ca^{2+} are spatially and temporally heterogeneous, and localized "hot spots" or "sparks" are observed, together with waves of Ca^{2+} that are propagated through the excited cell. These oscillations may represent a graded signal being converted into digital signals, the sequential activation of Ca^{2+}-demanding processes that require different timing of signals, or different concentrations of Ca^{2+}. Heterogeneity of Ca^{2+} mobilization likely serves as a mechanism that protects the cell against the deleterious consequences of persistently elevated Ca^{2+} levels.

Regulation of Cellular Calcium Stores

Sources. Two principal sources of Ca^{2+} are used in cellular signaling: (a) release from intracellular stores in the sarcoplasmic

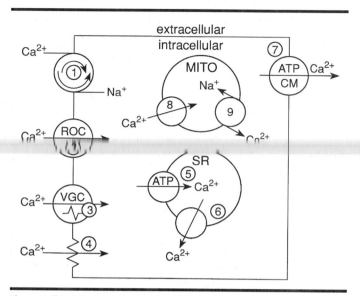

Figure A27.1. The regulation of cellular Ca^{2+} movements. (1) Na^+/Ca^{2+} exchanger; (2) receptor-operated (ligand-gated) channels; (3) voltage-gated channels; (4) store-operated channels; (5) adenosine triphosphate (ATP)–dependent Ca^{2+} uptake into sarcoplasmic reticulum; (6) Ca^{2+} release channel; (7) ATP-dependent pump across the plasma membrane; (8, 9) mitochondrial (MITO) transport processes. CM, calmodulin, ROC, receptor-operated channel; SR, sarcoplasmic reticulum; VGC, voltage-gated channel.

reticulum or equivalent structures and (b) entry across the plasma membrane. Ca^{2+} mobilization by either route can give rise to "elementary calcium events," representing the opening of single channels. These elementary events can be visualized as "sparks" and "puffs" in fluorescent dye–labeled cells.

Regulatory mechanisms. Ca^{2+} movements are tightly regulated. Various Ca^{2+} regulatory processes are depicted in **Figure A27.1**. These processes are not of equal importance in every cell type, but all cells maintain mechanisms that permit Ca^{2+} influx, efflux, storage, and mobilization and that are critical to the maintenance of overall cellular Ca^{2+} homeostasis. Adenosine triphosphate–dependent pumps direct Ca^{2+} to 2 principal reservoirs: the sarcoplasmic or endoplasmic reticulum and the extracellular space.

Ligand-gated channels. Plasma membrane signals increase intracellular Ca^{2+} through several processes. G protein–coupled receptors and tyrosine kinases typically mobilize Ca^{2+} (via the inositol triphosphate (IP_3) receptor, with subsequent Ca^{2+} release from the endoplasmic reticulum (see Chapters A28–A32). Ligand- (or receptor-operated) and voltage-gated Ca^{2+} channels mobilize Ca^{2+} from extracellular sources. These processes can be linked, as in Ca^{2+}-induced Ca^{2+} release events in which entry of Ca^{2+} stimulates the release of Ca^{2+} from intracellular stores.

Voltage-gated channels. Of particular importance to the cardiovascular system is Ca^{2+} mobilization through voltage-gated channels. Defects in Ca^{2+} regulation contribute to a variety of pathologic states, including the hyperreactivity of vascular smooth muscle in hypertension. A number of molecular diseases are associated with defects in Ca^{2+} channels, including

malignant hyperthermia (ryanodine receptor) and hypokalemic periodic paralysis (L-type voltage-gated Ca^{2+} channel).

Calmodulin

Expression of the intracellular Ca^{2+} signal requires the presence of intracellular sensors or receptors. Calmodulin and the other members (approximately 200) of this protein family bind calcium with micromolar affinity and undergo conformational changes linked to effector recruitment. These proteins share a common Ca^{2+}-binding motif: the EF hand (a helix-loop-helix structure).

Structure. Calmodulin is a 148-residue protein that contains 4 EF hands, 2 each at the C- and N-terminal domains, respectively. Calcium binding to these hands is a cooperative process that is accompanied by significant conformational changes of the protein structure. In these changes, the α-helical content of the protein increases, and the C- and N-terminal domains become separated and then connected via an α-helix to form a dumbbell-shaped structure. This helix allows calmodulin to interact with many different effector proteins that typically contain calmodulin-binding domains constituted by 9 to 26 amino acid residue amphipathic helices.

Function. Calmodulin is found in all smooth muscle and nonmuscle cells where it regulates large families of intracellular Ca^{2+}-dependent proteins, including cyclic nucleotide phosphodiesterase, adenylyl cyclase, Ca^{2+}-adenosine triphosphatase, phosphorylase kinase, phospholipase A_2, nitric oxide synthase, voltage-gated Ca^{2+} channels, IP_3 and ryanodine receptors, transcription factors including the cyclic adenosine monophosphate response element binding protein, serum response factor and CAAT-enhancer binding protein, and the several proteins involved in vesicle-driven neurotransmitter release.

Interactions. Calmodulin interacts reversibly with many targets with K_D values in the nanomolar range, but it also functions as an integral subunit with other targets, including inducible nitric oxide synthase and the ryanodine receptor. The dynamic association of calmodulin with its targets is determined by the limiting stoichiometric availability of the protein. This competition among targets facilitates cross-talk between multiple calmodulin-sensitive signaling pathways.

Ca^{2+}/Calmodulin-Dependent Protein Kinases

General properties. A major responsibility of calmodulin is the activation of members of the serine/tyrosine protein kinase family referred to as *Ca^{2+}/calmodulin-dependent protein kinases* or *CaM kinases*. This large family includes the CaM kinases I, II, III, and IV, phosphorylase kinase, and myosin light-chain kinase. These kinases share a similar domain structure but differ functionally according to whether they are multifunctional with several substrates (CaM kinase I, II, and IV) or have but a single substrate (phosphorylase kinase, myosin light-chain kinase, and CaM kinase III). The general domain architecture of these kinases is that of an N-terminal kinase domain followed by an autoinhibitory domain and a calmodulin-binding domain and, for phosphorylase kinase and CaM kinase II, a C-terminal oligomerization domain.

The role of Ca^{2+}/CaM is to bind to the protein and remove the autoinhibitory domain that functions as a pseudosubstrate, allowing substrate access.

Subtypes. CaM kinases are also distinguished by their localization and activation characteristics. The multifunctional CaM kinases I and II are ubiquitously expressed in the cytoplasm, whereas CaM kinase IV has a more limited nuclear and cytoplasmic localization. CaM kinase II, the best characterized of the CaM kinases is encoded by 4 separate genes—α, β, γ, and δ—and their alternate splicing yields a total of 24 subtypes; every cell contains at least 1 subtype of this kinase. Activation of the CaM kinases depends on their primary interaction with calmodulin but may also be further achieved by phosphorylation. CaM kinases I and IV are phosphorylated in the activation loop embedded within the catalytic domain and CaM kinase IV also undergoes autophosphorylation to achieve further activation. This autoregulatory process confers significant activity on CaM kinase II even in the absence of Ca^{2+}/CaM ("autonomous activity") and provides an ability to translate Ca^{2+} transient frequencies into graded levels of effector activation. The CaM kinases are themselves part of a regulatory cascade being activated by other kinases—that is, CaM kinase kinases. CaM kinase I and IV are activated by CaM kinase kinases α and β, which may themselves be activated by other upstream kinases.

Calcium Pumps

The 2 principal pumps involved in the control of poststimulus Ca^{2+} levels are located in the sarcoplasmic reticulum (or endoplasmic reticulum) and plasma membrane (Figure A27.1). Ca^{2+} activation of the pumps provides a critical link between Ca^{2+}-mobilizing processes and cellular recovery from elevated intracellular Ca^{2+} levels. The CaM-dependent adenosine triphosphatase of the plasma membrane is widely distributed across eukaryotic cells. In nonmuscle cells, the role of the plasma membrane pump is likely to be minor. Both pumps are of the P-type and can be distinguished from the multimeric F- and V-types. The P-type pumps form an energized acyl-phosphate intermediate that is coupled to Ca^{2+} transport through the interconversion of E1 and E2 states. The cardiac isoform of the pump is regulated by the inhibitory protein phospholamban which, when phosphorylated through adenosine monophosphate and CaM kinase, dissociates to relieve inhibition. Pump activity is also modulated by acidic phospholipids and polyunsaturated fatty acids, notably phosphatidylinositol and its phosphorylated derivatives. Additionally, inhibitors such as thapsigargin bind with subnanomolar affinity to the pump, trapping it in a "dead-end" conformation.

Calcium Channels

The 2 major types of calcium channels are widely distributed in excitable tissues. Those in are the voltage-sensitive (voltage-gated) channels and the (relatively) voltage-independent (ligand-gated) channels.

Voltage-gated Ca²⁺ channels. Voltage-gated Ca^{2+} channels, widely distributed in excitable tissues, are located in close spatial proximity to the vesicular neurotransmitter release mechanism, thus ensuring a tight temporal and spatial coupling between nerve impulse and transmitter release. Depletion of intracellular Ca^{2+} stores is also linked to the opening of store-operated Ca^{2+} channels in the plasma membrane.

Subclasses. At least 6 major classes of voltage-gated Ca^{2+} channels exist in the cardiovascular and nervous systems: T, L, N, P, Q, and R (Ca_V1, Ca_V2, and Ca_V3) classes. They are distinguished by their electrophysiologic and pharmacologic characteristics, their function, and their localization. The T- and L-type channels are of particular importance to the functional pharmacology of the cardiovascular system, and the L-type channel is the site of action of the therapeutically important Ca^{2+} channel blockers (including diltiazem, verapamil, nifedipine, and the second-generation 1,4-dihydropyridines such as amlodipine and isradipine).

Structure and function. Voltage-gated Ca^{2+} channels belong to an ion channel "superfamily" that includes Na^+ and K^+ channels. The channels have a heteromeric structure with the principal α-subunit possessing the channel pore and gating mechanisms as well as the drug binding sites. The properties of this channel subunit are substantially modified by the presence of other subunits, notably the β-subunit.

Regulation of activity. The activities of the voltage-gated Ca^{2+} channels are regulated by their association with calmodulin, parallel to the behavior of other ion channels, including Ca^{2+}-activated big conductance K^+ channels and cyclic nucleotide-gated channels. Calmodulin interacts at the IQ domain of the α-subunit of the voltage-gated Ca^{2+} channel of the L, P/Q, and R types, where the association with the permeant Ca^{2+} then mediates channel inactivation.

Voltage-independent (ligand-gated) Ca²⁺ channels. Some evidence suggests that ligand-gated and store-operated channels may belong to the same protein family—the transient receptor potential channel (TRP) type. α-Receptors and angiotensin II receptors are examples of this type of channel. Intracellular release of calcium is controlled by 2 classes of ligand-gated Ca^{2+} channels: IP3- and ryanodine-sensitive channels that are linked to G protein–coupled receptors and to Ca^{2+} influx, respectively. These channels are structurally related but exist in multiple subclasses that are expressed in tissue-specific manner. Both types of channels show biphasic sensitivity to Ca^{2+} with low concentrations of Ca^{2+} serving to activate and mediate Ca^{2+} release and high Ca^{2+} serving to blunt or inhibit activation. The low-dose stimulatory effect of Ca^{2+} underlies the phenomenon of "Ca^{2+}-induced Ca^{2+} release" (see Chapter A32).

SUGGESTED READING

1. Ashcroft FM. *Ion Channels and Disease*. London, UK: Academic Press; 2000.
2. Carafoli E, Klee C, eds. *Calcium as a Cellular Regulator*. New York, NY: Oxford University Press; 1999.
3. Elliott AC. Recent developments in non-excitable cell calcium entry. *Cell Calcium*. 2001;30:73–93.
4. Hook SS, Means AR. Ca^{2+}/CaM-Dependent kinases: from activation to function. *Annu Rev Pharmacol Toxicol*. 2001;41:471–508.
5. McFadzean I, Gibson A. The developing relationship between receptor-operated and store-operated calcium channels in smooth muscle. *Brit J Pharmacol*. 2002;135:1–13.

6. Means AR. Regulatory cascades involving calmodulin-dependent protein kinases. *Mol Endocrinol*. 2000;14:4–13.
7. Persechini A, Stemmer PM. Calmodulin is a limiting factor in the cell. *Trends Cardiovasc Med*. 2002;12:32–38.
8. Soderling TR, Chang B, Brickey D. Cellular signaling through multifunc-
tional Ca^{2+}/calmodulin-dependent protein kinase II. *J Biol Chem*. 2001;276:3719–3722.
9. Toutenhoofd SL, Strehler EE. The calmodulin multigene family as a unique case of genetic redundancy: multiple levels of regulation to provide spatial and temporal control of calmodulin pools? *Cell Calcium*. 2000;28:83–96.

Chapter A28

Receptors and Functions

Greti Aguilera, MD

KEY POINTS

- Receptors are protein complexes that recognize specific hormones and translate extracellular hormonal influences into intracellular events.

- The guanyl nucleotide protein–coupled receptor superfamily is the largest group of plasma membrane receptors.

- Hormone-ligand binding activates receptors acutely but usually downregulates receptor number or affinity chronically, thus reducing tissue sensitivity.

- Receptor binding properties and signaling efficacy can be modulated by protein-protein interactions between homologous or heterologous receptors or with other nonreceptor proteins.

See also Chapters A1, A3, A9, A12–A18, A29–A33, A75, A76, C140–C142, C145, and C148

General Properties of Receptors

Cell communication, an essential component of integrated physiologic function in multicellular organisms, is mediated largely through informational molecules such as hormones and neurotransmitters. These molecules, or "first messengers," are recognized by 2 types of receptor proteins in the target cell. Type 1 includes receptors for growth factors, catecholamines, cytokines, and prostaglandins that are located in the plasma membrane. Type 2 receptors, including receptors for steroids and iodothyronines, are located in the cytoplasm or nucleus of the cell. Receptors have 2 major functions: (a) recognition of a specific hormone ligand and (b) intracellular transmission of information leading to modification of cell function. Hormone analogs capable of binding the receptor without activating transduction mechanisms act as receptor antagonists.

Receptor Binding Properties

Binding kinetics. The use of radiolabeled ligands has made the identification and measurement of receptors for steroids, peptide hormones, and neurotransmitters in their target tissues possible. In general, each ligand-receptor interaction is rapid and reversible, consistent with the time course of the biologic effects of hormones. Binding kinetics depend on the rates of association and dissociation of the ligand-receptor complexes, which are affected by temperature and pH. The ratio between association and dissociation rates determines the association constant. The reciprocal of the association constant is the dissociation constant, which is usually expressed as the ligand concentration necessary to saturate the binding sites.

Affinity and receptor number. Receptor-ligand binding exhibits high affinity, which allows for significant binding despite low circulating levels of hormones. Receptor binding is always saturable, indicating a limited number of binding sites. Receptor affinity usually correlates well with tissue sensitivity to the biologic effect of the hormone, but in a number of systems, full biologic response is achieved with only partial receptor occupancy. The presence of excess or "spare" receptors may be important to maintain biologic effects of hormones in physiologic or pathologic conditions involving alterations of receptor number. Biologic activity of receptors is often modulated by receptor oligomerization or by association of receptors with other cell proteins.

Transduction Mechanisms

In general, a requisite for a receptor molecule is the ability to communicate information to effector molecules inside the cell. The informational transduction can be carried out by the receptor itself or through activation of intermediary signaling molecules.

Type 1 (cell surface) receptors. Interaction of hormones or neurotransmitters with cell surface receptors leads to modification of cell function through a chain of events involving the generation of "second-messenger" molecules. Cell surface receptors can be categorized into 2 major groups: (a) receptors with intrinsic enzymatic or ion channel activity (see Chapter A27) and (b) receptors coupled to cellular effector molecules through a transduction protein (see Chapter A29). Molecular cloning and characterization of these receptors show that they are anchored to the cell membrane through 1 or several hydrophobic amino acid sequences. In general, the structure of these receptors consists of an extracellular domain, transmembrane regions, and 1 or more intracellular regions responsible for catalytic activity or coupling to intermediary proteins.

Type 2 (intracellular) receptors. Intracellular receptors, such as steroid and thyroid hormone receptors, are dimeric proteins consisting of a hormone-binding subunit and a regulatory subunit. After ligand (first-messenger) binding, the regulatory subunit dissociates from the complex, and the activated hormone-binding subunit interacts with DNA, influencing gene transcription. Activated receptors interact with DNA-responsive elements in the form of homodimers. Receptor-DNA binding activity can be modulated through formation of heterodimers with other cellular proteins or transacting factors.

Intrinsic Activity of Cell Surface Receptors

Receptor intrinsic activity. Receptors for growth factors and insulin include a tyrosine kinase domain and 1 or more tyrosine phosphorylation sites as structural parts of the receptor molecule. Ligand interaction with these receptors results in receptor autophosphorylation, leading to binding of the phosphorylated receptor domains to signaling molecules such as phosphatidylinositol kinase, guanosine triphosphatase (GTPase)-activating factor, phospholipase C, src, or serine kinases.

Receptor-gated ion channels. Receptor-gated ion channels, in which the receptor is a structural component of the ion channel, also exhibit intrinsic activity. Examples of this type are γ-aminobutyric acid receptors associated with Cl^- and HCO_3^- transport; nicotinic acetylcholine receptors associated with Na^+, K^+, and Ca^{2+} transport; N-methyl-D-aspartate and non-NMDA glutamate receptors associated with Na^+, K^+, and Ca^{2+} transport; 5-hydroxytryptamine receptors associated with Na^+ and K^+ transport; and channel-opening adenosine triphosphate receptors associated with Ca^{2+}, Na^+, and Mg^{2+} transport.

Receptors without intrinsic activity. A second group of cell-surface receptors lacks intrinsic activity and uses an intermediary protein or enzyme such as adenylate cyclase, phospholipase C, ion channels, or tyrosine kinases for signaling to effectors. Two major types belong to this group: (a) the cytokine receptor superfamily, including growth hormone and prolactin receptors, which activate tyrosine kinases of the JAK family, and (b) the G protein receptor superfamily (GPCR).

G protein–coupled activation. G proteins are located on the intracellular side of the plasma membrane, in which they can interact with receptors as well as effector signaling systems. G proteins consist of three subunits, α, β, and γ, of which α has guanosine triphosphate (GTP) binding and GTPase activity properties (see Chapter A29). Occupancy of the receptor by its ligand causes conformational changes in the associated G protein, allowing binding of the α subunit to GTP and dissociation from the β/γ-complex. The activated α subunit activates an effector molecule, such as adenylyl cyclase or phospholipase C. This process is rapidly reversible on degradation of bound GTP by the intrinsic GTPase activity of the α subunit.

Nonagonist G protein interactions. Although ligand binding is responsible for hormonal activation of receptors, there is evidence that unligated GPCRs exist in at least 2 states: an inactive conformation and a constitutively active conformation with affinity for the G protein in the absence of agonist. Inverse agonists are ligand analogs that preferentially stabilize the receptor in the inactive conformation, thus decreasing basal receptor activity in the absence of ligand.

Receptor Regulation

The effectiveness of a hormone depends on its concentration, the number and affinity of receptors in the target tissue, and postreceptor events.

Receptor number. For a given set of conditions, changes in receptor number result in changes in the concentration of agonist needed to achieve an effect. In tissues containing "spare receptors," the effect may be achieved at very low agonist concentrations. When viewed from the perspective of the standard sigmoidal dose-response relationships observed with most ligands, the presence of spare receptors corresponds to a shift to the left of the dose-response curve. In contrast, if additional receptors are synthesized, the maximum (plateau) effect may increase.

Heterologous regulation. Although peptide hormone receptors undergo changes in number and affinity when exposed to their ligand (homologous regulation), the binding and activity of many receptors can be regulated by heterologous hormones. For example, thyroid hormone regulates the number of β receptors. Increased hormone levels usually result in receptor loss and desensitization of the biologic responses to the hormone. For example, β receptors are downregulated by epinephrine.

Downregulation. Several types of mechanisms lead to receptor downregulation. (a) Negative cooperativity occurs with the insulin receptor, in which partial receptor occupancy decreases the binding affinity of the remaining receptors. (b) Internalization and lysosomal degradation of hormone-receptor complexes occur with receptors for epidermal growth factor, human chorionic gonadotropin, gonadotropin-releasing hormone, and insulin. (c) Receptor phosphorylation can be heterologous via second messenger–dependent kinases or homologous via phosphorylation of agonist-occupied receptor by G protein receptor kinases. (d) Guanyl nucleotides reduce high-affinity binding in membrane preparations of a number of GPCRs, probably through conformational changes in the receptor protein. Some peptide hormone receptors, such as adrenal angiotensin II (Ang II), prolactin, and gonadotropin-releasing hormone receptors, have been shown to undergo upregulation after exposure to increased hormone levels.

Tissue sensitivity. In a number of conditions, receptor regulation can contribute to the sensitivity of the target tissue to a hormone. For example, downregulation of Ang II receptors could account for the low pressor responses to the peptide during sodium restriction and other clinical states of high renin secretion. Conversely, upregulation of Ang II receptors may contribute to the increases in sensitivity of the adrenal glomerulosa to Ang II during sodium restriction.

Protein-Protein Interactions and Receptor Function

Dimerization and oligomerization. There is increasing evidence that activity of the GPCRs can be modulated by interactions with other G protein receptors and various other proteins, effectors, or second messengers. Evidence from ligand binding, immunodetection, co-immunoprecipitation, and confocal microscopy (with fluorescent or bioluminescent energy transfer) demonstrate that some GPCRs function as homodimers or larger oligomers. GPCRs may also form heterodimers, either between subtypes of the same receptor family or between receptors of different families. Receptor homo- or heterodimerization modulates binding affinity, coupling to signaling systems, and agonist-mediated endocytosis.

Receptor-modulating proteins. In addition, certain G protein receptors can change their ligand binding specificities as a result of direct interactions with other intracellular and extracellular proteins. The most dramatic example occurs with the receptor for calcitonin gene-related peptide and adrenomedullin. The CGRP receptor interacts with novel proteins encoded by the same gene, called *receptor activity modifying proteins*. Interaction with different members of the receptor activity modifying protein family determines receptor specificity as the adrenomedullin or the calcitonin gene-related peptide receptor. Other proteins with specific receptor-modulating properties

are the AT_1 receptor-associated protein, shown to specifically downregulate AT_1 angiotensin receptors, and a 24 kd single transmembrane domain protein called *calcyon*, which modifies coupling of the dopamine D_1 receptor. Such protein-protein interactions allow a greater diversity of function for individual GPCRs within different cell backgrounds. The composition of the various protein complexes can also influence other receptor properties such as subcellular localization, binding affinity and specificity, and signaling and trafficking processes.

SUGGESTED READING

1. Bouvier M. Oligomerization of G-protein-coupled receptors. *Nat Rev Neurosci*. 2001;2:274–286.
2. Ferguson SS, Caron M. G-protein-coupled receptor adaptation mechanisms. *Semin Cell Dev Biol*. 1998;9:119–127.
3. Kahn RC, Smith RJ, Chin WW. Mechanism of action of hormones that act at the cell surface. In: Wilson JD, Foster DW, Kronenberg HM, Larsen PR, eds. *Williams Textbook of Endocrinology*. Philadelphia, PA: WB Saunders; 1998.
4. Milligan G, White JH. Protein-protein interactions at G-protein-coupled receptors. *Trends Pharmacol Sci*. 2001;22:513–518.
5. Rodbell M. The complex regulation of receptor-coupled G-proteins. *Adv Enzyme Regul*. 1997;37:427–435.
6. Wess J. Molecular basis of receptor/G-protein-coupling selectivity. *Pharmacol Ther*. 1998;80:231–264.

Chapter A29

Guanine Nucleotide Binding Proteins

James C. Garrison, PhD

KEY POINTS

- Guanine nucleotide binding proteins (G proteins) induce a wide variety of responses in differentiated target cells in response to ligands bound to receptor types with 7 transmembrane-spanning domains.

- G proteins communicate the signal of ligand binding by regulating the activity of intracellular effectors, such as adenylyl cyclase, phospholipase C-β, and ion channels, which in turn regulate the levels of second messengers such as cyclic adenosine monophosphate, inositol phosphates, diacylglycerol, and K^+ or Ca^{2+} ions.

- G proteins can be stimulatory or inhibitory; interactions of G protein receptors can counterregulate physiologic effects within single cells.

See also Chapters A1, A3, A12, A15, A17, A24, A28, and A30–A33

G Protein–Coupled Receptors

Many cell surface receptors regulate intracellular effectors through a family of signal-transducing proteins termed *guanine nucleotide binding proteins*, or *G proteins*, that are common to virtually all cells. The specificity of response in a given tissue is achieved by several linked factors: differential expression of the receptors that activate the signaling process, the nature of the intracellular signal [e.g., cyclic adenosine monophosphate (cAMP) or Ca^{2+}], the targets of these signals, and the downstream molecule(s) regulated by the signal. Because many of the targets of second messengers are protein kinases, the cellular response in certain tissues is also determined by the nature

of the intracellular substrates expressed for the relevant kinases (see Chapter A32).

Ligand types. G protein–coupled receptors are responsible for monitoring signals from neurotransmitters, hormones, autacoids, lipids such as lysophosphatidic acid or sphingosine-1 phosphate, chemokines, light, odorants, and other sensory stimuli in the extracellular environment. Approximately 60% of these receptors are involved in the sensory pathways of smell, vision, and taste. In the cardiovascular system, some of the major agonists for these receptors are acetylcholine (muscarinic receptors), serotonin, catecholamines, angiotensin, vasopressin, endothelin, histamine, bradykinin, prostaglandins,

Table A29.1. Properties of G Protein α Subunits

α SUBUNIT	TISSUE DISTRIBUTION	EFFECTOR (ACTION)	EFFECT ON MESSAGE
G_s family			
$G_s{}^a$	Wide	Adenylyl cyclase ($\uparrow$)	Increase cAMP
		Ca^{2+} channels ($\uparrow$)	Increase Ca^{2+} current
G_{olf}	Olfactory tissue	Adenylyl cyclase ($\uparrow$)	Increase cAMP
G_i family			
G_{i1}	Wide	Adenylyl cyclase ($\downarrow$)	Decrease cAMP
G_{i2}	Wide	Adenylyl cyclase ($\downarrow$)	Decrease cAMP
G_{i3}	Wide	Adenylyl cyclase ($\downarrow$)	Decrease cAMP
$G_o{}^a$	Neuronal	Ion channels ($\downarrow$)	Decrease Ca^{2+} current
		GRIN ($\uparrow$)	Increase neurite outgrowth
G_i and G_o via $\beta\gamma$		K^+ channels ($\uparrow$)	Increase K^+ current
		Phospholipase C-β ($\uparrow$)	Increase IP$_3$, DAG
		Ca^{2+} channels ($\downarrow$)	Decrease Ca^{2+} current
G_t	Rod and cone cells	cGMP phosphodiesterase ($\uparrow$)	Decrease cGMP
G_g	Tongue	cGMP phosphodiesterase ($\uparrow$)	Decrease cGMP
G_z	Brain	Adenylyl cyclase ($\downarrow$)	Decrease cAMP
G_q family			
G_q	Wide	Phospholipase C-β ($\uparrow$)	Increase IP$_3$, DAG
G_{11}	Wide	Phospholipase C-β ($\uparrow$)	Increase IP$_3$, DAG
G_{14}	Wide	Phospholipase C-β ($\uparrow$)	Increase IP$_3$, DAG
G_{15}	Hematopoietic cells	Phospholipase C-β ($\uparrow$)	Increase IP$_3$, DAG
G_{16}	Hematopoietic cells	Phospholipase C-β ($\uparrow$)	Increase IP$_3$, DAG
G_{12} family			
G_{12}	Wide	Rho GTP exchange factor, cyclase (?)	Activate Rho targets
G_{13}	Wide	Rho GTP exchange factor, Na$^+$/H$^+$ antiporter (?)	Activate Rho targets
		Na$^+$/H$^+$ Antiporter ($\uparrow$)	Change in cytoplasmic [ion]
		Radixin ($\uparrow$)	Increase transformation

cAMP, cyclic adenosine monophosphate; cGMP, cyclic guanosine monophosphate; DAG, diacylglycerol.
^{a}The G_s and G_o α subunits have multiple splice variants.

thrombin, lysophosphatidic acid, sphingosine-1 phosphate, and adenosine.

Receptor structure. G protein–coupled receptors share a characteristic structure composed of 7 membrane-spanning domains with 4 intracellular loops that are responsible for direct interaction with the G proteins. The intracellular segments most responsible for recognition of G proteins include the third intracellular loop between helices V and IV and the carboxyl-terminal domain. G protein–coupled receptors are monomeric proteins with molecular weights ranging from 35,000 to 70,000 kd and are members of the rhodopsin family. The receptors are activated by the binding of ligands to sites within the 7 transmembrane domains or to the extracellular loops of the molecule where ligand binding causes conformational changes in the transmembrane-spanning domains.

Receptor isoforms. It is common for multiple isoforms (or subtypes) of a receptor type to respond to a single ligand; for example, 5 isoforms of the muscarinic receptor all respond to acetylcholine. However, the different isoforms are commonly expressed in different tissues and couple to different G proteins. For example, the muscarinic M$_2$ receptor is expressed in cardiac tissue and regulates members of the G protein–activated inwardly rectifying potassium (GIRK) K$^+$ channels by coupling to the G$_i$ and G$_o$ α subunits (see Chapter A26) and releasing $\beta\gamma$ subunits, which activate the channel. The muscarinic M$_3$ receptor is expressed in smooth muscle and regulates contraction via the G$_q$ α subunit leading to activation of phospholipase C-β and the eventual release of Ca^{2+}.

Receptor networks. G protein–coupled receptors can form complex regulatory networks in which 1 receptor may couple to multiple G proteins and generate a variety of signals in a given cell. Conversely, multiple different types of receptors may interact with a single member of the G protein family and generate the same signal. The best-studied effectors regulated by this mechanism are adenylyl cyclase, cyclic guanosine monophosphate (cGMP) phosphodiesterase, phospholipase C-β, phosphatidylinositol 3-kinase, and certain members of the calcium, sodium, or potassium channel families.

G Protein Family

Basic structure and subunits. The heterotrimeric G proteins themselves are composed of three subunits: α subunits with molecular weights of 39 to 52 kd, β subunits with molecular weights of 35 to 39 kd, and γ subunits with molecular weights of 6 to 8 kd. The α subunits can bind 1 mol guanosine triphosphate (GTP) or guanosine diphosphate (GDP)/mol α subunit. The β and γ subunits form a functional unit, called the *$\beta\gamma$-dimer*, which cannot be dissociated without loss of activity.

Structural diversity. There is significant diversity in the subunits making up the heterotrimer. Currently, 17 genes are known to encode α subunits. Five encode β subunits and 12 encode γ subunits. Alternative splicing of the genes for the α subunit yields 22 different α subunits and splicing of the 5 β subunit genes yields 7 different β subunits. The genes for the 12 γ subunits do not appear to be alternatively spliced. Although some sensory cells express only a limited subset of α and $\beta\gamma$ subunits, most cells can express a majority of the known proteins that compose the heterotrimer (**Table A29.1**). Both the α and γ subunits are posttranslationally modified by lipid attachments, causing the heterotrimer to reside at the inner surface of the plasma membrane. The α subunit is modified by combination with palmitate or myristate. The γ subunits are modified by isoprenylation, farnesylation (in the case of γ-1, γ-8, and γ-11) or geranylgeranyl in all other γ subunits.

Heterotrimer families. The G protein heterotrimers are grouped into 4 families according to the similarity in their amino acid sequences or the function of their α subunits (Table A29.1).

Stimulatory. Members of the G_s (stimulatory) family include the G_s and G_{olf} proteins, which stimulate adenylyl cyclase to produce the second messenger cAMP.

Inhibitory. Members of the G_i (inhibitory) family are more diverse and include the G_t, G_{i1}, G_{i2}, G_{i3}, G_o, G_z, and G_g proteins. The α_i subunits inhibit adenylyl cyclase, regulate the gating of ion channels by releasing the βγ subunit, and the α_t or α_g subunits stimulate cGMP phosphodiesterases, especially those involved in the senses of vision (α_t) and taste (α_g). The G_o α subunit also has a specific effector (G protein–regulated inducer of neurite outgrowth), which induces formation of fine processes in cultured neuronal cells.

G_q Proteins. The G_q family includes G_q, G_{11}, G_{14}, G_{15}, and G_{16}. These α subunits stimulate phospholipase C-β to hydrolyze the membrane lipid phosphatidylinositol 4,5-biphosphate, leading to formation of the second messengers inositol trisphosphate (IP_3) and diacylglycerol (DAG).

G_{12} Proteins. The G_{12} family (including the G_{12} and G_{13} α subunits) can regulate the p115 Rho guanine nucleotide exchange factor (p115 Rho GEF), thus providing a direct link between cell surface receptors coupled to large G proteins and pathways regulated by small G proteins such as *Rho*. The G_{12} and G_{13} α subunits may also interact with proteins such as radixin, which interacts with cytoskeletal elements to affect events such as cell migration and transformation.

Activation of G Proteins by Receptors

Activation complexes and second messengers. The basal state of the G protein signaling system consists of the receptor α-GDP-βγ complex. When an agonist ligand binds to the receptor, the conformational change induced in the receptor causes the α subunit to release the bound GDP. The binding site becomes occupied with GTP from the cytoplasm, causing a conformational change in the α subunit and a reduction in its affinity for the βγ subunit. This activation process generates 2 active signaling molecules, the α-GTP complex and the βγ dimer. Both of these signals can activate effectors (**Figure A29.1**). The activated α-GTP complex regulates effectors such as adenylyl cyclase, the cGMP phosphodiesterase in the visual system, phospholipase C-β, or Na+ channels. Most of these interactions lead to an increase in the level of a second messenger in the cell, such as an increase in adenylyl cyclase activity causing a rise in cAMP levels, or an increase in phospholipase C activity causing a rise in IP_3, intracellular Ca^{2+}, and DAG.

Receptor occupancy and subunit interactions. As receptor occupancy increases, a greater number of α subunits is activated, causing a larger cellular response. βγ subunits also stimulate or inhibit adenylyl cyclase, phospholipase C-β, or muscarinic K+ channel (GIRK channels) in cardiac tissue, and

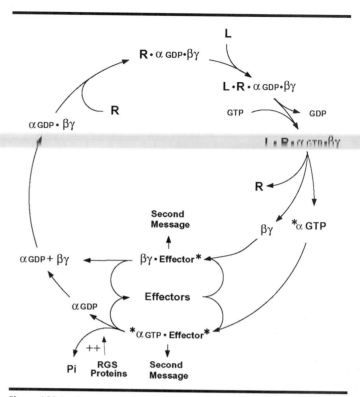

Figure A29.1. Sequence of activation and inactivation of G protein–coupled receptors and effectors. Binding of hormone or other ligand (L) to its receptor (R) causes dissociation of guanosine diphosphate (GDP) and binding of guanosine triphosphate (GTP) to the α subunit of the G protein heterotrimer. Ligand-receptor binding also causes dissociation of G protein subunits. Both the GTP-bound α subunit and βγ subunit regulate the activity of various effectors. Hydrolysis of GTP to GDP and inorganic phosphate (Pi) terminates participation of G protein subunits and leads to their reassociation into the inactive heterotrimer. The regulators of G protein signaling (RGS) proteins markedly increase the rate of GTP hydrolysis by the α subunit and speed termination of the signal.

inhibit L- and N-type Ca^{2+} channels in neural tissue. Because of the high concentrations of G_i and G_o in the plasma membrane, it is thought that the βγ dimers released from these α subunits may play the most significant regulatory roles in cell signaling. Thus, receptors coupled to G_i or G_o may regulate certain cell functions via the βγ dimer and others via the α subunit. Important examples of regulation via the βγ dimer in the cardiovascular system include modulation of the cardiac sinoatrial (SA) and atrioventricular nodes by muscarinic K+ channels and activation of phospholipase C-β in mast cells, leukocytes, neutrophils, and/or other white blood cells.

Signal termination and regulators of G protein signaling proteins. The G protein signal is terminated by the intrinsic guanosine triphosphatase activity of the α subunit, and the action of a family of proteins termed the *regulators of G protein signaling* (RGS proteins). The guanosine triphosphatase activity of the α subunit hydrolyzes bound GTP to GDP, which remains bound to the α subunit and converts it from the active to the inactive form. This hydrolysis is markedly stimulated (100- to 1000-fold) by RGS proteins. When bound GTP is hydrolyzed by the α subunit, the affinity of the α subunit for the βγ-dimer increases, and the GDP-bound form of the α subunit sequesters the βγ subunit. These 2 events return the system to the basal state. There are over 20 members of the RGS family, and many members of the family have other regulatory domains, implying that this family of proteins has multiple important functions. For example, the RGS proteins may be determinants of the specificity of signaling in a variety of tissues.

Regulation of Effectors

Effector activation.   The actions of the α-GTP complex and the $\beta\gamma$ dimer initiate complex signaling patterns with certain common features. The activation of effectors by the α-GTP complex or the $\beta\gamma$-dimer appears to occur by direct protein-protein interactions, causing the effector to shift to a more active state. Activation of these proteins changes the concentration of intracellular messengers such as cAMP, DAG, IP_3, Ca^{2+}, or K^+ ions. Adenylyl cyclase, ion channels, and phospholipase C-β are important effectors found in virtually all cells and regulate the response of organ systems to a large number of hormones, neurotransmitters, and autacoids. An important example of activation of adenylyl cyclase in the cardiovascular system is β-adrenergic stimulation of cardiac rate and force of contraction. β-Adrenergic receptors activate adenylyl cyclase via G_s and increase the level of cAMP in all cardiac tissues. The rise in cAMP activates cAMP-dependent protein kinase, which increases cardiac rate and force of contraction. Phospholipase C-β plays a very important role in regulating contraction of smooth muscle by controlling the level of Ca^{2+} in the cytoplasm of these cells. The α_1-adrenergic receptor that regulates vascular tone is coupled to the G_q α subunit. Activation of this receptor by norepinephrine produces an active G_q–α-GTP complex that markedly stimulates phospholipase C-β, leading to increases in IP_3, DAG, intracellular Ca^{2+} levels, and ultimately to contraction of smooth muscle.

Effector inhibition.   Adenylyl cyclase activity can also be inhibited by receptors coupled to the G_i α subunit in most cells. Examples of cardiovascular receptors that inhibit adenylyl cyclase include the muscarinic m_2, α_2-adrenergic, adenosine A_1, and angiotensin AT_1 receptors. As noted above, many second messengers generated by receptor activation lead to activation of protein kinases that produce a cellular response by increasing the phosphorylation state of important regulatory proteins in the target cells. This is the case for cAMP, Ca^{2+}, and DAG, which activate the cAMP-dependent protein kinase, members of the Ca^{2+}/calmodulin-dependent protein kinase family, and the multiple isoforms of protein kinase C, respectively.

Counterregulatory Effects of G Proteins

In many tissues, it is common to find 2 or more receptors acting to regulate important functions via opposing effects. In the SA node in the heart, the activity of the cardiac pacemaker cells is stimulated by norepinephrine acting on β_1-adrenergic receptors, which in turn stimulates adenylyl cyclase via the activated G_s α subunit. This raises the level of cAMP in the cells and increases pacemaker activity. However, the muscarinic potassium channel in the SA node directly opposes the actions of norepinephrine, inhibiting pacemaker activity by 2 mechanisms: the muscarinic m_2 receptor couples to the G_i protein to produce the activated G_i–α-GTP complex, which inhibits adenylyl cyclase and lowers cAMP, and the $\beta\gamma$ dimer directly activates the K^+ channel. Both the decrease in cAMP and the increase in K^+ conductance slow the heart and oppose the rate-increasing effects of norepinephrine.

SUGGESTED READING

1. Clapham DE, Neer EJ. G protein $\beta\gamma$ subunits. *Annu Rev Pharmacol Toxicol.* 1997;37:167–203.
2. Downes GB, Gautam N. The G protein subunit gene families. *Genomics.* 1999;62:544–552.
3. Hamm HE. The many faces of G protein signaling. *J Biol Chem.* 1998;273:669–672.
4. Milligan G, White JH. Protein-protein interactions at G protein–coupled receptors. *Trends Pharm Sci.* 2001;22:513–518.
5. Neer EJ. Heterotrimeric G proteins: organizers of transmembrane signals. *Cell.* 1995;80:249–257.
6. Ross ER, Wilkie TW. GTPase-activating proteins for heterotrimeric G proteins: regulators of G protein signaling (RGS) and RGS-like proteins. *Annu Rev Biochem.* 2000;69:795–827.

Cyclic Nucleotides

Kevin J. Catt, MD, PhD

KEY POINTS

- Seven transmembrane-domain receptors that couple to G_s and G_i regulate the activity of adenylyl cyclases and the production of cyclic adenosine monophosphate, a major second messenger. Calcium influx and phosphodiesterases also determine the intracellular cyclic adenosine monophosphate levels.

- Cyclic adenosine monophosphate activates protein kinase A isoforms that phosphorylate regulatory proteins in the plasma membrane, cytoplasm, and nucleus. It also opens cyclic nucleotide-gated channels in the cell membrane. A-kinase anchoring proteins determine the spatial distribution of protein kinase–dependent phosphorylation within the cell.

- Cyclic guanosine monophosphate is produced by cytoplasmic and membrane-associated guanylyl cyclases that are activated by nitric oxide and atrial natriuretic peptide, respectively. Cyclic guanosine monophosphate is also regulated by phosphodiesterases and stimulates protein phosphorylation by protein kinase G.

See also Chapters A1, A3, A12–A18, A24, A27–A29, and A31–A33

Numerous hormones, neurotransmitters, and growth factors act on their target cells by binding to highly specific receptor molecules that are embedded in the plasma membrane and locked in place by their hydrophobic transmembrane domains. Many of these cell-surface receptors are coupled through heterotrimeric guanine nucleotide regulatory proteins (G proteins) to enzymes [e.g., adenylyl cyclases (ACs) and phospholipases] that produce a variety of intracellular signaling molecules during agonist activation. The "second messengers" formed during agonist activation of G protein–coupled receptors include cyclic adenosine monophosphate (cAMP), inositol phosphates, diacylglycerol, calcium, and arachidonic acid.

Cyclic Nucleotides

Cyclic adenosine monophosphate. Many G protein–coupled receptors are linked through G_s to the activation of adenylyl cyclase and the formation of cAMP, a pervasive intracellular messenger in species ranging from bacteria to mammals. Most of the physiologic actions of cAMP are mediated by cAMP-dependent protein kinase (PKA), which controls multiple aspects of cell function through phosphorylation of protein substrates. cAMP also regulates certain guanine nucleotide exchange proteins (EPACs) and activates an important set of cyclic nucleotide-gated cationic channels (CNG channels) in the plasma membrane of several excitable cell types.

Cyclic guanosine monophosphate. Cyclic guanosine monophosphate (cGMP) is produced by 2 different systems: (a) the intrinsic guanylyl cyclases of plasma membrane receptors for natriuretic factors and (b) soluble guanylyl cyclases that are activated by nitric oxide (NO). cGMP is the major messenger in visual transduction in vertebrates and in signaling by natriuretic peptides. Virtually all of the enzymes involved in second

messenger generation and action exist as multiple isoforms, most of which are regulated by Ca^{2+}, protein phosphorylation, and interactions with specific phospholipids. The cGMP formed by activation of guanylyl cyclases has a restricted range of actions, largely expressed through protein phosphorylation mediated by cGMP-dependent protein kinase and through activation of CNG channels. cGMP has a central role in the visual system and is a major physiologic regulator of vasodilatation induced by atrial natriuretic peptides (ANPs), which activate membrane-associated guanylyl cyclase in smooth muscle, kidney, endothelial cells, and adrenal glands. Several hormones that stimulate phospholipid turnover also increase cGMP production, probably via the activation of guanylyl cyclase by protein kinase C (PKC) or arachidonic acid metabolites. The resulting increases in cGMP production are responsible for smooth muscle relaxation and vasodilatation via activation of protein kinase G (PKG) and phosphorylation of specific proteins involved in the contractile mechanism.

Adenylyl Cyclases

Subtypes. Several structurally related ACs are expressed in animal cells, and in mammals the ACs are encoded by 9 different genes. Most ACs contain 2 hydrophobic domains, each composed of 6 transmembrane helices associated with the plasma membrane and 2 cytoplasmic catalytic domains. AC1 is expressed in neural and adrenal medullary cells, AC2 in brain, skeletal muscle, and lung, AC3 in brain and olfactory cells, AC4 in the brain and elsewhere, and AC5 and AC6 in heart, brain, and other tissues. The major AC isoforms in the brain are the Ca^{2+}/calmodulin (CaM)-stimulated AC1, Ca^{2+}-insensitive AC2, and the Ca^{2+}-inhibited AC. All 9 of the AC enzymes are stimulated by $G_s\alpha$ and forskolin, and AC1 and AC4 are also activated by Ca^{2+}-CaM. The latter ACs are abundant in neural tissue and are sensitive to transmitter-induced changes in cytoplasmic Ca^{2+} concentration. In several cell types, Ca^{2+} exerts a direct inhibitory effect on the activity of AC4, whereas in others, the AC9 enzyme is inhibited by Ca^{2+}/calcineurin.

Regulation. Most Ca^{2+}-mobilizing hormones act primarily through stimulation of phosphoinositide hydrolysis and generation of inositol 1,4,5-triphosphate; this G_q-mediated effect is indirectly responsible for regulating the activities of the Ca^{2+}- and CaM-sensitive adenylyl cyclases. In neuronal cells, Ca^{2+}-sensitive ACs are often adjacent to plasma membrane channels (*N*-methyl-D-aspartate, L-type, and CNG) that regulate Ca^{2+} influx, and in nonexcitable cells are near the store-operated Trp channels that control capacitative Ca^{2+} entry. In addition to being regulated by G_s or G_i α subunits that activate or inhibit enzyme activity, some ACs are also regulated by βγ subunits. AC1, when stimulated by $α_s$ or Ca^{2+}-CaM, is inhibited by βγ. Conversely, stimulation of the AC2 and AC4 enzymes by $α_s$ is potentiated by βγ subunits. The βγ subunits that modulate AC activity are largely derived from G_i and G_o, which are abundant in the brain and elsewhere. The basal and $α_s$-stimulated activities of the AC2 enzyme are also increased by PKC during activation of G_q by calcium-mobilizing hormones. Thus, the activation of ACs by G_s can be potentiated or inhibited by other receptor-mediated pathways that operate through G_i, G_o, or G_q in the same cell type.

Multimeric and subcellular signaling. Recently, ACs have been found to dimerize or oligomerize via their hydrophobic domains, and they may thus participate in the formation of multimeric signaling complexes, a feature that is becoming apparent in a wide variety of intracellular signaling pathways and cascades. An unusual soluble adenylyl cyclase activated by bicarbonate is present in the testis and in fluid-transporting tissues such as the kidney. Because soluble adenylyl cyclase is not bound to the plasma membrane, it has the potential for participating in the formation of intracellular microdomains that are activated by bicarbonate and other intracellular regulatory factors.

Cyclic Adenosine Monophosphate–Dependent Protein Kinases

PKAs are present in all eukaryotic cells as the major mediators of the effects of cAMP. Cyclic nucleotide-dependent protein kinases are rapidly activated by the micromolar concentrations of cAMP or cGMP that occur in hormone-stimulated cells.

Regulatory subunits. Cyclic nucleotides bind to specific regulatory sites on the enzymes, which share several common structural features. In PKA, the regulatory and catalytic domains are expressed as 2 separate molecules that associate to form an inactive complex. In the cGMP-dependent enzyme (PKG), these domains are present in a single molecule.

The inactive form of PKA is a tetramer ($R_2 \cdot C_2$) composed of 2 regulatory (R) subunits and 2 catalytic (C) subunits. In the absence of cAMP, the subunits bind to each other with high affinity, and the regulatory subunits interact with the catalytic site to maintain the holoenzymes in their basal inactive state. Binding of cAMP to the regulatory subunits dissociates the

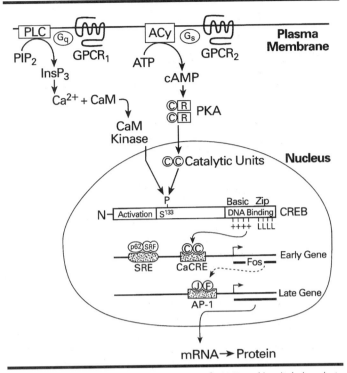

Figure A30.1. Receptor-mediated activation of cAMP and inositol phosphate signaling pathways. Diagram also illustrates manner in which both pathways converge on phosphorylation and activation of nuclear transcription factor, cAMP-responsive enhancer element-binding (CREB) protein. Activated CREB protein binds to CRE located in promoter of *fos* and other early-response genes. Increase in *fos* and formation of *fos-jun* heterodimers activates AP1 sites that promote expression of intermediate- and late-response genes. ATP, adenosine triphosphate; CaM, calmodulin; cAMP, cyclic adenosine monophosphate; CRE, cAMP-responsive enhancer element; GPCR, G protein–coupled receptor; InsP$_3$, inositol triphosphate; PKA, protein kinase; SRE, serum-response element.

inactive holoenzyme and releases catalytic subunits that phosphorylate intracellular substrates (**Figure A30.1**). The regulatory subunits released by cAMP-induced dissociation of protein kinase remain as R_2 dimers that can later undergo reassociation with free catalytic subunits. This sequence can be represented by the equation $R_2 \cdot C_2 + 4cAMP \rightleftharpoons R_2 \cdot cAMP_4 + 2C.$)

Catalytic subunits. The catalytic subunit is common to both major forms of PKA but the regulatory subunits show several differences. Two major forms of protein kinase are present in most tissues but their proportions vary in each cell type. The holoenzymes are generally similar in subunit composition ($R_2 \cdot C_2$) and molecular mass (≈ 170 kd). The regulatory subunits differ in their molecular masses, R_1 being smaller (49 kd) and more uniform in size than R_2 (52–56 kd). The R_1 and R_2 subunits exist in α- and β-isoforms that differ in size and tissue distribution. The α-isoforms are expressed constitutively in many tissues, but the β-isoforms have a more limited distribution and are most abundant in the nervous system. The selective regulation of these isoforms during differentiation and hormonal stimulation could mediate specific responses to the cAMP pathway. In some tissues, free R_1 and R_2 subunits are present in excess over the catalytic subunit and interact with other cellular proteins or structures. Selective increases in the

R_2 subunit occur in several tissues during cAMP-induced differentiation. The catalytic subunits are also encoded by multiple genes, giving rise to α, β, and γ isoforms. Because each regulatory subunit can associate with any of the C subunits, a wide variety of $R_2 \cdot C_2$ holoenzymes can exist in various tissues. The existence of at least 12 forms of PKA provides for a considerable degree of diversity in the tissue-specific expression, intracellular localization, and activation properties of the individual enzymes.

Clinical implications. There is considerable evidence that overactivity of the cAMP signaling system can be associated with significant aberrations of cell growth and proliferation.

Cyclic adenosine monophosphate signaling overactivity. Activating mutations of the *GNAS1* gene, which encodes the adenylyl cyclase-stimulatory α subunit of G_s, cause sporadic growth hormone–secreting pituitary tumors, as well as the McCune-Albright syndrome of precocious puberty associated with acromegaly, nodular adrenal hyperplasia, and functioning thyroid nodules.

Mutations. Mutations of the gene encoding the PKA R_1 α-subunit have been implicated in the genesis of the Carney complex, a rare form of multiple endocrine neoplasia. Recently, changes in PKA expression and in the normal $R_1 : R_2$ subunit ratio were found to occur in breast cancer and may promote neoplastic cell growth by affecting cells' sensitivity to estrogens. Furthermore, inhibitors of type I PKA can exert cooperative antineoplastic effects with certain cytotoxic drugs and epidermal growth factor–receptor inhibitors.

Role of anchoring proteins. In addition to the concentration of cyclic nucleotides in the cell, PKA spatial distribution and temporal profiles are important aspects of intracellular signaling. Earlier observations suggesting compartmentalization of cyclic nucleotides and more recent findings localizing PKAs to specific intracellular domains have lent support to this concept. A large and growing family of at least 20 A-kinase anchor proteins (AKAPs) is now known to determine the spatial distribution of PKA isoforms within the cell. This permits PKAs to remain near their target proteins, thereby increasing the efficiency and specificity of subcellular cAMP-dependent signaling in regions ranging from the cell membrane to the nucleus, including mitochondria, cytoskeletal elements, and vesicular systems. The ability of AKAPs to sequester PKA isoforms from the cytoplasm to the cell membrane, cytoskeleton, and organelles could be especially important in sperm, eggs, and polarized cells, including columnar epithelium and neurons.

Specific roles of AKAPs have been identified in insulin secretion, β-adrenergic receptor signaling, and uterine contraction. In pancreatic β-cells, AKAPs form complexes with PKA and protein phosphatase 2B that regulate insulin release, and with PKA and L-type Ca^{2+} channels at the plasma membrane. During β-adrenergic signaling, AKAP250 (or gravin) forms a complex with PKA, PKC, and phosphatase 2B. Gravin binds the complex to the cytoplasmic tail of the receptor, where it phosphorylates adjacent substrates and the receptor itself. This contributes to the processes of receptor desensitization and its subsequent endocytosis, during which the AKAP remains bound to the receptor and may facilitate its dephosphorylation and recycling to the cell surface.

Nuclear signaling by the cyclic adenosine monophosphate/ protein kinase pathway. Receptor-mediated activation of adenylyl cyclase activity is often followed by cAMP-mediated stimulation of gene transcription. This results from the phosphorylation by PKA of transcriptional regulatory proteins that bind to cAMP-responsive enhancer elements (CREs: TGACGTCA) located in the promoter regions of cAMP-regulated genes.

cAMP-responsive enhancer element binding proteins. CRE-binding (CREB) proteins that mediate transcriptional activation during stimulation of cAMP production include activators and inhibitors of gene expression. The CREB proteins belong to a superfamily of transcription factors that are characterized structurally as basic region leucine zipper (bZip) proteins, which interact via their leucine zipper domains to form specific homodimers and heterodimers with other family members. In some CREBs, the phosphorylation of a specific serine residue (Ser^{133}) by PKA promotes their transcriptional activation potential and stimulates gene expression. The same residue is also phosphorylated by Ca^{2+}-CaM–dependent protein kinases and thus serves to integrate signals from at least 2 distinct signaling pathways (Figure A30.1).

cAMP-responsive enhancer element modulator proteins. An important subset of the CREB family is the CRE-modulator (CREM) protein group, which is derived from a single gene by a variety of transcriptional and translational processes. CREM proteins possess specific activator or inhibitory functions, have specific tissue locations, and are important mediators of physiologic and neuroendocrine responses. CREMs are phosphorylated by PKA and Ca^{2+}-CaM–dependent kinases at the equivalent serine residue (Ser^{117}) as CREB, and also by PKC and mitogen-activated S6 kinase. CREM proteins are thus responsive to multiple signal transduction pathways, including those involved in mitogen-induced gene expression.

Guanylyl Cyclases

The guanylyl cyclases that catalyze the formation of cGMP from guanosine triphosphate exist as membrane-associated and soluble forms in most mammalian cells. The membrane-associated enzymes are located with the cytoplasmic regions of cell-surface receptors with a single transmembrane domain and an extracellular hormone-binding domain. These receptors are activated by ANPs, heat-stable *Escherichia coli* enterotoxin, and sea urchin egg peptides that stimulate sperm motility.

Membrane-associated guanylyl cyclases. The 3 major forms of receptor guanylyl cyclase (called *GC-A*, *GC-B*, and *GC-C*) contain a cysteine-rich extracellular domain for ligand binding and an intracellular catalytic domain that is highly conserved in guanylyl and adenylyl cyclases. The ANPs produced in the heart and brain act on GC-A and GC-B receptors, and enterotoxin probably acts on the GC-C receptor.

Soluble forms. Soluble guanylyl cyclases are present in most tissues and are abundant in lung and smooth muscle. They contain no membrane-spanning domains and are activated by NO, which interacts with a heme-binding region of the molecule. This effect of NO is responsible for the vasodilator actions of nitrate donors (nitroglycerin and nitroprusside) and accounts for the actions of endogenous vasodilators such as acetylcholine, bradykinin, and substance P, which stimulate NO synthesis in endothelial cells. Gaseous NO diffuses into the adjacent cells and activates soluble guanylyl cyclase, leading to activation of PKG, cGMP production, and smooth muscle relaxation.

Protein kinase G. PKGs are abundant in invertebrates but have a more limited distribution in mammalian tissues. Whereas PKAs regulate the activities of major metabolic pathways, including lipolysis, glycogenolysis, and steroidogenesis, the cGMP-dependent enzymes are involved in the control of gene expression, neuronal function, vascular tone, and platelet aggregation. Because PKGs are monomeric molecules, their activation does not involve the subunit dissociation that is typical of the cAMP-dependent enzyme. The marked amino acid sequence homologies between cGMP- and cAMP-dependent protein kinases, and predicted similarities in their structures suggest that the 2 enzymes have evolved from an ancestral phosphotransferase.

Cyclic Nucleotide–Gated Channels

In addition to their widespread actions through PKA and PKG, both cAMP and cGMP can activate nonselective voltage-dependent cation channels located in the plasma membrane of many neural and related cell types. These CNG channels, which act as sensors of cAMP and cGMP, are formed by 4 subunits that contain a 6-transmembrane-domain module similar to that of voltage-gated potassium channels. CNG channels are highly sensitive to cyclic nucleotides, especially those formed in submembrane microdomains. These channels are abundant in the rod and cone photoreceptors of the retina, and in ganglion, bipolar, and Muller glial cells, where they mediate light-induced neurotransmission. A mutation in the human CNG3 gene probably causes the loss of cone function leading to total color blindness in humans. CNG channels are also important in the control of pituitary hormone secretion, and may be involved in the regulation of pulsatile gonadotropin-releasing hormone release from the hypothalamus.

Cyclic Nucleotide Phosphodiesterases

Phosphodiesterase actions. The cyclic nucleotides produced at the plasma membrane in agonist-stimulated cells are released to a variable extent into the extracellular fluid, where they are rapidly inactivated by intracellular phosphodiesterases (PDEs), which have important roles in retinal phototransduction, smooth muscle contraction, insulin secretion, and fertility. Cyclic nucleotide levels within the cell are usually governed by changes in their rates of for-

mation, but in some tissues (e.g., retina), activation of PDEs is the major determinant of their concentration. Another important function of PDEs is to coordinate the activities of cyclic nucleotide and phosphoinositide signaling pathways, largely through the regulatory action of Ca^{2+}-CaM on PDE activity.

Subtypes. Mammalian cells contain about 50 PDEs that are classified into 11 families based on their amino acid sequences and functional properties. All possess a central catalytic domain and an N-terminal regulatory domain that binds Ca^{2+}-CaM and also contains binding sites for cGMP. PDEs 4, 7, and 8 are highly specific for cAMP, and PDEs 5, 6, and 9 are highly specific for cGMP. PDEs 1, 2, 3, 10, and 11 have dual specificity with variable degrees of preference for cAMP or cGMP. PDE1 enzymes are stimulated by Ca^{2+}-CAM and are activated by calcium-mobilizing agonists and inhibited by methylxanthines. PDE2 is stimulated by cGMP. The PDE7 enzymes are stimulated by cAMP and are activated by ANPs. PDE3 enzymes are inhibited by cGMP, which competes with cAMP at the catalytic site, and are regulated by insulin, glucagon, and dexamethasone. PDE4 enzymes are specific for cGMP and are activated by cAMP-stimulating agonists. PDE5 is specific for cGMP and is activated by NO; it is specifically inhibited by sildenafil, which is often effective in erectile dysfunction. PDE6 enzymes are specific for cGMP and include rod and cone isoforms that are activated by transducin. Agonist-induced increases in cAMP are accompanied by increased activity of the cGMP-inhibited PDEs as a result of their cAMP-dependent phosphorylation and by a transient decrease in the activity of the Ca^{2+}-CaM–dependent PDEs. Several hormones that stimulate cAMP production also increase the expression of the high-affinity cAMP-specific PDEs.

SUGGESTED READING

1. Hanoune J, Defer N. Regulation and role of adenylyl cyclase isoforms. *Annu Rev Pharmacol Toxicol.* 2001;41:145–174.
2. Hurley JH. The adenylyl and guanylyl cyclase superfamily. *Current Opin Struct Biol.* 1998;8:770–777.
3. Hurley JH. Structure, mechanism and regulation of mammalian adenylyl cyclase. *J Biol Chem.* 1999;274:7599–7602.
4. Lucas KA, Pitari GM, Kazerounian S, et al. Guanylyl cyclases and signaling by cyclic GMP. *Pharmacol Rev.* 2000;52:375–413.
5. Mehats C, Anderson CB, Filopanti M, et al. Cyclic nucleotide phosphodiesterases and their role in endocrine cell signaling. *Trends Endocrinol Metab.* 2002;1:29–35.
6. Michel JJ, Scott JD. AKA mediated signal transduction. *Annu Rev Pharmacol Toxicol.* 2002;42:235–257.
7. Schwartz JH. The many dimensions of cAMP signaling. *Proc Natl Acad Sci U S A.* 2001;98:13482–13484.
8. Stratakis CA, Cho-Chung YS. Protein kinase A and human disease. *Trends Endocrinol Metab.* 2002;13:50–53.

Inositol Phospholipids and Inositol Phosphates

Tamas Balla, MD, PhD

KEY POINTS

- Phosphoinositides are formed by phosphorylation of various ring positions of phosphatidylinositol by specific inositol lipid kinases in virtually every cell membrane.

- Phospholipase C–mediated hydrolysis of membrane phosphatidylinositol 4,5-biphosphate is a major signaling mechanism by which cell-surface receptors regulate cellular functions.

- Inositol 1,4,5-trisphosphate and diacylglycerol are the 2 primary messengers that regulate Ca^{2+} release and protein kinase C activity, respectively, on phospholipase C activation.

- Phosphoinositides also serve as localization signals for important regulatory proteins and, hence, contribute to the regulation of protein signaling complexes in specific membrane compartments.

- Some isoforms of phosphoinositides (e.g., the 3-phosphorylated forms) are not hydrolyzed by phospholipase C enzymes; inositol lipid phosphatases are critically important in regulating their levels.

See also Chapters A3, A12, A20, A21, A27–A30, and A32

General Properties of Phosphoinositides

The inositol phospholipids found in all cellular membranes correspond to only a small fraction of the total cellular phospholipids, yet they have remarkable importance in regulating a wide variety of cell functions. They are synthesized from phosphatidylinositol by phosphorylation of the various hydroxyls of the inositol ring to form polyphosphoinositides. These function as docking sites to promote formation of molecular signaling complexes or as precursors for soluble inositol polyphosphates that act as diffusible intracellular messengers. Phosphoinositides are involved in the control of many processes, including membrane traffic as well as endo- and exocytosis. They also regulate mitogenesis and apoptosis and are key components in the generation of cytosolic Ca^{2+} transients.

Phosphoinositides and Ca^{2+} Signaling

Phospholipase C products. The first recognized changes of inositol phospholipid metabolism were related to increased hydrolysis of phosphoinositides by phospholipase C (PLC) when certain cell-surface receptors were stimulated by their agonist ligands. The main substrate of PLC action is phosphatidylinositol 4,5-bisphosphate [$PI(4,5)P_2$], which is synthesized from phosphatidylinositol (PI) via phosphatidylinositol 4-phosphate [PI(4)P]. In agonist-stimulated cells, $PI(4,5)P_2$ is rapidly hydrolyzed by phospholipase C to form 2 powerful second messengers, inositol 1,4,5-trisphosphate [$Ins(1,4,5)P_3$ or IP_3] and diacylglycerol (DAG) **(Figure A31.1)**.

Inositol 1,4,5-trisphosphate and calcium transients. Ins(1,4, 5)P_3 binds to specific receptors in the endoplasmic reticulum to release stored calcium into the cytoplasm. The resulting "cal-

cium transient" initiates cellular responses such as exocytosis, contraction, and neurotransmission. However, the calcium release must be supplemented by entry of calcium from the extracellular fluid to maintain cellular responses during continued agonist stimulation. This calcium influx occurs through plasma-membrane calcium channels that are activated directly or indirectly by $Ins(1,4,5)P_3$, which thus serves to both initiate and maintain specific cellular responses.

Inositol 1,4,5-trisphosphate metabolism. After exerting its action on calcium mobilization, $Ins(1,4,5)P_3$ is rapidly degraded to lower inositol phosphates [$Ins(1,4)P_2$, $Ins(4)P$] and then to inositol, which is subsequently reincorporated into the biosynthetic pathway to form PI, PI(4)P, and $PI(4,5)P_2$.

In addition to being catabolized to inositol, $Ins(1,4,5)P_3$ is phosphorylated to form $Ins(1,3,4,5)P_4$, which may also participate in calcium regulation and contributes to a minor degree to the formation of higher inositol phosphates ($InsP_5$ and $InsP_6$) that are present in many cell types.

Diacylglycerol. The DAG formed by phospholipase C activation acts as a co-messenger with the $Ins(1,4,5)P_3$-induced rise of intracellular calcium to activate protein kinases, particularly certain isoforms of protein kinase C (PKC), that phosphorylate numerous key proteins, receptors, ion channels, and enzymes in cell membranes, cytoplasm, and nucleus.

Phospholipase C

Multiple forms of phospholipase C have been identified in various tissues. These have been designated as α, β, γ, δ, and contain several conserved regions interrupted by dissimilar amino acid sequences. Two such domains (X and Y) form the catalytic site of

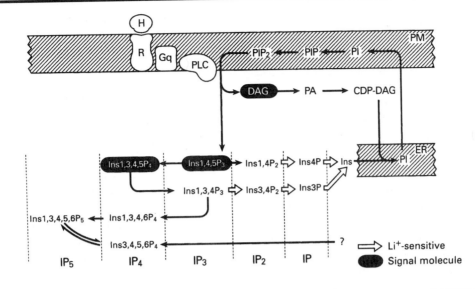

Figure A31.1. Pathways of inositol phosphates and diacylglycerol (DAG) in response to hormones (H) interacting with their receptors (R) in plasma membrane (PM) and metabolic pathways linking various inositol phosphates. Regeneration of phospholipid precursors occurs in endoplasmic reticulum (ER). CDP, cytidine diphosphate; PA, phosphatidic acid; PI, phosphatidylinositol; PLC, phospholipase C.

the enzyme, whereas others with homology with protein domains found in the *src* oncogene, called *SH2* and *SH3*, bind to phosphotyrosine residues and proline-rich sequences of specific proteins.

Activation of phospholipase C-β. Phospholipase C-β is activated by receptors of the G protein–coupled variety, which possess a rhodopsin-like structure with 7 transmembrane domains and which mediate the actions of numerous hormones and neurotransmitters. In contrast, phospholipase C-γ is activated by receptors for growth factors, such as platelet-derived growth factor and epidermal growth factor, that undergo tyrosine phosphorylation and thus bind to the SH2 domains of phospholipase C-γ and other signaling molecules. Within the calcium-phosphoinositide signaling system, phospholipases β and γ appear to be the major enzymes responsible for generating the second messengers that activate cell responses to hormones and growth factors.

β-Isozyme forms and actions. The β-isozyme of phospholipase C exists in 4 forms (β_1-β_4), 2 of which (β_1 and β_3) are activated by G protein α subunits and the other (β_2) by βγ-dimers derived from dissociation of the heterotrimeric proteins G_i/G_o, although βγ subunits can also stimulate the other isoforms to a lesser degree. Cells of hematopoietic origin contain relatively high amounts of the β_2 enzyme that is stimulated by the βγ subunits liberated from the abundant G_i/G_o proteins. This explains why pertussis toxin treatment almost completely eliminates PLC activation via their G protein–coupled receptors in such cells. In most cells, however, the G protein–coupled receptors activate PLC in a pertussis toxin-insensitive manner, via the α subunits of $G_{q/11}$ proteins.

Phospholipase C-γ forms and actions. PLCγ enzymes have 2 forms (γ_1 and γ_2) and are activated by receptor tyrosine kinases. These enzymes contain an extra stretch of regulatory sequence inserted in between the 2 parts of their conserved catalytic domains (X and Y). This insertion contains 2 SH2 domains and 1 SH3 domain sandwiched between the 2 halves of what appears to be a pleckstrin homology (PH) domain. PLCγ binds to phosphorylated tyrosines of several growth factor receptors or adaptor molecules, and is thereby recruited to the plasma membrane and phosphorylated on critical tyrosine residues. Membrane association and tyrosine phosphorylation increases the activity of the enzyme, probably through association with other regulatory proteins. An additional feature of PLCγ is its regulation by $PI(3,4,5)P_3$, which is especially prominent during $PLC\gamma_2$ activation in immune cells. This is believed to result from the increased recruitment of PLCγ to the plasma membrane via interaction of its PH domain with $PI(3,4,5)P_3$ molecules.

Phospholipase C-δ. All phospholipase C enzymes are activated by Ca^{2+} ions, but only the δ-isoform is believed to be regulated primarily by changes in the cytosolic Ca^{2+} concentration.

Inositol 1,4,5-Trisphosphate Receptors

Characteristics. $Ins(1,4,5)P_3$ formed during activation of phospholipase C binds with high affinity to specific intracellular receptors located in the endoplasmic (or sarcoplasmic) reticulum, which serves as the internal store of calcium released during agonist stimulation. In some cells, $Ins(1,4,5)P_3$ receptors might also be present in the plasma membrane. The receptor is a large protein of 260 to 300 kd in size that forms a tetramer and functions as a Ca^{2+} channel. After $Ins(1,4,5)P_3$ binding, Ca^{2+} moves through the $Ins(1,4,5)P_3$ receptor channel along its concentration gradient from the intracellular stores to the cytosol.

Molecular variants. Several forms of the $Ins(1,4,5)P_3$ receptor have been cloned (type I, type II, and type III) and show a great deal of sequence homology and similar domain structure. The type I $Ins(1,4,5)P_3$ receptor has several splice variants, some of which are only expressed in neurons, and others only in peripheral tissues. It is generally agreed that most tissues probably contain more than 1 form of the receptor that can even form heterotetramers.

Binding domains. Ins(1,4,5)P$_3$ receptors contain an N-terminal Ins(1,4,5)P$_3$-binding domain that binds the ligand even if expressed separately from the rest of the receptor channel. The C-terminal part of the molecule contains 6 transmembrane domains and functions as the channel domain. The region between the Ins(1,4,5)P$_3$-binding and the channel domains is the regulatory domain, which contains phosphorylation sites as well as binding sites for other regulators such as adenosine triphosphate, Ca^{2+}, calmodulin, or immunophilins.

Modulation of Ca^{2+}-induced Ca^{2+} release. In addition to Ins(1,4,5)P$_3$-induced Ca^{2+} release, the most unique feature of the Ins(1,4,5)P$_3$ receptor is its ability to modulate Ca^{2+}-induced Ca^{2+} release. In this respect, the receptor behaves like its structural relative, the ryanodine receptor channel, which is found in heart and striated muscle. This modulatory feature of the Ins(1,4,5)P$_3$ receptor is part of the process that allows a stimulatory effect of small Ca^{2+} increases (above resting cytosolic levels) on channel opening, whereas high Ca^{2+} concentrations (μmol/L range) cause channel inactivation. According to current models, Ins(1,4,5)P$_3$ determines the threshold level of Ca^{2+} at which Ins(1,4,5)P$_3$ channels open. Ca^{2+} increases in the absence of Ins(1,4,5)P$_3$ are not sufficient to open the channel, but once the channels are activated, Ins(1,4,5)P$_3$ concentrations have little additional influence on the amount of Ca^{2+} that is released. During channel activation, further Ca^{2+} release is governed primarily by the amount or filling-state of the Ca^{2+} pools (endoplasmic reticulum and extracellular space) and the inactivation of the channel by Ca^{2+} and Ins(1,4,5)P$_3$. This biphasic regulation of the Ins(1,4,5)P$_3$ receptor channel by Ca^{2+} is the underlying mechanism for the oscillatory cytosolic Ca^{2+} signals that are observed in many cells during stimulation with low agonist concentrations.

Inositol Polyphosphates

Highly phosphorylated inositols such as InsP$_5$ and InsP$_6$ are present in large amounts in mammalian as well as in avian and plant cells. Their relationship to the second messenger Ins(1,4,5)P$_3$ and its metabolite Ins(1,3,4,5)P$_4$ is not clear, although an enzymatic pathway leading to their formation has been identified by which Ins(1,3,4)P$_3$ [a metabolite of Ins(1,3,4,5)P$_4$] is converted to Ins(1,3,4,6)P$_4$ with subsequent production of InsP$_5$. Isotope labeling studies have showed that the labeling of the highly phosphorylated inositols with myoinositol is very slow and changes only after prolonged agonist stimulation. The labeling of InsP$_5$ and Ins(3,4,5,6)P$_4$/Ins(1,4,5,6)P$_4$ has been found to correlate with the growth rate of cells. Some highly phosphorylated inositols also contain pyrophosphate groups attached to their rings, and the more rapid turnover and regulation of these pyrophosphorylations may indicate that they could be involved in acutely regulated cellular responses.

Regulatory Role of Phosphoinositides in Cellular Membranes

Phosphoinositides not only serve as precursors of the second messengers Ins(1,4,5)P$_3$ and DAG but also function as regulators of signaling proteins on the surface of various membranes. Numerous regulatory proteins are stimulated by different isomers of inositol phospholipids, and several protein motifs that interact with inositides and mediate their regulatory influences have been identified. These include PH domains, phox-homology (or PX) domains, and others that can be found in many proteins. Because these domains can recruit proteins to the sites where inositides are formed in the membranes, local production and degradation of these lipids is an effective way to control the dynamics of protein signaling complexes in localized membrane compartments.

Phosphoinositide Kinases

Several groups of enzymes that can produce phosphoinositides have been isolated and identified. PI 4-kinases phosphorylate PI on the 4-position of the inositol ring to produce PI(4)P, some of which is converted to PI(4,5)P$_2$. However, PI(4) is probably also a regulator of the function of some proteins, as indicated by the several forms of PI 4-kinases (type II and type III forms) that have been shown to serve nonredundant functions.

Phosphatidylinositol 3-kinases. An important group of PI kinases (type I enzymes) phosphorylate inositol lipids on the 3 rather than the 4 or 5 position of the inositol ring and are regulated by growth factor receptors and oncogenic tyrosine kinases. The 3-phosphorylated inositides are not hydrolyzed by any known phospholipase C, and they exert their regulatory functions by binding to specific protein modules that are present in many signaling proteins. PI 3-kinases are classified into 3 groups.

Class I enzymes. Class I enzyme regulation is best understood. The activity and cellular localization of the 110 kd catalytic subunit of 3 of the 4 isoforms is dependent on a closely associated p85 regulatory subunit, which has 2 SH2 and 1 SH3 domains for interaction with tyrosine-phosphorylated and proline-rich sequences, respectively. Activation of growth factor receptors or soluble tyrosine kinases brings the p85/p110 complex to cellular membranes, where p85 undergoes tyrosine phosphorylation, leading to an increased catalytic activity of the complex. Smaller splice variants of p85 lacking the SH3 domain (p55 and p50) have also been described, but less is known about their specific regulatory features. A fourth and somewhat different member of the class I PI 3-kinase family is PI3Kγ, which has sequence similarities to the other members, but is primarily regulated by βγ subunits of heterotrimeric G proteins, either directly or via the adaptor protein p101.

Class II enzymes. Class II PI 3-kinases are larger (170–220 kd) proteins that contain the characteristic lipid kinase catalytic and lipid kinase unique domains but also possess a C-terminal C2 domain that could mediate Ca^{2+} and phospholipid regulation of the enzyme. Little is known about the regulation of the class II PI 3-kinases and the processes in which they play a regulatory role.

Class III enzymes. Class III PI 3-kinase only phosphorylates PI, and its function is crucial for vacuolar sorting in yeast. The mammalian enzymes are probably also involved at multiple steps in endocytic membrane trafficking.

Phosphatidylinositol phosphate kinases. Type I and type II phosphatidylinositol phosphate (PIP) kinases phosphorylate PI(4)P and PI(5)P, respectively, to form PI(4,5)P$_2$. Another group of enzymes, proposed to be termed *type III PIP kinases*, phosphorylate PI(3)P to PI(3,5)P$_2$, and the yeast homologue of this enzyme is also important in vacuolar sorting.

Phosphoinositide Phosphatases

Several enzymes have been found to dephosphorylate inositol lipids and inositol phosphates at specific positions of the inositol ring.

Group I 5-phosphatases. Group I 5-phosphatase can dephosphorylate only water-soluble Ins(1,4,5)P$_3$ and Ins(1,3,4,5)P$_4$, and it regulates the levels of these soluble messengers and, hence, Ca^{2+} signaling.

Group II 5-phosphatases. Group II 5-phosphatases can dephosphorylate the lipids [PI(4,5)P$_2$ and PI(3,4,5)P$_3$] in addition to the soluble inositol phosphates. One of these enzymes, the OCRL protein, is mutated in the X-linked human disease, the oculocerebrorenal syndrome of Lowe, which is characterized by renal tubular acidosis, mental retardation, early development of cataract, retinal degeneration, and renal failure. The OCRL protein is believed to be associated primarily with the trans-Golgi network and is also present in lysosomal membranes. At present, it is not clear how the defect in OCRL protein function leads to development of the features of Lowe's disease. Additional members of the group II 5-phosphatases are the synaptojanins, which are also believed to hydrolyze inositol lipids rather than inositol phosphates. These proteins have been implicated in synaptic vesicle trafficking, in association with other proteins important for the retrieval of exocytosed synaptic vesicles.

Group III 5-phosphatases. The group III 5-phosphatases, src-homology 2–containing inositide 5' phosphatase (SHIP) and SHIP2, hydrolyze substrates that contain a phosphate group at position 3 of the inositol ring [i.e., Ins(1,3,4,5)P$_4$ or PI(3,4,5)P$_3$] and serve as important negative regulators to terminate activation of PI(3,4,5)P$_3$-dependent pathways. Less is known about the group IV 5-phosphatases, which can also hydrolyze PI(3,4,5)P$_3$.

One of the tumor suppressor gene products, PTEN, has been recently shown to be an inositol lipid phosphatase that hydrolyzes the 3-phosphate group and has relatively broad substrate specificity. PTEN could exert its tumor suppressor action by hydrolyzing PI(3,4,5)P$_3$, acting similarly to SHIP and antagonizing the effects of growth factors that increase the level of this phosphoinositide.

Phosphatidylcholine Signaling

In addition to the lipid second messengers derived from phosphoinositides, agonist stimulation is associated with the hydrolysis of phosphatidylcholine by a variety of phospholipases [including phospholipase A$_2$, PLC, and phospholipase D (PLD)] to form DAG, phosphatidic acid, and arachidonic acid. Both G proteins and PKC have been implicated in the activation of PLD, leading to the release of phosphatidic acid and its subsequent conversion (via phosphatidic acid phosphohydrolase) to DAG.

In a given cell type, various agonists can stimulate the activation of PLC, PLD, or both. The proportion of DAG generated from phosphoinositide breakdown can lead to secondary activation of PLD through PKC, causing a further increase in DAG production from the hydrolysis of phosphatidylcholine and metabolism of phosphatidic acid.

Two major forms of phosphatidylcholine-specific PLD, PLD$_1$ and PLD$_2$, have been isolated and identified by molecular cloning. Both of these enzymes are regulated by phosphoinositides, especially PI(4,5)P$_2$. PLD$_1$ activity is also stimulated by the Arf family of small guanosine triphosphate binding proteins, as well as by PKC. Activation of PLD by cell-surface receptors has been well documented, but the enzyme's role in vesicular trafficking is also important. This suggests that these enzymes, like inositide kinases, control multiple processes at specific membrane compartments within the cells.

SUGGESTED READING

1. Berridge MJ. Inositol trisphosphate and diacylglycerol: two interacting second messengers. *Annu Rev Biochem.* 1987;56:159–193.
2. Exton JH. Phospholipase D-structure, regulation and function. *Rev Physiol Biochem Pharmacol.* 2002;144:1–94.
3. Fruman DA, Meyers RE, Cantley LC. Phosphoinositide kinases. *Annu Rev Biochem.* 1998;67:481–507.
4. Irvine RF, Schell MJ. Back in the water: the return of the inositol phosphates. *Nat Rev Mol Cell Biol.* 2001;2(5):327–338.
5. Lemmon MA, Ferguson KM. Signal-dependent membrane targeting by pleckstrin homology (PH) domains. *Biochem J.* 2000;350(Pt 1):1–18.
6. Majerus PW, Kisseleva MV, Norris FA. The role of phosphatases in inositol signaling reactions. *J Biol Chem.* 1999;274(16):10669–10672.
7. Martin TF. PI(4,5)P(2) regulation of surface membrane traffic. *Curr Opin Cell Biol.* 2001;13(4):493–499.
8. Simonsen A, Wurmser AE, Emr SD, Stenmark H. The role of phosphoinositides in membrane transport. *Curr Opin Cell Biol.* 2001;13(4):485–492.

Protein Phosphorylation

George W. Booz, PhD; Kenneth M. Baker, MD

KEY POINTS

- Protein phosphorylation plays an important role in the control of many cellular processes, including metabolism, membrane transport, volume regulation, protein synthesis, and gene expression.

- The sequential activation of protein kinases in distinct phosphorylation cascades is the principal means by which cells respond to external stimuli.

- The activity of transcription factors can be regulated by phosphorylation in several ways. Phosphorylation may control the cellular location of a transcription factor; modulate DNA-binding activity, transactivation potential, or both; or be required for recruitment of a coactivator.

- Protein phosphorylation is critically important in regulating protein synthesis. Control occurs primarily at the level of translation initiation, which is correlated with cell growth and is influenced by mitogens that activate the MAPK and/or PI3K cascades.

See also Chapters A24, A28–A31, and A33

For many cellular proteins, phosphorylation by a kinase triggers a conformational change that modifies activity or function. An important feature of this type of covalent modification is that it is reversible through the action of a phosphatase, thus allowing protein phosphorylation to serve as a molecular switch for turning proteins and cellular systems (e.g., channels) on and off. In general, phosphorylation acts like an on switch, but there are many examples of phosphorylation inhibiting the function of a protein, as with GSK-3 (see **Table A32.1** for abbreviations). Protein phosphorylation affects metabolism, membrane transport, volume regulation, protein synthesis, and gene expression.

Protein Kinases

The sequential activation of protein kinases in distinct phosphorylation cascades is the principal means by which cells respond to external stimuli. These cascades amplify and prolong an initial signal, allow for the integration of different signals, and often result in a sustained or permanent cellular response to a transient external stimulus. Protein phosphorylation cascades, in particular those involving the MAPKs, are critically important in development, growth, cellular survival, and programmed cell death or apoptosis. The importance of protein phosphorylation to the physiology of the cell is underscored by the fact that protein kinases are the largest known protein family, representing an estimated 1% to 3% of all mammalian genes.

Structure and function. Protein kinases are structurally related by having a catalytic domain that (a) binds and orients a substrate peptide/protein and a purine nucleotide triphosphate donor [adenosine triphosphate (ATP)/guanosine triphosphate (GTP)] as a complex with a divalent cation (Mg^{2+} or Mn^{2+}) and (b) facilitates the transfer of the γ-phosphate of the donor to a hydroxyl residue (serine, threonine, or tyrosine) of the substrate.

Groups. Based on the amino acid sequence of the catalytic domain, eukaryotic protein kinases can be organized into 4 groups that have related functions and share substrate preference. The AGC group phosphorylates serine/threonine residues near the basic residues arginine and lysine. The AGC group includes the cyclic nucleotide–dependent kinases PKA and PKG, PKCs, ribosomal S6Ks, PKB/Akt, and β-adrenergic receptor kinases. The CaMK group, containing the Ca^{2+}/calmodulin-regulated and related kinases, phosphorylates serine or threonine residues near basic amino acids. The CMGC kinases phosphorylate serine/threonine residues in proline-rich domains and include cyclin-dependent kinases, GSK-3, MAPKs, and Clk (Cdk-like) kinase. The PTK group includes both receptor kinases (e.g., receptors for EGF, PDGF, insulin, and FGF) and nonreceptor kinases (e.g., the Jak and Src families) that phosphorylate tyrosine residues. Several recently described kinases fall outside of these major subgroups, including MEKs, MEKKs, the Raf family, and MLKs.

Phosphorylation and Intracellular Signaling

Signaling cascades. Cells respond to external stimuli by a multitude of intracellular signaling cascades involving phosphorylation or dephosphorylation events linked to cell membrane receptors, channels, or integrins. These cascades serve to distribute a ligand's signal throughout the cell, resulting in short- and long-term responses. Signaling cascades can be activated by second messengers [e.g., cyclic adenosine monophosphate (cAMP), cyclic guanosine monophosphate (cGMP), Ca^{2+}, diacylglycerol] or by tyrosine kinase (both receptor and nonreceptor).

One stimulus generally activates multiple signaling cascades, both second messenger- and tyrosine kinase-dependent. A cascade may involve a simple second messenger-kinase pair (e.g., cAMP-PKA) or a series of sequentially activated kinases (e.g.,

Table A32.1. Selected Abbreviations and Acronyms

CaMK = Ca^{2+}/calmodulin regulated kinase
CBP = CREB-binding protein
CRE = cAMP response element
CREB = CRE-binding protein
EGF = epidermal growth factor
eIF = eukaryotic initiation factor
ERK = extracellular signal–regulated kinase
FGF = fibroblast growth factor
FH = forkhead (transcription factor)
FRAP = FKBP 12-rapamycin–associated protein
GEF = guanine nucleotide exchange factor
GPCR = G protein–coupled receptor
GSK-3 = glycogen synthase kinase-3
IKK = IκB kinase
IRS-1 = insulin receptor substrate-1
Jak = Janus kinase
JNK = c-Jun NH$_2$ terminal kinase
MAPK = mitogen activated protein kinase
MAPKAP = MAPK activated protein
MEK = MAPK kinase
MEKK = MEK kinase
MLK = mixed lineage kinase
Mnk = MAPK interacting kinase
mTOR = mammalian target of rapamycin
NFAT = nuclear factor of activated T cells
PDGF = platelet derived growth factor
PDK1 = 3-phosphoinositide–dependent protein kinase 1
PI3K = phosphoinositide 3 kinase
PKA = protein kinase A
PKB = protein kinase B
PKC = protein kinase C
PKG = protein kinase G
PTB = phosphotyrosine binding
PTK = protein tyrosine kinase
RTK = receptor tyrosine kinase
S6K = (ribosomal) S6 kinase
SAPK = stress-activated protein kinase
SH2 = Src-homology 2
Smad = contraction: Sma and Mad (mothers against decapentaplegic)
STAT = signal transducers and activators of transcription

MAPK cascades). Cascades can exhibit branching, and one cascade can initiate another via formation of a second messenger or via activation of a tyrosine or serine/threonine kinase. Cross-talk can occur between cascades at the level of the membrane transducers, signaling components, or effector proteins, resulting in synergistic or antagonistic effects (see Chapters A28 and A29).

Recruitment and spatial organization of kinases and effector proteins.
Two important regulatory mechanisms for the control of intracellular signaling are (a) the recruitment of kinases and effector proteins to a particular subcellular location such as a receptor and (b) the organization of kinases in a phosphorylation cascade into complexes or modules, before or after stimulation.

Ordering events. Ordering events confine a signal to the appropriate subcellular location, optimize the response time, and reinforce the specificity with which kinases interact with targets. Protein-protein or protein-lipid interactions form the basis of these ordering events, which are mediated by defined domains of 35 to 150 amino acids. Several domains important in protein-protein interactions recognize specific phosphoty-

rosine or phosphoserine/threonine motifs. SH2 domains bind to specific phosphotyrosine containing motifs, such as those found on receptors for cytokines, growth factors, and antigens. Specificity is conferred by the preference of the domain for the amino acids immediately following the phosphorylated tyrosine.

Conformational proteins. Numerous adaptor, scaffold, and docking proteins, enzymes, cytoskeletal proteins, inhibitory factors, and transcription factors contain 1 or more SH2 domains. PTB domains bind Asn-Pro-X-Tyr motifs, with some requiring phosphorylation of the tyrosine residue. The PTB domains of the docking proteins, IRS-1 and Shc, exhibit this requirement. The forkhead-associated domain, which is found primarily in eukaryotic nuclear proteins, binds specific motifs phosphorylated by serine/threonine kinases.

14-3-3 proteins. A family of proteins known as 14-3-3 proteins form homo- and heterodimeric cuplike structures that bind discrete phosphoserine containing motifs. 14-3-3 proteins function like adaptor or scaffold proteins and are involved in the regulation of mitogenesis, cell cycle progression, and apoptosis, by either enhancing or inhibiting the activity of the proteins they bind. Bad, the Rafs, various PKCs, MEKK1, and FH transcription factors are some of the proteins the 14-3-3 proteins bind.

Multisite phosphorylation and signal strength.
Phosphorylation of more than 1 site is a common feature of many proteins involved in intracellular signaling. Multisite phosphorylation of receptors or docking proteins allows for the activation of multiple signaling cascades by 1 agonist. Phosphorylation of a protein on multiple sites can also determine the strength and duration of a signal; allow for different agonists to have synergistic, antagonistic, or redundant effects; or raise the threshold required for the activation of a protein.

The regulation of phosphorylase kinase by both cAMP and Ca^{2+} signals in mammalian skeletal muscle is an example of multisite phosphorylation that is important in stimulating glycogenolysis during increased muscle activity. By increasing cAMP, adrenaline activates PKA, which phosphorylates the α- and β-regulatory subunits of phosphorylase kinase, thereby enhancing sensitivity of the catalytic subunit to regulation by the Ca^{2+}-regulated δ calmodulin subunit as well as its maximum kinase activity.

Mitogen activated protein kinase phosphorylation cascades.
MAPKs are a family of serine/threonine kinases that play a central role in many basic cellular processes, including proliferation, differentiation, and apoptosis (**Figure A32.1**). MAPKs affect cellular processes and gene expression by phosphorylating structural or functional proteins and transcription factors or by activating other kinases. There are 6 mammalian MAPK families linked to distinct signaling cascades that are organized hierarchically into 3-tiered modules. Activation of MAPKs requires phosphorylation of threonine and tyrosine residues by the family of cytosolic dual-specificity kinases (MAPKK). MAPKK activation in turn results from phosphorylation by serine/threonine kinases (MAPKKK). MAPKKKs are activated by small G proteins or other protein kinases, thus

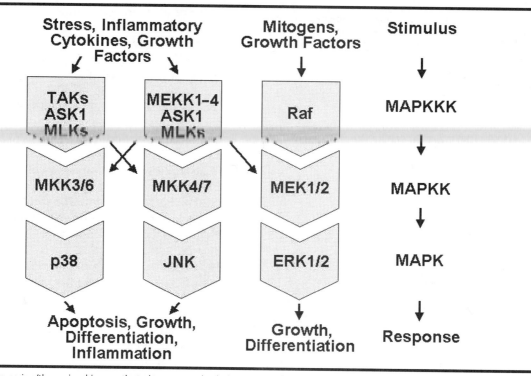

Figure A32.1. MAPKs are serine/threonine kinases that play a central role in many basic cellular processes. The 6 mammalian MAPK families are linked to distinct signaling cascades that are organized into 3-enzyme modules. MAPKs are phosphorylated and activated by MAPKKs, which are phosphorylated and activated by MAPKKKs. A particular MAPKKK may activate MAPKKs that are involved in different MAPK cascades. MAPKKKs are activated by small G proteins or other protein kinases, thus linking MAPK cascades to cell-surface receptors or external stimuli. The MAPK phosphorylation cascades that have received the most attention are those linked to the activation of ERK1/2, p38, and JNK/SAPK.

linking the MAPK module to a cell-surface receptor or external stimulus. Three phosphorylation cascades linked to the activation of ERK1/2, p38, and SAPK/JNK members of the MAPK family have received the most attention. The ERK1/2 MAPK cascade is activated by growth factors and mitogens and is involved in cellular growth and differentiation. The p38 and SAPK/JNK MAPK cascades, which are linked to a broad range of cellular responses such as growth, apoptosis, differentiation, or inflammation, are activated by growth factors (generally weakly and depending on cell type), inflammatory cytokines, and various stress stimuli (e.g., ultraviolet light, heat, reactive oxygen species, and protein synthesis inhibitors).

Receptor Coupling to the Extracellular Signal–Regulated Kinase Cascade

Tyrosine phosphorylation and docking. On ligand binding, RTKs undergo dimerization or conformational change, which results in the autophosphorylation of multiple tyrosine residues in the cytoplasmic region of the receptor. These phosphorylated tyrosine residues serve as docking sites for various proteins with 1 or more SH2 or PTB domains. One such protein is the nonenzymic adaptor protein Shc, which also has an SH3 domain that recognizes a left-hand polyproline type II helix domain in other proteins. Shc binds to the GEF protein, mSOS, directly by the SH3 domain or via an adaptor protein, GRB2. mSOS binds to and activates the small G protein Ras by catalyzing the release of guanosine diphosphate (GDP). Activated Ras in turn recruits the MAPKKK Raf to the membrane, thereby triggering the cascade that results in ERK1/2 activation.

G protein coupling. G protein–coupled receptors can couple to ERK1/2 activation by multiple means. For example, G_q/G_o-coupled receptors may stimulate the ERK cascade through Ras, by activating PKC, PI3K, or both, or by activating the nonreceptor protein tyrosine kinase, Pyk2, via increases in intracellular Ca^{2+}. Pyk2 in turn activates Src and/or leads to Shc phosphorylation. G_q/G_i-coupled receptors may also activate the ERK cascade independently of Ras, via PKC-mediated activation of Raf. G_i-coupled receptors may be linked to the ERK cascade via activation of the Src family tyrosine kinases, which results in Shc phosphorylation and formation of the Shc-GRB2-mSOS-Ras complex. Src family kinases are direct effectors of $G\alpha_i$ or may be activated indirectly via $G\beta\gamma$-mediated activation of PI3K. Finally, GPCRs may activate the ERK cascade via transactivation of the PDGF or EGF receptors by either Ca^{2+}-dependent or -independent mechanisms.

Phosphoinositide 3 Kinase Phosphorylation Cascade

Parallel pathways: mitogen activated protein kinase phosphoinositide 3 kinase. Agonists that stimulate MAPK activity commonly induce a parallel phosphorylation cascade that is linked to PI3K activation and has been implicated in enhancing protein synthesis, promoting cell survival and mediating many of the cellular actions of insulin (see Chapter A31). PI3K represents a family of membrane proteins, composed of an 85-kd regulatory subunit and a 110-kd catalytic subunit, that phosphorylate the 3'-OH position of the inositol ring in inositol phospholipids, and various proteins on serine and threonine, including IRS-1. Association of SH2 domains in the regulatory subunit with phosphorylated tyrosine residues activates PI3K. Ras and the βγ subunit of heterotrimeric G proteins may also activate the catalytic subunit (a 101-kd regulatory protein, which is found in certain mammalian cell types, is directly activated by G proteins).

Cellular effects. The phosphorylated lipid products of PI3K have been implicated in membrane ruffling and cytoskeletal changes, receptor endocytosis, activation of certain PKC isoforms, and in the translocation of PKB/Akt to the membrane, where it is activated through serine-threonine phosphorylation by PDK1 and a yet-to-be-identified kinase. There are numerous targets downstream of activated PKB/Akt, many of which impact cell survival and protein synthesis. For example, activated PKB promotes cell survival by activating IKK, and inhibiting Bad, caspase-9, and FH transcription factors. PKB activation promotes protein synthesis by activating FRAP/mTOR and inhibiting GSK-3. FRAP/mTOR may be activated independently of PKB and appears also to function as an intracellular sensor of amino acid levels.

Regulation of Transcription Factor Activity

Transcription factors can be regulated by changes in their concentration or activity. Concentration reflects the activity of multiple steps from transcription to translation, each of which may be regulated by protein phosphorylation. The activity of transcription factors can be regulated by phosphorylation in several ways.

Transcription factors. First, phosphorylation may control the cellular location of a transcription factor. Four examples of transcription factors under this type of control are the Smads, NFκBs, STATs, and cytoplasmic NFATs.
Smads. The Smads are latent cytoplasmic transcription factors that become active at cognate receptors, which have serine kinase activity and bind the transforming growth factor β superfamily of ligands. Serine phosphorylation of Smads results in an association with regulatory Smads and translocation to the nucleus.
NFκB. The NFκB proteins are found in the cytoplasm bound to the anchor protein IκB in the nonstimulated state. Phosphorylation of IκB by IKK, PKC, or PKA induces its proteolysis, thus liberating the transcription factor and allowing it to move into the nucleus.
Signal transducers and activators of transcription. The STATs are the only known transcription factors activated from a latent state by tyrosine phosphorylation. Cytoplasmic STATs are phosphorylated by the Jak or Src family of kinases, resulting in STAT dimerization (via intermolecular binding of their juxtaposed phosphorylated tyrosine residues and SH2 domains) and subsequent nuclear translocation.
Nuclear factor of activated T cells. The cytoplasmic NFATs are activated by agonists that increase cell calcium. Increased calcium activates the phosphatase calcineurin, which dephosphorylates the NFATs, resulting in nuclear translocation. The NFATs are phosphorylated by several kinases, including GSK-3 and JNK.

DNA-binding activity. Second, phosphorylation may modulate the DNA-binding activity or transactivation potential of a transcription factor. For example, JNKs phosphorylate 2 sites in the N-terminal transactivation domain of c-Jun, thereby enhanc-

ing transactivation potential, and ERKs phosphorylate an inhibitor domain in C/EBPβ, disrupting intramolecular binding with the transactivation domain and permitting DNA binding.

Coactivator recruitment. Last, phosphorylation (generally on serine) of a transcription factor may be required for recruitment of a coactivator. PKA-mediated CREB phosphorylation causes it to bind CBP, which is required for CREB to function as a transcription factor. A conserved serine residue modulates STAT transcriptional activity in an isoform-specific manner: Phosphorylation may enhance transcriptional activity through recruitment of coactivators, prolong tyrosine phosphorylation and DNA binding, or interfere with tyrosine phosphorylation and activation.

Regulation of Protein Synthesis

Protein phosphorylation is critically important in regulating protein synthesis. Control occurs primarily at the level of translation initiation, which is correlated with cell growth and is influenced by mitogens that activate the MAPK or PI3K cascades.

Translation initiation and eukaryotic initiation factors. Translation initiation is a multistep process whereby the 40S ribosome subunit is positioned at the AUG initiation codon of the messenger RNA (mRNA) transcript. Attachment of the ribosome to the transcript is facilitated by a cap structure [7-methyl guanosine triphosphate] found at the 5' terminus of all nuclear encoded eukaryotic mRNAs. Attachment requires the participation of eIFs and is initiated by eIF4F, which functions to unwind secondary structure in the 5' untranslated region of mRNA, thereby facilitating ribosome binding to the 5' end. eIF4F consists of 3 protein subunits: eIF4E, the cap-binding subunit which is present in rate-limiting amounts; eIF4A, an RNA helicase which (in synergy with eIF4B) exhibits bidirectional RNA unwinding activity; and eIF4G, a scaffold protein, that also binds to ribosome-associated eIF3 and thus functions as a link between ribosome and mRNA. The function of eIF4E is negatively regulated by 4E-BP binding proteins, which compete with eIF4G for a common binding site on eIF4E. Phosphorylation of 4E-BPs decreases the affinity for eIF4E, thereby allowing cap-dependent translation initiation to occur and resulting in enhanced protein synthesis.

Extracellular modulation of 4E-BP binding proteins. 4E-BP hyperphosphorylation is induced by extracellular stimuli such as insulin and various growth and survival factors via a signaling cascade involving the sequential activation of PI3K, PDK1, and PKB/Akt. 4E-BP hyperphosphorylation may be dependent on its initial phosphorylation by FRAP/mTOR. The phosphorylation states of eIF4G and eIF4B are also affected by this signaling cascade, but what significance this has on function has not been established. ERK activation may also result in 4E-BP hyperphosphorylation, after 4E-BP is initially phosphorylated by FRAP/mTOR. In addition to being under negative control via 4E-BP, eIF4E function appears to be positively regulated by phosphorylation on Ser209, after it is bound to eIF4G. In general, a strong correlation occurs between eIF4E phosphorylation and rates of protein synthesis and cell growth, but how Ser209 phosphorylation affects eIF4E function is not clear. Phosphorylation of eIF4E on Ser209 may play a key role in regulating *de novo* initiation of translation as opposed to reinitiation. Recent evidence indicates that the kinases responsible for eIF4E phosphorylation in the cell are Mnk1 and 2, which are substrates for the ERK1/2 and p38 MAPKs.

Ribosomal biogenesis upregulation.

Hormones and mitogens can also stimulate protein synthesis by inducing the upregulation of ribosome biogenesis, thereby increasing the translational capacity of the cell. Ribosome biogenesis is subject to a unique mechanism of translational regulation involving phosphorylation of the 40S ribosomal S6 protein by the serine/threonine protein kinase, p70 S6K. This phosphorylation enhances the ribosomal binding of mRNAs that contain a 5' terminal oligopyrimidine tract (5'TOP) adjacent to the cap, thereby enhancing translation. The mRNAs that encode much of the translational machinery, including numerous ribosomal proteins, elongation factors, and the poly(A) binding protein, contain a 5' terminal oligopyrimidine tract. The enzymatic activity of the S6Ks, which are members of the AGC superfamily, is regulated by phosphorylation. Two homologs encoded by different genes occur in mammals, S6K1 and S6K2. S6K enzymatic activity is regulated by the phosphorylation of multiple serine or threonine residues within the catalytic, linker, and pseudosubstrate domains. Phosphorylation of Thr229 and Thr389 in the catalytic and linker domains, respectively, is critical for kinase function of p70 S6K1 and occurs downstream of PI3K activation at 2 levels: FRAP/mTOR activation leads to Thr389 phosphorylation, which allows for the direct phosphorylation of Thr229 by PDK1. The atypical PKCs, PKCλ and PKCζ, which can be activated by PDK1, also appear to play a role in S6K1 activation. S6K2 is highly homologous to S6K1 but differs from S6K1 in the N- and C-terminal regions. S6K2 is primarily found in the nucleus and seems to be regulated in a similar manner as S6K1 but with stronger positive regulation by ERK1/2, which phosphorylates sites within the C-terminal pseudosubstrate region. Phosphorylation of these sites is thought to activate S6K by relieving pseudosubstrate suppression. Last, phosphorylation of the ribosomal DNA transcription factor upstream binding factor is another way in which ribosome biogenesis is positively regulated by mitogens and growth factors.

Translation modulation by eukaryotic initiation factor 2.

Protein phosphorylation is also important in the control of translation by eIF2, which functions to transfer the initiator methionyl–transfer RNA to the 40S subunit, thus forming the 43S preinitiation complex. In its function, eIF2 binds and hydrolyzes GTP. For eIF2 to participate in another round of initiation, GDP has to be exchanged for GTP in a process catalyzed by eIF2B. Amino acid deprivation, double-stranded RNA, and other stress stimuli activate kinases that phosphorylate eIF2, stabilize the eIF2-GDP-eIF2B complex, and inhibit protein synthesis. Also, phosphorylation by GSK-3 inhibits eIF2B. Blocking the function of eIF2 results in the inhibition of protein synthesis and can lead to apoptosis. Serine phosphorylation of GSK-3 by PKB-, p6K, or MAPKAP-K1 relieves the inhibitory effect of GSK-3 on eIF2B. Thus, eIF2B activity can be enhanced by growth factors via either the PI3K cascade (PKB, FRAP/mTOR and S6K activation) or ERK1/2 (MAPKAP-K1 and S6K activation) or by amino acids via FRAP/mTOR.

Messenger RNA release and peptide chain elongation.

Protein phosphorylation plays a role in the regulation of other aspects of protein synthesis, including the release of mRNA from the nucleus and peptide chain elongation. Recent studies have shown that RNA stability and premessenger RNA splicing are also controlled by phosphorylation events that are linked to the various kinase cascades activated by extracellular stimuli.

SUGGESTED READING

1. Brivanlou AH, Darnell JE. Signal transduction and the control of gene expression. *Science.* 2002;295:813–818.
2. Chang L, Karin M. Mammalian MAP kinase signalling cascades. *Nature.* 2001;410:37–40.
3. Cohen P. The regulation of protein function by multisite phosphorylation—a 25 year update. *Trends Biochem Sci.* 2000;25:596–601.
4. Gingras AC, Raught B, Sonenberg N. Regulation of translation initiation by FRAP/mTOR. *Genes Dev.* 2001;15:807–826.
5. Graves JD, Krebs EG. Protein phosphorylation and signal transduction. *Pharmacol Ther.* 1999;82:111–121.
6. Hanks SK, Hunter T. Protein kinases 6. The eukaryotic protein kinase superfamily: kinase (catalytic) domain structure and classification. *FASEB J.* 1995;9:576–596.
7. Kyriakis JM, Avruch J. Mammalian mitogen-activated protein kinase signal transduction pathways activated by stress and inflammation. *Physiol Rev.* 2001;81:807–869.
8. Pearson G, Robinson F, Beers Gibson T, et al. Mitogen-activated protein (MAP) kinase pathways: regulation and physiological functions. *Endocr Rev.* 2001;22:153–183.
9. Vanhaesebroeck B, Alessi DR. The PI3K-PDK1 connection: more than just a road to PKB. *Biochem J.* 2000;346:561–576.
10. Wilson KF, Cerione RA. Signal transduction and post-transcriptional gene expression. *Biol Chem.* 2000;381:357–365.

Chapter A33

Vascular Smooth Muscle Contraction and Relaxation

Brett M. Mitchell, PhD; Kanchan A. Chitaley, PhD; R. Clinton Webb, PhD

KEY POINTS

- Phosphorylation of myosin light chain regulates the interaction of myosin and actin, and thus modulates the contractile state of the vasculature.

- Regulation of myosin light-chain phosphatase by Ca^{2+}-dependent and Ca^{2+}-independent mechanisms dynamically determines the state of myosin light-chain phosphorylation and muscular contraction.

- After removal of a contractile stimulus, relaxation occurs as a result of decreased intracellular Ca^{2+} and increased myosin light-chain phosphatase activity.

See also Chapters A25–A32 and C146

Contractile Mechanism

The contractile state of vascular smooth muscle (VSM) is the primary determinant of lumen diameter and therefore of systemic vascular resistance. The process of VSM cell contraction, independent of membrane potential, is regulated by receptor and mechanical (stretch) activation of the contractile proteins myosin and actin. Phosphorylation of the 20-kd light chain of myosin enables the myosin-actin interaction. Energy released from myosin adenosine triphosphatase (ATPase) activity results in sliding of myosin crossbridges over actin, causing contraction. The initiation of crossbridge cycling is thus determined primarily by the phosphorylation state of myosin light chain (MLC) in a highly regulated process.

Ca²⁺-Dependent Contraction

Phosphorylation of MLC is initiated by the Ca^{2+}-calmodulin–dependent activation of MLC kinase (see Chapter A27). As the intracellular Ca^{2+} concentration ($[Ca^{2+}]_i$) increases, Ca^{2+} combines with calmodulin to activate MLC kinase (**Figure A33.1**). Cytosolic Ca^{2+} is increased through Ca^{2+} release from intracellular stores, predominantly the sarcoplasmic reticulum (SR), as well as from Ca^{2+} entry from the extracellular space. Agonist binding of vasoconstrictors such as norepinephrine or angiotensin II to heterotrimeric G protein–coupled receptors stimulates phospholipase C activity, resulting in the production of inositol trisphosphate and diacylglycerol (DAG) from phosphatidylinositol 4,5 bisphosphate (PIP_2) (see Chapter A31). The binding of inositol trisphosphate to receptors on the SR results in the release of Ca^{2+} into the cytosol. Ca^{2+} entry is also mediated by Ca^{2+} channels in the plasma membrane. Voltage-gated Ca^{2+} channels open in response to changes in cell membrane potential, and intracellular mediators such as DAG may activate signaling cascades to stimulate the opening of membrane Ca^{2+} channels.

Ca²⁺-Sensitization Mechanism for Contraction

Roles of phosphatases and kinases. In addition to the Ca^{2+}-dependent activation of MLC kinase, the state of MLC phosphorylation is further regulated by MLC phosphatase, which removes the high-energy phosphate from MLC, thus promoting vasorelaxation (Figure A33.1). MLC phosphatase consists of 3 major subunits: a 37-kd catalytic subunit, a 20-kd variable subunit, and a 110- to 130-kd myosin-binding subunit. The 110- to 130-kd myosin-binding subunit, when phosphorylated, inhibits the enzymatic activity of MLC phosphatase. The small G protein, RhoA, and its downstream target, Rho-kinase, play a direct role in the regulation of MLC phosphatase activity. Rho-kinase, a serine/threonine kinase, phosphorylates the myosin-binding subunit of MLC phosphatase, inhibiting its activity and promoting the phosphorylated state of MLC (Figure A33.1). Y-27632, a selective inhibitor of Rho-kinase, induces relaxation of isolated agonist-contracted blood vessels and lowers blood pressure in hypertensive but not normotensive rats. Recently, an increased vasodilator response to Rho-kinase inhibition in hypertensive humans has been demonstrated, suggesting that Rho-kinase contributes to elevated peripheral resistance in essential hypertension.

Other regulating influences. MLC kinase and MLC phosphatase are also regulated by other factors (Figure A33.1). Calmodulin-dependent protein kinase II decreases the sensitivity of MLC kinase for Ca^{2+}, promoting vasodilation. Additionally, MLC phosphatase activity is stimulated in phasic smooth muscle by telokin, a 16-kd protein, and inhibited by a downstream mediator of DAG and protein kinase C, CPI-17. Independent of MLC, various proteins such as caldesmon and calponin modulate actin and thus influence crossbridge cycling. Although these factors affect myosin and actin, their physiologic importance is not clear (Figure A33.1).

Decreased Intracellular Ca²⁺ and Vascular Smooth Muscle Relaxation

Vasodilation occurs as a result of decreased intracellular Ca^{2+} and increased MLC phosphatase activity. Several mechanisms involving the SR and the plasma membrane are implicated in removal of cytosolic Ca^{2+}. Deficiencies in mechanisms that sequester intracellular Ca^{2+} or increase MLC phosphatase

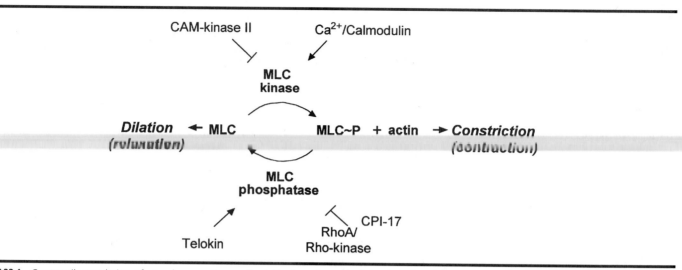

Figure A33.1. Contractile regulation of vascular smooth muscle. Activation of myosin light chain (MLC) kinase and MLC phosphatase (MLC-P) dynamically regulates the phosphorylation state of MLC and thus the interaction of myosin and actin for contraction. Various signaling molecules can affect MLC kinase and MLC phosphatase activation and thus modulate cellular contraction. CAM, calmodulin.

activity may contribute to enhanced vasoconstriction and hypertension.

Sarcoplasmic reticulum Ca²⁺ uptake and adenosine triphosphate hydrolysis. Ca^{2+} uptake into the SR is concomitant with ATP hydrolysis and is dependent on ATP and magnesium (Mg^{2+}). This SR Ca,Mg-ATPase, when phosphorylated, binds 2 Ca^{2+} ions that are subsequently translocated to the luminal side of the SR and released. Mg^{2+} binds to the catalytic site of Ca,Mg-ATPase to mediate the reaction. The SR Ca,Mg-ATPase is inhibited by vanadate, thapsigargin, cyclopiazonic acid, and phospholamban. Phosphorylation of phospholamban removes its inhibitory effect and stimulates ATP-dependent Ca^{2+} uptake. SR Ca^{2+}-binding proteins also contribute to decreased intracellular Ca^{2+} levels. In the last decade, calsequestrin and calreticulin have been identified in smooth muscle cells as SR Ca^{2+}-binding proteins.

Ca,Mg-adenosine triphosphatases. The plasma membrane also contains Ca,Mg-ATPases that aid in the removal of Ca^{2+} from the cell. These enzymes differ from the SR protein in that they have an autoinhibitory domain that can be bound by calmodulin and cause stimulation of the plasma membrane Ca^{2+} pump. Calmodulin consists of 4 homologous domains that each can bind 1 Ca^{2+} and 2 high-affinity and 2 low-affinity sites. Ca^{2+} binding to the 2 high-affinity sites increases binding of calmodulin to the plasma membrane Ca,Mg-ATPase, which then increases the affinity of the remaining Ca^{2+} binding sites for Ca^{2+}. The plasma membrane Ca,Mg-ATPase can be stimulated with phospholipids and inhibited by oxytocin.

Na⁺/Ca²⁺ exchangers. Calcium extrusion pumps located on the plasma membrane aid in decreasing intracellular Ca^{2+}. This low-affinity antiporter is closely coupled to intracellular Ca^{2+} levels and can be inhibited by amiloride and quinidine.

Blockade of voltage-gated Ca²⁺ channels. Voltage-dependent Ca^{2+} channels located in the plasma membrane are important for Ca^{2+} influx and VSM cell contraction as previously mentioned; inhibition of these channels also elicits or augments relaxation. The clinical significance of this mechanism is defined by the vasodilator properties of L-channel antagonists such as dihydropyridines, phe-

nylalkylamines, and benzothiazepines, which bind to distinct receptors on the channel protein and inhibit Ca^{2+} entry. L-channel blockade has been used clinically in controlling hypertension.

Increased Myosin Light-Chain Phosphatase Activity and Vascular Smooth Muscle Relaxation

Although MLC kinase and MLC phosphatase are constitutively active in phosphorylating and dephosphorylating MLC, respectively, lowering Ca^{2+} decreases the rate of myosin phosphorylation and increases MLC phosphatase activity. The increase in MLC phosphatase activity is potentiated by the phosphorylation of cytosolic inhibitor proteins that release the bound MLC phosphatase catalytic subunits. These catalytic subunits then bind with the targeting subunits and together increase the affinity for MLC. Dephosphorylation of MLC leads to detachment of actin-myosin crossbridges and relaxation.

Abnormal Contractile Regulation in Hypertension

As noted above, alterations in the regulatory processes maintaining intracellular Ca^{2+} and MLC phosphorylation have been proposed as possible mechanisms contributing to the increased vasoconstriction and impaired vasodilation characteristic of hypertension. In addition, alterations in upstream targets that impact Ca^{2+} and MLC phosphorylation have also been implicated. For example, changes in the affinity, number, or subtype of α-adrenergic receptors leading to enhanced vasoconstriction have been characterized in VSM cells in some types of hypertension. Impaired vasodilation may occur as the result of abnormal cyclic nucleotide-dependent signaling pathways coupled with reductions in receptor activation or agonist bioavailability (endothelium dysfunction, reduced nitric oxide, and cyclic guanine monophosphate). The complexity and redundancy of the cell signaling pathways regulating intracellular Ca^{2+} and MLC phosphorylation provide additional therapeutic potential for the treatment of hypertension.

SUGGESTED READING

1. Barany M. *Biochemistry of Smooth Muscle Contraction*. San Diego, CA: Academic Press; 1996.

2. Chitaley K, Weber DS, Webb RC. RhoA/Rho-kinase, vascular changes and hypertension. *Curr Hypertens Rep.* 2001;3:139–144.

3. Feletou M, Vanhoutte PM. Endothelium-dependent hyperpolarization of vascular smooth muscle cells. *Acta Pharmacol Sin.* 2000;21:1–18.

4. Meiss RA. Mechanics of smooth muscle contraction. In: Kao CY, Carsten ME, eds. *Cellular Aspects of Smooth Muscle Function.* New York, NY: Cambridge University Press; 1997:169–201.

5. Morgan K. The role of calcium in the control of vascular tone as assessed by the Ca^{++} indicator Aequorin. *Cardiovasc Drugs Ther.* 1990;4:1355–1362.

6. Solaro RJ. Myosin light chain phosphatase: a Cinderella of cellular signaling. *Circ Res.* 2000;87:173–175.

7. Somlyo AP, Somlyo AV. From pharmacomechanical coupling to G-proteins and myosin phosphatase. *Acta Physiol Scand.* 1998;164:437–448.

8. Uehata M, Ishizaki T, Satoh H, et al. Calcium sensitization of smooth muscle mediated by a Rho-associated protein kinase in hypertension. *Nature.* 1997;389:990–994.

9. Woodrum DA, Brophy CM. The paradox of smooth muscle physiology. *Mol Cell Endocrinol.* 2001;177:135–143.

Section 3. *Vasoregulatory Systems*

Chapter A34

Central Nervous System in Arterial Pressure Regulation

J. Michael Wyss, PhD

KEY POINTS

- Tonic activity of the sympathetic nervous system continuously and differentially regulates the constriction of peripheral resistance vessels and contributes to heart rate control and cardiac output.

- Nuclei in the medulla oblongata maintain tonic sympathetic nervous system activity based on sensory input from baroreceptors and chemoreceptors and modulation by other brain centers, including the hypothalamus.

- The hypothalamus coordinately regulates blood pressure by alterations in neurohormonal release and by regulation of the brainstem cardiovascular nuclei.

- Cerebral cortical and subcortical areas alter cardiovascular function to meet the demands of cortically driven behaviors.

See also Chapters A2, A35–A38, A40–A43, C120, C143, and C161

Although the cardiovascular system is capable of maintaining blood flow and cardiac function in the absence of any nervous system input, addition of neural control mechanisms allows very precise, short-term (second-to-second and minute-to-minute) cardiovascular regulation. Studies over the past 30 years have demonstrated that the nervous system also can contribute to long-term cardiovascular and blood pressure regulation. In several animal models and in subsets of human hypertensive patients, inappropriate regulation of the cardiovascular system by the nervous system appears to play a significant role in chronic hypertension and the resulting target organ damage. The final common pathway for the nervous system's contribution to chronic arterial pressure control is via the sympathetic and parasympathetic divisions of the autonomic nervous and neurohormonal systems that are primarily regulated by the hypothalamus. Most experimental evidence suggests that compared to the parasympathetic nervous system, the sympathetic nervous and neurohormonal systems contribute much more to the pathogenesis of hypertension.

Peripheral Autonomic Nervous System

Neuroanatomy. The autonomic nervous system includes sympathetic and parasympathetic divisions and the associated afferent (sensory) feedback that courses along with each division. Sympathetic and parasympathetic motor neuron cell bodies lie in peripheral ganglia. In the sympathetic nervous system, neuron cell bodies lie in ganglia that are immediately lateral to the spinal cord (paravertebral) or anterior to the vertebral column (prevertebral). The prevertebral neurons primarily innervate visceral organs, including the heart and kidney, whereas the paravertebral neurons project more prominently to blood vessels throughout the body. Irrespective of their location, all sympathetic ganglia neurons are innervated by preganglionic neurons that lie in the thoracic portion of the spinal cord. Parasympathetic motor neurons lie in ganglia that are very close to the organ that is innervated. These ganglion cells are innervated by neuronal cell bodies that lie in the medulla (for organs above the transverse colon) and the sacral spinal cord (for organs below the transverse colon). Sensory afferent feedback from the innervated tissue is projected back through the ganglia to the central nervous system (CNS). Most sympathetic afferents terminate in the spinal cord at the level that correlates with the ganglia through which they course (e.g., the kidney is innervated by the lower thoracic sympathetic ganglia, and the sensory feedback terminates in the lower thoracic spinal cord).

Parasympathetic sensory innervation follows the projection pattern of the motor fibers, and most of it terminates in the dorsal brain stem.

Cardiovascular monitoring systems.

Many studies have investigated the roles of baroreflex and chemoreflex abnormalities in hypertension, but no study has been able to prove conclusively that chronic arterial pressure elevations originate from reflex abnormalities (see Chapters A35 and A36).

Baroreceptors. The brain continuously monitors arterial pressure, primarily via stretch receptors (mechanoreceptors) attached to vagal and glossopharyngeal axons innervating the aortic arch and carotid bifurcation (aortocarotid or "high-pressure" baroreceptors). In parallel, blood volume is monitored by branches of the vagus nerve innervating the cardiac atria and ventricles (cardiopulmonary or "low-pressure" baroreceptors). Baroreceptors located elsewhere in the body (e.g., the kidney) serve a similar function.

Chemoreceptors. Chemoreceptors that are sensitive to vascular O_2 deficiency, CO_2 excess, and H^+ excess are found in the carotid bodies and adjacent to the aorta. These receptors are not as important to arterial pressure regulation as the mechanoreceptors under routine pathophysiologic conditions but appear to play a role in arterial pressure regulation during extreme conditions such as hypoxia.

Osmoreceptors. Osmoreceptors found in several areas of the brain and in the periphery can also modify arterial pressure; recent studies have highlighted the importance of hepatic osmoreceptors in cardiovascular regulation.

Modulation of neurotransmission.

Less conventional forms of synaptic transmission may be important to the sympathetic nervous system's role in arterial pressure regulation. Kopp and associates have demonstrated that neurotransmitters released from efferent (motor) nerve terminals in the kidney can alter the ability of neurons to send information to the CNS conduction of information in nearby afferent (sensory) axons. Similarly, Kruelen and associates have shown that some peripheral afferent nerves directly innervate neurons in the sympathetic ganglia and give rise to sensory feedback control that does not go through the CNS. Other neurotransmitters and neuromodulators released by sensory neurons can have profound effects on the target organs; perhaps the best example is calcitonin gene–related peptide (CGRP), which when released by the peripheral afferent neurons onto the blood vessels, causes potent vasodilation. Recent studies in the rat suggest that the release of CGRP is inhibited by α_2-adrenoreceptor activation. Thus, the overabundance of norepinephrine in a target tissue could increase vasoconstriction not only directly by stimulation of α_1-adrenoceptors, but also indirectly via inhibition of CGRP release.

Abnormalities in hypertension.

Whereas several aspects of peripheral sympathetic innervation may be primary contributors to some forms of hypertension, evidence available points to 2 peripheral anomalies in hypertensive animal models.

Increased neurons and varicosities. In some genetic models of hypertension in the rat, there is a greater than normal number of sympathetic postganglionic neurons or neuronal varicosities, the bead-like storage and release sites for norepinephrine that exist in sympathetic neurons. This is suggestive of an increased sympathetic drive to the organs and appears to be related to a failure of the nervous system to appropriately prune down the number of postganglionic neurons or varicosities during development.

Altered sensory feedback. Second, increased sensory feedback from vital organs or diminished baroreflex control appears to contribute to hypertension in some forms of the disease. Irrespective of cause, in several animal models of hypertension, an overactive sympathetic nervous system appears to promote greater vasoconstriction in the periphery and result in hypertension. In these models, the interaction appears to be most important during the development of the disease and much less important during the maintenance phase.

Regulation of Arterial Pressure by the Spinal Cord and Medulla

Integrated responses of the sympathetic nervous system.

Preganglionic neurons that lie in the thoracic spinal cord, primarily in the intermediolateral cell column are the final common pathway for CNS regulation of the peripheral sympathetic nervous system. Preganglionic neurons are directly regulated by descending inputs from the cervical spinal cord, brain stem, and diencephalons, and from sensory innervation of the spinal cord. Under usual physiologic conditions, the sympathetic nervous system is not regulated *en masse* but rather in regional or organ-related fashion and in patterns that meet the heterogeneous needs of the organism to react to its surroundings. For instance, during defense behaviors, blood flow is increased to the skin and skeletal muscle and decreased to the gut. Blood flow to individual capillary beds is differentially regulated according to local metabolic factors. Although the spinal cord components of the sympathetic nervous system may contribute to some aspects of hypertension, most research points to abnormalities at higher centers of the CNS as the primary neuronal contributors to hypertension.

Brain-stem control centers.

The medulla, the most caudal portion of the brain, contains 4 major neuronal complexes that are important for cardiovascular control (**Table A34.1**).

Nucleus tractus solitarius. The nucleus tractus solitarius (NTS) is the major site for the transfer of cardiovascular information to the brain from the periphery. The NTS is responsible for integrating signals from cardiopulmonary and aortocarotid baroreceptors and chemoreceptors and initiating appropriate responses. Additionally, the NTS receives input from cardiovascular receptors in the kidney, liver, and muscle as well as the forebrain and brainstem neurons involved in cardiovascular regulation. NTS projections directly modify sympathetic and parasympathetic tone and the release of vasopressin from the hypothalamus. Reis and his colleagues demonstrated that NTS lesions result in acute fulminating hypertension in rats and less severe hypertension in other species. Lesions of the NTS in cats and dogs increase lability of blood pressure but not the overall mean blood pressure. However, in rats and, perhaps, in humans, primary abnormalities in the NTS may contribute to hypertension by increasing sympathetic nervous system activity. Cardiovascular neurons in the NTS are organized in functionally distinct regions. Stimulation of the middle third of the

Table A34.1. Major Areas of the Central Nervous System That Modify Arterial Pressure and May Play a Role in Hypertension

LEVEL OF THE CENTRAL NERVOUS SYSTEM	AREA OF THE BRAIN	PRIMARY EFFECT ON ARTERIAL PRESSURE
Cerebral cortex	Neocortex and amygdala	Alterations in arterial pressure related to behavior and emotion
Hypothalamus	Anterior and preoptic nuclei	Primarily decrease arterial pressure
	Lateral and posterior nuclei	Primarily increase arterial pressure
	Paraventricular and supraoptic nuclei	Primarily increase arterial pressure and vasopressin release
Brain stem	Nucleus of the solitary tract	Receives baroreflex and related sensory input to the brain
	Rostroventrolateral medulla	Tonic sympathetic nervous system activation; tonic arterial pressure drive
	Caudal ventrolateral medulla	Modulates activity of the rostroventrolateral medulla
	Area postrema	Changes in arterial pressure related especially to circulating substances (e.g., angiotensin II)
Spinal cord	Intermediolateral cell column	Final central nervous system formatting for sympathetic nervous system control of blood pressure

NTS causes depressor and bradycardic responses, whereas stimulation of the midline region of the more posterior commissural NTS increases blood pressure and heart rate. Lesions of the commissural NTS prevent hypertension in several animal models. Other studies demonstrate that γ-aminobutyric acid A (GABA$_A$) and GABA$_B$ receptors are differentially located in the NTS, and stimulation of pre- versus postsynaptic receptors may differentially suppress baroreflex responses, contributing to hypertension in some animal models. Further, in the early stage of hypertension in hypertensive rats and in humans, blood pressure tends to rapidly rise during the waking hours and then fall to approximately normal levels during the sleeping hours. If the baroreflex resets to the higher and lower arterial pressures during each phase, then it may fail to appropriately buffer the rise and fall of arterial pressure during the 24-hour period. Such an effect could increase stress on the vessels during the early wake period, when sympathetic nervous system activity is high, worsening the hypertension.

Area postrema. In the rat, the area postrema, which lies dorsal to NTS, can monitor blood levels of hormones and neurotransmitters because it lacks a blood–brain barrier. Stimulation of area postrema neurons by circulating or local angiotensin II (Ang II) decreases baroreflex sensitivity and increases sympathetic activity. Conversely, arginine vasopressin binds to V$_1$ receptors in the area postrema, inhibiting sympathetic nervous system activity and increasing baroreflex sensitivity. The area postrema is critical for the development of hypertension in high renin models such as the mRen rat, but area postrema lesions normalize arterial pressure in some hypertensive animal models and the area postrema does not appear to modulate dietary salt-sensitive hypertension in rats.

Rostroventrolateral medulla. The rostroventrolateral medulla (RVLM) contains the motor neurons that provide tonic drive to the spinal cord preganglionic motor neurons that directly regulate sympathetic nervous system activity. Thus, the RVLM is the nodal point for the regulation of sympathetic nervous system outflow. Descending projections to the RVLM originate in lateral parabrachial nucleus and periaqueductal gray, paraventricular hypothalamic nucleus and in other parts of the forebrain. Activation of most of these inputs to the RVLM increases sympathetic nervous system activity and thereby elevates arterial pressure, primarily by increasing arterial resistance. Glutamate and AMPA receptors are the primary mode of activation of RVLM neurons, but acetylcholine (ACh) is used by excitatory inputs from the lateral parabrachial nucleus, posterior hypothalamus, and lateral septal area to RVLM. RVLM drive to the preganglionic sympathetic neurons provides the background of vasoconstriction, cardiac contractility, and catecholamine release that set the basal state of arterial pressure. Increased RVLM firing increases arterial pressure, whereas inhibition of the RVLM or its output decreases arterial pressure. Whereas the RVLM (like the preganglionic neurons) is known to play a permissive role in almost any form of CNS-driven hypertension, several studies suggest that its role contribution may be more primary. Inhibitory input to RVLM neurons is blunted in spontaneously hypertensive rats (SHRs), and angiotensin microinjections into this region elicit greater responses in SHRs than in normotensive control rats. Further, ACh content is elevated in RVLM of 2 models of hypertension (SHRs and DOCA-salt rats), and inhibition of ACh-esterase in the RVLM produces an exaggerated increase in arterial pressure in these models.

Caudal ventrolateral medulla. The caudal ventrolateral medulla (CVLM) is composed of neurons that are scattered in the ventral medulla from the RVLM to the spinomedullary junction. These neurons provide tonic and baroreflex-mediated inhibition to the RVLM neurons, likely via GABA-ergic projections. Although the role of CVLM in hypertension is unclear, the activity of CVLM neurons in young SHR is depressed, raising the possibility that loss of sympathoinhibition from this nucleus may contribute to some forms of hypertension.

Regulation of Arterial Pressure by the Hypothalamus

Whereas the medullary neurons are responsible for the sensory reception and final motor output by which the brain regulates arterial pressure, higher brain areas provide the descending integration that coordinates arterial pressure and behavioral responses (Table A34.1). A role for the hypothalamus in chronic hypertension has been inferred from experimentation with regional ablation, electric stimulation, and neuronal transplantation studies.

Lateral posterior hypothalamus. Transplantation of the hypothalamus from a genetically hypertensive rat induces hypertension in a genetically normotensive recipient. The lateral and posterior hypothalamus contain predominantly sympathoexcitatory neurons, whereas the anterior and preoptic regions tend to be sympathoinhibitory. In rats made hypertensive by administration of the steroid deoxycorticosterone acetate in conjunction with a high salt diet, stimulation of the posterior or lateral hypothalamus increases arterial pressure and heart rate, whereas lesions of the posterior hypothalamus reduce arterial pressure. In the posterior hypothalamus of SHRs, imbalances in norepinephrine, ACh, and GABA may contribute to hypertension.

Paraventricular nucleus. Many of the magnocellular neurons of the paraventricular nucleus (PVN) and the associated supraoptic nucleus synthesize and release vasopressin into the circulation. The parvocellular neurons in PVN project nerve fibers to several CNS cardiovascular control nuclei, including the RVLM, area postrema, NTS, and the intermediolateral nucleus of the spinal cord, and parvocellular neurons appear to alter cardiovascular function via these connections. Activity of parvocellular neurons in the PVN is influenced by glutamate and Ang II, both of which directly increase sympathetic activity. SHRs display abnormal regulation of parvocellular neurons in the PVN, and the interaction between PVN neurons and Ang II appears to be altered in several forms of hypertension. Leptin has been found to modify PVN neuronal activity, potentially contributing to arterial pressure elevations in obesity.

Anteroventral third ventricle. The anterior hypothalamus contains several areas that are important in cardiovascular control, including the anteroventral third ventricle. Lesions of the anteroventral third ventricle prevent the development of hypertension and attenuate established hypertension in several animal models. The median preoptic nucleus appears to underlie many of these cardiovascular effects; the inputs it receives from circumventricular organs and brainstem nuclei play a significant role in the cardiovascular function. Other preoptic nuclei regulate vasopressin release and water balance and contribute at least indirectly to arterial pressure control.

Anterior hypothalamus. The anterior hypothalamic nucleus, along with the preoptic area, provides important sympathoinhibitory influences, most of which are mediated by projections to sympathoexcitatory nuclei in the diencephalon and brain stem. Stimulation of these nuclei elicits a decrease in arterial pressure and heart rate, whereas lesions in the anterior hypothalamic area increase arterial pressure. In SHRs, diets high in salt exacerbate hypertension, at least in part by reducing sympathoinhibitory drive from the anterior hypothalamic nucleus.

Regulation of Arterial Pressure by the Basal Ganglia and Cerebral Cortex

Subcortical nuclei that may play a role in arterial pressure changes include the basal ganglia, the septal nuclei, and the amygdala (Table A34.1).

Amygdala. The amygdala regulates defense ("fight-or-flight") responses and has the closest potential linkage to hypertension. Stimulation of the amygdala results in elevated sympathetic activity and a corresponding increase in arterial pressure. Further, lesions of the amygdala attenuate the development of

hypertension in SHRs, whereas stress-induced glutamate release in the amygdala is enhanced in SHRs compared to controls.

Hippocampus. Experimental and clinical observations indicate that the cortex affects cardiovascular function and that several cortical regions are asymmetrically involved. The hippocampus contributes to arterial pressure regulation, in part, through opioid-mediated hypotensive effects. In the rat, 70% of insular cortex neurons display significant responses to baroreceptor manipulations, whereas less than 35% of neurons in the surrounding cortex show similar activity.

Insular cortex. Most of the insular cortex neurons that respond to baroreceptor changes are in the right (versus the left) posterior insular cortex. In the monkey, cardiovascular information also converges on insular cortex neurons, and approximately twice as many of the baroreceptor-sensitive neurons are in the right cerebral hemisphere. In humans, the left (compared to the right) insular cortex appears to dominate parasympathetic control of the cardiovascular system. Strokes that significantly involve the left insular cortex are associated with an increase in sympathetic tone and a decrease in the phase relationship between heart rate and blood pressure. These observations point to the potential importance of the insular cortex in both chronic and acute regulation of cardiovascular function and suggest that right-left asymmetries in the brain may be important in optimal cardiovascular control.

Infralimbic cortex. In addition to the insular cortex, other areas of the cerebral cortex contribute to cardiovascular control. Stimulation of infralimbic cortex (and to a lesser extent the prefrontal cortex) alters arterial pressure and many of its neurons project fibers to the lateral hypothalamus, the periaqueductal gray, and the medulla. These forebrain areas thus can also influence arterial pressure, heart rate, and baroreflex gain.

SUGGESTED READING

1. Colombari E, Sato MA, Cravo SL, et al. Role of the medulla oblongata in hypertension. *Hypertension.* 2001;38:549–554.
2. Esler M. Sympathetic nervous system: contribution to human hypertension and related cardiovascular diseases. *J Cardiovasc Pharmacol.* 1995;26(Suppl. 2):S24–S28.
3. Loewy AD. Anatomy of the autonomic nervous system. In: Loewy AD, Speyer KM, eds. *Central Regulation of Autonomic Functions.* New York, Oxford University Press; 1990:3–16.
4. Lopes HF, Silva HB, Consolim-Colombo FM, et al. Autonomic abnormalities demonstrable in young normotensive subjects who are children of hypertensive parents. *Braz J Med Biol Res.* 2000;33(1):51–54.
5. Mifflin SW. What does the brain know about blood pressure? *News Physiol Sci.* 2001;16:266–271.
6. Oparil S, Chen YF, Berecek KH, et al. The role of the central nervous system in hypertension. In: Laragh JH, Brenner BM, eds. *Hypertension: Pathophysiology, Diagnosis and Management.* 2nd ed. New York, NY: Raven Press; 1995:713–740.
7. Oppenheimer SM, Kedem G, Martin WM. Left-insular cortex lesions perturb cardiac autonomic tone in humans. *Clin Auton Res.* 1996; 6(3):131–140.
8. Osborn JW, Collister JP, Carlson SH. Angiotensin and osmoreceptor inputs to the area postrema: role in long-term control of fluid homeostasis and arterial pressure. *Clin Exp Pharmacol Physiol.* 2000;27:443–449.
9. Peng N, Wei CC, Oparil S, Wyss JM. The organum vasculosum of the lamina terminalis regulates noradrenaline release in the anterior hypothalamic nucleus. *Neuroscience.* 2000;99(1):149–156.
10. Zhang ZH, Dougherty PM, Oppenheimer SM. Characterization of baroreceptor-related neurons in the monkey insular cortex. *Brain Res.* 1998;796:303–306.

Arterial Baroreflexes

Mark W. Chapleau, PhD

KEY POINTS

- Stretch-sensitive baroreceptor nerve endings in the carotid sinuses and aortic arch rapidly detect changes in arterial pressure and initiate reflex circulatory adjustments to reduce or "buffer" blood pressure variability and its adverse consequences.

- Important determinants of baroreflex sensitivity include large artery compliance, the activity of mechanosensitive and voltage-dependent ion channels on the sensory nerve terminals, and central mechanisms that alter the coupling of baroreceptor afferent signals to autonomic efferent nerve activities.

- Rapid baroreflex resetting occurs during acute hypertension, a phenomenon that helps preserve baroreflex buffering at the ambient pressure level.

- Endothelial dysfunction, oxidative stress, platelet activation, and angiotensin II may contribute to decreased baroreflex sensitivity in patients with chronic hypertension and vascular disease.

See also Chapters A34, A36–A38, A40–A43, A60, C120, and C161

Arterial baroreceptors are stretch-sensitive sensory nerve endings located in carotid sinuses and aortic arch that function as arterial pressure sensors (**Figure A35.1**). Afferent (sensory) baroreceptor activity is transmitted to the nucleus tractus solitarii in the medulla oblongata, where the signals are integrated and relayed through a network of central neurons that determine parasympathetic and sympathetic nerve outflow to the heart, kidney, and vasculature.

Baroreflex Function

Cellular mechanisms of baroreceptor activation. Baroreceptors are activated as a result of their deformation during vascular distension. The mechanism of transducing deformation into membrane depolarization is thought to involve opening of mechanosensitive ion channels present on the sensory nerve terminals (**Figure A35.2**). The mechanically induced depolarization, if of sufficient magnitude, opens voltage-dependent Na^+ and K^+ channels, leading to generation of action potentials at the "spike initiating zone" near the peripheral endings (Figure A35.2).

Buffering of arterial pressure fluctuations. The arterial baroreflex is the primary mechanism for rapid buffering of acute fluctuations in arterial pressure that occur during postural changes, behavioral and physiologic stress, and changes in blood volume. Increases in pressure and baroreceptor activity trigger reflex parasympathetic activation, sympathetic inhibition, and decreases in heart rate (HR) and vascular resistance that oppose the rise in pressure. Conversely, baroreceptor activity decreases during a fall in pressure, producing reflex-mediated increases in HR and vascular resistance. The baroreflex also influences secretion of vasopressin and renin, which contribute to blood pressure regulation. Thus, the baroreflex pro-

vides moment-to-moment negative feedback regulation of arterial pressure that minimizes pressure lability. The extreme pressure lability observed in baroreceptor-denervated subjects underscores the importance of the reflex in buffering changes in pressure.

Tonic sympathoinhibitory function. In addition to responding to changes in pressure, ongoing baroreceptor activity under resting conditions tonically inhibits baseline sympathetic nerve activity and release of vasopressin and renin. The powerful tonic inhibitory influence of baroreceptor activity is easily appreciated by observing the profound autonomic changes and increase in blood pressure that occur acutely after baroreceptor denervation.

Baroreflex Resetting during Acute and Chronic Hypertension

Rapid baroreflex resetting. During a sustained increase in arterial pressure, baroreceptor activity declines or adapts over a period of seconds to minutes. The mechanism of adaptation involves mechanical viscoelastic relaxation and activation of 4-aminopyridine–sensitive K^+ channels. On return of pressure to lower levels after periods of acute hypertension (5 to 30 minutes), the baroreceptor pressure threshold is increased and baroreceptor activity is suppressed (**Figure A35.3**). Rapid baroreceptor resetting and the resulting rightward shift of the pressure-activity curve is caused in part by activation of an electrogenic Na^+ pump, which hyperpolarizes the baroreceptor nerve endings. Rapid resetting does not alter the slope of the pressure-activity curve or attenuate maximum baroreceptor activity (Figure A35.3). Rapid baroreceptor resetting is usually accompanied by resetting of the arterial pressure-HR and pressure-sympathetic nerve activity relations and allows effec-

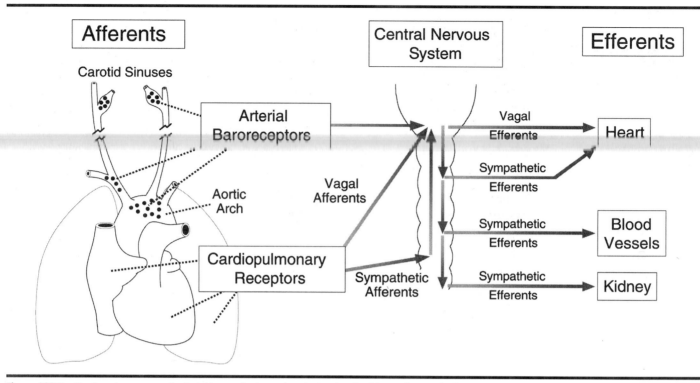

Figure A35.1.   Cardiopulmonary and arterial baroreflex neural pathways involved in cardiovascular homeostasis and blood pressure regulation. Locations of arterial baroreceptors are indicated by filled circles. For discussion of cardiopulmonary baroreflexes, see Chapter A36.

tive buffering of pressure fluctuations to persist at the new prevailing pressure level (Figure A35.3).

Chronic baroreflex resetting. In chronic hypertension, the baroreceptors are reset to higher pressures (Figure A35.3). The resting level of baroreceptor activity is relatively "normal"

despite the high pressure, but the slope of the curve (i.e., change in HR/change in pressure) may be decreased. Several mechanisms contribute to decreased baroreflex sensitivity and resetting in hypertension, including reduced vascular compliance of the carotid sinuses and aortic arch and impaired central mediation of the reflex.

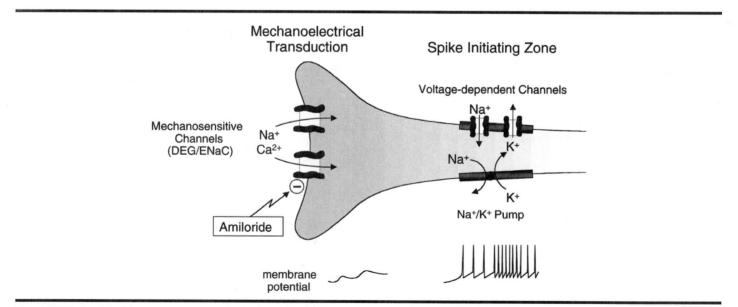

Figure A35.2.   Model of baroreceptor nerve terminal. Mechanosensitive ion channels are thought to mediate mechanoelectrical transduction. Evidence suggests that these channels are members of the DEG/ENaC gene family and are inhibited by amiloride. Opening of mechanosensitive channels allows Na$^+$ and Ca^{2+} influx and depolarization of the endings. Sufficient depolarization opens voltage-dependent Na$^+$ and K$^+$ channels at the "spike initiating zone," triggering action potentials at frequencies related to the magnitude of depolarization. An electrogenic Na$^+$ pump maintains Na$^+$ and K$^+$ gradients and influences membrane potential.

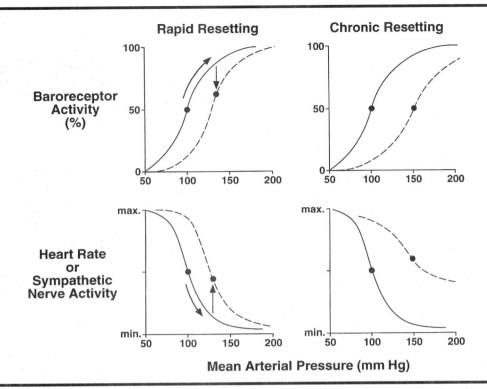

Figure A35.3. Shown are effects of acute and chronic hypertension on baroreceptor pressure–afferent activity **(top)** and pressure–heart rate (HR) or sympathetic activity **(bottom)** relations. **Left:** Initial responses to increased pressure are increased baroreceptor activity and reflex decreases in HR and sympathetic activity. Sustained acute hypertension results in baroreceptor adaptation, a return of HR and sympathetic activity toward control, and a shift in the baroreceptor function curves to the right. **Right:** In chronic hypertension, resting baroreceptor activity is relatively normal, function curves are shifted further to the right, and the slope and range of the curves may be decreased.

Neurohumoral and Paracrine Modulation of the Baroreflex

Hormones. Various hormones and autacoids can influence the baroreflexes. Angiotensin II (Ang II) resets the baroreflex function curve to higher pressures independently of its effect on arterial pressure. In contrast, vasopressin resets the baroreflex curve to lower pressures. These actions are mediated in part through effects of circulating Ang II and vasopressin on the area postrema, a circumventricular region that lacks a blood–brain barrier and contains neurons that project to the vasomotor control centers.

Diseases. Hypertension and heart failure are often associated with neurohumoral activation, including increases in angiotensin, vasopressin, or both. The magnitude and selectivity of the increases in these hormones, which may depend on the underlying cause of the disease, influence the net effect on the baroreflex. For example, renal hypertension associated with high levels of Ang II is characterized by pronounced baroreflex resetting, decreased slope of the pressure-HR relation, reduced maximum range of HR modulation, and increased sympathetic nerve activity at rest. The altered baroreflex results not only from the elevated pressure but also from the central nervous system actions of Ang II. In contrast, other types of hypertension may exhibit less baroreflex resetting and lower levels of sympathetic activity.

Paracrine factors. Paracrine factors produced near baroreceptor endings may alter baroreceptor afferent activity through effects on vascular tone or ion channels on the baroreceptor nerve terminals. Factors that act directly on baroreceptors to increase excitabil-

ity include norepinephrine and prostacyclin. Factors that decrease excitability include reactive oxygen species, factor(s) released from activated platelets, and nitric oxide. Therefore, antioxidants, antiplatelet agents, angiotensin-converting enzyme inhibitors, and angiotensin receptor antagonists have the potential to restore baroreflex sensitivity in patients with cardiovascular disease.

Clinical Implications

Family history studies. Baroreflex-mediated changes in sympathetic activity are decreased in normotensive subjects with a family history of hypertension. These and other data suggest that genetic factors may influence baroreflex sensitivity independently of blood pressure.

Antihypertensive drug effects. Changes in baroreflex function in chronic hypertension can be at least partially reversed by effective treatment of the hypertension. Rapid baroreflex resetting occurs during decreases as well as increases in pressure and is preserved in treated chronic hypertension. Therefore, the baroreflex function curve may be shifted to lower pressures soon after therapy is initiated. This resetting is expected to help maintain pressure at the lower level. Reversal of structural vascular changes with longer periods of treatment causes additional improvement in baroreceptor sensitivity.

Baroreflexes and sudden death after myocardial infarction. In addition to regulating arterial pressure, the baroreflex exerts a significant influence on the electrical properties of the heart through modulation of parasympathetic and sympathetic nerve activity. Ventricular arrhythmias are a common cause of death during myocardial ischemia and after myocardial infarction. Animal and clinical studies have demonstrated that decreased baroreflex sensitivity for control of HR predicts susceptibility to arrhythmias and sudden death after acute myocardial infarction, suggesting that the baroreflex may protect the heart from arrhythmias.

Future clinical developments. Assessment of baroreflex sensitivity may provide a valuable method of screening patients with cardiovascular disease. In addition to laboratory-based tests of baroreflex sensitivity, methods have been developed to assess spontaneous baroreflex sensitivity under "daily life" conditions using computer-based analysis of spontaneous variations in arterial pressure and HR. The use of these methods for the evaluation of patients with cardiovascular disease remains to be demonstrated.

SUGGESTED READING

1. Chapleau MW, Cunningham JT, Sullivan MJ, et al. Structural versus functional modulation of the arterial baroreflex. *Hypertension.* 1995;26:341–347.
2. Chapleau MW, Li Z, Meyrelles SS, et al. Mechanisms determining sensitivity of baroreceptor afferents in health and disease. In: Chapleau MW, Abboud FM, eds. *Neuro-Cardiovascular Regulation: From Molecules to Man. Ann N Y Acad Sci.* 2001;940:1–19.
3. Corey DP, Garcia-Anoveros J. Mechanosensation and the DEG/ENaC ion channels. *Science.* 1996;273:323–324.
4. Drummond HA, Price MP, Welsh MJ, Abboud FM. A molecular component of the arterial baroreceptor mechanotransducer. *Neuron.* 1998;21:1435–1441.
5. Korner PI. Cardiac baroreflex in hypertension: role of the heart and angiotensin II. *Clin Exp Hypertens.* 1993;17:423–459.
6. Kunze DL, Andresen MC. Arterial baroreceptors: excitation and modulation. In: Zucker IH, Gilmore JP, eds. *Reflex Control of the Circulation.* Boca Raton, FL: CRC Press; 1991:139–164.
7. La Rovere MT, Bigger JT Jr, Marcus FI, et al. Baroreflex sensitivity and heart-rate variability in prediction of total cardiac mortality after myocardial infarction. *Lancet.* 1998;351:478–484.
8. Mancia G, Mark AL. Arterial baroreflexes in humans. In: *Handbook of Physiology.* Section 2, vol III, part 2. Bethesda, MD: American Physiological Society; 1983:755–793.
9. Parati G, Di Rienzo M, Mancia G. How to measure baroreflex sensitivity: from the cardiovascular laboratory to daily life. *J Hypertens.* 2000;18:7–19.
10. Persson PB, Kirchheim HR. *Baroreceptor Reflexes: Integrative Functions and Clinical Aspects.* Berlin: Springer-Verlag; 1991.

Chapter A36

Cardiopulmonary Baroreflexes

Mark E. Dunlap, MD

KEY POINTS

- The cardiopulmonary baroreflex arc includes stretch fibers in the heart and lungs that act as volume sensors, relaying information about central blood volume to the brain stem, where signals are integrated with those from the arterial baroreflexes to modulate sympathetic nervous outflow.

- Cardiopulmonary baroreflexes exert potent tonic inhibitory influences over sympathetic outflow and play an important role in systemic blood pressure and volume homeostasis.

- Important interactions exist between cardiopulmonary baroreflexes and other neurohormonal systems.

See also Chapters A34, A35, A37, A38, A40, A42, and C155

Cardiopulmonary Baroreflex System

The cardiopulmonary baroreflex (CPBR) system is comprised of a set of sensory afferent fibers that respond to central (intrathoracic) volume signals to modulate the outflow of sympathetic efferent nerve fibers, thus contributing importantly to blood pressure and volume regulation (see Chapter A35 and Figure A35.1).

Reflex arcs controlling blood volume. CPBRs exert minimal effects on parasympathetic outflow. Myelinated and unmyelinated vagal afferent (sensory) fibers arise from the left ventricle, left atrium, and pulmonary veins, although the unmyelinated fibers mediate most of the baroreflex responses. The afferent cell bodies lie in the nodose ganglia, from which they send projections to the nucleus tractus solitarius (NTS) in the brain stem. NTS activity modulates the outflow of sympathetic nerve traffic from the brain-stem nuclei that control efferent sympathetic outflow to the heart, kidneys, and blood vessels (see Chapter A34). Blood volume, cardiac preload, cardiac output, and peripheral vasoconstriction are thus under direct control of the CPBR.

Afferent fibers. Cardiopulmonary receptors are activated by mechanical and chemosensitive stimuli acting through different sets of receptors.

Chemoreceptors. Chemosensitive receptors exert their primary effects during pathologic states, especially during ischemia, hypoxia, and heart failure. Activation of these receptors in the setting of an inferior myocardial infarction leads to bradycardia and hypotension owing to powerful inhibition of sympathetic outflow and stimulation of parasympathetic outflow, an effect known as the *von Bezold-Jarisch reflex.*

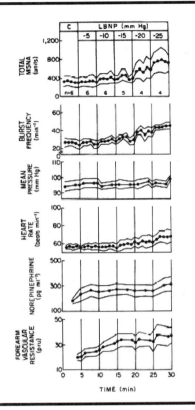

Figure A36.1. LBNP, lower body negative pressure; MSNA, muscle sympathetic nerve activity. (From Rowell LB. *Human Cardiovascular Control*. New York, NY: Oxford University Press;1993:95, with permission.)

Polymodal receptors. A parallel set of afferent fibers also course in the sympathetic nerves. These sympathetic afferent fibers exert excitatory influences over sympathetic outflow. Evidence from animal experiments suggests that these endings are polymodal and respond to chemical and mechanosensitive stimuli. Although efferent fibers play an important role during pathologic conditions (e.g., they mediate the sensation of angina during myocardial ischemia), the contribution of these fibers to tonic circulatory control is less clear.

Preload Reduction and Blood Pressure Control

Sympathetic response to acute preload reduction. During either assumption of upright posture or application of lower body negative pressure in humans, blood volume decreases in the central (intrathoracic) compartment, thereby decreasing central venous pressure and reducing right and left ventricular filling pressures or "preload." These reductions in filling pressure reduce the degree of distension of the left ventricle, thereby "unloading" or deactivating the cardiopulmonary baroreceptors and causing reflex increases in sympathetic outflow and vascular resistance (**Figure A36.1**). At low levels of pressure reduction (e.g., lower body negative pressure changes of 5–10 mm Hg), changes in sympathetic activity and vascular resistance occur before changes in blood pressure or heart rate, indicating that the arterial baroreflex system, which controls parasympathetic and sympathetic outflow, is not engaged. The CPBR is thus much more selective for sympathetic responses.

Integrated compensatory responses. With progressively greater decrements in filling pressure (as with severe dehydration or subacute hemorrhage), the cardiopulmonary baroreflex becomes more fully engaged, but other compensatory responses also occur. Cardiac output is diminished owing to decreased preload via the Frank-Starling mechanism, and the arterial baroreflex also becomes engaged, leading to increases in heart rate. The net increases in sympathetic outflow and vascular resistance protect against systemic hypotension, especially orthostatic hypotension. CPBR inactivation during zero gravity helps explain the transient orthostatic intolerance that is a common phenomenon after space flight.

Interactions of Cardiopulmonary Baroreflex and Other Neurohormonal Systems

Hormonal modulation. The CPBR is involved in controlling the release of several peptides involved in hemodynamic and volume homeostasis, including renin, vasopressin, and endothelin. The CPBR also is modulated by several other neurohormones. For example, vasopressin has been shown to sensitize the CPBR such that the sympathoinhibitory influence becomes augmented. Atrial natriuretic peptide, released by distension of the atria, exerts a net inhibitory effect on sympathetic outflow. Atrial natriuretic peptide also has other complex effects, including sensitization of vagal afferent fibers and probable neuromodulatory activity at other central or ganglionic sites.

Baroreflex interactions. Cardiopulmonary and arterial baroreceptors send projections to the NTS and other medullary sites and appear to converge on the same synapses and affect one another. For example, unloading of the CPBR improves carotid baroreflex control of blood pressure, with the greatest effects occurring after a certain threshold filling pressure is achieved. The significance of this finding is that arterial baroreflex sensitivity is heightened when humans are in the upright position, thus achieving the tightest beat-to-beat control over blood pressure.

Pain and other responses. There also appears to be an interaction between CPBR and central analgesic centers, because loading CPBR by leg elevation leads to lower pain scores in response to painful stimulation. Thus, there is convergence of neurons centrally of several different systems. These interplays among different neurohormonal systems underscore the redundant and sensitive mechanisms by which these reflexes are involved in controlling systemic pressure and volume homeostasis.

Age Effects

Resting sympathetic activity increases with advancing age in humans. This has led investigators to question whether age-associated alterations in CPBR might contribute to age-related sympathoexcitation. Indeed, vasodilatory responses to volume loading are attenuated in older people. However, when sympathetic nerve responses have been measured directly in humans, sympathoinhibitory responses provoked by CPBR are usually preserved in older subjects. Thus, the reduced vascular responses to volume changes that have been observed in the elderly are more likely the result of attenuated responses of the vasculature or alterations in ventricular compliance. It also seems unlikely that altered CPBR function causes the increased sympathetic activity with aging, unless the CPBR system becomes simultaneously hypersensitive to preload reduction and hyposensitive to volume loading. Such a pattern is not incompatible with the restrictive or blunting effects that might be caused by left ventricular hypertrophy, however.

Hypertension and Ventricular Hypertrophy

Early changes. CPBR function appears to be augmented in the early stages of hypertension in normotensive subjects with a family history of hypertension (compared to subjects without a family history of hypertension). CPBR reflexes are similarly increased in borderline hypertensive rats given a high salt diet. Saline loading itself augments CPBR sensitivity in normotensive subjects without a family history of hypertension.

Established hypertension and left ventricular hypertrophy. As hypertension progresses, CPBRs become blunted, an effect that becomes more pronounced as left ventricular hypertrophy (LVH) progresses and the cardiac walls become less distensible. Because some studies in humans have failed to demonstrate abnormal CPBR in fully developed hypertension, it is likely that the net response depends on the relative contributions of augmented responses and the degree of LVH present. LVH appears to attenuate the CPBR, possibly owing to altered ventricular compliance, and there is increased CPBR sensitivity with regression of LVH, suggesting that hypertension is associated with functional (not irreversible) alterations in the CPBR

function. This lends support to the importance of treating hypertension with agents that promote regression of cardiac hypertrophy because normalization of ventricular mass leads to improved sympathoinhibitory responses to CPBR stimulation.

SUGGESTED READING

1. Ertl AC, Diedrich A, Biaggioni I. Baroreflex dysfunction induced by microgravity: potential relevance to postflight orthostatic intolerance. *Clin Auton Res.* 2000;10(5):269–277.
2. Morgan JS. Sympathoinhibitory effects of atrial natriuretic factor in normal humans. *Circulation.* 1990;81:1860–1873.
3. Grassi G, Giannattasio C, Cleroux J, et al. Cardiopulmonary reflex before and after regression of left ventricular hypertrophy in essential hypertension. *Hypertension.* 1988;12(3):227–237.
4. Hasser EM, DiCarlo SE, Applegate RJ, Bishop VS. Osmotically released vasopressin augments cardiopulmonary reflex inhibition of the circulation. *Am J Physiol.* 1988;254(5 Pt 2):R815–R820.
5. Iwase N, Takata S, Ogawa J, et al. The effects of sodium loading on cardiopulmonary baroreflexes. *Clin Exp Pharmacol Physiol.* 1989;(Suppl. 15):109–111.
6. Pawelczyk JA, Raven PB. Reductions in central venous pressure improve carotid baroreflex responses in conscious men. *Am J Physiol.* 1989;257(5 Pt 2):H1389–H1395.
7. Rowell LB. *Human Cardiovascular Control.* New York, NY: Oxford University Press; 1993.
8. Rowell LB, Seals DR. Sympathetic activity during graded central hypovolemia in hypoxemic humans. *Am J Physiol.* 1990;259(4 Pt 2):H1197–H11206.
9. Tanaka H, Davy KP, Seals DR. Cardiopulmonary baroreflex inhibition of sympathetic nerve activity is preserved with age in healthy humans. *J Physiol.* 1999;515(Pt 1):249–254.
10. Ueda M, Nomura G, Shibata H, et al. Assessment of cardiopulmonary baroreflex function in hypertensive and normotensive subjects with or without hypertensive relatives. *Clin Exp Pharmacol Physiol.* 1989;(Suppl.15):89–92.

Chapter A37

Renal Nerves and Extracellular Volume Regulation

Jeffrey L. Osborn, PhD; Suzanne G. Greenberg, PhD

KEY POINTS

- Renal nerves control urinary sodium and chloride excretion by modulating renin release and tubular sodium reabsorption; acute and rapid adjustments in sodium excretion during changes in extracellular fluid volume are mediated by inverse changes in renal sympathetic outflow.

- Cardiac stretch receptors (cardiopulmonary baroreflexes) modulate renal sympathetic nerve activity.

- Renal sympathetic nerve activity accounts for approximately 35% of the short-term adjustment in sodium excretion after step changes in sodium intake.

- Edema-forming states such as heart failure or cirrhosis exhibit increased renal sympathetic activity, which functions to support the circulation.

See also Chapters A3, A13, A14, A16, A20, A34–A36, A38, A39, A41, and A42

Effects of Renal Nerve Stimulation

Activation of renal sympathetic nerves plays a critical role in the regulation of renal tubular function via preglomerular constriction, reduced glomerular filtration pressure, and stimulation of sodium reabsorption in the proximal convoluted tubules and medullary thick ascending limbs.

Effects on sodium transport. The cellular mechanism(s) responsible for neural regulation of tubular sodium excretion include: α_1-adrenergic stimulation of sodium-hydrogen exchange (with accompanying bicarbonate reabsorption) in the proximal convoluted tubule, activation of Na^+-K^+ATPase (proximal convoluted tubules) and stimulation

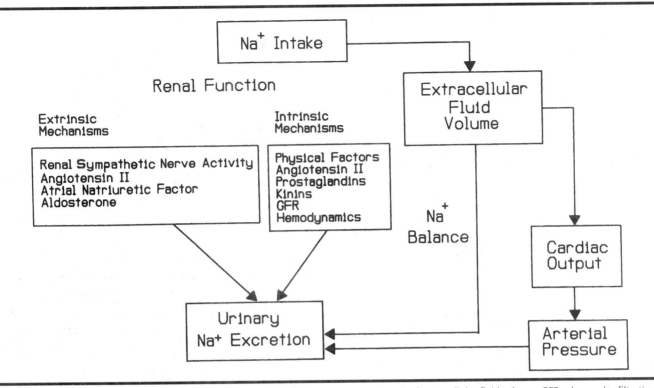

Figure A37.1. Major factors modulating urinary sodium excretion as a function of regulation of extracellular fluid volume. GFR, glomerular filtration rate.

of the $2Cl^- Na^+$-K^+ cotransporter of the thick ascending limb.

Other physiologic effects. In addition to direct effects of renal nerves on tubular transport, sodium balance is also critically influenced by activation of the renin-angiotensin-aldosterone axis, which is activated in parallel with the sympathetic nervous system via direct neural stimulation of renin release (β_1-adrenergic stimulation) and indirectly by α_2-adrenergic stimulation of tubular sodium reabsorption, which also promotes macula-densa cell-mediated renin release. In addition, there is α_1-mediated constriction of afferent arterioles, which tends to decrease glomerular filtration pressure, increase filtration fraction, and reduce the filtered load of sodium. These critical effects of renal neuroadrenergic stimulation on kidney function have led to the notion that elevation of renal sympathetic nerve activity vitally influences the regulation of sodium balance and consequently extracellular fluid volume (ECFV).

Afferent Control of Renal Sympathetic Nerve Activity

Neurogenic influences on the control of ECFV involve sodium intake and urinary sodium excretion. Behavioral factors and hypothalamic control of sodium intake are critical to the overall level of ingested sodium and consequently ECFV. Changes in ECFV, however, are predominantly controlled via urinary sodium excretion (**Figure A37.1**). Changes in efferent renal sympathetic tone occur inversely in response to both low-pressure (cardiopulmonary) baroreflex afferent input of the right atrial stretch receptors and high-pressure baroreflex mechanisms of the carotid sinus and aortic arch.

Aortocarotid baroreflexes. Basal efferent renal nerve activity is mediated predominantly by aortocarotid (high-pressure) baroreflexes. The pattern of sympathetic outflow exhibits an episodic "bursting" pattern coincident with the cardiac and respiratory cycles. Thus, renal nerve activity is low (and sometimes silent) during systole and peaks during diastole.

Cardiopulmonary and somatosensory afferent inputs. DiBona and colleagues have reported that efferent renal sympathetic responses are closely and inversely associated with increases and decreases in right atrial pressure after dietary changes in sodium intake, suggesting that low pressure cardiac vagal afferent nerve fibers leading to the central nervous system are significant in the "sensing" of ECFV and overall status of total body sodium. There is also significant input from numerous somatosensory afferent inputs as well as potential "sodium receptors" located in the hepatic and portal regions of the systemic circulation. The summation of numerous afferent inputs within the central nervous system provide specific and selective influences on urinary sodium excretion via control of renal sympathetic outflow.

Renal Sympathetic Nerve Activity and Sodium Balance

In the absence of renal nerve traffic, regulation of urinary sodium excretion is mediated solely by long-term controllers of ECVF, including humoral factors, renal blood flow, glomerular filtration rate, and physical forces (i.e., oncotic pressure).

Influence of renal sympathetic nerve activity. The renal efferent responses to increased or decreased sodium intake are associated with inverse changes in urinary sodium excretion. After a step decrease in sodium intake in conscious dogs (by IV

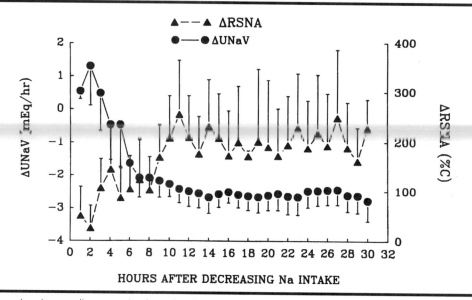

Figure A37.2.   Hourly changes in urinary sodium excretion (UNaV) and renal sympathetic nerve activity (RSNA) during the first 30 hours after a step decrease in Na intake.

infusion), renal efferent nerve activity increases, and this neurogenic activation is associated with a simultaneous decrease in urinary sodium excretion (**Figure A37.2**). The renal neurogenic response to a step decrease in sodium intake becomes maximal within 10 hours, approximately the same time period in which the antinatriuretic response is maximal. These rapid decreases in urinary sodium excretion are abolished by bilateral renal denervation. The neural and nonneural factors affecting sodium balance and regulation of ECFV have been semiquantitated in conscious animals with innervated and denervated kidneys 72 hours after a step increase in sodium intake. In the absence of renal nerves, the rate of achieving sodium balance is significantly delayed (**Figure 37.3**). The neural component of the summed controllers of sodium balance (and consequently ECFV) has been estimated at approximately 35% of the total sodium intake.

Integrated physiologic impact. Because the regulation of ECFV is vital to the functioning of the organism and in particular the cardiovascular system, numerous other intrinsic and extrinsic renal factors mediate changes in urinary sodium excretion and contribute substantially to the overall sodium balance. The sum total of these controllers thereby provide important redundancy to this regulatory system (Figure A37.1). Thus, renal efferent nerve traffic is primarily critical to the control of the rate at which sodium balance is achieved during increases and decreases in sodium intake, whereas other long-term controllers of sodium excretion maintain the appropriate level of sodium excretion.

Renal Sympathetic Nerve Activity and Edema-Forming States

There are several pathophysiologic conditions in which altered control of renal efferent sympathetic nerve activity contributes to an imbalance in the regulation of sodium excretion and to excess fluid and water retention. These major edema-forming states include congestive heart failure, cardiac tamponade, nephrotic syndrome, and cirrhosis of the liver. In each of these pathophysiologic conditions, one or a combination of the controllers of urinary sodium excretion (Figure A37.1) determines ECFV status. The activation of renal sympathetic outflow functions as a consequence of afferent sensory signals that respond to overall cardiovascular dysfunction. In this regard, the risk of complete cardiovascular collapse may be significantly decreased under conditions in which renal sympathetic outflow is substantially increased. Thus, even in these conditions in which overall cardiovascular function is declining, activation of renal sympathetic nerve activity tends to provide circulatory support.

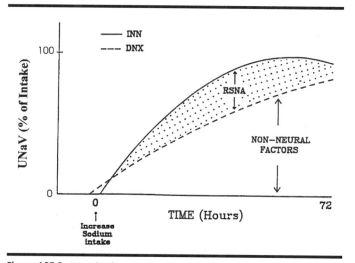

Figure A37.3.   Hourly changes in urinary sodium excretion (UNaV) in rats with innervated (INN) and denervated (DNX) kidneys for 72 consecutive hours after a step increase in sodium intake. The stippled area represents the sodium excretion response, which can be attributed to inhibition of renal sympathetic outflow. RSNA, renal sympathetic nerve activity.

SUGGESTED READING

1. Awazu M, Ichikawa I. Alterations in renal functions in experimental congestive heart failure. *Semin Nephrol.* 1994;14:401–411.

2. Greenberg SG, Tershner S, Osborn JL. Neurogenic regulation of rate of achieving sodium balance after increasing sodium intake. *Am J Physiol.* 1991;261:F300–F307.
3. Kopp UC, DiBona GF. The neural control of renal function. In: Seldin DW,

Giebisch G, eds. *The Kidney: Physiology and Pathophysiology.* 2nd ed. New York, NY: Raven Press; 1992:1157–1204.
4. Osborn JL. Relation between sodium intake, renal function, and the regulation of arterial pressure. *Hypertension.* 1991;17 (suppl I):I91–I96.

Chapter A38

Systemic Hemodynamics and Regional Blood Flow Regulation

Thomas G. Coleman, PhD; John E. Hall, PhD

KEY POINTS

- Regional blood flows are precisely and powerfully regulated to satisfy the metabolic needs of individual tissues, including relatively constant flow (e.g., brain) or highly variable flow (e.g., skeletal muscle for different activity levels or skin for temperature regulation).

- Regional blood flow regulation is relatively normal in essential hypertension, with most organs showing a normal flow and an elevated vascular resistance proportional to the increase in systemic pressure.

- Exercise-induced vasodilation is impaired in essential hypertension.

- The kidney often shows decreased blood flow in long-standing hypertension; this could be a sign of a renal defect that is contributing to the hypertension.

See also Chapters A34–A37, A41, A42, A46, and C117

The whole-body hemodynamic pattern seen most often in established essential hypertension, at least in supine humans, is one of increased total peripheral resistance and normal cardiac output. This flow and resistance pattern is determined by regional blood flow regulation, because cardiac output is equal to the mathematical sum of all regional blood flows, and total peripheral resistance is equal to the parallel sum of all regional vascular resistances (**Figure A38.1**).

Principles of Blood Flow Regulation

The metabolic state of a tissue is maintained by a stable relationship between metabolism and blood flow (**Figure A38.2**). The following discussion travels counterclockwise around Figure A38.2, beginning at top center. Blood flow through a tissue is equal to the pressure gradient across the tissue divided by the vascular resistance of the tissue. The pressure gradient is arterial pressure minus venous pressure; because this latter pressure is relatively small, it is often omitted. Thus,

(Equation 1) Blood flow = arterial pressure/vascular resistance

According to the theory of Poiseuille, vascular resistance is proportional to the viscosity of the blood and the length of the vessels, whereas resistance is inversely proportional to the radius of the vessels raised to the 4th power. Under normal conditions, the radius is the most important of these 3 factors.

$$\text{(Equation 2) Resistance} \propto (\text{viscosity} \times \text{length})/\text{radius}^4$$

The radius of small, high-resistance blood vessels is determined by the tension generated by the smooth muscle in the

vessel wall. Tension is influenced by local metabolic factors that are determined by the balance between metabolic need and nutrient transport.

Nutrient transport is a function of blood flow, completing the circular and stable relationship. In addition to local metabolic factors, smooth muscle tension can be modified by overriding neural and humoral factors. This is particularly important in the control of skin blood flow and in preserving blood flow to vital organs in cardiovascular crises, such as severe hemorrhage.

Normal Regional Blood Flow Regulation

Regional blood flow is highly varied and in some cases highly variable. Many tissues have a blood flow of 3 to 5 mL · min⁻¹ · 100 g⁻¹, a value that just meets basal metabolic demands. The brain and heart have flows of 50 to 100 mL · min⁻¹ · 100 g⁻¹ because of their relatively high rates of metabo-

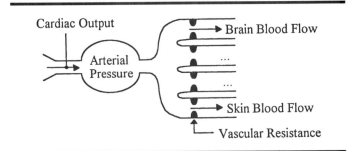

Figure A38.1. Flow and resistance.

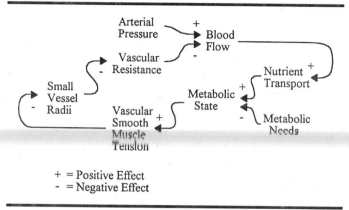

+ = Positive Effect
– = Negative Effect

Figure A38.2. Interrelationships between pressure, resistance, blood flow, and metabolic state.

Table A38.1.	**Kidney versus Brain Blood Flow and Oxygen Use**		
	OXYGEN USE (ML/MIN)	BLOOD FLOW (ML/MIN)	ORGAN WEIGHT (G)
Kidney	300	22	1,200
Brain	1,400	50	720

lism. The kidney has a blood flow of 350 mL · min^{-1} · 100 g^{-1}, a value that greatly exceeds its metabolic needs.

Cerebral blood flow. Cerebral blood flow is relatively constant because of autoregulation (see Chapter A39), yet it is very sensitive to CO_2 tension in the brain. CO_2 tension, in turn, is a function of blood flow, with increased flow washing out excess cerebral CO_2. This interrelationship tends to keep brain pH constant and, in general, provides a stable environment for cerebral neural function. The stimulatory effect of cerebral CO_2 on ventilation and the ability of ventilation to remove excess CO_2 provide an additional stabilizing factor for the cerebral environment as well as other tissues.

Myocardial blood flow. Myocardial blood flow is proportional to myocardial oxygen use, which, in turn, is proportional to myocardial workload. Under normal conditions, the heart extracts <50% of the oxygen delivered to it. This percentage is close to the practical maximum and is approximately twice the whole-body oxygen extraction. Thus, it is not increases in extraction but rather increases in coronary blood flow that satisfy myocardial oxygen demands during increased myocardial workload.

Skeletal muscle blood flow. Muscular flow is proportional to skeletal muscle workload and generally to cardiac output, ranging from a low of 4 mL · min^{-1} · 100 g^{-1} at rest to nearly 100 mL · min^{-1} · 100 g^{-1} during strenuous exercise. Because a trained athlete's body typically contains >20 kg of skeletal muscle, total muscle blood flow can approach 20 L per min in these individuals during strenuous exercise. Flow delivers enough oxygen, fatty acids, and glucose to maintain adequate muscle phosphocreatine stores.

Skin blood flow. Cutaneous and subcutaneous flow regulates heat loss from the body by metering the flow of heat from the core to the surface of the body, where heat is lost to the environment. Skin blood flow is controlled by the central nervous system via sympathetic nerves. Normal skin blood flow is <250 mL · min^{-1} · m^{-2} of surface area, but marked increases and decreases from that value occur as needed. Even with severe vasoconstriction, skin blood flow is usually great enough to meet the basic metabolic demands of the skin.

Renal blood flow. Renal blood flow is relatively constant and very large, averaging approximately 20% of cardiac output. On a unit weight basis, the kidney has twice the oxygen consumption

of the brain but 7 times the blood flow (**Table A38.1**). A high renal blood flow makes possible a high rate of glomerular filtration. The kidney generally filters 125 mL/min from a renal plasma flow of 660 mL/min. The total plasma volume is processed (i.e., filtered and reabsorbed) more than 60 times each day.

Control of Salt and Water Excretion (Natriuresis)

Renal sodium excretion rises or falls in a very precise way to match dietary sodium intake; the half-time of the response is <2 days. Renal blood flow, in partnership with renal nerve activity and the renin-angiotensin system, helps to implement control of sodium excretion while keeping glomerular filtration relatively steady. When dietary sodium intake is decreased, renal blood flow decreases; this is associated with decreased sodium filtration and excretion and increased sodium reabsorption, renin secretion, angiotensin formation, and renal vascular resistance (**Figure A38.3**). As mentioned in the section Renal Blood Flow, the very high and relatively fixed kidney blood flow supports the basic functions of the kidney: filtering unwanted metabolites and controlling sodium balance. High, fixed flow may also be related in some way to erythropoiesis, by which the kidney is able to detect with great precision not only hypoxemia but also anemia.

Importance of Systemic Pressure in Regional Blood Flow Regulation

Responses to exercise. Regional blood flow regulation requires an adequate systemic arterial pressure, as illustrated by the response to physical exercise in patients with autonomic dysfunction. As the normal person begins to exercise, skeletal muscle resistance decreases, whereas cardiac output and skeletal muscle flow increase markedly; arterial pressure remains relatively constant. As persons with autonomic dysfunction begin to exercise, skeletal muscle resistance decreases, but cardiac output and skeletal muscle blood flow increase only modestly. Consequently, arterial pressure plummets, exercise is not well tolerated, and syncope is common.

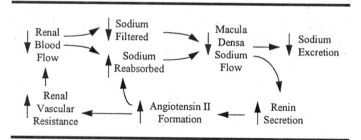

Figure A38.3. Events occurring when dietary sodium intake, and thus renal blood flow, is decreased.

Table A38.2. Cerebral Hemodynamics in Essential Hypertension

	CEREBRAL BLOOD FLOW (MM HG)	VASCULAR RESISTANCE (ML · MIN^{-1} · 100 G^{-1})	MEAN ARTERIAL PRESSURE (MM HG · ML^{-1} · MIN^{-1} ·100 G^{-1})
Normal subjects	86	54	1.6
Essential hypertension	159	54	3.0

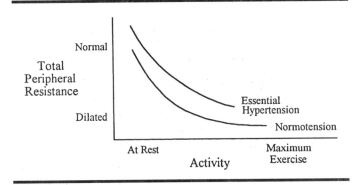

Figure A38.4. Relationship between total peripheral resistance and physical activity in normotensive and hypertensive individuals.

Determinants of arterial pressure. Arterial pressure is determined by the balance between the filling effect of cardiac output and the draining effect of regional blood flow (Figure A38.1). Tissue dilation drains additional blood from the arterial tree. If arterial pressure is to be held constant, this blood must be replaced by an increase in cardiac output. Several mechanisms make important contributions. The vasodilation itself increases venous return and, therefore, cardiac output. Repetitive contractions of skeletal muscle pump blood back to the heart, and venous valves prevent backflow. The autonomic nervous system increases venous pressure, heart rate, and myocardial contractility. These factors combine to provide the cardiac output and arterial pressure needed for proper regional flow regulation. When cardiac outflow is inadequate, as in heart failure or hypovolemia, neural and humoral factors produce systemic vasoconstriction that overrides normal flow control in many organs. This response initially keeps arterial pressure and blood flow to the brain and heart from falling too low; eventually, however, chronic hypoperfusion leads to the syndrome of heart failure.

Essential Hypertension

Regional hemodynamics. The hemodynamic pattern seen at rest most often in essential hypertension is normal blood flow with elevated vascular resistance. This pattern suggests that regulation of regional blood flow is generally not impaired. Oxygen consumption is normal. Cerebral blood flow shows a normal value of <50 mL · min^{-1} · 100 g tissue^{-1} in essential hypertension (**Table A38.2**). Coronary blood flow is elevated in essential hypertension in proportion to the prevailing amount of myocardial hypertrophy. Blood flow per unit weight of heart muscle is normal, with a value of <80 mL · min^{-1} · 100 g^{-1}. Splanchnic blood flow is slightly reduced in essential hypertension, having a typical value of 750 mL · min^{-1} · m^{-2} of surface area compared with 800 mL · min^{-1} · m^{-2} in normotensive subjects. Skin blood flow is normal.

Control of skeletal muscle blood flow is for the most part normal in essential hypertension, but several peculiarities have been identified. The ability of skeletal muscle to dilate is less than normal in essential hypertension, as characterized by the minimum attainable vascular resistance. This impairment is probably due to structural limitations imposed by vessel wall hypertrophy. In addition, skeletal muscle blood flow per gram of tissue at rest is somewhat elevated.

Exercise responses. The hemodynamic response to exercise is altered in hypertension. The maximum level of exercise, quantified by oxygen uptake, is depressed in proportion to the severity of hypertension. Arterial pressure is high before exercise and goes even higher during exercise. In the presence of the dilation defect noted above, elevated blood pressure boosts blood flow through the skeletal muscle (Equation 1), but it also creates a detrimental increase in cardiac afterload that limits cardiac output and exercise performance. At each level of exercise below maximum, cardiac output and skeletal muscle blood flow is identical to normotensive subjects but is achieved at a higher vascular resistance (**Figure A38.4**) and higher arterial pressure; the resistance and pressure influences cancel each other (Equation 1) to yield a normal flow.

Renal hemodynamics. Renal blood flow has been observed to be increased, normal, or decreased in essential hypertension. These flow data must be interpreted with regard to the special functional needs of the kidney. For instance, dietary protein, dietary sodium, and weight gain all require increases in renal blood flow, whereas nephron damage and nephron loss lead to decreases. Renal blood flow tends to be normal or increased early in hypertension, particularly in obese subjects, whereas flow is generally reduced in longer-standing hypertension and nonobese subjects. It has been repeatedly postulated that inadequate renal blood flow is a pathophysiologic factor in essential hypertension.

Renovascular Hypertension

In experimental renal artery stenosis, increased renal preglomerular resistance produces a predictable rise in arterial pressure that is proportional to the severity of the constriction. The immediate response to preglomerular vasoconstriction is a decrease in renal blood flow (Equation 1). A secondary increase in arterial pressure then follows, which is due to a combination of increased renin secretion and renal sodium retention, with hyperreninemia having an important early role and sodium retention having an important chronic role. The eventual hemodynamic picture is elevated total peripheral resistance, normal cardiac output and plasma renin activity, and decreased renal blood flow (see Chapter A48).

SUGGESTED READING

1. Amery A, Julius S, Whitlock LS, Conway J. Influence of hypertension on the hemodynamic response to exercise. *Circulation.* 1967;36:231–237.
2. Bevegård S, Jonsson B, Karlöf I. Circulatory responses to recumbent exercise and head-up tilting in patients with disturbed sympathetic cardiovascular control (postural hypotension). *Acta Med Scand.* 1962;172:623–636.

3. Coleman TG, Guyton AC, Young DB, et al. The role of the kidney in essential hypertension. *Clin Exp Pharmacol Physiol.* 1975;2:571–581.
4. Goldblatt H, Lynch J, Hanzal RF, Summerville WW. Studies on experimental hypertension, I: the production of persistent elevation of systolic blood pressure by means of renal ischemia. *J Exp Med.* 1934;59:347–379.
5. Hollenberg NK, Merrill JP. Intrarenal perfusion in the young "essential" hypertensive: a subpopulation resistant to sodium restriction. *Trans Assoc Am Physicians.* 1970;83:93–101.
6. Kety SS, Hafkenschiel JH, Jeffers WA, et al. The blood flow, vascular resistance, and oxygen consumption of the brain in essential hypertension. *J Clin Invest.* 1948;27:511–514.
7. Ljungman S, Aurell M, Hartford M, et al. Blood pressure and renal function. *Acta Med Scand.* 1980;208:17–25.
8. Rowe GG, Castillo CA, Maxwell GM, Crumpton CW. A hemodynamic study of hypertension including observations on coronary blood flow. *Ann Intern Med.* 1961;54:405–412.
9. Wilkins RW, Culbertson JW, Rymut AA. The hepatic blood flow in resting hypertensive patients before and after splanchnicectomy. *J Clin Invest.* 1952;31:529–531.

Chapter A39

Autoregulation of Blood Flow

Richard J. Roman, PhD

KEY POINTS

- Local or regional autoregulation of blood flow, especially in the renal and cerebral circulations, allows flow to remain relatively constant over a wide range of arterial pressure.

- Autoregulation involves 2 major mechanisms: myogenic activation of vascular smooth muscle via altered shear stress on vascular walls and metabolically stimulated release of mediators (e.g., nitric oxide, prostacyclin, epoxyeicosatrienoic acids) from the vascular endothelium and surrounding tissues.

- Vascular resistance is elevated in hypertension, and the range of blood flow autoregulation is shifted toward higher pressures.

- Impaired autoregulation of blood flow contributes to the neurologic deficits associated with hemorrhagic and ischemic stroke and the development of hypertension and diabetic-induced glomerulosclerosis.

See also Chapters A16, A20, A26, A33, A37, A38, A68, A69, A71, and C160

Blood flow in the renal, cerebral, splanchnic, and skeletal muscle vascular beds remains relatively constant despite fluctuations in mean arterial pressure from 70 to 120 mm Hg. This phenomenon is known as *autoregulation*; the range of constant perfusion is referred to as the *autoregulation plateau* (**Figure A39.1**).

Mechanisms of Autoregulation of Blood Flow

Two general mechanisms contribute to the autoregulation of blood flow: myogenic regulation of precapillary arterioles and metabolic regulation of blood flow.

Myogenic activation of precapillary arterioles.

Elevations in transmural pressure locally induce constriction of resistance arterioles through calcium influx through voltage-sensitive calcium channels, a rise in intracellular calcium, and depolarization of vascular smooth muscle. Recent studies have indicated that the myogenic response is triggered by activation of stretch-activated cation channels with subsequent calcium influx and activation of protein kinase C and phospholipase A_2, which promotes the release of arachidonic acid from the membrane. Arachidonic acid is converted locally by cytochrome P450 into the vasoconstrictor metabolite, 20-hydroxyeicosatetraenoic acid (20-HETE), which depolarizes the cell by blocking calcium-activated potassium channels and opening voltage sensitive calcium channels (see Chapter A20). Inhibitors of the formation of 20-HETE block pressure-induced contraction of isolated arterioles *in vitro* and autoregulation of renal and cerebral blood flow *in vivo*.

Metabolic regulation of blood flow.

When perfusion pressure and blood flow are reduced in a vascular bed, the tissue becomes hypoxic. Hypoxia triggers the release of vasodilator mediators such as nitric oxide, prostacyclin, prostaglandins, epoxyeicosatrienoic acids (EETs), endothelial-derived hyperpolarizing factor (EDHF), and adenosine from the vascular endothelium and surrounding parenchymal tissues. The fall in tissue PO_2 associated with reductions in perfusion pressure reduces the formation of 20-HETE, which serves as an endogenous inhibitor of potassium channels in vascular smooth muscle cells. Hypoxia-induced falls in intracellular pH and PO_2 can also directly hyperpolarize vascular smooth muscle cells by increasing the opening of potassium channels. In partial compensation, local increases in blood flow serve to wash out the vasodilators and promote vasoconstriction. In addition, elevations in tissue PO_2 enhance the formation of 20-HETE in vascular smooth muscle cells. Inhibitors of the formation of 20-HETE have recently been shown to

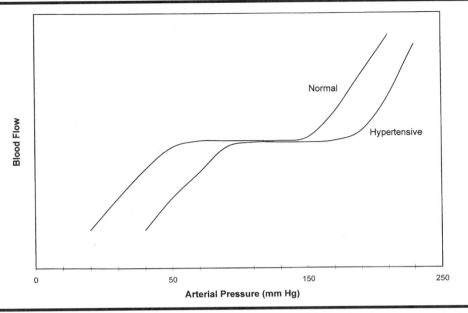
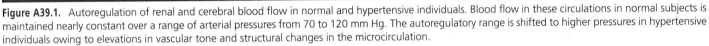

Figure A39.1. Autoregulation of renal and cerebral blood flow in normal and hypertensive individuals. Blood flow in these circulations in normal subjects is maintained nearly constant over a range of arterial pressures from 70 to 120 mm Hg. The autoregulatory range is shifted to higher pressures in hypertensive individuals owing to elevations in vascular tone and structural changes in the microcirculation.

block the vasoconstrictor response of isolated arterioles to elevations in both PO_2 *in vitro* as well as the vasoconstrictor response to elevations in tissue PO_2 in a variety of skeletal muscle beds *in vivo*.

Shear Stress and Blood Flow Regulation

Determinants of shear stress. Shear stress represents the frictional forces acting on the intimal surface of vessels in response to blood flow. Shear stress can be calculated by the following equation:

$$\text{Shear stress} = 8\eta V/R$$

where η is the viscosity of blood, V is the flow velocity, and R is the inner diameter of the vessel. Shear stress is directly dependent on the velocity of flow in a vessel and is inversely proportional to vascular diameter.

Release of vasoactive substances. Increases in shear stress stimulate the release of vasodilator mediators from the endothelium as summarized in **Figure A39.2**. These products include nitric oxide, prostaglandin E_2, prostacyclin, EETs, and perhaps another still-to-be-defined EDHF that dilates vessels by opening potassium channels in vascular smooth muscle cells and lowering intracellular calcium.

Signaling pathways. Each vasoactive substance uses a different signal transduction pathway. Nitric oxide stimulates the formation of cyclic guanosine monophosphate and inhibits the formation of 20-HETE in vascular smooth muscle cells. Both effects open potassium channels to hyperpolarize the cell and diminish calcium entry through voltage-sensitive channels. Prostacyclin and prostaglandin E_2 act on a receptor to promote vasodilation via a cyclic adenosine monophosphate–dependent pathway. EETs are potent vasodilators that also open potassium channels in vascular smooth muscle cells. Recent data suggest that EETs stimulate the formation of cyclic adenosine diphosphate ribose in vascular smooth muscle

cells. In coronary arteries and other vascular beds, EETs have been identified to be EDHF. However, in other vessels, blockade of the formation of EETs does not fully block the response to endothelial dependent vasodilators in the presence of cyclooxygenase and nitric oxide synthase inhibitors. This has led to the view that there are likely other EDHF molecules that can be released from the endothelium.

Physiologic integration. In general, shear stress stimulates the release of endothelial-derived relaxing factors that act as negative modulators of autoregulatory responses. For example, acute elevations in perfusion pressure promote myogenic responses in vessels to autoregulate blood flow. The reduction in vascular diameter, however, increases shear stress, which promotes the release of nitric oxide and other endothelial-derived relaxing factors, thus opposing further vasoconstriction. Besides acting as a negative modulator of myogenic responses, shear force-related

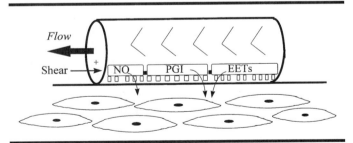

Figure A39.2. Effects of shear stress on the release of vasoactive mediators from the vascular endothelium. Increases in flow within a vessel increase shear stress, which promotes the release of nitric oxide (NO), prostacyclin (PGI), and epoxyeicosatrienoic acids (EETs) and perhaps another endothelial-derived hyperpolarizing factor from the vascular endothelium. All of these factors are potent vasodilators that open potassium channels in vascular smooth muscle cells through different signal transduction pathways.

changes in vascular tone also play an important role in dilating large vessels and augmenting blood flow to skeletal muscle during exercise or in response to increases in metabolic demand. The accumulation of metabolic products during exercise lowers vascular resistance in the skeletal muscle microcirculation and increases blood flow. Increased blood flow and flow velocity in the larger upstream vessels then stimulates the release of nitric oxide and other mediators to dilate these vessels and promote increased flow and delivery of oxygen to the bed.

Renal Autoregulation

Autoregulatory mechanisms are especially well developed in the kidney to allow for the maintenance of a relatively constant glomerular capillary pressure, glomerular filtration rate, and clearance of metabolic wastes over a wide range of arterial pressure. Two mechanisms are predominantly responsible for the autoregulation of blood flow in the kidney.

Afferent arteriolar pressure. Myogenic activation of preglomerular arterioles caused by elevations in transmural pressure in the afferent arterioles (vessel diameters of 20 μm) causes counterregulatory changes via mechanisms similar to those in larger arteries.

Tubuloglomerular feedback. Tubuloglomerular feedback (TGF) acts in concert with the myogenic response by sensing changes in the chloride concentration of the urine reaching macula densa cells in the distal tubule and adjusting the diameter of the afferent arteriole accordingly. Acute elevations in renal arterial pressure and flow initially increase glomerular capillary pressure and glomerular filtration rate, which in turn increase tubular flow rate and the concentration of chloride reaching the macula densa. The rise in chloride concentration, which is sensed by an unknown mechanism, causes contraction of the portion of the afferent arteriole adjacent to the juxtaglomerular apparatus, completing the feedback loop. TGF is an effective autoregulatory mechanism because the chloride concentration of the fluid reaching the macula densa is dependent on urine flow rate, which in turn is directly related to the rate of glomerular filtration and to the mean glomerular capillary pressure. The nature of the constrictor substance released by the macula densa remains to be fully defined, but data suggest that it may be adenosine triphosphate (ATP) or adenosine. Adenosine acts on adenosine 1 receptors, and ATP stimulates a purogenic receptor to constrict the afferent arteriole. Data also suggest that ATP (and possibly adenosine as well) stimulate the formation of 20-HETE in the afferent arteriole and that 20-HETE contributes to the TGF-mediated response by blocking potassium channels and enhancing calcium influx into these cells. In this regard, blockade of cytochrome P450 metabolism of arachidonic acid has been found to block autoregulation of renal blood flow and TGF-mediated responses in the rat *in vivo*. Similarly, knockout of adenosine receptors in the mouse and pharmacologic blockade of ATP receptors in the rat attenuate TGF responses.

Salt-sensitivity and renal deterioration in hypertension. In addition to the increase in renal vascular resistance in angiotensin II–dependent and essential hypertensive patients, altered autoregulation of renal blood flow also accompanies salt-sensi-

tive forms of hypertension. For example, TGF responses and autoregulation of glomerular filtration rate and glomerular capillary pressure are impaired in Dahl salt-sensitive rats and in rats treated with mineralocorticoids and salt. These animals have elevated glomerular capillary pressure, endothelial dysfunction and damage, and rapid development of proteinuria and glomerulosclerosis. A similar abnormality in glomerular capillary hemodynamics associated with dilation of the renal afferent arteriole is thought to contribute to the rapid development of glomerulosclerosis in black and diabetic hypertensive patients.

Cerebral Autoregulation

In the brain, autoregulatory mechanisms are well developed to maintain adequate perfusion, oxygenation, and substrate delivery as blood pressure varies. Two major mechanisms contribute to the autoregulation of cerebral blood flow: the myogenic behavior of larger cerebral arteries and metabolic autoregulatory adjustments of small arterioles in the cerebral cortex.

Large arterial mechanisms. The large cerebral arteries originating from the circle of Willis and the smaller pial arteries on the surface of the brain are highly myogenically active, accounting for a major fraction of total cerebral vascular resistance. Their myogenic responses increase cerebral vascular resistance sufficiently to minimize changes in blood flow and pressure in downstream elements of the cerebral circulation.

Arteriolar mechanisms. The remainder of the autoregulatory adjustments in cerebral vascular resistance occur at the level of the small arterioles supplying capillary networks in the cerebral cortex. In these arterioles, changes in vascular resistance are mediated by the release of vasoactive metabolites from metabolically active neural tissue and the vascular endothelium in response to small alterations in pH, PCO_2, and PO_2. Elevations in blood or tissue pH or PCO_2 or hypoxia increase cerebral blood flow and impair autoregulation. The nature of the metabolites that mediate the changes in cerebral vascular resistance remain to be fully identified, but there is evidence that nitric oxide, prostacyclin, prostaglandins, EETs, and adenosine play a role. In addition, changes in intracellular pH and PO_2 have direct effects on tone in cerebral vascular smooth muscle cells.

Impaired autoregulation in stroke. Autoregulation of cerebral blood flow is impaired after ischemic or hemorrhagic stroke, in which there is a generalized loss of the ability of the vasculature to dilate in response to nitric oxide and other vasodilators. Impaired vasodilation may be related to increased production of superoxide radical and subsequent inactivation of nitric oxide or to changes in the expression of potassium channels and second messenger pathways in cerebrovascular smooth muscle cells. Regardless of the mechanism involved, impairments in vasodilator pathways do contribute to the neurologic deficits and ischemic brain injury associated with hemorrhagic and ischemic stroke.

Autoregulation in Hypertension

Elevations in vascular resistance, especially in the renal and cerebral vascular beds, are characteristic of hypertension (see Chapter A38).

Autoregulatory shift. The autoregulatory plateaus for renal and cerebral blood flow in hypertension are shifted to higher pressure ranges, with the magnitude of the shift dependent on the severity and duration of the hypertension (Figure A39.1) and the accompanying degree of hypertrophy and thickening of the wall of arterioles, endothelial dysfunction, and potentiation of myogenic responses.

Antihypertensive drug effects. Generally, autoregulatory relationships in moderate hypertension are near-normal, and arterial pressure can be lowered into the normotensive range without compromising renal or cerebral perfusion. However, in patients with severe or long-standing hypertension, the hypertrophic structural changes in the cerebral and renal circulations may be severe, and it may not be possible to lower blood pressure to the normotensive range quickly without compromising blood flow. Under these conditions, persistent therapy with a gradual reduction in blood pressure is recommended so that regression of vascular hypertrophy (i.e., vascular remodeling) can occur, with a shift in the autoregulatory curve back toward the normal range.

SUGGESTED READING

1. Cohen RA, Vanhoutte PM. Endothelium-dependent hyperpolarization: beyond nitric oxide and cGMP. *Circulation.* 1995;92:3337–3349.
2. Faraci FM, Heistad DD. Regulation of the cerebral circulation: role of endothelium and potassium channels. *Physiol Rev.* 1998;78:53–97.
3. Heistad DD, Kontos JP. Cerebral circulation. In: Berne RM, Sperelakis N, eds. *Handbook of Physiology: The Cardiovascular System.* Bethesda, MD: American Physiological Society; 1979.
4. Navar LG, Inscho EW, Majid SA, et al. Paracrine regulation of the renal microcirculation. *Physiol Rev.* 1996;76:425–536.
5. Roman RJ. P-450 metabolites of arachidonic acid in the control of cardiovascular function. *Physiol Rev.* 2002;82:131–185.
6. Strandgaard S, Paulson OB. Cerebral blood flow and its pathophysiology in hypertension. *Am J Hypertens.* 1989;2:486–492.

Chapter A40

Respiration and Blood Pressure

Gianfranco Parati, MD, FAHA, FESC; Joseph L. Izzo, Jr, MD; Benjamin Gavish, PhD

KEY POINTS

- Cyclic respiratory movements cause variability in heart rate and blood pressure at the respiratory frequency.

- The mechanisms of respiratory-induced cardiovascular variability are mechanical, neural, and metabolic, involving volume alterations, cardiopulmonary and arterial baroreceptors, and chemoreceptors.

- A number of pathologic conditions, including congestive heart failure, chronic obstructive pulmonary disease, obstructive sleep apnea, and cardiac tamponade, are characterized by significant respiration-induced changes in blood pressure and heart rate.

- Chronic use of slow-breathing exercises reduces sympathetic activity, vasodilates, and lowers blood pressure.

See also Chapters A34–A36, A55, and C129

Successful maintenance of tissue perfusion and adequate transport of O_2 and CO_2 into cells under variable metabolic conditions demands a continuous interplay between respiratory, cardiac, and vascular systems. Respiratory movements and the resulting ventilation stimulate a number of sensory systems integrated in the brain stem that lead to modulation of sympathetic nervous outflow and physiologic variability in the cardiovascular system.

Blood Pressure and Heart Rate Effects of Respiration

In 1733, Hales first noticed the occurrence of oscillations in the level of blood pressure in phase with respiration, oscillations subsequently defined as *Traube-Hering waves.* Ludwig first described the respiratory variations in heart rate [i.e., respiratory sinus arrhythmia (RSA)] in 1847 by noting that heart rate increases during inspiration and decreases during expiration. During phasic breathing, blood pressure varies with each phase of the respiratory cycle in humans according to the rate and depth of breathing, the abdominal or thoracic pattern of respiration, the subject's posture, and the presence or absence of RSA. At moderate breathing rates, blood pressure falls during most of inspiration, whereas at slow rates, a rise in pressure characterizes inspiration. At respiratory rates above 6 breaths/min, the amplitude of respiratory-induced blood pressure oscillations is inversely proportional to the respiratory rate. Respiratory oscillations of blood pressure are enhanced in the upright posture (**Figure A40.1**).

Heart rate control mechanisms. The effects of respiration on heart rate are almost solely dependent on neural mechanisms. Three mechanisms are generally proposed to explain RSA, which are not mutually exclusive: central, baroreflex, and chemoreflex.

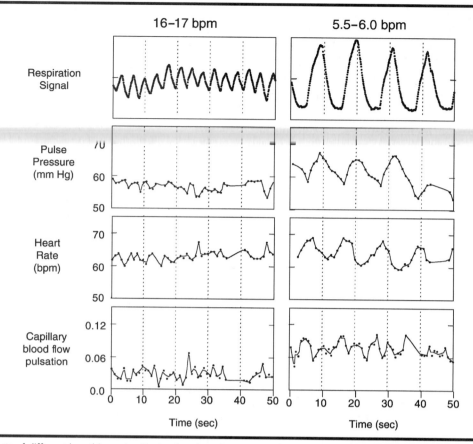

Figure A40.1.   Acute effects of different breathing rates. Fluctuations in pulse pressure, heart rate, and capillary blood flow were monitored noninvasively in a normotensive subject. Synchronization of changes in pulse pressure and heart rate with the respiration signal occurs along with increased amplitude of changes at slow breathing. The trend toward opposite changes in pulse pressure and heart rate is probably owing to baroreflex influences. The capillary blood flow pulsations (derived from analysis of skin laser Doppler signal) increase considerably during the slow breathing. Chronic effects differ in that reduced blood pressure appears to result from reduction of sympathetic outflow that has been entrained by the slow breathing exercise. bpm, beats per minute.

Central mechanisms. RSA originates from a direct effect of respiratory oscillations in medullary neuron firing rates on cardiomotor neurons. This old theory is mostly supported by animal studies and has not always been confirmed in humans. **Baroreflex mechanisms.** Blood pressure changes secondary to respiratory movements influence heart rate through the arterial baroreflex. The important involvement of this mechanism in generating RSA is also suggested by the evidence that the arterial baroreflex input-output relationship is not constant during the respiratory cycle and is affected by inputs from the cardiopulmonary stretch receptors. This implies that baroreflex sensitivity may vary as a function of the respiratory phase, at least at lower breathing rates. In normal human subjects, reflex mechanisms seem to play a predominant role in generating RSA. **Chemoreflex mechanisms.** Reflexes other than the arterial baroreflex (e.g., the cardiopulmonary reflex) and local stretch of the sinus node (responsible for a change in the spontaneous depolarization rate of cardiac pacemaker cells), and respiratory-related oscillations in $PaCO_2$ and arterial pH, act with a time constant longer than normal breathing.

Respiration and Blood Pressure

Hemodynamic responses to variations in intrathoracic pressure.
Cyclic changes in ventilation due to phasic breathing have mechanical effects through changes in intrathoracic pressure. Venous return to the right heart is increased during inspiration and reduced during expiration. There is also during inspiration a compression of the abdominal venous compartment by the descending diaphragm, which facilitates blood movement toward the heart. These respiration-related changes in venous return, delayed and dampened while passing through the lungs, lead to reciprocal changes in the venous flow to the right and left heart chambers during inspiration and expiration. This results in regular falls and rises in blood pressure due to respiratory-related changes in left ventricular venous return, which are responsible for reductions (inspiration) and increases (expiration) in stroke volume. Moreover, during inspiration, increased "afterload" to the left ventricle (owing to a reduction in intrathoracic pressure) also leads to a temporary reduction in cardiac output and blood pressure in absence of changes in ventricular contractility. The blood pressure reduction during inspiration may be particularly pronounced in specific pathologic conditions, leading to the so-called pulsus paradoxus (see the section Pulsus Paradoxus).

Neural control mechanisms
Chemoreceptors. Blood gas changes have both a direct action on peripheral vascular resistance and a reflex effect on the heart and peripheral circulation through changes in peripheral arterial chemoreceptor activity.

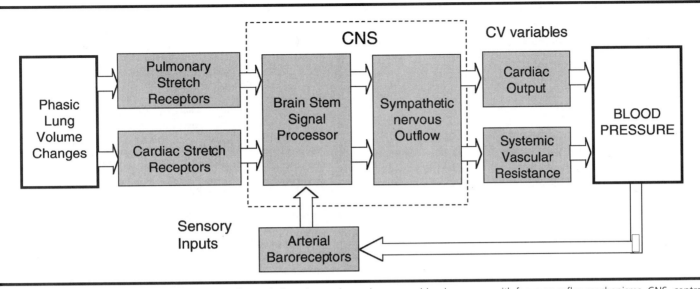

Figure A40.2. Scheme illustrating the modulating effects of phase lung volume changes on blood pressure, with focus on reflex mechanisms. CNS, central nervous system; CV, cardiovascular.

Cardiopulmonary and arterial baroreflexes. The heart and peripheral vessels are strongly influenced by central respiratory centers and reflexes originating from cardiopulmonary stretch receptors and arterial baroreceptors (see Chapters A35 and A36), which in turn lead to reflex changes in heart rate, sympathetic activity, and total peripheral resistance (**Figure A40.2**). It has also been shown that the neural effects of cyclic variations in respiratory activity may influence the afferent signals coming from other peripheral vascular receptors and directed to the central nervous system.

Syndromes of Disordered Breathing

Changes in respiratory activity characterize a number of pathologic conditions in humans, ranging from chronic obstructive pulmonary disease to chronic congestive heart failure and obstructive sleep apnea. Under these conditions, changes in the features of phasic breathing may importantly affect cardiac and vascular function, and thus contribute to patients' cardiovascular risk.

Cheyne-Stokes respiration. In patients with severe congestive heart failure, marked periodic swings in blood pressure synchronous with the periodic breathing pattern are characteristic of Cheyne-Stokes respiration. This syndrome has been shown to carry an adverse prognosis.

Obstructive sleep apnea syndrome. Recurrent episodes of upper airway obstruction during sleep lead to sleep fragmentation, arterial blood oxygen desaturation, chemoreflex stimulation, reduction in arterial baroreflex sensitivity, increase in sympathetic neural activity, and periodic increases in blood pressure (see Chapter A55). All these changes may contribute to the increased rate of cardiovascular complications in obstructive sleep apnea syndrome patients. In severe obstructive sleep apnea syndrome, the assessment of the transfer function between changes in arterial oxygen saturation and the associated blood pressure swings may help in quantifying the increase in cardiovascular risk typical of this condition.

Pulsus paradoxus. An exaggerated reduction in the amplitude of the arterial pulse during *inspiration* (often defined as a systolic blood pressure decrease exceeding 12 mm Hg) is observed in cases of severely impaired cardiac filling rate in a condition known as *pulsus paradoxus*. Pulsus paradoxus is an important physical finding of cardiac tamponade and results from the marked inspiratory decline of left ventricular stroke volume owing to a markedly decreased end-diastolic volume. Due to the increased intrapericardial pressure, the intraventricular septum shifts towards the left ventricle during inspiration, further decreasing left ventricular preload in addition to the expected reduction in venous return that occurs during this breathing phase. Other clinical conditions associated with pulsus paradoxus besides cardiac tamponade are chronic obstructive pulmonary disease and, more rarely, constrictive pericarditis, pulmonary embolism, pregnancy, marked obesity, and partial obstruction of the superior vena cava.

Effects of Slow Breathing on Cardiovascular Control Mechanisms

Respiratory-induced reflex modulation of sympathetic activity and peripheral resistance can be affected by breathing rate. Reducing the breathing rate (from 15–20 to 6–10 breaths/min) increases tidal volume while maintaining minute ventilation. There is increased cardiopulmonary stretch-receptor stimulation, which in turn reduces sympathetic efferent fibers discharge, resulting in vasodilation. This process is accompanied by a shift from the smaller-amplitude "thoracic breathing" to larger-amplitude "abdominal breathing," which in terms of energy consumption is more favorable at slow rates. Moreover, arterial baroreflex sensitivity at breathing rates of 3 to 12 breaths/min is enhanced during expiration. This expiratory enhancement is not evident at higher breathing rates. Of special interest is slow-breathing at a rate around 6 breaths/min (0.1 Hz), a rate that overlays spontaneous fluctuations in sympathetic neural traffic and peripheral vascular tone (also occurring at a frequency around 0.1 Hz). These fluctuations may play an important role in controlling peripheral vascular resistance. Breathing at 0.1 Hz (i.e., once every 10 seconds) may thus enhance and further synchronize the well-known spontaneous blood pressure oscillations at this frequency, known as *Mayer waves*. Breathing at very low frequencies (slower than 4 breaths/min) is usually inconvenient and is associated with a drop in PO_2 and an increase in PCO_2, which activate chemoreceptors to accelerate the breathing rate.

Therapeutic Effects of Slow Breathing

Syndromes characterized by systemic vasoconstriction can in theory be improved by using the slow breathing exercise to reduce sympathetic outflow and allow systemic vasodilation.

Blood pressure lowering. Slow breathing exercises, especially with prolonged expiration, have now been studied in clinical trials. When used daily for 15 minutes, a device that guides the slow breathing exercise (RESPeRATE) was found to help lower systolic blood pressure by approximately 5 to 10 mm Hg. The device has been approved for use as an adjunct to lifestyle modifications and drug therapy.

Other benefits. Beneficial effects of slow breathing on the cardiovascular system, including sensitizing the arterial baroreflex, activating the cardiopulmonary reflex, reducing vascular resistance, and increasing peripheral blood flow, have potential applications in other areas of cardiovascular medicine, especially as a nonpharmacologic approach to aid patients with heart failure.

SUGGESTED READING

1. Castiglioni P, Bonsignore MR, Insalaco G, et al. Signal processing procedures for the evaluation of the cardiovascular effects in the obstructive sleep apnea syndrome. *Comput Cardiol.* 2001;28:221–224.
2. Daly M de B. Interactions between respiration and circulation. In: Cheniack NS, JG Widdicombe, eds. *Handbook of Physiology.* Bethesda, MD: American Physiological Society; 1986:529–594.
3. Eckberg DL, Nerhed C, Wallyn G. Respiratory modulation of muscle sympathetic and vagal cardiac outflow in man. *J Physiol.* 1985;365:181–196.
4. Eckberg DL, Orshan CR. Respiratory and baroreceptor reflex interactions in man. *J Clin Invest.* 1977;59:780–785.
5. Gottlieb Tirala L. *The Cure of High Blood Pressure by Respiratory Exercises.* New York, NY: Westerman Inc.; 1936.
6. Guyton AC, Hall JE. *Textbook of Medical Physiology.* 9th ed. Philadelphia, PA: Saunders; 1996.
7. Hirsch JA, Bishop B. Respiratory sinus arrhythmia in humans: how breathing pattern modulates heart rate. *Am J Physiol.* 1981;241:H620–H629.
8. Pinski MR. Cardiopulmonary interactions associated with airflow obstruction. In: Hall JB, Corbridge TC, Rodrigo C, Rodrigo G, eds. *Acute Asthma—Assessment and Management.* New York, NY: McGraw-Hill; 2000:105–123.
9. Triedman JK, Saul JP. Blood pressure modulation by central venous pressure and respiration. Buffering effects of heart rate reflexes. *Circulation.* 1994;89:169–179.

Section 4. *Pathophysiology of Primary and Secondary Hypertension*

Chapter A41

Experimental Models of Hypertension

Ralph E. Watson, MD, FACP; Donald J. DiPette, MD

KEY POINTS

- Because human hypertension is heterogeneous, several animal models have been developed to mimic its many facets.

- Hypertension can be produced by various vascular, renal, adrenal, neural, and genetic manipulations.

- Newer molecular techniques have become increasingly important in the development of animal models to determine the involvement of a particular gene or genetic locus in hypertension.

See also Chapters A34, A46, A48–A51, A54, A71, and A74–A76

The difficulty in studying a disease process such as hypertension begins with the fact that the etiology of hypertension is heterogeneous. Hypertension can be primary ("essential") or secondary to a defined process, such as renal artery stenosis. The pathophysiology of essential hypertension is also heterogeneous and varies by renin status, sodium dependency, etc. Therefore, a spectrum of experimental animal models of hypertension has been developed to aid in the investigation of essential hypertension and secondary forms of hypertension.

Inbred Rat Models of Essential Hypertension

Genetic models of experimental hypertension that have been developed to approximate the pathogenesis of human essential hypertension include the spontaneously hypertensive rat (SHR), the SHR–stroke-prone (SHR-SP) substrain, Dahl salt-sensitive and salt-resistant rat strains, Milan hypertensive and normotensive rat strains, and Lyon hypertensive and normotensive rat strains. Although these inbred strains may differ in genetics, cellular alterations, or neurohumoral mechanisms, under appropriate conditions they all share 1 thing: the spontaneous development of an elevation of blood pressure. The 2 most commonly studied are the SHR and the Dahl salt-sensitive and salt-resistant strains.

Spontaneously hypertensive and stroke-prone rats. Both the SHR and the SHR-SP rat strains develop hypertension and target organ damage similar to that seen in human essential hypertension. The pathogenesis of hypertension in the SHR appears to be heterogeneous; cellular, central nervous system, neurohumoral, and renal abnormalities have been proposed. The SHR is a "normal-renin" model, and its blood pressure is relatively sodium-independent. More recently, a substrain of SHR that is salt-sensitive has been developed. There has been intense debate over the applicability of the SHR to human essential hypertension. Part of this debate revolves around the appropriate normotensive control for the SHR strain. Most investigators use the normotensive Wistar-Kyoto (WKY) rat, as the SHR was originally derived from a WKY colony. However, normotensive WKY rats vary genetically among differing colonies and suppliers and exhibit different degrees of phenotypic expression of a given trait. The model remains useful in studies of the target organ complications of hypertension, in screening of potential pharmacologic antihypertensive agents, and in the investigation of genetic determinants of high blood pressure. At least 3 gene loci are thought to be involved, 1 of which may be in close association with the angiotensinogen gene. It has been speculated that a similar multiple gene interaction is involved in human essential hypertension.

Dahl rats. In contrast to the SHR, the Dahl salt-sensitive strain requires administration of increased dietary sodium for the rapid and full development of its blood pressure elevation. When the Dahl salt-sensitive and salt-resistant strains are placed on a high-salt diet (8% NaCl in the drinking water), the resistant strain develops only a small elevation of blood pressure, whereas the sensitive strain exhibits a substantial blood pressure rise within 4 to 6 weeks.

Renal Artery Stenosis

Two classic animal models of renovascular disease have been developed in multiple species by constriction of 1 or both of the renal arteries. These models are named after the pioneering work of Goldblatt and colleagues and are classified as *two-kidney, one-clip* (2K-1C) or *one-kidney, one-clip* (1K-1C) Goldblatt hypertension models (see Chapter A48).

Two-kidney, one-clip model. In the 2K-1C model, both native kidneys are intact, but a constricting clip (to resemble a clinical stenosis) is placed on 1 renal artery (usually the left renal artery in the rat model). In the absence of damage to the contralateral nonclipped kidney, this model is a classic renin-dependent model, at least in its early phases.

One-kidney, one-clip model. In the 1K-1C model, unilateral nephrectomy is followed by a constricting renal artery clip on the remaining kidney. This model resembles patients who have only a solitary kidney and a significant renal artery stenosis in that remaining kidney. This model may also approximate the pathophysiology of bilateral renal artery stenosis. In contrast to the 2K-1C model, in which plasma renin activity is significantly elevated and the hypertension is clearly renin-dependent, in the 1K-1C

model, the plasma renin activity is increased only in the first few days after renal artery constriction. After this initial phase, plasma renin activity decreases into the normal range. Furthermore, during this chronic phase, blockade of the renin-angiotensin system does not significantly lower blood pressure. Aggressive diuresis with accompanying sodium depletion renders the model renin-dependent again. Thus, in this model, there is interplay between early activation of the renin-angiotensin system and sodium retention in that both are required for the full development and maintenance of hypertension.

Renal Parenchymal Hypertension

Renal mass reduction salt-induced model. Clinically, the most common secondary cause of hypertension is a loss of renal function from any cause. The animal model that most closely approximates this clinical condition is the renal mass reduction salt-induced model, most commonly studied in the rat and dog. In this model, a renal mass reduction of >85% is required. To accomplish this, a unilateral nephrectomy is followed by surgical removal of two-thirds of the remaining kidney. By itself, this degree of renal mass reduction results in only a slight blood pressure increase compared to sham-operated, normotensive control animals. A further increase in blood pressure is provoked when excess salt is administered in the drinking water or in the diet. In the renal mass reduction salt-induced hypertensive model, plasma renin activity is low and hypertension is salt-dependent, but interestingly, blockade of the renin-angiotensin-aldosterone system (RAAS) with angiotensin-converting enzyme or AT-1 receptor antagonists results in a lowering of blood pressure. Explanations for this apparent paradox include effects of anti-RAAS drugs on tissue RAAS, sympathetic nervous system activity, vasopressin, or an increase in vasodilators, such as calcitonin gene-related peptide or substance P.

Other renal models. Although not as commonly used for experimental purposes, there are many other renal animal models of experimental hypertension, such as renal ischemic models, perinephric ("renal wrap") hypertension, and the chronic administration of angiotensin II (angiotensin-induced hypertension).

Adrenal Steroid Models

Mineralocorticoid hypertension. The most common adrenal model studied is the mineralocorticoid-salt or deoxycorticosterone-salt model. This model resembles the clinical situation of aldosterone excess. Hypertension is produced by a surgical uninephrectomy followed by administration of a mineralocorticoid (usually deoxycorticosterone) and excess salt (usually 0.9% NaCl drinking water). Blood pressure then rises within a few weeks into the hypertensive range. If left untreated, the hypertension progresses, and the animals develop weight loss and target-organ damage. If a more gradual blood pressure rise is desired, the kidneys can be left intact. This is a sodium-dependent, low-renin model. As in other models, nonsodium mechanisms have been suggested to play a role in the full development of the hypertension, including activation of the sympathetic nervous system, local renin-angiotensin production, and vasopressin activation. This model, in conjunction with the renin-dependent 2K-1C Goldblatt model, is useful in studying the dependency on the renin-angiotensin system of a therapeutic agent.

Glucocorticoid hypertension. Excess production of glucocorticoids, such as cortisol (Cushing's syndrome or disease), also clinically leads to secondary hypertension. The glucocorticoid-induced hypertension model is produced by the administration of excess glucocorticoid to normotensive animals. The rat has been the most commonly used species. Unlike some of the other models, no other manipulation, such as surgery or salt administration, is necessary. The mechanism of the blood pressure elevation is most likely multifactorial and is extremely difficult to treat pharmacologically, often requiring blockade of multiple pressor systems.

Pheochromocytoma and adrenal regeneration. The adrenal medulla produces the catecholamines epinephrine and norepinephrine. Excess catecholamine production accompanied by hypertension is seen in the clinical syndrome of pheochromocytoma. Models of pheochromocytoma include the chronic exogenous administration of catecholamines and the New England Deaconess Hospital pheochromocytoma tumor-bearing rat. There are other models of adrenal experimental hypertension, such as that accompanying adrenal regeneration.

Neurogenic Models

The brain is a major target organ of the hypertensive process, and it also plays a major role in blood pressure regulation and the pathophysiology of hypertension. Neurogenic models of experimental hypertension involve the surgical manipulation of specific brain areas, such as the periventricular (AV3V) region, and peripheral sinoaortic deafferentation. Recently, borderline hypertension has been modeled as well. The stroke-prone SHR is often used to investigate the pathophysiology of cerebrovascular disease. For example, in this model, dietary potassium supplementation has been shown to decrease the frequency of stroke, independently of blood pressure.

Molecular Models

A great deal of recent investigation of hypertension has been devoted to dissecting the molecular basis of hypertension. Human essential hypertension is clearly polygenic (i.e., caused by small phenotypic effects of common genetic variations found throughout the population). Any one of these variations may not be sufficient to result in a blood pressure increase, but their additive effect may produce hypertension.

Gene titration. Using gene titration, the expression of a chosen gene product is varied by generating animals with different numbers of copies of the gene coding for the specific protein. This model of genetic overexpression allows determination of causation by testing the effects on a phenotype of changes in expression of the altered gene and can be performed in a variety of animal species. Reduplication of the angiotensinogen gene in rodents causes hypertension.

Transgenic and knockout models. There has been a rapid development of transgenic manipulations and specific gene knockouts, both permanent and conditional, in the mouse. Transgenic animals have foreign DNA introduced into their genome using embryonic stem cell methodology, thus creating a new strain that expresses the gene of interest. Examples of transgenic rat strains are those in which the mouse and human renin gene and the human angiotensinogen gene were incorporated into the rat genome, and the mouse that overexpresses the renin gene. There is also a knockout mouse model of the angiotensin AT_2-receptor. The latest developments in knockout technology allow for the control of the spatial and temporal onset of the gene modification of interest.

Congenic models. Congenic methodology uses repetitive inbreeding, resulting in a generation of animals that is almost entirely devoid of or entirely contains a certain genetic locus. Thus, the blood pressure phenotype can be correlated with the presence or absence of a certain locus. For example, manipulation of nitric oxide, particularly its inhibition with $N^{[\omega]}$-nitro-L-arginine methyl ester, has led to newer models of experimental hypertension, including pregnancy-induced hypertension.

SUGGESTED READING

1. Bohr DF, Dominiczak AF. Experimental hypertension. *Hypertension.* 1991;17(suppl I):I39–I44.
2. DiPette DJ, Simpson K, Rogers A, Holland OB. Haemodynamic response to magnesium administration in mineralocorticoid-salt and two-kidney, one-clip renovascular hypertension. *J Hypertens.* 1988;6:413–417.
3. Gavras H, Brunner HR, Thurston H, Laragh JH. Reciprocation of renin dependency with sodium volume dependency in renal hypertension. *Science.* 1975;188:1316–1317.
4. Kreutz R, Higuchi M, Ganten D. Molecular genetics of hypertension. *Clin Exp Hypertens.* 1992;14:15–34.
5. Mockrin SC, Dzau VJ, Gross KW, Horan MJ. Transgenic animals: new approaches to hypertension research. *Hypertension.* 1991;17:394–399.
6. Phillips MI. Gene therapy for hypertension: the preclinical data. *Hypertension.* 2001;38(pt 2):543–548.
7. Takahashi N, Smithies O. Gene targeting approaches to analyzing hypertension. *J Am Soc Nephrol.* 1999;10:1598–1605.
8. Tobian L. Salt and hypertension: lessons from animal models that relate to human hypertension. *Hypertension.* 1991;17(suppl I):I52–I58.
9. Yagil Y, Yagil C. Genetic models of hypertension in experimental animals. *Exp Nephrol.* 2001;9:1–9.
10. Yamori Y. Overview: studies from spontaneous hypertension: development from animal models toward man. *Clin Exp Hypertens.* 1991;13:631–644.

Chapter A42

Sympathetic Nervous System in Human Hypertension

Tomas J. Kara, MD; Virend K. Somers, MD, PhD

KEY POINTS

- The sympathetic nervous system is a key mediator of acute changes in blood pressure and heart rate and may contribute importantly to initiation and maintenance of high blood pressure in essential and secondary hypertension.

- Impairment or potentiation of cardiovascular reflexes are important mechanisms for heightened sympathetic drive in hypertensive patients.

- Sympathetic activation may contribute to high blood pressure not only by vasoconstriction but also via enhanced sodium retention, trophic effects on blood vessels, and abnormalities in ion transport.

- Sympathetic activation in response to vasodilators may oppose the fall in blood pressure as well as the end-organ protection conferred by the blood pressure reduction.

See also Chapters A43, A46, A48–A51, A57, A58, C143, and C152

The sympathetic nervous system (SNS) is the primary mediator of acute changes in blood pressure and also contributes importantly to long-term blood pressure regulation. Short-term changes in blood pressure and blood pressure variability are governed by sympathetically mediated increases in arterial and venous constriction and cardiac output. In the longer term, sympathetic activation causes renal vasoconstriction and contributes to increased renal sodium retention, thickening of blood vessel walls, increased vascular resistance, and inhibition of the Na^+/K^+ pump, with consequent decreased cellular sodium efflux. There is a positive feedback interaction between the sympathetic and the renin-angiotensin system; angiotensin II acts peripherally and centrally to increase sympathetic drive. For all these reasons, overactivity of the SNS is an attractive candidate mechanism to explain human hypertension.

Sympathetic Nervous System in Essential Hypertension

Responses to sympatholytic drugs. Ganglionic blockade induces a greater decrease in blood pressure in hypertensive than in normotensive individuals. This observation led to the concept of "neurogenically mediated" hypertension owing to excessive sympathetic drive or increased vascular sensitivity to norepinephrine. The reliable blood pressure–lowering effect of agents that inhibit sympathetic drive at different levels, such as ganglionic blockers, reserpine, clonidine, and adrenoceptor blockers, is evidence of the importance of sympathetic activation in maintaining elevated blood pressure levels.

Catecholamine concentrations. Plasma catecholamines are nevertheless not consistently elevated in hypertension. This may reflect in part selective sympathetic activation to specific vascular beds such as the kidney. Oparil and colleagues have

suggested that patients with essential hypertension often have increased renal vascular resistance secondary to renal vasoconstriction mediated by sympathetic neural mechanisms.

Catecholamine turnover. Cardiac and renal norepinephrine spillover are increased in hypertension, particularly in young hypertensives younger than 40 years of age. These findings are consistent with the concept of early hyperkinetic hypertension, in which tachycardia, increased cardiac output, and renal vasoconstriction are present. This condition may evolve into established hypertension in which increased blood pressure may be maintained by structural vascular changes.

Nerve traffic recordings. Microneurographic intraneural recordings of sympathetic traffic to muscle blood vessels suggest increased sympathetic drive in hypertensive patients (**Figure A42.1**) but are also not consistent.

Difficulties in Interpretation of Studies

There remains a lack of consensus on the role of the SNS in essential hypertension that may reflect several factors.

Heterogeneity of hypertension. Essential hypertension is itself a remarkably heterogeneous disease. The clinical, neural, and biochemical profile can be influenced substantially by coexisting conditions such as obesity and level of physical conditioning. Occult disease conditions such as left ventricular dysfunction, obstructive sleep apnea, and glucose intolerance may also affect sympathetic neural drive. The heterogeneity of the hypertensive disease process is evident not only across individuals but applies also to the evolution of the disease condition within the same individual. Early hyperkinetic hypertension, in which sympathetic activation and its consequences are readily apparent, may develop over the long term into established hyper-

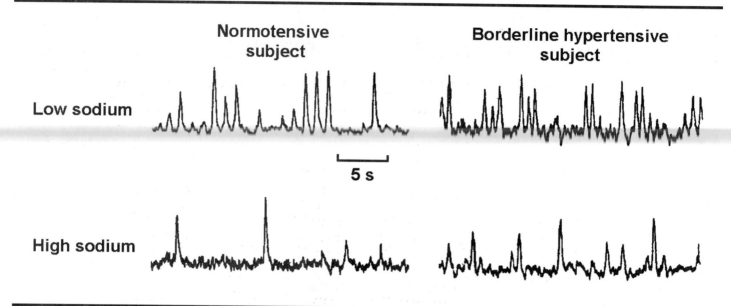

Figure A42.1. Recordings of muscle sympathetic nerve activity in a normotensive subject and in a borderline hypertensive subject on both low and high sodium diets. Sympathetic nerve activity was higher in the borderline hypertensive subject independent of diet. A similar conclusion was supported by the summary data on the 2 groups of subjects. (From Anderson EA, Sinkey CA, Lawton WJ, Mark AL. Elevated sympathetic nerve activity in borderline hypertensive humans: evidence from direct intraneural recordings. *Hypertension.* 1989;14:177–183, with permission.)

tension in which sympathetic activation may be less clear or less important in maintaining blood pressure levels. At any given time, there is also heterogeneity in the level of sympathetic drive to different vascular beds. For example, high sympathetic traffic to renal blood vessels may have important consequences not reflected in measurements of plasma catecholamines or sympathetic traffic to other vascular beds.

Reflex abnormalities. Assumption of the upright posture markedly stimulates the SNS. Studies of responses to orthostatic stress suggest that elevated levels of sympathetic drive in hypertensive patients may be masked when these individuals are in the supine position because of an enhanced sympathetic inhibition in response to activation of the cardiopulmonary receptors. Also important is the idea that any increase in blood pressure would be expected to act through baroreflexes to suppress sympathetic activity. Thus, in a hypertensive patient, the presence of "normal" sympathetic drive may in fact reflect a relative increase in sympathetic activity that is not suppressed fully by the impaired baroreflex mechanism (see Chapters A35 and A36).

Sympathetic Nervous System in Secondary Hypertension

Another argument that the SNS is important in chronic hypertension derives from observations of SNS overactivity in secondary forms of hypertension.

Pheochromocytoma. The classic example of catecholamine-mediated secondary hypertension is pheochromocytoma. In humans and animals with pheochromocytoma, early removal of the chromaffin tumor restores blood pressure to normal.

Renovascular hypertension. Increased sympathetic nervous activity (increased plasma norepinephrine and muscle sympathetic activity) also occurs in humans and animals with renovascular hypertension (**Figure A42.2**), at least early in the condition.

In renovascular hypertension, central effects of angiotensin II are thought to increase sympathetic outflow and to potentiate the peripheral effect of norepinephrine. Sympathetic activation decreases several days after successful renal angioplasty.

Cyclosporin-induced hypertension. Hypertension in patients receiving cyclosporine is associated with increased sympathetic nerve traffic. After cardiac transplantation, the level of sympathetic traffic appears to be linked to the severity of hypertension. However, not all studies of transplant recipients have shown high sympathetic drive. Time after transplantation and the presence of cardiac reinnervation may also modulate the level of sympathetic activation in heart transplant recipients.

Preeclampsia. In patients with preeclampsia, increased blood pressure and vascular resistance are accompanied by 3-fold increases in SNS traffic compared to control subjects and twice the level seen in nonpregnant women with hypertension. After delivery, blood pressure and sympathetic nerve activity decrease.

Aldosteronism. In contrast to the examples mentioned in the section Preeclampsia, patients with primary aldosteronism do not demonstrate marked increases in plasma or urinary catecholamines (Figure A42.2). However, "normal" SNS traffic in the setting of severe hypertension may be more closely related to accompanying baroreflex abnormalities, which do not fully suppress SNS outflow. Animals and humans with mineralocorticoid hypertension respond briskly to central or peripheral sympatholytic agents, which also suggests that the SNS plays some role in mineralocorticoid hypertension.

Sympathetic Activation as a Mediator of End-Organ Damage

The role of the SNS in hypertension may extend beyond serving merely as a mechanism for increasing blood pressure and may directly participate in structural and functional consequences of

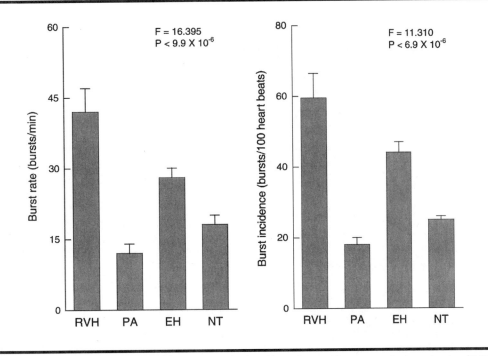

Figure A42.2. Muscle sympathetic nerve activity in normotensive subjects (NT) and in patients with renovascular hypertension (RVH), primary aldosteronism (PA), and essential hypertension (EH). Sympathetic burst frequency was higher in renovascular hypertension and essential hypertension than in normal individuals. Sympathetic activity was, however, decreased in patients with primary aldosteronism. (From Miyajima E, Yamada Y, Yoshida Y, et al. Muscle sympathetic nerve activity in renovascular hypertension and primary aldosteronism. *Hypertension*. 1991;17:1057–1062, with permission.)

heightened intravascular pressure. Catecholamines are an important mediator of trophic processes that may enhance pressor-mediated vascular and myocardial cell hypertrophy. Pressor effects of neural vasoconstriction are amplified by thicker vessel walls and narrow lumens. Cardiac sympathetic activation exacerbates dispersion of electric refractoriness and instability consequent to left ventricular hypertrophy, predisposing to arrhythmias. In heart failure, there is a clear and compelling association between elevated plasma catecholamines and poorer prognosis.

Sympathetic Activation by Antihypertensive Medications

Vasodilator medications such as hydralazine or amlodipine lower blood pressure but also result in increases in heart rate and sympathetic activity. In contrast, vasodilation with angiotensin-converting enzyme inhibitors or angiotensin receptor blockers is not accompanied by significant reflex sympathetic activation, perhaps because decreasing angiotensin's action reduces sympathetic activation, resets the baroreflex, or both.

SUGGESTED READING

1. Blood Pressure Lowering Treatment Trialists' Collaboration. Effects of ACE inhibitors, calcium antagonists, and other blood-pressure-lowering drugs: results of prospectively designed overviews of randomized trials. *Lancet*. 2000;356:1955–1964.
2. de Champlain J, Karas M, Nguyen P, et al. Different effects of nifedipine and amlodipine on circulating catecholamine levels in essential hypertensive patients. *J Hypertens*. 1998;16(9):357–369.
3. DiBona GF. Sympathetic nervous system influences on the kidney: role in hypertension. *Am J Hypertens*. 1989;2(suppl):119S–124S.
4. Esler M, Jennings G, Biviano B, et al. Mechanism of elevated plasma noradrenaline in the course of essential hypertension. *J Cardiovasc Pharmacol*. 1986;8:S39–43.
5. Goldstein DS. Plasma catecholamine and essential hypertension: an analytical review. *Hypertension*. 1983;5:86–99.
6. Izzo JL Jr. Sympathetic nervous system in acute and chronic blood pressure elevation. In: Oparil S, Weber MA, eds. *Hypertension: A Companion to Brenner & Rector's the Kidney*. Philadelphia: WB Saunders; 2000:42–58.
7. Pahor M, Psaty BM, Alderman MH, et al. Health outcomes associated with calcium antagonists compared with other first-line antihypertensive therapies: a meta-analysis of randomised controlled trials. *Lancet*. 2000;356:1949–1954.
8. Scherrer U, Vissing SF, Morgan BJ, et al. Cyclosporine-induced sympathetic activation and hypertension after heart transplantation. *N Engl J Med*. 1990;323:693–699.
9. Somers VK, Narkiewicz K. Sympathetic neural mechanisms in hypertension. In: Mathias CJ, Bannister R, eds. *Autonomic Failure: A Textbook of Clinical Disorders of the Autonomic Nervous System*. 4th ed. Oxford, NY: Oxford University Press; 1999:468–476.
10. Staessen JA, Wang J-G, Thijs L. Cardiovascular protection and blood pressure reduction: a meta-analysis. *Lancet*. 2001;358:1305–1315.

Chapter A43

Stress Responses and Blood Pressure Reactivity

Joseph L. Izzo, Jr, MD

KEY POINTS

- An individual's blood pressure responsiveness (i.e., blood pressure reactivity) to external stimuli depends on several factors, including the degree of activation of the sympathetic nervous system, pathologic alterations in the vasculature (endothelial dysfunction and arterial stiffness), psychological and behavioral characteristics such as coping skills, and cultural factors.

- Blood pressure reactivity is relatively reproducible within individuals but highly variable between individuals; blood pressure reactivity correlates only weakly with resting (basal) blood pressures or hypertension status.

- Hemodynamic responses are stimulus-specific but are modified by disease; for example, mental stress causes increased cardiac output in normotensives, but in hypertensives, vascular resistance increases as well.

- Increased blood pressure reactivity may be associated with higher cardiovascular risk in hypertension.

See also Chapters A34–A36, A38, A40, A42, A56, A60, A66, A76, B81, B88, B98, B100, B101, C112, C113, C117, C129, and C130

Blood pressure (BP) is intrinsically variable because adjustments in pressure and flow are important features of an individual's ability to adjust to acute and chronic changes in the environment. BP variability has been commonly viewed as "background noise" in the diagnosis of chronic hypertension, but a closer view reveals that BP variability and reactivity have distinct physiologic and perhaps pathophysiologic significance.

Modulation of Sympathetic Nervous Output

The coordination of acute stress responses was correctly attributed by Bernard to the nervous system, whose orchestration of responses to environmental changes he considered to be adaptive or "sympathetic." Selye believed that sympathetic nervous responses were essentially "all or nothing" or "fight or flight" responses. Today, it is known that the sympathetic system directs a variety of different patterns of multiple organ-specific responses that also involve other neurohormones. These specialized responses allow precise, energy-conserving adaptations to a wide variety of environmental stimuli (see Chapter A34).

Strength and duration of stimulus. Life-threatening stimuli (e.g., cardiogenic shock) cause a global sympathoadrenal response that involves massive release of catecholamines from sympathetic nerve terminals and the adrenal medulla. Less threatening stimuli such as mild hypoglycemia involve predominantly adrenal epinephrine release. Mild mental stress may involve only modest neuronal norepinephrine release. Stimuli also have intrinsically different relative durations, so the total responses and amounts of catecholamine released per stress episode differ widely. In hypertension, painful stimuli such as the cold pressor test cause exaggerated catecholamine release and a supranormal BP response.

Modulation of sympathetic responses. The sympathoadrenal system is capable of orchestrating a series of patterned, organ-specific neural responses. Because there are separate nerves controlling the heart and blood vessels, BP and heart rate responses also vary. Certain stimuli cause predictable differences in hemodynamics, such as an increase in cardiac output during mental stress or hypoglycemia or an increase in vasoconstriction in response to cold. Disease states can modify these stimulus-specific patterns; aerobic exercise or mental stress tend to increase cardiac output in normotensive individuals but tend to cause a combined flow-resistance increase in hypertensives. Concomitant stimulation of other hormones such as vasopressin or angiotensin II cause further modulation of the systemic response and help redirect blood flow to the organs most directly involved in the response.

Baroreflexes. Acute BP increases in normotensives are truncated by activation of aortocarotid baroreflexes (see Chapter A35), which directly limit sympathetic outflow. Blunting of the aortocarotid baroreflexes occurs in hypertension and in older individuals with carotid arteriosclerosis. In people with autonomic neuropathy (diabetics or those with autonomic insufficiency), BP responses can be exaggerated because of baroreflex dysfunction.

Vascular Modulation of Blood Pressure Reactivity

Patterns of blood pressure response. Pathophysiologic changes in large and small blood vessels associated with hypertension and aging alter the pattern of systolic and diastolic BP responses to environmental stressors. In normotensives and younger hypertensives, acute stress responses that involve increased cardiac stroke volume manifest themselves as an increase in pulse pressure (increased systolic and decreased diastolic). Responses that are predominantly vasoconstrictive are generally associated with increased diastolic pressure with variable systolic responses.

Vascular stiffness (arteriosclerosis) and pulse pressure variability. In older people and long-standing hypertensives, there is increased variability or "lability" of systolic pressure and decreased variability of diastolic pressure. This phenomenon occurs because arterial stiffness (which also contributes to baroreflex blunting and increased sympathetic outflow) creates a situation in which *only* systolic BP can vary in response to stimulation. In older people with stiff blood vessels (arteriosclerosis), variations in stroke volume tend to widen pulse pressure as they do in younger normotensives. However, in the arteriosclerotic individual, changes in vascular resistance have less effect on diastolic pressure because diastolic flow is already very low. In these people, increases in vascular resistance are more likely to increase systolic BP because of the phenomenon of increased wave reflection and late-systolic augmentation (see Chapter A60).

Endothelial dysfunction and increased vasoreactivity. Individuals with conditions causing endothelial dysfunction (e.g., hypercholesterolemia, insulin resistance) exhibit exaggerated BP responses to mental arithmetic or isometric exercise that are mediated via increased systemic vascular resistance. Treatment of dyslipidemia with statins (**Figure A43.1**) or insulin resistance with thiazolidinediones (insulin sensitizers) decreases the risk factor and the magnitude of the BP reactivity proportionally. It is likely that improved nitric oxide availability is the underlying mechanism for the beneficial effect of these drugs on exaggerated vasoreactivity (see Chapter A66).

Physical Deconditioning. Exercise conditioning tends to blunt BP reactivity, and it is likely that physical inactivity has the opposite effect. Beneficial effects of exercise on BP reactivity probably involve multiple mechanisms including improved baroreflex sensitivity, improvements in endothelial function, and greater sense of personal command.

Behavioral Aspects of Blood Pressure Reactivity

Neurophysiology. Emotional responses and some conscious behaviors are integrated by the hypothalamus, which in turn modulates activity of the medullary control centers that govern sympathetic nerve firing rates and catecholamine release. Through these pathways, cognitive and behavioral influences can modulate BP reactivity.

Anger and hostility. Several studies have found a correlation between anger or hostility (2 closely related parameters) and BP reactivity to various stressors. In addition, those with high anger or hostility scores demonstrate significantly longer persistence of the BP elevations caused by the experimental stressor.

Stress perception, coping, and locus of control. An individual's perception of a given stimulus and the nature of the individual's ability to cope with that particular challenge can significantly influence BP reactivity. A prevalent theory of stress modulation involves the concept *coping ability*, which is a measure of an individual's ability to use available resources to cope with stressful situations. Some psychologists have related coping skills to another concept, *locus of control*, which is another measure of individual environmental control. An example of the power of enhanced coping skills is provided by a study in which patients undergoing ambulatory ophthalmologic surgery were either allowed to listen to the music of their choice via headphones or allowed no music (**Figure A43.2** and **Figure A43.3**). The "no-music" group demonstrated significant BP reactivity to the stress of surgery, whereas the music group had virtually no BP elevations during surgery (Figure A43.2). Music recipients reported less stress and greater coping ability than those who did not receive music (Figure A43.3).

Social support. Closely related to coping ability is the degree of social support, which enhances coping. The physiologic independence of the mechanisms controlling resting and reactive BP changes can be demonstrated in psychophysiologic experiments. Allen and coworkers randomly allocated hypertensives to angiotensin-converting enzyme (ACE) inhibition alone or ACE inhibition plus pet acquisition (a form of nonevaluative social support). ACE inhibitors lowered resting home BPs equally in both groups but had no effect on BP reactivity to mental arithmetic or to a stressful speech task. In contrast, pet acquisition markedly diminished BP reactivity.

Racial and Cultural Aspects of Blood Pressure Reactivity

Differences in BP reactivity have been attributed to race and societal acculturation or "urbanization." Responses to mental stress in blacks are greater than those of white controls, and stress responses tend to increase in individuals who move from primitive or rural settings to cities. The apparent racial differences may represent genetic traits, but it seems more likely that they are the result of differences in levels of anger/hostility, social support, or a general imbalance between the amount of environmental stress and the individual's coping skills.

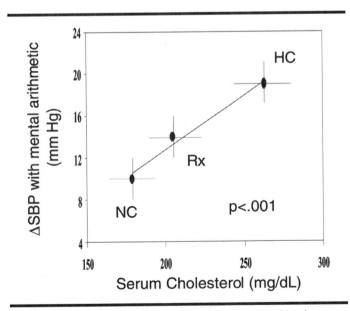

Figure A43.1. Relationship of serum cholesterol to systolic blood pressure (SBP) reactivity to mental stress. Despite similar baseline blood pressure (BP) values, hypercholesterolemic subjects (HC) have greater BP reactivity than normocholesterolemic controls (NC). Treatment of HC with a statin (Rx) for 6 weeks proportionally lowered BP reactivity and total cholesterol. Error bars are 1 SD. (Modified from Sung BH, Izzo JL Jr, Wilson MF. Effects of cholesterol reduction on BP response to mental stress in patients with high cholesterol. *Am J Hypertens*. 1997;10:592–599, with permission.)

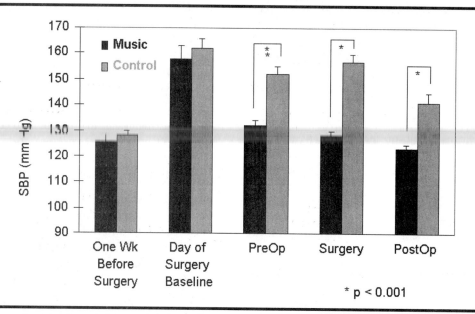

Figure A43.2. Blood pressure responses to ambulatory ophthalmologic surgery in individuals provided access to music and controls without music access. SBP, systolic blood pressure. (Modified from Allen K, Golden LH, Izzo JL Jr, et al. Normalization of hypertensive responses during ambulatory surgical stress by perioperative music. *Psychosom Med.* 2001;63:487–492.)

Clinical Impact of Stress-Induced Blood Pressure Variation

Population variation. Interindividual differences in stress responses can be quite marked. In a revealing study, Mancia and coworkers studied intraarterial BP responses to the act of taking a cuff BP in hospitalized subjects and found that the cuff measurement itself increased BP by an average of 27/14 mm Hg. What was more striking, however, was the range of reactivity that was observed: from 0 to 50 mm Hg systolic pressure. Furthermore, there was substantial variation in the time required for the stress-induced BP increases to return to baseline.

Lack of relationship to resting blood pressure. It has been erroneously assumed that all BPs within a given individual are proportional to that individual's resting level. Although there is a trend toward increased BP variability in those with the highest BPs, an individual's BP response to stress is largely independent of resting pressure level, with extremely wide variation. This point is of particular relevance when it is realized that the usual techniques of BP measurement in clinical settings reflect some degree of environmental stress and therefore tend to have greater variability across the population than corresponding home BPs.

Clinical and research impact. In the typical office setting, BP is measured after a few minutes in the seated position. For the vast majority of individuals, this represents a "low-stress"

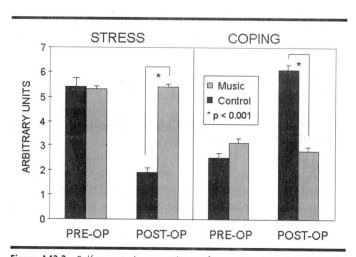

Figure A43.3. Self-reported perceptions of stress and coping levels in individuals provided headphone music compared to controls. (See Figure A43.2.)

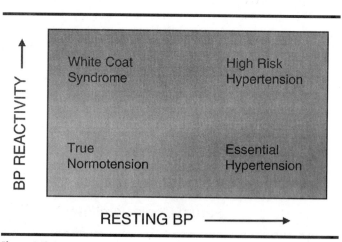

Figure A43.4. An integrated model of hypertension and blood pressure (BP) reactivity. Resting BP is controlled by different factors than those that affect BP reactivity. Neurogenic factors, vascular factors (especially vascular stiffness and endothelial dysfunction), and behavioral factors contribute to enhanced BP reactivity. The addition of exaggerated BP reactivity to resting hypertension leads to high-risk hypertension, whereas increased BP reactivity alone causes the "white-coat syndrome," a condition of low cardiac risk.

state owing to the orthostatic stimulus of sitting and to emotional and behavioral factors. Wide variability in "stress-decay" time enhances variation further. Accordingly, the reliability of a given set of BPs in the physician's office is limited. There are several consequences of this variation, including confusion in diagnosis and management of individual patients. Low reliability of individual BP values in clinical trials creates the need to use relatively large and expensive sample sizes to achieve statistical significance. The greater variability of systolic compared to diastolic BP, especially in older subjects, has been an important hidden barrier (because the cost of sample size increases) to the study of systolic hypertension.

Integrated Model of Hypertension and Blood Pressure Reactivity

BP is a highly complex physiologic variable, so it is not surprising that casual BP measurements are only loose surrogates for subclinical or clinical cardiovascular disease. BP variability itself may relate to increased organ damage and may also reflect the presence of other risk factors. For example, arteriosclerosis and endothelial dysfunction are markers of diffuse vascular disease that may predispose to increased stress reactivity of BP. An integrated model is presented in **Figure A43.4**.

SUGGESTED READING

1. Allen K, Golden LH, Izzo JL Jr, et al. Normalization of hypertensive responses during ambulatory surgical stress by perioperative music. *Psychosom Med.* 2001;63:487–492.
2. Allen K, Shykoff BE, Izzo JL Jr. Pet ownership, but not ACE inhibitor therapy, blunts home blood pressure responses to mental stress. *Hypertension.* 2001;38(4):815–820.
3. Fredrickson BL, Maynard KE, Helms MJ, et al. Hostility predicts magnitude and duration of blood pressure response to anger. *J Behav Med.* 2000;23:229–243.
4. Head GA. Baroreflexes and cardiovascular regulation in hypertension. *J Cardiovasc Pharmacol.* 1995;26(Suppl 2):S7–S16.
5. Mancia G, Bertinieri G, Grassi G, et al. Effects of blood-pressure measurement by the doctor on patient's blood pressure and heart rate. *Lancet.* 1983;2:695–698.
6. Mancia G, Grassi G. Mechanisms and clinical implications of blood pressure variability. *J Cardiovasc Pharmacol.* 2000;35:S15–S19.
7. Raven PB, Potts JT, Shi X. Baroreflex regulation of blood pressure during dynamic exercise. *Exerc Sport Sci Rev.* 1997;25:365–389.
8. Sung BH, Izzo JL Jr, Dandona P, Wilson MF. Vasodilatory effects of troglitazone improve blood pressure at rest and during mental stress in type 2 diabetes mellitus. *Hypertension.* 1999;34:83–88.
9. Sung BH, Izzo JL Jr, Wilson MF. Effects of cholesterol reduction on BP response to mental stress in patients with high cholesterol. *Am J Hypertens.* 1997;10(6):592–599.
10. van Rooyen JM, Huisman HW, Eloff FC, et al. Cardiovascular reactivity in black South-African males of different age groups: the influence of urbanization. *Ethn Dis.* 2002;12:69–75.

Chapter A44

Obesity

Lewis Landsberg, MD

KEY POINTS

- Hypertension and obesity are closely linked: Blood pressure increases with increasing body weight, and the incidence of hypertension among obese people approaches 50%.

- Obesity and hypertension occur frequently in a "metabolic syndrome" or risk factor constellation that includes insulin resistance and a characteristic dyslipidemia (low high-density lipoprotein cholesterol, high triglycerides).

- The pathophysiology of obesity-related hypertension is complex and involves insulin resistance, leptin, salt sensitivity, and inappropriately elevated sympathetic nervous system activity.

See also Chapters A11, A42, A45, A46, A53, A55, B81, B93, B97, B98, C118, C129, C130, C162, and C172

Epidemiology and Clinical Importance

The relationship between hypertension and obesity is well documented. As shown in **Figure A44.1** from the Framingham Heart Study, the prevalence of hypertension in men and women as a function of age increases substantially with increases in relative weight, so that the prevalence of hypertension is almost 50% in the most obese groups. This association is not the result of "cuff artifact" imposed by increased arm circumference, and the relationship does not depend on increased salt intake in the obese. Recent weight gain, however, is a very important factor in the development of hypertension. In the Framingham study, obesity or recent weight gain accounted for 70% of new-onset hypertension. It is abundantly clear, therefore, that obesity is a major factor in the development of hypertension. Both obesity and the associated metabolic syndrome have shown an alarming increase in prevalence over the last decade—an increase that affects both the developed and developing world. Projections indicate that at the present rate of growth, more than 40% of the population of the United States will be obese (body mass index >30) by 2015.

Body Fat Distribution Patterns

Body fat distribution plays a critical role as a risk factor for hypertension. Vague observed >50 years ago that the cardiovas-

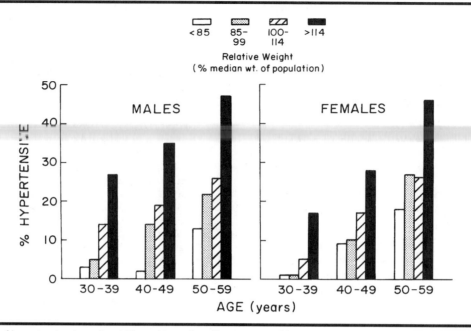

Figure A44.1. Prevalence of hypertension (systolic >160 mm Hg or diastolic >95 mm Hg) by age and sex in 4 relative weight groups at the first Framingham Heart Study examination. All trends are significant at $p = .05$. (Reprinted from Kannel et al. The relation of adiposity to blood pressure and development of hypertension: the Framingham study. *Ann Intern Med.* 1967;67:48–59, with permission.)

cular and metabolic consequences of obesity were most marked in individuals with the abdominal or upper-body form of obesity ("apples" vs. "pears"). These observations were confirmed in the mid-1980s by large-scale epidemiologic studies in Scandinavia. An increase in waist to hip ratio or abdominal circumference (**Figure A44.2**), surrogate markers for the upper-body fat pattern, is an independent risk factor for the development of high blood pressure and other cardiovascular risk factors.

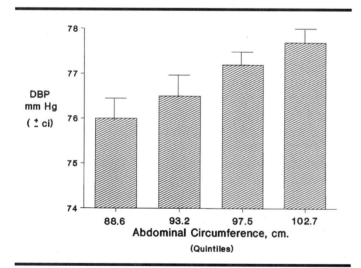

Figure A44.2. Diastolic blood pressures ±95% confidence intervals (ci) are shown for 1972 subjects from the Normative Aging Study as a function of abdominal circumference. Note that blood pressure and abdominal girth increased together. (Data from Cassano PA, Segal MR, Vokonas PS, Weiss ST. Body fat distribution, blood pressure, and hypertension: a prospective cohort study of men in the normative aging study. *Ann Epidemiol.* 1990;1:33–48. Figure reprinted from Landsberg L. Obesity and hypertension: experimental data. *J Hypertens.* 1992;10:S195–S201, with permission.)

Risk Factor Constellation (Metabolic Syndrome, Insulin Resistance Syndrome, Metabolic Syndrome X)

Both obesity and hypertension independently increase cardiovascular risk. Hypertension and upper body obesity are part of a larger risk factor constellation that includes additional major manifestations, including insulin resistance, characteristic dyslipidemia (low high-density lipoprotein cholesterol and high triglycerides with small, dense, atherogenic low-density lipoprotein), type 2 diabetes mellitus, salt sensitivity, microalbuminuria, and prothrombotic coagulation abnormalities (see Chapter A45). These additional factors increase the likelihood of adverse cardiovascular events, thereby accentuating the danger imposed by both obesity and hypertension. The prevalence of the metabolic syndrome, moreover, is increasing. It has been recently estimated that more than 20% of adults in the United States has the metabolic syndrome, with a striking increase in the younger population.

Pathophysiology of Obesity-Related Hypertension

Hemodynamics. The relationship between obesity and blood pressure is not explained adequately by hemodynamics. Although it is true that the obese tend to have increased blood volume and increased cardiac output compared with lean individuals, these differences disappear when corrected for the increased body mass. Peripheral resistance is elevated in obese hypertensives compared with obese normotensives.

Salt sensitivity hyperinsulinemia and sympathetic overactivity. Intake of sodium in the obese is frequently greater than in lean individuals, but increased sodium intake is not a sufficient explanation for the hypertension because weight loss in obese hypertensive individuals decreases blood pressure even when salt intake is unchanged. Salt sensitivity in obese people, with enhanced renal sodium reabsorption and the accompanying shift in the pressure-natriuresis curve, may be secondary to the effects of increased insulin levels, increased sympathetic nervous system activity, or both. Insulin levels track with hypertension in the obese, and insulin has been demonstrated to be antinatriuretic. Obese persons have increased sympathetic nervous system activity; renal sympathetic activation causes salt retention, and, at the level of the vasculature, sympathetic vasoconstriction increases vascular resistance. The origin of sympathetic hyperactivity in obesity is related, at least in part, to hyperinsulinemia, because insulin stimulates the sympathetic nervous system, but factors such as leptin may contribute importantly as well (see Chapter A11).

SUGGESTED READING

1. Ford ES, Giles WH, Dietz WH. Prevalence of the metabolic syndrome among US adults. *JAMA.* 2002;287:356–359.

2. Grassi G, Seravalle G, Cattaneo BM, et al. Sympathetic activation in obese normotensive subjects. *Hypertension.* 1995;25:560–563.
3. Haynes WG, Morgan DA, Walsh SA, et al. Receptor-mediated regional sympathetic nerve activation by leptin. *J Clin Invest.* 1997;100:270–278.
4. Kannel WB, Brand N, Skinner JJ Jr, et al. The relation of adiposity to blood pressure and development of hypertension: the Framingham study. *Ann Intern Med.* 1967;67:48–59.
5. Kopelman PG. Obesity as a medical problem. *Nature.* 2000;404(6778):635–643.
6. Krieger DR, Landsberg L. Obesity and hypertension. In: Laragh JH, Brenner BM, eds. *Hypertension: Pathophysiology, Diagnosis, and Management.* 2nd ed. New York, NY: Raven Press Ltd; 1995:2367–2388.
7. Reaven GM, Lithell H, Landsberg L. Hypertension and associated metabolic abnormalities: the role of insulin resistance and the sympathoadrenal system. *N Engl J Med.* 1996;334:374–381.
8. Reisin E, Abel R, Modan M, et al. Effect of weight loss without salt restriction on the reduction of blood pressure in overweight hypertensive patients. *N Engl J Med.* 1978;298:1–6.
9. Tuck ML, Sowers J, Dornfeld L, et al. The effect of weight reduction on blood pressure, plasma renin activity, and plasma aldosterone levels in obese patients. *N Engl J Med.* 1981;304:930–933.

Chapter A45

Insulin Resistance and Hypertension

Helmut O. Steinberg, MD

KEY POINTS

- Insulin resistance is a risk factor for the development of hypertension and cardiovascular disease.

- The prevalence of insulin resistance in the United States is approximately 20% and continues to rise.

- Insulin resistance is almost always associated with a cluster of cardiovascular risk factors, including obesity, dyslipidemia, dysfibrinolysis, endothelial dysfunction, salt sensitivity, and hypertension.

- Insulin resistance is associated with increased sympathetic nervous activity, hyperleptinemia, impaired endothelial function, and increased vascular reactivity.

See also Chapters A11, A42, A44, A46, A47, A53, A57, A66, A67, B81, B90, B97, C127, C129, C130, C149, and C162

Insulin resistance (IR) is a potent risk factor for the development of cardiovascular diseases. *IR* is defined as the inability of the body to achieve normal rates of glucose uptake in response to insulin. IR occurs at multiple organ sites, including the liver, fat, endothelial, and skeletal muscle cells, the last of which is most important on a quantitative basis. The "gold standard" for quantification of IR is the euglycemic hyperinsulinemic clamp technique, which under steady-state conditions, measures the glucose uptake into skeletal muscle. With IR progression, there is increasing fasting hyperinsulinemia—another hallmark of IR.

Prevalence and Associated Abnormalities

IR often occurs in association with a cluster of other metabolic abnormalities: impaired glucose tolerance, type 2 diabetes mellitus, obesity, low high-density lipoprotein cholesterol, elevated triglyceride and free fatty acid levels, and hypertension.

This clustering of cardiovascular risk factors has been named the *insulin resistance syndrome, metabolic syndrome X,* or the *cardiovascular dysmetabolic syndrome*; it is associated with a 2- to 3-fold increase in rates of cardiovascular morbidity and mortality. IR and essential hypertension are common in the U.S. population. More than 45 million subjects exhibit IR, which is seen mostly in obese and type 2 diabetic subjects; hypertension is found in nearly 60 million Americans. Whether IR is one cause of hypertension or whether both conditions result from a more basic defect remains unanswered.

Association of Insulin Resistance and Hypertension

IR and essential hypertension are polygenic conditions. The expression of both hypertension and IR is modified by environmental factors, such as diet and degree of physical activity. If IR and hypertension are independent genetic traits, one would expect the incidence of the combination of IR and hypertension to equal that predicted by chance. Prospective studies, however, have demonstrated that hypertension develops more often in subjects with hyperinsulinemia than in subjects with normal insulin levels. Furthermore, cross-sectional studies also have shown that IR is accompanied by hypertension more often than expected by chance alone; IR is found in up to 50% of hypertensive subjects, and nearly 50% of obese subjects exhibit hypertension. Taken together, these findings provide evidence that IR and hypertension are strongly linked. The link between IR and hypertension is further supported by the observation that worsening of IR because of weight gain or sedentary lifestyle is associated with a higher incidence of hypertension. Conversely, maneuvers that decrease IR, such as weight loss or exercise, diminish blood pressure levels. Furthermore, drugs that improve insulin sensitivity (such as the thiazolidinedione or "glitazone" class of insulin sensitizers) have been reported to lower blood pressure, at least in some individuals, independent of weight loss or increased levels of exercise.

Mechanisms of Hypertension

Cellular effects of insulin. The cellular mechanism by which IR predisposes to hypertension remains unknown. It was originally believed that elevated insulin levels per se caused blood pressure elevation. This idea was based on *in vitro* observations that insulin can directly stimulate Na,K adenosine triphosphatase and a number of ion channels and pumps, thereby increasing intracellular sodium and calcium concentrations. Intracellular Ca^{2+} is a major determinant of vascular smooth muscle cell tension and contractility in response to vasopressor substances. However, recent data indicate that Ca^{2+} flux into vascular smooth muscle cells and into platelets is actually decreased by insulin. Thus, IR and impaired insulin action to reduce Ca^{2+} influx could contribute to the development of hypertension.

Vasodilator effects of insulin. Elevated insulin levels thus are not likely to cause hypertension because insulin is a powerful vasodilator. Insulin administered to normal subjects even in high pharmacologic doses does not cause blood pressure elevation; in fact, it usually causes a small but significant decrease in blood pressure because of its vasodilatory action. Furthermore, insulin attenuates the pressor effects of norepinephrine and angiotensin II in normal insulin-sensitive subjects but not in IR subjects. The vasodilator action of insulin is mediated via its own receptor on the endothelial cell, in part through the release of nitric oxide. Nitric oxide displays a host of antiatherogenic

properties, suggesting that decreased production or release of endothelial nitric oxide in IR could explain, at least in part, the higher rates of hypertension and macrovascular diseases in IR.

Increased leptin and sympathetic activity. At the level of the whole organism, both insulin and leptin (a hormone produced by fat cells in proportion to fat mass; see Chapter A11) cause increased sympathetic nervous system activity. Obese IR (hyperinsulinemic and hyperleptinemic) subjects exhibit higher sympathetic nervous system activity, which leads to elevation of cardiac output and peripheral vasoconstriction and increased blood pressure.

Antinatriuresis. Another possible mechanism thought to be responsible for the development of hypertension is the ability of insulin to cause acute sodium and water retention as has been demonstrated during acute dosing studies in animals and humans. The acute effects are mediated by direct actions of insulin on renal tubular transport. It remains unclear whether these effects persist in the chronic condition, however.

Proposed integrated mechanism. IR could cause hypertension via the following hypothetical steps. Early in the course of IR, the production or release of nitric oxide decreases, and responses to pressor hormones become exaggerated. Later, progressive obesity, worsening IR, hyperinsulinemia, and hyperleptinemia occur, resulting in increased sympathetic nervous system activity and, perhaps, sodium and water retention. It is also possible that increasd catecholamine levels in hypertensives exacerbate IR. In either case, the vasodepressor system would be impaired in IR, and the unopposed higher sympathetic nervous system activity, the heightened reactivity to pressors, and the retention of sodium and water could exacerbate hypertension. However, this hypothetical scenario has not yet been fully experimentally confirmed.

SUGGESTED READING

1. Baron AD. Hemodynamic actions of insulin. *Am J Physiol.* 1994;267:E187–E202.
2. Ferrannini E, Buzzigoli G, Bonadonna R, et al. Insulin resistance in essential hypertension. *N Engl J Med.* 1987;317:350–357.
3. Haffner SM, Valdez RA, Hazuda HP, et al. Prospective analysis of the insulin-resistance syndrome (syndrome X). *Diabetes.* 1992;41:715–722.
4. Jiang ZY, Lin YW, Clemont A, et al. Characterization of selective resistance to insulin signaling in the vasculature of obese zucker (fa/fa) rats. *J Clin Invest.* 1999;104:447–457.
5. Reaven GM. Banting lecture 1988: role of insulin resistance in human disease. *Diabetes.* 1988;37:1595–1607.
6. Steinberg HO, Chaker H, Leaming R, et al. Obesity/insulin resistance is associated with endothelial dysfunction: implications for the syndrome of insulin resistance. *J Clin Invest.* 1996;97:2601–2610.

Salt Sensitivity

Myron H. Weinberger, MD

KEY POINTS

- Increased dietary salt intake does not raise blood pressure in all hypertensive persons; those whose blood pressures rise in response to high salt diets or fall with salt restriction are termed *salt sensitive*.

- Factors influencing salt sensitivity include obesity, age, race, plasma renin level, sympathetic nervous system activity, and the presence of concomitant diseases such as diabetes mellitus and renal insufficiency.

- Variants in genes encoding α-adducin and angiotensinogen are associated with increased blood pressure and salt sensitivity.

- Salt sensitivity in normotensives is associated with an increased risk for the development of hypertension, cardiovascular events, and death.

See also Chapters A4, A36–A38, A42, A44, A45, A47, A49, A75–A78, B93, B94, B97, C129, and C139

Studies in large groups of hypertensives and normotensives show a variable relationship between dietary salt intake and blood pressure (BP). However, BP in some individuals is responsive (or "sensitive") to variation of dietary sodium, whereas others show little or no BP response to changes in sodium balance.

Clinical Studies

Epidemiologic associations. Anecdotal observations relating excessive salt intake to increased BP were followed by population studies confirming the relationship. Populations that typically ingest an average of less than 100 mEq/day of sodium (or chloride) generally have a lower incidence of hypertension and its cardiovascular consequences than populations in which sodium chloride intake is higher. Other characteristics that may differentiate these groups are physical activity, body mass, genetic factors, calcium and potassium intake, stress, and other lifestyle components.

Dietary interventions. Despite epidemiologic associations, interventional studies have not consistently demonstrated a decrease in BP when dietary sodium intake is reduced. Interventions typically involve only short-term dietary salt reduction, whereas epidemiologic observations relate to lifelong exposure, so it would be inappropriate to conclude that sodium is not an important factor in the pathogenesis of essential hypertension. Dietary factors also interact, further confounding interpretation. In the DASH trial of sodium restriction and potassium enhancement, a small effect of salt restriction was observed independent of caloric or potassium intake changes.

Pathophysiology

Salt resistance and impaired counterregulation. An easily measured and consistent abnormality, relative renin suppression (low-renin hypertension), is associated with an enhanced BP response to sodium depletion (i.e., salt sensitivity). A subnormal renin response to volume depletion may explain the enhanced fall in BP with a low-salt diet, but it does not account for the rise in BP during salt loading.

Neurogenic features of salt sensitivity. Some studies suggest that salt-sensitive subjects have enhanced sympathetic nervous system activity that is associated with a failure to suppress sympathetic outflow during salt loading. It is also possible that there is an influence of sodium balance on vascular responses to vasoactive substances. Reduced natriuresis may result from reduced activity of the renal dopaminergic system, which has been proposed to have a role in modulating renal sodium excretion and the BP response to sodium loading.

Role of chloride ion. It has been suggested that it is the chloride rather than sodium that is responsible for the rise in BP in salt-sensitive subjects. However, sodium and chloride track closely because 95% of the dietary sources of sodium is in the form of sodium chloride.

Techniques for Evaluating Salt Sensitivity

Salt sensitivity of BP is a reproducible response in an individual, regardless of how it is assessed. BP responses to sodium can be studied experimentally by manipulating sodium balance under standardized conditions. Regardless of the method used to alter sodium balance, the degree of BP change defining salt sensitivity is arbitrary. BP responses are continuously distributed, so salt sensitivity simply means that BP changes by more than a specified increment.

Controlled dietary manipulation. Kawasaki and colleagues studied BP responses during 1 week of low sodium intake (9 mEq/day) followed by 1 week of high sodium intake (249 mEq/day). Subjects who had a mean arterial BP on the last day of the high-sodium period 10% greater than that on the last day of the low sodium intake were defined as *salt sensitive*; the remainder were called *salt insensitive*. BP at the end of the high-salt period was not significantly different from that observed during a normal-sodium (109-mEq/day) diet in either group, emphasizing that normal sodium intake in Westernized societies is far in excess of biologic requirements. In this study, the difference between salt-sensitive and salt-insensitive hypertensives was primarily the degree of BP reduction during the low-salt diet compared to their normal salt intake.

Acute saline infusion. Weinberger and colleagues examined the BP responses of 375 normotensives and 192 essential hypertensives after rapid extracellular volume expansion. Intravenous infusion of 2 L of normal (0.9%) saline over a 4-hour period was followed on the next day by sodium and volume depletion induced by a low-sodium (10-mEq/day) diet and enhanced by 3 doses of 40 mg of furosemide. The mean arterial BP on the morning after sodium and volume depletion was compared with that after the saline infusion. A decrease in mean arterial pressure of ≥10 mm Hg was designated as salt sensitive, and a decrease of ≤5 mm Hg (or an increase in mean arterial pressure) after sodium and volume depletion was defined as salt resistant. Decreases in mean arterial pressure of 6 to 9 mm Hg were deemed indeterminate. The responses to this protocol are similar to those of longer periods of dietary sodium manipulation and are reproducible.

Genetic Markers of Salt Sensitivity

To date, 2 genes show promise as markers of salt sensitivity: α-adducin and angiotensinogen (see Chapters A75 and A76).

α-Adducin. α-Adducin, a heterodimeric protein thought to regulate cell signal transduction by interacting with the actin cytoskeleton, acts on proximal renal tubular cells to modulate sodium reabsorption. Genetic linkage studies have identified the α-adducin gene as candidate for hypertension, and subsequent studies have identified a mutation (substitution of tryptophan for glycine at amino acid residue 460). Salt sensitivity in hypertensives has been characterized by α-adducin genotype: BP fell more in response to salt restriction in hypertensives with the Trp allele (Trp/Trp and Trp/Gly) than in Gly/Gly homozygotes. Institution of early salt restriction in individuals with the Trp allele could possibly result in prevention of hypertension or at least in a delay in its onset.

Angiotensinogen. Hunt and coworkers directly examined a polymorphism (A vs. G) at the (−6) nucleotide of the promotor region of the angiotensinogen in the genotypes of 1,509 participants in phase II of the Trials of Hypertension Prevention. If sodium intake was not altered, subjects with the AA genotype had a higher incidence of hypertension after 3 years than those with the GG genotype (44.6% vs. 31.5%, respectively), although the difference was not statistically significant. If sodium intake was reduced, subjects with the AA genotype had a significantly lower incidence of hypertension (relative risk = 0.57; confidence interval, 0.34–0.98) than those with the GG genotype (relative risk = 1.2; confidence interval, 0.79–1.81). Such studies suggest that there are genetic-environment interactions in these traits and that responsiveness to specific life-

Table A46.1. Clinical Predictors of Salt Sensitivity

Older age
Low-renin hypertension (including blacks)
Insulin resistance/diabetes
Renal failure
Increased sympathetic activity

style interventions varies across the population of people with hypertension.

Clinical Correlations

Clinical associations. Clinical groups with salt sensitivity are shown in **Table A46.1**. It has been suggested that impaired renal sodium handling in these populations may be responsible for salt sensitivity of BP, but this possibility has not been convincingly demonstrated.

Prediction of cardiovascular risk in normotensives. In addition to the greater prevalence of salt sensitivity in older individuals, salt sensitivity in normotensive subjects is associated with a significantly greater age-related increase in BP than in salt-resistant normotensive subjects, implying that the age-related rise in BP may be a reflection of salt sensitivity. A follow-up study of 708 normotensive and hypertensive subjects, in whom salt sensitivity was initially characterized as long as 25 years ago, indicates that salt-sensitive normotensive subjects had a survival rate that was not significantly different from that of hypertensive subjects and that the majority of deaths were related to cardiovascular disease. These findings suggest that salt sensitivity of BP is a marker for future cardiovascular events.

SUGGESTED READING

1. Campese VM, Romoff MS, Levitan D, et al. Abnormal relationship between sodium intake and sympathetic nervous system activity in salt-sensitive patients with essential hypertension. *Kidney Int.* 1982;21:371–378.
2. Gill JR Jr, Grossman E, Goldstein DS. High urinary dopa and low urinary dopamine-to-dopa ratio in salt-sensitive hypertension. *Hypertension.* 1991;18:614–621.
3. Kawasaki T, Delea CS, Bartter FC, Smith H. The effect of high-sodium and low-sodium intakes on blood pressure and other related variables in human subjects with idiopathic hypertension. *Am J Med.* 1978;64:193–198.
4. Kurtz TW, Al-Bander HA, Morris RC Jr. "Salt-sensitive" essential hypertension in men: is the sodium ion alone important? *N Engl J Med.* 1987;317:1043–1048.
5. Rankin LI, Luft FC, Henry DP, et al. Sodium intake alters the effects of norepinephrine on blood pressure. *Hypertension.* 1981;3:650–656.
6. Weinberger MH. Salt sensitivity of blood pressure in humans. *Hypertension.* 1996;27:481–490.
7. Weinberger MH, Fineberg NS. Sodium and volume sensitivity of blood pressure: age and pressure change over time. *Hypertension.* 1991;18:67–71.
8. Weinberger MH, Fineberg NS, Fineberg SE, Weinberger M. Salt sensitivity, pulse pressure, and death in normal and hypertensive humans. *Hypertension.* 2001;37[part 2]:429–432.
9. Weinberger MH, Miller JZ, Fineberg NS, et al. Association of haptoglobin with sodium sensitivity and resistance of blood pressure. *Hypertension.* 1987;10:443–446.
10. Weinberger MH, Miller JZ, Luft FC, et al. Definitions and characteristics of sodium sensitivity and blood pressure resistance. *Hypertension.* 1986;8(suppl II):II127–II134.

Chapter A47

Divalent Cations in Hypertension

Lawrence M. Resnick, MD

KEY POINTS

- Hypertension, arterial stiffness, cardiac hypertrophy, insulin resistance, obesity, and type 2 diabetes are all characterized by similar elevations in cytosolic free calcium and reductions in cytosolic magnesium.

- According to the divalent cation hypothesis, blood pressure is determined by reciprocating contributions of extracellular calcium-dependent (low-renin, salt-sensitive, high α-adrenergic activity, insulin-resistant) and intracellular calcium release–dependent (high-renin, salt-insensitive, insulin-sensitive) pressor mechanisms.

- Dietary salt and dietary calcium have opposite effects on blood pressure owing to their opposite, hormone-mediated promotion and suppression, respectively, of cellular calcium uptake.

- The predominant operative calcium-dependent mechanism predicts blood pressure responsiveness to dietary and antihypertensive drug therapies.

See also Chapters A25–A27, A33, A41, A45, A46, A61, B96, B97, and C144–146

Abnormal steady-state cellular ion activity is an attractive hypothesis in an integrative model that includes hypertension as one manifestation of a more generalized cellular ionic defect that also involves insulin resistance, hyperinsulinemia, left ventricular hypertrophy, increased arterial stiffness, abnormal platelet aggregation, enhanced sympathetic nerve activity, and accelerated atherosclerotic disease. All of these features are components of what has been previously called the *cardiovascular-dysmetabolic syndrome*, *metabolic syndrome X*, or the *insulin resistance syndrome*. Furthermore, the activity of ion-active hormone systems appears to identify individual blood-pressure responsiveness to dietary minerals, nutrients, and antihypertensive drugs.

Cellular Calcium Flux and Cardiovascular Physiology

Vascular smooth muscle contraction. In vascular smooth muscle, plasma membrane depolarization-induced Ca^{2+} current and subsequent Ca^{2+} release from the sarcoplasmic reticulum elevates cytosolic free Ca^{2+} ($[Ca^{2+}]_i$) levels and triggers a cascade of molecular rearrangements of calmodulin and myosin light-chain kinase, ultimately leading to myofilament shortening and vasoconstriction (see Chapter A27). Conversely, vasorelaxation restores basal $[Ca^{2+}]_i$ levels via cellular Ca^{2+} egress and Ca^{2+} reuptake into sarcoplasmic reticulum stores.

Cardiac function, hormone release, and ion transport. As has been experimentally verified, blood pressure (BP) and $[Ca^{2+}]_i$ levels are directly related. Similar Ca-dependent events also regulate a wide spectrum of cellular responses, including cardiac function, hormone secretion, renal ion excretion, and neural excitation. Furthermore, a reciprocal relation exists between levels of $[Ca^{2+}]_i$ and intracellular free Mg ($[Mg^{2+}]_i$),

the most prevalent intracellular divalent cation. Mg^{2+} buffers the constrictor effects of $[Ca^{2+}]_i$, and cellular Mg deficiency leads to enhanced Ca-induced cell vasoconstriction.

Glucose and Insulin as Intracellular Ion Regulators

Increased extracellular glucose concentrations, *in vivo* or *in vitro*, raise $[Ca^{2+}]_i$ and lower $[Mg^{2+}]_i$ levels, a pattern similar to the abnormal ionic profile found in diabetes and hypertension. Fasting glucose and HbA_{1c} levels in nondiabetic and diabetic subjects predict fasting $[Ca^{2+}]_i$, $[Mg^{2+}]_i$, and BP levels, so it is possible that small increases in glucose concentrations, even within the normal range, may affect basal $[Ca^{2+}]_i$ and $[Mg^{2+}]_i$ content and, thus, basal vascular tone. Insulin, independent of glucose, also stimulates ion flux, raising $[Mg^{2+}]_i$ and, under some circumstances, $[Ca^{2+}]_i$ in vascular and other tissues. In hypertension, these ionic actions are blunted in direct proportion to the deviation of basal $[Ca^{2+}]_i$ and $[Mg^{2+}]_i$ values from normal. Insulin resistance is thus at least partly an ionic phenomenon that is part of a more generalized pattern of cell responses to different stimuli.

Cardiovascular-Dysmetabolic Syndrome (Insulin Resistance)

In clinical situations, elevated $[Ca^{2+}]_i$ levels or suppressed $[Mg^{2+}]_i$ levels are observed in essential hypertension, insulin resistance, obesity, and type 2 diabetes. Quantitatively, the higher the $[Ca^{2+}]_i$ and the lower the $[Mg^{2+}]_i$, the more elevated the BP, cardiac hypertrophy, arterial stiffness, hyperinsulinemia, insulin resistance, and abdominal visceral fat mass. Hence, each of the above aspects of hypertensive disease appears to reflect a shared cellular ionic lesion defined at least in part by

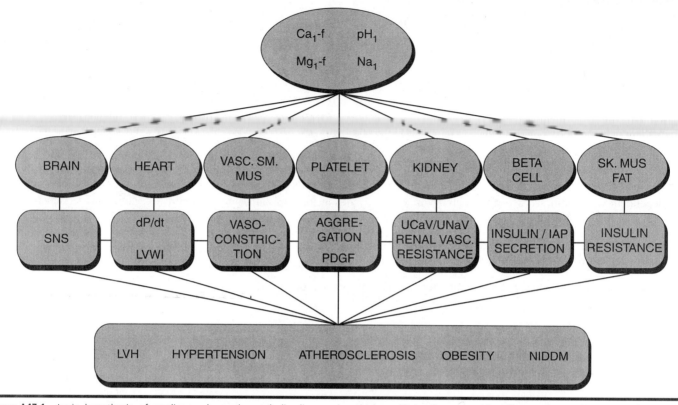

Figure A47.1. Ionic hypothesis of cardiovascular and metabolic disease, in which multiple disease entities **(bottom)** are clinical manifestations of underlying cellular ion abnormalities shared in common **(top)** but expressed differently in different organ systems **(middle)** (see text). dP/dt, upstroke pattern on apex cardiogram; IAP, islet-activating protein; LVH, left ventricular hypertrophy; LVWI, left ventricular work index; NIDDM, non–insulin-dependent diabetes mellitus; PDGF, platelet-derived growth factor; SK MUS FAT, skeletal muscular fat; SNS, sympathetic nervous system; UCaV, urinary calcium volume; UNaV, urinary sodium volume; VASC, vascular; VASC SM MUS, vascular smooth muscle.

excess steady-state $[Ca^{2+}]_i$ and reciprocally suppressed $[Mg^{2+}]_i$ levels. One consequence of this ionic approach is that rather than hypertension "causing" insulin resistance, or conversely, insulin resistance and hyperinsulinemia causing hypertension, it is more likely that each represents an altered response of different tissues to the same alteration of the cellular ionic environment **(Figure A47.1)**.

Extracellular Ion Regulation

The intracellular ionic environment common to hypertension and the other conditions mentioned in the section Cardiovascular-Dysmetabolic Syndrome (Insulin Resistance) is influenced by extracellular environmental factors that affect ion-active hormone systems **(Table A47.1)**. Low-renin hypertensive subjects exhibit significantly lower serum ionized Ca^{2+} and calcitonin levels and reciprocally higher serum Mg^{2+}, parathyroid hormone, and 1,25-dihydroxyvitamin D (1,25D) concentrations when compared to normotensive or other hypertensive subjects. High-renin subjects exhibit oppositely skewed values. These deviations in both directions away from normotensive values suggest an extracellular Ca^{2+} deficiency in low-renin subjects, and in high-renin subjects, a Ca^{2+} surfeit.

Dietary Salt and Intracellular Divalent Cations

Because $[Ca^{2+}]_i$ levels reflect the steady-state equilibrium between extracellular Ca and intracellular Ca stores, elevated $[Ca^{2+}]_i$ in hypertension implies, by definition, an altered con-

tribution of at least 1 of these 2 Ca^{2+} equilibria, which vary within and between subjects **(Figure A47.2)**. Volume excess and high-salt diets transiently lower extracellular Ca^{2+}, increasing levels of Ca^{2+} hormones such as 1,25D, along with other factors such as ouabain-like molecules and parathyroid hypertensive factor. Ca^{2+}-active hormones stimulate extracellular Ca uptake, thereby promoting vasoconstriction and suppressing renal renin release. In salt-sensitive subjects, salt loading reproduces the cellular ionic-hormonal profile of the low-renin subject, with decreased extracellular Ca^{2+} levels owing to 1,25D, digitalis-like factor, and/or α-adrenergic activity–mediated shifts of Ca^{2+} intracellularly, increased $[Ca^{2+}]_i$, and thus elevated BP.

Cellular Ca^{2+} Balance and Blood Pressure Regulation

Despite uniform elevations of $[Ca^{2+}]_i$ levels in all types of hypertension, there are heterogeneous deviations, both higher and lower than normotensive values, of extracellular Ca^{2+} and Mg^{2+} ion and hormone levels among different subjects. BP remains relatively constant as long as steady-state $[Ca^{2+}]_i$ levels remain unchanged. BP and cellular Ca^{2+} homeostasis are coordinately regulated in a see-saw fashion. If the incremental increase in extracellular Ca^{2+} during a high-salt diet is offset by an equal and opposite suppression of angiotensin II–dependent intracellular Ca^{2+} release, BP again remains constant. Conversely, with a low dietary salt intake and the associated positive Ca^{2+} balance, there is a transient rise of extracellular Ca^{2+} and a physiologic fall

Table A47.1. Evidence of Altered Divalent Cation Metabolism in Hypertension

Epidemiology
　Increased incidence/prevalence of hypertension with decreased dietary Ca and/or Mg intake
　Influence of dietary salt on BP preferentially in subjects with low calcium intakes
　Increased urinary Ca relative to Na in hypertension
Pathophysiology
　Intracellular
　　Elevated steady-state fasting $[Ca^{2+}]_i$/suppressed $[Mg^{2+}]_i$
　　BP directly proportional to $[Ca^{2+}]_i$, inversely to $[Mg^{2+}]_i$
　Extracellular
　　Low-renin hypertension
　　　Decreased Ca-io, calcitonin, increased Mg-o, parathyroid hormone, 1,25D
　　High-renin hypertension
　　　Increased Ca-io, calcitonin, decreased Mg-o, parathyroid hormone, 1,25D
　Salt-sensitive hypertension
　　ΔBP directly proportional to Δ1,25D, $\Delta[Ca^{2+}]_i$, inversely to $\Delta[Mg^{2+}]_i$, and ΔCa-io
　Other risk factors in hypertension are directly proportional to fasting $[Ca^{2+}]_i$, and inversely to $[Mg^{2+}]_i$
　　Left ventricular mass
　　Arterial stiffness
　　Abdominal visceral fat
　　Insulin resistance
　　Glycosylated hemoglobin and fasting blood sugar in normal and type 2 diabetic subjects
Therapy
　Oral calcium can lower BP.
　　Preferentially effective in low-renin, salt-sensitive, elderly subjects
　　Lowers 1,25D, $[Ca^{2+}]_i$
　　ΔBP directly related to Ca-io, plasma renin activity, inversely related to 1,25D, urinary volume of sodium
　All antihypertensive drugs lower elevated $[Ca^{2+}]_i$, and/or elevate the decreased $[Mg^{2+}]_i$ of hypertension.
　　ΔBP directly related to $\Delta [Ca^{2+}]_i$, inversely to $\Delta [Mg^{2+}]_i$

Δ, change; 1,25D, 1,25-dihydroxyvitamin D; BP, blood pressure; $[Ca^{2+}]_i$, cytosolic free intracellular calcium; Ca-io, extracellular ionized calcium; $[Mg^{2+}]_i$, intracellular free Mg.

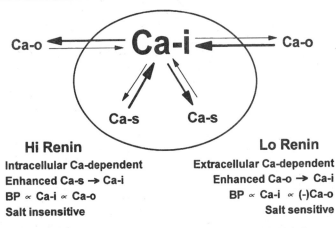

$$BP \propto (Ca\text{-}i) = f(Ca\text{-}o) + g(Ca\text{-}s)$$

Figure A47.2. Dual Ca mechanisms in hypertension, in which an inappropriate excess cytosolic free Ca (Ca-i) can result alternatively from enhanced (e.g., salt-dependent) extracellular Ca (Ca-o, *right*) transport intracellularly, from enhanced (e.g., angiotensin II–mediated) intracellular Ca release from intracellular Ca stores (Ca-s, *left*), or both. Primary increases in Ca-i from either source may be at least partially offset by a secondary increase in Ca extrusion from cytosol into Ca stores (*right*) or into extracellular space (*left*). Altogether, the net blood pressure (BP) is proportional to the ambient steady-state $[Ca^{2+}]_i$ level, which is, in turn, determined by reciprocating contributions of each Ca source, defined here as $f(Ca\text{-}o)$ and $g(Ca\text{-}s)$ **(bottom)** (see text).

Table A47.2. Equivalent Descriptions of Blood Pressure (BP) Homeostasis[a]

Clinical/physiologic level
　BP = volume × vasoconstriction
　(salt) × (renin)
Tissue/organ level
　BP = cardiac output × peripheral resistance
　(cardiac output) × (total peripheral resistance)
Cellular/ionic level
　$BP = k[Ca^{2+}]_i = k\{f(Ca\text{-}o) \times g(Ca\text{-}s)\}$
　(extracellular Ca) × (cellular Ca stores)

$[Ca^{2+}]_i$, cytosolic free intracellular calcium; Ca-o, extracellular ionized calcium; Ca-s, intracellular Ca stores; k, proportionality factor [either a constant or a function of other non-calcium (e.g., magnesium-related variables)] describing BP as a function of $[Ca^{2+}]_i$ (and thus BP) level.
[a]At each level of description in this table, the 2 terms on the right, which define BP, are reciprocally related, elevations of one calling forth a reduction in the other, the resulting BP normally remaining constant (see text).

in Ca^{2+}-regulating hormones. Overall, BP homeostasis remains intact unless an increase in extracellular Ca^{2+} entry or intracellular Ca^{2+} release exceeds the limits of physiologic compensation **(Table A47.2)**. In such conditions as primary aldosteronism, low-renin essential hypertension, unilateral renal artery stenosis, and renin-secreting tumors, there is an imbalance favoring hypertension. In such conditions as normal-high renin or non-modulating hypertension, bilateral renal artery stenosis, pre-eclampsia, or malignant hypertension, there may be a failure of reciprocal suppression of the counterregulatory mechanism.

Hypotensive Conditions

The importance of extracellular Ca^{2+} and Ca^{2+} hormones in hypertension is further demonstrated by hypotensive responses in elderly, low-renin, and/or salt-sensitive subjects to (a) oral Ca^{2+} supplementation, which physiologically suppresses Ca^{2+} ionophoric hormones such as 1,25D and parathyroid hypertensive factor; (b) Ca^{2+} antagonists, which directly block extracellular Ca^{2+} uptake; and (c) α-adrenergic antagonists, which reverse the ionic and BP effects of salt.

SUGGESTED READING

1. Barbagallo M, Gupta RK, Bardicef O, et al. Altered ionic effects of insulin in hypertension: role of basal ion levels in determining cellular responsiveness. *J Clin Endocrinol Metab.* 1997;82:1761–1765.
2. Barbagallo M, Gupta RK, Dominguez LJ, Resnick LM. Cellular ionic alterations with age: relation to hypertension and diabetes. *J Am Geriatrics Soc.* 2000;48:1111–1116.
3. Erne P, Bolli P, Bürgissen E, Bühler FR. Correlation of platelet calcium with blood pressure: effect of antihypertensive therapy. *N Engl J Med.* 1984;310:1084–1088.
4. Hunt SC, Williams RR, Kuida H. Different plasma ionized calcium correlations with blood pressure in high and low renin normotensive adults in Utah. *Am J Hypertens.* 1991;4:1–8.

5. Resnick LM. Ionic disturbances of calcium and magnesium metabolism in essential hypertension. In: Laragh JH, Brenner BM, eds. *Hypertension: Pathophysiology, Diagnosis, and Management.* 2nd ed. New York, NY: Raven Press; 1995:1169–1193.
6. Resnick LM. The cellular ionic basis of hypertension and allied clinical conditions. *Prog Cardiovasc Dis.* 1999;42:1–22.
7. Resnick LM, Gupta RK, DiFabio B, et al. Intracellular ionic consequences of dietary salt loading in essential hypertension: relation to blood pressure and effects of calcium channel blockade. *J Clin Invest.* 1994;94:1269–1276.

8. Resnick LM, Gupta RK, Laragh JH. Intracellular free magnesium in erythrocytes of essential hypertension: relation to blood pressure and serum divalent cations. *Proc Natl Acad Sci U S A.* 1984;81:6511–6515.
9. Resnick LM, Laragh JH, Sealey JE, Alderman MH. Divalent cations in essential hypertension: relations between serum ionized calcium, magnesium, and plasma renin activity. *N Engl J Med.* 1983;309:888–891.
10. Resnick LM, Müller FB, Laragh JH. Calcium-regulating hormones in essential hypertension: relation to plasma renin activity and sodium metabolism. *Ann Intern Med.* 1986;105:649–654.

Chapter A48

Pathophysiology of Renovascular Hypertension

L. Gabriel Navar, PhD; David W. Ploth, MD

KEY POINTS

- Reduced renal perfusion pressure resulting from stenosis of the arteries of 1 or both kidneys causes unilateral or bilateral renovascular hypertension through the interaction of inappropriate activity of the renin-angiotensin-aldosterone system and impaired salt and water excretion.

- In bilateral (symmetric) renal artery stenosis, early activation of the renin-angiotensin-aldosterone system gives way to impaired pressure-induced natriuresis in the chronic phase.

- In unilateral (asymmetric) renal artery stenosis, the hypertension is primarily due to persistence of systemic and renal angiotensin II–dependency, with secondary impairment of pressure-natriuresis.

- Renin-angiotensin-aldosterone system blocking drugs can temporarily reduce glomerular filtration in patients with renal artery stenosis; this phenomenon is a clinical clue to the presence of renovascular hypertension.

See also Chapters A5, A8, A37, A38, A41, A49, A71, C110, C123, and C168

Increased arterial pressure caused by stenosis, constriction, or lesions of the renal arteries involving one or both kidneys is categorized as renovascular hypertension. The derangements may be quite variable, ranging from overt renal arterial stenosis of one or both renal arteries to subtle microvascular lesions that are not easily detectable clinically.

Subtypes and Animal Models

There are 2 main categories of renovascular hypertension in conditions in which 2 kidneys are present: unilateral (asymmetric) and bilateral (symmetric) renovascular involvement. In animals, these conditions are represented respectively by models in which a constricting clip is applied to 1 or both renal arteries to create the two-kidney, one-clip (2K-1C) (Goldblatt) model and the two-kidney, two-clip (2K-2C) model. A third model that corresponds to renovascular hypertension in a single kidney, as in renal transplant patients, is the one-kidney, one-clip (1K-1C) model, which shares many features of the 2K-2C model. Renal artery stenosis can be caused by arteriosclerotic vascular disease of the renal artery, fibromuscular dysplasia, external compression by a tumor, or stenosis at the anastomosis in transplanted kidneys. Even

microvascular lesions owing to diffuse arteriosclerosis or arteritis of the intrarenal vasculature can participate in this process.

Mechanisms of Hypertension

There are 2 main mechanisms of hypertension in renovascular disease: activation of the renin-angiotensin-aldosterone system (RAAS) and impaired salt and water excretion owing to reduced pressure beyond the stenosis. The extent to which these 2 mechanisms contribute to the chronic blood pressure elevation of renovascular hypertension depends on the anatomy of the condition.

Bilateral renal artery stenosis and stenosis in a single renal artery. Hypertension owing to bilateral renal artery stenosis (and the 2K-2C model) or stenosis of the artery to a solitary kidney (and the 1K-1C model) share the same fundamental mechanisms. Although there is an inappropriate increase in the activity of the RAAS in these conditions, impaired salt and water excretion is the most prominent mechanism of chronic hypertension.

Renin-angiotensin activation (early phase). The critical initiating event is the decrease in renal perfusion pressure, with or without marked or sustained reductions in renal blood flow

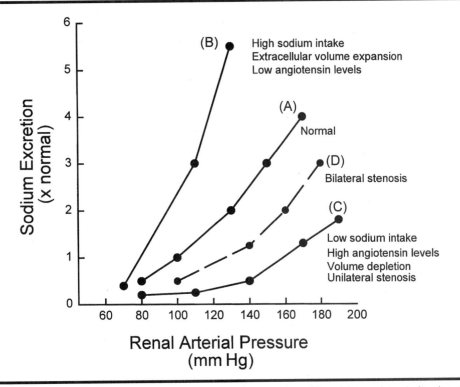

Figure A48.1. Relationship between renal arterial pressure and sodium excretion for normal conditions, high angiotensin (Ang) states, and reduced Ang states. The increase in sodium excretion in response to an increase in renal arterial pressure is referred to as *pressure natriuresis* and serves as the critical link between the regulation of arterial pressure and the renal regulation of sodium balance and extracellular volume. In bilateral renal vascular hypertension, the curve is shifted to the right (*curve D*) because of the reduced intrarenal perfusion pressure. In unilateral renovascular hypertension, the curve for the stenotic kidney is shifted to the right (*curve D*), and the relationship in the nonstenotic kidney remains inappropriately suppressed because of elevated intrarenal Ang II levels (*curve C*).

and glomerular filtration rate (GFR). Release of renin occurs in response to (a) decreased perfusion pressure at the juxtaglomerular apparatus of the afferent arterioles and (b) decreased sodium and chloride delivery to the macula densa segment of the ascending loop of Henle. Increased intrarenal and systemic concentrations of renin lead to increased systemic and intrarenal generation of angiotensin I (Ang I) and Ang II. Ang II has many pressor effects throughout the body (see Chapter A3). Over time, the hyperreninemia subsides because of the increased systemic and intrarenal pressure.

Salt and water retention (late phase). With time, Ang II–dependency of the systemic hypertension also becomes attenuated because of progressive retention of salt and water, leading to a relative expansion of extracellular fluid/blood volume and an increase in cardiac preload and stroke volume. Reductions in renal arterial pressure (down to the range of 70 to 80 mm Hg) do not always cause sustained decreases in renal blood flow and GFR because renal autoregulatory mechanisms are able to maintain renal hemodynamic function. Nevertheless, the reduced intrarenal perfusion pressure markedly compromises sodium excretory capability (**Figure A48.1**). When the degree of stenosis results in marked lowering of intrarenal perfusion pressure, the kidneys are unable to maintain adequate renal excretion of water and electrolytes. As a result, sodium retention and expansion of extracellular fluid volume occur similar to the pattern observed in chronic renal insufficiency, with measurable decreases in renal blood flow and GFR.

Resetting of pressure-natriuresis. Because functional renal mass is subjected to reduced perfusion pressure, there is a direct

reduction in pressure-dependent sodium excretion, sometimes called *resetting* of the pressure-natriuresis phenomenon (Figure A48.1). For any given hormonal and neural setting, there is a direct relationship between arterial pressure and the rate of sodium excretion. In the presence of bilateral renal arterial stenosis (2K-2C) or stenosis in a solitary kidney, the reduced renal arterial pressure lowers sodium excretion and minimizes sodium excretory responsiveness to natriuretic stimuli activated by volume expansion. Furthermore, increased intrarenal Ang II activity elicits vasoconstrictor effects on the kidney, directly stimulates net tubular sodium reabsorption, and increases sodium retention via increased aldosterone levels. These changes are synergistic with the direct effects of reduced perfusion pressure to cause sodium and water retention, expansion of the extracellular and intravascular compartments, and increased cardiac preload. Chronically, salt and water balance is restored at the expense of systemic hypertension. Even if the pressure-natriuresis relationship is restored to the normal profile, the entire relationship is shifted to a higher systemic pressure because of the pressure gradient caused by the stenotic lesions (curve A of Figure A48.1). This situation is represented by curve D in Figure A48.1, showing that the extent of the shift is dependent on the degree of stenosis.

Asymmetric (Goldblatt) Renovascular Hypertension

Persistence of abnormal renin-angiotensin stimulation.
In experimental asymmetric renovascular hypertension, an early neurogenic phase occurs, during which the administration of

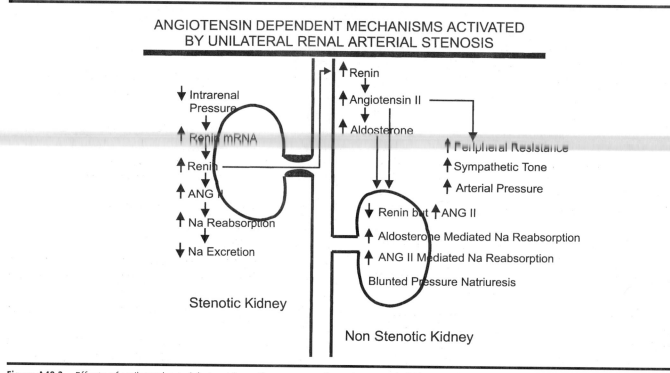

ANGIOTENSIN DEPENDENT MECHANISMS ACTIVATED BY UNILATERAL RENAL ARTERIAL STENOSIS

Figure A48.2.   Effects of unilateral arterial stenosis on the responses from the stenotic kidney and on the changes in the systemic circulation and on the contralateral nonstenotic kidney. ANG II, angiotensin II; mRNA, messenger RNA.

antibody to nerve growth factor blunts subsequent blood pressure elevations. This phenomenon is due to the systemic actions of Ang II (see Chapter A3). The important difference between hypertension caused by unilateral versus bilateral renal arterial stenosis is the persistent Ang-dependency in unilateral stenosis. The pressure distal to the stenosis is apparently never completely restored, so there is continuous renin stimulation and elevated circulating Ang II levels (**Figure A48.2**). In response to relatively subtle but sustained increases in circulating Ang II concentrations, there is accumulation of Ang II in the kidney by an AT_1 receptor–mediated internalization mechanism. In addition, the nonstenotic kidney has augmented angiotensinogen messenger RNA levels with increased or maintained local production of Ang II although the renin activity is markedly diminished. These elevated intrarenal Ang II levels can be maintained even when the circulating Ang II concentrations are only slightly increased.

Role of the normal kidney.   Although a single normal kidney is sufficient to maintain fluid and electrolyte balance at normotensive arterial pressures, an uninvolved kidney cannot prevent hypertension in unilateral renal arterial stenosis. The pathophysiology of hypertension in this model (2K-1C) depends on progressive changes in the hormonal, neural, and hemodynamic influences caused by the stenotic kidney (Figure A48.2). Although the nonstenotic kidney is not an initial causative factor, it develops inappropriately enhanced sodium reabsorption, resulting in an expanded extracellular fluid volume, that can be counteracted only by the elevated arterial pressure. Reduced perfusion pressure in the affected kidney causes increased unilateral renin production and release, resulting in elevated circulating levels of Ang I and Ang II. Unlike the situation in bilateral stenosis, however, the nonstenotic kidney remains exposed to the elevated systemic arterial pressure and should therefore be able to increase sodium excretion as long

as the pressure-natriuresis mechanism remains intact. However, increased circulating and intrarenal Ang II levels and the associated increases in aldosterone blunt the expected natriuresis elicited by increased renal perfusion pressure. In the presence of sustained elevations in Ang II and associated aldosterone levels, the pressure-natriuresis relationship of the nonstenotic kidney becomes markedly suppressed, as shown in curve C of Figure A48.1. Elevated circulating Ang II levels influence the nonstenotic kidney through multiple mechanisms, including (a) renal vasoconstrictor effects on both afferent and efferent arterioles that reduce renal plasma flow and GFR; (b) enhanced proximal and distal tubule sodium reabsorption; and (c) over the long term, afferent arteriolar hypertrophy and nephrosclerosis. Furthermore, prolonged elevations of intrarenal Ang II levels in the presence of hypertension activates several proliferative and inflammatory factors and cytokines that exacerbate the injury caused by the elevated arterial pressure. Once this occurs, repair of the vascular stenosis or even nephrectomy of the stenotic kidney will not restore arterial pressure to normal, probably because of progressive damage in the nonstenotic kidney caused by the combination of hypertension, nephrosclerosis, and increased intrarenal Ang II levels. Thus, it is essential to detect and treat or surgically correct the hypertension due to renal vascular lesions at the earliest possible time.

Antihypertensive Drug Effects

Pseudotolerance mechanisms.   The interactive balance between volume-dependent and Ang II–dependent components of the hypertension in bilateral renal artery stenosis leads to intrinsic limitations to the effects of monotherapeutic regimens of antihypertensive drugs. Vasodilator or Ang antagonist therapy reduces systemic arterial pressure but also lowers renal perfusion pressure and causes further volume retention and volume-dependent hypertension. On the other hand, diuretic therapy enhances sodium excretion and favors relative volume depletion but also causes further RAAS activation. These "pseudoresistance" or "pseudotolerance" effects are minimized by combining diuretics with anti-RAAS drugs.

Effects on glomerular filtration. In the extreme case, volume-depleted subjects can become extremely sensitive to reductions in arterial pressure and may respond to blood pressure-lowering drugs by exhibiting reductions in creatinine clearance or even by developing acute renal failure. Treatment with Ang-converting enzyme inhibitors or AT_1-receptor antagonists may cause temporary deterioration of renal function depending on the severity of the bilateral stenosis. If renal perfusion pressure is at or below the lower limit of the autoregulatory range, maximal constriction of the efferent arterioles becomes critical for the maintenance of glomerular capillary pressure and glomerular filtration. If Ang II levels are decreased by Ang-converting enzyme inhibitors or blocked by AT_1-receptor antagonists, efferent arteriolar constriction is diminished and glomerular capillary pressure and GFR are reduced, sometimes to levels below those necessary to maintain GFR. In this setting, the kidney continues to be perfused and generally does not suffer from ischemic damage or acute tubular necrosis. Subsequent withdrawal of the anti-RAAS agent is met with a restoration of GFR and urine flow.

SUGGESTED READING

1. Guan S, Fox J, Mitchell KD, Navar LG. Angiotensin and angiotensin-converting enzyme tissue levels in two-kidney, one clip hypertensive rats. *Hypertension.* 1992;20:763–767.
2. Imamura A, Mackenzie HS, Hutchison FN, et al. Effects of chronic treatment with angiotensin converting enzyme inhibitor or an angiotensin receptor antagonist in two-kidney, one-clip hypertensive rats. *Kidney Int.* 1995;47:1394–1402.
3. Laragh JH. The modern evaluation and treatment of hypertension: the causal role of the kidneys. *J Urol.* 1992;147:1469–1477.
4. Martinez-Maldonado M. Pathophysiology of renovascular hypertension. *Hypertension.* 1991;17:707–719.
5. Mitchell KD, Navar LG. Intrarenal actions of angiotensin II in pathogenesis of experimental hypertension. In: Laragh JH, Brenner BM, eds. *Hypertension: Pathophysiology, Diagnosis, and Management.* New York, NY: Raven Press; 1995:1437–1450.
6. Navar LG, Harrison-Bernard LM, Nishiyama A, Kobori H. Regulation of intrarenal angiotensin II in hypertension. *Hypertension.* 2002;39:316–322.
7. Navar LG, Hamm LL. The kidney in blood pressure regulation. In: Wilcox CS, ed. *Atlas of Diseases of the Kidney. Hypertension and the Kidney.* Vol 3. Philadelphia, PA: Current Medicine; 1999:1.1–1.22.
8. Ploth DW. Renovascular hypertension. In: Jacobson HR, Striker GE, Klahr S, eds. *The Principles and Practice of Nephrology.* 2nd ed. St. Louis, MO: Mosby-Year Book; 1995:379–386.
9. Pohl MA. Renal artery stenosis, renal vascular hypertension and ischemic nephropathy. In: Schrier RW, Gottschalk CW, eds. *Diseases of the Kidney.* 6th ed. Boston, MA: Little, Brown and Company; 1997:1367–1423.
10. Wolf G, ed. The renin-angiotensin system and progression of renal diseases. In: *Contrib Nephrol.* 2001;135(theme issue):1–268.

Chapter A49

Pathophysiology of Renal Parenchymal Hypertension

Vito M. Campese, MD

KEY POINTS

- Excessive intravascular volume is a major pathogenetic factor in the hypertension associated with renal failure; dietary sodium restriction, administration of diuretics, or removal of excessive fluids with dialysis are important adjuncts in the management of these patients.

- Another central feature of the hypertension of renal failure is increased sympathetic nerve activity due to altered afferent stimuli from the injured kidneys to the brain, reduced central dopaminergic tone, reduced baroreceptor sensitivity, abnormal vagal function, increased intracellular Ca^{2+} concentration, and increased plasma β-endorphin and β-lipotropin.

- Excessive renin secretion in relation to the state of sodium/volume balance is another important interactive factor in the pathogenesis of hypertension in renal failure.

- Endothelial dysfunction, perhaps owing to inhibition of nitric oxide synthesis or excessive oxidative burden, may also contribute to hypertension in renal failure.

See also Chapters A34, A36–A38, A41, A58, A71, B84, C124, and C159

Clinical Impact of Hypertension in Renal Disease

The association between hypertension and chronic renal disease has been recognized since the pioneering work of Richard Bright in 1836. Renal disease is by far the most common cause of secondary hypertension, and hypertension is present in more than 80% of patients with chronic renal failure. Hypertension also directly contributes to the progression of renal disease, which further exacerbates hypertension.

Cardiovascular disease is the leading cause of death in patients with end-stage renal disease, especially in the first year of treatment. Hypertension is the single most important pre-

Table A49.1. Factors Implicated in the Pathogenesis of Hypertension in End-Stage Renal Disease

Sodium and volume excess
Renin-angiotensin-aldosterone system
Adrenergic system and baroreceptor activity
Endothelium-derived vasodepressor substances
Endothelium-derived vasoconstrictor substances
Erythropoietin
Oxidative stress
Divalent cations and parathyroid hormone
Structural changes in the arteries
Preexistent essential hypertension
Miscellaneous
    Arteriovenous fistula
    Vasopressin
    Serotonin
    Thyroid function
    Calcitonin gene-related peptide

dictor of coronary artery disease in uremic patients, even more predictive than cigarette smoking or dyslipidemia. The nocturnal dipping of blood pressure is significantly blunted in these patients, probably because of autonomic dysfunction or alteration of sleeping patterns, and this factor also has been associated with increased cardiovascular morbidity. Measurement of blood pressure only during the day may lead to the erroneous impression of good antihypertensive control.

Pathogenetic Factors

Several factors have been implicated in the pathophysiology of hypertension in renal patients (**Table A49.1**).

Sodium and volume excess. Excessive intravascular volume is a major pathogenetic factor and dietary sodium restriction, administration of diuretics, or removal of excessive fluids with dialysis are important adjuncts in the management of hypertension in these patients. The mechanisms by which sodium excess may lead to arterial hypertension in the uremic patient are complex. In early phases, sodium excess leads to volume expansion, increased cardiac preload, and increased cardiac output. Later, hypertension is sustained by increased peripheral vascular resistance. Restriction of dietary sodium intake to 1 g per day helps to control the volume status in these patients.

Renin-angiotensin system activation. The role of excessive renin secretion in relation to the state of sodium/volume balance has long been recognized as an important factor in the pathogenesis of hypertension in patients with renal parenchymal diseases. Several factors support this notion. First, there is an abnormal relationship between exchangeable sodium or blood volume and plasma renin activity or plasma angiotensin II. This finding suggests that even "normal" plasma concentrations of renin are inappropriately high in relation to the state of sodium and volume balance. Second, a direct relationship between plasma renin activity and blood pressure frequently can be found. Third, blood pressure can be effectively reduced in most of these patients by the administration of angiotensin-converting enzyme inhibitors or angiotensin II blockers. Finally, bilateral nephrectomy results in normalization of blood pressure in most patients with renal disease.

Sympathetic nervous system overactivity. The kidney is not only an elaborate filtering device but also a sensory organ richly innervated with afferent and efferent sympathetic nerves. There are 2 main functional types of renal sensory receptors and afferent nerves: renal baroreceptors, which increase their firing in response to changes in renal perfusion and intrarenal pressure, and renal chemoreceptors, which are stimulated by ischemic metabolites or uremic toxins. Activation of renal chemoreceptors or baroreceptors and renal afferent nerves (that disinhibit integrative nuclei of the central nervous system) can activate efferent sympathetic pathways and raise blood pressure.

Rat models. Acute renal injury caused by an intrarenal injection of phenol in the rat increases the secretion of norepinephrine from the posterior hypothalamic nuclei, stimulates renal efferent sympathetic nerve activity, and raises blood pressure. These effects are permanent and occur in the absence of any change in renal function. Thus, an injury to a limited portion of 1 kidney may cause a permanent elevation of noradrenergic activity and blood pressure.

Human hypertension. In patients with chronic renal failure, plasma norepinephrine levels are usually increased. Direct microelectrode recordings of postganglionic sympathetic action potentials in peroneal nerves of chronic hemodialysis patients (with and without bilateral nephrectomy) have shown that the rate of sympathetic nerve discharge is much higher in dialysis patients with their native kidneys than in those who have undergone bilateral nephrectomy or in controls. In both groups of uremic patients, plasma norepinephrine levels varied widely, and no correlation was found between those levels and sympathetic nerve discharge in the peroneal nerves. In patients with bilateral nephrectomy, the decrease in sympathetic nerve firing was associated with lower regional vascular resistance and mean arterial pressure. Other mechanisms potentially responsible for the increase in sympathetic nerve activity in uremic patients include reduced central dopaminergic tone, reduced baroreceptor sensitivity, abnormal vagal function, increased $[Ca^{2+}]_i$ concentration, and increased plasma β-endorphin and β-lipotropin.

Endothelial dysfunction

Nitric oxide synthesis. In rats, chronic inhibition of nitric oxide (NO) synthesis causes systemic hypertension, marked renal vasoconstriction and hypoperfusion, a fall in glomerular filtration rate, an increase in filtration fraction, a rise in plasma renin levels, focal arteriolar obliteration, and segmental fibrinoid necrosis of the glomeruli. Administration of an NO synthase inhibitor increased renal sympathetic nerve activity and systemic blood pressure in male rats. *In vitro* and *in vivo* NO synthesis can also be inhibited by an endogenous compound, N^G,N^G-dimethylarginine [asymmetrical dimethylarginine (ADMA)]. Significantly higher plasma levels of ADMA and lower plasma arginine to dimethylarginine ratios have been observed in some uremic patients on chronic hemodialysis, suggesting that endogenous ADMA contributes to hypertension.

Endothelin. Compelling evidence that endothelin (ET)-1 might play a role in the pathophysiology of hypertension was reported in 2 cases of hemangioendothelioma, a rare malignant vascular neoplasm. In these cases, plasma levels of ET were 10-fold to 15-fold greater than those of normal or essential hypertensive subjects. Surgical removal of the tumor led to resolution of hypertension in both cases. In 1 patient, recurrence of the tumor was accompanied by a rise in plasma ET levels and in blood pressure. Hypertensive patients with chronic renal failure have higher plasma ET-1 levels than normotensive subjects. Elevated plasma ET-1 and ET-3 levels have also been observed in hemodialysis patients, along with a positive correlation between blood pressure and ET-1 serum levels.

Erythropoietin. Recombinant human erythropoietin (rHu-EPO), which is currently widely used to treat anemia in patients with chronic renal failure, can worsen hypertension and increase the requirement for antihypertensive drugs. The rise in blood pressure during treatment with rHu-EPO has not been observed in patients receiving rHu-EPO for other reasons, suggesting that renal disease may confer a particular susceptibility to the hypertensive action of rHu-EPO. The rise in blood pressure during rHu-EPO administration occurs within weeks to months. Patients who are at greater risk for developing hypertension during rHu-EPO therapy are those with severe anemia, those whose anemia is corrected too rapidly, or those with preexisting hypertension. Anemia itself causes a hyperdynamic state characterized by increased cardiac output and decreased total peripheral vascular resistance (TPR). Correction of the anemia with rHu-EPO leads to a decrease in cardiac output and a rise in TPR. Patients who become hypertensive or experience an exacerbation of hypertension during rHu-EPO therapy either have an exaggerated rise of TPR in response to the increase in hematocrit or do not suppress cardiac output to the same extent as patients who remain normotensive. The increase in blood viscosity during rHu-EPO therapy correlates with the increase in TPR but not with blood pressure changes. Hypertension induced by rHu-EPO therapy could also be a result of enhanced pressor responsiveness to norepinephrine and angiotensin II, an increase in cytosolic free calcium, or an increase in ET-1 secretion.

Divalent ions and parathyroid hormone. Chronic renal failure is associated with secondary hyperparathyroidism and increased $[Ca^{2+}]_i$ in many organs, including the myocardium and platelets. Correlations between: (a) platelet or lymphocyte $[Ca^{2+}]_i$ and blood pressure, (b) serum parathyroid hormone (PTH) and platelet $[Ca^{2+}]_i$, and (c) platelet $[Ca^{2+}]_i$ or PTH and

mean blood pressure have been found. In patients with high serum PTH receiving nifedipine, platelet $[Ca^{2+}]_i$ was not increased. In patients with hyperparathyroidism, treatment with a vitamin D metabolite caused proportional reductions in serum PTH, platelet $[Ca^{2+}]_i$, and mean blood pressure, suggesting that increased serum PTH may be responsible for the rise in $[Ca^{2+}]_i$ and the increase in blood pressure in these patients.

Oxidative stress and hypertension. Considerable attention has been given to the effects of short-lived reactive oxygen species and reactive nitrogen species on blood pressure and cardiovascular toxicity. Reactive oxygen species are increased in uremic rats, and they react with NO, producing and other cytotoxic reactive nitrogen species capable of nitrating proteins and damaging cells. Antioxidant therapy ameliorates the hypertension of chronic renal disease, improves vascular tissue NO production, and lowers tissue nitrotyrosine.

SUGGESTED READING

1. Baumgart P, Walger P, Gemen S, et al. Blood pressure elevation during the night in chronic renal failure, hemodialysis, and renal transplantation. *Nephron.* 1991;57:293–298.
2. Baylis C, Mitruka B, Deng A. Chronic blockade of nitric oxide synthesis in the rat produces systemic hypertension and glomerular damage. *J Clin Invest.* 1992;90:278–281.
3. Campese VM, Chervu I. Hypertension in dialysis subjects. In: Henrich WL, ed. *Principles and Practice of Dialysis.* Baltimore, MD: Williams & Wilkins; 1994:148–169.
4. Converse RL Jr, Jacobsen TN, Toto RD, et al. Sympathetic overactivity in patients with chronic renal failure. *N Engl J Med.* 1992;327:1912–1918.
5. Katholi RE. Renal nerves and hypertension: an update. *Fed Proc.* 1985;44: 2846–2850.
6. Raine AEG, Bedford L, Simpson AW, et al. Hyperparathyroidism, platelet intracellular free calcium and hypertension in chronic renal failure. *Kidney Int.* 1993;43:700–705.
7. Shichiri M, Hirata Y, Ando K, et al. Plasma endothelin levels in hypertension and chronic renal failure. *Hypertension.* 1990;15:493–496.
8. Steffen HM, Brunner R, Müller R, et al. Peripheral hemodynamics, blood viscosity, and the renin-angiotensin system in hemodialysis patients under therapy with recombinant human erythropoietin. *Contrib Nephrol.* 1989;76:292–298.
9. Vaziri ND, Oveisi F, Ding Y. Role of increased oxygen free radical activity in the pathogenesis of uremic hypertension. *Kidney Int.* 1998;53:1748–1754.
10. Ye S, Ozgur B, Campese VM. Renal afferent impulses, the posterior hypothalamus, and hypertension in rats with chronic renal failure. *Kidney Int.* 1997;51:722–727.

Chapter A50

Pathophysiology of Adrenal Cortical Hypertension

Naftali Stern, MD; Michael Tuck, MD

KEY POINTS

- Hypertension related to adrenal steroids generally results from overproduction of adrenal cortical steroids with mineralocorticoid or glucocorticoid properties.

- The final common pathways in the pathogenesis of adrenal cortical hypertension converge on excessive activation of mineralocorticoid receptors or glucocorticoid receptors.

- Aldosterone causes elevations in blood pressure by direct rapid nongenomic effects as well as via classic mineralocorticoid receptors in renal tubular cells.

- Hyperaldosteronism in one of its many forms is increasingly recognized as a relatively common cause of secondary hypertension.

See also Chapters A3, A9, A10, A42, A77, C110–C113, C118, C128, and C170

MINERALOCORTICOID EFFECTS

Regulation of Mineralocorticoid Secretion in the Adrenal Cortex

Angiotensin II and potassium. Circulating angiotensin II (Ang II) and serum K^+ are the major regulators of aldosterone (Aldo) secretion (see Chapter A10). They enhance release of prestored Aldo, promote the conversion of cholesterol to pregnenolone, and increase the activity of Aldo synthase (AS), the adrenal cortical enzyme expressed exclusively in glomerulosa cells. Ang II upregulates its AT_1 receptor, providing sustained secretory Aldo responses. Aldo synthesis increases linearly as K^+ concentrations rise, and there is a synergistic interaction between K^+ and Ang II such that each stimulus augments the response to the other. This may be related, in part, to K^+-mediated activation of an intraadrenal renin-angiotensin system. Modulation of Aldo secretion in response to changes in volume or sodium status is exerted by changes in renin release, whereas changes in K^+ balance act directly on Aldo secretion.

Adrenocorticotropic hormone. Adrenocorticotropic hormone (ACTH) is a potent short-term secretagogue of Aldo secretion and also controls its circadian rhythm, which parallels that of cortisol. However, continued stimulation with ACTH results in suppression of Aldo via accumulation of 11-deoxycorticosterone (DOC). DOC has approximately 3% of the mineralocorticoid activity of Aldo and is synthesized in the zona fasciculata under control of ACTH. Excess DOC leads to salt and water retention, which in turn suppresses renin and Ang II, the dominant regulators of Aldo. Chronic exposure to ACTH inhibits AS expression and induces 17α-hydroxylase activity in the zona glomerulosa. This effect diverts the Aldo biosynthetic pathway towards cortisol production.

Other hormonal modulation. Atrial natriuretic peptide (ANP), a peptide released from the atria in response to hypervolemia, suppresses Aldo secretion *in vivo* by inhibiting basal and stimulated Aldo secretion, sympathetic nervous outflow, and renin secretion. Other hormones that have paracrine or autocrine modulatory effects on Aldo release include the inhibitors dopamine, adrenomedullin, and nitric oxide and the stimulants epinephrine, acetylcholine, and endothelin.

Renal Effects of Mineralocorticoid Action

Renal mineralocorticoid receptors. Mineralocorticoid receptors (MR) in the kidney are the primary targets for mineralocorticoid action (see Chapter A11). After binding to the MR, Aldo rapidly stimulates the expression of sgk, which, in turn, phosphorylates and thereby disengages Nedd4 proteins from the Na channel, thus allowing enhanced Na^+ channel surface expression and reduction in its ubiquination and degradation. Aldo promotes the reabsorption of NaCl and the secretion of K^+ in the principal cells in the cortical collecting tubule. Aldo increases Na^+ reabsorption but does not directly enhance K^+ secretion in the papillary (inner medullary) collecting tubules. It also stimulates NaCl reabsorption in the distal tubule by increasing the number of Na^+-Cl^- co-transporters in the luminal membrane. If distal tubular sodium delivery remains high, there is secondary enhancement of the exchange of Na^+ for K^+ and H^+. Overall, Aldo leads to increased renal reabsorption of sodium, kaliuresis, and increased hydrogen ion excretion, resulting in metabolic alkalosis (with or without hypokalemia). MRs are not specific and can be activated by Aldo, DOC, or cortisol.

Renal tubular sodium channels. Aldo-mediated sodium reabsorption in renal tubular cells depends on increasing the number of open amiloride-sensitive Na$^+$ channels by opening inactive Na$^+$ channels and insertion of new channels in the luminal membrane. Aldo also increases the number of open K$^+$ channels in the apical (luminal) membrane, and Na$^+$,K$^+$-ATPase (adenosine triphosphatase) activity in the basolateral membrane by *de novo* synthesis of new Na$^+$-K$^+$ pump units. Increased Na$^+$-K$^+$ pump activity allows shifting of Na$^+$ (which entered tubular cells via open Na$^+$ channels) from within the cell to the interstitial fluid at the basal aspect of the cell and further, by passive diffusion, into the systemic circulation. A number of Aldo-sensitive genes have been identified, including serum and glucocorticoid (GC)-inducible kinase and small, monomeric Ras guanosine triphosphate–binding proteins. Another Aldo-inducible regulator of Na$^+$ channel activity is prostasin, a serine protease that is expressed in epithelial tissues, which are known as *sites of amiloride-sensitive transepithelial Na transport*. Aldo increases prostasin expression, which increases the activity of the epithelial sodium channel. Urinary prostasin levels are high in patients with Aldo-producing adenomas.

Kaliuresis. The electrogenic effect of the inward movement of Na$^+$ into tubular cells through Na$^+$ channels is neutralized by either passive Cl$^-$ reabsorption via the paracellular pathway or by K$^+$ secretion from the cell into the tubular lumen. K$^+$ excretion is also enhanced by Aldo-stimulated Na$^+$,K$^+$-ATPase activity, which increases K$^+$ entry across the basolateral membrane. The ensuing rise in cell K$^+$ concentration permits continued K$^+$ secretion into the tubular fluid at the luminal aspect of the cell.

Acid-base balance. Direct MR-dependent stimulation of H$^+$ secretion at the intercalated cells in the renal cortex and in the tubular cells in the outer medulla via increases in H$^+$-ATPase protein expression and activity in the apical membrane. Increased anion delivery to the distal tubule and the accompanying luminal negative potential result from Na$^+$ entry to the principal tubular cells and a favorable electric gradient for the counter-diffusion of H$^+$ to the lumen.

Aldosterone escape. Despite hypervolemia, edema is absent owing to an Aldo escape phenomenon, a physiologic response to continued exposure to high concentrations of Aldo that limits the volume expansion and sodium retention. After an initial weight gain, spontaneous diuresis ensues, reducing the retained volume to a minimal excess. This escape phenomenon reflects the effect of increased secretion of ANP, which increases glomerular filtration rate and diminishes sodium reabsorption in the inner medullary-collecting duct. The elevation of arterial blood pressure also leads to pressure natriuresis; increase in the production of renal dopamine, which augments natriuresis; and glomerular filtration. A decrease in the thiazide-sensitive Na-Cl co-transporter units, which enhance sodium reabsorption in the distal tubule, also limits sodium retention.

Interaction of cortisol with mineralocorticoid receptors: 11β-hydroxysteroid dehydrogenase type II enzyme. The MR has roughly equal affinities for cortisol and Aldo. Because the renal concentration of cortisol is 1,000-fold higher than Aldo, it would be expected that high cortisol should be the predominant influence on MRs. Protection of the MR from activation by cortisol is provided by the 11β-hydroxysteroid dehydrogenase type II (11βHSD2) enzyme, which is co-expressed with the MR and rapidly catalyzes the conversion of cortisol into cortisone. Because cortisone is unable to bind to the MR, the receptor remains largely under the control of Aldo (see Chapter A11). In rare cases of overwhelming cortisol excess, the capacity of this enzyme to metabolize cortisol is exceeded by inordinately high cortisol concentrations such as those found in Cushing's syndrome owing to ectopic ACTH secretion. Excessive MR stimulation also occurs in the monogenic disorder of apparent mineralocorticoid excess in which there is a genetic defect in 11βHSD2 (see Chapter A77). Several agents, such as licorice (active metabolite glycyrrhetinic acid) and carbenoxolone, directly inhibit 11βHSD2. High doses of furosemide may also affect the enzyme.

Cardiovascular Effects of Aldosterone

Genomic effects

Interaction with angiotensin II. Aldo upregulates AT$_1$-receptor expression in cardiac myocytes and in vascular smooth muscle cells (VSMCs); the Aldo antagonist spironolactone and the Ang II blocker losartan block this effect. Aldo also prevents Ang II–mediated downregulation of AT$_1$ receptors and inositol phosphate signaling. Hence, Aldo may potentiate Ang II effects in cardiac and vascular tissue.

Induction of fibrosis. Cardiac myocytes, endothelial cells, and VSMCs contain high-affinity MRs. Cardiac fibroblasts and VSMCs also contain the enzyme 11βHSD2. Chronic Aldo infusion in uninephrectomized rats on a high-salt diet causes myocardial accumulation of interstitial and perivascular collagen that can be prevented by spironolactone. Increased cardiac accumulation of collagen is found in primary aldosteronism and in experimental activation of the renin-angiotensin system, which produce the same pathology. Spironolactone also prevents aortic collagen accumulation in spontaneously hypertensive rats. In patients with congestive heart failure, spironolactone may improve outcomes by reducing levels of procollagen type III N-terminal aminopeptide.

Stimulation of active cation transport in vascular cells. Aldo induces an increase in the expression of the α$_1$ subunit and β$_1$-messenger RNA (mRNA) of the Na$^+$,K$^+$-ATPase contributing to Na$^+$-K$^+$ pump activation. It also increases active cation transport in VSMC.

Nongenomic vascular effects.
Aldo can produce direct rises in systemic vascular resistance independent of its effect on salt and fluid balance. Because these effects are characterized by rapid onset of action within minutes, insensitivity to inhibitors of transcription and protein synthesis, and insensitivity to MR antagonists, they are considered to be nongenomic in nature. After binding of Aldo to a putative membrane receptor, several second messenger cascades are activated such as adenyl cyclase, increased phosphorylation of cyclic adenosine monophosphate-response element binding protein, and the formation of inositol 1,4,5-triphosphate, diacylglycerol, intracellular Ca^{2+}, and protein kinase C activity. In humans, there is an increase in systemic vascular resistance as early as 5 min after the injection of 0.5 mg Aldo. Nongenomic effects of Aldo provide potential mechanisms for intracellular cross-talk with other vasoactive hormones. For example, operating via cyclic adenosine mono-

phosphate, Aldo sensitizes VSMC to the effects of β-adrenergic agonists and the autonomic nervous system. The importance of the direct vascular mineralocorticoid effects are evident in studies in 11βHSD2 knockout mice, in which decreased endothelium-dependent vasodilation and increased contractile response to norepinephrine are seen, independent of total body sodium balance.

Central Nervous System Effects

Central nervous system effects of mineralocorticoids operate via MRs localized in the hippocampus, amygdala, lateral septum, and hypothalamus, particularly in the periventricular regions. Central administration of Aldo in rats and dogs at doses that are too low to affect peripheral Aldo results in increased blood pressure, which can be inhibited by spironolactone administered to the central nervous system. Intracerebroventricular administration of Aldo antagonists improves volume regulation and reduces sympathetic drive in experimentally induced heart failure and reduced blood pressure in the deoxycorticosterone acetate–salt hypertensive rat. Ablation of the anteroventral third ventricle area and central sympathectomy prevents the development of deoxycorticosterone acetate–salt hypertension. Mineralocorticoids also act on the brain to enhance sodium intake. Because there is evidence for *de novo* synthesis of steroids within the brain, paracrine activation of MRs by locally synthesized steroids possessing mineralocorticoid properties could contribute to blood pressure regulation.

Molecular Pathogenesis

Primary hyperaldosteronism. The fundamental abnormality leading to primary hyperaldosteronism (PHA) remains unknown and several forms may exist (see Chapter A77). An activating somatic mutation in the Gs alpha gene has been identified in a single case. Mutations in several candidate genes such as the AS gene and the AT1R are not found in PHA. However, idiopathic hyperaldosteronism (IHA) may be linked to polymorphisms in the Aldo synthase (CYP11B2) gene (−344C, *CYP11B2* intron2 sequence) or to overexpression of CYP11B2 mRNA as found in the mononuclear leukocytes of patients with IHA. Gene expression analysis of Aldo-producing adenoma (APA) reveals greater ACTH receptor mRNA in functional compared to nonfunctioning adrenal adenomas or androgen secreting adrenal carcinomas. Additionally, the level of CYP11B2 mRNA is higher in the adenomatous portion than in the nonadenomatous portion of adrenal glands harboring aldosteronomas. Aldosteronoma cells expressed adrenomedullin and adrenomedullin-sensitive receptors; adrenomedullin reportedly promotes growth in these cells. The only example of a well-understood monogenic form of primary hyperaldosteronism is familial hyperaldosteronism (FH) type I, also known as *GC-remediable aldosteronism*, results from a chimeric gene formed as a result of unequal crossover at meiosis between the highly homologous 11β-hydroxylase (CYP11B1) and AS (CYP11B2) gene on chromosome 8q24.3 (see Chapters A11 and A77). FH type II is another rare form of hyperaldosteronism in which a genome-wide search has revealed linkage with a locus in chromosome 7, but the underlying mechanism remains unknown.

Congenital Adrenal Hyperplasia

Syndromes associated with hyperplasia of the adrenal, usually without hypertension, are caused by genetic defects in hydroxylase enzymes (see Chapters A10 and A77).

11β-Hydroxylase (CYP11B1) deficiency. 11β-hydroxylase (CYP11B1) deficiency disorder is the second most common cause of congenital adrenal hyperplasia (CAH) (1 in 100,000 live births) and is more common in Jews of Moroccan ancestry (1 per 5,000 births). It may present in the postnatal period or during adolescence or in early adulthood ("late-onset" form). Inheritance is autosomal recessive, and the affected CYP11B1 gene is on chromosome 8q21-q22. Diminished ability to convert 11-deoxycortisol (compound S) to cortisol results in a compensatory rise in ACTH, leading to accumulation of steroid precursors such as DOC, which possesses mineralocorticoid capacity. There is also a shift in the steroid biosynthetic pathway toward excessive production of adrenal androgens. In these subjects, there are elevated concentrations of DOC, a low plasma renin activity (PRA) and Aldo, and increased levels of dehydroepiandrosterone, dehydroepiandrosterone sulfate, and testosterone. In the severe form of this disease, hypertension occurs in early life in association with hypokalemia, ambiguous genitalia and virilization in females, and penile enlargement in boys, or later on as precocious puberty and short stature. Acne, hirsutism, and menstrual irregularities may be the presenting symptoms in the late-onset forms, in which hypertension is less common. Hypertension can be severe, yet the correlation between arterial pressure and 11-DOC levels is weak. Blood pressure often remains high despite an apparently adequate suppression of DOC and adrenal androgen production and normalization of PRA levels. One potential explanation for this phenomenon is that the use of high doses of GCs to attain ACTH suppression invoke a GC-dependent form of hypertension.

17α-Hydroxylase (CYP17) deficiency. 17α-Hydroxylase (CYP17) deficiency is a rare autosomal recessive form of CAH caused by mutations of the CYP17 gene on chromosome 10. The 17-hydroxylase protein has dual 17-hydroxylase (hydroxylation) of progesterone to 17α-hydroxyprogesterone and 17,20-lyase activities. Defective CYP17 protein impairs cortisol production and the formation of C-18 steroids (i.e., androgens and estrogens). Although most afflicted patients display the results of the combined 17-hydroxylase/17,20-lyase defects, some develop syndromes reflecting the absence of only 1 enzymatic activity. Hypertension evolves primarily as a result of 17-hydroxylase deficiency, leading to a reduced cortisol production with a shift of progesterone biosynthesis towards the mineralocorticoid pathway (which does not require 17-hydroxylation) and a compensatory hypersecretion of ACTH, with accumulation of progesterone, pregnenolone, DOC, corticosterone, and 18-hydroxy-DOC. Increased overall mineralocorticoid activity leads to hypertension and hypokalemia with suppressed PRA and Aldo levels. The 17,20-lyase deficiency leads to low androgen and estrogen concentrations and hypogonadism (pseudohermaphroditism in males and primary amenorrhea with absent secondary sexual features in females).

Clinical Features of Primary Hyperaldosteronism

PHA may be more common than previously believed; some estimates suggest that the condition occurs in 10% to 14% of unselected hypertensive patients.

Subtypes. There are several forms of PHA: (a) adrenal APA (60%); (b) IHA with bilateral micronodular hyperplasia of the adrenals (40%); (c) unilateral micronodular adrenal hyperplasia (1–2%); (d) FH type I, also known as *GC-remediable hyperaldosteronism* (see Chapter A77); (e) FH type II, a new variety of familial primary aldosteronism with autosomal dominant inheritance not suppressible with dexamethasone that often involves adrenocortical adenoma formation; (f) Aldo-producing adrenal carcinoma (rare); and (g) ectopic (extraadrenal) Aldo producing adenoma (rare).

Clinical and laboratory features. In general, excessive Aldo-induced reabsorption of sodium and water causes volume expansion, hypertension, and low PRA. Enhanced renal excretion of K^+ and H^+ ions promotes hypokalemic metabolic alkalosis. The hypertension is a universal finding ranging from mild to severe, but hypokalemia is not always present, with as many as 50% being normokalemic. Severe hypokalemia, which is more common in APA than in IHA, can cause muscle weakness, fatigue, cramping, muscle paralysis, a renal concentrating defect, polyuria/polydipsia (sometimes resistant to vasopressin), widened QT interval with U waves, myocardial fibrosis and left ventricular hypertrophy, impaired insulin secretion, diminished glucose tolerance, blunted circulatory reflex responses with postural hypotension, and bradycardia. Mild hypomagnesemia may be present and appears to result from decreased tubular reabsorption of magnesium.

Differential points. There are differences among the major forms of PHA. Hypertension and hypokalemia are generally more severe in APA than in IHA. Levels of 18-hydroxycorticosterone, an intermediary product of Aldo synthase, are higher in APA than IHA. Aldo secretion is extremely sensitive to Ang II in IHA, but most cases of APA are sensitive to ACTH and relatively insensitive to Ang II. Thus, if challenged by the 4-hour upright posture test, IHA patients demonstrate an increase in Aldo, whereas APA patients typically show a decline in plasma Aldo. Yet, 10% to 30% of APA patients remain Ang II–sensitive, with increased Aldo secretion after postural challenge.

GLUCOCORTICOIDS

GCs increase blood pressure in human subjects, although this effect is highly variable. The administration of GCs results in enhanced sensitivity to pressor hormones such as catecholamines and Ang II. There is an interaction of GC with MRs and glucocorticoid receptor at multiple sites, including the vasculature, kidney, and brain in GC-induced hypertension.

Mechanisms of Hypertension

Vascular effects. GC increases the number of α-adrenergic, Ang II, and vasopressin receptors in vascular tissue. GCs also increase Ang II production and upregulate angiotensin-converting enzyme expression, amplifying the effect on Ang II receptors by facilitating Ang II formation. There is a glucocorticoid receptor–mediated upregulation of Na^+,K^+-ATPase expression in VSMC, which leads to hyperpolarization and downregulation of calcium-dependent potassium channels. This effect lowers membrane potential. Chronic GC treatment downregulates the expression of the Na^+-Ca^{2+} exchanger, favoring increased cytosolic calcium and vasoconstriction. GCs also decrease cyclic guanosine monophosphate formation in response to ANP, impair endothelial-dependent vasodilator, block the expression of inducible nitric oxide synthase, and inhibit estradiol-induced expression of endothelial nitric oxide synthase.

Renal effects. GCs increase glomerular filtration rate by poorly understood mechanisms. Such "hyperfiltration" with the ensuing increased glomerular pressure could impair renal function. GCs do not usually induce clinically significant salt retention unless they activate renal MRs (owing to genetic or functional impairment in renal 11βHSD2), but they do exert several tubular effects conducive to increased sodium reabsorption, including upregulation of Ang II receptor number, increased Na^+,K^+-ATPase activity in the basolateral membrane, and increased apical membrane Na^+-H^+ exchanger activity in proximal tubular cells, all of which are likely offset by the increase in filtration rate, thus resulting in little net change in overall sodium balance.

Cushing's Syndrome

Clinical features. Hypertension (80%) and hypokalemia are the most common presenting symptoms in Cushing's syndrome, particularly in cases of ectopic ACTH syndromes characterized by very high circulating ACTH levels. The very high level of cortisol may exceed the neutralizing capacity of the 11βHSD2 that normally converts cortisol to inactive cortisone. Diminished inactivation of cortisol by ring A reductase has also been described in ectopic ACTH syndrome. These mechanisms, although independent of ACTH, may also be operative in adrenal carcinoma. In Cushing's disease owing to a pituitary adenoma producing ACTH, PRA and Aldo levels are normal. In Cushing's syndrome secondary to ectopic ACTH secretion, high plasma DOC induces a mineralocorticoid-excess syndrome that can precede the manifestations of GC excess and can include a phase of hypertension associated with hypervolemia, suppression of PRA, and normal or low plasma Aldo.

Subclinical disease and adrenal "incidentalomas." More subtle forms of hypercortisolism are being detected with increasing frequency as adrenal "incidentalomas." The excess production of cortisol in these patients often occurs in the absence of clinical signs of Cushing's syndrome. Adrenal incidentalomas can be associated with severe hypertension and other features of the metabolic syndrome such as glucose intolerance or diabetes, obesity, and dyslipidemia.

SUGGESTED READING

1. Bernini G, Moretti A, Argenio G, Salvetti A. Primary Aldosteronism in normokalemic patients with adrenal incidentalomas. *Eur J Endocrinol.* 2002;146:523–529.
2. Funder JW. Non-genomic actions of Aldosterone: role in hypertension. *Curr Opin Nephrol Hypertens.* 2001;10:227–230.

3. Ganguly A. Prevalence of primary Aldosteronism in unselected hypertensive populations: screening and definitive diagnosis. *J Clin Endocrinol Metab.* 2001;86:4002–4004.

4. Geller DS, Farhi A, Pinkerton N, et al. Activating mineralocorticoid receptor mutation in hypertension exacerbated by pregnancy. *Science.* 2000;289:119–123.

5. Lifton RP, Dluhy RG, Powers M, et al. Hereditary hypertension caused by chimaeric gene duplications and ectopic expression of Aldosterone synthase. *Nat Genet.* 1992;2:66–74.

6. Moneva MH, Gomez-Sanchez CE. Pathophysiology of adrenal hypertension. *Semin Nephrol.* 2002;22:44–53.

7. Rossi GP, Di Bello V, Ganzaroli C, et al. Excess Aldosterone is associated with alterations of myocardial texture in primary Aldosteronism. *Hypertension.* 2002;40:23–27.

8. Rossi R, Tauchmanova L, Luciano A, et al. Subclinical Cushing's syndrome in patients with adrenal incidentaloma: clinical and biochemical features. *J Clin Endocrinol Metab.* 2000;85:1440–1448.

9. Rossier BC, Pradervand S, Schild L, Hummler E. Epithelial sodium channel and the control of sodium balance: interaction between genetic and environmental factors. *Annu Rev Physiol.* 2002;64:877–897.

10. White PC. 11-beta-hydroxysteroid dehydrogenase and its role in the syndrome of apparent mineralocorticoid excess. *Am J Med Sci.* 2001;322:308–315.

Chapter A51

Pathophysiology of Pheochromocytoma

William M. Manger, MD, PhD; Ray W. Gifford, Jr, MD, MS; Graeme F. Eisenhofer, PhD

KEY POINTS

- Pheochromocytoma is a rare catecholamine-secreting neural crest tumor that can arise in the abdomen, pelvis, chest, or neck and can be multicentric; histopathology cannot determine if a tumor is benign or malignant, but approximately 10% are invasive or metastatic.

- Approximately 20% are familial and may be associated with the multiple endocrine neoplasia syndrome that includes tumors or hyperplasia of the thyroid and parathyroid glands and other neuroectodermal tumors; chromosome abnormalities permit detection of familial disease.

- Clinical and laboratory manifestations are caused mainly by excess circulating catecholamines, although pheochromocytomas may also secrete peptides that cause additional manifestations.

- Diagnosis can almost always be made by determining plasma or urinary catecholamines or metanephrines; if not recognized and appropriately treated, pheochromocytomas can cause lethal cardiovascular complications.

See also Chapters A1, A2, A13, A41, A52, C110, C128, and C169

Pheochromocytoma is a rare catecholamine-secreting tumor that causes systolic and diastolic hypertension in less than 0.05% of hypertensive subjects. It may be cured by surgical resection in approximately 90% of patients, but, if unrecognized, it almost invariably causes lethal cerebrovascular or cardiovascular complications from excess circulating catecholamines.

Genetics and Associated Syndromes

Approximately 20% of pheochromocytomas are familial with an autosomal dominant mode of inheritance and may be associated with multiple endocrine neoplasms (MENs), von Hippel-Lindau (VHL) disease, carotid body or multiple paragangliomas, and neurofibromatosis type 1. Susceptibility to familial paraganglioma and familial pheochromocytoma appears to be associated with genetic mutations in mitochondrial succinate dehydrogenase enzymes.

Multiple endocrine neoplasia syndromes. Coexistence of pheochromocytoma with medullary thyroid carcinoma (MTC), C-cell hyperplasia, or parathyroid neoplasms or hyperplasia constitutes MEN type 2a. Coexistence of pheochromocytoma with MTC, mucosal neuromas, thickened corneal nerves, alimentary tract ganglioneuromatoses, and often a marfanoid habitus constitutes MEN type 2b. Hyperparathyroidism occurs in approximately half of patients with MEN type 2a but rarely in type 2b. MTC almost always precedes pheochromocytoma in these MEN syndromes. Genetic mutations (e.g., *RET* protooncogene on chromosome 10 for MEN type 2a and 2b syndromes and chromosome 11q for carotid body and multiple paragangliomas) are involved in the pathogenesis of familial pheochromocytoma.

Neurofibromatosis. von Recklinghausen's peripheral neurofibromatosis, often with café au lait spots, is found in approximately 5% of patients with pheochromocytoma, whereas pheochromocytoma occurs in 1% of persons with neurofibromatosis. Chromosome 17q mutations have been found in this syndrome.

von Hippel-Lindau syndrome. Pheochromocytomas coexist in 14% of patients with VHL disease, which is characterized by hemangioblastoma of the cerebellum or other parts of the central nervous system, retinal angioma, renal and pancreatic cysts, renal carcinoma, and cystadenoma of the epididymis. Chromosome 3p mutations have been found in this syndrome.

Embryology and Anatomic Locations

Pheochromocytomas arise from neuroectodermal chromaffin cells. Embryologically related diseases arising from neural crest maldevelopment (e.g., pheochromocytoma, neuroblastoma, neurofibromatosis, MTC, carcinoid, and MEN) have been designated *neurocristopathies*. Some of these tumors are capable of *a*mine *p*recursor *u*ptake and *d*ecarboxylation (the APUD system), and they may secrete catecholamines and a variety of peptides. The vast majority of pheochromocytomas (98%) occur in the abdomen or pelvis, the major site being the adrenal medullae (85%). In adults, approximately 15% of pheochromocytomas are extraadrenal, originating in the organ of Zuckerkandl, the urinary bladder, or paraganglia chromaffin cells, which are found associated with sympathetic nerves and plexuses. Extraadrenal and multiple pheochromocytomas are approximately twice as common in children. Occasionally, tumors occur in the chest (<2%) in a paraspinal location or intrapericardially, in the neck (<0.1%), and rarely in other locations (e.g., base of the skull extending intracranially through the jugular foramen, middle ear, or spermatic cord).

Histopathology

Pheochromocytomas average 5 cm in diameter but may be microscopic or weigh up to 4 kg. Tumors are usually encapsulated and rarely contain calcium. Tumor cells are usually pleomorphic and polygonal or spheroidal, and they harbor multiple storage vesicles containing norepinephrine or epinephrine. Ten percent of adrenal and up to 40% of extraadrenal tumors metastasize or invade adjacent structures. Malignancy cannot be determined histologically, but a normal flow cytometric DNA pattern of pheochromocytoma cells predicts benignancy, whereas an abnormal pattern (polyploidy) portends malignancy in up to 39% of cases. Malignancy is more frequent in tumors secreting dopamine or its precursor dihydroxyphenylalanine. Rarely, benign tumors are multicentric.

Other Vasoactive Substances Secreted

Many substances have been identified in some pheochromocytomas: chromogranins, vasoactive intestinal peptide, enkephalins, β-endorphin, dynorphin, α-melanocyte–stimulating hormone, adrenocorticotropic hormone, neuropeptide Y, neuron-specific enolase, atrial natriuretic factor, corticotropin-releasing factor, growth hormone releasing factor, somatostatin, parathyroid hormone, calcitonin, substance P, synaptophysin, gastrin-releasing peptide, neurotensin, insulin-like growth factor, gastrin, cholecystokinin, serotonin, motilin, interleukin-6, erythropoietin-like substance, adrenomedullin, angiotensin II, and angiotensin-converting enzyme. Some of these may be released into the circulation and cause physiologic effects with diverse manifestations.

Clinical Manifestations

Symptoms and signs of pheochromocytoma are mainly caused by hypercatecholaminemia.

Blood pressure patterns. Approximately 50% of pheochromocytomas present with sustained hypertension. Paroxysmal hypertension occurs in approximately 45%. Because of episodic secretion of catecholamines, manifestations may appear suddenly and mimic other diseases. Approximately 5% remain normotensive, especially those with familial tumors. Symptomatic hypertensive attacks caused by pheochromocytoma usually occur one or more times weekly and usually last for less than 1 hour. Rarely, patients with predominantly epinephrine-secreting tumors have hypertension alternating with hypotension, which may be severe. Orthostatic hypotension is occasionally a sign of pheochromocytoma in patients with sustained hypertension that probably results from desensitized adrenergic receptors and hypovolemia.

Hypercatecholaminemic symptoms. Severe headaches, generalized sweating, palpitations with tachycardia (rarely reflex bradycardia), or a combination of these symptoms occur in up to 95% of persons with functioning pheochromocytomas. Anxiety, fear of death, and pallor (rarely flushing) are frequent during paroxysmal attacks. Hypercatecholaminemia may cause hyperglycemia, elevated triglycerides, and hyperreninemia (by stimulating renal β_1-adrenoreceptors). Hypercatecholaminemia can cause hypermetabolism and weight loss, severe constipation, or pseudo-obstruction because catecholamines inhibit peristalsis. Rarely, ischemic enterocolitis with intestinal necrosis may complicate intense mesenteric artery vasoconstriction. Fine tremors and slight fever (rarely hyperpyrexia) may occur. Polydipsia, polyuria, and convulsions are not uncommon in children. Transient arrhythmias or electrocardiogram (ECG) changes suggesting ischemia or strain during hypertensive episodes or sudden heart failure may occur, and catecholamine cardiomyopathy, hypertension, and coronary atherosclerosis can cause permanent damage with persistent ECG changes.

Symptoms due to other hormones. Secretion of vasoactive intestinal peptide, serotonin, or calcitonin from a pheochromocytoma or secretion of calcitonin, serotonin, or prostaglandin from a coexisting MTC can cause diarrhea accompanied by hypokalemia and hypochlorhydria or achlorhydria. Rarely, pheochromocytomas or coexisting hemangioblastomas secrete erythropoietin and cause polycythemia. Approximately 2% of patients harboring pheochromocytomas present with unexplained shock, abdominal pain, pulmonary edema, and intense mydriasis unresponsive to light; 1% develop pheochromocytoma multisystem crisis (i.e., multiple organ system failure, hyperpyrexia, encephalopathy, with severe hypertension, hypotension), sometimes associated with lactic acidosis and, rarely, disseminated intravascular coagulation. Severe retinopathy can occur with sustained but not paroxysmal hypertension.

Diagnostic testing. All patients with sustained or paroxysmal hypertension and manifestations suggesting pheochromocytoma should be screened for the tumor. Asymptomatic patients with unexplained hypertension should be screened if they have laboratory or ECG abnormalities that may be caused by hypercatecholaminemia or radiographic or magnetic resonance imaging suggesting pheochromocytoma, or if they have diseases sometimes coexisting with this tumor. Imaging studies are usually only indicated after biochemical determinations have established the likelihood of a pheochromocytoma.

Catecholamines and metabolites. In the setting of sustained or during paroxysmal hypertension, plasma free (unconjugated) metanephrine and normetanephrine, plasma catecholamines, 24-hour urinary catecholamines, and 24-hour urinary metanephrine and normetanephrine are almost invariably elevated in pheochromocytoma and are considered to be the preferred diagnostic tests. The increased reliability of free metanephrine and normetanephrine may be due to the fact that these metabolites are continuously produced within pheochromocytoma cells and continuously enter the circulation, whereas catecholamine release is sometimes episodic. Plasma free metanephrine and normetanephrine are less influenced than catecholamines by physiologic activation of the sympathoadrenal system. Normal concentrations of plasma free metanephrine and normetanephrine, even in the absence of hypertension, can be used to rule out sporadic and familial pheochromocytomas with a sensitivity of 99% and 97%, respectively. More traditional indicators such as 24-hour urinary total metanephrine and vanillylmandelic acid are less sensitive and less specific; total urinary metanephrine and vanillylmandelic acid have respective sensitivities of only 60% and 46% for detecting familial pheochromocytoma and 88% and 77% for detecting sporadic pheochromocytoma. With few exceptions (e.g., heart failure, neuroblastoma, baroreflex failure, severe physiologic or pathologic stress), plasma catecholamines >2,000 pg/mL are diagnostic of pheochromocytoma.

Familial screening. If familial disease is established, first-degree relatives should be investigated for genetic mutations. Patients with pheochromocytomas should be screened for evidence of MTC, hyperparathyroidism, and VHL, and patients with the latter diseases or neurofibromatosis and hypertension should be screened for pheochromocytoma.

SUGGESTED READING

1. Bravo EL. Evolving concepts in the pathophysiology, diagnosis, and treatment of pheochromocytoma. *Endocr Rev.* 1994;15:356–368.
2. Eisenhofer G, Huynh T-T, Hiroi M, Pacak K. Understanding catecholamine metabolism as a guide to the biochemical diagnosis of pheochromocytoma. *Rev Endocr Metab Disord.* 2001;2:297–311.
3. Lenders JWM, Pacak K, Walther MM, et al. Biochemical diagnosis of pheochromocytoma: which test is best? *JAMA.* 2002;287:1427–1434.
4. Manger WM, Gifford RW Jr. Pheochromocytoma: a clinical overview. In: Laragh JH, Brenner BM, eds. *Hypertension: Pathophysiology, Diagnosis and Management.* 2nd ed. New York, NY: Raven Press; 1995:2225–2244.
5. Manger WM, Gifford RW Jr. *Clinical and Experimental Pheochromocytoma.* 2nd ed. Cambridge, MA: Blackwell Science; 1996.
6. Manger WM, Gifford RW Jr. Pheochromocytoma: diagnosis and treatment. *J Clin Hypertens.* 2002;4:62–72.
7. Pacak K, Linehan WM, Eisenhower G, et al. Recent advances in genetics, diagnosis, localization and treatment of pheochromocytoma. *Ann Int Med.* 2001;134:315–329.

Chapter A52

Hypertension Caused by Thyroid and Parathyroid Abnormalities, Acromegaly, and Androgens

Yoram Shenker, MD

KEY POINTS

- Hypothyroidism is often associated with diastolic hypertension, increased catecholamine levels, and increased vascular resistance; replacement of thyroid hormone usually normalizes these parameters.

- Thyrotoxicosis is often associated with systolic hypertension due to increased cardiac output and decreased peripheral resistance; treatment of thyrotoxicosis normalizes blood pressure.

- Hypertension in hyperparathyroidism is multifactorial and may be related to cellular effect of calcium, effects of parathyroid hormone, renal insufficiency, or changes in the renin-angiotensin-aldosterone system.

- Approximately 50% of acromegalic patients are hypertensive with increased cardiac output and left ventricular hypertrophy induced by a direct effect of growth hormone.

See also Chapters A1, A3, B96, C110, and C171

THYROID AND HYPERTENSION

Clinical Aspects

Hypothyroidism. The reported prevalence of hypertension in hypothyroidism varies between 0% and 50%. Hypothyroidism has been identified as a cause of hypertension in as many as 3% of hypertensive patients. Many hypertensive hypothyroid patients have predominantly diastolic hypertension, and the degree of severity of hypothyroidism seems to be correlated with diastolic blood pressure. On the other hand, a recent study found no increase in prevalence of hypertension in hypothyroid geriatric patients as compared to euthyroid geriatric population and no association between thyroid-stimulating hormone (TSH) level and diastolic blood pressure. Thyroid hormone replacement in hypertensive hypothyroid patients decreases systolic and diastolic blood pressure, but

Table A52.1. Endocrine and Cardiovascular Changes in Thyroid Disorders

ENDOCRINE/ CARDIOVASCULAR FUNCTIONS	HYPOTHYROIDISM	THYROTOXICOSIS
Catecholamine levels	Increased	Normal/ decreased
Density of β-adrenergic receptors	Decreased	Increased
Plasma renin activity levels	Decreased	Increased
Aldosterone levels	Decreased	Increased
Blood volume	Decreased	Increased
Cardiac output	Decreased	Increased
Stroke volume	Decreased	Increased
Heart rate	Decreased	Increased
Peripheral vascular resistance	Increased	Decreased

normalization of blood pressure is less likely in older patients and in those with more long-standing hypertension.

Hyperthyroidism. The prevalence of hypertension in thyrotoxicosis is probably in the range of 20% to 30%. Systolic hypertension dominates because of the increased cardiac indices and decreased peripheral resistance; high diastolic blood pressure is uncommon in thyrotoxicosis. The prevalence of hypertension in thyrotoxic patients is particularly increased in patients <49 years old. Treatment of thyrotoxicosis and restoration of the euthyroid state usually leads to normalization of systolic blood pressure, particularly in younger patients.

Mechanisms of Hypertension

Cellular effects of thyroid hormone. Most of the effects of thyroid hormones are mediated through activation of specific nuclear receptors, which increase transcription of a specific messenger RNA and increase production of proteins that mediate the function of the thyroid hormones in different organ systems. Some of the effects of thyroid hormones, including cardiovascular effects, occur very rapidly and appear to be directly related to nongenomic effects (**Table A52.1**).

Hemodynamic variations. Thyrotoxicosis or excess administration of thyroid hormones is associated with increased cardiac output, stroke volume, heart rate, and contractility. It also leads to increased blood volume, decreased peripheral vascular resistance, and a widened pulse pressure (decreased diastolic pressure and increased systolic blood pressure).

Conversely, hypothyroidism is associated with low cardiac output and increased total peripheral resistance, which may be partially related to acceleration of structural changes in vascular tissue caused by thyroid hormone deficiency. Total blood volume is decreased in hypothyroidism.

Autonomic interactions. The cardiovascular manifestations of thyrotoxicosis closely resemble those caused by infusion of epinephrine, and many of the symptoms of thyrotoxicosis are controlled by β-blockers. Yet, catecholamine levels in thyrotoxicosis are either low or normal. One possible explanation is increased sensitivity to catecholamines, which may be related to increased density of β-adrenergic receptors, as has been found

in heart tissue and leukocytes. The absence of increased response to adrenergic agonists in thyrotoxicosis, however, casts some doubt on the receptor sensitivity hypothesis. Hypothyroid patients have high plasma norepinephrine levels, particularly when they are hypertensive, along with high muscle sympathetic nerve activity. The number of β-adrenergic receptors in hypothyroid patients is decreased, leading to increased α-adrenergic responses, a possible explanation for the increase in peripheral vascular resistance and hypertension of hypothyroidism.

Renin-angiotensin system. Plasma renin activity (PRA) is low in hypothyroidism; it increases when thyroxine is replaced. Aldosterone secretion rate and the response of aldosterone to other secretagogues are also diminished. This suggests that the renin-aldosterone system does not play a role in hypertension of hypothyroidism. PRA is increased in thyrotoxicosis, which may be related to thyroid hormone–induced hepatic synthesis of renin substrate (angiotensinogen), which is similar to the effects of estrogen and cortisol, and which leads to stimulation of the entire renin-aldosterone system. Administration of angiotensin II antagonists in thyrotoxic patients does not necessarily reduce blood pressure, which casts doubt on the role of the renin-aldosterone system in thyrotoxic hypertension.

PARATHYROIDS AND HYPERTENSION

Clinical Aspects

Hypertension is frequently associated with primary hyperparathyroidism (caused by adenoma or hyperplasia of the parathyroid gland), pseudohypoparathyroidism [caused by resistance to the parathyroid hormone (PTH)], or secondary hyperparathyroidism (most often caused by advanced renal failure). The prevalence of hypertension in selected groups with primary hyperparathyroidism varies from 10% to >70%. Patients with pseudohypoparathyroidism have a 40% to 50% prevalence of hypertension.

Mechanisms of Hypertension in Hyperparathyroidism

Hypertension in different forms of hyperparathyroidism is probably multifactorial. The possibility of coexisting essential hypertension and hyperparathyroidism cannot be ignored, considering the high prevalence of both conditions in the elderly population.

Serum calcium and blood pressure. Acute infusion of calcium into normotensive patients usually leads to increased peripheral vascular resistance. Conditions of non–PTH-dependent hypercalcemia are also quite frequently associated with hypertension. These observations have led to the hypothesis that hypercalcemia causes increased free intracellular calcium, which is known to increase vascular smooth muscle contractility, and thus leads to hypertension. Conversely, some studies do not support the idea of hypertensive effects of hypercalcemia. Hypocalcemia has also been associated with hypertension, and multiple studies have shown the beneficial effects of calcium supplementation on systolic blood pressure in essential hypertension.

Parathyroid hormone and hypertension. Patients with pseudohypoparathyroidism (who are hypocalcemic with high

PTH levels) have as much hypertension as patients with primary hyperparathyroidism, suggesting that increased PTH itself may be responsible for hypertension. Moreover, patients with pseudohypoparathyroidism and hypertension remain hypertensive after correction of hypocalcemia. In a long-term study, PTH infusion in normotensive subjects led to hypertension, possibly related to adrenocorticotropic hormone–stimulated cortisol and aldosterone secretion. Conversely, other acute studies have shown vasodilatory and hypotensive effects of high PTH levels.

Parathyroid hormone–induced renal disease and hypertension. Most studies have shown that the prevalence of hypertension is much higher in patients with hyperparathyroidism who have renal insufficiency than in hyperparathyroid patients without renal dysfunction.

Renin-aldosterone system in hyperparathyroidism. Many studies have shown increased PRA and aldosterone levels in hyperparathyroidism. In a recent small study, hypertensive hyperparathyroid patients were compared with normotensive hyperparathyroid patients and normal control subjects. PRA and plasma aldosterone levels were higher in the hypertensive hyperparathyroid patients, who also had a greater pressor response to infused norepinephrine. Parathyroidectomy normalized blood pressure, PRA, plasma aldosterone, and pressor responsiveness to norepinephrine in 8 out of 10 subjects.

Response of Hypertension to Parathyroidectomy

According to different reports, 20% to 100% of patients with hypertension and hyperparathyroidism experience normal or improved blood pressures after undergoing parathyroidectomy. No known factor can predict which patient with hypertension will respond favorably to parathyroidectomy. Some studies suggest that the effect of decreased blood pressure after such surgery usually does not last more than 3 years. At present, the consensus is that hypertension alone is not a reason to perform a parathyroidectomy in a hyperparathyroid patient.

ACROMEGALY AND HYPERTENSION

Clinical Features

Acromegaly is a disease of adults caused by chronic excess of growth hormone (GH). Gigantism is a similar condition associated with increased height that develops before puberty and closure of the epiphyses. The vast majority of cases of acromegaly are due to GH-producing pituitary adenomas (usually macroadenomas, which by definition are larger than 1 cm). Another cause of acromegaly is an excess of GH-releasing hormone secreted either eutopically by a hypothalamic tumor or ectopically from a carcinoid or islet cell tumor. Ectopic GH secretion is extremely rare, with only 1 well-documented case of a GH-producing pancreatic islet cell tumor. Hypertension is very common in acromegaly. In the largest series ever published, 51% of 500 acromegalic patients were hypertensive, with half of these having borderline hypertension and half having frank hypertension.

Mechanisms of Hypertension

Cardiac stroke volume is increased in active acromegaly before the onset of high blood pressure. Hypertensive acromegalics also have a reduction in end systolic stress, which is an index of afterload. These changes result in increased cardiac output, which may be involved in the development of hypertension. An increase in left ventricular mass, apparently due to a direct trophic effect on cardiomyocytes, is a very frequent finding in acromegaly. Recently, impaired circadian blood pressure profile was found in hypertensive as well as in some normotensive acromegalics. The nondipping profile was associated with higher GH levels. The structural and functional cardiovascular abnormalities of acromegaly respond to treatment when GH levels are successfully controlled. In many cases, such treatment also leads to cure or at least amelioration of hypertension, particularly if patients are diagnosed and treated relatively early in the course of the disease.

ANDROGENS AND HYPERTENSION

The fact that men are at greater risk for cardiovascular disease and have higher blood pressure than age-matched premenopausal women raises questions about the possible role of androgens or lack of estrogens in hypertension. Hormone replacement therapy does not usually cause significant reduction in blood pressure, suggesting that loss of estrogen in postmenopausal women is not the predominant factor in their high blood pressure. Based on rat models, androgens blunt the pressure-natriuresis relationship through activation of the renin-angiotensin system, but currently there is no human evidence for this hypothesis.

SUGGESTED READING

1. Akpunonu BE, Mulrow PJ, Hoffman EA. Secondary hypertension: evaluation and treatment: thyrotoxicosis and hypertension [published correction appears in *Dis Mon.* 1997;43:62]. *Dis Mon.* 1996;42:689–703.
2. Bergus GR, Mold JW, Barton ED, Randall CS. The lack of association between hypertension and hypothyroidism in a primary care setting. *J Hum Hypertens.* 1999;13:231–235.
3. Ezzat S, Forster MJ, Berchtold P, et al. Acromegaly: clinical and biochemical features in 500 patients. *Medicine.* 1994;73:233–240.
4. Gennari C, Nami R, Gonnelli S. Hypertension and primary hyperparathyroidism: the role of adrenergic and renin-angiotensin-aldosterone systems. *Miner Electrolyte Metab.* 1995;21:77–81.
5. López-Velasco R, Escobar-Morreale HF, Vega B, et al. Cardiac involvement in acromegaly: specific myocardiopathy or consequence of systemic hypertension? *J Clin Endocrinol Metab.* 1997;82:1047–1053.
6. Pietrobelli DJ, Akopian M, Olivieri AO, et al. Altered circadian blood pressure profile in patients with active acromegaly. Relationship with left ventricular mass and hormonal values. *J Hum Hypertens.* 2001;15:601–605.
7. Reckelhoff JF. Gender differences in the regulation of blood pressure. *Hypertension.* 2001;37:1199–1208.
8. Saito I, Saruta T. Hypertension in thyroid disorders. *Endocrinol Metab Clin North Am.* 1994;23:379–386.

Polycystic Ovary Syndrome

Caren G. Solomon, MD, MPH; Ellen W. Seely, MD

KEY POINTS

- Polycystic ovary syndrome is associated with obesity and insulin resistance, known risk factors for hypertension and cardiovascular disease.

- Women with polycystic ovary syndrome have higher blood pressures and a higher prevalence of hypertension than women with regular menstrual cycles.

- It remains uncertain whether the increased risk for hypertension in polycystic ovary syndrome is explained by the greater tendency to obesity in affected women.

See also Chapters A44–A46, B86, B97, and C162

Clinical Aspects

Polycystic ovary syndrome (PCOS) affects approximately 5% of women of reproductive age. Although there is no universally accepted definition for PCOS, it is frequently defined as the combination of anovulation (fewer than 6 periods a year) and androgen excess that is not due to another endocrine disorder. Characteristic clinical features of PCOS include irregular menstrual cycles, hirsutism, acne, and infertility (**Table A53.1**). An elevated serum level of testosterone is central to the diagnosis and may be seen in the absence of signs of androgen excess on physical examination. The ovaries typically have multiple cysts, which may be visualized on ultrasound examination, but this finding may also be seen in normally cycling women and is thus not diagnostic of PCOS.

Obesity as a Contributing Factor

Obesity, in particular central obesity, is extremely common, although up to 20% of women with this syndrome are not obese. There are substantial data to support a relationship between PCOS and elevated blood pressure. A number of reports suggest a 2- to 3-fold increased prevalence of hypertension among women with this syndrome. However, these studies did not adjust for body mass index or look specifically at the subgroup of lean women with PCOS. Whether blood pressure is increased in women with PCOS independent of obesity is not clear. Some data support an association between PCOS and higher blood pressure, measured in the office or using ambulatory monitoring, even after adjustment for body mass index. However, other investigators have failed to find an independent association using either of these techniques. Available data have not convincingly demonstrated higher blood pressures among lean women with PCOS, suggesting that obesity may explain the overall higher risks for hypertension associated with this syndrome.

Insulin Resistance

A hallmark of PCOS is insulin resistance out of proportion to the magnitude of obesity. Even lean women with PCOS have been documented to be insulin resistant as compared with weight-matched controls. Insulin resistance may be the central cause of PCOS and may also contribute to the associated hypertension. These possibilities are supported by observations that improvement in insulin sensitivity in women with PCOS following weight loss or use of insulin sensitizers (e.g., metformin or a thiazolidinedione) can correct the clinical manifestations of PCOS and lower blood pressure. The elevated testosterone levels found in PCOS may also contribute to the hypertension.

Associated Risks

Hypertension in pregnancy. PCOS may also be associated with a higher risk of new-onset hypertension in pregnancy. However, as with essential hypertension, it remains controversial whether this risk is wholly explained by greater body mass index, a recognized risk factor for hypertension associated with pregnancy (see Chapter A57).

Coronary risk factors. Several coronary risk factors associated with hypertension are also more common in women with PCOS. Type 2 diabetes mellitus is 2 to 3 times more frequent in women with PCOS than in weight-matched controls. Women with PCOS also have increased levels of triglycerides and lower

Table A53.1. Manifestations of Polycystic Ovary Syndrome

CLINICAL	LABORATORY
Oligomenorrhea/amenorrhea	Elevated testosterone
Infertility	Insulin resistance/hyperinsulinemia
Hirsutism	Hyperglycemia
Acne	Hypertriglyceridemia and low high-density lipoprotein-cholesterol
Central obesity	
Type 2 diabetes mellitus	
Hypertension	
Dyslipidemia	
Pregnancy-related hypertension and diabetes	
Cardiovascular disease (not definitive)	
Endometrial hyperplasia/cancer	

levels of high-density-lipoprotein cholesterol relative to normally cycling women, and endothelial dysfunction has been described in these women. The combination of these metabolic derangements would be expected to increase cardiovascular risk in this population. Several reports have suggested increased atherosclerosis in PCOS, but further confirmation is needed.

SUGGESTED READING

1. Conway GS, Agrawal R, Betteridge DJ, Jacobs HS. Risk factors for coronary artery disease in lean and obese women with polycystic ovarian syndrome. *Clin Endocrinol.* 1992;37:119–125.

2. Dahlgren E, Janson PO, Johannson S, et al. Women with polycystic ovary syndrome wedge resected in 1956 to 1965: a long-term follow up focusing on natural history and circulating hormones. *Fertil Steril.* 1992;57:505–513.
3. Solomon CG. The epidemiology of polycystic ovary syndrome: prevalence and associated disease risks. *Endocrinol Metab Clin North Am* 1999;28:247–263.
4. Talbott E, Guzick D, Clerici A, et al. Coronary heart disease risk factors in women with polycystic ovary syndrome. *Arterioscler Thromb Vasc Biol.* 1995;15:821–826.
5. Urman B, Sarac E, Dogan L, et al. Pregnancy in infertile PCOD patients: complications and outcome. *J Reprod Med.* 1997;42:501–505.

Chapter A54

Coarctation of the Aorta

Albert P. Rocchini, MD

KEY POINTS

- Coarctation of the aorta is the most common congenital cardiovascular cause of hypertension.

- Coarctation is identified by the presence of higher blood pressures in the arms (usually the right arm) than in the legs.

- Coarctation can be corrected with surgery or balloon angioplasty.

- Despite successful repair of coarctation, many individuals have persistent cardiovascular problems, including chronic hypertension, coronary artery disease, aortic aneurysms, and stroke.

See also Chapters A41, A61, C110, and C128

Coarctation of the aorta is the most common congenital cardiovascular cause of hypertension and the fourth most frequent (7.5%) form of congenital heart disease that requires cardiac catheterization or surgery during the first year of life, affecting men more often than women (1.7:1.0). It is usually sporadic in occurrence but has been reported in monozygotic twins concordant for the anomaly and in 1 family in an autosomal dominant pattern. It is common in children with Turner's syndrome (35%). The poor prognosis of untreated patients with coarctation of the aorta is well known: 20% of patients die between the first and second decade of life, and 80% expire before age 50.

Mechanisms of Hypertension

There are 3 different types of hypertension associated with coarctation of the aorta: prerepair hypertension, postrepair paradoxical hypertension, and late postrepair hypertension.

Prerepair hypertension. Hypertension associated with coarctation of the thoracic aorta prerepair is relatively poorly understood. The 3 main theories to explain the hypertension are the mechanical theory, the neural theory, and the Goldblatt-type phenomenon.

Mechanical theory. The mechanical theory, first suggested in 1948, was based on the notion that the hypertension proximal to the coarcted segment is a function of the high resistance to left ventricular output imposed by the narrowing itself. The finding that many patients with coarctation have hypertension below as well as above the narrowing along with the fact that hypertension persists despite the presence of large collateral channels has cast doubt on this theory.

Neural theory. The neural theory proposes that hypertension is the result of readjustment of the baroreceptors in the aortic arch such that the increased proximal pressure is necessary to insure an adequate blood supply to the organs distal to the obstruction. There have been no objective data to support or refute this theory.

Goldblatt-type phenomenon. The third and most likely explanation for the hypertension observed in patients with coarctation of the aorta is the Goldblatt-type phenomena. This theory suggests that the narrowed aortic segment causes renal hypoperfusion, which in turn causes stimulation of the renin-angiotensin-aldosterone system. The studies of Scott and Bahnson strongly support this theory. These investigators created coarctation in dogs and showed that hypertension could be prevented if 1 kidney is transplanted above the coarctation and the other kidney is removed. Until recently, the major criticism of the renal hypoperfusion theory was that children with coarctation who were hypertensive did not have elevated plasma renin activity and did not have decreased renal blood flow. However, when coarctation patients are volume depleted, plasma renin activity is dramatically increased, and their blood pressures become very responsive to antagonists of the renin-angiotensin system. A similar situation has been documented in experimental models of one-kidney, one-clip Goldblatt hypertension.

Postrepair paradoxical hypertension. Severe hypertension frequently occurs during the first week after surgical repair of coarctation of the aorta. The sympathetic nervous system and the renin-angiotensin system have been shown to be important mediators of this "paradoxical hypertension." Because balloon angioplasty is not associated with paradoxical hypertension, it appears that some aspect of the surgical repair such as the unintentional disruption of some of the afferent thoracic sympathetic nerve fibers occurs, leading to a loss of the normal balance of excitatory and depressor sympathetic mechanoreceptors and the development of a net increase in sympathetic activity. This increased sympathetic activity in turn stimulates renin release and leads to the development of paradoxical hypertension. Paradoxical hypertension can be prevented or reversed with β-blockers, angiotensin-converting enzyme inhibitors, or angiotensin receptor blockers.

Late postrepair hypertension. Many individuals with good hemodynamic repairs (with no resting gradients) develop significant upper extremity hypertension with treadmill exercise. Markel et al. demonstrated that exercise hypertension is not observed with arm exercise and that these patients have increased vascular reactivity to norepinephrine in the right arm, normal norepinephrine reactivity in the legs, and abnormal baroreceptor activity. It has thus been postulated that the resting and exercise systolic hypertension that frequently occurs in many subjects late postoperatively is owing to an abnormal compliance and responsiveness of the vessels in the vascular bed proximal to the original coarctation. Children or adults who have minimal resting arm-leg gradient and hypertension (resting or exercise-induced) should be treated with antihypertensive medications such as angiotensin-converting enzyme inhibitors or calcium channel blockers that improve arterial compliance.

Clinical Correlation

Diagnosis. The physical findings that are diagnostic of coarctation are diminished femoral pulses and a systolic pressure gradient between right arm and the legs. A grade 2 or 3 over 6 systolic murmur, usually heard best in the posterior left interscapular area, is a common sign that is important in localizing the coarctation to the thoracic aorta. Among patients with well-developed collateral blood flow, systolic or continuous murmurs may be heard over the left and right sides of the chest. Noninvasive conformation of the diagnosis can be made by chest x-ray and echocardiogram. On the frontal projection of the chest x-ray, a discrete thoracic coarctation may show a *3 sign*, comprised of the borders of the proximal aorta, the coarcted segment, and post-stenotic dilated segment. Barium swallow may reveal indentations of the same structures on the esophagus in a *reverse 3* configuration. Echocardiogram and Doppler determinations are useful in localizing the site of the coarctated segment, in assessing the anatomy of the aortic arch, and in estimating the pressure gradient across the coarctation. Cardiac catheterization should be reserved for those infants and children in whom the echocardiogram or physical examination suggests abnormal location of the coarctation (i.e., abdominal aorta), the presence of other car-

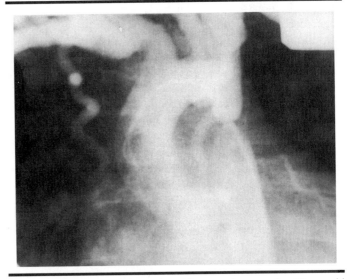

Figure A54.1. This is a left anterior oblique angiogram of a 10-year-old boy with a discrete thoracic coarctation of the aorta.

diac lesions, or abnormal aortic arch anatomy. Catheterization can also be used to enable nonsurgical treatment with balloon angioplasty (**Figure A54.1**).

Repair techniques. The 2 general current approaches used to treat coarctation of the aorta are thoracic surgery or balloon angioplasty, with or without placement of an intravascular stent. Surgical techniques include resection and extended end-to-end anastomosis, left subclavian flap angioplasty, synthetic patch angioplasty, or (rarely) the use of a tube interposition graft. The incidence of restenosis depends more on the age at the time of repair than the type of surgical repair (occurring in up to 20% of children operated on younger than 1 year of age and only occurring in 3% of children older than 3 years of age). Balloon angioplasty can be used for the initial treatment of coarctation of the aorta and for treatment of restenosis after surgical repair, but in some patients, it may be unsuccessful due to elastic recoil of the vessel or unfavorable anatomy (long-segment narrowing or arch hypoplasty). In an attempt to reduce the limitations of balloon angioplasty, intravascular balloon expandable stents have been used to treat individuals with native coarctation. This technique is usually reserved for adults or older adolescents, individuals with recurrent coarctation in whom balloon angioplasty does not effectively relieve the obstruction, or those with restenosis of a repaired hypoplastic aortic arch.

Prognosis. Coarctation of the aorta should be treated as early in childhood as possible. On the surface, it would appear that if the coarctation is successfully treated, long-term survival should approach that of the general population. However, based on recent reports, this does not seem to be the case. Many individuals with repaired coarctation of the aorta do not have a normal life expectancy. They can suffer from significant cardiovascular problems, including ischemic heart disease, cerebral hemorrhage, aortic aneurysms, and persistent hypertension. In 254 survivors of coarctation repair performed between 1948 and 1976, 95% of patients were alive at 10 years, 89% at 20 years, 82% at 30 years, and 79% at 40 years after operation. The mean age at death among those 45 individuals who died late was 34 years. Predictors of survival were age at operation ($p = .004$), and the blood pressure at the first post-operative visit ($p < .001$). Age at the time of initial surgical repair significantly affected long-term survival: 30-year survival rate after successful correction of coarctation was 93% in individuals operated on at younger than 5 years of age, 91% in individuals operated on between 5 and 10 years of age, and 76% in individuals operated on after age 10. Coronary artery disease was the most common cause of late death, occurring in 10 patients at the mean age of death of 55 years, all of whom were greater than 10 years of age at the time of their coarctation repair. Other causes of death were second cardiac operation (7), sudden death (7, 6 of whom were older than 10 years of age at the time of the coarctation repair), and ruptured ascending aortic aneurysm (7).

SUGGESTED READING

1. Cambell M. Natural history of coarctation of the aorta. *Br Heart J.* 1970;32:63–69.

2. Clarkson P, Nicholson M, Barratt-Boyes B, et al. Results after repair of coarctation of the aorta beyond infancy. A 10- to 28-year follow-up with particular reference to late systemic hypertension. *Am J Cardiol.* 1983;51:1481–1488.

3. Cohen M, Fuster V, Steele P, et al. Coarctation of the aorta. Long-term follow-up and prediction of outcome after surgical correction. *Circulation.* 1989;80:840–845.

4. Gidding SS, Rocchini AP, Beekman RH, et al. Therapeutic effect of propranolol on paradoxical hypertension after repair of coarctation of the aorta. *N Engl J Med.* 1985;312:1224–1228.

5. Markel H, Rocchini AP, Beekman RH, et al. Exercise-induced hypertension after repair of coarctation of the aorta: arm versus leg exercise. *J Am Coll Cardiol.* 1986;8:165–171.

6. Salazar O, Steinberger J, Carpenter B, et al. Predictors of hypertension in long-term survivors of repaired coarctation of the aorta. *J Am Coll Cardiol.* 1996;27(Suppl A):35A.

7. Scott HW, Bahnson HT. Evidence for a renal factor on the hypertension of coarctation of the aorta. *Surgery.* 1951;30:206–217.

8. Stewart A, Ahmed R, Travill C, Newman C. Coarctation of the aorta life and health 20–44 years after surgical repair. *Br Heart J.* 1993;69:65–70.

Chapter A55

Pathophysiology of Sleep Apnea

Barbara J. Morgan, PhD

KEY POINTS

- In a large proportion of middle-aged adults, apnea and hypopnea during sleep result in sleep fragmentation, intermittent asphyxia, sympathetic nervous activation, and marked transient blood pressure elevations.

- A dose-response relationship exists between severity of sleep-disordered breathing and the degree of daytime blood pressure elevation.

- The causal link between sleep-disordered breathing and hypertension in animal models further suggests that sleep-disordered breathing may be an underlying pathophysiologic factor in chronic hypertension.

See also Chapters A34, A42, A44, B97, C112, C113, C162, and C172

Epidemiology

The estimated prevalence of clinically significant sleep-disordered breathing (≥ 5 apneas or hypopneas per hour of sleep plus complaints of daytime sleepiness) in middle-aged adults is 2% for women and 4% for men. Although daytime hypersomnolence is the predominant symptom reported by those affected, frequent traffic accidents, declines in cognitive function, and increased incidence of psychiatric disorders have also been reported. Sleep apnea syndrome is associated with long-term cardiovascular morbidity from systemic and pulmonary hypertension, myocardial infarction, and stroke, and also with metabolic disorders such as glucose intolerance and insulin resistance.

Pathophysiology

Airway obstruction and hypoxia. The onset of sleep is associated with a decrease in neural drive to the muscles of the respiratory pump and to those that stiffen and maintain patency of the upper airway. Loss of muscle tone reduces airway caliber, thereby increasing transpulmonary resistance and rendering the airway more collapsible. In individuals with anatomic compromise (e.g., pharyngeal fat deposition, enlargement of the soft palate or tongue, or craniofacial abnormalities), sleep-induced loss of muscle tone predisposes to complete collapse of the upper airway, or apnea. Both apneas and hypopneas (episodes of partial airway collapse) produce transient hypoxemia, hypercapnia, acidosis, and, in most cases, arousal from sleep. Each event triggers marked increases in sympathetic nervous system activity and blood pressure (**Figure A55.1**). Individuals with obstructive sleep apnea syndrome may experience hundreds of these events throughout the course of a single night's sleep. In these patients and also in individuals with less severe sleep-disordered breathing, the normal sleep-related decline in blood pressure and heart rate is greatly attenuated or even absent.

Sympathetic nervous activation. Enhanced sympathetic nervous system activity appears to be centrally involved in the hypertension associated with sleep apnea. A rat model that pro-

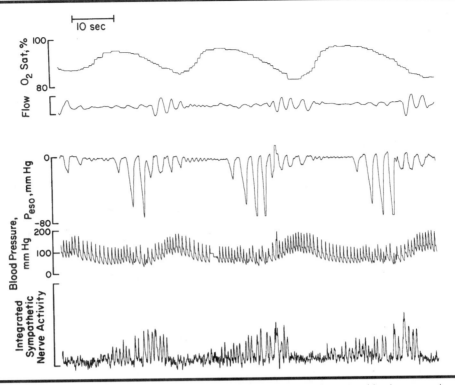

Figure A55.1. Mixed (central and obstructive) sleep apneas produce marked sympathoexcitation and transient blood pressure elevations in a patient with sleep apnea syndrome. P_{eso}, esophageal pressure; Sat, saturation. (From Skatrud JB, Badr MS, Morgan BJ. Control of breathing during sleep and sleep disordered breathing. In: Altose M, Kawakami Y, eds. *Control of Breathing in Health and Disease*. New York, NY: Marcel Dekker; 1999:379–422, with permission.)

duces intermittent hypoxia during sleep causes persistent daytime hypertension with as few as 5 weeks of exposure, but only in animals with an intact sympathetic nervous system. Augmented sympathetic activity during wakefulness (when breathing is stable) is observed in individuals with sleep apnea syndrome, although the mechanisms responsible for conversion of acute, apnea-induced episodes of sympathetic stimulation to chronic sympathetic overactivity are not known.

Renin-angiotensin system. The renin-angiotensin system contributes importantly to hypertension in rats exposed to intermittent hypoxia during sleep. In this model, renal nerve denervation, angiotensin II receptor blockade, and suppression of the renin-angiotensin system by high salt diet all prevent the rise in blood pressure. In a seeming paradox, plasma renin activity is reduced, not elevated, in humans with sleep apnea syndrome. However, sleep apnea and hypoxia increase plasma levels of atrial natriuretic peptide, a hormone known to inhibit renin release.

Endothelial dysfunction. There is growing evidence that sleep apnea, probably via the resultant hypoxia, interferes with the function of vascular endothelium. In rats exposed to hypoxia and in patients with sleep apnea syndrome, plasma endothelin levels are increased and circulating nitric oxide levels are depressed. Endothelium-dependent vasodilatation, an important mechanism in regulation of vascular tone, is impaired in rats exposed to chronic episodic hypoxia and in humans with sleep apnea syndrome (**Figure A55.2**).

Antihypertensive drug effects. Amelioration of some types of sleep-disordered breathing has been observed after treatment

of high blood pressure. This finding raises the possibility that the acute and chronic hypertension caused by sleep-disordered breathing can, in turn, exacerbate sleep-disordered breathing. The question of whether the 2 conditions could be linked by a positive feedback mechanism awaits further exploration.

Sleep Apnea and Hypertension

Established hypertension and sleep apnea. Hypertension is highly prevalent (50% to 90%) in individuals with sleep apnea syndrome. Although some of the blood pressure elevation may be attributed to comorbid obesity, several lines of evidence suggest that the relationship between sleep apnea and hypertension is potentially causal. First, blood pressure decreases in some individuals when sleep apnea is successfully treated. Second, a dose-response-type relationship with the appropriate temporal sequence has been observed between sleep-disordered breathing and daytime blood pressure elevation in a large, population-based study. Finally, evidence obtained in an animal model strongly supports the notion of a cause-and-effect relationship. Persistent daytime hypertension has been produced by frequent tracheal occlusions during nocturnal sleep in a canine model (**Figure A55.3**). In parallel experiments, sleep fragmentation produced by acoustic stimuli failed to affect daytime blood pressure, suggesting that the chemical or mechanical consequences of the occlusions contributed more importantly to the hypertensive effect of this intervention.

Sleep-disordered breathing and borderline hypertension. Most clinical investigations linking sleep-disordered breathing and hypertension have focused on individuals with obstructive

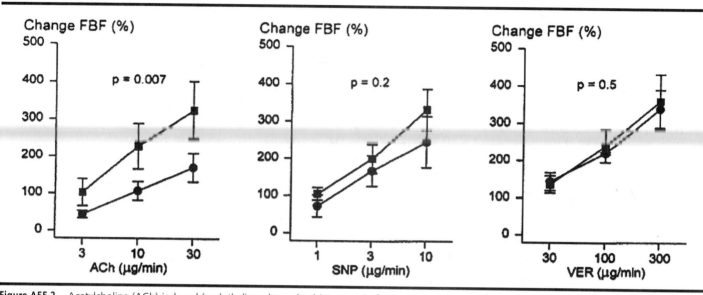

Figure A55.2. Acetylcholine (ACh)-induced (endothelium-dependent) increases in forearm blood flow (FBF) were attenuated in 8 patients with obstructive sleep apnea (*circles*) versus 9 age- and weight-matched control subjects (*squares*), whereas endothelium independent increases evoked by sodium nitroprusside (SNP) and verapamil (VER) were comparable in the 2 groups (means ± standard error). (From Kato M, Roberts-Thomson P, Phillips BG, et al. Impairment of endothelium-dependent vasodilation of resistance vessels in patients with obstructive sleep apnea. *Circulation.* 2000;102:2607–2610, with permission.)

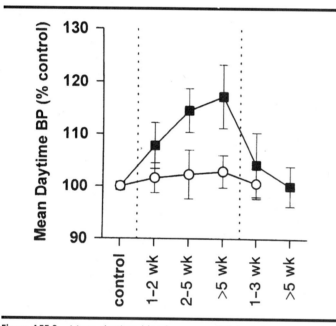

Figure A55.3. Mean daytime blood pressure (BP) in 4 dogs exposed to intermittent tracheal occlusions during sleep (*filled squares*) and sleep fragmentation (*open circles*) (means ± standard error). The vertical dashed lines represent the durations of the exposures. (From Brooks D, Horner RL, Kozar LF, et al. Obstructive sleep apnea as a cause of systemic hypertension. *J Clin Invest.* 1997;99:106–109, with permission.)

sleep apnea syndrome (i.e., those who represent the severe end of the sleep-disordered breathing spectrum). It has recently been appreciated that marked fluctuations in systolic and diastolic pressure accompany mild to moderate as well as severe sleep-disordered breathing. These less severe events (hypopneas and infrequent apneas) are very common in the undiagnosed population, and they contribute to small but statistically significant elevations in daytime blood pressure. The health risks associated with mild to moderate sleep-disordered breathing and the effects of early intervention in this group of individuals remain to be elucidated.

SUGGESTED READING

1. Carlson JT, Hedner J, Elam M, et al. Augmented resting sympathetic activity in awake patients with obstructive sleep apnea. *Chest.* 1993;103:1763–1768.
2. Fletcher EC. Physiological consequences of intermittent hypoxia: systemic blood pressure. *J Appl Physiol.* 2001;90:1600–1605.
3. Mayer J, Weichler U, Herres-Mayer B, et al. Influence of metoprolol and cilazapril on blood pressure and on sleep apnea activity. *J Cardiovasc Pharmacol.* 1990;16:952–961.
4. Morgan BJ, Dempsey JA, Pegelow D, et al. Blood pressure perturbations caused by subclinical sleep disordered breathing. *Sleep.* 1998;21:737–746.
5. Peppard P, Young T, Palta M, Skatrud JB. Prospective study of the association between sleep-disordered breathing and hypertension. *N Engl J Med.* 2000;342:1378–1384.
6. Young T, Palta M, Dempsey J, et al. The occurrence of sleep-disordered breathing among middle-aged adults. *N Engl J Med.* 1993;328:1230–1235.

Chapter A56

Affective Illness and Hypertension

Joseph L. Izzo, Jr, MD

KEY POINTS

- The prevalence of depression is high in hypertensive patients.

- Subcortical white matter lesions and cognitive impairment are found in increased levels in individuals with depression and hypertension.

- Blood pressure lowering per se does not cause depression.

- The incidence of depression is very low with most antihypertensive drugs.

See also Chapters A2, A17, A70, B100, and C173

Clinical experience suggests an inverse association between affective illness (depression) and blood pressure. Major factors that could contribute to this inverse relationship include linked differences in central nervous system (CNS), monoamine metabolism between the 2 conditions, or diverse effects of antihypertensive or antidepressant drugs.

Neurochemical Aspects of Affective Illness

Serotonin depletion and selective serotonin reuptake inhibitors. The central role of 5-hydroxytryptamine (5-HT or serotonin) in affective illness has been amply demonstrated. Defects in CNS availability of 5-HT cause mood disturbances, principally in the form of unipolar depression. The clinical importance of central 5-HT depletion is demonstrated by the dramatic mood improvements achieved with selective serotonin reuptake inhibitors (SSRIs), of which paroxetine (Prozac) was the prototype drug. Clinical experience with SSRIs has taught us that it is unlikely that CNS serotonin depletion plays a causal role in hypertension because SSRIs have little effect on blood pressure.

Norepinephrine depletion and other antidepressants. The linkage between serotonin and norepinephrine metabolism in the CNS is complex. Both monoamines are metabolized by monoamine oxidases (MAOs). Nonspecific inhibitors of MAOs were the first effective antidepressants. It has been assumed that these agents act by potentiating CNS monoamine availability, which tends to raise mood and lower blood pressure simultaneously. Cardiovascular control centers in the medulla oblongata and other subcortical brain regions are highly sensitive to norepinephrine content (see Chapter A34). When norepinephrine release is diminished within the CNS, blood pressure tends to rise. Conversely, intraventricular administration of norepinephrine or α_2-agonists such as clonidine diminishes sympathetic nervous outflow and lowers blood pressure (see Chapters A34 and A42). Tricyclic antidepressants (imipramine, etc.), which are relatively unselective inhibitors of neuronal amine reuptake, are

reasonably effective antidepressants. In some cases, tricyclics lower blood pressure, but the effect is inconsistent.

Thus, whether CNS norepinephrine depletion plays any role in depression is unclear, but it may play a role in the pathogenesis of hypertension.

Neuroanatomic Changes in Depression

Individuals with late-onset depression demonstrate a greater number of subcortical white matter hyperintensities and smaller basal ganglia than nondepressed individuals. These age-related changes are similar to those attributed to atherosclerosis (lipohyalinosis) and tend to increase with duration of hypertension. Increased subcortical white matter lesions are also found in individuals with cognitive impairment, but potential relationships among cerebral microcirculatory abnormalities, neurochemical deficits, cognitive impairment, and depression have not been systematically studied.

Clinical Aspects

Stress, depression, and hypertension. It has been estimated that between 10% and 15% of men and 20% and 27% of women with hypertension manifest depressive symptoms. Rabkin found the incidence of major depression to be 3 times greater in hypertensives than normotensives, irrespective of age, gender, other chronic medical illnesses, or medication history. Psychosocial stress may be associated with both depression and blood pressure elevation. In many cases, feelings of fatigue, exhaustion, and emotional distress coexist. Whether such feelings are driven by a fundamental biochemical abnormality of norepinephrine or serotonin metabolism remains to be determined.

Well-being and blood pressure control. Despite previous conjecture to the contrary, better blood pressure control improves (not worsens) general well-being, including mood scores. The first study to demonstrate this point used the angiotensin-converting enzyme inhibitor captopril. Since then, other studies such as the dihydropyridine-based Hypertension Optimal Treatment trial have confirmed that lower blood pressure is associated with better quality of life, suggesting that hypertension is not an asymptomatic disorder and that it is the control of hypertension and not the specific drug class used that is beneficial.

Depression and cardiovascular mortality. There is a strong association between depressive symptoms and cardiac mortality. Studies of patients postmyocardial infarction have revealed a much poorer survival rate in individuals with clinical depression. The underlying mechanisms for this phenomenon are not presently known.

Pharmacologic Implications

Hypertensive reactions to antidepressant drug combinations. Hypertensive crisis occurs rarely when clomipramine, fluoxetine, beroxitene, or sertraline are used alone; mechanisms remain unknown. The combination of MAO inhibitors and SSRI drugs is contraindicated, in part owing to the potential for severe hypertension. Venlafaxine may increase blood pressure in normotensive patients by a few mm Hg but does not tend to increase blood pressure in people with coexistent depression and hypertension. Another well-known interaction is that of guanethidine with tricyclic antidepressants; by interfering with the neuronal uptake of guanethidine, tricyclic antidepressants may precipitate a rapid increase in blood pressure.

Antihypertensive drugs and depression. The rate of depression caused by antihypertensive drugs has never been systematically studied, but the maximal incidence rate of depression is no more than a few percent of patients treated. The neuronal norepinephrine-depleting drug reserpine has been most often associated with reversible depression, but the vast majority of

patients treated with reserpine have no depressive symptoms. β-blockers and central sympatholytic agents such as methyldopa or clonidine also have been reported to cause low incidence rates of depression. Lower doses of tricyclic antidepressants may be required when diltiazem or verapamil are used because tricyclics inhibit oxidation of the calcium antagonists by CYP3A4 enzymes.

SUGGESTED READING

1. Applegate WB, Pressel S, Wittes J, et al. Impact of the treatment of isolated systolic hypertension on behavioral variables. *Arch Intern Med.* 1994;154: 2154–2160.
2. Feighner JP. Cardiovascular safety in depressed patients: focus on venlafaxine. *J Clin Psychiatry.* 1995;56:574–579.
3. Fuller BF. DMS-III depression and hypertension in two psychiatric outpatient populations. *Psychosomatics.* 1988;29:417–423.
4. Krishnan KR, McDonald WM, Doraiswamy PM, et al. Neuroanatomical substrates of depression in the elderly. *Eur Arch Psychiatry Clin Neurosci.* 1993;243:41–46.
5. Palombo V, Scurti R, Muscari A, et al. Blood pressure and intellectual function in elderly subjects. *Age Aging.* 1997;26:91–98.
6. Patten SB, Williams JV, Love EJ. Case-control studies of cardiovascular medications as risk factors for clinically diagnosed depressive disorders in a hospitalized population. *Can J Psychiatry.* 1996;41:469–476.
7. Rabkin JG, Charles E, Kass F. Hypertension and DMS-III depression in psychiatric outpatients. *Am J Psychiatry.* 1983;140:1072–1074.
8. Simonsick EM, Wallace RB, Blazer DG, Berkman LF. Depressive symptomatology and hypertension-associated morbidity and mortality in older adults. *Psychosom Med.* 1995;57:427–435.
9. Todarello O, Taylor GJ, Parker JD, Fanelli M. Alexithymia in essential hypertensive and psychiatric outpatients: a comparative study. *J Psychosom Res.* 1995;39:987–994.
10. Wells KB, Rogers W, Burnam MA, Camp P. Course of depression in patients with hypertension, myocardial infarction, or insulin-dependent diabetes. *Am J Psychiatry.* 1993;150:632–638.

Chapter A57

Pathophysiology of Preeclampsia

Ellen W. Seely, MD; Marshall D. Lindheimer, MD

KEY POINTS

- Preeclampsia is a multisystem disorder of pregnancy characterized by hypertension, proteinuria, and variable abnormalities in liver function and coagulation.

- Hypertension in preeclampsia is caused by marked increases in systemic vascular resistance.

- The etiology of preeclampsia is probably multifactorial.

See also Chapters A3, A41, A42, A47, and C165

Preeclampsia is a hypertensive condition limited to pregnancy which, along with its convulsive phase (eclampsia), remains a leading cause of maternal and fetal morbidity and death. There are still no definitive means for its prevention, and the approach to its treatment remains controversial.

Epidemiology

Preeclampsia complicates over 3% of all pregnancies and approximately 7% of nulliparous gestations in the United States. The disorder is more apt to occur in several "high-risk" populations (women with diabetes, twins, chronic hypertension, underlying renal disease, and previous preeclampsia, in which the incidence is between 20% to 25%). The disorder may also occur more frequently in patients with thrombotic disorders, such as populations manifesting factor V Leiden, protein C and S deficiency, and increased antiphospholipid antibody titers, as well as those with certain angiotensinogen gene variants and hyperhomocystinemia. In the absence of superimposed preeclampsia, most other forms of hypertension complicating pregnancy have a relatively benign course.

Etiology and Pathophysiology

Preeclampsia is a complex disorder whose etiology and pathophysiology are not fully understood. There are 3 schools of current thought: (a) that preeclampsia is of placental origin, (b) that the etiology resides in factors initiated in the maternal environment, and (c) that pathology related to the placenta and to the mother must interact to cause the disease.

Abnormal placentation. The possibility of failed remodeling of the spiral arteries is currently the focus of intense investigation. Many believe that compromised placental blood flow and the hypoxic uteroplacental environment leads to the release of many factors that may enter the maternal circulation and are toxic to maternal endothelium. There is evidence that in preeclampsia cytotrophoblast cells fail to express a normal vascular adhesion phenotype, and adhesion molecules are believed to be crucial to the process of vascular remodeling. Others suggest that women with the angiotensinogen gene variant (T235) may have abnormalities of the local renin-angiotensin system in placental vessels leading to inappropriate angiogenesis and possible clotting in very small vessels. Other areas of investigation include factors affecting apoptosis, the role of the human leukocyte antigen G (a leukocyte antigen that may play a role in maternal tolerance to the placenta) as well as alterations in the production of trophoblast growth factors and other placental proteins. Finally, there is a growing literature documenting excessive trafficking of fetal DNA, cells, and trophoblastic debris across the placenta into the maternal circulation, perhaps owing to alteration in the placental maternal fetal barrier.

Abnormal vascular reactivity. Increased maternal vascular reactivity to endogenous pressor substances may explain the blood pressure lability seen in some patients and may be a cause of the peripheral vasoconstriction seen in preeclampsia. Current theories propose that preeclampsia is preceded or accompanied by alterations in the balance of vasodilating prostanoids and other pressor systems such as endothelin and angiotensin II (Ang II), their receptor density in tissues, and autoantibodies that are agonist to the AT_1 receptor. A failure of production of nitric oxide synthase and nitric oxide–dependent and –independent vasodilation may occur. Maternal endothelial dysfunction may also be caused by increased levels of cytokines, altered autocoid systems, vitamin and mineral deficiencies, or oxidative stress. There is evidence that the balance between circulating oxidant and antioxidant activity is challenged by the gravid state; if circulating oxidant activity dominates, endothelial damage occurs, leading to preeclampsia. A host of substances that stimulate, temporize, or counterbalance the production of free radicals (e.g., serum iron, xanthine oxidase, low-density lipoproteins, isoprostanes, and vitamin C) are being investigated.

Insulin resistance and sympathetic overactivity. Insulin resistance is postulated to play a role in the pathophysiology of essential hypertension (see Chapter A45). Insulin resistance is a hallmark of normal pregnancy, but some studies have shown greater insulin resistance preceding preeclampsia and in postpartum women who had preeclamptic pregnancies. The increase in sympathetic nervous system tone described in preeclampsia may be mediated by hyperinsulinemia and could explain the vasoconstriction seen in this disorder.

Increased activity of the renin-angiotensin-aldosterone system. Disordered regulation of the renin-angiotensin-aldosterone system (RAAS) appears to play a role in the pathophysiology of preeclampsia. Unlike the activation of this system seen in normotensive pregnancy, women with preeclampsia have lower levels of all circulating components of this system. At the same time, there appears to be activation of cellular and tissue RAAS components, including those of the developing placental vasculature. RAAS suppression in preeclampsia in the face of decreased plasma volume has been used as an argument to support the presence of disordered volume sensing. The characteristic lack of a pregnancy-associated blunting of Ang II responsiveness in preeclampsia may be owing to excessive upregulation of Ang II receptors in a variety of tissues. Polymorphisms of the angiotensinogen gene are seen in increased frequency in women with preeclampsia.

Immunologic changes. An immune response to paternal antigen in the fetoplacental unit is proposed as an etiology of preeclampsia. This may explain the occasional reports of inflammatory responses associated with preeclampsia, including activation of circulating leukocytes. The propensity of preeclampsia to occur in the first pregnancy supports the immune hypothesis. Preeclampsia usually decreases in frequency with subsequent pregnancies; however, if the father is new, the incidence is similar to that of the first pregnancy. However, this concept has been recently challenged by the finding that a longer interval between pregnancies (with the same partner) is also associated with preeclampsia.

Genetic factors. Inheritance of a gene or genes that predispose to the development of preeclampsia is suggested by the familial nature of preeclampsia. Maternal transmission was first described by Chesley in the 1960s. Evidence for paternal transmission of the risk of preeclampsia has also been described. There have been reports of several specific allelic substitutions that have been associated with preeclampsia. Gene variants associated with essential hypertension, thrombophilia, endothelial function, and vasoactive hormones have been investigated with mixed results.

Abnormal calcium metabolism. Hypocalciuria is another characteristic finding in women with preeclampsia. Low urinary calcium is associated with lower levels of 1,25-dihydroxyvitamin D [$1,25(OH)_2$] and higher parathyroid hormone levels than in normal pregnancy. Despite the finding of hypocalciuria, trials to decrease the incidence of preeclampsia by means of calcium supplementation have not been successful.

Other circulating substances. There is an extensive literature relating to serum factors that are altered in preeclamptics, but most findings are very preliminary. Placental proteins (e.g., activin and inhibin A), circulating inhibitors of cell membrane pumps, atrial peptides, various growth factors, adhesion molecules, and activators of white blood cells and platelets may be important.

Effects on Organ Systems

Cardiovascular System. Hypertension in overt preeclampsia is primarily due to a marked reversal of the vasodilation characteristic of normal gestation. Even when peripheral edema is marked, most investigators find cardiac output to be decreased or normal and pulmonary capillary wedge pressure low or low normal. Intravascular volumes are decreased compared to normal gestation, usually manifested clinically by a rise in hematocrit. Another feature of the disease is a reversal of the tendency of normal gravidas to resist the pressor effects of infused angiotensin.

Kidney. In contrast to the normal pattern of renal vasodilation in pregnancy, there is renal vasoconstriction with reduced glomerular filtration rate and renal plasma flow in preeclampsia. The decrement in renal hemodynamics is usually minimal (approximately 25%), but, on occasion, preeclampsia may be associated with acute renal failure requiring renal replacement therapy. Functional changes are accompanied by a microscopic renal lesion characterized by hypertrophy of the glomerular capillary endothelial and mesangial cells, termed *glomerular endotheliosis*, which is associated with proteinuria, a hallmark of preeclampsia. The severity of these vascular lesions correlates best with the magnitude of proteinuria and hyperuricemia.

Brain. The greatest clinical concern in women with preeclampsia is that it may progress to eclampsia and convulsions. Eclampsia is frequently preceded by premonitory symptoms and signs, including hyperreflexia, visual disturbances, and severe headaches but may also occur suddenly and without warning. Fatal cases of preeclampsia demonstrate various degrees of cerebral bleeding from microscopic petechiae to gross hemorrhage. Coagulopathy may occur with preeclampsia, as fibrin deposition has been noted in the brain at autopsy. Other researchers have suggested similarities to hypertensive encephalopathy, a view contested in the older literature. More recently, using Doppler techniques have suggested 2 forms of eclampsia: one characterized by cerebral underperfusion (consistent with severe vasoconstriction) and the other by overperfusion (suggesting loss of autoregulation, as in hypertensive encephalopathy). Reports using imaging techniques describe transient localized hemorrhage or edema. The latter may be due to iatrogenic volume loading, as it was not a feature of a large autopsy series in the older literature.

Liver. The liver involvement found in preeclampsia is characterized by periportal lesions with cell necrosis and at times associated with infarction and fibrin deposition. There are also periportal hemorrhages, which may become confluent and develop into hematomas. Subcapsular bleeding that leads to a rupture is a serious complication of preeclampsia.

Placenta. Abnormal placentation is a characteristic feature of preeclampsia, the major lesions being a failure of the uterine spiral arteries to undergo normal remodeling and dilate and the pathologic finding termed *acute atherosis*. Preeclampsia is associated with intrauterine growth restriction attributed to decreased placental perfusion, but surprisingly as many as one-fourth of preeclamptics deliver babies that are large for gestational age. The frequent need for preterm delivery makes preeclampsia a leading cause of premature delivery in the United States.

Clinical Correlation

Diagnosis. Preeclampsia typically presents after gestational week 20, most cases occurring in nulliparas and presenting late in the third trimester. It is a multisystem disease, affecting primarily the cardiovascular system, kidneys, brain, and placenta. Preeclampsia is diagnosed by the *de novo* appearance of hypertension ($\geq$140/90 mm Hg) and proteinuria ($\geq$300 mg/day), mainly after gestational week 20. In addition to the hallmark of proteinuria, other common clinical and laboratory manifestations include facial edema, hemoconcentration, thrombocytopenia, hypoalbuminemia, hyperuricemia, liver enzyme abnormalities, and hypocalciuria.

Differential diagnosis. When the multisystem involvement described in the section Diagnosis is present, a diagnosis of preeclampsia is clear. When hypertension is the only clinical manifestation, preeclampsia is difficult to diagnose; the National High Blood Pressure Education Program has recently stressed that a diagnosis of preeclampsia requires the presence of both *de novo* hypertension and proteinuria. In the absence of proteinuria, preeclampsia should still be considered when symptoms of headaches, blurring of vision, abdominal pain, elevated liver function test, or falling platelet count are present. Other findings that support a diagnosis of preeclampsia include increasing or elevated serum uric acid or creatinine, hypoalbuminuria, hypocalciuria, or the sudden appearance of edema.

The diagnosis is also difficult in women with preexisting chronic hypertension, in whom "superimposed preeclampsia" may be heralded when systolic or diastolic blood pressure levels suddenly increase, proteinuria appears, protein excretion increases dramatically, or if any of the less common signs and symptoms appear.

Clinical course. Regardless of its severity, the disorder resolves postpartum, and blood pressure usually normalizes within 10 days. Most of the morbidity occurs when the disease presents before gestational week 36, called *early preeclampsia* or *preeclampsia remote from term*. Left untreated, preeclampsia can progress to a life-threatening convulsive form termed *eclampsia*. A particularly dangerous form of preeclampsia is the HELLP syndrome (*h*emolysis *e*levated *l*iver function tests and *l*ow *p*latelets). This variant is characterized by the sudden appearance of a microangiopathic hemolytic anemia, a rapidly falling platelet count, and increments in bilirubin and liver enzymes; HELLP is an emergency that often requires interruption of the pregnancy to avoid progression to renal failure, sepsis, eclampsia with cerebral hemorrhage, and death.

SUGGESTED READING

1. Esplin MS, Fausett MB, Fraser A, et al. Paternal and maternal components of the predisposition to preeclampsia. *N Engl J Med.* 2001;344:867–872.
2. Kupferminc MJ, Eldoer A, Steinman N, et al. Increased frequency of genetic thrombophilia in women with complications of pregnancy. *N Engl J Med.* 1999;340:9–13.

3. Lindheimer MD, Roberts JM, Cunningham FG, eds. *Chesley's Hypertensive Disorders in Pregnancy*. 2nd ed. Stamford, CT: Appleton & Lange; 1999.

4. Report of the National High Blood Pressure Education Program Working Group on high blood pressure in pregnancy. *Am J Obstet Gynecol.* 2000;183:S1–S22.

5. Roberts JM, Cooper DW. Pathogenesis and genetics of pre-eclampsia. *Lancet.* 2001;357:53–56.

6. Roberts JM, Lain KY. Recent insights into the pathogenesis of preeclampsia. *Placenta.* 2002;23:359–372.

7. Smith GCS, Pell JP, Walsh D. Pregnancy complications and maternal risk of ischaemic heart disease: a retrospective cohort study of 129,290 births. *Lancet.* 2001;357:2002–2006.

8. Skjaerven R, Wilcox AJ, Lie RT. The interval between pregnancies and the risk of preeclampsia. *N Engl J Med.* 2002; 346:33–38.

9. Solomon CG, Seely EW. Brief review: hypertension in pregnancy; a manifestation of the insulin resistance syndrome? *Hypertension.* 2000;17:1072–1077.

10. Walker JJ. Pre-eclampsia. *Lancet.* 2000;356:1260–1265.

Chapter A58

Hypertension and Transplantation

Stephen C. Textor, MD

KEY POINTS

- Hypertension is a regular feature in solid organ transplantation because of preexisting conditions and vascular effects of immunosuppressive calcineurin inhibitors (cyclosporine and tacrolimus).

- Clinical features include reversal of circadian blood pressure pattern and interaction with corticosteroids.

- Interaction of hypertension with other major risk factors, including renal failure, diabetes, and preexisting atherosclerosis, makes control of posttransplant hypertension important.

See also Chapters A41, A42, A46, A49, A50, A66, A71, C112, C113, and C174

Pretransplant Cardiovascular Diseases

Transplantation regularly occurs in individuals with preexisting cardiovascular disease, including hypertension. Renal transplantation for end-stage renal disease in the United States is most commonly associated with diabetes and hypertensive arteriolar disease (arteriolosclerosis and nephrosclerosis). Cardiac transplantation often is associated with preexisting atherosclerosis. Pancreas transplantation in diabetes also carries a pretransplant burden of vascular disease before the addition of immunosuppression.

Posttransplant Hypertension

Hypertension after renal transplantation is recognized as a risk factor for graft failure. Levels of blood pressure 1 year after an allograft predict survival of the kidney over subsequent years. Early rises in blood pressure predict acute rejection. A major limitation to long-term success of cardiac allografts is the development of vascular injury designated *allograft vasculopathy*, which can appear as smooth, accelerated diffuse atherosclerotic disease affecting the coronaries. Although hypertension represents an important "non-immunologic" mediator of graft injury, whether effective blood pressure control can reduce these manifestations specific to the transplant environment is not yet proven in clinical trials.

Immunosuppression therapy (cyclosporin and tacrolimus).
Posttransplant hypertension occurs as a result of several factors. In addition to preexisting diseases, the combined effects of corticosteroids, calcineurin inhibition, and reduced renal function together produce a rise in blood pressure in 65% to 100% of solid organ transplant recipients. Most of the studies have identified cyclosporine-based immunosuppression as a major predisposing factor in posttransplant hypertension. Tacrolimus shares the final common pathway of calcineurin inhibition but differs in potency and the magnitude of specific side effects. Both agents cause hypertension, although weight gain, the rate of rise of blood pressure, and accelerated cardiovascular risk are more prominent with cyclosporine. Changes in lipids are less striking with tacrolimus, but nephrotoxicity and glucose intolerance appear to be greater. Glomerular filtration and renal blood flow predictably fall within hours of calcineurin inhibitor administration. Studies in normal volunteers indicate that a rise in arterial pressure can occur within hours and days of starting cyclosporine, even before sustained changes in renal function or sodium retention can be detected.

De novo hypertension or acceleration of previous hypertension occurs within weeks to months after solid organ transplantation (**Figure A58.1**). Different organ transplants have variable features of preexisting cardiovascular morbidity, blood pressure, and kidney function.

Salt sensitivity. Studies in renal and cardiac allograft recipients indicate that the degree and rate of blood pressure rise is affected by salt intake. Postoperative volume expansion combined with diminished glomerular filtration commonly leads to a rise in blood pressure soon after surgery in these settings. Efforts to limit sodium intake or use of diuretics to reduce arterial pressure may also contribute to rising serum creatinine

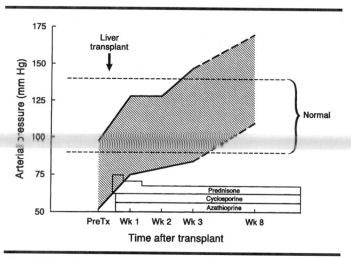

Figure A58.1. Arterial pressures during the first weeks after liver transplantation. Doses of immunosuppressive drugs, including glucocorticoids (prednisone) and cyclosporine, are highest immediately after transplantation. The progressive rise of arterial pressure over several weeks was accompanied by a reduction in cardiac output and increased system vascular resistance. PreTx, pretransplant.

levels. Salt and water depletion are especially problematic in patients with pancreas allografts connected to bladder drainage; these patients are susceptible to substantial volume depletion and orthostatic hypotension.

Hemodynamics. Over a period of a few weeks after transplant, hyperdynamic cardiac output levels fall to normal, and systemic vascular resistance rises from below normal levels to widespread vasoconstriction. These changes occur particularly during administration of cyclosporine but develop more gradually during tacrolimus administration. Postoperative volume expansion resolves gradually with pressure-induced natriuresis, despite reduced renal blood flows and glomerular filtration rates.

Alterations in vascular tone. Chronic posttransplant hypertension is associated with increased vascular resistance, mostly owing to the use of calcineurin inhibitors (**Table A58.1**). Early after transplantation, plasma renin activity is low in humans. Over time, plasma renin rises, possibly related to renal parenchymal injury and arteriolar disease ("hyalinosis"). Endothelium-derived vasoconstrictors, including endothelin and thromboxane, are increased, in systemic and local organ circulations. Impaired vasodilatation during exposure to calcineurin inhibitors reflects several abnormalities. Endothelium-derived prostacyclin falls in response to cyclosporine and to steroid administration. The activity of nitric oxide falls after exposure to cyclosporine or tacrolimus. Under some conditions these

changes appear to be reversible, but after long-term administration, hyaline thickening of arteriolar walls becomes fixed. It is likely that pathways determining the generation of oxygen free radicals shift toward greater degrees of oxidative stress.

Increased sympathetic nervous activity. Direct nerve traffic recordings in humans have confirmed animal data suggesting increased sympathetic nervous traffic associated with cyclosporin use. Sympathetic traffic is also increased after cardiac transplantation.

Interaction with corticosteroids. Most transplant regimens include oral corticosteroids, which alter sodium excretion and vascular reactivity, particularly when kidney function is diminished. When combined with calcineurin inhibitors, steroids regularly magnify the rise in arterial pressure posttransplantation. Recent trends to limit or withdraw steroid immunosuppression after liver transplantation have been associated with reductions in the prevalence and intensity of posttransplant hypertension.

Calcineurin nephrotoxicity. Tacrolimus and cyclosporine induce transient, intense vasoconstriction within the kidney soon after administration. This can sometimes be reversed on discontinuing or lowering the dose of drug. During sustained administration, however, vascular and interstitial changes develop ("striped interstitial fibrosis"), which eventually become irreversible despite drug withdrawal. During long-term calcineurin inhibition, nephrotoxicity can cause end-stage renal disease in up to 10% of cardiac and liver allograft recipients. As renal function deteriorates, hypertension commonly worsens, as with any other form of renal insufficiency.

Clinical Manifestations of Posttransplant Hypertension

Accelerated hypertension. Clinical manifestations of hypertension vary widely after transplantation (**Table A58.2**). Episodes of accelerated hypertension are occasionally associated with intracranial hemorrhage and microangiopathic hemolytic uremic syndrome with cyclosporine or tacrolimus. These processes can be reversed after withholding the drug temporarily, after which the drug usually can be restarted with effective antihypertensive therapy.

Circadian reversal. A striking and regularly observed feature is the reversal of circadian blood pressure regulation. Daytime blood pressures are often the lowest of the 24-hour period, with a loss of

---

Table A58.1. Proposed Mechanisms of Hypertension after Clinical Transplantation

Endothelial dysfunction with disturbed vasomotor systems
   Reduced nitric oxide production
   Reduced prostacyclin excretion
   Increased endothelin release
   ?Increased thromboxane
Renal dysfunction with impaired sodium excretion
Increased sympathetic neural activity

Table A58.2. Clinical Manifestations of Hypertension after Transplantation

Rapid rise in arterial pressure after introduction of cyclosporine/
   steroid immunosuppression
Vasoconstriction in most vascular beds
Accelerated hypertension if untreated
   Encephalopathy
   Microangiopathic hemolysis
   Intravascular thrombosis
   Intracranial hemorrhage
   Reversal of circadian blood pressure patterns
   Acceleration of atherosclerosis

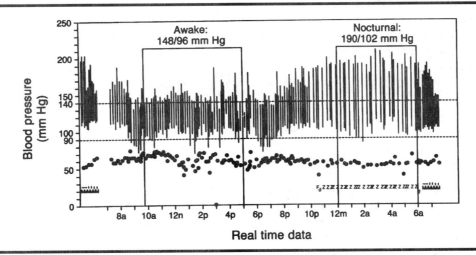

Figure A58.2. Ambulatory blood pressure monitoring in a young woman 4 months after transplantation. Pressures when the patient is awake underestimate the average 24-hour pressure because of a paradoxic nocturnal rise in pressure. This is sometimes associated with a distinctive syndrome of nocturia, headache, and disturbed sleep. a, AM; m, midnight; n, noon; p, PM. (From Textor SC, Taler SJ, Canzanello VJ, Schwartz L. Cyclosporine, blood pressure, and atherosclerosis. *Cardiol Rev.* 1997;5:141–151, with permission.)

nocturnal blood pressure fall and, occasionally, a considerable nocturnal rise (**Figure A58.2**). Patients sometimes describe a reversed day-night pattern of urination with profound nocturia. Occasionally there are nocturnal episodes of accelerated hypertension, headache, and encephalopathy that may be unrecognized. Circadian reversal has been observed after renal, liver, and cardiac transplantation, most commonly during the first year. It may reflect the effects of corticosteroids, disturbed autonomic regulation, or other mechanisms. Although nearly universal during the first year after transplant, restoration of more normal circadian patterns can develop over subsequent years.

Long-term blood pressure trends. Generally, posttransplant hypertension persists despite gradual reduction of immunosuppression after the first year. The intensity and antihypertensive requirements may stabilize or diminish with time. These observations argue for some degree of dose-dependency related to calcineurin inhibitors and steroid use. Some cases of posttransplantation hypertension have resolved entirely after several years, despite stable graft function and persistent calcineurin effect on the kidney. This most often occurs in younger women.

Importance of aggressive blood pressure control. Considering the pretransplant comorbid cardiovascular disease burden associated with organ failure, particularly from diabetes, the importance of preventing additional cardiovascular disease after transplantation cannot be overstated. Death from cardiovascular disease with a functioning kidney is now among the most common causes of graft loss after kidney transplantation.

SUGGESTED READING

1. Canzanello VJ, Schwartz L, Taler SJ, et al. Evolution of cardiovascular risk after liver transplantation: a comparison of cyclosporine A and tacrolimus (FK506). *Liver Transpl Surg.* 1997;3:1–9.
2. Cosio FG, Pelletier RP, Pesavento TE, et al. Elevated blood pressure predicts the risk of acute rejection in renal allograft recipients. *Kidney Int.* 2001;59:1158–1164.
3. Mange KC, Cizman B, Joffe M, Feldman HI. Arterial hypertension and renal allograft survival. *JAMA.* 2000;283:633–638.
4. Sander M, Victor RG. Hypertension after cardiac transplantation: pathophysiology and management. *Curr Opin Nephrol Hypertens.* 1995;4:443–451.
5. Taler SJ, Textor SC, Canzanello VJ, et al. Role of steroid dose in hypertension early after liver transplantation with tacrolimus (FK506) and cyclosporine. *Transplantation.* 1996;62:1588–1592.
6. Textor SC, Taler SJ, Canzanello VJ, et al. Posttransplantation hypertension related to calcineurin inhibitors. *Liver Transpl.* 2000;6:521–530.
7. Textor SC, Wiesner R, Wilson DJ, et al. Systemic and renal hemodynamic differences between FK506 and cyclosporine A in liver transplant recipients. *Transplantation.* 1993;55:1332–1339.
8. van de Borne P, Leeman M, Primo G, Degaute JP. Reappearance of a normal circadian rhythm of blood pressure after cardiac transplantation. *Am J Cardiol.* 1992;69:794–801.

Aging, Hypertension, and the Heart

Edward G. Lakatta, MD

KEY POINTS

- The incidence of hypertension and resultant heart failure increase dramatically with age.

- Human, animal, cellular, and molecular perspectives indicate that hypertension and aging both cause similar patterns of altered heart structure and function and gene expression.

- The interaction of mechanisms that underlie cardiac and vascular aging with those that cause hypertension substantially modifies the hypertensive phenotype as organisms age.

See also Chapters A35, A36, A38, A41, A60–A62, A78, B83, C118, C119, C151, C155, and C156

Hypertension, Aging, and Heart Failure

It is estimated that by the year 2035, nearly 1 in 4 individuals in the United States will be 65 years of age or older. Hypertension and resultant complications, including chronic heart failure (see Chapter B83), reach epidemic proportions among older persons. In older individuals, specific pathophysiologic mechanisms that underlie hypertension and heart failure become superimposed on heart and vascular substrates that are modified by an aging process, per se. Thus, an understanding of how aging modifies cardiovascular structure and function is critical to an understanding of hypertension in the geriatric population.

Aging-Hypertension Continuum

Heart structure and function at rest. A unified interpretation of cardiac changes that accompany advancing age in otherwise healthy persons without clinical hypertension suggests that the observed changes are at least in part adaptations to age-related arterial changes (**Figure A59.1**; see also Chapter A60). The major age-related change affecting the heart is large arterial stiffening, which leads to increased pulse wave velocity and early reflected pulse waves, which produce late-systolic augmentation in arterial pressure, with a reduced or maintained diastolic pressure. There is usually a mild increase in systemic vascular resistance (SVR) and an increase in pulse pressure, accompanied by aortic dilatation and wall thickening. Increased left ventricular (LV) wall thickness, largely due to an increase in ventricular myocyte size, results in part from increased vascular impedance and acts to moderate the increase in LV wall tension. Modest focal increases in collagen also occur with aging.

Prolonged contractile activation of the thickened LV wall maintains a normal ejection time in the presence of the late augmentation of aortic impedance, preserving systolic cardiac pump function at rest. A downside of prolonged contractile activation is that at the time of the mitral valve opening, myocardial relax-

ation is less complete in older than in younger individuals, and early LV filling rate tends to be reduced. Structural changes and functional heterogeneity occurring within the LV with aging may also contribute to this reduction in peak LV filling rate. However, concomitant age-related cardiac adaptations, especially left atrial enlargement and an enhanced atrial contribution to ventricular filling, compensate for the reduced early diastolic filling and act to maintain end-diastolic volume. Potential age-associated changes in the concentrations or sensitivities to pressor hormones, growth factors, and cytokines, (catecholamines, angiotensin II, endothelin, transforming growth factor β, and fibroblast growth factor) that influence myocardial or vascular cells or their extracellular matrices, may also have a role in the cardiac adaptive changes as depicted in Figure A59.1.

Impaired cardiovascular reserve. Impaired LV ejection, heart rate, and reserve capacity are accompanied by an acute modest increase in LV end-diastolic volume in healthy, community dwelling persons (**Table A59.1**). Mechanisms that underlie the age-associated reduction in maximum ejection fraction are multifactorial and include (a) a reduction in intrinsic myocardial contractility, (b) an increase in afterload, (c) a diminished effectiveness of the autonomic modulation of LV contractility and arterial afterload, and (d) mismatching of arterial-ventricular loading. Although these age-associated changes in cardiovascular reserve, per se, are insufficient to produce clinical heart failure, they do affect the clinical presentation of heart failure by modifying the threshold for symptoms and signs and the severity and prognosis of heart failure.

Deficient catecholamine-modulation of cardiovascular function. Multiple lines of evidence support the idea that the efficiency of postsynaptic β-adrenergic signaling declines with aging, most likely due in part to desensitization of the β-receptor signaling cascade. All of the factors that have been identified to play a role in the deficient cardiovascular reserve with aging,

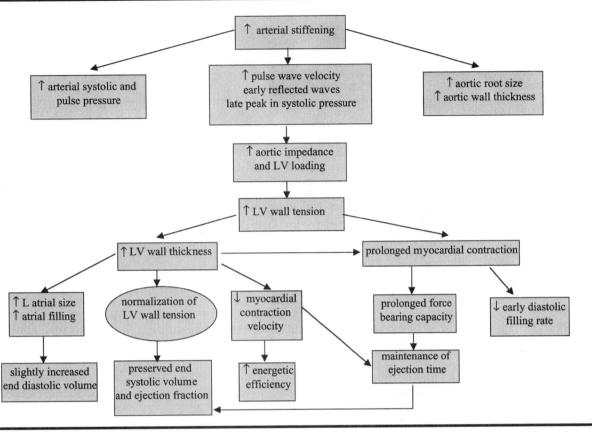

Figure A59.1. Arterial and cardiac changes that occur with aging in healthy humans. One interpretation of the constellation (*flow of arrows*) is that vascular changes lead to cardiac structural and functional alterations that maintain cardiac function. ↓, decrease; ↑, increase; LV, left ventricular. [From Lakatta EG. Cardiovascular regulatory mechanisms in advanced age. *Physiol Rev.* 1993;73(2):413–465, with permission.]

reduced heart rate, prolonged filling time, increased afterload (cardiac and vascular), reduced myocardial contractility, and redistribution of blood flow reflect a deficient response to sympathetic stimulation. Apparent deficits in sympathetic modulation of these functions during acute stress in older persons may occur in the presence of exaggerated plasma levels of norepinephrine and epinephrine.

Chronic hypertension mimics accelerated aging. Parallel structural and functional changes in the large arteries (stiffness), cardiac mass (hypertrophy), and myocardial relaxation and filling (diastolic dysfunction) occur in normotensive aging and hypertension at any age. This continuum of age-related change is simply accelerated in individuals with chronic hypertension, so that the same changes occur at an earlier age or to an exaggerated degree. In this regard, the traditional clinical distinction between normotension and hypertension is quite arbitrary, although it may be useful with regard to cardiovascular risk stratification. In fact, the similarities between aging and hypertension are so striking that aging can be considered to be "muted hypertension," while hypertension can be likened to "accelerated aging."

Some differences exist, however, between hypertension and aging. For example, in contrast to a modest increase in SVR in normotensive aging, in hypertension, SVR increases more substantially. Increased SVR plays a greater role in vascular loading of the heart in hypertensives than in normotensives. Additionally, in older hypertensives, resting stroke volume and cardiac output are not maintained at levels seen in younger hypertensives.

Cellular Mechanisms of Cardiac Aging: Perspectives from Animal Models

Many age-associated changes in cardiac structure and function observed in humans also occur across a wide range of species. The vast majority of studies of cardiac cellular aging have employed rodent models (**Table A59.2**).

Table A59.1. Exhaustive Upright Exercise: Reduction in Aerobic Capacity and Cardiac Regulation Between Ages of 20 and 80 Years in Healthy Men and Women

Oxygen consumption	↓ (50%)
(Arteriovenous) O_2	↓ (25%)
Cardiac index	↓ (25%)
Heart rate	↓ (25%)
Stroke volume	No change
Preload	
End-diastolic volume	↑ (30%)
Afterload	↑
Vascular (pulmonary vascular resistance)	↑ (30%)
Cardiac (end-systolic volume)	↑ (275%)
Cardiac (end-diastolic volume)	↑ (30%)
Contractility	↓ (60%)
Ejection fraction	↓ (15%)
Plasma catecholamines	↑
Cardiac and vascular responses to β-adrenergic stimulation	↓

↓, decrease; ↑, increase.

Table A59.2. Myocardial Changes with Adult Aging in Rodents

STRUCTURAL Δ	FUNCTIONAL Δ	IONIC, BIOPHYSICAL/BIOCHEMICAL MECHANISM(S)	MOLECULAR MECHANISMS
Myocyte size Myocyte number	Prolonged contraction	Prolonged cytosolic Ca^{2+} transient	
		↓ Sarcoplasmic reticulum Ca^{2+} pumping rate	↓ Sarcoplasmic reticulum Ca^{2+} pump mRNA
		↓ Pump site density	No Δ calsequestrin mRNA
	Prolonged action potential	↓ Calcium influx inactivation	↑ Na-Ca exchanger mRNA
		↓ Transient outward K^+ current density	
	Diminished contraction velocity	↓ α MHC protein	↓ α MHC mRNA
		↑ β MHC protein	↑ β MHC mRNA
		↓ Myosin ATPase activity	No Δ Actin mRNA
		↓ RXRβ1 and γ mRNA	↓ RXRβ1 and γ mRNA
		↓ RXRβ1 and γ protein	
		↓ Thyroid receptor protein	
	Diminished β-adrenergic contractile response	↓ Coupling β-adrenergic receptor-acylase	↓ $β_1$AR mRNA
		No Δ inhibitory G protein activation	No Δ β-adrenergic receptor kinase mRNA
		No Δ β-adrenergic receptor kinase activity	
		↓ Troponin-I pholpholamban	
		↓ Phospholamban phosphorylation	
		↓ Calcium influx augmentation	
		↓ Intracellular calcium transient augmentation	
		↑ Enkephalin peptides	↑ Proenkephalin mRNA
↑Y Matrix connective tissue	↑ Myocardial stiffness	↑ Hydroxyline proline content	↑ Collagen mRNA
		↑ Activity of myocardial renin-angiotensin system	↑ Fibronectin mRNA
			↑ Angiotensin AT-1 receptor mRNA
		↑ Atrial natriuretic peptide	↑ Atrial natriuretic peptide mRNA
	↓ Growth response		↓ Induction of immediate early genes
	↓ Heat shock response		↓ Activation of heat shock factor

↓, decrease; ↑, increase; Δ, change; ATPase, adenosine triphosphatase; MHC, myosin heavy chain; mRNA, messenger RNA; RXR, retinoid X-receptor.

Left ventricular structure. Even in the absence of hypertension, the hearts of senescent rats (24–30 months of age) exhibit moderate LV hypertrophy (25%) compared to hearts from young and middle-aged animals. Matrix and myocyte volume increase. The average LV collagen content doubles between adulthood and senescence and the level of fibronectin is also markedly increased. The average volume of individual cardiomyocytes approximately doubles over the adult range, whereas the number of myocytes generally decreases with aging, due primarily to apoptosis with some increase in necrosis.

Excitation-contraction-relaxation. The kinetics of cellular reactions that underlie cardiac automaticity are reduced in senescent versus younger adult rodent hearts. There is prolongation of the action potential, the transient increase in cytosolic Ca^{2+} evoked by the action potential, and the ensuing contraction (Table A59.2). This altered pattern of Ca^{2+} regulation allows the myocardium of older hearts to generate force for a longer time after excitation. The prolonged isovolumic relaxation period in the healthy human heart with aging may, in part, be attributable to prolonged contractile protein Ca^{2+} activation, enabling the continued ejection of blood during late systole, a beneficial adaptation with respect to enhanced vascular stiffness and early reflected pulse waves (Figure A59.1).

Ca^{2+} loading. Excess cardiomyocyte Ca^{2+} loading can lead to dysregulation of Ca^{2+} homeostasis, impaired diastolic and systolic function, arrhythmias, and cell death. In the senescent heart during high pacing rates, the excess of cytosolic Ca^{2+} promotes incomplete relaxation and favors increased diastolic tone. The senescent heart also exhibits a reduced threshold for pathologic manifestations of excess Ca^{2+} loading during conditions (physiologic and pharmacologic) that increase Ca^{2+} influx such as neurotransmitter stimulation, postischemic reperfusion, or oxidative stress. Causes of reduced Ca^{2+} tolerance of the older cardiocytes, compared to those of the younger adult heart, include (a) changes in Ca^{2+} regulatory protein levels (Table A59.2) and (b) alterations in the composition of membranes in which Ca^{2+} regulatory proteins reside, including an increase in membrane $\omega_6{:}\omega_3$-polyunsaturated fatty acids with aging. It is believed that ω_3-polyunsaturated fatty acid promotes cardiac calcium dysregulation and enhances the likelihood of intracellular generation of reactive oxygen species.

Adrenergic receptors. Studies in isolated LV muscle in individual rat ventricular cardiomyocytes, similar to recent studies in humans, indicate that a reduced response to β-adrenoceptor (βAR) stimulation occurs with aging. The most remarkable change within the βAR system with aging appears to be the decrease in the efficacy of coupling of the βAR receptor to the postreceptor signal transduction system that generates the contractile response. Aging is also accompanied by a striking increase in ventricular messenger RNA and protein levels of atrial natriuretic peptide, proenkephalin, and adenosine. Negative effects of opioid peptides and adenosine on cardiac contraction parameters may also contribute to age-associated reduction in the βAR responsiveness of the heart.

Integrated view. Coordinated changes in several key steps of excitation-contraction coupling and its regulation by cell-surface receptors occur with aging. These changes, which are at the structural, biochemical, biophysical, and molecular, result in a prolonged Ca^{2+} transients and prolonged contraction. The resultant altered Ca^{2+} homeostasis permits prolonged and efficient force-bearing capacity in the older heart, but renders it more prone to spontaneous Ca^{2+} oscillations and Ca^{2+}-dependent arrhythmias. β-Adrenergic modulation of excitation-contraction coupling mechanisms also becomes impaired.

Pressure overload in young rats mimics normotensive aging.
Many of the age-associated changes in structure, function, and gene expression that occur with aging also occur in the hypertrophied myocardium of younger animals with experimentally induced chronic hypertension. Additionally, similar reductions in cellular RNA concentration and the rate of protein synthesis are observed with aging and chronic myocardial overload in the rat model. It is tempting to speculate that this nearly identical pattern of change in gene expression in young hypertensive and older normotensive rodents may indicate that a common set of transcription factors regulates cardiac cellular adaptation during pressure-overload hypertrophy and aging. This particular constellation of shifts in gene expression appears to be adaptive, in that it allows for an energy-efficient and prolonged contraction. In the hypertensive rodent heart, it can be inferred that these changes in gene expression permit functional adaptations in response to an increased vascular "afterload." Specifically, the capacity for molecular adaptation to hemodynamic overload, ischemia, or both is diminished in aged hearts.

Heart failure at older ages in hypertensive rats.
With advancing age in the spontaneously hypertensive rat (SHR), chronic hypertension and cardiac hypertrophy eventually give way to heart failure and normotension. Young adult and middle-aged SHRs exhibit compensated cardiac hypertrophy. Depressed contractile function and increased fibrosis are observed in advanced age, beginning at approximately 18 months. The transition from compensated hypertrophy to failure with aging in the SHR seems to demonstrate quite well the consequences of interactions between "normal aging" and disease. This transition is characterized by a progressive impairment of LV function and ventricular dilatation in the absence of an additional increase in LV mass. The pattern of altered gene expression that accompanies the transition to heart failure during advanced age in the SHR supports the notion that total contractile protein decreases whereas total connective tissue protein increases and suggests that these processes are regulated at a pretranslational level. Although the accumulated effects of long-term hypertension and the genetic nature of the model cannot be dismissed, it seems appropriate to hypothesize that the effects of normal aging reduce the reserve capacity of the heart for adaptation in the SHR and conspire with hypertension to decrease the chances of survival.

Therapeutic Implications
Alterations in cardiovascular function that exceed the identified limits for age-associated changes for healthy elderly individuals are most likely manifestations of interactions of aging with age-associated changes of severe physical deconditioning or with other cardiovascular diseases. Specific cardiovascular changes that occur during aging in health perhaps should not truly be considered to reflect a normal process because they are so similar to those seen with hypertension and other risk factors that merit intervention. Lifestyle changes such as regular vigorous exercise have already been shown to be effective in retarding the speed of cardiac aging, including improvements in ventricular ejection capacity and reductions in cardiac afterload via reduced arterial stiffness.

SUGGESTED READING
1. Lakatta EG. Cardiovascular regulatory mechanisms in advanced age. *Physiol Rev.* 1993;73:413–465.
2. Lakatta EG. Cardiovascular aging research: the next horizons. *J Am Geriatr Soc.* 1999;47:613–625.
3. Lakatta EG. Age-associated cardiovascular changes in health: impact on cardiovascular disease in older persons. *Heart Failure Rev.* 2002;7:29–49.
4. Lakatta EG, Schulman SP, Gerstenblith G. Cardiovascular aging in health and therapeutic considerations with respect to cardiovascular disease in older patients. In: Fuster V, Alexander RW, King S, et al, eds. *Hurst's The Heart.* New York, NY: McGraw-Hill; 2001:2329–2355.
5. Lakatta EG, Sollott SJ, Pepe S. The old heart: operating on the edge. In: Bock G, Goode JA, eds. *Aging Vulnerability: Causes and Interventions.* Novartis Foundation Symposium 235. Chichester, NY: John Wiley and Sons; 2001:172–201.

Chapter A60

Aging, Hypertension, and Arterial Stiffness

Stanley S. Franklin, MD, FACP, FACC; Joseph L. Izzo, Jr, MD

KEY POINTS

- Increased central arterial stiffness is caused by functional and structural changes in the contractile-elastic units of the vessel wall media.

- Central arterial stiffness and systolic pressure are major determinants of cardiovascular risk in older people (>50 years of age), whereas increased systemic vascular resistance and diastolic pressure predominate in younger adults.

- Central arterial stiffness and early wave reflection increase peak aortic systolic blood pressure and left ventricular workload.

- As arteries stiffen and pulse wave amplification decreases with aging, there is a gradual shift from diastolic to systolic and eventually to pulse pressure as predictors of cardiovascular risk.

See also Chapters A38, A59, A61–A63, A78, B81–B84, C119, and C151

Physiology of Pulsatile Flow

The arterial system has dual interrelated functions: (a) to provide a sufficient quantity of blood to various tissues of the body (the conduit function) and (b) to convert highly pulsatile flow into more continuous flow at the level of the small arteries (the cushioning, compliance, or capacitance function). The conduit function allows the maintenance of relatively constant mean arterial blood pressure (MAP) between the ascending aorta and the peripheral arteries and is achieved by the mechanical and neural integration of cardiac output and systemic vascular resistance. MAP, in the presence of a constant cardiac output, represents the static or steady-state component of the circulation during diastole and is a reasonable surrogate for systemic vascular resistance. The pulsatile load is borne primarily by elastic-containing central arteries—the thoracic aorta and its branches, which fulfill the bulk of the cushioning function by expanding during systole to store some but not all of each stroke volume and then contracting during diastole to facilitate peripheral run-off of the stored blood. The cushioning function thus supports diastolic blood flow to peripheral tissues.

Determination of Systolic and Pulse Pressure

The amount of rise in systolic blood pressure (SBP) during systole depends on 3 major factors: (a) left ventricular performance, (b) the stiffness of the central conduit arteries, and (c) the degree of systemic resistance. The minimum diastolic blood pressure (DBP) in a given individual is most heavily dependent on 2 major factors: (a) the duration of diastole and (b) the rate of aortic outflow, both of which are determined by systemic resistance and the magnitude of stiffness of the thoracic aorta (**Figure A60.1**). Most important, DBP rises with increased resistance but falls with increased stiffness. Pulse pressure (PP), the difference between peak SBP and end-DBP, represents a surrogate measurement of central elastic artery stiffness in the presence of a constant cardiac output and heart rate. Thus, the central arterial stiffening is manifested by 3 factors: (a) a rise in SBP, (b) a fall in DBP, and (c) a resulting increase in PP.

Structural Relations within the Arterial Wall

The elastic behavior of the arterial wall depends primarily on the composition and arrangement of the materials that make up the tunica media or middle layer of the arterial wall. In the media of the thoracic aorta and its immediate branches are large attachments of elastic lamellae to smooth muscle cells, constituting the contractile-elastic units, which are arranged in an alternating oblique pattern that exerts maximum force in a circumferential direction. This arrangement is important for the balance of normal changes in intraluminal pressure and tension that occur during systole and diastole. In a normal young healthy person, the medial fibrous elements of the thoracic aorta contain a predominance of elastin over collagen, but as one proceeds distally along the arterial tree there is a rapid reversal of the proportion, with more collagen than elastin in the peripheral muscular arteries. Thus, the thoracic aorta and its immediate branches (such as carotid arteries) show greater elasticity, whereas more distal vessels become progressively stiffer.

Pulse Wave Amplification

The intrinsic changes in the vascular tree mentioned above, along with the tapering of the aorta, lead to the phenomenon of pulse wave amplification. Pulse wave amplification causes central aortic pulse pressure to be lower than peripheral vascular pulse pressure (**Figure A60.2**). This phenomenon is clinically important in that blood pressures determined at intermediate sites such as the brachial artery are intrinsically different from pressures measured simultaneously at the aortic root or in peripheral arteries. Thus, brachial blood pressure is intrinsically limited in its ability to assess pulsatile pressure loads within the vascular tree.

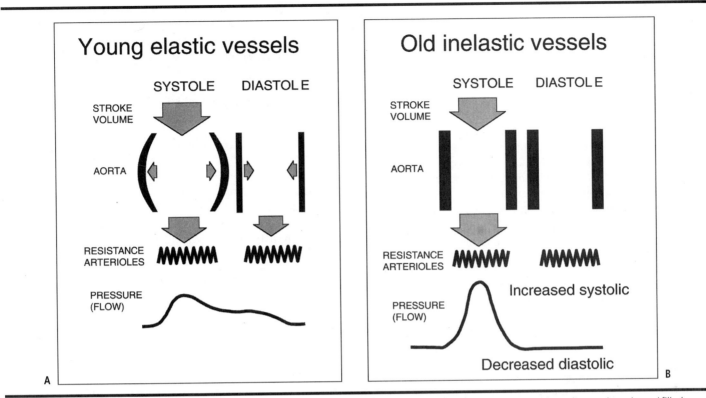

Figure A60.1.   Pathogenesis of wide pulse pressure. **A:** In a younger subject whose aorta has a high elastin content, each cardiac stroke volume (*filled arrow at top*) distends the aorta, which has a reservoir or capacitance function. As a result, not all of each stroke volume is transmitted through the distal resistance arterioles during systole. Elastic recoil of the aorta during diastole causes the remnant of the original stroke volume to be transmitted distally. The result is a relatively smooth arterial pulse contour and narrow pulse pressure. **B:** In an aorta of an older person, loss of elastin and gain of collagen increases stiffness and destroys the capacitance function. In this example, the entire stroke volume is transmitted through the resistance arterioles during systole, with no diastolic flow. The result is a direct increase in systolic pressure, a decrease in diastolic pressure, and a widening of pulse pressure. In this example, stroke volume, systemic resistance, and mean arterial pressure are equal in the younger and older subject. (Adapted from Izzo JL. *J Am Geriatr Soc.* 1981;29:520–534.)

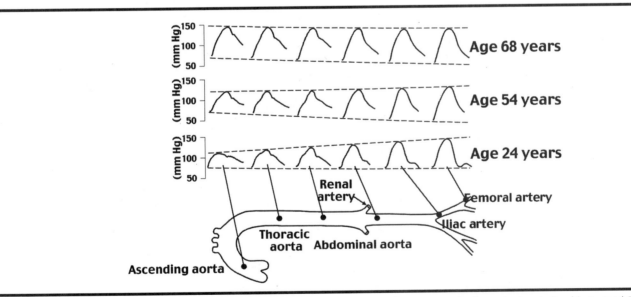

Figure A60.2.   Pressure wave recorded along the arterial tree from the proximal ascending aorta to the femoral artery in 3 subjects aged 24, 54, and 68 years. (From Nichols WW, Avolio AP, Kelly RP, O'Rourke MF. Effect of age and of hypertension on wave travel and reflections. In: O'Rourke MF, Safar ME, Dzau V, eds. *Arterial Vasodilation: Mechanisms and Therapy.* London: Edward Arnold; 1993, with permission.)

Hypertension and Arterial Stiffness (Arteriosclerosis)

Hypertension can produce arterial stiffness by functional and structural mechanisms. With the development of hypertension and increased intramural pressure, the load-bearing elastic lamellae stretch and become functionally stiffer. Constriction also tends to favor increased stiffness.

Heterogeneity of changes. Importantly, not all arteries become stiff with age. Although there are long-standing structural changes with aging that cause increased stiffness of the thoracic aorta and its branches, the more peripheral muscular arteries (such as the brachial artery) retain their normal or even increased elasticity in people with hypertension. Thus, studies of compliance of peripheral vessels in hypertension cannot be interpreted as reflectors of a uniform change in arterial elastic properties.

Loss of elastin. Central arterial elasticity is critically dependent on normal content and function of the matrix protein elastin, which, with a half-life of 40 years, is one of the most stable proteins in the body. Despite this stability, fatigue of elastin fibers and lamellae can occur by the sixth decade of life from the accumulated cyclic stress of more than 2 billion aorta expansions during ventricular contraction. Long-standing cyclic stress in the media of elastic-containing arteries produces fatigue and eventual fracturing of elastin along with structural changes of the extracellular matrix that include proliferation of collagen and deposition of calcium. Humoral factors, cytokines, and oxidative metabolites may also play a role. This degenerative process, classically termed *arteriosclerosis*, is the pathologic process that results in increased central arterial stiffness. Hypertension left untreated accelerates the rate of development of conduit artery stiffness. This, in turn, can perpetuate a vicious cycle of accelerated hypertension and further increases in stiffness.

Atherosclerosis versus Arteriosclerosis

Disease processes such as diabetes, chronic renal failure and generalized atherosclerosis can accelerate aging of the aorta and central arteries with earlier development of arterial stiffness. Arteriosclerosis is often confused with atherosclerosis, but these 2 disease states are independent, frequently overlapping, conditions (**Table A60.1**). Atherosclerosis is primarily focal, starts in the intima, and tends to be occlusive. Arteriosclerosis tends to be diffuse, starts in the media, and frequently results in a dilated and tortuous aorta. Moreover, the pathophysiology of atherosclerosis is that of inflammatory disease with lipid-containing plaques and predominantly downstream ischemic disease. Arteriosclerosis represents degenerative large arterial disease, which results in increased thoracic aortic stiffness and elevated left ventricular workload.

Pulse Wave Propagation and Reflection

Pulse wave velocity. It is a fundamental principle that pulse waves travel faster in stiffer arteries, and therefore measurement of pulse wave velocity is a clinical surrogate for large arterial stiffness. Given that peripheral arteries are usually stiffer than central arteries, however, an intrinsic limitation of the method is its heterogeneity. Pulse wave velocity has been shown to be a predictor of cardiovascular morbidity and mortality, but it remains a research tool at present.

Pulse wave morphology. The morphology of any pulse wave results from the summation of incident (forward-traveling) and reflected (backward-traveling) pressure waves (**Figure A60.3**). Pulse wave propagation and reflection varies considerably according to age. In young adults with full height and maximum elasticity of their central arteries, the summation of the incident (forward-traveling) arterial pressure wave with the reflected (backward-traveling) wave results in progressive pulse pressure amplification so that SBP is 20 to 30 mm Hg higher at the brachial artery than at the ascending aorta. This contrasts with MAP and DBP, surrogates for peripheral resistance, which fall minimally with distance from the heart in vessels at all ages.

Wave reflection and ventricular load. The degree of wave reflection and the pulse wave morphology are directly dependent on aging and arterial stiffness. The development of increasing arterial stiffness and increased wave reflection with aging and hypertension completely abolishes the difference between central and peripheral pulse pressure by age 50 to 60 years (Figure A60.2). Arterial stiffness impacts the left ventricle in 2 ways: (a) the ejection of the stroke volume from the left ventricle into a stiff aorta generates a higher early systolic pressure and (b) the increased velocity of the aortic pulse wave allows the reflected waves to return to the aortic root earlier, during late systole, in which the reflected waves summate with the forward-traveling wave to create an increase or "augmentation" of central systolic pressure and ventricular load (Figure A60.3). In elderly persons with isolated systolic hypertension, aortic systolic pressure can be increased by as much as 30 to 40 mm Hg as a result of the early return of wave reflection. This increased ventricular load is essentially "wasted" cardiac work. Left ventricular workload is thus ultimately dependent on 3 major components: (a) systemic vascular resistance, (b) early systolic impedance increases to the forward-traveling wave caused by proximal aortic stiffening, and (c) late systolic impedance increases caused by early return of the reflected (backward-traveling) pressure wave. Cardiovascular risk is thus more closely related to peak SBP in the central ascending aorta, which is the principal determinant of left ventricular workload, than by simultaneously recorded SBP readings in peripheral arteries.

Table A60.1. Differential Features of Arteriosclerosis and Atherosclerosis

FEATURES	ATHEROSCLEROSIS	ARTERIOSCLEROSIS
Distribution	Focal	Diffuse
Location	Intima	Media, adventitia
Geometry	Occlusive	Dilatory
Pathology	Plaque	↓ Elastin, ↑ collagen, Ca^{2+}
Physiology	Inflammation	Large artery stiffness
Hemodynamics	Ischemia	↑ Left ventricular workload

↓, decrease; ↑ increase.

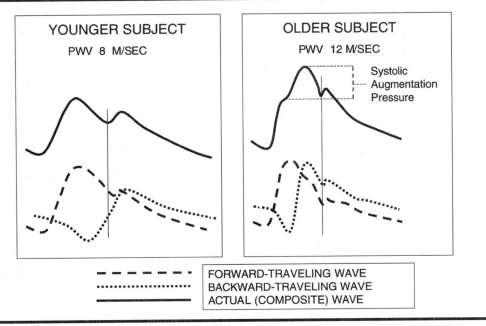

Figure A60.3. Effect of age on peak systolic pressure. All arterial waveforms are composite waves (*heavy line*) composed of forward-traveling (*dashed line*) and backward-traveling (*dotted line*) reflected waves. Vertical line represents aortic valve closure. Left panel represents the arterial waveform in a younger subject with pulse wave velocity (PWV) 8 m/sec; the reflected wave returns to the aortic root in early diastole in which it augments diastolic pressure and improves coronary filling. Right panel represents the arterial waveform in an older subject with PWV 12 m/sec. PWV is directly proportional to arterial stiffness. In the older subject with stiffer arteries, the reflected wave returns to the aortic root in late systole, in which it augments peak systolic pressure, increases ventricular loading, and promotes ventricular hypertrophy. (Modified from Asmar R. *Arterial Stiffness.*)

Clinical Impact of Arteriosclerosis

Age-related change in blood pressure. Both cross-sectional and longitudinal population studies show that SBP rises progressively beginning in adolescence. In contrast, DBP initially increases with age, levels off at approximately age 50 years, and decreases after age 60 years. Thus, PP begins to increase after age 50. The rise in SBP and DBP up to age 50 years can best be explained by the dominance of peripheral vascular resistance in systemic hemodynamics (**Table A60.2**). The transition age of 50 to 60 years when DBP levels off constitutes a near balancing of increased resistance and increased thoracic aortic stiffness as hemodynamic determinants. After age 60 years, the fall in DBP and the rapid widening of PP become surrogate indicators of central arterial stiffening. Indeed, after age 60 years, central arterial stiffness, rather than systemic vascular resistance, becomes the dominant hemodynamic factor in normotensive and hypertensive individuals.

Relation to coronary heart disease risk. SBP is superior to DBP as a predictor of coronary heart disease (CHD) risk after the age of 50 years (**Figure A60.4**). However, many recent studies, generally in older individuals, have shown PP to be slightly superior to SBP in predicting risk. When both SBP and DBP were included in a dual Cox model in individuals 50 to 79 years of age from the original Framingham cohort, CHD risk was inversely related to DBP at any given level of SBP, suggesting that PP predicted risk better than either SBP or DBP alone. A far greater increase in CHD risk occurred with increments in PP at a constant SBP than did parallel increments in SBP and DBP at a constant PP. From the age of 20 to 79 years, there was a continuous, graded shift from DBP to SBP and eventually to PP as predictors of CHD risk. In individuals less than 50 years of age, DBP was the strongest predictor. Age 50 to 59 years was a transition period when all 3 blood pressure indexes were comparable predictors, and from 60 years of age onward, DBP was negatively related to CHD risk so that PP became superior to SBP. Overall, the power of diastolic pressure to predict risk disappears by middle age and is supplanted by systolic pressure in individuals more than age 50 (Figure A60.4). CHD events are therefore related more to the pulsatile stress of central elastic arterial stiffness during systole than to the steady-state stress of peripheral arteriolar resistance during diastole.

Table A60.2. Hemodynamic Patterns of Age-Related Changes in Blood Pressure

AGE (YR)	DIASTOLIC BLOOD PRESSURE (MM HG)	SYSTOLIC BLOOD PRESSURE (MM HG)	MEAN ARTERIAL PRESSURE (MM HG)	PULSE PRESSURE (MM HG)	HEMODYNAMICS
30–49	↑	↑	↑	→↑	R>S
50–59	→	↑	→	↑↑	R = S
≥60	↓	↑	→↓	↑↑↑↑	S>R

↓, decrease; ↑, increase; →, no change; R, small-vessel resistance; S, large-vessel stiffness.

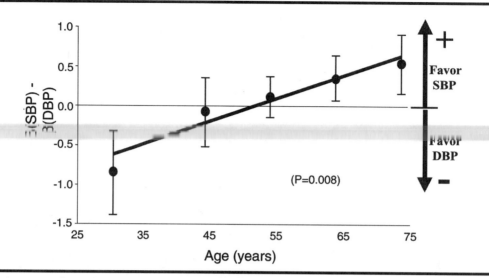

Figure A60.4.   Difference in coronary heart disease prediction between systolic blood pressure (SBP) and diastolic (DBP) as function of age. Difference in β coefficients (from Cox proportional-hazards regression) between SBP and DBP is plotted as function of age, obtaining this regression line: β(SBP) − β(DBP) = −1.49848 + 0.0290 × age ($p = .008$). (From Franklin SS, Larson MG, Khan SA, et al. Does the relation of blood pressure to coronary heart disease risk change with aging? The Framingham Heart Study. *Circulation.* 2001;103:1245–1249, with permission.)

Limitations of Pulse Pressure as a Risk Marker

Increased PP may be a surrogate marker for several possible pathologic mechanisms, all originating from underlying increased central arterial stiffness and contributing to disorders of the myocardium. Increased aortic pulsatile load elevates left ventricular systolic wall stress, decreases coronary flow reserve, impairs left ventricular relaxation, and may lead to diastolic dysfunction. Increased aortic pulsatile load is the major factor in the development of left ventricular hypertrophy with increased coronary blood flow requirements. Simultaneously, the decrease in DBP further compromises the oxygen supply to demand ratio by reducing coronary flow. Furthermore, increased pulsatile stress leads to endothelial dysfunction with a greater propensity for coronary atherosclerosis and for rupture of unstable atherosclerotic plaques. Conversely, wide PP may simply serve as a marker for diffuse atherosclerosis. PP becomes an even stronger predictor of risk in middle-aged and older populations with risk factors such as diabetes or dyslipidemia, with target-organ damage such as left ventricular hypertrophy or albuminuria, and in persons with prior cardiovascular events such as myocardial infarction, ventricular dysfunction, heart failure, or end-stage renal disease. However, cuff PP cannot replace SBP as a single measure of cardiovascular risk, because PP may significantly underestimate systemic vascular resistance. PP is also a late manifestation of change and, as such, becomes manifested at a time when interventions to retard arteriosclerosis may be less effective. PP per se is also not a useful marker of therapeutic responsiveness to antihypertensive therapy. Systolic pressure falls disproportionately in individuals with isolated systolic hypertension when vasodilators are used. In this setting, the narrowed posttreatment PP is simply a reflection of peripheral vasodilation rather than an intrinsic change in arterial stiffness. To date, no clinical trials have been conducted to identify the value of pharmacologic manipulation of PP.

Clinical Strategies to Assess Arterial Stiffness

The best current strategy for assessing risk in the elderly begins with determining the level of SBP elevation and is followed by the adjustment of risk upward when wide PP (i.e., discordantly low DBP) is present. Because of the limitations of PP, alternative methods for estimating stiffness have been developed (see Chapter C119). Central artery stiffness, whether estimated by aortic or carotid waveforms, centrally transformed radial artery waveforms, or by indirect measurement of pulse wave velocity, represents an early independent risk factor for the development of cardiovascular disease. Measurement of central elastic artery stiffness may allow better assessment of cardiovascular risk before hypertension develops and long before the onset of cardiovascular complications.

SUGGESTED READING

1. Benetos A, Adamorpoulos C, Bureau JM, et al. Determinants of accelerated progression of arterial stiffness in normotensive subjects and in treated hypertensive subjects over a 6-year period. *Circulation.* 2002;105:1202–1207.
2. Boutouyrie P, Tropeano AI, Asmar R, et al. Aortic stiffness is an independent predictor of primary coronary events in hypertensive patients: a longitudinal study. *Hypertension.* 2002;39:10–15.
3. Franklin SS, Gustin WG, Wong ND, et al. Hemodynamic patterns of age-related changes in blood pressure: the Framingham Heart Study. *Circulation.* 1997;96:308–315.
4. Franklin SS, Khan SA, Wong ND, et al. Is pulse pressure useful in predicting risk for coronary heart disease? The Framingham Heart Study. *Circulation.* 1999;100:353–360.
5. Franklin SS, Larson MG, Khan SA, et al. Does the relation of blood pressure to coronary heart disease risk change with aging? The Framingham Heart Study. *Circulation.* 2001;103:1245–1249.
6. Izzo JL Jr, Levy D, Black HR for the Coordinating Committee, National High Blood Pressure Education Program, National Heart, Lung, and Blood Institute. Clinical advisory statement: importance of systolic blood pressure in older Americans. *Hypertension.* 2000;35:1021–1024.
7. Mitchell GF, Moye LA, Braunwald E, et al. Sphygmomanometrically determined pulse pressure is a powerful independent predictor of recurrent events after myocardial infarction in patients with impaired left ventricular function. *Circulation.* 1997;96:4254–4260.
8. Nichols WW, O'Rourke MF. *McDonald's Blood Flow in Arteries.* 4th ed. London, UK: E Arnold; 1998.

9. Staessen JA, Gasowski J, Wang JG, et al. Risk of untreated and treated isolated systolic hypertension in the elderly: meta-analysis of outcome trials.
Lancet. 2000;355:865–872.

10. Wilkinson IB, Franklin SS, Hall IR, et al. Pressure amplification explains
why pulse pressure is unrelated to risk in young subjects. *Hypertension.*
2001;38:1461–1466.

Chapter A61

Pathogenesis of Hypertensive Left Ventricular Hypertrophy and Diastolic Dysfunction

Edward D. Frohlich, MD

KEY POINTS

- Left ventricular hypertrophy is an independent risk factor for premature cardiovascular morbidity and mortality that is associated with impaired coronary hemodynamics, increased vulnerability to cardiac dysrhythmias, sudden death, predisposition to systolic or diastolic dysfunction, cardiac failure, and accelerated coronary atherosclerosis.

- Left ventricular hypertrophy is associated with increased wall tension and myocardial oxygen demand, endothelial dysfunction of the myocardium and coronary vessels, reduced coronary blood flow and flow reserve, and angina pectoris with or without occlusive atherosclerotic coronary artery disease.

- Left ventricular hypertrophy is a heterogeneous condition in which individual myofibrils can increase their circumferential diameter (concentric hypertrophy) or length (eccentric hypertrophy).

- Histologically, left ventricular hypertrophy is characterized by increased myocyte mass (hypertrophy) and increased extracellular matrix deposition (fibrosis), both of which may be at least partially reversed by effective antihypertensive therapy.

See also Chapters A38, A54, A59, A60, A62, A66, A67, A78, B83, C115–C118, C155, and C156

Natural History of Hypertensive Left Ventricular Hypertrophy

As the left ventricle progressively hypertrophies in response to the aging process and the pressure overload imposed by chronic hypertension (see Chapter A59), its contractile (systolic) pumping reserve becomes diminished until eventually, cardiac failure supervenes unless arterial pressure is controlled. Even before systolic dysfunction becomes clinically evident, the hypertrophic left ventricle becomes "stiffer" (less distensible), and diastolic filling becomes impaired as a result of ventricular fibrosis. In response to increased ventricular stiffness, the left atrium enlarges and thickens to provide a "booster pump" that acts to maintain diastolic filling. Increased left atrial size is notable in the development of a fourth heart sound, P-wave changes on electrocardiogram, and corresponding echocardiographic findings. Hypertensive patients with left ventricular hypertrophy (LVH) (especially elderly, black, diabetic, and ischemic heart disease patients) may develop diastolic dysfunction and experience cardiac failure despite apparent normal systolic function. Angina pectoris may occur in response to the increased wall tension, myocardial oxygen demand, and endothelial dysfunction associated with collagen deposition and ventricular ischemia that results from perivascular fibrosis, hypertensive coronary arteriolar disease, or concomitant occlusive atherosclerotic disease of the epicardial coronary arteries.

Etiology of Left Ventricular Hypertrophy

The primary factors responsible for the development of LVH are pressure and volume overload, but a number of non-hemodynamic factors may also contribute, including a variety of humoral mechanisms and growth factors (e.g., catecholamines, angiotensin II, endothelins) that promote vascular and cardiac myocyte growth. Other clinical considerations include stage of hypertensive disease, demographic factors (e.g., age, gender, race), existence of comorbid diseases (e.g., obesity, diabetes mellitus, atherosclerotic coronary arterial disease), and coincident pharmacologic therapies.

Eccentric versus Concentric Hypertrophy

LVH is a heterogeneous condition that has been characterized by the changes in individual myofibrils, which can increase their circumferential diameters (concentric hypertrophy), lengths (eccentric hypertrophy), or both. Left ventricular (LV) end-diastolic volume thus tends to be increased in conditions of eccentric hypertrophy such as the athlete's heart, asymmetric septal hypertrophy, and, of course, volume overload. Concentric hypertrophy occurs most commonly in hypertension or early in aortic stenosis and tends to be associated with normal or reduced LV end-diastolic volume. The mixed pattern of LVH results from combined chronic pressure and volume overload. When hypertension is associated with increased preload, the structural abnormality may be more eccentric in nature, especially in patients with obesity or chronic renal insufficiency. In untreated hypertension, progression from LVH to heart failure is associated with eccentric and concentric hypertrophy.

Systolic versus Diastolic Dysfunction

Impaired left ventricular systolic function is a common consequence of LVH, particularly in the untreated patient. Diastolic dysfunction occurs in the absence of systolic dysfunction but when systolic dysfunction already exists, there is almost always some degree of impaired diastolic function. When diastolic dysfunction exists in the absence of systolic dysfunction, it usually occurs in elderly patients with ventricular collagen deposition, fibrosis, and ischemia.

Pathogenesis of Increased Cardiovascular Risk

The precise explanation for the increased risk associated with LVH is not known, but a number of mechanisms clearly contribute. LVH is associated with progressive impairment in coronary blood flow and flow reserve and increased minimal coronary vascular resistance, fibrosis of the extracellular matrix, and perivascular fibrosis, as well as endothelial dysfunction. Epicardial and microvascular arteriolar disease are exacerbated by the atherogenic process in patients with hypertensive disease and LVH. Progressive contraction of intravascular (plasma) volume, in conjunction with increasing arterial pressure and vascular resistance, may further alter the rheology and viscosity abnormalities of the coronary microcirculation in patients with LVH. These changes contribute to the development of congestive heart failure, coronary arterial insufficiency, angina pectoris, cardiac dysrhythmias, and sudden death. Compounding these factors is increased deposition of collagen and fibrosis that increases stiffness of the ventricular chamber and the likelihood of developing ventricular dysfunction and eventual cardiac failure.

Clinical Correlation

Comparison of diagnostic techniques. Detection of LVH may be accomplished by various techniques. The chest x-ray is not nearly as sensitive as the electrocardiogram (ECG) and may be associated with changes that not only reflect LVH but ventricular chamber dilation as well. For the routine evaluation of the patient with hypertension, the ECG remains the most useful and cost effective method, but it also falls short of detecting early LVH. The most useful and sensitive clinical means for detecting early LVH and associated changes in left ventricular function is the echocardiogram. Recently, less costly limited echocardiography has been suggested for increased LV mass in carefully selected patients, particularly in those with stage I blood pressure levels and no other evidence of LVH. It should not be used routinely in all patients with hypertension, because increased LV mass can be detected by the electrocardiogram. Other more costly techniques that provide a more clear-cut definition of LVH are magnetic resonance and positron emission imaging techniques. The existence of a fourth heart sound and the presence of at least 2 ECG criteria of left atrial abnormality are highly concordant with early development of left atrial enlargement and LVH on echocardiogram.

Electrocardiogram criteria. There are 30 or more indices that have been proposed for the diagnosis of LVH by the ECG. The most commonly used criteria are the Sokolow-Lyons criteria (sum of the negative deflection in V_1 and positive deflection in V_5 or V_6 greater than 35 or 38 mV) and the Cornell voltage criteria (product of the QRS duration and the sum of the positive deflection in aVL and negative deflection in V_3 greater than 2,440 mV/msec). Highly sensitive is the McPhee index (sum of the tallest precordial R wave and deepest S wave ≥4.5 mV), and the LV strain pattern (i.e., the QRS complex and T wave vectors are 180 degrees apart) that cause few false-negative diagnoses. The latter strain pattern is associated with severely diminished vascularity of the hypertrophied ventricle and with coronary arteriography evidence of ischemic disease. Enhancing the diagnostic ability of the ECG, particularly in early LVH, are left atrial (P wave) abnormalities. Among these latter criteria are the following: P wave ≥0.12 second in duration, bipeak interval "notched" P waves ≥0.04 second, P wave duration to PR segment ratio of ≥1.6 in lead II, and terminal atrial forces (V_1) ≥0.04 second. Presence of 2 or more of these criteria is highly concordant with the presence of cardiac dysrhythmias, echocardiographic evidence of left atrial enlargement, and LVH.

Echocardiogram. The M-mode, 2-D echocardiogram (with or without Doppler flow measurements) provides a highly precise means of detecting LVH clinically. Interventricular septal hypertrophy (≥1.0 cm) may be the first finding, and the increased width of the LV free wall to ≥1.1 cm indicates LVH. Increased LV mass suggests LVH, but this index takes into consideration LV diastolic volume, which is different between men and women (<100 and ≥131 g/m², respectively) and even varies with intravascular and ventricular volume (which change with weight reduction). Also important are changes in early and late ventricular filling (E-A wave reversal) that correlate strongly with increases in left atrial pressure.

Treatment Effects

The best treatment for LVH is prevention; this means early treatment of hypertension. Treatment of systolic and diastolic dysfunction results in reduction of LV mass along with improved diastolic distensibility and relaxation. All forms of antihypertensive therapy reduce LV mass. Treatment of systolic functional impairment may also improve to some degree the diastolic dysfunction. The major objective in treatment is the fastidious control of systolic and diastolic arterial pressure (<140 and <90 mm Hg, respectively). Despite some concern about reducing arterial pressures to levels of 80 to 85 mm Hg for fear of impairing coronary arterial blood flow in diastole (the so-called J-curve), recent prospective studies (i.e., SHEP, STOP-Hypertension, MRC, SAVE, SOLVD) have not consistently identified increased coronary risk at low diastolic pressures.

A number of experimental studies have demonstrated the efficacy of the angiotensin-converting enzyme inhibitors, angiotensin receptor antagonists, and calcium antagonists may reduce the hydroxyproline and collagen contents and fibrosis of the ventricle. Well-controlled trials have yet to be concluded to demonstrate the benefit that reversal (of LVH) improves morbidity and mortality. Reduction of risk from LVH reversed must be disassociated from the pharmacologic actions of reducing pressure, improving coronary blood flow and flow reserve, or even preventing dysrhythmias.

SUGGESTED READING

1. Dunn FG, Pringle SD. Sudden cardiac death, ventricular arrhythmias, and hypertensive left ventricular hypertrophy. *J Hypertens.* 1993;11:1003–1010.
2. Frohlich ED. Is reversal of left ventricular hypertrophy in hypertension beneficial? *Hypertension.* 1991;18(suppl I):33–38.
3. Frohlich ED. Risk mechanisms in hypertensive heart disease. *Hypertension.* 1999;34:782–789.
4. Frohlich ED, Apstein C, Chobanian AV, et al. The heart in hypertension. *N Engl J Med.* 1992;327:998–1008.
5. Levy D, Larson MG, Vasan RS, et al. The progression from hypertension to congestive heart failure. *JAMA.* 1996;275:1557–1562.
6. Roman MJ, Saba PS, Pina R, et al. Parallel cardiac and vascular adaptation in hypertension. *Circulation.* 1992;86:1909–1918.
7. Sheps SG, Frohlich ED. Limited echocardiography for hypertensive left ventricular hypertrophy. *Hypertension.* 1997;29:560–563.
8. Siscovick DS, Raghunathan TE, Psaty BM, et al. Diuretic therapy for hypertension and the risk of primary cardiac arrest. *N Engl J Med.* 1994;330:1852–1857.
9. Strauer BE. Repair of coronary arterioles after treatment with perindopril in hypertensive heart disease. *Hypertension.* 2000;36:220–225.
10. Treasure CB, Klein JL, Vita JA, et al. Hypertension and left ventricular hypertrophy are associated with impaired endothelium-mediated relaxation in human coronary resistance vessels. *Circulation.* 1993;87:86–93.

Chapter A62

Pathogenesis of Chronic Heart Failure

Thierry H. Le Jemtel, MD; Farhana Latif, MD

KEY POINTS

- The cardiovascular background of patients with left ventricular diastolic and systolic dysfunction differs.

- Inhibition of the renin-angiotensin-aldosterone system is the most potent intervention to reverse abnormal left ventricular remodeling (concentric hypertrophy) in patients with diastolic dysfunction.

- β-blockade is the most potent intervention to reverse abnormal left ventricular remodeling (dilation and eccentric hypertrophy) in patients with systolic dysfunction.

- Alterations in the skeletal muscle mass, peripheral vascular structure and function, and tissue metabolism are responsible for the symptoms of left ventricular systolic dysfunction.

See also Chapters A59, A65–A67, A78, B81, B106, C115, C116, C121, C155, and C156

Left ventricular (LV) dysfunction is more prevalent in older people (see Chapter A59) and is usually preceded by a clinical history of hypertension, coronary artery disease (CAD), diabetes mellitus, substance or alcohol abuse, or valvular heart disease. Rarely, LV dysfunction in younger individuals occurs in the absence of these preexisting conditions. The primary problem is usually myocyte loss, but myocyte dysfunction can be observed in patients with viral myocarditis or in familial or idiopathic dilated cardiomyopathy.

Comorbidities and Patterns of Cardiac Dysfunction

The prevalence of cardiovascular conditions and the pattern of LV remodeling differ in patients with diastolic and systolic dysfunction.

Coronary artery disease and diabetes. CAD is present in only one-third of patients with diastolic dysfunction, whereas significant CAD is found in two-thirds of patients with systolic dysfunction. The greater occurrence of diabetes mellitus in patients with diastolic dysfunction is probably related to the increased prevalence of obesity in diabetics and the strong association of obesity and LV diastolic dysfunction.

Hypertension. In contrast to CAD and diabetes mellitus, hypertension is present in roughly equal proportions, ranging from 65% to 75%, in patients with diastolic or systolic dysfunction. The association of hypertension, diabetes, and obesity that is frequently observed in patients with diastolic dysfunction suggests that diastolic dysfunction may be a late manifestation of the cardiovascular dysmetabolic syndrome (insulin resistance).

Left Ventricular Hypertrophy and Diastolic Dysfunction

Pressure overload and myocyte hypertrophy. Chronic exposure to pressure overload leads to LV concentric hypertrophy, most commonly in patients with hypertension or severe aortic stenosis. According to the law of Laplace (Wall tension = Pressure × Radius/Wall Thickness × 2), the LV wall thickens to normalize increased LV wall tension resulting from chronic elevation of systemic pressure. Cardiac myocytes become larger circumferentially (concentric hypertrophy) and additional sarcomeres are added in parallel (eccentric hypertrophy).

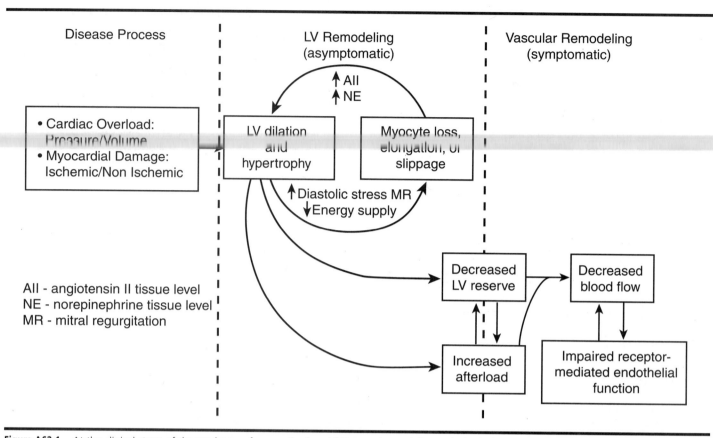

Figure A62.1. At the clinical stage of the syndrome of congestive heart failure owing to left ventricular (LV) systolic dysfunction that is characterized by LV dilatation, LV reserve is exhausted and cardiac output is reduced at rest as cardiac afterload rises owing to excessive vasoconstriction. Decreased regional blood flow and increased oxidative stress result in vascular endothelial dysfunction that, in turn, is responsible for disturbances at the microvasculature level and impaired oxygen delivery. Symptoms are also related to peripheral vascular abnormalities.

Molecular and contractile changes. At the molecular level, concentric hypertrophy is associated with a switch from α to β myosin heavy chain, resulting in slower energy-saving contractions. There is downregulation of sarcoplasmatic reticulum Ca^{2+}-ATPase, resulting in increased concentration of Ca^{2+} at end-diastole and impaired myocyte relaxation. The stimuli that are responsible for hypertrophic growth are still under investigation but are believed to include mechanical sensors and local activation of the renin-angiotensin-aldosterone and sympathetic nervous systems, as well as overexpression of various growth factors and cytokines. The superiority of angiotensin receptor blockade over β-blockade in reversing ventricular hypertrophy in the Losartan Intervention For Endpoint (LIFE) trial can be interpreted as evidence for a role of the renin-angiotensin-aldosterone system in LV hypertrophy. A common pathway to several of the stimuli that trigger LV hypertrophy appears to be the $Gq\alpha$ subunit of the heteromeric G protein; overexpression of $Gq\alpha$ predisposes to apoptosis.

Matrix proteins. The number of fibroblasts also increases in left ventricular hypertrophy, enhancing the production of collagen that may contribute to LV diastolic dysfunction. In addition to collagen, excess osteopontin and fibronectin deposition occurs.

Myocardial stiffness and cardiac filling. Myocyte hypertrophy, fibroblast hyperplasia, and increased collagen production promote global LV diastolic function that is characterized by inadequate LV filling despite elevated diastolic pressure. More-

over, a normal or even supranormal LV ejection fraction is not able to overcome the decrease in stroke volume resulting from the progressive reduction in end-diastolic volume. As a maladaptive compensatory measure, heart rate increases to maintain an adequate cardiac output. However, this rise in heart rate tends to further compromise the filling of an already stiff left ventricle by further reducing cardiac filling time during diastole. Chronic elevation of the LV filling pressure results in increasing left atrial pressure, followed by atrial dilatation and, eventually, atrial fibrillation. Chronic elevation of the LV filling pressure also results in moderate to severe pulmonary hypertension that leads to right ventricular dilatation, further limiting LV filling owing to septal displacement.

Left Ventricular Dilatation and Systolic Dysfunction

Volume overload. Dilatation predominates over hypertrophy when volume overload is the predominant stimulus to LV remodeling (**Figure A62.1**). Volume overload, presumably owing to increased venous return or functional mitral regurgitation, is a common consequence of significant myocyte loss, especially after myocardial infarction. Volume overload also constitutes the main hemodynamic burden of severe valvular regurgitation.

Cellular changes. Reactive LV hypertrophy associated with myocyte dysfunction or loss is characterized by addition of contracting units in series (sometimes called *eccentric hypertrophy*) and slippage of myofibrils and myocardial fibers. Myocyte elongation is limited to 2.2 mm, and side-to-side slippage of myocytes greatly contributes to LV dilatation. Of note, myocyte elongation can initiate a program of cell death (apoptosis), thereby promoting further myocyte loss and LV dilation. Progressive LV dilation causes increasing resting LV wall tension, which adds a component of diastolic dysfunction and indicates a poor prognosis. Diastolic dysfunction and functional mitral insufficiency promote pulmonary artery hypertension and elevation in right ventricular filling pressure.

Impaired coronary flow reserve. Coronary blood flow reserve is reduced in patients with dilated left ventricles, independently from the presence of significant epicardial CAD. When the metabolic demands are increased by stress, exercise, or administration of a positive inotropic agent such as dobutamine, the demand on oxygen can outstrip its delivery. Myocardial ischemia and angina pectoris thus can occur even in the absence of overt CAD. Part of the pathogenesis of impaired coronary flow reserve is impaired endothelium-dependent vasodilation owing to impaired bioavailability of nitric oxide (see Chapter A66) and functional as well as anatomic decreases in capillary density.

Impact of β-blockade. β-Adrenergic blockade frequently reverses LV dilation and improves LV performance in patients with systolic dysfunction. Because β-adrenergic blockade has no significant impact on the number of cardiac myocytes, it presumably improves LV systolic performance and reverses remodeling by enhancing myocyte function. This observation suggests that myocyte dysfunction (rather than loss) is a major factor in LV remodeling in a substantial cohort of patients. The exact mechanisms that mediate the reversal of myocyte dysfunction by β-adrenergic blockade are presently unknown.

Future approaches. Newer drugs that selectively enhance myocardial contractility without raising intracellular Ca^{2+} concentration appear very promising. An alternative approach to enhance LV systolic performance and reverse remodeling in patients with LV systolic dysfunction is to increase the number of cardiac myocytes by mobilizing stem cells from the bone marrow.

Systemic Maladaptations and Heart Failure Symptoms

Neurohumoral activation. Local activation of the renin-angiotensin system directly mediates many of the above-mentioned myocardial maladaptations, whereas systemic activation of the renin-angiotensin and sympathetic nervous systems contributes to abnormalities in the peripheral circulation and skeletal muscles that are responsible for the progression of symptoms in patients with systolic dysfunction. To date, peripheral circulatory alterations have not been extensively investigated in patients with LV diastolic dysfunction.

Physical deconditioning. Weakness and poor exercise tolerance in patients with severe heart failure (HF) owing to advanced LV systolic dysfunction cannot be differentiated from those reported in muscles of patients with severe chronic lung disease. Decreased physical activity is a common denominator between HF and chronic lung disease and may

be another major factor responsible for peripheral muscular and circulatory alterations in addition to systemic activation of the renin-angiotensin-aldosterone and sympathetic nervous systems. From a therapeutic standpoint, an issue of considerable interest is the reversibility of these peripheral alterations. The disappointing effects of cardiac transplantation and LV assist devices on functional capacity point out that peripheral alterations may not be fully reversible at late stages of HF despite substantial enhancement of LV systolic function.

Skeletal muscle alterations. In severe HF, skeletal muscle mass, capillary to fiber ratio, and mitochondrial volume are decreased, whereas the amount of fibrosis, number of lipid deposits, and activity of acid phosphatases are increased. Skeletal muscle metabolism evaluated by phosphorus 31–nuclear magnetic resonance is altered during exercise, as evidenced by an increased inorganic phosphate to creatine phosphate ratio and rapid fall in pH. The increase in glycolysis and decrease in oxidative metabolism is secondary to a switch in myosin heavy chain isoforms from myosin heavy chain type I to II b/x in skeletal muscle, whereas the reverse (type II b/x to I) occurs in the diaphragm.

Oxidative stress and systemic vascular impairment. When the compensatory limit of LV remodeling is reached, the LV becomes unable to maintain an adequate cardiac output, and thus fails to meet the metabolic demands of the body. Compromised regional blood flow and increased oxidative stress reduce nitric oxide production and increase nitric oxide degradation. Consequently, endothelium-dependent vasodilatation is impaired to a greater extent during exercise, when oxidative stress increases, as compared to resting conditions, when oxidative stress is less (see Chapters A65 and A66). Inadequate skeletal muscle perfusion leads to focal necrosis and inflammation, with release of cytokines, growth factors, and inflammatory markers that in turn promote vascular endothelial dysfunction, inflammatory responses in skeletal muscles, and fibrosis. Physical training can lower oxidative stress by building up antioxidant defenses but cannot reverse skeletal muscle fibrosis. Thus maintenance of adequate physical activity is an important adjunct to the management of HF patients.

SUGGESTED READING

1. Colombo PC, Ashton AW, Celaj S, et al. Biopsy coupled to quantitative immunofluorescence: a new method to study the vascular endothelium. *J Appl Physiol.* 2002;92:1331–1338.
2. Dahlof B, Devereux RB, Kjeldsen SE, et al. Cardiovascular morbidity and mortality in the losartan intervention for endpoint reduction in hypertension study (life): a randomised trial against atenolol. *Lancet.* 2002;356:995–1003.
3. Eichorn EJ, Bristow MR. Medical therapy can improve the biological properties of the failing heart: a new era in the treatment of heart failure. *Circulation.* 1996;94:2285–2296.
4. Ennezat PV, Malendowicz SL, Testa M, et al. Physical training in patients with chronic heart failure enhances the expression of genes encoding antioxidative enzymes. *J Am Coll Cardiol.* 2001;38:194–198.
5. Gasdker HB, Wouters EFM, van der Vusse GJ, Schols AMWJ. Skeletal muscle dysfunction in chronic obstructive lung disease and chronic heart failure; underlying mechanisms and therapy perspectives. *Am J Clin Nutr.* 2000;73:1033–1047.

6. Hunter JJ, Chien KR. Signaling pathways for cardiac hypertrophy and failure. *N Engl J Med.* 1999;341:1276–1283.
7. Patel MB, Kaplan IV, Patni RN, et al. Sustained improvement in flow-mediated vasodilatation after short-term administration of dobutamine in patients with severe congestive heart failure. *Circulation.* 1999;99:60–64.

8. Reaven GM, Lithell H, Landsberg L. Hypertension and associated metabolic abnormalities—the role of insulin resistance and the sympathoadrenal system. *N Engl J Med.* 1996;334:374–381.
9. Schrier RW, Abraham WT. Hormones and hemodynamics in heart failure. *N Engl J Med.* 1999;341:577–585.

Chapter A63

Mechanisms of Vascular Remodeling

Gary L. Baumbach, MD

KEY POINTS

- Vascular remodeling describes a variety of changes in vascular structure, including hypertrophy.

- Hypertrophic inward remodeling represents a decrease in lumen diameter associated with an increase in vessel wall material.

- Eutrophic inward remodeling refers to a decrease in lumen diameter without a change in the composition or amount of vessel wall material.

- Hypertrophic remodeling involves cell division and enlargement, whereas eutrophic remodeling involves cell migration and rearrangement.

See also Chapters A3, A12, A16, A19, A24, A34, A38, A60, A64–A66, A68–A71, and A78

Mechanisms and Terminology

Study of the alterations in vascular structure that occur during chronic hypertension has been ongoing for nearly 2 centuries.

Wall to lumen ratio. In recent times, a common approach to the study of arterial wall pathophysiology has been to measure the wall to lumen (W/L) ratio of vessels. The W/L ratio, however, is physiologically sensitive. A vessel that dilates acutely exhibits an increase in lumen diameter and a slight attenuation of wall thickness, causing a marked decrease in W/L ratio; the opposite pattern accompanies physiologic vasoconstriction. It also follows that the W/L ratio by itself cannot fully describe chronic structural changes in peripheral vessels and that other concepts and terminology are required.

Definitions of hypertrophy and remodeling. *Hypertrophy* of the vessel wall was thought to be the structural change primarily responsible for altered vascular responses in chronic hypertension until the 1980s, when the concept of remodeling was introduced. *Remodeling* was initially defined as a reduction in diameter of arterioles during chronic hypertension that could not be attributed to altered distensibility. It soon became apparent, however, that a further refinement in terminology was needed because the term *remodeling* is often used in a more general sense to describe a variety of changes in vascular structure, including hypertrophy of the vessel wall. Consequently, it has been proposed that modifiers be added to more precisely define the meaning of remodeling. For example, *eutrophic inward remodeling* refers to a decrease in lumen diameter without a change in the thickness of the arterial wall or the characteristics of the material within the vessel wall. In contrast, *hypertrophic inward remodeling* is defined as a decrease in

lumen diameter associated with an increase in wall thickness and vessel wall material. In the context of this review, *hypertrophy* refers to hypertrophic inward remodeling and *remodeling* refers to eutrophic inward remodeling (**Figure A63.1**).

Mechanisms of Hypertrophy

Intravascular pressure. Pharmacologic approaches using responses to blood pressure–lowering drugs have inherent limitations in the study of vascular pathology, especially because these drugs also affect hormones and other potential determinants of vascular hypertrophy. An approach that avoids the limitations of antihypertensive treatment is to reduce arterial pressure locally by ligation of upstream vessels. After arterial ligation, neurohumoral factors are similar in blood vessels downstream from the ligation and in control vessels. Based on arterial ligation studies, it is clear that increases in arterial pressure during chronic hypertension contribute to vascular hypertrophy. An unanticipated outcome of these studies was the finding that pulse pressure may contribute more to the development of hypertrophy than mean pressure, systolic pressure, or wall tension (see Chapter A60). This possibility is supported by the finding that cyclic stretching increases DNA synthesis and rate of growth of vascular smooth cells in culture.

Sympathetic nerves. Sympathetic nerves play a role in the development of cerebral vascular hypertrophy during chronic hypertension. W/L ratio and cross-sectional areas of the vessel walls are reduced in cerebral arterioles of spontaneously hypertensive stroke-prone rats (SHRSP) after sympathetic denerva-

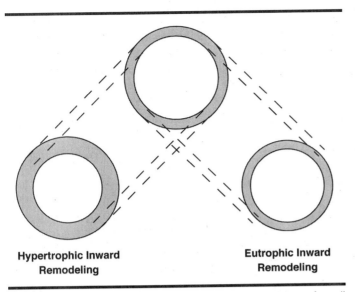

**Hypertrophic Inward
Remodeling**

**Eutrophic Inward
Remodeling**

Figure A63.1. Hypertrophic and eutrophic inward remodeling of small resistance arteries and arterioles. *Inward remodeling* refers to a structural reduction in the vascular lumen. When lumen reduction is owing to encroachment on the lumen by an increase in vessel wall mass (i.e., hypertrophy), it is referred to as *hypertrophic inward remodeling*. When, on the other hand, lumen reduction is owing to an overall decrease in vessel caliber (i.e., reduced external diameter) without an increase in wall mass, it is referred to as *eutrophic inward remodeling*.

tion. Denervation reduces the content of all components in the arteriolar wall (smooth muscle, elastin, collagen, basement membrane, and endothelium), but its effect is greatest on smooth muscle. Sympathetic denervation further reduces, rather than increases, external diameter of cerebral arterioles in SHRSP. Thus, in contrast to their contribution to vascular hypertrophy, sympathetic nerves do not appear to contribute to cerebral vascular remodeling during chronic hypertension.

Angiotensin II. In vascular smooth muscle cells in culture, angiotensin II (Ang II) stimulates hyperplasia and hypertrophy. Hypertrophy of cremaster arterioles is attenuated by doses of an angiotensin-converting enzyme (ACE) inhibitor that do not reduce arterial pressure in experimental Goldblatt hypertension in rats. Thus, vascular hypertrophy may be stimulated by Ang II independent of its pressor effect. This hypothesis, however, is not without controversy because there is also evidence that effects of ACE inhibitors on vascular structure may depend primarily on their effects on blood pressure.

Genetic factors. A genetic predisposition to increased sympathetic nerve activity and hypertrophy of peripheral resistance vessels may exist. Increases in W/L ratio in mesenteric arteries, as well as increases in tissue norepinephrine and hindlimb minimal resistance, precede development of hypertension in spontaneously hypertensive rats (SHR). Thus, genetic factors may influence development of vascular hypertrophy in chronic hypertension. On the other hand, vascular hypertrophy has been found in a variety of models of secondary hypertension, which suggests that genetic factors are not required for the development of hypertrophy.

Endothelin-1. Studies relating endothelin-1 (ET-1) to alterations in vascular structure in chronic hypertension have yielded conflicting results. Treatment of SHR with bosentan, an endothelin receptor blocker, does not inhibit hypertrophy in

small mesenteric, coronary, renal, or femoral arteries. In contrast, bosentan prevents hypertrophy in cerebral arterioles of SHRSP. Several factors may account for the different findings. First, ET-1 may contribute to hypertrophy of cerebral vessels but not mesenteric, coronary, renal, or femoral vessels. Second, the contribution of ET-1 to vascular hypertrophy may vary with vessel size. Third, ET-1 may contribute to hypertrophy only when arterial pressure increases above a critical threshold. This possibility is suggested by observations that arterial pressure is somewhat higher in SHRSP than in SHR and bosentan lowers arterial pressure in SHRSP but not in SHR.

Nitric oxide. Nitric oxide (NO) suppresses mitogenesis and proliferation of vascular smooth muscle cells in tissue culture, but inhibition of NO synthase (NOS) has no effect on serum-stimulated DNA synthesis in carotid and renal arteries in organ culture. Hypertension induced in Sprague-Dawley rats by administration of N^{G}-nitro-L-arginine methyl ester (L-NAME), an inhibitor of NOS, results in hypertrophy of cerebral arterioles that is not prevented by carotid ligation. Thus, NO deficiency may be a determinant of cerebral vascular hypertrophy during chronic hypertension. Alternative interpretations include indirect effects of NOS inhibition such as altered production of endothelin or increased activity of the renin-angiotensin system.

Oxidative stress. Evidence of exaggerated superoxide (O_2^-) production in hypertension has been obtained using indirect measurements (e.g., reduction of nitroblue tetrazolium) in animals made acutely hypertensive by infusion of vasoconstrictors. Interestingly, endothelium-dependent vasorelaxation was found to be markedly impaired at the same time. These observations have led to the suggestion that O_2^- may play a key role in pathologic changes of vascular reactivity induced by hypertension. Superoxide dismutase prevents vascular damage and increases survival in hypertensive rats. A mechanism by which oxidative stress may influence vascular growth is by reducing availability of NO in the vessel wall. NO inhibits growth of vascular smooth muscle in tissue culture. The bioactivity of NO depends, in part, on its interaction with reactive oxygen species, particularly O_2^-. Because O_2^- inactivates NO *in vivo*, it has been suggested that inactivation of NO by O_2^- contributes to impaired vascular function under several pathophysiologic conditions. Thus, oxidative stress during chronic hypertension may contribute to hypertrophy of the vascular wall by inactivating NO and thus diminishing its growth inhibitory influence (**Figure A63.2**). O_2^- also may contribute to vascular growth through alterations in cell signaling. Hydrogen peroxide in particular has been shown to mediate Ang II–induced activation of epidermal growth factor–receptors, p38 mitogen activated protein kinase, and protein kinase β (see Chapter A65). In addition, exposure of vascular smooth muscle cells to hydrogen peroxide results in increases in cell volume and intracellular incorporation of tritiated leucine. Furthermore, inhibition of hydrogen peroxide by overexpression of human catalase inhibits vascular smooth muscle proliferation.

Mechanisms of Remodeling

Intravascular pressure. Antihypertensive treatment with hydralazine or carotid ligation normalizes cerebral arteriolar

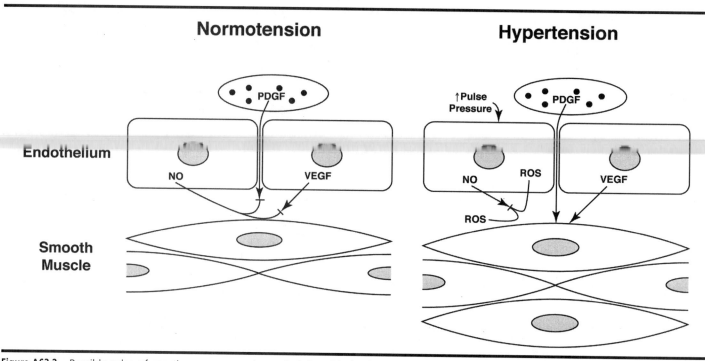

Figure A63.2. Possible roles of reactive oxygen species and nitric oxide (NO) in development of vascular hypertrophy in response to increases in arterial pulse pressure during chronic hypertension. Under normotensive conditions, NO may prevent hypertrophy by inhibiting trophic responses of vascular muscle to growth promoters, such as platelet-derived growth factor (PDGF) and vascular endothelial growth factor (VEGF). Chronic hypertension increases oxidative stress in the vessel wall. Reactive oxygen species (ROS), and in particular superoxide, react with NO to yield peroxynitrite ($ONOO^-$), thereby reducing levels of available NO. Reduced levels of NO may contribute to hypertrophy owing to removal of its growth inhibitory influence.

pulse pressure in cerebral arterioles of SHRSP, but neither treatment prevents arteriolar remodeling. Importantly, both treatments fail to normalize cerebral arteriolar mean pressure in SHRSP. Thus, although pulse pressure can be excluded as a mechanism of cerebral vascular remodeling, a role for mean pressure cannot be ruled out.

Angiotensin II. Treatment with an ACE inhibitor, but not hydralazine, prevents remodeling of cerebral arterioles in SHRSP. In addition, treatment with a selective AT_1-receptor antagonist attenuates remodeling of cerebral arterioles in SHRSP. In contrast to sympathetic nerves and intravascular pulse pressure, therefore, angiotensin may be a determinant of cerebral vascular remodeling, as well as hypertrophy, during chronic hypertension.

Genetic factors. In contrast to the questionable role of genetic factors in relation to development of vascular hypertrophy, 2 lines of evidence suggest genetic factors' important contribution to development of vascular remodeling in chronic hypertension. First, remodeling occurs in several types of genetic hypertension, including SHR, SHRSP, and Dahl S/JR hypertensive rats. Furthermore, remodeling rather than medial hypertrophy is responsible for reductions in lumen diameter and increases in media to lumen ratio in renal afferent arterioles in SHR and small subcutaneous arteries from human essential hypertensives. The second line of evidence is that vascular remodeling has not been observed in models of secondary hypertension, such as renal hypertension or hypertension secondary to inhibition of NO synthesis. Thus, remodeling does not appear to be secondary to hypertension per se and may involve genetic factors.

Endothelin. ET-1 influences eutrophic remodeling in small mesenteric arteries in deoxycorticosterone acetate–salt hypertensive rats. However, treatment with bosentan has no effect on remodeling of cerebral arterioles, suggesting that ET-1 probably does not contribute to remodeling of cerebral arterioles in SHRSP. There are at least 2 possible reasons for this apparent discrepancy. First, determinants of remodeling may vary in different vascular beds. Second, and perhaps more likely, deoxycorticosterone acetate–salt hypertension may reduce external diameter of small mesenteric arteries in rats as a consequence of reduced distensibility rather than remodeling.

Nitric oxide and eutrophic outward remodeling. Treatment of Sprague-Dawley rats with L-NAME does not result in a reduction of external diameter in cerebral arterioles and in fact results in an increase in external diameter. In other words, treatment with L-NAME produces eutrophic outward remodeling, in cerebral arterioles, rather than inward remodeling. This finding suggests that reductions in availability of NO do not play a role in eutrophic inward remodeling of resistance arteries during chronic hypertension.

Synthesis

A host of potential mechanisms may contribute to hypertrophy and remodeling of small resistance arteries and arterioles during chronic hypertension. Many of the factors that play a role in hypertrophy of cerebral arterioles (such as arterial pulse pressure, sympathetic nerves, and endothelial factors) do not appear to contribute to eutrophic remodeling. One reason for this apparent discrepancy is that the mechanisms of hypertrophy and eutrophic remodeling are likely quite different (cell division and increased cell size, as opposed to cell migration and rearrangement). To expand our understanding of the mechanisms involved in eutrophic remodeling will likely require exploring new paradigms. Two areas that show some promise in this regard are apoptosis and matrix metalloproteinases. With respect to mechanisms of hypertrophy, the 2 areas that show promise of furthering our understanding are endothelial-dependent mechanisms and oxidative stress.

SUGGESTED READING

1. Baumbach GL, Heistad DD. Remodeling of cerebral arterioles in chronic hypertension. *Hypertension.* 1989;13:968–972.
2. Baumbach GL, Heistad DD. Mechanisms involved in the genesis of cerebral vascular damage in hypertension. In: Hansson L, Birkenhager WH, eds. *Handbook of Hypertension: Assessment of Hypertensive Organ Damage.* New York, NY: Elsevier Science; 1997:249–268.
3. Dzau VJ. Vascular remodeling—the emerging paradigm of programmed cell death (apoptosis): the Francis B. Parker lectureship. *Chest.* 1998;114:91S–99S.
4. Folkow B. Physiological aspects of primary hypertension. *Physiol Rev.* 1982;62:347–504.
5. Griendling KK, Sorescu D, Ushio-Fukai M. NAD(P)H oxidase: role in cardiovascular biology and disease. *Circ Res.* 2000;86:494–501.
6. Intengan HD. Vascular remodeling in hypertension: roles of apoptosis, inflammation, and fibrosis. *Hypertension.* 2001;38:581–587.
7. Irani K. Oxidant signaling in vascular cell growth, death, and survival: a review of the roles of reactive oxygen species in smooth muscle and endothelial cell mitogenic and apoptotic signaling. *Circ Res.* 2000;87:179–183.
8. Mulvany MJ, Baumbach GL, Aalkjaer C, et al. Vascular remodeling. [See comments.] *Hypertension.* 1996;28:505–506.

Chapter A64

Microvascular Regulation and Dysregulation

Andrew S. Greene, PhD

KEY POINTS

- Microvascular abnormalities in hypertension are functional (increased vascular sensitivity and constriction) and structural (increased vessel wall thickness and loss of capillaries rarefaction).

- Microcirculatory rarefaction is associated with metabolic abnormalities such as insulin resistance and altered organ function.

- Long-term normalization of blood pressure, especially with renin-angiotensin blocking drugs, ameliorates large vessel and microcirculatory structural changes.

See also Chapters A24, A34, A63, A66, and A70–A72

The microcirculation is involved in the genesis and maintenance of hypertension and plays a major role in many of the functional changes that take place. Because the microcirculation is the site of much of the systemic vascular resistance as well as virtually all of the oxygen and nutrient exchange function, changes in microcirculatory function and structure would be expected to have a significant impact on systemic hemodynamics and organ function (**Figure A64.1**).

Microcirculatory Structural Changes in Hypertension

Remodeling. Associated with the rise in pressure in chronic hypertension is dramatic remodeling of the microcirculatory architecture, including the vascular connections and the blood vessels themselves. Increased growth of the media of arterioles, owing primarily to vascular smooth muscle hypertrophy rather than hyperplasia, results in an increased wall to lumen ratio (see Chapter A63). When the muscular wall is hypertrophic, peripheral resistance tends to increase because thicker-walled vessels tend to have reduced luminal diameters, especially during neurogenic or humoral vasoconstriction. Medial hypertro-phy is thought to develop as a response to increased flow velocity and shear stress, which is a signal for arteriolar remodeling. In this capacity, the hypertrophic response acts to normalize shear stress in arterioles. Increased shear forces in the microcirculation appear to be vasodilatory and angiogenic. In normal situations, neoformation of capillaries promotes a restoration of normal shear forces. In hypertension, reverse angiogenesis of small arterioles and capillaries (rarefaction) may occur.

Rarefaction. Rarefaction, resulting in a vessel loss of up to 50% of microvessels, may be due either to hemodynamic factors or to the action or depletion of locally acting trophic or growth factors such as angiotensin II, insulin, fibroblast growth factor, transforming growth factor-β, platelet-derived growth factor, or others. Ultimately, rarefaction in chronic hypertension is thought to be mediated via degenerative changes in microvessels, such as atrophy of vascular smooth muscle cells (VSMCs) through apoptosis and attenuation of the endothelium. Yet, some evidence exists that microcirculatory rarefaction precedes the development of chronic hypertension and thus may play a role in causality.

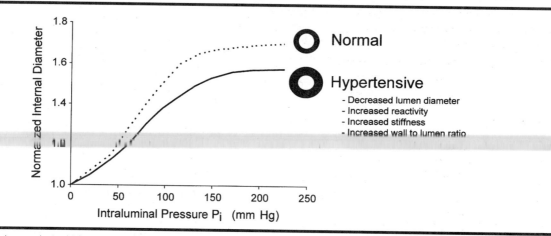

Figure A64.1. Hypertension results in thickening of vascular wall, which shifts pressure-diameter relationship of arterioles in such a way that internal diameter is reduced. This hypertrophic response to increased pressure results in decreased lumen diameter, increased vascular reactivity, and decreased compliance. Recent studies suggest that only through aggressive long-term normalization of blood pressure can these structural changes be reversed. P_i, intraluminal pressure.

Cellular changes. In addition to the postgrowth remodeling of established microvascular networks, a series of other morphologic abnormalities can be seen. VSMCs may be retracted or atrophic with extensive rough endoplasmic reticulum and other organelles, suggesting modulation of some VSMCs toward a secretory phenotype. Vessels undergoing hypertrophy have an increased number of polyploid VSMCs. Endothelial cells may be attenuated, separated from VSMCs, or detached from their basement membrane, whereas pericytes are frequently absent from capillaries. These changes in endothelial cell morphology may impact dramatically on the permeability of the microvasculature, resulting in alterations in the transport of metabolites, interstitial matrix injury, and end-organ damage. Thrombi, neutrophils, and prephagocytic cells may also be present in the microcirculatory

vessels during the early stages of some experimental forms of hypertension. Interestingly, many degenerative structural changes associated with arteriolar rarefaction are similar to those that occur during ischemic injury; however, no inflammatory phagocytic response is observed during the development of hypertension compared with that normally seen in ischemic injury.

Functional Consequences of Microcirculatory Damage

Functional impact of structural changes. Functional abnormalities of the microcirculatory vessels arise in part from anatomic changes. Microvascular compliance and capacity are reduced because of an increased collagen to elastin ratio in

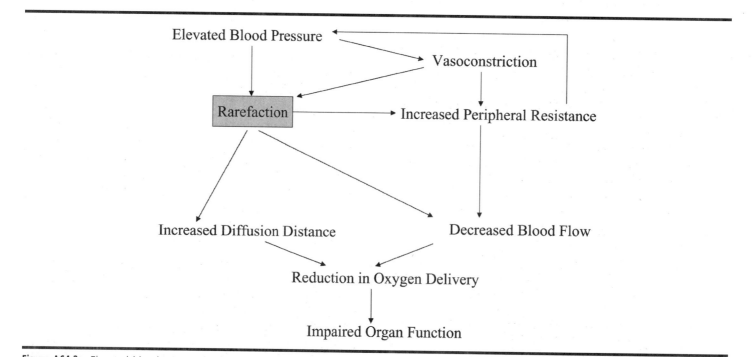

Figure A64.2. Elevated blood pressure and associated neuroendocrine changes cause vasoconstriction and a reduction in microvessel density, both of which increase peripheral resistance and decrease tissue blood flow. Rarefaction further compounds this decreased perfusion by increasing diffusion distance and further reducing oxygen delivery, resulting in impaired organ function.

microvessels as well as a reduced number of vessels. Increased myogenic tone, which contributes to reduced capacity, is due in part to vascular wall hypertrophy.

Role of the autonomic system. Damage to the blood–brain barrier, which occurs primarily in capillaries and small venules, may be linked to increases in central sympathetic drive. In addition to increased autoregulatory tone, microvascular diameters may also be decreased because of elevated sympathetic nerve activity. Although much of the evidence for participation of a neural component in high systemic resistance has been obtained by indirect approaches such as neural ablation, experimental evidence suggests that a primary genetic abnormality may exist in control of the peripheral sympathetic outflow, resulting in increased sympathetic drive in many forms of hypertension. Increased levels of adrenergic stimulation and of circulating pressor hormones contribute to increased peripheral resistance during the development of essential hypertension.

Other changes. Abnormal responses to constrictor and dilator stimuli are exacerbated by impairment in endothelial function. Permeability of capillaries is increased throughout the body, with a resulting redistribution of protein and water from plasma to the interstitial space. Changes in the population of hormone receptors on VSMCs and endothelial cells can augment the constrictor and hypertrophic effects of endocrine, paracrine, and autocrine fac-

tors. In addition to the enhanced sensitivity to vasoconstrictor agents, the arterioles of hypertensive individuals appear to be more sensitive to increased levels of oxygen and less responsive to vasodilatory stimuli, including hypoxia, than those of normotensive control subjects. The enhanced constriction of arterioles in response to increased oxygen availability may indicate heightened autoregulatory responsiveness, whereby small increases in total blood volume or decreases in vascular compliance could result in chronic elevation of systemic resistance (**Figure A64.2**).

SUGGESTED READING

1. Cannon RO III. The heart in hypertension: thinking small. *Am J Hypertens.* 1996;9:406–408.
2. Cowley AW Jr. Long-term control of arterial blood pressure. *Physiol Rev.* 1992;72:231–300.
3. Draaijer P, Le Noble JL, Leunissen KM, Struyker-Boudier HA. The microcirculation and essential hypertension. *Neth J Med.* 1991;39:158–169.
4. Drexler H. Endothelial dysfunction: clinical implications. *Prog Cardiovasc Dis.* 1997;39:287–324.
5. Hutchins PM, Lynch CD, Cooney PT, Curseen KA. The microcirculation in experimental hypertension and aging. *Cardiovasc Res.* 1996;32:772–780.
6. Rieder MJ, Roman RJ, Greene AS. Reversal of microvascular rarefaction and reduced renal mass hypertension. *Hypertension.* 1997;30:120–127.
7. Schiffrin EL. The endothelium of resistance arteries: physiology and role in hypertension. *Prostaglandins Leukot Essent Fatty Acids.* 1996;54:17–25.
8. Sullivan JM, Prewitt RL, Josephs JA. Attenuation of the microcirculation in young patients with high-output borderline hypertension. *Hypertension.* 1983;5:844–851.

Chapter A65

Oxidative Stress and Hypertension

David G. Harrison, MD; Kathy K. Griendling, PhD

KEY POINTS

- Reactive oxygen species are produced as a by-product of numerous cellular metabolic processes.

- Normal and abnormal cellular processes are influenced by reactive oxygen species, including cellular growth and hypertrophy, inflammation, remodeling, lipid oxidation, and modulation of vascular tone.

- Increased vascular production of superoxide ($O_2^{\cdot-}$), which occurs in several diseases, modulates the bioactivity of nitric oxide and is partially dependent on angiotensin II.

- Nicotinamide adenine dinucleotide phosphate oxidases are major vascular sources of reactive oxygen species. Production of superoxide ($O_2^{\cdot-}$) by nicotinamide adenine dinucleotide phosphate oxidases may contribute to the pathogenesis of hypertension, promote target organ damage, activate other oxidative enzymes, and impair antioxidant defenses.

See also Chapters A3, A15, A19, A38, A43, A59, A60, A63, A64, A66, and A67

Reactive Oxygen Species

There is growing interest in the role of oxidative stress as a component of many human diseases, particularly vascular diseases. The term *oxidative stress* implies a state in which cells are exposed to high concentrations of molecular oxygen or chemical derivatives of oxygen called *reactive oxygen species* (ROS). In

the process of normal cellular metabolism, oxygen undergoes a series of univalent reductions, leading sequentially to the production of superoxide anion ($O_2^{\cdot-}$), hydrogen peroxide (H_2O_2), and H_2O (**Figure A65.1**). Other important oxidants that have relevance to vascular biology include hypochlorous acid, hydroxyl radical ($OH^{\cdot}$), reactive aldehydes, lipid peroxides,

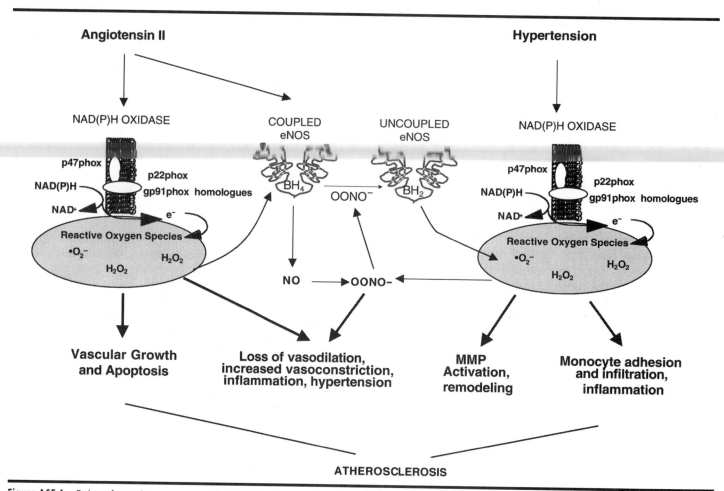

Figure A65.1. Roles of reactive oxygen species (ROS) in the vessel wall. Two major sources of superoxide seem to be important in hypertension. The nicotinamide adenine dinucleotide phosphate [NAD(P)H] oxidase is activated by several pathophysiologic stimuli, including angiotensin II and hypertension to produce $O_2^{\cdot-}$. Superoxide in turn serves as a source of other ROS, leading to downstream signaling events and promoting oxidation. Formation of peroxynitrite and other oxidants may lead to "uncoupling" of the endothelial nitric oxide synthase (eNOS) by causing oxidation of tetrahydrobiopterin. The consequences of oxidative stress include alteration of vasomotor tone, altered gene expression, inflammatory responses, and vascular remodeling. Ultimately, these processes, which are activated in hypertension, predispose to formation of atheroma. BH_2, dihydrobiopterin; BH_4, tetrahydrobiopterin; MMP, matrix metalloproteinase; NO, nitric oxide.

lipid radicals, and nitrogen oxides (see Chapter A19). Several of these, including $O_2^{\cdot-}$, $OH^{\cdot}$, and nitric oxide ($NO^{\cdot}$), are radicals with an unpaired electron in their outer orbital. Others are oxidants and quite biologically active, but are not radicals.

Sources of reactive oxygen species. Sources of ROS include components of mitochondrial electron transport, xanthine oxidase, cyclooxygenases, lipoxygenases, nitric oxide (NO) synthase, heme oxygenases, peroxidases, hemoproteins such as heme and hematin, and nicotinamide adenine dinucleotide (NADH) oxidases. One of the best-characterized sources of ROS is the phagocytic nicotinamide adenine dinucleotide phosphate [NAD(P)H] oxidase. This enzyme system is capable of producing very large, cytotoxic amounts of oxygen radicals. A major source of ROS in blood vessels is a membrane-associated NADPH oxidase expressed by endothelial cells, vascular smooth muscle cells (VSMCs) and fibroblasts that bear some similarity to the phagocytic oxidase.

Oxidative stress and redox state. The terms *oxidative stress* and *redox state* are often used loosely and interchangeably, without attention to their true meaning. The redox state or redox potential of a cell refers to the chemical environment within the cell as it relates to the number of reducing equivalents available, which can be estimated by examining ratios of so-called redox couples, such as lactate/pyruvate, $NADH/NAD^+$, and reduced/oxidized glutathione. Exposure of cells to oxidizing conditions may alter redox couples by consuming reducing equivalents, but redox state may also be altered in other ways. For example, exposure of cells to lactate can markedly increase the levels of NADH by conversion of NAD^+ to NADH via the activation of lactate dehydrogenase. Conversely, exposure to high concentrations of pyruvate produces the opposite effect. Redox state may also be altered by oxidative stress, but altered redox state may not necessarily change the oxidative environment.

Vascular Processes Affected by Reactive Oxygen Species

Reactive oxygen species in cell signaling and growth. ROS are not simply toxic by-products of cellular metabolism; they also participate in normal cellular signaling and function in very important ways. Growth of vascular smooth muscle is stimulated by H_2O_2, a process that is dependent on the expression and binding of the transcription factors c-*fos* and c-*jun*.

More important, hormone- and growth factor–stimulated proliferation and hypertrophy are mediated by and require intracellular H_2O_2. There are multiple molecular targets of ROS that mediate the growth response, including Ras, calcium calmodulin kinase II, c-Src, Akt, p38 mitogen-activated protein kinase, and protein tyrosine phosphatases. The ways in which these factors interact and are affected by ROS likely involve direct modifications of the enzymes or modulation of signaling complex formation.

Regulation of gene expression. Oxidative stress is also important as a modulator of gene expression. For example, it seems to play a critical role in initiating expression of proinflammatory molecules such as vascular cell adhesion molecule-1 and monocyte chemotactic protein-1, early events in atherogenesis. An important mediator of transcription of these genes is the nuclear transcription factor NFκB. This factor exists in the cytoplasm as a heterotrimer and is stimulated by ROS via dissociation of an inhibitory subunit (IκB) from a p50-p65 complex that translocates to the nucleus to mediate gene transcription. ROS also modulate gene expression via transcription factors binding to AP-1, SP-1, antioxidant response elements, and other *cis*-acting elements.

Modulation of extracellular matrix. An important component of vascular growth and remodeling is degradation and resynthesis of extracellular matrix. Specialized enzymes known as *matrix metalloproteinases* (MMPs) mediate the degradation process. MMP-2 and MMP-9 are involved in degradation of basement membrane and elastin, respectively. Both are converted from inactive zymogens to their active forms by several ROS (including H_2O_2 and peroxynitrite) via a direct effect of the oxidant on the proenzyme, probably via an interaction with a cysteine in the inhibitory domain of the proenzymes. Such an activation process may be quite important in matrix degradation in regions of vessels exposed to high levels of oxidant stress, such as the shoulder regions of vulnerable plaques. The decrease of aortic elastin content related to aging and the resultant increase in vascular stiffness may be other pathogenetic effects of oxidative stress.

Oxidation of lipoproteins. A particularly important pathophysiologic event related to ROS is oxidation of lipids, and in particular low-density lipoprotein (LDL). Under normal circumstances, native LDL cycles in and out of the vessel wall, although its uptake may be enhanced under certain conditions. It is now clear that changes in the oxidative environment in the vessel wall can lead to modification of the LDL particle. These modifications result in formation of a spectrum of oxidized lipoproteins. LDL receptors are able to differentiate between LDL and oxidized LDL (oxLDL). In oxLDL, several "new" biologically active molecules are formed; oxLDL contains phospholipase A_2–like enzymatic activity, and within the LDL particle, the active conversion of phosphatidylcholine to lysophosphatidylcholine causes numerous untoward biologic effects on the endothelium. Linoleic acid and other fatty acids are oxidized to their respective hydroperoxides, which can participate in radical chain reactions, resulting in transfer of electrons to other molecules and the formation of additional radicals.

Modulation of the biologic activity of nitric oxide. Of particular importance to hypertension and vascular biology is the interaction between $O_2^{\cdot -}$ and $NO^{\cdot}$. Because $O_2^{\cdot -}$ and $NO^{\cdot}$ are radicals that contain unpaired electrons in their outer orbitals, they can undergo extremely rapid, diffusion-limited radical-radical reactions with rates similar to those of $O_2^{\cdot -}$ and superoxide dismutases (SODs). These nonenzymatic reactions can be 10,000 times faster than reactions between $O_2^{\cdot -}$ and common "scavenger" antioxidants such as vitamins A, E, and C. Given these considerations, it is not at all surprising that several recent large trials have failed to show that vitamins improve event rates in subjects with coronary artery disease, largely because the vitamins employed are poor antioxidants.

Peroxynitrite. A major product of the $O_2^{\cdot -}$ and $NO^{\cdot}$ interaction is peroxynitrite anion ($OONO^-$). Peroxynitrite is a weak vasodilator compared to $NO^{\cdot}$, and thus this reaction markedly impairs the vasodilator capacity of $NO^{\cdot}$. Many of the beneficial effects of $NO^{\cdot}$ (inhibition of platelet aggregation and smooth muscle cell growth, inhibition of vascular cell adhesion molecule-1 expression, etc.) are lost when $OONO^-$ is present.

Superoxide and nitric oxide interactions in vascular disease. The rapidity of the reactions between $O_2^{\cdot -}$ and $NO^{\cdot}$ and $O_2^{\cdot -}$ and SODs suggests that in compartments in which these 3 entities coexist, their interactions could alter the amounts or activities of available $O_2^{\cdot -}$, SOD, or $NO^{\cdot}$. Indeed, this seems to be the case. In the normal vessel, the balance between $NO^{\cdot}$ and $O_2^{\cdot -}$ favors the net production of $NO^{\cdot}$, permits a state of basal vasodilatation, and the maintenance of normal blood pressure.

The critical balance between $NO^{\cdot}$ and $O_2^{\cdot -}$ is altered in the setting of numerous common disease states. These include atherosclerosis, hypertension, diabetes, cigarette smoking, and aging. In hypercholesterolemia, vessels produce excess quantities of $O_2^{\cdot -}$, leading to destruction of $NO^{\cdot}$ and impaired endothelium-dependent vascular relaxation. Treatment of vessels or animals with membrane-targeted forms of SOD markedly improves endothelium-dependent vascular relaxation. Likewise, infusion of antioxidant vitamins transiently improves endothelium-dependent vasodilatation as has been shown in forearm vessels in human subjects with diabetes and cigarette smokers.

Reactive Oxygen Species in Hypertension

Role of nicotinamide adenine dinucleotide phosphate oxidases. Membrane-bound, NAD(P)H-dependent oxidases are major sources of $O_2^{\cdot -}$ in vascular tissues. Several laboratories have shown that the endothelial, vascular smooth muscle, and adventitial cells contain membrane-associated oxidases that use NADPH as substrates for electron transfer to molecular oxygen. On a molecular level, vascular oxidases share limited homology with neutrophil respiratory burst oxidase. Many of the neutrophil components, including p22phox, p47phox, and the small guanosine triphosphatase Rac-1, are present in vascular cells. During the past few years, a family of proteins (NOXs) with homology to the neutrophil oxidase catalytic subunit, gp91phox, was discovered and has been shown to play a critical role in smooth muscle and endothelial cell function. Functionally, vascular NADPH oxidases differ from neutrophil oxidase in many respects. The neutrophil oxidase releases massive amounts of $O_2^{\cdot -}$ in bursts, whereas the vascular oxidases produce $O_2^{\cdot -}$ at low levels in a continuous fashion. The $O_2^{\cdot -}$ generated in VSMCs appears to be mostly intracellular, with only a limited amount of $O_2^{\cdot-}$ released to the exterior of the cell, as occurs in phagocytes. In endothelial cells, $O_2^{\cdot-}$ is released both intra- and extracellularly. Recent data from our laboratory indicate that although the vascular NAD(P)H oxidases produce $O_2^{\cdot-}$, they produce approximately 4-fold greater amounts of H_2O_2.

Regulation of oxidase activity by angiotensin II in hypertension. A particularly important aspect of the vascular NAD(P)H oxidases is that angiotensin II (Ang II) and certain cytokines regulate their activities. Ang II increases H_2O_2 production by 2- to 3-fold in VSMCs, and this leads to activation of specific growth-related signaling pathways, which in turn mediate hypertrophic growth responses to Ang II. The effect of Ang II on activity of the NAD(P)H oxidases is important *in vivo*. In aortas of rats made hypertensive by Ang II infusion, there is increased NAD(P)H oxidase activity and expression of several NAD(P)H oxidase subunits, including nox1, gp91phox, and p22phox. A critical role of $O_2^{\cdot-}$ in the hypertension caused by Ang II has been demonstrated by several studies showing that membrane-targeted forms of SOD dramatically lower blood pressure in this model. Recently, it has been shown that mice lacking p47phox, a critical subunit for vascular and neutrophil oxidases, have a dramatically reduced hypertensive response to chronic Ang II infusion. Taken together, these data provide unequivocal evidence that the ROS derived from NAD(P)H oxidases play a central role in Ang II-induced hypertension.

Reactive oxygen species and uncoupling of nitric oxide synthase: role of tetrahydrobiopterin oxidation. The nitric oxide synthases can produce large amounts of $O_2^{\cdot-}$ when deprived of their critical cofactor (tetrahydrobiopterin) or their substrate (L-arginine). In this state, referred to as *NOS uncoupling*, electron flow through the enzyme results in reduction of molecular oxygen to form $O_2^{\cdot-}$ at the prosthetic heme site rather than formation of NO˙. In aortas of mice with deoxycorticosterone acetate-salt hypertension, $O_2^{\cdot-}$ production from NO˙ synthase is markedly increased, and tetrahydrobiopterin oxidation is evident. In this model, initial production of ROS from the NAD(P)H oxidase leads to oxidation of tetrahydrobiopterin, uncoupling of endothelial NO synthase, decreased NO˙ production, and increased superoxide production from endothelial NO synthase. Treatment of deoxycorticosterone acetate-salt mice with oral tetrahydrobiopterin reduces vascular $O_2^{\cdot-}$ production, increases NO˙ production, and blunts the increase in blood pressure. These recent studies suggest that treatment strategies that increase tetrahydrobioprotein or prevent its oxidation may prove useful in treatment of hypertension.

Effects on vascular reactivity. $O_2^{\cdot-}$ and other ROS can have effects on vascular reactivity that are independent of NO˙. In vascular smooth muscle, intracellular calcium levels may be increased by ROS by interference with calcium reuptake by the sarcoplasmic reticulum. ROS can react with omega fatty acids in the membrane to produce isoprostanes, which can be detected in the blood of humans in whom oxidative stress is increased (e.g., subjects with hypercholesterolemia, diabetics, and cigarette smokers). These oxidatively modified fatty acids act on prostaglandin H/thromboxane receptors to enhance vasoconstriction.

Treatment Strategies Altering Reactive Oxygen Species

Several commonly employed treatment strategies impact the production of ROS by vascular cells. Both angiotensin-converting enzyme inhibitors and Ang II receptor antagonists dramatically reduce activation of the NAD(P)H oxidases in animal models of hypertension and hypercholesterolemia. Likewise, hydroxymethylglutaryl coenzyme A–reductase inhibitors inhibit activation of the small G-protein Rac-1 by preventing production of geranyl-geranyl pyrophosphate, crucial for its membrane association. These agents have also been shown to inhibit activity of the NAD(P)H oxidases in vascular and myocardial cells. It is very likely that a portion of the beneficial effects of these agents in the setting of hypertension and other forms of vascular disease relates to their ability to inhibit a major source of oxidant stress.

SUGGESTED READING

1. Mollnau H, Wendt M, Szocs K, et al. Effects of angiotensin II infusion on the expression and function of NAD(P)H oxidase and components of nitric oxide/cGMP signaling. *Circ Res.* 2002;90:E58–E65.
2. Griendling KK, Sorescu D, Lassègue B, et al. Modulation of protein kinase activity and gene expression by reactive oxygen species and their role in vascular physiology and pathophysiology. *Arterioscler Thromb Vasc Biol.* 2000;20:2175–2183.
3. Landmesser U, Harrison DG. Oxidative stress and vascular damage in hypertension. *Coron Artery Dis.* 2001;12:455–461.
4. Burdon RH. Superoxide and hydrogen peroxide in relation to mammalian cell proliferation. *Free Radic Biol Med.* 1995;18:775–794.
5. Laursen JB, Somers M, Kurz S, et al. Endothelial regulation of vasomotion in apoE-deficient mice: implications for interactions between peroxynitrite and tetrahydrobiopterin. *Circulation.* 2001;103:1282–1288.
6. Wolin MS. Interactions of oxidants with vascular signaling systems. *Arterioscler Thromb Vasc Biol.* 2000;20:1430–1442.
7. Freeman JL, Lambeth JD. NADPH oxidase activity is independent of p47phox in vitro. *J Biol Chem.* 1996;271:22578–22582.
8. Nickenig G, Harrison DG. The AT(1)-type angiotensin receptor in oxidative stress and atherogenesis: Part II: AT(1) receptor regulation. *Circulation.* 2002;105:530–536.
9. Nickenig G, Harrison DG. The AT(1)-type angiotensin receptor in oxidative stress and atherogenesis: Part I: oxidative stress and atherogenesis. *Circulation.* 2002;105:393–396.
10. Diaz MN, Frei B, Vita JA, et al. Antioxidants and atherosclerotic heart disease. *N Engl J Med.* 1997;337:408–416.

Chapter A66

Endothelial Function and Cardiovascular Disease

Julian P. J. Halcox, MA, MRCP; Arshed A. Quyyumi, MD, FACC, FRCP

KEY POINTS

- The endothelium is an active organ that modulates activity of vascular smooth muscle and guards against unwanted thrombosis by elaborating several vasoactive substances, most notably nitric oxide.

- Endothelial dysfunction is a precursor of atherosclerosis and is associated with conventional risk factors such as hyperlipidemia, hypertension, excess angiotensin II, and oxidative stress.

- Several novel risk factors for endothelial dysfunction have been discovered, including insulin resistance, lipoprotein (a), depression, and certain infections.

- Endothelial dysfunction is an independent cardiovascular risk factor and strategies to improve endothelial dysfunction may improve prognosis.

See also Chapters A16, A19, A24, A39, A43, A60, A62–A65, A67, A68, A71, and A72

The vascular endothelium is the largest "organ" in the body, comprising over 14,000 square ft of surface area and weighing 2 to 3 kg. Vascular endothelial cells are extremely active and play a critical role in the regulation of blood vessel tone and cellular activity in the vascular wall (see Chapter A16). Endothelial cells modulate underlying blood vessel tone by secreting a variety of dilator and constrictor substances. Dilator substances include nitric oxide (NO), prostacyclin, and endothelium-derived hyperpolarizing factor (EDHF); constricting agents include endothelin, superoxide anions, vasoconstrictor prostanoids, and locally generated angiotensin II (**Figure A66.1**). In addition to their influence on vascular tone, these agents and other factors produced by the endothelium may modify platelet aggregation, thrombogenicity of the blood, vascular inflammation and oxidative stress, and more importantly over the long-term, cell migration and proliferation, with subsequent development of atherosclerosis and its complications.

Normal Endothelial Cell Function and Nitric Oxide

In 1980, Furchgott and Zawadski described a labile substance secreted from endothelial cells that dilated rabbit aortic rings. This substance was initially termed *endothelium-derived relaxing factor* and was subsequently identified as NO. NO is a diatomic molecule produced from L-arginine by the constitutive action of endothelial NO synthase (eNOS) (see Chapter A16). Under healthy conditions, tonically released NO diffuses into vascular smooth muscle cells, where it causes activation of G protein–bound guanylyl cyclase, increased intracellular cyclic guanosine monophosphate (GMP) levels, and subsequent smooth muscle relaxation. NO can also inhibit platelet adhesion and, to a lesser extent, suppress platelet aggregation. NO is also able to modulate transcription of several genes that are involved in inflammatory processes in the vascular wall, including inhibition of P-selectin and MCP-1 gene expression, thus suppressing inflammatory activity. Furthermore, endothelial NO attenuates the generation of the vasoconstrictor endothelin, which itself promotes inflammation and proliferation.

Endothelial Cell Dysfunction

Abnormal nitric oxide and superoxide metabolism. Traditional cardiovascular risk factors such as hypertension, hyperlipidemia, insulin resistance/diabetes, and tobacco use are associated with endothelial dysfunction. Reduced bioavailability of NO in the setting of increased superoxide anion levels, largely owing to increased nicotinamide adenine dinucleotide phosphate oxidase activity, is a common underlying abnormality in these conditions. Increased levels of free radicals in the vascular wall lead to NO oxidation to nitrite, nitrate, and peroxynitrite metabolites, that lead to further generation of free radicals and cytokine activation. Reduction in basal NO activity may be paradoxically accompanied by excess generation of NO after stimulation and catabolism to higher nitrogen oxides. NO bioavailability can be enhanced by administration of antioxidants that scavenge oxygen free radicals (such as ascorbic acid, probucol, or vitamin E), or with superoxide dismutase, angiotensin II receptor antagonists, angiotensin-converting enzyme inhibitors, and endothelin receptor antagonists. In renal failure, eNOS activity may be attenuated by naturally occurring L-arginine analogs (e.g., asymmetric dimethyl L-arginine) that compete for L-arginine binding sites, or by reduced cofactors such as tetrahydrobiopterin that uncouple eNOS and generate superoxide anion. As NO bioavailability decreases, transcriptional factors such as NFκB, which are inactive in normal endothelial cells, become activated and translocate to the nucleus, where they transcribe genes that generate a cascade of events characterized by activation of cytokines (e.g., interleukin-1 or tumor necrosis factor-α) and expression of adhesion molecules (e.g., E-selectin, vascular cell adhesion

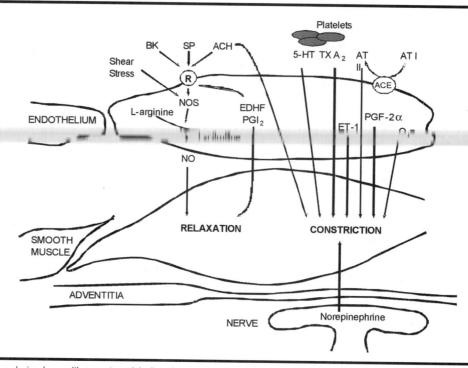

Figure A66.1. Endothelium-derived vasodilators. Acetylcholine (ACH), bradykinin (BK), and substance P (SP) stimulate endothelial cells to release vasodilator substances via activation of specific receptors on the endothelial cell surface. Acetylcholine binds to M_1 or M_3 muscarinic receptors, BK binds to B_2 kinin receptors, and SP binds to NK1 neurokinin receptors. Shear stress activates nitric oxide synthase (NOS) but does not release prostacyclin (PGI_2). Nitric oxide and PGI_2 also have inhibitory effects on platelet aggregation and adhesion.

Endogenous vasoconstrictors. Angiotensin generated in circulating blood and by tissue-bound angiotensin-converting enzyme (ACE) causes vasoconstriction via activation of smooth muscle AT_1-receptors. Endothelin vasoconstricts by activating ET_A- and ET_B-receptors on vascular smooth muscle. Platelet-derived serotonin, thromboxane A_2 (TxA_2), and norepinephrine from sympathetic nerve terminals stimulate smooth muscles via 5-hydroxytryptamine (serotonin, 5-HT), TxA_2, and α_1-adrenergic receptors, respectively. AT I, angiotensin I; AT II, angiotensin II; EDHF, endothelium-derived hyperpolarizing factor; ET-1, endothelin-1; O_2^-, superoxide ion; PGF-2α, prostaglandin F-2α; R, receptor.

molecule-1, and intercellular adhesion molecule-1) on the surface of the endothelial cells. These processes stimulate inflammatory activity in the vessel wall by enhancing the binding and transendothelial migration of leukocytes, thus initiating and facilitating the progression of atherogenesis.

Hormonal influences. Basal release of NO from the vascular endothelium is also closely regulated by other endothelial-derived peptides and mediators. Bradykinin appears to modulate vascular NO activity at rest and on stimulation. Inhibition of bradykinin β_2 receptors causes constriction and inhibits flow-mediated vasodilation, indicating its crucial role in modulating resting coronary vascular tone and function. Blockade of the endothelin ET_A receptor improves endothelial dysfunction in patients with risk factors for atherosclerosis. Other local modulators of endothelial NO are probably angiotensin II, substance P, EDHF, and others.

Genetic predisposition. How family history plays an important and independent role in predisposing to coronary artery disease can be appreciated by understanding the impact of the individual's genotype on the vascular phenotype. Polymorphisms in several genes (**Table A66.1**) are likely to modulate protein expression in diverse molecular pathways and alter endothelial function.

Thrombosis. NO diffuses from the endothelium toward the smooth muscle cell where it stimulates platelet cyclic GMP

Table A66.1. Conventional and Novel Risk Factors

Conventional risk factors for endothelial dysfunction	
Sedentary status/obesity	
Males	
Hypertension	
Hypercholesterolemia	
Type 1 and type 2 diabetes	
Smoking	
Aging	
Postmenopausal status	
Heart failure	
Novel risk factors for endothelial dysfunction	
Insulin resistance	
Homocysteine	
Lipoprotein(a)	
Asymmetric dimethylarginine	
Depression	
Chronic infections	
Inflammatory factors	C-reactive protein
	Interleukin-1
	Interleukin-6
	Tumor necrosis factor-α
Genetic factors	Endothelial nitric oxide synthase
	Angiotensin-converting enzyme I/D
	Angiotensinogen
	Interleukin-6 promoter
	Chemokine receptors
Impaired repair	Low endothelial progenitor activity

activity, thereby preventing platelet aggregation to the blood vessel surface. The endothelium-independent inhibition of platelet adhesiveness and aggregation are enhanced in patients with endothelial dysfunction. The increased local activity of platelet-derived growth aggravates inflammation and promotes atherosclerosis. The vascular endothelium is important in maintaining the balance of the fibrinolytic system. Release of tissue plasminogen activator, which helps protect against endogenous thrombosis, is depressed in conditions associated with endothelial dysfunction, whereas generation of its endogenous inhibitor plasminogen activator inhibitor is increased (see Chapter A23). The mechanisms underlying this relationship have not yet been clearly elucidated; however, bradykinin and angiotensin II appear to play an important role. Thus, endothelial dysfunction leads to an increase in platelet activation and ability to aggregate and a shift in the intrinsic fibrinolytic balance towards a prothrombotic state, which may predispose to acute thrombotic cardiovascular events.

Endothelial Repair and Regeneration

When endothelial denudation and apoptosis occur, repair and replacement depends on the release and delivery of bone marrow–derived stem cells of endothelial lineage, called *endothelial progenitor cells* (EPCs). EPCs can be isolated and grown from peripheral blood samples and constitute a bone marrow–derived population of stem cells that differentiate from a common hemangioblast precursor. They contribute to postnatal neovascularization and may play a key role in ongoing endothelial repair. The number of EPCs in peripheral blood is reduced in patients with coronary artery disease and correlates inversely with the number of risk factors to which patients are exposed. Endothelial function and EPC counts are inversely correlated, independent of traditional risk factors. This raises the intriguing possibility that bone marrow–derived EPCs repair damaged endothelial cells, and endothelial dysfunction occurs as a result of the interaction of risk factors and depletion of reparative EPCs. Finally, there is evidence to indicate that statin therapy increases EPC counts, thus raising the possibility that drugs that improve endothelial function do so partly by stimulating EPC activity.

Clinical Assessment of Coronary Endothelial Function

The most commonly employed techniques for assessing endothelial function are measurement of the vasodilator responses of muscular arteries to vasodilators that release NO (e.g., including acetylcholine, bradykinin, and substance P). Alternately, flow-mediated vasodilator responds to increased shear stress or the response to blockers of eNOS.

Acetylcholine responses. In human studies, the integrity of the endothelium was originally defined by the presence of a preserved vasodilator response to acetylcholine. Abnormal function is characterized by a reduced dilator response or a constrictor response, resulting from smooth muscle muscarinic receptor stimulation that overwhelms the depressed or absent dilating effect of endothelium-derived NO. Most of the observed epicardial dilation and part of the coronary microvascular dilation in response to acetylcholine, substance P, and

bradykinin are due to release of NO, but the remainder appears to be secondary to release of an EDHF, believed to be an epoxide generated from arachidonic acid by the action of cytochrome P450. Patients with angiographically normal coronary arteries and one or more conventional risk factors for atherosclerosis exhibit depressed responses to acetylcholine and other endothelium-dependent vasodilators. The degree of depression of the vasodilator response correlates with the number of risk factors.

L-Arginine analogs. Short-term administration of the L-arginine analog, N^G-monomethyl-L-arginine, a competitive inhibitor of eNOS, elevates systemic blood pressure, reduces coronary blood flow, and constricts epicardial coronary arteries, indicating that tonic basal release of NO in the normal human circulation contributes to resting coronary and peripheral vasodilator tone, at least over the short term. This effect is significantly attenuated in subjects with atherosclerosis or its risk factors, consistent with reduced bioavailability of NO in these individuals.

Peripheral Vascular Endothelial Function: Correlation with Coronary Vascular Function

Endothelium-dependent vasodilator function in muscular arteries can be assessed using 2-D ultrasound. Brachial arterial responses to increased shear stress can be quantitated before and after the hyperemic phase of reperfusion that follows 5 minutes of forearm ischemia. Microvascular endothelium-dependent vasodilator function is measured by assessing the increase in forearm blood flow in response to the endothelium-dependent probes acetylcholine, bradykinin, or substance P. As in the coronary circulation, peripheral endothelium-dependent vasodilation is depressed in the presence of conventional risk factors for atherosclerosis and is predominantly NO dependent, with EDHF playing a larger role in resistance vessel dilation. Studies that have examined the relationship between peripheral and coronary endothelial vasodilator function show a reasonably high correlation.

Serum Markers of Endothelial Dysfunction

The Framingham Heart Study has found that the risk of developing clinically apparent atherosclerosis is only partially accounted for by the presence of conventional risk factors such as hyperlipidemia, hypertension, smoking, aging, and diabetes. Although there is a correlation between the number of conventional risk factors and endothelial dysfunction, this by no means accounts for all the variability observed. Novel risk factors for endothelial dysfunction (Table A66.1) include hyperhomocystinemia, sedentary lifestyle, and exposure to multiple pathogens, including *Chlamydia pneumoniae*, cytomegalovirus, herpes simplex viruses, *Helicobacter pylori*, and hepatitis virus. Mediators of endothelial activation and inflammation can be measured in the circulation and have been studied as indicators of increased risk of future cardiovascular events. Serum levels of C-reactive protein (CRP), an acute-phase reactant produced in response to inflammatory cytokines such as interleukin-6, appears to be a marker of systemic microinflammation. Levels of CRP are raised in association with diabetes, hypertension, hyperlipidemia, and acute coronary syndromes. Moreover, intervention trials with statins have demonstrated that benefit is greatest in those who have high CRP levels, suggesting that individuals with vascular inflammation are likely to experience the greatest benefit. Baseline levels of CRP, serum amyloid A, interleukin-6, and intercellular adhesion molecule-1 appear to independently predict increased cardiovascular risk in healthy patients and in those with acute coronary syndromes.

Clinical Consequences of Endothelial Dysfunction

Endothelial nitric oxide, coronary vasomotion, and myocardial ischemia. Coronary vasodilation in response to stimuli such as exercise, cardiac pacing, or pain (coldpressor) is depressed in subjects with atherosclerosis and in subjects with risk factors for atherosclerosis, in part due to reduced NO bioavailability. Similarly, reduced forearm vasodilation in response to reactive hyperemia in high-risk individuals reflects reduced NO bioavailability. Endothelial dysfunction and reduced coronary vasodilation during physiologic stress can cause myocardial ischemia and angina, even in the presence of normal epicardial coronary arteries, as has been corroborated by several angiographic studies. The mechanism underlying the paradoxical coronary arterial constriction during physiologic stress is considered to be impaired endothelial NO release and activation of AKT kinases in response to increased shear stress. The pathogenesis of coronary artery disease is discussed in Chapter A67.

Treatment to Improve Endothelial Function

Numerous therapeutic strategies have been developed to improve endothelial dysfunction with promising results. Physical exercise reliably improves endothelial dysfunction in the coronary and peripheral circulations of sedentary individuals. Substitution of ω_3-fatty acids in the diet also improves vascular dysfunction, whereas a high fat meal is able to temporarily abrogate endothelial function. L-arginine has shown promise in some studies where oral administration with 5 to 9 g daily has been associated with improvement in function, particularly in those conditions with elevated levels of asymmetric dimethyl L-arginine. Risk factor modification has proven to be an effective approach; for example, several trials of lipid lowering, particularly with statins, have demonstrated significant and sustained

improvement of endothelial dysfunction and increase in EPC activity. Similarly, antihypertensive therapy, particularly with angiotensin-converting enzyme inhibitors and angiotensin receptor antagonists, and, in certain trials, with calcium antagonists, have been associated with improvement in endothelial function. Thiazolidinediones appear to improve endothelial dysfunction in diabetics and in those with insulin resistance compared to sulphonlyureas. Antioxidant vitamins such as vitamins C and E, although able to improve dysfunction when given acutely in high concentrations, do not appear to improve function after chronic oral therapy. Phosphodiesterase inhibitors that decelerate metabolism of cyclic GMP produced as a result of NO release may also improve endothelial dysfunction. New investigative approaches could employ endothelin receptor antagonists, neutral endopeptidase inhibitors, phosphodiesterase type 5 antagonists, novel antiinflammatory agents (e.g., tumor necrosis factor-α antagonists), new generation thiazolidinediones, or cell therapy.

SUGGESTED READING

1. Barnes PJ, Karin M. Nuclear factor-κB: a pivotal transcription factor in chronic inflammatory diseases. *N Engl J Med.* 1997;336:1066–1071.
2. Cai H, Harrison DG. Endothelial dysfunction in cardiovascular diseases: the role of oxidant stress. *Circ Res.* 2000;87:840–844.
3. Diodati JG, Dakak N, Gilligan DM, Quyyumi AA. Effect of atherosclerosis on endothelium-dependent inhibition of platelet activation in humans. *Circulation.* 1998;98(1):17–24.
4. Fichtlscherer S, Rosenberger G, Walter DH, et al. Elevated C-reactive protein levels and impaired endothelial vasoreactivity in patients with coronary artery disease. *Circulation.* 2000;102:1000–1006.
5. Halcox JPJ, Quyyumi AA. Coronary vascular endothelial function and myocardial ischemia: why should we worry about endothelial dysfunction. *Coron Artery Dis.* 2001;12:475–484.
6. Jern S, Wall U, Bergbrant A, et al. Endothelium-dependent vasodilation and tissue-type plasminogen activator release in borderline hypertension. *Arterioscler Thromb Vasc Biol.* 1997;17(12):3376–3383.
7. Ludmer PL, Selwyn AP, Shook TL, et al. Paradoxical vasoconstriction induced by acetylcholine in atherosclerotic coronary arteries. *N Engl J Med.* 1986;315:1046–1051.
8. Quyyumi AA, Dakak N, Andrews NP, et al. Nitric oxide activity in the human coronary circulation. Impact of risk factors for coronary atherosclerosis. *J Clin Invest.* 1995;95:1747–1755.
9. Schachinger V, Britten MB, Zeiher AM. Prognostic impact of coronary vasodilator dysfunction on adverse long-term outcome of coronary heart disease. *Circulation.* 2000;101:1899–1906.

Chapter A67

Atherogenesis and Coronary Artery Disease

Thomas D. Giles, MD

KEY POINTS

- Atherosclerosis is a complex degenerative condition initially characterized by endothelial dysfunction and lipid accumulation in the endothelium and media, followed by wall thickening and outward remodeling, and later by luminal encroachment, thrombosis, and occlusion.

- Atherosclerotic plaque formation involves the interaction of genetic predisposition and environmental risk factors (e.g., dyslipidemia, hypertension, insulin resistance, smoking, infections) with diffuse vascular injury caused by hemodynamic (shear) stress, cellular proliferation, chronic low-grade inflammation, and thrombosis.

- Hypertension promotes or accelerates all phases of the development of atherosclerotic lesions, from plaque formation to rupture.

- Plaque instability and deterioration lead to sudden events such as erosion, fracture, or thrombosis, with or without vessel occlusion, that cause acute myocardial infarction and sudden death.

See also Chapters A16, A23, A24, A65, A66, B81, B85, C115, C116, and C154

Atherosclerosis is a degenerative disorder that includes vascular cell proliferation, medial expansion of conduit arteries, ischemia, and, ultimately, ischemic necrosis of myocardium. This major disease is a dominating worldwide source of morbidity and mortality, expressing itself not only as coronary heart disease, but as cerebrovascular and peripheral arterial disease. The risk of atherosclerosis is significantly amplified by the presence of hypertension, insulin resistance, smoking, and lack of exercise.

Metabolic Factors in Atherogenesis

Low-density lipoprotein and apo-lipoproteins. Epidemiologic studies have established that elevated total cholesterol, increased low-density lipoprotein (LDL) and decreased high-density lipoprotein (HDL) are major risk factors associated with atherosclerosis and its major consequences. Dietary lipids are transported by the portal circulation to the liver as triglycerides in chylomicrons. The liver loads triglycerides into very-low-density lipoprotein, which interacts with LDL and HDL to transport lipids to and from peripheral tissues. LDL particles consist of a phospholipid coat enclosing cholesterol and carrying a unique protein apolipoprotein B-100 (Apo-B). In industrialized societies, circulating LDL increases dramatically in the first 2 decades of life. Abnormalities of other components, including lipoprotein(a), which surrounds the lipid center and serves as a transport mechanism, also exist in individuals with coronary disease.

Low-density lipoprotein metabolism and receptor action. The N-terminal domain of Apo-B is recognized by specific LDL receptors that allow hepatic uptake. Approximately 75% of LDL is removed from the circulation by the liver by LDL receptors that are regulated by specific genes controlled by transcription factors sensitive to circulating LDL levels. Decreased blood or tissue LDL leads to upregulation of LDL receptors that enhance LDL removal and turnover. Upregulation of LDL receptors is a major part of the beneficial effects of hydroxymethylglutaryl coenzyme A reductase inhibition. Apo-B is also recognized by LDL receptors on endothelial cells and hepatocytes. The removal rate of LDL from the circulation depends on the number and availability of LDL receptors. LDL can accumulate in the arterial wall when serum concentrations are high.

High-density lipoprotein metabolism. HDL is a unique protein secreted into the plasma by the liver and intestines that binds to circulating cholesterol. HDL prevents the oxidation of LDL by binding to transitional metal ions in the intima. HDL serves as a reservoir for apolipoproteins and is the major factor controlling cholesterol uptake by the liver. When HDL interacts with cell membranes, lecithin cholesterol acyltransferase combines cholesterol and phosphatidyl choline to make cholesteryl ester, which is then transported to the liver. HDL contains a phospholipid coat with an Apo E protein, which affects reverse cholesterol transport and can also function as an antioxidant that controls subsequent inflammatory responses. Thus, in contrast to LDL, high HDL levels help prevent atherosclerosis.

Oxygen radicals and nitrate metabolism. Oxidation and oxidized LDL itself lead to a continuous local excess of oxygen free radicals that play an important pathogenic role in atherosclerosis (see Chapter A65). Excess free radicals bind to nitric oxide (NO) to produce peroxynitrite. When free radicals are generated in the presence of peroxynitrite, there is a reduction in the activity of endothelial NO synthase (eNOS). The appearance of abnormal substrates that compete for eNOS, including asymmetric dimethylarginine, impair the ability of DNA and messenger RNA to code for the production of eNOS and also cause abnormal binding between eNOS and caveolin, a membrane-bound protein that further disables the enzyme. All of these mechanisms lead to impairment of endothelium-dependent dilation and other vascular protective properties.

Low-density lipoprotein oxidation and vascular scavenger pathways. LDL is protected from oxidation in the blood, but if it is present in sufficient excess to penetrate the extracellular matrix in the vessel wall, it is subsequently oxidized by a variety of enzymatic and nonenzymatic mechanisms, including myeloperoxidase, 15-lipoxygenase, and nicotinamide adenine dinucleotide phosphate oxidase. Lipid oxidation is amplified in diabetes, insulin resistance, smoking, and hypertension. In atherogenesis, the lysine component of the LDL particle is modified so that it is no longer recognized by the classic LDL receptor. At the same time, lipoprotein scavenger receptors appear on vascular and inflammatory cells. Oxidized LDL (oxo-LDL) is taken up by macrophages and foam cells via the scavenger receptors at a rate up to 10 times faster than LDL receptors can process. Thus, activation of vascular scavenger receptors leads to preferential accumulation of oxo-LDL within cells, a process that is central to the progression of atherosclerosis. Oxo-LDL is also a potent chemoattractant for circulating macrophages, and when ingested by macrophages, inhibits their motility, leads to sequestration of macrophages in the intima of arterial wall, and exhibits cytotoxicity in endothelial cells. Glycated LDL is highly immunogenic and LDL-immune complexes are rapidly phagocytized by macrophages. The unique Apo-B protein associated with LDL also becomes fragmented and immunogenic.

Vascular Susceptibility to Atherosclerosis

There is wide variation in the clinical expression of atherosclerosis that is explained in part by differences in individual blood vessels.

Endothelial dysfunction. Early impairment of endothelium-dependent NO-dependent vasodilation (see Chapter A66) appears in the younger relatives of patients with arterial disease. This clinical observation is consistent with outcomes from a wide range of genetic knockout experiments involving LDL receptors, interleukin-10, Apo-A1 receptors, and other receptors that lead to impairment of the protective mechanisms in the arterial wall and amplify atherosclerosis. The endothelium normally exhibits a slow turnover rate, and there are adequate anticoagulant defenses, including adequate production of tissue plasminogen activator (tPA) and heparans and limited production of plasminogen activator inhibitor (PAI-1) and thrombomodulin. The healthy endothelium also maintains adequate constitutive local production of NO, which maintains optimum lumen area, limits the impact of shear forces, and contributes to the local defense against coagulation.

Hemodynamic factors and shear stress. Local physical forces are important in the pathogenesis and location of initial fatty streak development and early atherosclerotic lesions. Typically, the outer walls of arterial bifurcations and inner walls of arterial curvatures are most affected. Low shear stress promotes vasoconstriction, inhibits vasodilation, and promotes clotting. These processes are probably mediated through release of growth factors such as platelet-derived growth factor, transforming growth factor-β, and fibroblast growth factor-2, as well as through local release of inflammatory mediators such as vascular cell adhesion molecule-1 (VCAM-1), intercellular adhesion molecule-1 (ICAM-1), and monocyte chemotactic peptide (MCP-1). At the same time, vascular synthesis of NO and tPA are reduced and thrombosis is promoted through the release of thrombomodulin. Atherogenesis appears to be heightened at branch points and at flow dividers in conduit arteries. There is clinical evidence of early endothelium-dependent vasodilator dysfunction at these sites. There is also experimental evidence of the augmented activation of transcription factors such as NFκB that code for genes that initiate inflammation at susceptible branch points.

Vascular smooth muscle cells. During atherogenesis, vascular smooth muscle cells alter their phenotypic state. They migrate and proliferate locally, while accumulating oxo-LDL. Vascular smooth muscle cells exhibit proinflammatory mechanisms and secrete additional matrix that contribute to intimal-medial thickening and vascular stiffness.

Mononuclear cells. Abnormal and immunogenic protein epitopes on oxo-LDL provoke a response that resembles the normal reaction to infective agents. The expression of adhesion molecules, at first E-selectin and then ICAM and VCAM, attract then bind mononuclear cells to endothelial cell membranes. The bound monocytes are then subject to enhanced LDL oxidation via expression of ligands that bind MCP-1, which permits bound monocytes to take up more oxo-LDL via scavenger pathways. MCP-1 also impairs cholesterol efflux and binds to proteoglycans, subintimal collagen, and fibrin. Local inflammation is further enhanced when bound monocytes produce tumor necrosis factor-α, MCP-1, interleukins, chemoattractants, and chemokines. Monocyte-macrophages also present oxo-LDL antigens to T lymphocytes, contributing to the appearance of circulating antibodies to these altered proteins.

Inflammation. The presence of excess oxidant stress leads to activation of transcription factors such as NFκB, which cause upregulation of genes that initiate inflammation. Inflammation is exacerbated by the presence of certain intermediates of cholesterol synthesis, including mevalonate and geranyl-pyrophosphate, which interact with oxo-LDL to facilitate the isoprenylation (activation) of small proteins (e.g., rho GGP and geranyl rho-kinase) that regulate the inflammatory processes leading to atherogenesis and plaque formation. The above processes lead to impairment of endothelium-dependent dilation, in part because of the loss of available NO, as well as propagation of chronic low-grade inflammation, with the further differentiation of monocytes into macrophages in the blood vessel wall. Inflammation plays a role in every stage of atherosclerosis, including increased serum C-reactive protein, a marker of inflammation. Hypertension itself, a prominent risk factor for atherosclerosis, is associated with an enhanced inflammatory process that may be partly dependent on the actions of angiotensin II, which is thought to promote hypertensive end-organ damage via enhanced production of superoxide anion, increased expression by arterial smooth muscle cells of proinflammatory cytokines (e.g., interleukin-6 and MCP-1) and adhesion molecules (e.g., VCAM-1, ICAM, and P-selectin) by endothelial cells.

Coagulation. The proinflammatory mediators that cause inflammation also lead to the development of a procoagulant endothelial vascular interface that favors thrombosis. A deficiency of tPA relative to the available amount of PAI-1 enhances these procoagulant tendencies (see Chapter A23).

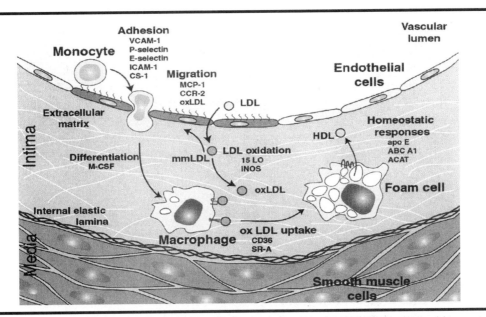

Figure A67.1. Early cell biology of atherosclerosis. Low-density lipoprotein (LDL) passes into the subintimal space and becomes oxidized. This leads to activation of the endothelium, where chemoattractants such as macrophage chemoattractant protein-1 serve to attract inflammatory cells. Activation of the endothelial surface includes expression of adhesion molecules such as vascular cell adhesion molecule-1 (VCAM-1), P-selectin, E-selectin, and intercellular adhesion molecule-1 (ICAM-1). These initiate monocyte transport into the subintima where macrophage colony stimulating factor facilitates transformation into a macrophage. Further uptake of oxidized LDL (OxLDL) occurs under the influence of specific receptors (CD36 and SR-A) in foam cell formation. (From Glass CK, Witzum JL. Atherosclerosis: the road ahead. *Cell*. 2001;104:503–516.)

Infection. Evidence continues to mount that infectious agents may contribute to atherogenesis. In particular, *Chlamydia pneumoniae* and cytomegalovirus exacerbate lesion development in animal models of atherosclerosis and restenosis. The risk of atherosclerosis related to infections is probably additive to other atherogenic stimuli to which an individual is exposed.

Progression of Coronary Atherosclerosis

Angioscopic and pathologic studies in humans have clearly shown that patients with clinically manifest coronary artery disease almost always have multiple plaques throughout their epicardial coronary arteries at different stages of development, with many exhibiting the features of high risk. The focal stenoses seen in conventional coronary angiography under-represent the degree of intimal thickening and plaque formation that occur in susceptible coronary arteries. Each plaque has its own history of growth, activation, erosion, fracture, thrombosis, and healing.

Early lesions. The early lesions (**Figure A67.1**) can be described morphologically as fatty dots or streaks associated histologically with the presence of isolated macrophage foam cells and multiple foam cell layers within the arterial intima. Accumulation of lipid in the arterial intima occurs when levels of oxo-LDL and blood pressure exceed threshold levels. Oxidized lipoproteins are then internalized by macrophages and intimal smooth muscle cells that change into characteristic foam cells. The integrity of the endothelium plays a key role in the rate at which lipids accumulate in the intima. When the endothelium is functionally impaired, as in dyslipidemia or insulin resistance, atherogenesis proceeds faster. Typically, smooth muscle cells and macrophages accumulate with some preference for the outer edges of branch points and flow dividers.

Arterial remodeling. Arterial remodeling is the result of the response of the arterial wall to the atherosclerotic process. In the past, atherosclerosis was thought to cause only progressive luminal encroachment. However, intravascular ultrasound studies have confirmed the model of progression proposed by Glagov and colleagues; accumulation of lipid in the arterial wall initially causes adventitial ("eutrophic outward") remodeling, with preservation of the arterial lumen. Only in advanced stages of atherogenesis does arterial narrowing occur.

Advanced lesions. The connection between minimal and advanced atherosclerosis resides principally in the formation of pools of extracellular lipid and the local fibrotic responses to the associated chronic inflammation (**Figure A67.2**). Local oxidant stress maintains continuous monocyte activation and results in production of tissue factor, impairment of cholesterol efflux, and appearance of several mechanisms mediating apoptosis (death receptors, protooncogenes, and tumor suppressor genes). These mechanisms may also be responsible for increased collection of debris in an expanding plaque. Extracellular lipid is mostly derived from macrophage foam cells that have died. As the lesions advance, the central core of the atheroma lesion is replaced by lipid, and there is disruption of the plaque surface layer ("fibrous cap"), with local hematoma and thrombus formation and, often, distal embolization. Disruption occurs where the shear forces are greatest, at the shoulder of the fibrous cap of the plaque. Activated cellular processes result in the formation of new connective tissue matrix, but these lesions do not tend to narrow the arterial lumen until the process is far advanced. Activated macrophages at these sites produce matrix metalloproteinases that are capable of digesting collagen-1, leaving behind weak and fragmented collagen fibers. Neovascularization in the intima appears to be another

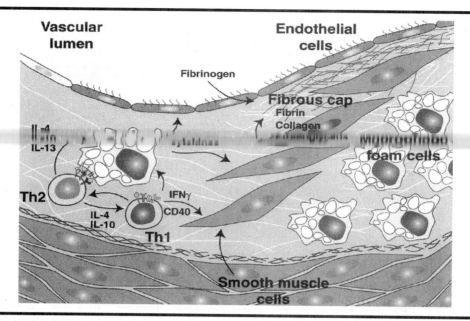

Figure A67.2. Plaque formation in atherosclerosis. The activated endothelium under the influence of oxidized low-density lipoprotein continues to permit the subintimal collection of inflammatory cells. In concert with T lymphocytes (Th2) and local production of chemokines [interleukin (IL)-1, IL-6, and IL-10], this chronic low-grade inflammation attracts activated smooth muscle cells that deposit collagen in the intima. The collection of the macrophage, foam cells, smooth muscle cells, matrix, and collagen as shown make up the development of the plaque. IFNγ, interferon gamma; Th1, T helper cell 1. (From Glass CK, Witzum JL. Atherosclerosis: the road ahead. *Cell*. 2001;104:503–516.)

late phenomenon, likely in response to repeated cycles of local rupture, hemorrhage, thrombosis, and healing, which all appear to be characterized by local accumulation of proteases.

Vulnerable plaques. Any plaque that is susceptible to disruption is said to be vulnerable (**Figure A67.3**). With further progression of the atherosclerotic process, calcification occurs. When 50% or more of the cross-sectional area of an atheroscle-

rotic lesion is mineralized, the lesion is termed *calcified*. Narrowing may occur abruptly with plaque disruption. The vulnerability of a plaque does not correlate well with its appearance at angiography. The most vulnerable plaques are usually those with large lipid cores, thin fibrous caps, and less calcium, so the determination of the degree of calcification (often semiquantitated using computerized tomography) may mislead one into underestimating the severity of the atherosclerotic plaque.

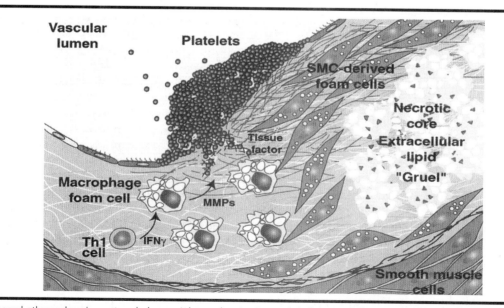

Figure A67.3. Advanced atherosclerosis: ruptured plaque. Advanced activation and dysfunction of the endothelium results in a procoagulant surface that attracts platelet and fibrin thrombi. In the atherosclerotic plaque, foam cells undergo programmed cell death to form a necrotic core. At the edge of the plaque, activated macrophages and foam cells continue to propagate low-grade inflammation and produce matrix metalloproteinases (MMPs) and tissue factor that enhance plaque rupture, hemorrhage, and thrombosis. IFNγ, interferon γ; SMC, smooth muscle cell; Th1, T helper cell. (From Glass CK, Witzum JL. Atherosclerosis: the road ahead. *Cell*. 2001;104:503–516, with permission.)

Clinical Correlations: Coronary Syndromes

Occlusive coronary disease and stable angina. With plaques of the stable variety, stenoses grow slowly without sudden deterioration. The progressive lumen narrowing impairs laminar flow and stress-induced increases in blood flow velocity. A pressure gradient eventually appears, there is progressive failure to increase flow on demand, and finally, episodic decreases in flow, in part due to the loss of endothelium-dependent dilation and abnormal reflex constriction. Transient decreases in coronary blood flow contribute to episodes of regional myocardial ischemia and a pattern of relatively stable angina pectoris that appears predictably at a given level of myocardial work.

Unstable angina and infarction. In contrast to stable angina, unstable angina (progressive or Prinzmetal's angina) is caused by vulnerable plaques, which have episodic local inflammatory flares, erosion, rupture, and thrombosis (with or without occlusion). Often, the acute event is minor and is followed by a degree of healing. When an unstable plaque suddenly deteriorates, major consequences are also common and acute alterations in regional coronary blood may lead to unstable angina, acute myocardial infarction, or death. The same pathogenic risk factors that cause chronic inflammation in each plaque remain actively involved throughout the development of the disease. Vulnerable plaques and complex lesions that acutely degenerate are often not visible with conventional angiography.

Atherosclerotic Markers

The appreciation of the relationship between the cell biology and clinical syndromes in atherosclerosis has encouraged the exploration of markers or surrogates to detect disease activity, estimate risk, and monitor therapies. These efforts include the imaging of atherosclerosis by optical coherence tomography or magnetic resonance. Blood tests to assess insulin resistance, C-reactive protein, PAI-1, and ICAM-1 have been employed in clinical studies, but none of these promising new endeavors has been shown to be uniquely sensitive or specific in primary or secondary prevention.

SUGGESTED READING

1. Epstein SE, Zhou YF, Zhu J. Infection and atherosclerosis: emerging mechanistic paradigms. *Circulation.* 1999;100:e20–e28.
2. Fuster V, Badimon L, Badimon JJ, Chesebro JH. The pathogenesis of coronary artery disease and the acute coronary syndrome. *N Engl J Med.* 1992;326:242–250.
3. Glagov S, Weisenberg E, Zarins CK, et al. Compensatory enlargement of human atherosclerotic coronary arteries. *N Engl J Med.* 1987;316:1371–1375.
4. Glass CK, Witzum JL. Atherosclerosis: the road ahead. *Cell.* 2001;104:503–516.
5. Kinlay S, Selwyn AP, Delagrange D, et al. Biological mechanisms for the clinical success of lipid-lowering in coronary artery disease and the use of surrogate end-points. *Curr Opin Lipidol.* 1996;7:389–397.
6. Lee RT, Libby P. The unstable atheroma. *Arterioscler Thromb Vasc Biol.* 1997;17:1859–1867.
7. Libby P, Ridker PM, Maseri A. Inflammation and atherosclerosis. *Circulation.* 2002;105:1135–1143.
8. Malek AM, Alper SL, Izumo S. Hemodynamic shear stress and its role in atherosclerosis. *JAMA.* 1999;282:2035–2042.
9. Selwyn AP, Kinlay S, Libby P, Ganz P. Atherogenic lipids, vascular dysfunction, and clinical signs of ischemic heart disease. *Circulation.* 1997;95:5–7.
10. Stary HC. Evolution and progression of atherosclerotic lesions in coronary arteries of children and young adults. *Arteriosclerosis.* 1989;9:119–132.

Chapter A68

Pathogenesis of Stroke

J. David Spence, MD, MBA; Patrick Pullicino, MD, PhD

KEY POINTS

- Blood pressure–related strokes caused by hyaline degeneration (lipohyalinosis) of the arteries at the base of the brain can be reduced markedly by good blood pressure control.

- Strokes may also be caused when an artery is occluded by an atheromatous plaque with or without an associated thrombus or by an embolus from a proximal source.

- Emboli may consist of atheromatous debris, platelet aggregates (white thrombus), or *in situ* (red) thrombus and may arise from an artery, the aorta, the heart, or the venous system by way of a patent foramen ovale; identification is important because treatment depends on the specific cause of stroke.

- Cerebral ischemic injury is not an "all-or-none" phenomenon, and the degree and duration of cerebral hypoperfusion are important in determining its severity.

- Clinical features may help localize the cerebral ischemic injury but are not reliable indicators of underlying pathogenesis; imaging studies are important for the appropriate management of a stroke patient.

See also Chapters A38, A60, A63, A64, A69, A70, B82, C125, and C160

The term *brain attack* has been proposed to replace *stroke* to stress the similarities between brain and heart ischemia and to emphasize the need for emergent treatment. The 3 main differences between stroke and heart attacks are

- Embolism is a major cause of stroke but an uncommon cause of heart attack.
- Occlusion of carotid or large intracranial arteries produces focal ischemic necrosis less frequently in the brain than coronary occlusion does in the heart because of the greater collateral circulation through the circle of Willis and cortical anastomoses.
- Hemorrhage secondary to arterial rupture is a frequent cause of stroke (<10%) but not of heart attack.

Cardiac ischemia is loosely related to stroke because subsequent atrial fibrillation and low cardiac output predispose to cerebral embolism. In addition, depending on the population used, 0.5% to 8.0% of cerebral infarctions are due to embolism related to recent myocardial infarction.

Pathogenetic Mechanisms of Cerebrovascular Disease

Hypertension. Hypertension is the most potent risk factor for cerebrovascular disease and contributes directly to the occurrence of stroke in at least 3 major ways and indirectly by exacerbating several other degenerative processes.

Lipohyalinosis, lacunar infarcts, and cerebral hemorrhage. Hypertension is associated with focal damage to small intracerebral arteries (lipohyalinosis) that causes the arteries to occlude. Ischemic necrosis then can give rise to small cavities in the brain (lacunar infarcts). Lipohyalinosis is also associated with rupture of small intracerebral arteries, which causes cerebral hemorrhage. The most vulnerable areas at the base of the brain collectively have been called the *vascular centrencephalon* (basal ganglia, thalamus, internal capsule, brain stem, and cerebellum). In this territory, short straight arteries with few branches transmit the pressure load directly to the resistance vessels, which can be mechanically damaged. In contrast, the arteries to the cortex are relatively long and have many branches, so the pressure load is dissipated to a greater degree. Blood pressure control reduces stroke by 40% and virtually eliminates strokes due to hypertensive small vessel disease.

Arteriolar hypertrophy, ischemic rarefaction, and dementia. Hypertension causes hypertrophy and thickening of the media of small intracerebral arteries, which favors diffuse hypoperfusion and ischemic rarefaction of white matter, especially in the periventricular "watershed" areas of the brain. White matter ischemic rarefaction (or subcortical arteriosclerotic encephalopathy) is present in almost all patients with long-standing hypertension and may give rise to a dementia syndrome called *Binswanger's disease* (see Chapter A69).

Berry aneurysms and subarachnoid hemorrhage. Hypertension is a risk factor for the rupture of larger berry aneurysms and associated subarachnoid hemorrhage.

Embolism. Emboli arise either from the heart or from proximal arteries. High-risk and medium-risk sources of embolism were identified as part of the TOAST study (**Table A68.1**).

Cardiac emboli. Cardiac emboli arise from cardiac thrombi in the left side of the heart secondary to abnormal intracardiac hemodynamics (e.g., dilated left atrium in atrial fibrillation) or from paradoxic embolism due to thrombi arising in the sys-

Table A68.1. **Trial of Org 10172 in Acute Stroke Treatment (TOAST) Classification of High- and Medium-Risk Sources of Cardioembolism**

High-risk sources
  Mechanical prosthetic valve
  Mitral stenosis with atrial fibrillation
  Atrial fibrillation (other than lone atrial fibrillation)
  Left atrial/atrial appendage thrombus
  Sick sinus syndrome
  Recent myocardial infarction (<4 wk)
  Left ventricular thrombus
  Dilated cardiomyopathy
  Akinetic left ventricular segment
  Atrial myxoma
  Infective endocarditis
Medium-risk sources
  Mitral valve prolapse
  Mitral annulus calcification
  Mitral stenosis without atrial fibrillation
  Left atrial turbulence (smoke)
  Atrial septal aneurysm
  Patent foramen ovale
  Atrial flutter
  Lone atrial fibrillation
  Bioprosthetic cardiac valve
  Nonbacterial thrombotic endocarditis
  Congestive heart failure
  Hypokinetic left ventricular segment
  Myocardial infarction (>4 wk, <6 mo)

From Adams HP Jr, Bendixen BH, Kappelle LJ, et al., and the TOAST Investigators. Classification of subtype of acute ischemic stroke: definitions for use in a multicenter clinical trial. *Stroke.* 1993;24:35–41, with permission.

temic veins and traversing to the left side of the heart through a patent foramen ovale (4% of ischemic strokes).

Arterial emboli. Arterial emboli are dislodged fragments of atherosclerotic debris or thrombi arising in an area of stagnant flow distal to a stenosis or secondary to atherosclerosis or dissection. Arteriogenic emboli frequently arise from the internal carotid artery near the carotid bifurcation and from the vertebral artery near its origin or termination. A tight stenosis can give rise to tiny arteriogenic emboli of platelet clumps that may produce recurrent transient focal cerebral or ocular ischemia. Embolization of atheromatous debris from a site of severe carotid stenosis can be prevented by endarterectomy.

Coagulation disorders. Coagulation disorders, including hyperhomocystinemia and factor V Leiden, predispose to cardioembolic stroke; factor V Leiden probably underlies the early excess of thromboembolic events in women treated with hormone replacement therapy.

Atherosclerosis. Atherosclerosis may become symptomatic by 3 major mechanisms.

Arteriogenic embolism. Atheroembolization of platelet aggregates (white thrombus) or atheromatous debris with or without white or red thrombus occludes arteries lying more distally. Quantitation of the surface area or volume of plaque in the carotid artery can be used to predict future stroke.

Hypoperfusion. Occlusion of an artery secondary to plaque rupture or intraplaque hemorrhage causes hemodynamic obstruction and produces distal cerebral hypoperfusion. The term *cerebral thrombosis* is often used for this process but may be somewhat misleading if it is interpreted as meaning that cerebral arter-

ies are typically occluded by primary thrombus formation. In actuality, the high blood flow velocity in cerebral arteries does not allow time for polymerization of fibrin to produce red thrombus. Arterial thrombosis occurs more commonly after the artery occludes, or rarely in the heart, in the setting of low blood flow due to atrial fibrillation or ventricular aneurysm. The distinction between white and red thrombus may be clinically useful. A white thrombus is treated preventively with antiplatelet agents, whereas red thrombus is treated acutely with anticoagulants.

Atherosclerotic occlusion. Atherosclerosis may occlude small penetrating arteries less than 1 mm in diameter (microatheroma) and may contribute to the formation of cavitary (lacunar) infarcts. Critical narrowing of small penetrating arteries may also cause recurrent episodes of transient hypoperfusion distally, presenting clinically as transient ischemic attacks.

Cortical hemorrhage. Hemorrhages in the cerebral cortex itself or in subcortical areas (not at the base of the brain) are much more commonly due to vascular malformations or to amyloid angiopathy rather than hypertension.

Clinical Aspects of Ischemic Stroke

Figure A68.1 gives relative frequency of ischemic stroke subtypes. With current levels of blood pressure control, lacunar strokes are approximately equal in frequency to embolic and large-vessel strokes.

Disease spectrum. Ischemic stroke is not an all-or-none phenomenon as was once thought. Reduction of cerebral blood flow due to arterial stenosis or occlusion may produce any degree of tissue injury, varying from isolated neuronal dropout to rarefaction of all tissue elements to complete cavitary necrosis. The 2 factors that appear to be most important in determining the severity of injury secondary to arterial occlusion are (a) the efficiency of the collateral circulation and (b) overall blood flow, which is related to cardiac output. The clinical manifestations of occlusion of a specific artery vary according to how the interplay of these factors affects local brain perfusion. A spectrum of clinical syndromes therefore exists, although a minor degree of hypoperfusion is often asymptomatic (**Figure A68.2**). More severe ischemia results in a reversible symptomatic loss of function (transient ischemic attack) but not tissue injury. Marked hypoperfusion and prolonged ischemia causes tissue necrosis with persistent clinical sequelae (irreversible stroke). Imaging techniques (magnetic resonance imaging, single-photon emission computed tomography, or transcranial Doppler) help define lesion extent and degree of cerebral perfusion, thereby improving therapy.

Acute stroke and the ischemic penumbra. It has been realized that moderate reduction of blood flow may not produce injury if reversed quickly but will progress to infarction if allowed to persist for 2 to 3 hours (Figure A68.2). Many strokes have a central core of severe reduction of blood flow with permanent infarction surrounded by a rim of tissue with moderate reduction of blood flow in which the dysfunction is potentially reversible. This surrounding area is called the *ischemic penumbra*. Restoration of normal flow to the penumbra within a few hours can result in restoration of function and clinical improvement. The ability of anticoagulants and thrombolytics and brain protective agents to improve outcome after a stroke appears to depend on the presence of an ischemic penumbra.

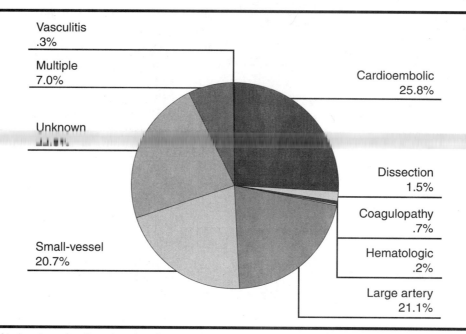

Vasculitis
.3%

Multiple
7.0%

Unknown

Small-vessel
20.7%

Cardioembolic
25.8%

Dissection
1.5%

Coagulopathy
.7%

Hematologic
.2%

Large artery
21.1%

Figure A68.1.   Subtypes of ischemic stroke. (Based on data from Grau AJ, Weimar C, Buggle F, et al. Risk factors, outcome and treatment in subtypes of ischemic stroke. *Stroke.* 2001;32:2559–2566.)

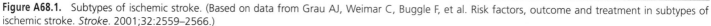

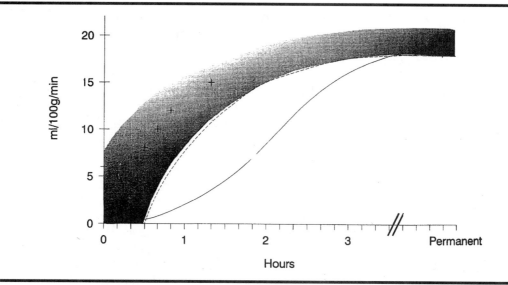

Figure A68.2.   Graph showing time-intensity relationship of ischemia and incomplete infarction. Area above curves represents combination of duration and intensity of ischemia that is tolerated without development of infarction, whereas points below curves result in infarction. Shaded area represents ischemic injury without infarction. (From Helgason CM, Wolf PA. American Heart Association Prevention Conference IV: prevention and rehabilitation of stroke. *Stroke.* 1997;28:1498–1526, with permission.)

Watershed (border-zone, low-flow) ischemia. An uncommon form of cerebral injury secondary to hypoperfusion often occurs in "watershed zones" between cerebral arterial territories. These low-flow or border-zone infarcts occur in the deep white matter adjacent to the lateral ventricle and are frequently associated with ipsilateral carotid occlusion.

Dementia and Stroke

The Nun Study showed a strong interaction between stroke and expression of Alzheimer's disease. Among some 700 nuns followed prospectively with testing of cognitive function, those with Alzheimer's disease at autopsy were 20 times as likely to have been demented in life if they had even 1 or 2 small lacunar infarcts (see Chapter A69).

SUGGESTED READING

1. Spence JD. Cerebral consequences of hypertension. In: Laragh JH, Brenner B, eds. *Hypertension: Pathophysiology, Diagnosis, and Management.* New York, NY: Raven Press; 1995:741–753.
2. SHEP Cooperative Research Group. Prevention of stroke by antihypertensive drug treatment in older persons with isolated systolic hypertension. Final results of the Systolic Hypertension in the Elderly Program (SHEP). *JAMA.* 1991;265:3255–3264.
3. Snowdon DA, Greiner LH, Mortimer JA, et al. Brain infarction and the clinical expression of Alzheimer disease. The Nun Study. *JAMA.* 1997;277:813–817.
4. Grau AJ, Weimar C, Buggle F, et al. Risk factors, outcome and treatment in subtypes of ischemic stroke. *Stroke.* 2001;32:2559–2566.
5. Adams HP Jr, Bendixen BH, Kappelle LJ, et al. and the TOAST Investigators. Classification of subtype of acute ischemic stroke: definitions for use in a multicenter clinical trial. *Stroke.* 1993;24:35–41.
6. Bronner LL, Kanter DS, Manson JE. Primary prevention of stroke. *N Engl J Med.* 1995;333:1392–1400.

7. Caplan LR. *Stroke: A Clinical Approach*. Boston, MA: Butterworth–Heine-mann; 1993.
8. Garcia JH, Lassen NA, Weiller C, et al. Ischemic stroke and incomplete infarction. *Stroke*. 1996;27:761–765.
9. Pullicino PM, Caplan LR, Hommel M. *Cerebral Small Artery Disease*. New York, NY: Raven Press; 1993.
10. Whisnant JP. Effectiveness versus efficacy of treatment of hypertension for stroke prevention. *Neurology*. 1996;46:301–307.

Chapter A69

Pathogenesis of Acute Hypertensive Encephalopathy

Donald D. Heistad, MD; William J. Lawton, MD; William T. Talman, MD

KEY POINTS

- Sympathetic nerves and local arteriolar constriction normally protect the cerebral microvasculature from hypertensive damage.

- Hypertensive encephalopathy is most likely due to "breakthrough" of cerebral autoregulation, with marked cerebral vasodilation disruption of the blood–brain barrier, and permeability increases, particularly in postcapillary venules.

- Breakthrough of autoregulation may be, in part, an active process mediated by calcium-dependent potassium channels.

- Hypertensive encephalopathy, a medical emergency usually accompanied by severe hypertension, headache, and other neurologic symptoms, responds clinically to blood pressure reduction.

See also Chapters A26, A34, A39, C125, C153, and C160

Hypertensive encephalopathy is a syndrome of severe hypertension with cerebral dysfunction and neurologic impairment. The diagnosis may be in doubt until neurologic improvement occurs as a result of pharmacologic reduction of arterial pressure. However, improvement may not occur until several days after reduction of arterial pressure (**Table A69.1**).

Pathophysiology

Role of exaggerated vasodilation. It was thought in the past that hypertensive encephalopathy is produced by cerebral ischemia resulting from spasm of cerebral blood vessels. This suggestion was based in part on the finding that, during acute hypertension in experimental animals, cerebral arterioles resemble a "sausage string," with segments of constricted and dilated blood vessels. A similar sausage-string appearance may be seen in retinal vessels of patients with hypertensive encephalopathy. There is now considerable evidence that the constricted portion of the sausage string represents the normal segments of the arterioles and the dilated portions represent the abnormal segments. The normal response of cerebral arterioles to acute hypertension is constriction, as the vessels "autoregulate" and prevent increases in blood flow during periods of increased blood pressure. Hypertension beyond the autoregulatory range causes small arteries and arterioles to dilate, blood flow to increase or "breakthrough," and microvascular pressure to increase.

Disruption of blood–brain barrier. With breakthrough of autoregulation, the blood–brain barrier may be impaired. The initial site of disruption of the blood–brain barrier during acute hypertension appears to be cerebral venules, not capillaries or arterioles. Cerebral arterioles are protected by a layer of smooth muscle cells, and wall stress in capillaries may not increase greatly because their diameter is small. In contrast, cerebral venules may be most vulnerable to increases in wall stress during acute hypertension, because their diameters are rather large and because venules do not have a layer of smooth muscle cells. Abnormal permeability may also occur.

Neurovascular dysregulation and abnormal ion transport. Sympathetic neural discharge, which normally has little effect on cerebral blood vessels, constricts cerebral vessels during acute hypertension, causing a shift in the autoregulation curve and setting the breakthrough point to higher levels of arterial pressure. Thus, activation of sympathetic nerves acts to attenuate increases in cerebral blood flow during acute hypertension and protects against disruption of the blood–brain barrier in downstream vessels.

Other mechanisms. Evidence suggests that activation of calcium-dependent potassium channels may also contribute to breakthrough of autoregulation. The finding suggests that breakthrough of autoregulation may involve an active process, with activation of potassium channels, and may not be simply a passive phenomenon that occurs when arterial pressure exceeds the autoregulatory capacity of cerebral blood vessels. This process may, in part, be mediated by parasympathetic innervation of cerebral vessels. Therefore, a balance between sympathetic and parasympathetic influences appears to modulate cerebral blood flow during acute hypertension. During chronic hypertension, hypertrophy of vessels, augmented by a trophic effect of sympathetic nerves, further reduces vascular wall stress and

Table A69.1. Hypertensive Encephalopathy

Triad
    Severe hypertension
    Encephalopathy
    Rapid resolution with treatment
Usually associated with malignant hypertension
Pathophysiology
    Cerebral vasodilatation
    Disruption of blood–brain barrier
Etiology
    Untreated essential hypertension
    Renal disease
    Renal vascular disease
    Pheochromocytoma
    Eclampsia
Differential diagnosis
    Central nervous system lesion, including tumor and stroke
    Drugs, vasculitis, uremia

protects the vessels. As cerebral blood flow increases during acute hypertension and the blood–brain barrier is disrupted, focal cerebral edema follows. Edema and local changes in ions and neurotransmitters probably contribute to impaired neuronal function and encephalopathy.

Clinical Features of Hypertensive Encephalopathy

Hypertensive encephalopathy occurs in the setting of acute increases in arterial pressure and consists of a triad of hypertension, signs of diffuse or multifocal cerebral dysfunction, and resolution of cerebral signs after effective treatment of hypertension. Resolution of symptoms should not be expected immediately, but may instead occur over several days.

Clinical presentation. In most patients with hypertensive encephalopathy, arterial pressure is extraordinarily high (often >250/150 mm Hg), but in some patients, especially pediatric patients, pregnant women, or those with recent onset of hypertension, the syndrome may occur with modest increases in arterial pressure. In patients with chronic hypertension, the preexisting shift in the autoregulatory curve tends to protect against encephalopathy except at very high levels of pressure. In contrast, in patients in whom the development of hypertension is rapid, such as occurs during acute glomerulonephritis or eclampsia, there is not sufficient time for a shift in the autoregulatory curve. In these circumstances, encephalopathy may occur during acute but quantitatively modest elevations of arterial pressure, especially in children.

Signs and symptoms. Encephalopathy may be manifested by a variety of symptoms. Headache, sometimes with restlessness, typically occurs early in the syndrome. Nausea, projectile vomiting, and visual blurring or blindness may be followed by drowsiness, confusion, and seizures. Papilledema, usually with retinal hemorrhages and exudates, may be observed, and retinal arteries may exhibit a sausage-string appearance. Papilledema, however, is not a *sine qua non* of hypertensive encephalopathy.

Imaging. Compression of the lateral ventricles on computerized tomographic scans or magnetic resonance imaging suggests cerebral edema, and the presence of cerebellar and brain stem edema may indicate hypertensive encephalopathy. Hypodense areas of white matter, presumably secondary to edema, have been observed during hypertensive encephalopathy and typically clear after treatment. The propensity for edema in the occipital lobes, with associated cortical blindness in hypertensive encephalopathy, has led to the use of the term *posterior leukoencephalopathy syndrome.*

Etiology. The most common underlying cause of hypertensive encephalopathy in adults is untreated or poorly treated essential hypertension. In many patients, however, and especially in children, hypertensive encephalopathy and malignant hypertension are due to underlying treatable diseases such as parenchymal renal disease, renal vascular hypertension, pheochromocytoma, and eclampsia. These possibilities should be evaluated after the clinical condition of the patient becomes stable.

Differential diagnosis. Intracerebral hemorrhage, subarachnoid hemorrhage, brain tumor, subdural hematoma, cerebral infarction, acute nephrotic syndrome, herpes simplex encephalitis, or seizures may produce hypertension and generalized or multifocal cerebral symptoms. These disorders often manifest characteristic neurologic findings and, with the exception of acute stroke or seizures, generally can be distinguished from hypertensive encephalopathy by magnetic resonance imaging examination. Antihypertensive therapy should not be delayed for brain imaging if the diagnosis of hypertensive encephalopathy is probable. However, if acute stroke is likely or cannot be distinguished from hypertensive encephalopathy, reduction of blood pressure generally should be avoided. Lumbar puncture is not generally indicated unless other causes of encephalopathy are being considered and should be avoided if a mass lesion is suspected.

Associated conditions and drug effects. Patients with hypertensive encephalopathy usually have other findings that are suggestive of malignant hypertension. In addition to papilledema, patients may have left ventricular hypertrophy, congestive heart failure, or renal insufficiency. Urinalysis may reveal hematuria, proteinuria (sometimes >3 g protein), and casts. Microangiopathic hemolytic anemia also may be present. Drugs, especially intravenous amphetamines and cocaine, can produce vasculitis and hypertension with symptoms that are similar to hypertensive encephalopathy. In patients who are taking monoamine oxidase inhibitors, such foods as cheddar cheese that contain tyramine may produce acute hypertension with stroke or hypertensive encephalopathy. Oral contraceptives have been associated with malignant hypertension. Withdrawal from clonidine treatment may produce acute hypertension and symptoms and signs consistent with hypertensive encephalopathy, as may treatment with cyclosporine or tacrolimus in transplant patients. Vasculitis from lupus erythematosus or polyarteritis may be associated with moderate or severe hypertension and cerebritis. Uremic encephalopathy may occur when serum creatinine exceeds 10 mg/dL, and the clinical presentation may be difficult to distinguish from hypertensive encephalopathy.

Clinical course. Reduction in blood pressure usually produces rapid clinical improvement. Approaches to antihypertensive therapy include intermediate target values for blood pressure and appropriate pharmacologic agents, as discussed elsewhere.

Anticonvulsant agents are not necessary for hypertensive encephalopathy. Seizures in affected patients cease with normalization of blood pressure and do not indicate a primary seizure disorder.

SUGGESTED READING

1. Baumbach GL, Heistad DD. Cerebral circulation in chronic arterial hypertension. *Hypertension.* 1988;12:89–95.
2. Blumenfeld JD, Laragh JH. Management of hypertensive crises: the scientific basis for treatment decisions. *Am J Hypertens.* 2001;14:1154–1167.
3. Healton EB, Brust JC, Feinfeld DA, Thomson GE. Hypertensive encephalopathy and the neurologic manifestations of malignant hypertension. *Neurology.* 1982;32:127–132.
4. Mayhan WG, Heistad DD. Permeability of blood–brain barrier to various sized molecules. *Am J Physiol: Heart Circ Physiol.* 1985;17:H712–H718.
5. Paternò R, Heistad DD, Faraci FM. Potassium channels modulate cerebral autoregulation during acute hypertension. *Am J Physiol: Heart Circ Physiol.* 2000;47:H2003–H2007.
6. Schwartz RB, Feske SK, Polak JF, et al. Preeclampsia-eclampsia: clinical and neuroradiographic correlates and insights into the pathogenesis of hypertensive encephalopathy. *Radiology.* 2000;217:371–376.
7. Strandgaard S, Paulson OB. Hypertensive disease and the cerebral circulation. In: Laragh JH, Brenner BM, eds. *Hypertension: Pathophysiology, Diagnosis, and Management.* New York, NY: Raven Press, 1990;1:399–416.
8. Talman WT, Nitschke-Dragon D. Parasympathetic nerves influence cerebral blood flow during hypertension in rat. *Brain Res.* 2000;873:145–148.
9. Vaughan CJ, Delanty N. Hypertensive emergencies. *Lancet.* 2000;356:411–417.
10. Wright RR, Mathews KD. Hypertensive encephalopathy in childhood. *J Child Neurol.* 1996;11:193–196.

Chapter A70

Pathogenesis of Mild Cognitive Impairment and Mixed Dementia

Linda A. Hershey, MD, PhD

KEY POINTS

- *Mild cognitive impairment* refers to a transitional state between normal aging and mild dementia.
- *Mixed dementia* is a term used to describe patients who at autopsy show the microscopic changes of cerebrovascular disease and Alzheimer's disease.
- Midlife blood pressure elevations are predictors of late-life subcortical white matter changes, brain atrophy, and cognitive decline.
- Blood pressure control in clinical trials with thiazide–angiotensin-converting enzyme inhibitor combinations or calcium antagonists reduces the risk of stroke and cognitive decline in chronic hypertension, but angiotensin-converting enzyme inhibitors and β-blockers may be more effective in protecting against demyelination.

See also Chapters A63, A64, A67, A68, C125, and C160

Hypertension and Cognitive Decline

Several recent epidemiologic studies have shown that midlife blood pressure elevation is a predictor of subcortical demyelination, brain atrophy, and cognitive decline in later years. These findings are independent of age, educational level, and baseline levels of cognition. Diabetes and hyperlipidemia are other major vascular risk factors in addition to hypertension (HTN) associated with cognitive decline in late life. Smoking status does not appear to appreciably influence later-life cognitive test scores.

The risk of developing cognitive deterioration and significant demyelination of subcortical white matter in patients with chronic HTN can be reduced by normalizing blood pressure with antihypertensive medications. In the Systolic Hypertension in Europe (Syst-EUR) study, dihydropyridine calcium antagonists reduced the rate of stroke and cognitive decline. The Perindopril Protection against Recurrent Stroke Study (PROGRESS) trial with thiazide–angiotensin-converting enzyme inhibitor combinations reduced the rate of recurrent stroke and cognitive decline. In smaller studies, therapy with β-blockers and angiotensin-converting enzyme inhibitors was associated with less white matter deterioration and less cognitive decline than with calcium antagonists or loop diuretics.

Mild Cognitive Impairment

Mild cognitive impairment (MCI) refers to a transitional state between the cognition of normal aging and mild dementia (**Table A70.1**). Patients with MCI complain of memory problems and have impaired memory function when tested. Nevertheless, they do not meet criteria for dementia because they are not functionally disabled. MCI patients can still perform instrumental activities of daily living, such as driving, balancing a checkbook, preparing meals, shopping, and remembering to take their medicines. Those with amnestic MCI have only memory complaints, whereas other MCI patients may have mild impairments in other cognitive domains, such as language or executive function.

Table A70.1. Clinical Spectrum between Normal Aging and Dementia

	NORMAL AGING	MILD COGNITIVE IMPAIRMENT	MILD DEMENTIA
Memory complaint	±	+	+
Memory impairment	–	+	+
Another cognitive complaint	–	±	+
Some loss of independence in IADLs	–	–	+

–, not present; +, present; ±, may or may not be present; IADLs, instrumental activities of daily living (driving, shopping, balancing a checkbook, etc.).

Table A70.3. Radiographic Features of the Vascular Dementias

	BINSWANGER'S DISEASE	MULTIINFARCT DEMENTIA	LACUNAR DEMENTIA
Multiple cortical infarcts	–	±	–
Multiple lacunar infarcts	+	–	±
Periventricular white matter changes	■	■	■

–, not present; +, present; ±, may or may not be present.

Ischemic Vascular Dementia

Pathogenesis. Patients with "pure" vascular dementia have evidence of infarcts, arteriolosclerosis (small vessel disease), and atherosclerosis (large vessel disease) in their brains at autopsy, but there are insufficient numbers of plaques and tangles for them to meet the pathologic criteria for Alzheimer's disease (AD). Clinically, vascular dementia patients differ from mixed dementia (MIX) and AD patients in that they are more likely to have a fluctuating or stable course, whereas MIX and AD patients usually progress slowly over time (**Table A70.2**). Vascular and MIX patients are more likely to have a history of HTN and diabetes than those with AD. The white matter changes in frontal lobes of vascular and MIX patients are the best explanations for their incontinence, emotional lability, lower-extremity hyperreflexia, and wide-based gait.

Subtypes of vascular dementia. There are 3 subtypes of vascular dementia: Binswanger's disease, multiinfarct dementia, and lacunar dementia (**Table A70.3**). Clinically, Binswanger's disease, multiinfarct dementia, and lacunar dementia share similar natural histories that typically include fluctuating courses with long plateaus, unlike the progressive deterioration seen in AD.

Binswanger's disease. Binswanger's disease is also known as *subcortical arteriosclerotic encephalopathy* because it is associated with sclerosis of the long penetrating (lenticulostriate) arterioles. There are periventricular white matter changes on brain imaging studies in Binswanger's disease, typically seen as lucencies on computerized tomography and hyperintensities on magnetic resonance imaging.

Multiinfarct and lacunar dementia. Multiinfarct dementia is more likely to develop when the total volume of tissue loss from cerebral infarction is greater than 100 mL. The rarest form of vascular dementia, known as *lacunar dementia*, is seen when strategically placed small infarcts result in global cognitive decline (bilateral infarcts in the mesial dorsal nuclei of the thalamus, for example). If imaging studies of demented patients with lacunar infarcts show signs of AD (widening of Sylvian fissures, enlargement of temporal horns, and atrophy of mesial temporal lobes), then the diagnosis is more likely to be MIX.

Mixed Dementia

General features. "Pure" vascular dementias account for only 5% to 10% of all dementing illnesses, but a much larger proportion of patients (20% to 30%) are afflicted with MIX. At autopsy, patients with MIX show microscopic changes of infarction, arteriolosclerosis, and atherosclerosis in addition to plaques, tangles, and the other degenerative changes of AD. MIX is the second most common cause of dementia in North America and Western Europe. In Asia, MIX and vascular dementia are more common than AD.

Therapy. It is important to recognize patients with MIX, because future strokes can be prevented and progression of dementia slowed by advising patients to (a) take aspirin, or if aspirin is not tolerated, clopidogrel (Plavix) and (b) to keep blood pressure tightly controlled (diastolic blood pressure within the 75 to 85 mm Hg range). Cognitive function and behavioral changes in patients with MIX have been reported to improve, or at least stabilize, with cholinesterase inhibitor therapies such as donepezil (Aricept), rivastigmine (Exelon), and galantamine (Reminyl).

Table A70.2. Clinical Features of Dementing Illnesses

	ISCHEMIC VASCULAR DEMENTIA	MILD DEMENTIA	ALZHEIMER'S DEMENTIA
Fluctuations	+	±	–
History of hypertension	+	±	–
Focal signs	+	±	–
Incontinence	+	±	–
Emotional lability	+	±	–
Hyperreflexia	+	±	–
Wide-based gait	+	±	–

–, not present; +, present; ±, may or may not be present.

SUGGESTED READING

1. Charletta D, Gorelick PB, Dollear TJ, et al. CT and MRI findings among African-Americans with Alzheimer's disease, vascular dementia, and stroke without dementia. *Neurology.* 1995;45:1456–1461.
2. Dufouil C, deKersaint-Gilly A, Besancon V, et al. Longitudinal study of blood pressure and white matter hyperintensities. *Neurology.* 2001;56:921–926.
3. Elias MF, D'Agostino RB, Elias PK, Wolf PA. Neuropsychological test performance cognitive functioning, blood pressure, and age: the Framingham Heart Study. *Exp Aging Res.* 1995;21:369–391.
4. Glynn RJ, Beckett LA, Hebert LE, et al. Current and remote blood pressure and cognitive decline. *JAMA.* 1999;281:438–445.

5. Heckbert SR, Longstreth WT Jr, Psaty BM, et al. The association of antihypertensive agents with MRI white matter findings and with Modified Mini-Mental State Examination in older adults. *J Am Geriatr Soc.* 1997;45:1423–1433.

6. Kivipelto M, Helkala E, Hanninen T, et al. Midlife vascular risk factors and late-life mild cognitive impairment. *Neurology.* 2001;56:1683–1689.

7. Knopman D, Boland LL, Mosley T, et al. Cardiovascular risk factors and cognitive decline in middle-aged adults. *Neurology.* 2001;56:42–48.

8. Launer LJ, Masaki K, Petrovich H, et al. The association between mid-life blood pressure levels and late-life cognitive function. The Honolulu-Asia Aging Study. *JAMA.* 1995;274:1846–1851.

9. Peterson RC, Doody R, Kurz A, et al. Current concepts in mild cognitive impairment. *Arch Neurol.* 2001;58:1985–1992.

10. Swan GE, DeCarli C, Miller BL, et al. Association of midlife blood pressure to late-life cognitive decline and brain morphology. *Neurology.* 1998;51:986–993.

Chapter A71

Pathogenesis of Hypertensive Renal Damage

Sharon Anderson, MD

KEY POINTS

- Elevated glomerular capillary pressure and glomerular ischemia lead to focal glomerulosclerosis, the form of glomerular capillary dropout that is the hallmark lesion of all forms of progressive renal disease.

- Hypertension is a cause and a consequence of glomerulosclerosis.

- Glomerular changes in hypertensive nephrosclerosis are essentially indistinguishable from changes seen in other forms of glomerulosclerosis.

- Elevated cholesterol, cigarette smoking, and hypertension act synergistically to accelerate glomerulosclerosis and renal failure.

See also Chapters A37, A48, A49, A63–A66, A78, B84, C124, C159, and C174

Progressive sclerosis of glomeruli is the final common pathway of a number of otherwise dissimilar renal diseases. The gross and microscopic appearance of the end-stage kidney that results from almost every form of renal disease is that of a shrunken and scarred mass of sclerotic glomeruli with tubulointerstitial fibrosis. At end stage, the initial renal insult often cannot be identified.

Hypertension and Progressive Renal Disease

Vicious cycle. Hypertension is integrally related to progressive renal failure, and hypertensive nephrosclerosis cannot be easily distinguished from other forms of glomerulosclerosis. Hypertension is both a cause and a consequence of renal disease, and systemic hypertension is one of the most important risk factors for progressive loss of renal function. Previously normotensive patients usually develop systemic hypertension as renal function deteriorates. Thus, a vicious cycle of progressive hypertension and progressive renal injury accelerates the development of end-stage renal disease (ESRD) in patients with intrinsic renal disease and accelerates age-related loss of renal function in individuals with otherwise normal kidneys. Although hypertension may initiate renal disease, the incidence of "pure" hypertensive nephropathy, in which hypertension is the only known etiologic factor, is difficult to quantify. Often, the coexistence of hypertension and chronic renal disease leads to a presumptive diagnosis of hypertensive nephropathy

although the underlying problem may be renovascular or parenchymal renal disease.

High-risk individuals. The incidence and prevalence of ESRD presumably secondary to essential hypertension are considerable (**Figure A71.1**) and are particularly high in blacks (**Figure A71.2**). The incidence of hypertension as a presumptive cause of ESRD is increasing, with highest rates seen in elderly and black populations. Because ESRD data come from analyses of persons receiving dialysis or kidney transplantation, changes in ESRD rates may reflect, in part, changing patterns of referral to ESRD therapy, poor control of hypertension, or failure of antihypertensive treatment to limit target-organ damage. The impressive reductions in morbidity and mortality from stroke and coronary artery disease resulting from modern antihypertensive therapy have not been reflected in commensurate reductions in ESRD. In chronic renal failure and in diabetic nephropathy, there are higher waking blood pressures and absence of the usual nocturnal decline in blood pressure, so that the hypertensive burden is more continuously present.

Morphology of Hypertensive Renal Injury

Typically, the kidney in hypertensive nephrosclerosis is shrunken, scarred, and coarsely granular. Vascular lesions are notable, including intimal thickening and fibrosis, reduplication

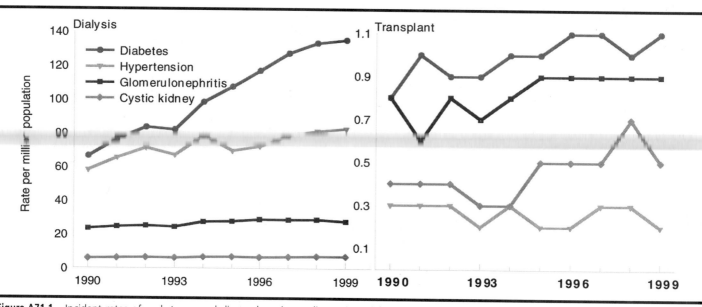

Figure A71.1. Incident rates of end-stage renal disease by primary diagnosis and first modality, adjusted for age, gender, and race. (From 2001 USRDS Annual Data Report. Available at: http://www.usrds.org/adr_2001.htm. Accessed on October 18, 2002.)

of the internal elastic lamina in arcuate and interlobular arteries, and hyalinization of arterioles (arteriolosclerosis). Glomerular injury is initially focal in nature and consists of tuft shrinkage with loss of cellularity. Eventually, sclerosis becomes more generalized, and associated tubules are frequently atrophic or fibrotic.

Mechanisms of Hypertensive Renal Injury

Hemodynamics and ischemia. Hypertension causes renal damage by multiple mechanisms, which may differ in various forms of renal injury. One such mechanism is ischemia, with glomerular hypoperfusion causing glomerulosclerosis and subsequently tubulointerstitial fibrosis. It is likely that ischemia is operative in patients with renovascular hypertension and diffuse intrarenal small vessel disease and may occur in patients

with hypertensive renal disease as well. In contrast, in hypertension secondary to intrinsic renal disease, glomerular capillary hyperperfusion and hypertension (rather than ischemia) appear to be the major pathogenetic mechanisms.

Protective role of afferent arteriolar constriction. The degree of afferent arteriolar constriction determines the degree of transmission of systemic pressure to the glomerular capillary network. The autoregulatory response of the normal kidney to increased perfusion pressure is an increase in afferent arteriolar (preglomerular) resistance, so that the increased systemic pressure is not fully transmitted to the glomerulus (**Figure A71.3**). However, if reflex afferent arteriolar constriction is impaired by disease or by drugs, the kidney cannot protect itself from increased systemic pressure, which is then freely transmitted into

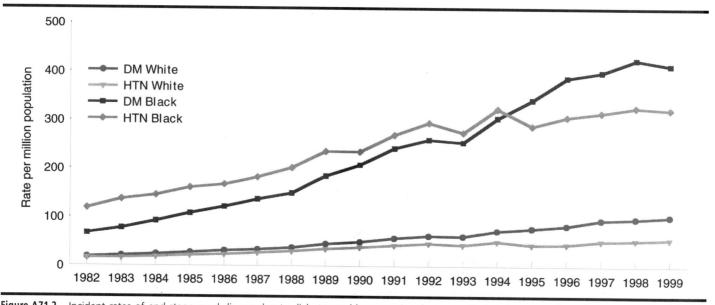

Figure A71.2. Incident rates of end-stage renal disease due to diabetes and hypertension, by race, adjusted for age and gender. DM, diabetes mellitus; HTN, hypertension. (From 2001 USRDS Annual Data Report. Available at: http://www.usrds.org/adr_2001.htm. Accessed on October 18, 2002.)

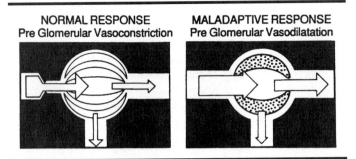

Figure A71.3. Preglomerular adaptations to increased systemic blood pressure. (From Keane WF, Anderson S, Aurell M, et al. Angiotensin converting enzyme inhibitors and progressive renal insufficiency. Current experience and future directions. *Ann Intern Med.* 1989;111:503, with permission.)

the glomerular capillary network, resulting in glomerular capillary hypertension. In humans, a physiologic situation of high systemic pressures with normal intraglomerular capillary pressures may explain the relatively low incidence of ESRD among the millions of patients with essential hypertension, particularly when hypertension is not severe. Renal manifestations in patients with essential hypertension may be similar to those in the spontaneously hypertensive rat (SHR). In the SHR, despite very high systemic blood pressure, afferent arteriolar vasoconstriction prevents excessive transmission of flow and pressure into the glomerular capillary network, and glomerular capillary pressure (P_{GC}) remains nearly normal. Despite high pressures, renal injury is modest and late to develop. The importance of afferent arteriolar vasoconstriction in conferring protection to the glomerular microvasculature is clearly demonstrated by uninephrectomy in the SHR, which results in lowering of afferent arteriolar resistance in the remaining kidney and elevation of P_{GC}. This latter hemodynamic alteration is associated with a large increase in proteinuria and acceleration of glomerular sclerosis.

Afferent arteriolar dilation and glomerular capillary hypertension. In contrast to the protective afferent arteriolar vasoconstriction in the SHR, other forms of renal disease are characterized by primary afferent arteriolar vasodilation and elevation of P_{GC} with coexisting systemic hypertension. This persistent afferent vasodilation can sometimes lead to glomerular hypertension, even when systemic blood pressure is normal, as in the rat with early diabetes. In animals with chronic renal failure, afferent and efferent arteriolar resistances are reduced. Because the reduction in afferent resistance exceeds that in efferent resistance, however, there are net increases in P_{GC} and persistent glomerular capillary hypertension. Reduction of P_{GC} by dietary protein restriction or pharmacologic intervention [angiotensin-converting enzyme (ACE) inhibition or angiotensin receptor blockade] consistently slows the rate of loss of renal function and limits development of proteinuria and glomerulosclerosis. Indirectly, clinical studies are consistent with the notion that afferent arteriolar vasodilation and consequent glomerular capillary hypertension are present in diabetes and other progressive renal disease. Increased glomerular pressures or renal plasma flow rates affect the growth and activity of glomerular component cells, inducing the elaboration or expression of cytokines and other mediators, which then stimulate mesangial matrix production and promote structural injury (**Figure A71.4**).

Other Mechanisms of Injury

Additional mechanisms of injury act synergistically with high systemic and glomerular capillary pressures to accelerate glomerulosclerosis. Although they are well described in experimental models, the role of these factors in clinical hypertensive renal disease is not yet fully defined.

Endothelial cell dysfunction. Fibrinoid material is found within the glomerulus in many forms of injury, suggesting that glomerular injury is promoted by endothelial cell dysfunction, a process similar to systemic atherosclerosis. Abnormal hemodynamic stresses and intracapillary thrombosis also occur and

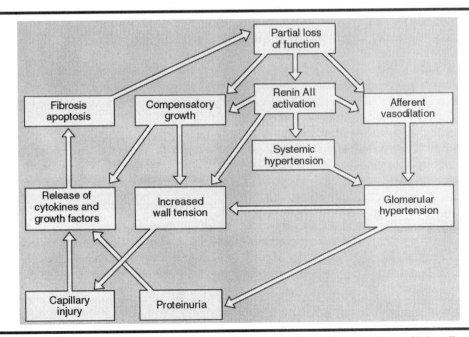

Figure A71.4. Relationships among systemic hypertension, glomerular capillary hypertension, and progressive renal injury. (From Dworkin et al. In: Schrier RW, ed. *Atlas of Diseases of the Kidney.* Philadelphia: Current Medicine; 1999, with permission.)

may be triggered by endothelial dysfunction. The vascular endothelial cell is an important source of vasoactive peptides (e.g., endothelin) and nitric oxide, which modulate the tone of the subjacent vascular smooth muscle, affect vascular reactivity, and influence cellular injury. Drugs that ameliorate endothelial dysfunction, such as antiplatelet agents and ACE inhibitors, may confer some of their beneficial effects via this mechanism.

Cholesterol oxidation. It is increasingly recognized that hypercholesterolemia, which is also associated with endothelial dysfunction, is a risk factor for progression of renal disease. Dietary cholesterol supplementation accelerates glomerular injury in experimental animals, and antihyperlipidemic therapy slows disease progression. When systemic hypertension and hyperlipidemia coexist, the combination induces more glomerular injury than either risk factor alone. As with atherosclerosis, oxidation of low-density lipoprotein may be a critical injury-promoting step. It is widely postulated that reactive oxygen species contribute to glomerulosclerosis.

Cigarette smoking. Epidemiologic studies confirm that cigarette smoking is a risk factor for progressive renal disease, particularly in patients with diabetes. Mechanisms and risk factors relevant to atherosclerosis appear to be equally relevant to glomerulosclerosis and equally aggravated by smoking.

Proteinuria. Elevated P_{GC} leads to enhanced traffic of macromolecules into the mesangial region and the urinary space. Increased macromolecular flux into the mesangium may stimulate the synthesis of matrix components by these cells. It has been suggested that persistent proteinuria may accelerate glomerular and tubular cell injury, consequently accelerating glomerulosclerosis. Indirect evidence in support of this notion derives from intervention trials in which antiproteinuric therapy is associated with slowing of disease progression.

Diagnosis of Hypertensive Nephropathy

Although a number of clinical features support a diagnosis of hypertensive nephrosclerosis (**Table A71.1**), this diagnosis can seldom be made with confidence. Prospective clinical follow-up, with observed progression from normal to impaired renal function over many years, improves diagnostic accuracy. Urinalysis is helpful to exclude other conditions. A low degree of proteinuria (usually <1.5 to 2.0 g/day) may be found, but there should not be evidence of active renal disease (cells or casts). Recently, it has been recognized that a subset of patients (perhaps 15%) with essential hypertension exhibit microalbuminuria (e.g., >20 mg/day), which is below that detected by standard dipstick. Microalbuminuria predicts increased cardiovascular risk, but its prognostic value in essential hypertension is not yet known, and its presence does not

confirm the diagnosis of hypertensive nephropathy. Renal imaging studies are also not helpful, other than to exclude alternative causes, such as obstruction, kidney stones, and renal artery stenosis. Even renal biopsy may not confirm the diagnosis because the morphologic findings are not pathognomonic. Accordingly, the diagnosis of hypertensive nephropathy is usually only presumptive and can be made with reasonable confidence only when other causes of chronic renal failure are excluded.

Role of Antihypertensive Therapy in Disease Progression

Given that hypertension hastens loss of kidney function, aggressive antihypertensive therapy is clearly mandatory. There is strong evidence that lowering blood pressure slows disease- and age-related loss of renal function. The Hypertension Detection and Follow-up Program Cooperative Group and the Multiple Risk Factor Intervention Trial (MRFIT) studies found accelerated loss of renal function in patients with persistent hypertension. As outlined in the *Sixth Report of the Joint National Committee on Prevention, Detection, Evaluation, and Treatment of High Blood Pressure*, renal insufficiency mandates more aggressive treatment and lower target blood pressure: ≤130/85 mm Hg in diabetic patients with proteinuria and >1 g/day and ≤120/75 mm Hg in renal failure. Different antihypertensive drug classes appear to differ in their ability to lower proteinuria and slow the progression of renal disease in hypertensive patients with renal disease. Of the available agents, drugs that block the renin-angiotensin system (ACE inhibitors and angiotensin receptor blockers) are the most potent antiproteinuric agents and have also been shown to be the most effective in slowing the progression of renal disease. Dihydropyridine calcium antagonists have not been found to be renoprotective in the African American Study of Kidney Disease and Hypertension (AASK) study and are not generally antiproteinuric. In contrast, nondihydropyridine calcium antagonists may have a favorable effect on proteinuria.

SUGGESTED READING

1. Dworkin LD, Shemin DG. The role of hypertension in progression of chronic renal disease. In: Schrier RW, ed. *Atlas of Diseases of the Kidney*. Vol 3. Philadelphia, PA: Current Medicine, 1999. Available at://www.kidneyatlas.org. Accessed on October 18, 2002.
2. Joint National Committee. The sixth report of the Joint National Committee on Prevention, Detection, Evaluation, and Treatment of High Blood Pressure (JNC VI). *Arch Intern Med*. 1997;157:2413–2446.
3. Meyrier A, Hill GS, Simon P. Ischemic renal diseases: new insights into old entities. *Kidney Int*. 1998;54:2–13.
4. Mountokalakis TD. The renal consequences of arterial hypertension. *Kidney Int*. 1997;51:1639–1653.
5. Rennke HG, Anderson S, Brenner BM. Structural and functional correlations in the progression of renal disease. In: Tisher CC, Brenner BM, eds. *Renal Pathology*. 2nd ed. Philadelphia, PA: JB Lippincott; 1994:116–142.
6. Silverman M, Bakris GL. Treatment of renal failure and blood pressure. *Curr Opin Nephrol Hypertens*. 1997;6:237–242.
7. Smith MC, Rahman M, Dunn MJ. Hypertension associated with renal parenchymal disease. In: Schrier RW, ed. *Diseases of the Kidney*. 7th ed. Philadelphia, PA: Lippincott Williams & Wilkins; 2001:1363–1397.
8. Weir MR, Dworkin LD. Antihypertensive drugs, dietary salt, and renal protection: how low should you go and with which therapy? *Am J Kidney Dis*. 1998;32:1–22.
9. U.S. Renal Data System. *USRDS 2001 Annual Data Report: Atlas of End-Stage Renal Disease in the United States*. Bethesda, MD: National Institutes of Health, National Institute of Diabetes and Digestive and Kidney Diseases; 2001. Available at: http://www.usrds.org. Accessed on October 18, 2002.
10. Whelton PK, He J, Perneger TV, Klag MJ. Kidney damage in benign essential hypertension. *Curr Opin Nephrol Hypertens*. 1997;6:177–183.

Table A71.1. Clinical Features Consistent with Hypertensive Nephrosclerosis

---

Black race
Positive family history; onset of hypertension between ages 25 and 45 yr
Long-standing or very severe hypertension
Evidence of hypertensive retinal damage
Evidence of hypertensive left ventricular hypertrophy
Onset of hypertension before development of proteinuria
Absence of any cause for primary renal disease
Biopsy evidence: degree of glomerular ischemia and fibrosis compatible with degree of arteriolar and small arterial vascular disease

The Eye in Hypertension

Robert N. Frank, MD

KEY POINTS

- The 3 circulations of the posterior portion of the eye (retinal, choroidal, and optic nerve) are all affected by hypertension.

- Diabetes and other diseases also affect the ocular circulations, often in ways similar to hypertension.

- Clinical descriptions of ophthalmoscopic changes in hypertension are important and should include specific observations about the 3 ocular circulations rather than a nonspecific grade.

- Although the classic changes of severe hypertension in the retina, choroid, and optic nerve have become less common, hypertension may accelerate other retinal disease processes, including diabetic retinopathy, retinal vein occlusions, and neovascular age-related macular degeneration.

See also Chapters A38, A60, A63, A64, A67, and C110

Figures A72.1 through A72.6 are found on the back cover of the *Hypertension Primer*.

The retina is the only tissue in the body in which blood vessels can be observed directly. Examination of the ocular fundi therefore provides an opportunity to observe the effects of hypertension in a unique vascular bed. In humans and other species with vascularized retinas, the rates of retinal glucose consumption and oxygen use are 3-fold higher than in any other tissue in the body. The retinal circulation is therefore highly sensitive to local tissue metabolic needs and is susceptible to damage from circulatory dysfunction.

Ocular Circulations and Hypertensive Changes

The retina and optic nerve in humans are supplied by 3 circulations, all of which derive from branches of the ophthalmic artery.

Retinal circulation. The retinal circulation is composed of the central retinal artery, the central retinal vein, and their respective branches.

Normal anatomy and physiology. The central retinal artery supplies the inner retinal layers and usually divides into 4 principal branches at the anterior surface of the optic nerve. Anterior to the lamina cribrosa of the optic nerve head, the retinal arteries and veins have no autonomic innervation but are controlled by autoregulation in response to local metabolic signals, especially partial pressure of oxygen, partial pressure of carbon dioxide, and intraocular pressure. Tight junctions between adjoining endothelial cells in the retinal vessels form 1 part of the blood–retinal barrier, which strictly governs the passage of molecules into the neural tissue of the retina. Breakdown of this barrier is an important pathologic change.

Changes in hypertension. Changes in the retinal blood vessels are the most common vascular lesions of systemic hypertension in the eye. There have been a number of classifications of hypertensive retinopathy, of which the best known are those of Keith, Wagener, and Barker, first proposed in 1939 and those of Scheie

proposed in 1953. Although these classifications are of historic interest, they are less useful clinically than a careful description of the lesions existent in the eye. Hypertensive retinopathy is actually a continuum, and certain types of lesions may be found in various combinations. Some lesions are relatively specific for hypertensive retinopathy [e.g., "copper wiring" of arterioles, "arteriovenous (A-V) nicking" and related crossing changes, and arterial macroaneurysms]. Other "hypertensive" lesions found in a number of disorders include the "cotton-wool spots" of diabetic retinopathy, systemic lupus erythematosus, retinal vein occlusions, and acquired immune deficiency syndrome. Flame-shaped intraretinal hemorrhages occur also in diabetic retinopathy, retinal vein occlusions, profound anemia, the leukemias, and other blood dyscrasias. Arterial "silver wiring" may occur in diabetic retinopathy, collagen-vascular diseases, and arterial occlusive diseases.

Choroidal circulation. The choroidal circulation includes the short posterior ciliary arteries and their branches in the choroid.

Normal anatomy and physiology. In humans, there are 2 external layers of arteries and veins and an inner layer, the choriocapillaris, which lies just outside the pigment epithelium of the retina. The portion of the choriocapillary endothelium immediately adjacent to the pigment epithelium is thin and fenestrated, and small molecules and even larger proteins readily pass in and out of these vessels. However, tight junctions connecting the cells of the retinal pigment epithelium form the second part of the blood–retinal barrier, governing the ingress of nutrient molecules and the egress of waste products. The choroidal vessels have an autonomic nerve supply that can regulate choroidal blood flow, which is substantially greater than that of the retina. The choroidal circulation supplies the retinal pigment epithelium and the photoreceptor layers of the retina, which are rich in mitochondria and are therefore responsible for the very active metabolism of the retina.

Changes in hypertension. Hypertensive choroidopathy occurs most frequently in younger individuals with acute, severe hypertensive episodes such as malignant hypertension or toxemia of pregnancy. Hypertensive changes in the choroidal vessels are observed much less frequently than hypertensive changes in the vessels of the retina. In theory, hypertensive choroidopathy occurs because the short choroidal arteries, which are most commonly affected by hypertensive changes, feed at right angles into the choroidal capillaries, allowing direct transmission of systemic blood pressure to the capillaries. Initial changes may include focal regions of choriocapillary nonperfusion owing to fibrinoid necrosis of the vessels. Clinically, this may be recognized initially only by special techniques such as intravenous fluorescein angiography. Subsequently, the retinal pigment epithelium over these nonperfused regions may develop a yellowish coloration, the Elschnig spot, which later becomes a scar with a pigmented center and an atrophic surrounding halo.

Optic nerve circulation.
The third circulation is that of the optic nerve.

Normal anatomy and physiology. Anteriorly, the optic nerve circulation is composed of branches of the central retinal artery, and posteriorly of branches of the short posterior ciliary vessels and of vessels supplying the pia mater. Blood flow in these vessels is highly influenced anteriorly by the intraocular pressure and posteriorly by intracranial pressure transmitted through the subarachnoid space.

Changes in hypertension. Hypertensive changes in the optic nerve are also relatively uncommon. The principal optic nerve lesion of hypertension is disc edema (Figure A72.1). The cause of this lesion is unclear because, as noted earlier, the optic nerve in the orbit receives a different blood supply in its anterior and posterior portions. Some investigators believe that a combination of ischemia (caused by vascular changes and increased intraocular or intracranial pressure) and diminished axoplasmic flow in the optic nerve fibers causes hypertensive optic nerve swelling.

Ophthalmoscopy in Hypertension

Arteriolar changes.
Arteriolar changes are the most common manifestations of hypertensive retinopathy.

Terminology. The central retinal artery and its 4 major branches are commonly called *arteries*, whereas smaller branches are termed *arterioles*, irrespective of the actual microscopic anatomy. However, this terminology is not used by all writers, and anatomically, the vessels that are visible in the retina by ophthalmoscopy are arterioles.

Arteriolar diameter changes. The initial visible change in the retinal vessels in hypertension is arteriolar narrowing. The median ratio of retinal arteriolar to venular diameters in non-hypertensive individuals has recently been determined, by an elaborate digital photographic method, to be 0.84. Owing to arterial remodeling, this ratio progressively decreases with increasing mean arterial blood pressure. Progressive arteriosclerotic changes also produce an increase in the central light reflex and a decrease in the width of the blood column seen on either side of the light reflex. As these changes progress, the normally yellowish-white light reflex becomes reddish-brown,

giving rise to the term *copper-wire* change. As thickening of the wall progresses, visibility of the blood column diminishes and eventually disappears, leading to the appearance of the artery as a white thread, the silver-wire change (Figure A72.2). Arterial silver wiring does not always mean that the vessel is no longer perfused, because blood flow can often be demonstrated by fluorescein angiography.

Arteriovenous nicking. An additional ophthalmoscopically visible change produced in the retinal vessels by hypertension and arteriosclerosis is A-V nicking. Ocular vessels are contained in an adventitial sheath. At those points where branch arteries cross over veins, the sheaths are essentially shared. The artery with its thickened wall and increased luminal pressure, together with proliferation of perivascular glia, externally compresses the low-pressure, thin-walled vein causing a tapered or "nicked" junction. In more long-standing hypertension, the vein changes direction where the artery crosses it, producing a right-angled bend. The most serious consequence of A-V nicking is actual occlusion of the vein.

Atherosclerosis versus arteriosclerosis. Changes in the retinal arterial wall in hypertension represent true arteriosclerosis, with thickening of the wall represented histopathologically by multiple internal elastic laminae and replacement of the muscle layer by collagen. By contrast, atherosclerosis is demonstrated in the retinal vessels only when cholesterol emboli lodge in the central retinal artery or one of its branches, where they may become visible ophthalmoscopically (Figure A72.3).

Central vein occlusion.
Central retinal vein occlusion can occur at the point where the central retinal artery and vein come in continuity with one another within the substance of the optic nerve. It is characterized by sudden, severe loss of vision and a "blood-and-thunder" fundus appearance, with dilated and tortuous veins and extensive hemorrhages in all 4 quadrants around the nerve head (Figure A72.4). Branch vein occlusion may cause vision loss if the macular portion of the retina is affected. A wedge-shaped cluster of hemorrhages, with its apex pointing at the responsible A-V crossing, is always present. After diabetic retinopathy, retinal vein occlusion is the second most common vascular disorder of the retina and is an important cause of visual loss. Although several causal factors may be involved, systemic hypertension is one of the most important.

Cotton-wool spots.
Reduced blood flow produced by sclerosis or fibrinoid necrosis of small retinal arterioles may lead to regions of infarction, which eventually become evident as round to oval white patches with soft borders, the so-called cotton-wool spots, or cytoid bodies (Figure A72.5). Because these lesions are the result of infarction, not exudation, they should not be termed *soft exudates*.

Aneurysms.
Lesions induced by excessive transmural pressure in the retinal vascular wall in hypertensive retinopathy include capillary microaneurysms and arterial (or arteriolar) macroaneurysms. Capillary microaneurysms are fusiform or berry-shaped outpouchings of the retinal capillaries. Although capillary microaneurysms are usually considered to be classic lesions of diabetic retinopathy, they may also occur in hypertensive retinopathy, in retinal vein occlusions (even in the absence of

hypertension), and in the retinopathy produced by leukemias and other blood dyscrasias. Arteriolar macroaneurysms, however, are characteristic of hypertension alone. They are berry-shaped dilations of a retinal artery or arteriole (Figure A72.6), which may be surrounded by hemorrhage or retinal edema with a circumferential ring of lipid exudate. Although macroaneurysms are dramatic in appearance, they are usually benign in behavior, because they often thrombose spontaneously. Evidence of hemorrhage or substantial retinal edema may be indications for laser photocoagulation.

Flame hemorrhages. Hypertensive retinopathy may also lead to a breakdown in the blood–retinal barrier, as demonstrated by intraretinal hemorrhages that are often flame-shaped. In the retinopathy of malignant hypertension, there is profound leakage of plasma from the capillaries within the macula. This condition may lead to loss of vision from the resultant macular edema and to the precipitation of lipid exudate in the form of radial deposits, the so-called macular star figure surrounding the fovea at the center of the macula.

Clinical Significance

The ocular lesions of systemic hypertension convey important information about the duration and severity of the hypertensive state and the efficacy of treatment. Because several of these lesions may have adverse consequences, the clinician should carefully examine the ocular fundi of all hypertensive patients as a regular part of the initial examination and at periodic follow-up visits. Individuals with suspicious regions of the fundus, acute, severe hypertensive episodes, or accelerated or malignant hypertension merit consultation with an ophthalmologist. Classic hypertensive retinopathy in its malignant stages has become less frequent owing to more effective treatment of systemic hypertension. Yet systemic hypertension remains a major contributor to several other vision-threatening ocular disorders. In addition to the risk of retinal vein occlusion, diabetic retinopathy (at least in individuals with type 2 diabetes) progresses more rapidly in individuals whose blood pressures are not controlled. The Macular Photocoagulation Study, a national randomized controlled clinical trial of laser photocoagulation for the neovascular form of age-related macular degeneration, showed better outcomes in normotensive patients than in hypertensives.

SUGGESTED READING

1. The Eye Disease Case-Control Study Group. Risk factors for branch retinal vein occlusion. *Am J Ophthalmol.* 1993;116:286–296.
2. The Eye Disease Case-Control Study Group. Risk factors for central retinal vein occlusion. *Arch Ophthalmol.* 1996;114:545–554.
3. Frank RN. Vascular disease of retina. In: Tso MOM, ed. *Retinal Diseases.* Philadelphia, PA: JB Lippincott; 1987:138–164.
4. Hubbard LD, Brothers RJ, King WN, et al. Atherosclerosis Risk in Communities Study Group. Methods for evaluation of retinal microvascular abnormalities associated with hypertension/sclerosis in the Atherosclerosis Risk in Communities Study. *Ophthalmology.* 1999;106:2269–2280.
5. Keith NM, Wagener HP, Barker NW. Some different types of essential hypertension: their course and prognosis. *Am J Med Sci.* 1974;268:336–345.
6. Knowler WC, Bennett PH, Ballintine EJ. Increased incidence of retinopathy in diabetics with elevated blood pressure: a six-year follow-up study in Pima Indians. *N Engl J Med.* 1980;302:645–650.
7. Macular Photocoagulation Study Group. Laser photocoagulation for juxtafoveal choroidal neovascularization: five-year results from randomized clinical trials. *Arch Ophthalmol.* 1994;112:500–509.
8. Scheie HG. Evaluation of ophthalmoscopic changes of hypertension and arteriolar sclerosis. *Arch Ophthalmol.* 1953;49:117–138.
9. UK Prospective Diabetes Study Group. Tight blood pressure control and risk of macrovascular and microvascular complications in type 2 diabetes: UKPDS 38. *BMJ.* 1998;317:703–713.
10. Wagener HP, Clay GE, Gipner JF. Classification of retinal lesions in presence of vascular hypertension: report submitted by committee. *Trans Am Ophthalmol Soc.* 1947;45:57–75.

Retinal Findings in Hypertension

Figures A72.1 through A72.6 are found on the back cover of the *Hypertension Primer*.

Figure A72.1.   (Upper left) Edema of the optic disc in a severely hypertensive, 20-year-old woman. Note also the markedly dilated retinal veins.

Figure A72.2.   (Upper middle) This photograph of the ocular fundus of a 48-year-old hypertensive woman shows several of the changes associated with hypertension and arteriosclerosis. The arteries and arterioles are severely narrowed, and there are "copper-wire" (*arrowhead*) and "silver-wire" (*arrow*) changes.

Figure A72.3.   (Upper right) This fundus photograph of a 57-year-old woman shows a cholesterol plaque lodged in a branch retinal artery (*arrowhead*). This finding is evidence of atherosclerosis.

Figure A72.4.   (Lower left) This 74-year-old man has had a central retinal vein occlusion, as demonstrated by multiple blot and flame-shaped hemorrhages surrounding his optic nerve head in all 4 quadrants and extending out into the retinal periphery. Central retinal vein occlusions are usually associated with profound and irreversible loss of vision.

Figure A72.5.   (Lower middle) Multiple cotton-wool spots (*arrowheads*) surrounding the optic nerve head of a 57-year-old hypertensive man.

Figure A72.6.   (Lower right) A retinal arterial macroaneurysm (*arrow*) presents as a large, berry-shaped, yellowish dilation of a retinal branch artery (*arrowhead*). The lesion is surrounded by hemorrhage.

Section 6. *Basic Genetics*

Basic Principles of Genetics

Nicholas J. Schork, PhD

KEY POINTS

- Genetics is the study of the transmission of biologic information from parents to offspring encoded in DNA according to Mendel's laws and related algebraic principles.

- DNA is distributed on 23 pairs of chromosomes in humans and is collectively referred to as a *genome*.

- A genomic site that varies in its DNA content across individuals is known as a *polymorphic locus*, which can be studied in sophisticated ways to identify disease-predisposing genes, assess ancestry, and human population differences.

See also Chapters A74–A78 and C114

Basic Genetics

Genetics, broadly stated, concerns the mechanisms responsible for the resemblance of individuals sharing parentage or ancestry—i.e., that siblings, parents, and offspring tend to share similar characteristics to a greater degree than unrelated individuals. DNA, the ultimate biologic entity responsible for this resemblance, not only transmits genetic information at fertilization (i.e., the generation of offspring) but also influences one's "phenotypic profile" or physical characteristics (e.g., traits such as height, blood pressure level, or diabetes susceptibility).

Phenotypes and heritability. The phenotypic profile of an individual is determined to a high degree by the DNA that he or she inherits. The reason that one's phenotypic profile is not completely dictated by parental DNA is that environmental forces (e.g., food intake, lifestyle, exposure to toxic substances) interact with one's DNA to ultimately shape the phenotype of an individual during his or her development and life history (see Chapter A76). The degree to which inherited DNA influences a particular phenotype over-and-above environmental stimuli is referred to as the *heritability* of that phenotype.

DNA, genes, and chromosomes. DNA is comprised of 4 basic nucleotides or "bases" that are held together on a sugar phosphate backbone. These bases are strung together in long sequences divided into 23 pairs of chromosomes in humans. Other species have different numbers of chromosomes and pairings. Because humans possess pairs of chromosomes, they are known as a *diploid* species. The chromosome pairs are known as *homologs*, and each parent in a human mating pair contributes 1 chromosome of these homologous pairs to each offspring. In healthy individuals, DNA is organized in a segmental fashion on chromosomes. Exceptions to this organized structure are often highly deleterious in nature, causing a variety of genetic diseases. Various segments of DNA associated with individual chromosomal locations (genetic loci) encode

information that is ultimately translated into the synthesis of proteins that form the building blocks of living organisms and ultimately work together to form or build individual phenotypes. Segments of DNA containing information that guides the formation of a protein are known as *genes*. Not all DNA, however, is associated with a gene that encodes information about a protein. Some segments of DNA dictate how much protein is made (i.e., influence gene "expression"), other segments dictate how the information about a protein is extracted from a gene (i.e., influence gene "splicing"), and other segments have no identifiable function.

Genomics. The totality of DNA possessed by an individual is known as his or her *genome*; *genomics*, as distinct from genetics, is the study of the organization and evolutionary history of DNA. The total human genome is approximately 3 billion bases long or, when considered as the product of 2 parental genomes, as 3 billion base pairs long (i.e., as roughly 6 billion "bits" of information divided up into pairs).

Genetic variation and polymorphisms. Mutation is the process whereby a single nucleotide or stretch of DNA sequence is altered. If such alterations affect DNA transmitted to an offspring and the mutated sequence ultimately influences some aspect of a gene and its encoded protein, then that offspring might have a different characteristic or phenotypic feature than the parent or another sibling. Genomic sequence sites often vary across individuals owing to mutations and the transmission of the offending mutations from parents to offspring. Alternative forms of the sequence (variously referred to as *alleles*, *genetic variants*, or simply as *variants*) found in greater than 1% of the population are referred to as *polymorphisms*, and their positions in the genome are known as *polymorphic loci*. Thus, DNA sequence variation ultimately contributes to differences in the phenotypic profiles or traits of individuals.

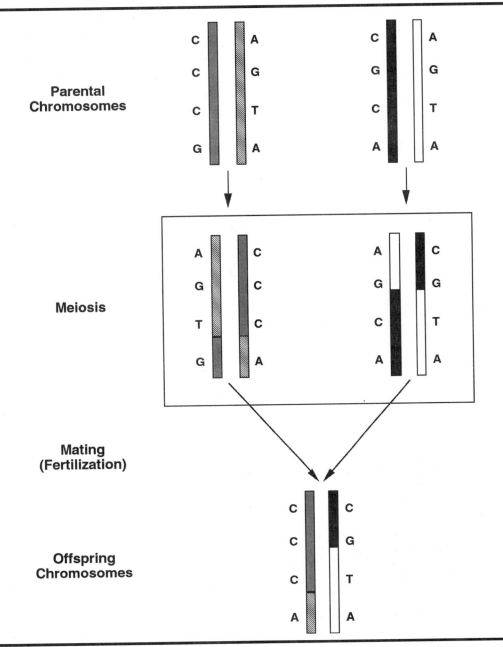

Figure A73.1. Simplified representation of the phenomena of recombination and the transmission of recombined chromosomes (resulting from meiosis) from parents to offspring. The shading patterns represent different parental chromosomes, and the letters next to each chromosome represent sequence variants or alleles present at particular genomic loci. During meiosis, homologous chromosomes pair up and exchange material resulting in 2 new recombined chromosomes. One of these recombined chromosomes is transmitted to an offspring during fertilization. An offspring thus shares DNA with each parent but has a chromosomal structure different from each parent.

Kinship, Meiosis, and Recombination

Kinship. The fact that siblings have DNA from the same parents contributes to their phenotypic resemblance. The *kinship* between any 2 individuals essentially refers to how much DNA they share. Obviously, the greater the number of recent, common ancestors any 2 individuals share, the greater the kinship between them and the more DNA they share. Individuals who share more DNA are also more likely to be similar phenotypically than individuals who share less DNA. The combination of variants at a particular genomic locus is referred to as the *genotype* of that individual. However, except for monozygotic twins, siblings do not share all of their DNA. This is due not only to very rare unique mutations that could arise in a parent's DNA between

matings but also to fundamental DNA recombination differences during meiosis.

Meiosis and recombination. Meiosis is of fundamental importance for generating phenotypic differences in related individuals. Meiosis is essentially the reductive replication of germ line cells that contain the DNA to be transmitted to offspring. In addition to producing gametes, meiosis leads to genomic changes that ultimately result in the creation of unique combinations of homologous chromosomes. During meiosis, an individual's homologous chromosomes pair up and exchange material. This exchange involves the actual merger of segments from each chromosome of a homologous pair and is known as *recombination*. The result of recombination is 2 new chromosomes that contain segments from

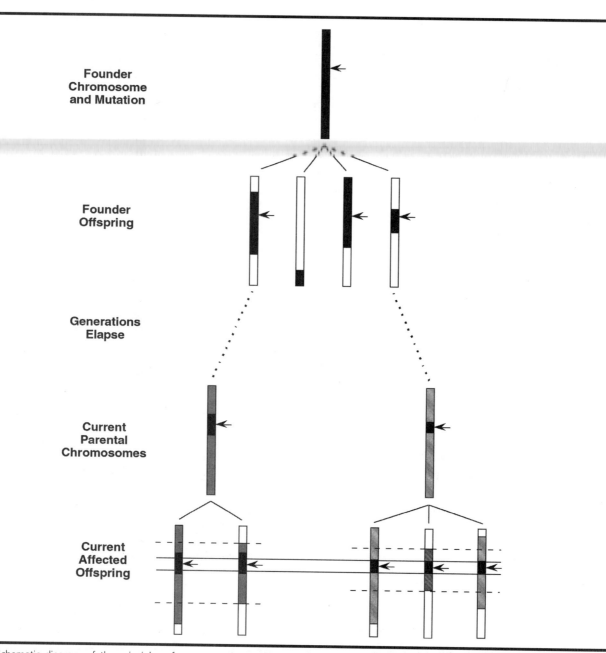

Figure A73.2. Schematic diagram of the principles of gene mapping and the assessment of co-segregation phenomena within and between families. A "founder" introduces a new mutation into a population. The dark-shaded chromosome is the chromosome on which the mutation arose. The site of the disease-conferring mutation is denoted by the arrow. For simplicity, only a single chromosome for each individual is drawn because emphasis is on tracing the history of the chromosome on which the mutation arose. The founder has 4 offspring, each of whom receives a segment of the chromosome harboring the mutation. Owing to recombination, only 3 offspring actually inherited a segment harboring the mutation. These offspring start lines of descent (i.e., have offspring) of their own. Over time, recombination breaks up the original ancestral chromosome harboring the mutation (i.e., the shaded chromosome) into smaller pieces, such that individuals inheriting the mutation in the latest generations possess only small pieces of the original ancestral chromosome flanking the site of the mutation. However, affected siblings share larger pieces of parental chromosomes harboring the mutation (*dashed horizontal lines*). This chromosomal material is different for different families because the parental chromosomes are likely to be unique. Individuals in different families share small segments of the original ancestral (founder) chromosome harboring the mutation (*solid horizontal lines*). Linkage studies attempt to exploit the identification of (large) shared chromosomes within families, whereas linkage disequilibrium or association studies attempt to exploit the identification of (small) shared chromosomes across families.

the original homologous pair possessed by an individual. One of these "new" chromosomes is transmitted (with 50% probability) to an offspring during fertilization and forms half of that offspring's own unique homologous chromosomal pair. The other chromosome of this pair comes from the other parent (**Figure A73.1**). Thus, it is true to say that individuals do not actually inherit parental genes, but rather combinations of parental chromosomal segments that harbor genes. The size of these altered chromosomal segments is dictated by the location of the recombination events.

Recombination frequency and chromosome distance.
Although the process of recombination is a complicated one, the shorter the distance between 2 loci on a chromosome, the less likely there is to be a recombination event occurring between them. In addition, other chromosomes are not affected by recombination events involving a particular chromosome pair, and there is a 50% chance that a chromosome resulting from the recombination of a homologous pair will be transmitted to an offspring during fertilization.

These facts are consistent with Mendel's laws and characterize the algebraic patterns of inheritance that geneticists have studied for years.

Sequence Variation and Genetic Maps

DNA sequence variation can arise as a result of mutation. This variation is sustained in a population if it is transmitted to subsequent generations of offspring. This variation, along with environmental stimuli, is responsible for phenotypic differences possessed by individuals. The recent near completion of the sequencing of the entire human genome has greatly facilitated resequencing studies, in which individual genomes are compared to identify polymorphic loci.

Polymorphisms. There are many kinds of polymorphisms, including simple base changes, deletions of small stretches of sequence, insertions of small stretches of sequence, and repetitions of small stretches of sequence that vary from individual to individual. Of these forms of polymorphism, the most abundant are simple base changes or *single nucleotide polymorphisms* (SNPs for short), in which 1 of the 4 bases is replaced by another. In addition to being the most abundant form of polymorphism, many of these single nucleotide polymorphisms are functionally significant in that they influence a particular phenotype or set of phenotypes.

Genetic maps. Major resources that have been developed as a result of the study of polymorphisms are genetic maps. When the genes responsible for a particular phenotype (e.g., height, cancer predisposition, blood pressure) are not known, genetic researchers often attempt to identify them by exploiting genetic maps, sequencing and genotyping technologies, and Mendel's and related laws. Gene identification can be pursued by collecting families that "segregate" the phenotype (i.e., have members with and without the phenotype of interest), by "genotyping" the variants each individual in the family possesses at various loci and then assessing evidence of co-segregation (i.e., the apparent simultaneous transmission from parents to offspring) of variants at those genetic loci with the phenotype of interest. If evidence for co-segregation is found using statistical methods, the locus harboring variants that actually influence the phenotype of interest is inferred to be located near the marker locus whose variants co-segregate with the phenotype. The marker locus need not cause a phenotype, but it must be associated with the locus under investigation to be

mapped. **Figure A73.2** offers a simplified schematic diagram for some of these principles.

Genome scans. By assessing evidence for co-segregation of marker locus at systematic intervals over the entire genome, it is possible to identify the genomic location of variants influencing a phenotype without any *a priori* knowledge of its location. Systematic studies of this sort are known as *genome scans* or *genome-wide searches* and can be pursued with methods that investigate co-segregation phenomena within families or across families.

Linkage analysis. Although the distinction is somewhat technical, co-segregation studies that exploit associations observed within families are known as *linkage analysis studies*, whereas co-segregation studies that exploit associations across families or even unrelated individuals are referred to as *linkage disequilibrium* or *association* studies. Mapping efforts of either sort are rendered difficult by the fact that there can be several genomic loci that contribute to a given trait and several environmental factors that can influence the contribution of each locus. This complexity can, in effect, obscure the contribution of any locus. Phenotypes with many determinants are often referred to as *complex, polygenic,* or *multifactorial* traits and present many challenges to geneticists, especially in the context of mapping and identifying their genetic determinants.

SUGGESTED READING

1. Cavalli-Sforza LL, Bodmer WF. *The Genetics of Human Populations.* San Francisco, CA: W. H. Freeman and Company; 1971.
2. Collins FS, Geyer MC, Chakravarti A. Variations on a theme: cataloguing human DNA sequence variation. *Science.* 1997;278:1580–1581.
3. Lander ES, Linton LM, Birren B, et al. Initial sequencing and analysis of the human genome. *Nature.* 2001;409:860–921.
4. Lander ES, Weinberg RS. Genomics: journey to the center of biology. *Science.* 2000;287:1777–1782.
5. Lander ES, Schork NJ. The genetic dissection of complex traits. *Science.* 1994;265:2037–2048.
6. Schork NJ, Chakravarti A. A non-mathematical overview of gene mapping techniques applied to human diseases. In: Mockrin SC, ed. *Molecular Genetics and Gene Therapy of Cardiovascular Disease.* New York, NY: Marcel Dekker; 1996:79–109.
7. Schork NJ, Thiel B, St. Jean P. Linkage analysis, kinship, and the short-term evolution of chromosomes. *J Exp Zool.* 1998;281:133–149.
8. Schork NJ, Fallin DF, Lanchbury JS. Single nucleotide polymorphisms and the future of genetic epidemiology. *Clin Genet.* 2000;58:250–264.
9. Wang DG, Fan JB, Siao CJ, et al. Large-scale identification, mapping, and genotyping of single-nucleotide polymorphisms in the human genome. *Science.* 1998;280:1077–1082.
10. Venter JC, Adams MD, Myers EW, et al. The sequence of the human genome. *Science.* 2001;291:1304–1351.

Genetics of Hypertension: Investigative Strategies

George T. Cicila, PhD

Blood Pressure as a Quantitative Trait

Blood pressure is a quantitative trait with continuous variation from low to high values in outbred populations of humans or animals. As with most quantitative traits, differences in blood pressure result from the contributions of many genes (i.e., blood pressure is a polygenic trait) interacting with each other and the environment. In outbred human populations, blood pressure values show a skewed normal distribution with values over a certain arbitrary threshold defined as *hypertension.*

Family studies. The influence of genes on hypertension was initially studied by comparing adopted children with biologic children, identical and nonidentical twins, and by assessing kindreds (see Chapter A75). Such studies have indicated, however, that half or less of the blood pressure variation in the general population is explained by genetic factors. Recently, mutations that cause a number of human diseases have been identified by first detecting chromosomal regions in which genetic markers co-segregate with the disease trait in families and then using positional cloning to identify the single defective gene responsible for the disease. This approach has been useful in identifying genes that cause rare, monogenic forms of heritable hypertension (see Chapter A77).

Polygenic Interactions in Human Essential Hypertension

The vast majority (98–99%) of patients with essential hypertension, in whom the cause is not due to obvious lesions in a single gene, are in a highly complex situation. Here, the many genetic alterations responsible for high blood pressure would be expected to be subtle, such as upregulated or downregulated expression of an active gene or point mutations that may alter but not abolish the activity of a protein. Because human essential hypertension is a polygenic disorder that is intrinsically genetically heterogeneous, different patients carry different subsets of genes that lead to elevated blood pressure. These genes that affect blood pressure can be described as having alternate (or allelic) variant forms associated with either increased or decreased blood pressure. The genetic components of essential hypertension are thought to be largely additive in nature, such that the blood pressure observed in a particular patient is dependent on the interaction of the environment with the balance between the number and relative strength of the low and high blood pressure alleles present. Epistasis, or the interaction between 2 or more nonallelic genes (i.e., those located at different positions in the genome), can lead to nonadditive effects, which complicates identification of disease-related genes by linkage analysis. Understanding of the molecular basis of blood pressure regulation is further complicated by the existence of genes that have no direct effect on blood pressure but that influence blood pressure in a specific environmental context, such as a high dietary salt intake.

Studying the Genetics of Human Essential Hypertension

Linkage analysis of extended families and positional cloning approaches are unlikely to identify genes that cause essential hypertension because they require the presence of a single major disease gene with a specific mode of inheritance. Headway can be made in the understanding of a polygenic trait by simplifying the analysis or the system or both. One way to identify genes involved in heritable forms of hypertension is to ignore quantitative differences in blood pressure and substitute a dichotomous, qualitative threshold criterion to define which individuals are affected such as blood pressure in hypertensive subjects.

Affected sib-pair analysis. Affected sib-pair analysis searches for increased levels of similarity in polymorphic genetic markers that differ greatly in size or sequence and thus allow the identification of different alleles in pairs of affected siblings. In this analysis, chromosomal regions showing higher degrees of marker similarity in hypertensive siblings (presumably from inheritance of the same alleles) are assumed to be more likely to contain alleles that affect blood pressure.

Genome scans. Polymorphic genetic markers, initially examined for candidate genes, can also be examined at regular distances along each chromosome. Thus, the whole genome can be scanned for chromosomal regions having elevated levels of genetic marker similarity. Genome scanning approaches now dominate the study of polygenic determinants of traits like blood pressure, particularly in animal models of genetic hypertension. Computer programs are used to identify chromosomal regions most likely to contain genes (or loci) associated with variation in blood pressure. Genes that control quantitative traits like blood pressure (i.e., traits with values having a continuous distribution) are known as *quantitative trait loci* (QTLs).

Association studies. Association studies are complementary to linkage analysis. Their main use is in identifying a particular gene as a strong candidate after a chromosomal region has already been linked to the trait. Frequencies of the different alleles for the proposed locus are examined in hypertensive patients and normotensive control subjects who have been carefully matched for confounding factors such as age, sex, and race. Linkage disequilibrium occurs when combinations of alleles at different loci (haplotypes) are observed at frequencies significantly higher than expected from chance association alone. If alleles have strikingly different frequencies in patients compared with unaffected control subjects, the differences could arise from causal involvement of the gene in disease susceptibility or from linkage disequilibrium. Although linkage disequilibrium can arise from several sources including recent admixtures of groups within a population, selection for a specific allele, or random genetic drift, disequilibrium occurring between tightly linked loci is expected to be more robust. In this way, linkage disequilibrium between a genetic marker and a disease or trait locus could lead to identifying 1 of the genes responsible for susceptibility to high blood pressure.

Animal Models of Genetic Hypertension

Identification of QTLs in animal models is a powerful method for simplifying and dissecting the genetic basis of human polygenic traits, such as blood pressure. Indeed, in some crossbred animal populations, ≥60% of the variation in blood pressure can be explained by genetic factors.

Selective breeding. Selectively bred rat strains have been developed that are divergent for a polygenic quantitative trait such as blood pressure. After systematic blood pressure measurement of a large heterogeneous population, several pairs of rats with the highest blood pressures are selected for mating to produce a high blood pressure strain, as has been accomplished with the spontaneously hypertensive rat strain. Blood pressures of progeny are measured, and several pairs of rats with the highest blood pressures are selected for mating. Repetition of this procedure further concentrates alleles associated with high blood pressure. At some point, further selection does not result in progeny with higher blood pressures than their parents, and the selectively bred strain is then inbred to fix the genes responsible for the trait. After brother-sister mating of rats from the selectively bred strain has occurred for at least 20 additional generations, more than 99% of the loci become homozygous (i.e., have 2 copies of the same allele) and the inbred strain is considered genetically homogeneous. Creation of inbred strains results in homozygous alleles at virtually all loci, including genes that are not involved in the genetic determination of blood pressure. Different selectively bred strains do not carry

identical sets of genes that affect blood pressure. The spontaneously hypertensive rat was developed to concentrate high blood pressure alleles, but other strains have been developed that will not become hypertensive without alteration of an environmental factor. Some strains are environmentally sensitive such as the Sabra hypertension-sensitive strain, which develops elevated blood pressure only when fed an excessive intake of dietary NaCl. The inbred Dahl salt-sensitive rat is spontaneously hypertensive and sensitive to excessive intake of dietary NaCl, whereas the Dahl salt-resistant rat does not develop high blood pressure even when fed a high NaCl diet.

Blood pressure quantitative trait loci in animal models. Studying inbred rats rather than human populations has several advantages. In such a population, a single set of genetic factors (the segregating alleles carried by each of the inbred strains that were crossbred) makes all polymorphic genetic markers fully informative for the genotype at all chromosomal loci.

Gene-environment interactions. The environment in which a segregating population is maintained can be controlled for nutritional, pharmacologic, or other interventions so that the observed phenotypic variation in blood pressure can be attributed directly to genetic components. Segregating populations are bred by mating inbred rats with contrasting phenotypes to produce first filial generation (F_1) animals that are genetically identical but heterozygous for every locus (i.e., carrying an allele from each parent at every locus). Hence, phenotypic variation observed in F_1 animals is due to environmental factors. Populations in which all alleles are segregating can be produced either by intercrossing male and female F_1 rats or by backcrossing F_1 rats with 1 of the parental strains.

Genome scanning. Genome scanning approaches have been used to identify blood pressure QTLs in segregating populations bred by crossing hypertensive rats from a number of different genetic models with contrasting normotensive strains. To date, blood pressure QTLs have been identified on many rat chromosomes, confirming the complex polygenic nature of blood pressure regulation in this species. One blood pressure QTL in the Dahl rat model contains a gene, steroid 11β-hydroxylase (*Cyp11b1*), with allelic variants encoding proteins with amino acid sequence differences that co-segregate with enzymatic activity and blood pressure differences. As with human patients, blood pressure QTLs identified in crossbred rodent populations can be only crudely localized to regions of 10 to 30 centimorgans (approximately 20 to 60 million base pairs) that contain many genes. Studies showing blood pressure QTLs have often been difficult to replicate in animal and human populations, adding significant uncertainty to their findings.

Using congenic strains to study blood pressure. Chromosomal regions containing either a "low" or "high" blood pressure QTL allele can be genetically transferred from one strain (donor) to another inbred (recipient) strain by selective breeding. F_1 (donor X recipient) rats are backcrossed to the appropriate parental strain, and the resulting progeny are examined for polymorphic genetic markers present in a selected chromosomal region. Progeny heterozygous for markers in this region are backcrossed to the recipient strain, with the process repeated until rats are identified that carry only the selected region of donor chromosome on a background of alleles from the recipient strain. The chosen rats are then brother-sister mated to become inbred congenic strains that are homozygous for the selected donor strain alleles. Congenic strains carry a small portion of donor chromosomal material on an otherwise uniform background of recipient strain alleles. Significant blood pressure differences between the congenic and recipient strains confirm the presence of a blood pressure QTL allele in the introgressed chromosomal region and define physical limits for the location of the QTLs. In the Dahl rat model alone, 8 blood pressure QTLs have been confirmed by use of congenic strains, including the rat chromosome 7 region containing *Cyp11b1*. Further selective breeding can be used to develop congenic substrains carrying a blood pressure QTL allele in a reduced portion of introgressed donor chromosome. These congenic substrains eliminate many genes not located in the congenic region from consideration as candidates and facilitate the subsequent identification and positional cloning of genes responsible for the development of hypertension. Differential gene expression between a congenic strain and the parental strain from which it was derived may be useful in identifying a strong candidate gene for a blood pressure QTL.

SUGGESTED READING

1. Aitman TJ, Glazier AM, Wallace CA, et al. Identification of Cd36 (*Fat*) as an insulin-resistance gene causing defective fatty acid and glucose metabolism in hypertensive rats. *Nat Genet.* 1999;21:76–83.
2. Cicila GT. Strategy for uncovering complex determinants of hypertension using animal models. *Curr Hypertens Rep.* 2000;2:1–10.
3. Cicila GT, Garrett MR, Dene H, Rapp JP. High resolution mapping of the blood pressure QTL on chromosome 7 using Dahl rat congenic strains. *Genomics.* 2001;72:51–60.
4. Cicila GT, Rapp JP, Wang J-M, et al. Linkage of 11 [beta] hydroxylase mutations with altered steroid biosynthesis and blood pressure in the Dahl rat. *Nat Genet.* 1993;3:346–353.
5. Falconer DS, Mackay TFC. *Introduction to Quantitative Genetics.* 4th ed. New York, NY: Longman, 1996.
6. Julier C, Delépine MBK, Terwilliger J, et al. Genetic susceptibility for human familial essential hypertension in a region of homology with blood pressure linkage on rat chromosome 10. *Hum Mol Genet.* 1997;6:2077–2085.
7. Rapp JP. Genetic analysis of inherited hypertension in the rat. *Physiol Rev.* 2000;8:135–172.
8. Siffert W, Rosskopf D, Siffert G, et al. Association of human G-protein [beta]3 subunit variant with hypertension. *Nat Genet.* 1998;18:45–48.
9. Stoll M, Cowley AW Jr, Tonellato PJ, et al. A genomic-systems biology map for cardiovascular function. *Science.* 2001;294:1723–1726.
10. Weeks DE, Lathrop GM. Polygenic disease: methods for mapping complex disease traits. *Trends Genet.* 1995;11:513–519.

Chapter A75

Genetics and Family History of Hypertension

Steven C. Hunt, PhD

KEY POINTS

- Blood pressure levels and hypertension have a quantifiable genetic component, and family history is related to hypertension risk.

- Genome-wide linkage analyses have identified chromosomal regions that may harbor genes related to hypertension and to the concordance of hypertension and dyslipidemia.

- Genes with the strongest evidence of a relation to hypertension include angiotensinogen and α-adducin.

- Controlling or removing behavioral risk factors appears to confer greater benefit in individuals with the greatest genetic risk.

See also Chapters A4, A14, A44–A46, A73, A74, A76–A78, and C114

There is evidence of a significant genetic component of blood pressure level in humans and of several intermediate phenotypes closely associated with hypertension that are directly related to specific genes. Intermediate phenotypes are quantifiable biologic traits (such as angiotensinogen levels or salt sensitivity) that, in appropriate combinations, account for a fraction of the overall risk for the development of hypertension.

Family History of Hypertension

A family history of hypertension is a commonly used measure of the familial aggregation of hypertension and can be used as a surrogate measure for undefined risk factors that may be shared by the family. A proper family history of older adults (roughly age 40 and older) includes listing all first-degree relatives and their age, sex, and current blood pressure status. For younger adults and youths, first-degree relatives of the parents should be identified.

Adults. Family history of hypertension significantly predicts the future onset of hypertension in family members. The strength of the prediction depends on the definition of a positive family history and on the age of the person at risk (**Table A75.1**). Having a single first-degree relative with hypertension is only a weak predictor of future hypertension, whereas a finding of ≥2 relatives with hypertension at an early age (<55 years) identifies a smaller subset of families who are at much higher

Table A75.1. Relative Risks of Hypertension for Different Definitions of a Positive Family History of Hypertension for Men and Women[a]

DEFINITIONS OF +FHx	% WITH +FHX	AGE GROUP				
		20–39	40–49	50–59	60–69	≥70
Men						
≥1 Affected	53	2.5	1.8	1.7	1.2	0.9
≥1 Before age 55 yr	32	2.8	2.1	1.8	1.1	0.8
≥2 Affected	24	3.8	2.4	2.3	1.2	0.6
≥2 Before age 55 yr	11	4.1	2.5	2.4	1.0	0.8
Women						
≥1 Affected	—	2.8	2.0	1.5	1.0	0.8
≥1 Before age 55 yr	—	3.2	2.3	1.5	1.0	0.8
≥2 Affected	—	3.8	2.4	2.3	1.2	0.6
≥2 Before age 55 yr	—	5.0	3.5	1.5	0.7	0.8

+FHx, family history of hypertension.
[a]Relative risks are based on 13 years of follow-up in a retrospective cohort study of 94,292 persons in 15,200 families and are relative to persons without any first-degree relatives with hypertension.

risk for the development of hypertension. At the same time, older persons in families with a strong family history of hypertension have a risk of developing hypertension similar to that of the general population, suggesting that these "protected" individuals do not share the genetic or environmental factors associated with early onset hypertension in their families. The presence of stroke or coronary artery disease in family members is another modifying factor when the significance of a positive family history of hypertension is evaluated.

Children and adolescents. Although family history definitions work reasonably well for adults, youths generally have first-degree relatives too young to have hypertension. In this setting, children have often been categorized by family history groups on the basis of the number of parents (0, 1, or 2) with hypertension. An alternative is to use medical history information on their second-degree relatives (first-degree relatives of the parents). In longitudinal studies of children, those with a positive family history of hypertension have higher blood pressures than those without a positive family history. Young adults with a systolic blood pressure reading higher than the age- and sex-specific ninetieth percentile have a greater prevalence of a positive family history of hypertension and more relatives with ischemic heart disease and stroke.

Correlative Studies

Intraclass correlation coefficients of blood pressure are low (in the 0.1 to 0.3 range) in most family studies. The correlations between brother pairs are generally similar to those of sister pairs and brother-sister pairs. Parent-offspring correlations tend to be slightly weaker than sib-sib correlations. Overall, heritability estimates cluster at 20% to 40% for family studies but are higher (50–70%) when twins are used. Adoption studies have also provided evidence for the genetic contribution to blood pressure and provide some insight into the question of genetic and environmental contributions. In families with natural children, adoptive children, or both natural and adoptive children, the intraclass correlation for systolic blood pressure

between adopted siblings was 0.16 compared with 0.38 between natural siblings. For diastolic blood pressure, the adoptee and natural sibling correlations were 0.29 and 0.53, respectively. The parent-adoptee correlations were much smaller than the parent–natural child correlations.

Intermediate Phenotypes and Hypertension Genes

Individual common susceptibility genes associated with essential hypertension can explain only a small proportion of blood pressure variation. This is expected because hypertension and blood pressure are considered to be polygenic phenotypes with complex environmental interactions (see Chapter A76). An advantage of identifying families with a positive family history of hypertension for studies of genetics is that these families tend to have the necessary collection of genes and behavioral habits that lead to hypertension. Such families can be used to study gene-gene and gene-environment interactions on blood pressure and the intermediate phenotypes (traits) that control blood pressure.

Aggregation of traits associated with insulin resistance and hypertension. The traits that comprise the cardiovascular metabolic syndrome are also associated genetically.

Obesity and hypertension. Several prospective studies have shown that measures of central obesity, particularly subscapular skinfold thickness, are strong predictors of the development of hypertension. Body mass index has also been shown in large population studies to be partially determined by major genes. Weight and obesity are responsible for part of the familial aggregation of blood pressure found between siblings and between spouses. Therefore, a gene that significantly increases a person's body weight would also tend to increase that person's blood pressure and promote clustering of high blood pressure in that family.

Dyslipidemia and hypertension. The clustering of abnormal lipids and insulin resistance has been well described in non-obese and obese individuals. These abnormalities have a strong familial component and tend to precede the development of increased blood pressure. In a population-based sample of hypertensive siblings, the most striking sibling aggregation of risk factors occurred for reduced high-density lipoprotein cholesterol (3.9 times more often than expected) and elevated triglyceride levels (3.0 times more often than expected). The sibship aggregation of these abnormalities was much higher than expected ($p < .0001$), with 40% of the 58 hypertensive sibships showing concordance for ≥1 lipid abnormalities. These hypertensive siblings were also significantly more obese than the general population and had elevated fasting insulin levels, smaller low-density lipoprotein particle size, and increased apolipoprotein B levels. The aggregation of hypertension and familial lipid abnormalities has been estimated to occur in 12% to 16% of all hypertensive patients and 1% to 2% of the general population. The familial aggregation of the dyslipidemic hypertension syndrome has been verified in a large twin study. Dyslipidemic hypertension was concordant 3 times more often among identical twins than among nonidentical twins ($p = .06$). In identical twin pairs discordant for this syndrome, the affected twin was often obese, whereas the unaffected twin had more normal weight. Thus, a nongenetic (environmental) factor influencing obesity may affect the expression of familial dyslipidemic hypertension and confound efforts to detect a gene for this syndrome. In addition, twins with both hypertension and lipid abnormalities had a much greater than expected coronary heart disease mortality compared with twins with only hypertension or lipid abnormalities. In another study, at least 21% of all sibling pairs with coronary heart disease had both hypertension and lipid abnormalities.

Insulin resistance and sympathetic activity. In a Japanese study, the heritability of the insulin resistance trait in families was found to be greater than that of early sympathetic activation. Both characteristics were predictive of blood pressure increases after 10 years of follow-up, but progressive increases in plasma norepinephrine were most closely related to the final blood pressure, suggesting a genetic-environmental interaction.

Age, gender, and salt intake. In isolated populations in which salt intake is low, blood pressure does not seem to increase with age. In most industrialized countries, however, blood pressure does increase with age. It has been suggested that there is an underlying unknown major gene for hypertension that is affected by age, genotype, and gender. According to this model, women with the putative high blood pressure gene have larger increases in systolic blood pressure with age. Approaches like this suggest the importance of simultaneously investigating environmental and genetic risk factors because a person's genotype may determine different environmental responses that could be missed if genotype were ignored.

Candidate Genes

Numerous linkage analyses using 300 to 500 markers spread over all chromosomes have suggested several locations for hypertension genes. Some of the more consistent areas are on chromosome arms 1q, 2p, 2q, 8p, 17q, and 18q. Several of these regions also have evidence for linkage of lipid-related traits in the area. Other less consistent regions may still harbor important hypertension genes. Genes involving the renin-angiotensin system have been most systematically scrutinized.

Renin-angiotensin-aldosterone genes and hypertension. The expression of these genes as traits or intermediate phenotypes can exhibit strong environmental modulation. This is especially true for those genes relating to the interaction of salt intake or salt sensitivity and activity of the renin-angiotensin-aldosterone system. Of special interest is the interaction of angiotensinogen gene variants with blood pressure sensitivity to dietary sodium; these interactions are discussed in detail in Chapters A45 and A76. To date, genes encoding angiotensinogen expression appear to be most closely related to hypertension but other genes possibly related to hypertension include the β_2-adrenoceptor, aldosterone synthase, the β_3 subunit of a G protein, and the angiotensin II AT_1 receptor.

Kallikrein. Kallikrein is an enzyme that converts inactive kininogen to bradykinin. An amino acid change (R53H) in the kallikrein gene has been shown to be associated with a 50% reduction in kallikrein levels. Also, a major gene has been statistically identified for low urinary kallikrein levels that explains 39% of the variance of urinary kallikrein and interacts with

Table A75.2. Polygenic Heritability Estimates of Some Hypertension Intermediate Phenotypes

PHENOTYPE	HERITABILITY
Height	75
Body mass index	24
Scapular skinfold	32
Waist circumference	25
Hip circumference	36
Cholesterol	44
Triglycerides	37
High-density lipoprotein cholesterol	45
Plasma insulin	45
Serum creatinine	23
Serum calcium	14
Serum potassium	23
Serum magnesium	57
Serum uric acid	31
Na-Li countertransport	65
Li-K cotransport	30
Na leak	43

potassium levels. If verified, this suggests that a decrease in dietary potassium in heterozygotes (50% of the population) would result in kallikrein levels similar to those of the low-kallikrein homozygotes, increasing the risk of hypertension. An increase in dietary potassium would be expected to raise kallikrein levels near the high-kallikrein homozygote mean, reducing the risk of hypertension.

Transport abnormalities. Biochemical and anthropometric variables with the strongest polygenic effects (many genes with additive, small effects) are shown in **Table A75.2.** Some of these phenotypes also show evidence of major gene control.

α-Adducin. α-Adducin is a membrane cytoskeletal protein that is involved with membrane transport. Markers at this locus have been genetically linked to hypertension, and association studies have found a variant within the gene that is associated with higher blood pressures. Persons with this variant have increased maximal Na,K-ATPase pump activity and increased renal tubular sodium reabsorption. Patients with the variant have a greater blood pressure response to diuretic treatment and also have a greater blood pressure decrease after acute sodium depletion by diet and furosemide.

Na-Li countertransport. Twin and pedigree studies have shown significant genetic control of erythrocyte Na-Li countertransport that probably represents *in vivo* Na-H exchange. A study in Italy suggested possible major gene inheritance of Na-K cotransport, especially in hypertensive families. Segregation analysis suggests that intraerythrocytic sodium levels are partially determined by a major gene with 4 alleles explaining 29% of the variance, whereas polygenes explained another 55%.

Ouabain-binding sites. Recessive inheritance of a major gene for a higher number of ouabain-binding sites explained 14% of the variance in the number of binding sites, and polygenic inheritance explained another 63%. Individuals with the major gene had lower intraerythrocytic Na^+ levels, in accordance with observations that higher Na^+,K^+-ATPase activity decreases intracellular Na^+ levels.

Uric acid. Uric acid has been shown in multivariate analyses to predict the future onset of hypertension, with relative risks in the range of 1.8 to 2.2, and uric acid has been related to hypertension and blood pressure in cross-sectional studies and within families.

SUGGESTED READING

1. Hunt SC, Hopkins PN, Lalouel J-M. Hypertension. In: King RA, Rotter JI, Motulsky AG, eds. *The Genetic Basis of Common Diseases*. 2nd ed. New York, NY: Oxford Press; 2002 (*in press*).
2. Hunt SC, Williams RR, Barlow GK. A comparison of positive family history definitions for defining risk of future disease. *J Chron Dis*. 1986;39:809–821.
3. Jeunemaitre X, Soubrier F, Kotelevtsev Y, et al. Molecular basis of human hypertension: role of angiotensinogen. *J Nephrol*. 1997;10:172–178.
4. Manunta P, Cerutti R, Bernardi L, et al. Renal genetic mechanisms of essential hypertension. *J Nephrol*. 1997;10:172–178.
5. Masuo K, Mikami H, Ogihara T, Tuck ML. Familial hypertension, insulin, sympathetic activity, and blood pressure elevation. *Hypertension*. 1998;32:96–100.
6. Pérusse L, Moll PP, Sing CF. Evidence that a single gene with gender- and age-dependent effects influences systolic blood pressure determination in a population-based sample. *Am J Hum Genet*. 1991;49:94–105.
7. Selby JV, Newman B, Quiroga J, et al. Concordance for dyslipidemic hypertension in male twins. *JAMA*. 1991;265:2079–2084.
8. Ward R. Familial aggregation and genetic epidemiology of blood pressure. In: Laragh JH, Brenner BM, eds. *Hypertension: Pathophysiology, Diagnosis, and Management*. New York, NY: Raven Press Ltd; 1990:81–100.
9. Williams GH, Dluhy RG, Lifton RP, et al. Non-modulation as an intermediate phenotype in essential hypertension. *Hypertension*. 1992;20:788–796.
10. Williams RR, Hunt SC, Hopkins PN, et al. Familial dyslipidemic hypertension: evidence from 58 Utah families for a syndrome present in approximately 12% of patients with essential hypertension. *JAMA*. 1988;259:3579–3586.

Chapter A76

Gene-Environment Interactions

Sharon L. R. Kardia, PhD

KEY POINTS

- Gene-by-environment interactions between genetic variations and environmental factors such as stress, diet, and physical activity contribute to the development of essential hypertension.

- Gene-by-salt interactions define subtypes of experimental and human hypertension.

- Knowledge of gene-by-environment interactions may lead to improved therapy that matches specific interventions with specific genetic subgroups (gene-by-drug interactions).

See also Chapters A4, A6, A45, A46, A73–A75, A78, and C114

General Background

On a fundamental level, it can be argued that all variation in blood pressure results from the interaction of genes and environment and that failure to consider this inextricably intertwined relationship leads to false dichotomization of genetic or environmental etiologies. However, it is quite difficult to quantitate how environmental variation combines with molecular genetic processes (within an individual) or with genetic variations (across individuals) to give rise to the wide spectrum of blood pressures observed in a population.

Historical aspects. The earliest demonstration and definition of a gene-environment interaction was the observation of a nonlinear relationship between variation in food availability and variation in body allometry (i.e., proportional growth of one character relative to another character) in different strains of *Hyalodaphnia*. Such variation is termed a *norm of reaction* and is essentially identical to the concept of gene-environment interaction; the norm of reaction is the set of phenotypes (e.g., weight) that is associated with environmental variation for a particular genotype or genome-type.

Allelic variation. Researchers are somewhat limited in their abilities to investigate the underlying causes of gene-environment interactions in humans. It is evident that environment-dependent gene expression is affected by allelic variation, which can influence how well signals from the environment are transduced to direct gene expression, as well as influencing how well the expressed gene's product performs its functional role. A genotype that responds to changes in the environment is classified broadly as being *sensitive*, whereas a phenotype that is not influenced by its environment is *insensitive*.

Gene-by-Salt Interactions

Salt sensitivity. Multiple interconnected homeodynamic mechanisms regulate the relationship between salt and water intake and resultant blood pressure levels within an individual. This relationship is known to be heterogeneous among individuals, who can be broadly categorized as *salt-sensitive* or *salt-resistant*. Two rare, monogenic forms of hypertension known as *glucocorticoid-remediable aldosteronism* and *apparent mineralocorticoid excess* are salt-sensitive volume expansion forms of hypertension (see Chapter A77).

α-Adducin. Another gene thought to be associated with increased renal tubular absorption of sodium is the α-adducin gene that was identified in Milan hypertensive rats, a volume-

Table A76.1. Studies Assessing the Role of Gene-by-Salt Interactions on Blood Pressure (BP)

GENE (POLYMORPHISM)	ENVIRONMENT	ASSOCIATION WITH BP RESPONSE	REFERENCES
Aldosterone synthase (C344T)	Dietary salt (220 mmol/d vs. 20 mmol/d)	None.	Brand. *J Hypertens.* 1999;17:1563.
Angiotensinogen (Met235Thr)	Dietary salt (220 mmol/d vs. 20 mmol/d)	None.	Schorr. *J Hypertens.* 1999;17:475.
	Dietary salt (260 mmol/d vs. 50 mmol/d)	None.	Giner. *Hypertension.* 2000;35:512.
	Low-sodium mineral salt vs. table salt	Thr235 shows greater BP decreases after sodium intervention.	Hunt. *Am J Hypertens.* 1999;12:460.
Angiotensin-converting enzyme (insertion/deletion)	Dietary salt (260 mmol/d vs. 50 mmol/d)	Insertion shows greater BP elevation on high-salt diet.	Giner. *Hypertension.* 2000;35:512.
α-Adducin (Gly460Trp)	Saline infusion followed by furosemide	Trp460 shows 2 times greater BP response.	Cusi. *Lancet.* 1997;349:1353.

expanded, salt-sensitive form of hypertension. In humans, an amino acid substitution in the α-adducin gene from glycine to tryptophan at codon 460 (*Gly460Trp*) has been associated with increased hypertension risk. In an acute salt-sensitivity test (saline infusion for the salt-loading phase followed by furosemide administration for the salt-depletion phase), Cusi and colleagues found that the decrease in mean arterial pressure was 2 times greater in the *Gly/Trp* heterozygotes than in the *Gly/Gly* homozygotes (**Table A76.1**). The α-adducin *Gly460Trp* variation also appears to be associated with the response of patients to the diuretic hydrochlorothiazide. *Gly/Trp* heterozygotes have twice the blood pressure reduction than the *Gly/Gly* homozygotes after 8 weeks of therapy. Overall, hypertensives carrying the *Trp460* variant may require higher renal perfusion pressure to excrete a sodium load. They also have enhanced renal tubular reabsorption of sodium, activation of Na,K-ATPase, lower plasma renin activity, and more profound decreases in blood pressure after acute sodium depletion or diuretic therapy.

Renin-angiotensin system.
The renin-angiotensin system is also known to play a major role in sodium-water balance, which influences blood pressure. Hypertensives with low renin often exhibit a greater blood pressure response to sodium loading, and salt-sensitive hypertensives show a blunted RAS response when there is a shift from low to high sodium in the diet. Several genes involved in this system, namely the angiotensinogen (*AGT*), angiotensin-converting enzyme (*ACE*), and angiotensin II type 1 receptor have been investigated for their association with hypertension, as well as salt sensitivity.

Angiotensinogen polymorphisms. The *AGT* gene has 2 well-studied polymorphisms: an A-to-G substitution at the −6 nucleotide position of the gene's promoter (denoted *−6 A/G*) and a methionine to threonine amino acid substitution at codon 235 (*Met235Thr*). The frequency of these variations is correlated in the general population (i.e., they are in linkage disequilibrium). The *Thr235* allele has been demonstrated to be weakly, but significantly, associated with hypertension in a wide variety of populations. Carriers of the *Thr235* variation also appear to have greater blood pressure response to sodium reduction, as do carriers of the *A* variant at the −6 position within the promoter of that gene. A final AGT example of a specific genotype-by-environment interaction study serves as a prototype for what is likely to be the next wave of gene-

environment studies in hypertension research. Briefly, Hunt and colleagues conducted a study testing whether the −6 A/G polymorphism in the promoter of the angiotensinogen gene was related to incidence of hypertension, and whether its presence could predict the blood pressure response to sodium reduction or weight loss. Participants were randomized in a 2 × 2 factorial design to sodium reduction, weight loss, combined intervention, or usual care. In the usual care group, individuals with the AA genotype at the −6 position had a higher incidence of hypertension than those with the GG genotype (**Figure A76.1**). In comparison, the blood pressure was significantly lower after sodium reduction for the AA group compared to the GG individuals. Similar genotype-by-environment interaction effects were observed for the influence of weight reduction on risk of hypertension.

Angiotensin-converting enzyme polymorphisms. The *ACE* gene has 1 widely studied polymorphism resulting from an insertion/deletion in intron 16. Although linkage evidence implicates this gene in hypertension risk, many more studies have

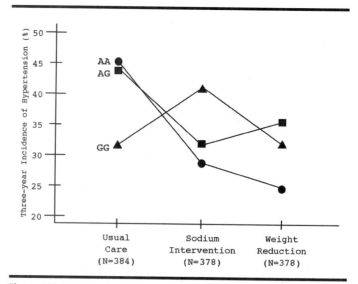

Figure A76.1. Example of an interaction between angiotensinogen *−6A/G* polymorphism and different t interventions on 3-year incidence of hypertension. (Adapted from Hunt SC, Cook NR, Oberman A, et al. Angiotensinogen genotype, sodium reduction, weight loss, and prevention of hypertension: trials of hypertension prevention phase II. *Hypertension.*1998;32:393–401.)

Table A76.2. Genetic Polymorphisms Associated with Blood Pressure (BP) Response to Antihypertensive Drug Therapy in Patients with Essential Hypertension

GENE (POLYMORPHISM)	ANTIHYPERTENSIVE MEDICATION	ASSOCIATION	REFERENCES
α-Adducin (Gly460Trp)	Thiazide Diuretics	Trp460 shows 2 times greater BP reduction	Cusi. *Lancet*. 1997;349:1353.
Angiotensinogen (Met235Thr)	ACE inhibitors Calcium antagonist β-Blocker ACE inhibitor	T235 shows greater BP reduction None	Hingorani. *J Hypertens*. 1995;13:1602. Dudley. *J Hypertens*. 1996;14:259.
ACE (insertion/deletion)	Calcium antagonist β-Blocker ACE inhibitor	None	Dudley. *J Hypertens*. 1996;14:259.
	ACE inhibitors ACE inhibitor	None None	Hingorani. *J Hypertens*. 1995;13:1602. Sasaki. *J Hypertens*. 1996;14:1403.
G protein α-Subunit [FokI (±)] β-Subunit (C825T)	β-Blockers Diuretic	FokI shows greater BP reduction C825T shows greater BP reduction	Jia. *Hypertension*. 1999;34:8. Turner. *Hypertension*. 2001;37:739.

ACE, angiotensin-converting enzyme.

demonstrated that the presence of the *D* variant is more closely associated with the microvascular and macrovascular sequelae of hypertension. With respect to its influence on salt sensitivity, the *I* variant confers greater blood pressure increases associated with changes from a low-salt (50 mmol/day) to high-salt (260 mmol/day) diet.

Gene-by-Drug Interactions

It is well known that hypertensives respond heterogeneously to antihypertensive drugs. This heterogeneity probably reflects a wide variety of factors, including differences in pharmacodynamic and pharmacokinetic properties and differences among individuals in the pathophysiologic traits influencing blood pressure levels. Pharmacogenetics, the study of genetic variations that influence responses to pharmacologic agents, is an emerging field whose main foundation is gene-environment interaction.

Pharmacogenetics and antihypertensive drug metabolism.
Traditional pharmacogenetics has focused on understanding variations in drug effects across individuals associated with variation in drug metabolizing enzymes. Specifically, the metabolism of certain therapeutic agents is well known to involve several phase I (dehydrogenases, esterases, *CYP450*s) and phase II enzymes. The *CYP450* enzymes have been reasonably well characterized, with over 150 different *CYP450* isoforms identified as products of more than 30 *CYP450* genes. Two notable polymorphisms affecting drug metabolism are the *CYP2D2* and the *N*-acetyltransferase 2 variants. Studies of the impact of the *CYP2D2* gene polymorphism on the metabolism of alprenolol, bufuralol, carvedilol, metoprolol, propranolol, and timolol indicate that mutations cause poor metabolism and excessive β-blockade in carriers. Carriers of the "rapid acetylator" *N*-acetyltransferase 2 polymorphism require higher doses of hydralazine to control blood pressure. Traditional pharmacogenetic phenomena as found for drug metabolizing enzymes are not likely to explain the majority of the variation in blood pressure response to antihypertensive therapy for a variety of reasons including their low gene frequency and because their effect on the pharmacokinetic effects are not well correlated with the blood pressure–lowering capabilities within or between antihypertensive classes.

Pharmacogenetics and population variation in drug responses.
Differences in blood pressure response to different antihypertensives is also thought to be associated with differences in the underlying pathophysiologic etiology of hypertension. For example, the impact of *AGT* and *ACE* genetic variations on blood pressure responsiveness to ACE inhibitors, β-blockers, and calcium antagonists has recently been studied during 4-week trials, which has found some variation in patient responses to these antihypertensive therapies. Variants in several other candidate genes, including the α-adducin, angiotensinogen, angiotensin-converting enzyme, β₁-adrenergic receptor, and β₂-adrenergic receptor, are likely to be associated with differences in the pathophysiology of hypertension, differential risk of developing hypertension, and variability in blood pressure response to antihypertensives (**Table A76.2**). Variants of the β₃ subunit of G proteins (GNβ3) may also influence blood pressure variation. In particular, a C-to-T substitution (*C825T*) has been shown to be associated with hypertension and responsiveness to hydrochlorothiazide. The *825T* variant causes a splice site mutation that results in a shortened protein that has increased signal transduction responsiveness to vasoactive and growth-promoting cellular factors.

SUGGESTED READING

1. Cusi D, Barlassina C, Azzani T, et al. Polymorphisms of α-adducin and salt sensitivity in patients with essential hypertension. *Lancet*. 1997;349:1338–1339.
2. Hunt SC, Cook NR, Oberman A, et al. Angiotensinogen genotype, sodium reduction, weight loss, and prevention of hypertension: trials of hypertension prevention phase II. *Hypertension*. 1998;32:393–401.
3. Laragh JH, Lamport B, Sealey J, Alderman MH. Diagnosis ex juvantibus. Individual response patterns to drugs reveals. *J Hypertens*. 1988;12:223–226.
4. Motulsky A. Drug reaction, enzymes and biochemical genetics. *JAMA*. 1957;165:835–837.
5. Turner ST, Schwartz GL, Chapman AB, Boerwinkle E. C825T polymor-

phism of the G protein α_3-subunit and antihypertensive response to a thiazide diuretic. *Hypertension.* 2001;37:739–748.

6. Turner ST. Pharmacogenetic markers of hypertension pathogenesis and

responses to therapy. In: Epstein M, ed. *Calcium Antagonists in Clinical Medicine.* Philadelphia, PA: Hanley & Belfus; 2002.

7. Weber WW. *Pharmacogenetics.* New York: Oxford University Press; 1997.

Chapter A77

Monogenic Determinant of Blood Pressure

Robert G. Dluhy, MD

KEY POINTS

- Monogenic (single-gene) forms of human hypertension involve gain-of-function mutations that result in overproduction of mineralocorticoids or increased mineralocorticoid activity.

- Clinical phenotypes usually include severe hypertension from birth, apparent volume expansion, suppression of plasma renin activity, and variable hypokalemia.

- Autosomal dominant and recessive renal salt-wasting syndromes result from loss-of-function mutations in the renin angiotensin system or renal ion transporters, with blood pressure dependent on intake of dietary sodium.

See also Chapters A9, A50, A73, C111, C114, and C170

Progress has recently been made in identifying the genetic mutations of mendelian, or single-gene, forms of human hypertension (**Table A77.1**). Monogenic hypertensive syndromes are caused by mutations in genes resulting in gain-of-function of transporters in the distal nephron, as well as various components of the renin-angiotensin-aldosterone system that result in excessive renal sodium retention. These syndromes can be divided into overproduction of mineralocorticoids versus increased mineralocorticoid activity. Identification of these mutated genes has also permitted targeted antihypertensive therapies.

Hypertension with Overproduction of Mineralocorticoids

Glucocorticoid-remediable aldosteronism.
Glucocorticoid-remediable aldosteronism (GRA), an autosomal dominant disorder characterized by moderate to severe hypertension in affected patients from birth onward, is the most common form of monogenic human hypertension. Because the majority of patients with GRA are not hypokalemic, the serum potassium level lacks sensitivity as a screening test for this disorder. Early hemorrhagic stroke (mean age, 32 years) is characteristic of GRA pedigrees. In a recent study, 48% of all GRA pedigrees and 18% of all GRA patients had cerebrovascular complications. In GRA, aldosterone secretion is positively and solely regulated by adrenocorticotropic hormone (ACTH), not by angiotensin II or potassium. As a consequence, exogenous low-dose glucocorticoid administration (which potently suppresses ACTH) profoundly suppresses aldosterone secretion in affected subjects, reversing the syndrome. As in other causes of primary aldosteronism, plasma renin levels are suppressed.

Aldosterone synthase gene duplication. Genetic analysis of GRA kindreds has revealed linkage of GRA to a mutation in the aldosterone synthase gene, which is closely related to steroid 11β-hydroxylase, a second gene involved in adrenal steroidogenesis. Both genes are 95% identical in DNA sequence, have identical intron-exon structures, and are located in close proximity on chromosome 8. In all GRA kindreds, affected subjects have 2 normal copies of genes encoding aldosterone synthase and 11β-hydroxylase. In addition, they have a novel gene duplication: a hybrid, or chimeric, gene duplication containing the 5' regulatory sequences conferring ACTH responsiveness of 11β-hydroxylase fused to more distal coding sequences of aldosterone synthase, the result of an unequal crossing-over between these 2 homologous genes (**Figure A77.1A**). In GRA kindreds, the sites of crossing-over are variable, indicating that in different pedigrees, the gene duplications arise independently rather than from a single ancestral mutation. In addition, the sites of crossing-over are all upstream of exon 5 of aldosterone synthase, suggesting that encoded amino acids in exon 5 are essential for aldosterone synthase enzymatic functions (Figure A77.1B). Gene duplication appears to explain all of the known physiologic and biochemical features previously reported in GRA. First, the promoter region of this chimeric gene contains regulatory sequences of 11β-hydroxylase and is regulated by ACTH. In addition, the chimeric gene allows ectopic expression of aldosterone synthase enzymatic activity in the ACTH-regulated zona fasciculata, which normally secretes only cortisol. Finally, the sole regulation of aldosterone secretion by ACTH and the suppression of aldosterone secretion by glucocorticoids in GRA is explained by the fact that aldosterone synthase gene is abnormally regulated by ACTH promoter sequences.

Table A77.1. Monogenic Forms of Human Hypertension

DISORDER	SITE OF ALTERATION IN KIDNEY OR RENIN-ANGIOTENSIN-ALDOSTERONE SYSTEM	GENES MUTATED
Glucocorticoid-remediable aldosteronism	Adrenal (aldosterone)	Aldosterone synthase
11β-Hydroxylase, 17α-hydroxylase deficiencies	Adrenal (mineralocorticoids)	CYP11B1; CYP17
Hypertension exacerbated in pregnancy	Renal (MR)	MR
Liddle's syndrome	Renal epithelial Na⁺ channel (ENaC)	β- or γ-subunit of ENaC genes
Syndrome of apparent mineralocorticoid excess	Renal (MR)	11β-Hydroxysteroid dehydrogenase (renal isoform) gene
Pseudohypoaldosteronism type II	Renal (distal nephron)	WNK kinases

ENaC, amiloride sensitive epithelial sodium channel; MR, mineralocorticoid receptor.

Genetic screening. Direct genetic screening for the presence of the gene duplication in GRA is 100% sensitive and specific for diagnosing GRA and is recommended for patients with primary aldosteronism without radiographic evidence of tumors, for young hypertensive individuals with suppressed levels of plasma renin activity (especially children), and for at-risk individuals in affected families. Directed treatments with low-dose glucocorticoids, amiloride, or spironolactone effectively treat the elevated blood pressure of GRA.

Disorders of steroid hormone biosynthesis (congenital adrenal hyperplasia). Various abnormalities of hydroxylase enzymes of the P450 class have been identified. These include C21, C17, and C11 hydroxylases, which are important steps in steroidogenesis. Disordered volume regulation and hypertension are usually not the presenting symptoms in the majority of patients with congenital adrenal hyperplasia (CAH). Rather, excessive androgenic effects in female patients or hypogonadism in male patients are more characteristic of the clinical phenotypes. 21-Hydroxylase deficiency, resulting from a mutated gene encoding P450C21 and accounting for >90% of the CAH genetic disorders, is not associated with hypertension but rather with sodium wasting in the severe clinical variant presenting in childhood.

P450C11β deficiency. P450C11β deficiency causes a hypertensive variant of CAH, in which hypertension and hypokalemia variably occur because impaired conversion of 11-deoxycorticosterone to corticosterone results in the accumulation of 11-deoxycorticosterone, a potent mineralocorticoid. Increased shunting into the androgen pathway leads to ambiguous exter-

nal genitalia at birth in girls (female pseudohermaphroditism) or hirsutism, virilization, or both in girls in the postnatal period. P450C11β deficiency is an uncommon cause of CAH in individuals of European ancestry but accounts for 15% of cases in Moslem and Jewish Middle Eastern populations. Mutations causing P450C11β deficiency cluster in exons 6 to 8 of the CYP11B1 gene.

P450C17α deficiency. P450C17α deficiency is characterized by hypogonadism, hypokalemia, and hypertension. This rare disorder causes decreased production of cortisol and shunting of precursors into the mineralocorticoid pathway; usually, 11-deoxycorticosterone production is elevated. Because P450C17α hydroxylation is required for biosynthesis of adrenal and gonadal testosterone and estrogen, this defect is associated with sexual immaturity, high urinary gonadotropin levels, and low urinary 17-ketosteroid excretion. Female patients have primary amenorrhea and lack of development of secondary sexual characteristics. Because of deficient androgen production, male patients have either ambiguous external genitalia or a female phenotype (male pseudohermaphroditism). Exogenous glucocorticoids can correct the hypertensive syndrome, and treatment with appropriate gonadal steroids results in sexual maturation. A large number of random mutations can cause 17α-hydroxylase deficiency, making genetic diagnosis difficult.

Hypertension with Increased Mineralocorticoid Activity

Syndrome of apparent mineralocorticoid excess. *In vitro,* cortisol and aldosterone are potent activators of renal mineral-

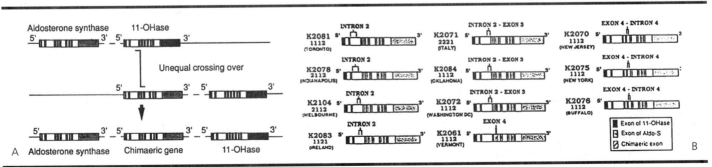

Figure A77.1. A: The chimeric gene duplication in glucocorticoid-remediable aldosteronism, a result of unequal crossing-over between the homologous 11β-hydroxylase and aldosterone synthase genes. The chimera fuses the 5'-regulatory sequences of the 11β-hydroxylase gene and the 3'-coding sequences of the aldosterone synthase gene. **B:** Crossover breakpoints in 11 glucocorticoid-remediable aldosteronism pedigrees. The sites of crossing-over are all upstream of exon 5 of aldosterone synthase. (From Lifton RP, Dluhy RG, Powers M, et al. Hereditary hypertension caused by chimaeric gene duplications and ectopic expression of aldosterone synthase. *Nat Genet.* 1992;2:66–74, with permission.)

GLUCOCORTICOID SHUTTLE

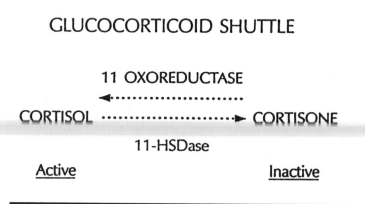

Figure A77.2. The glucocorticoid shuttle whereby the 2 isoforms of the 11β-hydroxysteroid dehydrogenase (11β-HSD) enzyme act as a reductase in the liver (cortisone to cortisol, 11β-HSD1) or a dehydrogenase in the kidney (11β-HSD2).

Table A77.2. Loss-of-Function Mutations with Renal Salt Wasting

DISORDER STATUS	GENES MUTATED	POTASSIUM[a]
Autosomal dominant pseudohypoaldosteronism type I	Mineralocorticoid receptor	Hyperkalemia[a]
Autosomal recessive (AR) pseudohypoaldosteronism type I	Sodium epithelial channel	Hyperkalemia
Gitelman's syndrome (AR)	Thiazide-sensitive Na-Cl cotransporter in distal convoluted tubule	Hypokalemia[a]
Bartter's syndrome (AR)	Ion transporters in thick ascending loop of Henle	Hypokalemia

AR, autosomal recessive inheritance.
[a]In all of these disorders, aldosterone levels are markedly elevated as a result of activation of the renin-angiotensin system owing to salt wasting, but in the pseudohypoaldosteronism type I syndromes, increased mineralocorticoid action is blocked owing to loss-of-function mutations of mineralocorticoid receptor and sodium epithelial channel.

ocorticoid receptors (MRs). Yet, aldosterone is the primary regulator of renal mineralocorticoid activity *in vivo*, because cortisol is normally excluded from occupying renal MRs by the enzyme 11β-hydroxysteroid dehydrogenase (11β-HSD) (see Chapter A11). There are 2 isoforms of the 11β-HSD enzyme. The first, 11β-HSD1, is nicotinamide adenine dinucleotide phosphate–preferring and active primarily as a reductase of cortisone to cortisol in the liver. The other, 11β-HSD2, is nicotinamide adenine dinucleotide–requiring and active as a dehydrogenase in the kidney (**Figure A77.2**). Normally, cortisol is metabolized to biologically inactive cortisone by 11β-HSD2 in the kidney, a feature that "protects" the MR from activation by cortisol. In states of 11β-HSD deficiency, the enzyme deficiency allows cortisol to reach and activate the type I renal MR, causing sodium retention and suppression of the renin-angiotensin-aldosterone system (see Chapter A11). The syndrome of apparent mineralocorticoid excess (AME) occurs as an autosomal recessive disorder and is the result of mutations in the gene coding for the kidney-specific isoform 11β-HSD2. Patients with congenital or acquired (licorice-ingestion) AME syndrome characteristically exhibit an increased ratio of cortisol to cortisone metabolites in the urine. The plasma half-life of cortisol is also prolonged in patients with AME.

Liddle's syndrome. Liddle's syndrome, a rare autosomal dominant disorder with variable penetrance, is characterized by hypertension, excessive sodium retention, hypokalemia (usually), and low plasma renin activity. Aldosterone levels are undetectable, and antagonism of the MR with spironolactone has no effect on blood pressure or serum potassium. The syndrome is ameliorated by amiloride, which blocks sodium reabsorption and potassium excretion by MR-independent mechanisms. The defect in Liddle's syndrome results from constitutive activation of amiloride-sensitive epithelial sodium channels (ENaC) on distal renal tubules, which causes excess sodium reabsorption. This channel is composed of at least 3 subunits and is normally regulated by aldosterone. The mutations causing Liddle's syndrome have been localized to genes on chromosome 16 that encode the β- and γ-subunits of ENaC. These gain-in-function mutations prolong the half-life of

ENaC at the renal distal tubule apical cell surface, resulting in increased channel number.

Hypertension exacerbated in pregnancy. An autosomal dominant mutation in the ligand binding portion of the MR results in activation of MR by progesterone and early onset hypertension that is markedly exacerbated during pregnancy. Hypertension is further accelerated during pregnancy by the elevated progesterone levels of the gravid state.

Pseudohypoaldosteronism type II. The phenotype of pseudohypoaldosteronism type II patients includes hypertension, suppressed plasma renin activity, normal renal function, and impaired potassium and H+ excretion. Mutations in genes encoding the WNK family of serine-threonine kinases in the distal nephron cause pseudohypoaldosteronism type II.

Normotensive Syndromes

A diverse group of loss-of-function mutations in ENaC, MR, and in renal tubule ion transporters results in sodium wasting and a tendency to hypotension unless compensated by a high sodium intake. Potassium levels are low or elevated depending on whether the mineralocorticoid activity of the elevated aldosterone levels is expressed (**Table A77.2**).

SUGGESTED READING

1. Curnow KM, Slutsker L, Vitek J, et al. Mutations in the CYP11β 1 gene causing congenital adrenal hyperplasia and hypertension cluster in exons 6, 7, and 8. *Proc Natl Acad Sci U S A.* 1993;90:4552–4556.
2. Funder JW, Pearce PT, Smith R, Smith AI. Mineralocorticoid action: target tissue specificity is enzyme, not receptor, mediated. *Science.* 1988;242:583–585.
3. Geller DS, Farhi A, Pinkerton N, et al. Activating mineralocorticoid receptor mutation in hypertension exacerbated by pregnancy. *Science.* 2000;289:119–123.
4. Lifton RP. Molecular genetics of human blood pressure variation. *Science.* 1996;272:676–680.
5. Lifton RP, Dluhy RG, Powers M, et al. A chimaeric 11β-hydroxylase/aldosterone synthase gene causes glucocorticoid-remediable aldosteronism and human hypertension. *Nature.* 1992a;355:262–265.

6. Lifton RP, Dluhy RG, Powers M, et al. Hereditary hypertension caused by chimaeric gene duplications and ectopic expression of aldosterone synthase. *Nat Genet.* 1992b;2:66–74.

7. Mune F, Rogerson FM, Nikkila H, et al. Human hypertension is caused by mutations in the kidney isozyme of 11β-hydroxysteroid dehydrogenase. *Nat Genet.* 1995;10:394–399.

8. Shimkets RA, Warnock DG, Bositis CM, et al. Liddle's syndrome: heritable human hypertension caused by mutations in the β subunit of the epithelial sodium channel. *Cell.* 1994;79:407–414.

9. Wilson FH, Disse-Nicodeme S, Choate KA, et al. Human hypertension caused by mutations in WNK kinases. *Science.* 2001;293:1107–1112.

10. Yanase T, Simpson ER, Waterman MR. 17α-Hydroxylase/17,20 lyase deficiency: from clinical investigation to molecular definition. *Endocrinol Rev.* 1991;12:91–108.

Chapter A78

Heritability of Hypertension and Target Organ Damage

Donna K. Arnett, MSPH, PhD

KEY POINTS

- Hypertension and blood pressure levels aggregate in families, suggesting a strong genetic component.

- Target organ damage to the heart and kidney is heritable, independent of hypertension.

- Quantitative markers such as left ventricular mass and measures of cardiac and renal function are useful intermediate phenotypes for determining the genetic basis of the complex blood pressure/hypertension phenotype.

- Chromosomes 2, 3, 4, 17, and 18 are consistently reported to influence the interindividual variation in blood pressure–related phenotypes.

See also Chapters A61, A71, A73–A77, B81, C114, C155, and C159

Blood pressure (BP) and hypertensive target organ damage have a significant genetic component, yet the identity of hypertension genes and the characteristics of the contributing DNA variation within hypertension genes are largely unknown. Multiple genetic pathways and environmental factors influence BP and its sequelae. This complexity provides a significant challenge to efforts to localize genes with major effects on BP regulation. Still, several genomic regions have been identified that are linked with BP and its consequences.

Heritability of Hypertension

A family history of hypertension is a commonly used index of familial aggregation of hypertension (see Chapter A75). First-degree relatives of hypertensives are at a 2-fold greater risk of hypertension compared to the general population. This risk increases to 4-fold when 2 or more family members have a history of hypertension.

Race. Race influences the risk for hypertension strongly; in blacks, a parental history of hypertension is a potent determinant of hypertension risk: A parental history of hypertension confers a 9-fold increased risk of hypertension.

Age. The strength of the association between family history and incidence of hypertension is dependent on the age of onset of hypertension in the family member and the age of the individual at risk. An early parental history of hypertension (before age 60 years) invokes a greater risk of hypertension in the offspring. Having 2 parents with hypertension before age 60 years increases the odds of hypertension to 5.3 in women and 7.8 in men. The younger the individual at risk, the greater the risk imposed by a positive family history of hypertension. At older ages (i.e., greater than 70 years), the hypertension odds associated with a positive family history is equal to the odds of hypertension in the general population.

Blood pressure correlation studies and heritability. The correlation coefficients for systolic BP level range from 0.15 to 0.60 across family studies. Diastolic BP follows a similar pattern, with correlation coefficients ranging from 0.3 to 0.6. The correlation coefficient for sibling pairs (generally between 0.4 and 0.6) is higher than for parent-offspring pair (generally approximately 0.2). In fact, the parent-offspring correlation is quite similar to that observed in spousal pairs (0.05 to 0.2 for systolic BP and 0.3 for diastolic BP), suggesting that shared family environment is also a strong determinant of BP. Among monozygotic twins, the correlation for systolic and diastolic BP approaches 0.7. The overall heritability of BP estimated from family studies is approximately 20% compared to the 60% heritability estimates observed in twin studies.

Genes versus environment: adopted versus natural children. Inferences regarding the role of genetics in the family aggregation of BP are problematic because the shared genetic information within a family is confounded with the shared family environment (see Chapters A75 and A76). Studies incorporating measures of BP in spouses sharing similar environments often report small but significant spousal correlation of BP level.

Table A78.1. Heritability Estimates of Left Ventricular (LV) Structural and Functional Traits Evaluated in Hypertensive Sib-Pairs

	BLACKS	WHITES
LV structural measures		
LV mass	0.70	0.26
Relative wall thickness	0.18	0.45
Posterior wall thickness	0.21	0.39
LV internal dimension	0.52	0.31
Aortic root diameter	0.62	0.32
LV systolic functional measures		
Stress-corrected mid-wall shortening	0.30	0.26
Fractional shortening	0.24	0.30
LV diastolic filling indices		
Mitral E wave	0.56	0.64
Mitral A wave	0.60	0.66
Isovolumic relaxation time	0.28	0.30

A powerful method to assess the unique contribution of the genetic control of BP is to measure families with both natural and adoptive children. Studies of adopted children have demonstrated much stronger sibling correlations in natural compared to adoptive siblings. Likewise, the parent–natural child BP correlations were stronger than those observed in parents and adoptive children, suggesting the observed familial correlation of BP is at least partially determined by shared genes.

Heritability of target organ damage. Hypertension is associated with damage to the heart, the kidney, and the brain. Because the major causes of morbidity and mortality among hypertensives are due to the cardiovascular, cerebrovascular, and renal manifestations of hypertension, and not the level of BP *per se*, understanding the genetic susceptibility of the target organs to the effects of hypertension is a matter of intense interest.

Left ventricular hypertrophy and related cardiac phenotypes. Left ventricular (LV) hypertrophy profoundly affects morbidity and mortality from cardiovascular diseases. LV hypertrophy prevalence ranges from 22% to 60% in hypertensive individuals. Data from twin studies and cohort studies report the heritability of LV mass to be 22% to 70%, independent of the effects of body size, BP, gender, and age. The heritability of LV functional and structural phenotypes is also high (Table A78.1). There is considerable interindividual variation in the response of the heart to hypertension. At equal BP levels, some individuals develop LV hypertrophy, whereas others do not, suggesting a genetic susceptibility to its expression. The genetic architecture of LV hypertrophy is likely structured by 3 separate pathways: genes that exert pleiotropic effects on hypertension and LV mass, genes that cause hypertension that in turn cause LV hypertrophy, and unique LV hypertrophy genes. Genetic mutations in sarcomeric proteins lead to severe, monogenic forms of hypertrophy. However, there is little information about the genetic contribution to the common, less severe form of LV hypertrophy that occurs in the majority of the individuals with hypertrophy.

Renal complications and end-stage renal disease. Renal disease is a complex phenotype that may result from hypertension or lead to its development. Numerous studies implicate hypertension in the etiology of renal disease. Hypertension is the second leading cause of end-stage renal disease (ESRD) in the United States. Chronic renal failure may be as high as 20% to 30% among individuals with untreated primary hypertension. Sustained elevations in BP cause nephrosclerosis and glomerulosclerosis (see Chapter A71) via hypertrophy hyalinization, and sclerosis of the walls of the preglomerular (afferent) arterioles. The blood supply to the nephron results in a decreased glomerular filtration rate and eventually focal ischemia and ESRD. Hemodynamic alterations in the kidney before the onset of

Table A78.2. Chromosomal Regions Showing Suggestive or Significant Evidence of Linkage for Blood Pressure (BP)– Related Phenotypes in 2 or More Populations

CHROMOSOME	SAMPLING DESIGN	PHENOTYPE	CENTIMORGAN	MARKER	LOGARITHM OF ODDS/ PROBABILITY VALUE
2	Extreme discordant	Systolic BP	57	D2S1788	$p < .009$
	Pedigree	Diastolic BP	97	D2S1790	3.9
	Nuclear families	Systolic BP	97	D2S1790	2.2
	Nuclear families	Systolic BP	103	D2S2972	2.3
	Affected sib-pair	Hypertension	141	D2S112	1.8
	Affected sib-pair	Hypertension	154	D2S2324	1.7
	Affected sib-pair	Hypertension	161	D2S142	1.3
	Pedigrees	Diastolic BP	217	D2S364	3.4
	Affected sib-pair	Hypertension	222	D2S2848	3.0
3	Low BP concordant	Systolic BP	4	D3S8287	$p < .002$
	Sib-pairs	Creatinine clearance	66	D3S2432	4.66
11	Sib-pairs	Left ventricular systolic function	53	D11S1993	4.0
	Discordant sib-pairs	Systolic BP	58	D11S2019	2.1
	Affected sib-pairs	Systolic BP	126	D11S934	$p < .004$
15	Discordant sib-pairs	Systolic BP	105	D15S657	2.7
	Discordant sib-pairs	Diastolic BP	113	D15S203	3.8
17	Concordant sib-pairs	Systolic BP	24	D17S1303	2.2
	Nuclear families	Systolic BP	67	D17S1299	4.7
	Nuclear families	Diastolic BP	74	D17	2.1
18	High BP sib-pairs	Postural change in BP	80	D18S585	2.6
	Pedigrees	Diastolic BP	155	D18S844	2.1

hypertension also affect pressure-natriuresis relationships (see Chapter A49), thereby raising BP. A growing body of evidence in humans and animal models supports the influence of genetic factors in the complex mechanisms affecting renal damage and suggests that the genetic basis for hypertensive nephropathy results from the interaction of BP genes and genes unique to renal damage. Familial aggregation of ESRD is observed in blacks and whites. Several studies have reported variation in candidate genes such as plasma kallikrein and transforming growth factor β. Other studies have identified linkage to a region on chromosome 10 that contains growth factor receptor genes interleukin-2 receptor α and interleukin-15 receptor α.

Chromosomal Linkages to Hypertension

To date, only genetic mutations for rare forms of hypertension have been identified. Altered salt homeostasis is the final common pathway for all the monogenic forms of abnormal BP discovered (see Chapter A77). Limited progress has been achieved in identification of susceptibility to polymorphisms in specific chromosomal regions or candidate genes for the common forms of hypertension, leading researchers to speculate that multiple interactions among genes and environments contribute to the prevalence of hypertension in the population (see Chapter A76). Given the number of intermediate phenotypes that contribute to the hypertensive phenotype, variation in a multitude of genes can potentially influence the expression of hypertension (**Table A78.2**).

Nevertheless, certain genomic regions appear to contribute to a host of BP-related traits. Although in individual studies the linkage signals may be only suggestive, when integrated across multiple studies, populations, and ethnic groups, the evidence points to a number of potentially important genomic areas contributing to BP phenotypes. At least 9 suggestive or significant loci on chromosome 2 have been linked to hypertension or related phenotypes in several populations using study designs with different sampling strategies. Chromosomes 3, 11, 17, and 18 have demonstrated suggestive or significant linkage to 1 or more BP phenotypes across various study populations and sampling designs.

SUGGESTED READING

1. Arnett DK, Devereux RB, Kitzman D, et al. Linkage of left ventricular contractility to chromosome 11 in humans: The HyperGEN Study. *Hypertension.* 2001;38:767–772.
2. Arnett DK, Hong Y, Bella JN, et al. Sibling correlation of left ventricular mass and geometry in hypertensive African-Americans and whites: the HyperGEN study. Hypertension Genetic Epidemiology Network. *Am J Hypertens.* 2001;14:1226–1230.
3. DeWan AT, Arnett DK, Atwood LD, et al. A genome scan for renal function among hypertensives: the HyperGEN study. *Am J Hum Genet.* 2001;68:136–144.
4. Doris P. Hypertension genetics, single nucleotide polymorphisms, and the common disease: common variant hypothesis. *Hypertension.* 2002;39:323–331.
5. Freedman BI, Bowden DW. The role of genetic factors in the development of end-stage renal disease. *Curr Opin Nephrol Hypertens.* 1995;4:230–234.
6. Harrap SB, Wong ZY, Stebbing M, et al. Blood pressure QTLs identified by genome-wide linkage analysis and dependence on associated phenotypes. *Physiol Genomics.* 2002;8:99–105.
7. Krushkal J, Ferrell R, Mockrin SC, et al. Genome-wide linkage analyses of systolic blood pressure using highly discordant siblings. *Circulation.* 1999;99:1407–1410.
8. Levy D, DeStefano AL, Larson MG, et al. Evidence for a gene influencing blood pressure on chromosome 17. Genome scan linkage results for longitudinal blood pressure phenotypes in subjects from the Framingham Heart Study. *Hypertension.* 2000;36:477–483.
9. Lifton RP, Gharavi AG, Geller DS. Molecular mechanisms of human hypertension. *Cell.* 2001;104:545–556.
10. Thomas J, Semenya K, Neser WB, et al. Parental hypertension as a predictor of hypertension in black physicians: the Meharry Cohort Study. *J Natl Med Assoc.* 1990;82:409–412.

Part B. POPULATION SCIENCE

Section 1. *Cardiovascular Risk in Populations and Individuals*

Chapter B79

Geographic Patterns of Hypertension: A Global Perspective

Richard S. Cooper, MD

KEY POINTS

- Geographic patterns of hypertension primarily reflect the level of economic and social development, as mediated by local cultural practice, rather than climate or natural phenomena.

- Mass migrations over the past century demonstrate that the role of intrinsic (genetic) susceptibility is clearly secondary to social conditions.

- Interpreting cross-cultural variation in blood pressure is inherently difficult, given the problems of standardizing survey methods and the overlay of ethnicity and social factors.

- The determinants of geographic variation in hypertension that have been quantified are obesity, sodium and fat intake, and black ancestry.

See also Chapters B80, B88–B95, and B100

Hypertension accounts for 6% of adult deaths worldwide and is common to all human populations except those few thousand individuals surviving in cultural isolation. Unlike coronary heart disease, for which studies of "geographic pathology" were so instructive about the underlying cause, regional variation in blood pressure (BP) remains poorly understood. Global influences, such as a temperature gradient leading away from the equator, have been suggested, but BP patterns are determined primarily by social and cultural factors at the local level.

Population Variation in Blood Pressure

Substantial problems confront attempts to sort out causal processes that determine BP variation among population groups. These include lack of standardization of BP measurements, potential bias introduced by variable treatment rates, and potential confounding effects of age. Despite these obvious problems, it is surprising that no databases exist that summarize in a standardized manner the prevalence of hypertension in the international community.

Genes versus Environment

The interaction of race, ethnicity, and environmental factors has further limited our ability to extract meaningful etiologic insights. At the very least, mass migrations over the past century have demonstrated that the role of intrinsic (genetic) susceptibility is clearly secondary to social conditions. Several of the putative factors that lead to hypertension are also extremely difficult to measure, particularly physical activity and psychosocial stress.

Patterns of Variation

Primitive societies. Populations can be separated into groups at 4 levels of risk (**Table B79.1**). Only a handful of "no hypertension" societies still exist, primarily confined to the Amazon basin. In these groups, BP does not rise with age and perhaps declines from age 18 years onward, following the pattern assumed to be "normal" for our species. In other regions of the tropics where subsistence agriculture remains the way of life, mean systolic pressure rises <10 mm Hg over the life course, and hypertension does occur. Moderate rates of hypertension also characterize most parts of Asia and the Indian subcontinent, with the notable exception of Japan.

Industrialized societies. Industrialized countries of Europe, North America, and the Pacific have hypertension rates that are similar overall, but subpopulations within these regions experience much greater risk. The extraordinary health burden imposed by hypertension in blacks is well recognized. Surprisingly, however,

Table B79.1. Categories of Hypertension Prevalence in Populations

CATEGORY	EXEMPLARY GROUPS	PREVALENCE, %[a]
Absent	Yanomami, Xingu	0
Low	Rural Africa and South China	7–15
Usual	Europe, U.S. whites, Japan	15–30
High	U.S. blacks, Russia, Finland	30–40

[a]Assumes a population structure with even distribution among 10-year age groups from 25 to 74 years.

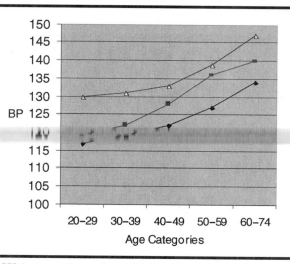

Figure B79.1. Comparison of systolic blood pressure—results from the Health Survey for England, 1998 and from the third National Health and Nutrition Examination Survey from 1991 in the United States. BP, blood pressure; ◆, U.S. white men; ■, U.S. black men; △, English men.

little attention has been given to similar observations in Slavic countries and Finland, however. Local surveys, as well as a major U.S.-U.S.S.R. cooperative study that used a standardized methodology demonstrate virtually identical levels of BP and hypertension prevalence among Finns, Russians, Poles, and U.S. blacks. Recent analyses suggest that most European countries have BPs that are higher than those reported in North America (**Figure B79.1**). Hypertension at these levels has also been reported from northern rural areas in Japan. In these societies, the high prevalence of hypertension has been attributed to a high intake of sodium or of alcohol. Cardiovascular sequelae occur at similarly high rates among all these groups.

Latitude. At the global level, a north-south hypertension gradient is apparent, although this most likely reflects parallel economic and industrial development. Increasing hypertension with distance from the equator has also been documented in China. The cause is unlikely to be climate or temperature, given the reverse pattern in the United States.

United States. Geographic variation within the United States is limited. The exception has always been the rural South, particularly the Southeast, where during the 1950s and 1960s, blacks were found to have among the highest BPs in the world. The regional variation in BP has left an indelible imprint on rates of cardiovascular disease. Specifically, migrants from the South carry with them a substantial excess risk. Although available survey data lack direct comparability, it appears that BPs have declined in the United States over the past 3 decades and that this secular trend may have been most prominent in the rural South. No obvious amelioration of risk factors can explain this phenomenon, and for obesity, the trends are in the opposite direction.

Role of Covariation in Risk Factors

Geographic patterns in hypertension are influenced by the overall variation in risk factors across the spectrum of economic development and specific local conditions. The high-fat diet of Finland and Russia, for example, has been suggested to be the cause of the exceptionally high prevalence of hypertension in that region. Blacks share the excess risk associated with lower socioeconomic status in industrialized societies and are exposed to additional psychosocial stressors. Given these complex patterns, it is virtually impossible to isolate variation in genetic predisposition across groups.

Intrinsic (genetic) factors have often been postulated as the cause of higher BPs among blacks. From the global perspective, however, populations of African origin are predominantly at low risk, given the level of economic development in most of

Africa and the Caribbean. The recent International Collaborative Study on Hypertension in Blacks (ICSHIB) documents the wide variation in hypertension prevalence across the course of the African diaspora. Body mass index, a measure of obesity and a proxy for the industrialized lifestyle, is virtually co-linear with hypertension prevalence in community samples from rural West Africa, the Caribbean, and the United States (**Figure B79.2**). A similar gradient in sodium and potassium intake exists across these populations, and, as shown by the International Study of Salt and Blood Pressure (INTERSALT), also explains some of the population variance. Factors that remain unaccounted for are psychosocial stressors and the direct effect of physical activity. Local variation among ethnic groups within a society may reflect various combinations of these risk factors.

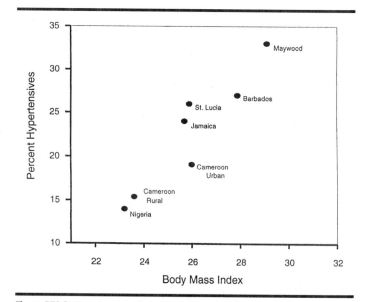

Figure B79.2. Prevalence of hypertension by body mass index in 7 populations of the African diaspora.

SUGGESTED READING

1. Cooper R, Rotimi C, Ataman S, et al. The prevalence of hypertension in seven populations of West African origin. *Am J Public Health.* 1997;87:160–168.
2. Kaufman JS, Owaje EE, James SA, et al. The determinants of hypertension in West Africa: contribution of anthropometric and dietary factors to urban-rural and socio-economic gradients. *Am J Epidemiol.* 1996;143:1203–1218.
3. McDonough R, Garrison GE, Hames CG. Blood pressure and hypertensive disease among negroes and whites in Evans County, Georgia. In: Stamler J, Stamler R, Pullman TN, eds. *The Epidemiology of Hypertension.* New York, NY: Grune & Stratton; 1967:167–187.
4. People's Republic of China–United States Cardiovascular and Cardiopulmonary Epidemiology Research Group. An epidemiological study of cardiovascular and cardiopulmonary disease risk factors in four populations in the People's Republic of China. *Circulation.* 1992;85:1083–1096.
5. Primatesta P, Brooks M, Poulter NR. Improved hypertension management and control: results from the health survey for England 1998. *Hypertension.* 2001;38:827–832.
6. Tyroler HA, Gasunov IS, Deev AD. *A Comparison of High Blood Pressure Prevalence and Treatment Status in Selected US and USSR Populations. First Joint US-USSR Symposium on Hypertension.* Bethesda, MD: National Institutes of Health Dept. of Health, Education, and Welfare; 1972. Publication 79–1272.

Chapter B80

Geographic Patterns of Hypertension in the United States

Edgar R. Miller III, MD, PhD

KEY POINTS

- The "stroke belt" includes states with a stroke mortality more than 10% above the national mean.

- Ten of the 11 states in the stroke belt are in the southeastern United States where the prevalence of hypertension is generally higher than the remainder of the nation.

- In the stroke belt, the excess risk of stroke mortality occurs in whites as well as blacks and in women as well as men.

See also Chapters A44, A45, A68, A71, B79, B81, B82, B84, B88, B89, B93–B95, and B98

Hypertension in the Southeastern United States

The prevalence of hypertension is higher in the southeastern United States compared to other regions. **Table B80.1** compares the prevalence of hypertension in the South with corresponding prevalence estimates in the rest of the nation, categorized by gender and race. The prevalence is higher for black men and women, but also higher for white men and, to a lesser degree, white women residing in the South. Among hypertensives, the level of blood pressure (BP) is higher in the South.

Several factors (genetic, sociodemographic, and environmental) may be responsible for this geographic pattern. For example, blacks born in the Southeast have a higher age-adjusted stroke mortality than blacks living in but born outside the Southeast, suggesting that indigenous rather than acquired factors are involved. Southern-born blacks residing in New York City have substantially higher cardiovascular disease mortality than do Northeast-born blacks residing in New York City. The beneficial impact of being born outside of the Southeast appears to be greater for blacks than for whites and is larger in men than in women; age, education, and socioeconomic status do not appear to be responsible. It is noteworthy that the higher stroke mortality rates in the southeastern United States documented over the last 6 decades are evident across demographic groups and cannot be attributed to race alone.

Table B80.2 compares the hypertension awareness, treatment, and control rates in the South with those in other regions of the United States by gender and ethnicity. Hypertension awareness rates exceed 50% and are similar in the South and the remainder of the country. Hypertension treatment rates are similar in women but lower in men residing in the South. Overall hypertension control rates are poor in the South, especially in men.

Consequences of Hypertension in the Southeastern United States

Stroke. Stroke mortality is also relatively high in the southeastern United States. Based on 1980 data, 11 states had stroke death rates more than 10% higher than the national average. These "stroke-belt" states form a contiguous cluster in the Southeast, with Indiana jutting upward from the cluster (**Figure B80.1**). Ten of the 11 states in the stroke belt are in the Southeast. **Table B80.3** provides a summary of the national rank and the age-adjusted stroke mortality rate for these states.

End-stage renal disease. The Southeast has one of the highest rates of end-stage renal disease (ESRD) in the nation, with 10 of the top 15 states in this area. Hypertension and diabetes are the 2 leading causes of ESRD. The 1995 sex- and age-

Table B80.1. Age-Adjusted Prevalence of Hypertension in the South

	SOUTH (%)	OTHER REGIONS (%)[a]
Black men	35.0	33.0
Black women	34.7	27.8
White men	26.5	24.3
White women	21.5	21.0

[a]Northeast, Central, and West

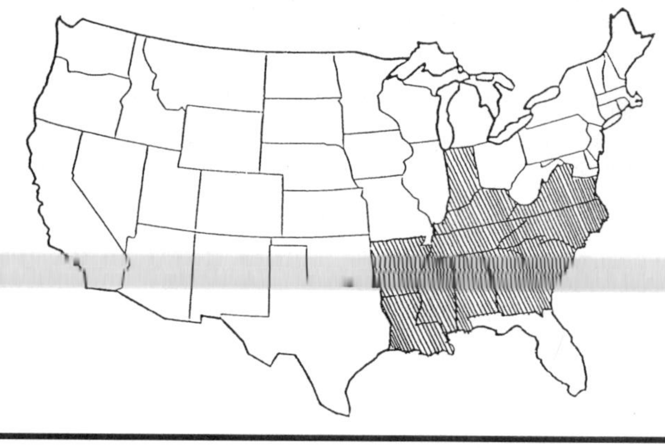

Figure B80.1. States that comprise the "stroke belt."

adjusted incidence of hypertension-related ESRD is 6-fold higher in blacks (237/million) than in whites (39/million). Fifty-four percent of U.S. blacks reside in the Southeast, a fact that undoubtedly influences the high prevalence of ESRD in the region. Racial differences in the incidence of ESRD are confounded by socioeconomic status. In Alabama, a clear relation has been reported between the number of patients with treated ESRD and the number of households with per capita incomes less than $7,500 within individual zip codes. Others have reported an independent inverse association between socioeconomic status and the incidence of treated ESRD. The high incidence in blacks is only partially explained by lower socioeconomic status.

Heart failure. Hypertension is a critical risk factor for heart failure. The prevalence and hospitalization rates for heart failure are increasing annually, and heart failure is now the most common hospital discharge diagnosis among individuals 65 years or older. The 5 states with the highest age-adjusted 1990 death rates for heart failure are all in the southern United States.

All-cause mortality. In a 15-year follow-up study of 11,936 hypertensive male veterans, all-cause mortality was 23% higher in the Southeastern stroke belt than other regions of the country. Access to medical care was equal for black and white veterans, and no racial difference in mortality was observed.

Possible Causes for the High Prevalence and Poor Control of Hypertension in the Southeastern United States

Obesity. Obesity is a strong and independent risk factor for hypertension in all racial and socioeconomic groups. Weight gain also contributes to much of the rise in BP with aging, and obesity may be one of the best predictors for the risk of developing hypertension later in life. Weight loss reduces BP in normotensive and hypertensive subjects. Even modest weight loss can lower BP or decrease the number of antihypertensive medications necessary for treating hypertensive individuals. National trends in obesity indicate that even after adjustment for age, the prevalence of obesity in U.S. adults has increased from 25% to 33% during the past decade. Six of the 15 states with the highest prevalence of obesity are in the southeastern region. The highest national prevalence of obesity (44%) occurs in black women; in the Southeast, 71% of black women are obese.

Physical inactivity. The prevalence of hypertension is increased in individuals with a low level of physical fitness. Physical inactivity is directly associated with an increase in

Table B80.2. Awareness, Treatment, and Control Rates (% of Total) for Hypertension in the South

	SOUTH	OTHER REGIONS[a]
Aware		
White men	61.8	62.9
Black men	68.6	68.8
White women	76.4	74.5
Black women	81.2	74.7
Treated		
White men	43.8	45.0
Black men	44.3	49.5
White women	60.1	59.8
Black women	65.3	65.0
Controlled[b]		
White men	18.5	19.3
Black men	19.3	22.3
White women	30.1	26.7
Black women	32.3	24.1

[a]Northeast, Central, and West.
[b]Blood pressure <140/90 mm Hg.

Table B80.3. Crude and Age-Adjusted Stroke Mortality in the Southeast by State and Rank

MORTALITY/100,000	RANK[a] (1986)	RANK (1998)	RATE[b] (1998)	AGE-ADJUSTED RATE[c] (1998)
South Carolina	1	1	75.6	37.0
Georgia	2	6	54.4	31.6
North Carolina	3	4	72.1	33.1
Alabama	4	7	67.3	30.6
Tennessee	5	5	72.9	32.6
Mississippi	6	3	66.0	33.4
Virginia	7	15	56.2	27.2
Arkansas	8	2	98.8	35.3
Kentucky	11	13	63.2	27.6
Louisiana	12	8	57.8	30.0
District of Columbia	19	10	60.2	28.4
Maryland	25	25	51.3	25.1
Florida	41	41	67.6	22.0
National median	—	—	58.6	25.1

[a]Rank among 50 states and the District of Columbia.
[b]Crude stroke mortality rates per 100,000.
[c]Age-adjusted stroke mortality rates per 100,000.

mortality from cardiovascular disease. Approximately one-fourth of U.S. adults (more so in women) report a sedentary lifestyle with no leisure-time physical activity. Physical inactivity is highly prevalent in the Southeast, affecting 25% to 43% of adults. Seven of the 10 states with the highest reported rates of no leisure-time physical activity are in the Southeast.

Salt intake. Excessive dietary salt intake has been suspected as a cause of the high prevalence of hypertension in the Southeast, especially in blacks. In the Southeast, the estimated average sodium intake ranges from approximately 140 to 180 mEq/day (i.e., 3,200 to 4,000 mg/day sodium, or 8 to 10 g/day salt). A high dietary salt intake clearly contributes to the risk of hypertension. High salt intake also antagonizes the BP-lowering effect of most antihypertensive drugs. In the Southeast, where obesity and salt sensitivity are very prevalent, high salt intake might have even greater therapeutic and public health implications than elsewhere in the United States. The International Study of Salt and Blood Pressure (INTERSALT) noted an association between high dietary salt intake and stroke mortality that was even stronger than the association between salt intake and the level of BP.

Potassium intake. In the Southeast, there is a relatively low dietary intake of potassium, ranging from approximately 34 to 55 mEq/day (i.e., 1,300 to 2,000 mg/day). Low dietary potassium intake may contribute to the risk of hypertension and stroke.

Low birth weight. Low birth weights, in particular those less than 2,500 to 3,000 g, have been associated with a number of cardiovascular risk factors, including hypertension. In the

Southeast, approximately 14% of black babies and 6% of white babies weigh less than 2,500 g. These rates of low-birth-weight infants are higher than race-matched rates of low-birth-weight infants in the United States as a whole.

SUGGESTED READING

1. Burt VL, Whelton P, Roccella EJ, et al. Prevalence of hypertension in the US adult population: results from the Third National Health and Nutrition Examination Survey, 1988–1991. *Hypertension.* 1995;25:305–313.
2. Fang J, Madhavan S, Alderman MH. The association between birthplace and mortality from cardiovascular causes among black and white residents of New York City. *N Engl J Med.* 1996;335:1545–1551.
3. Gaines K. Regional and ethnic differences in stroke in the southeastern United States population. *Ethn Dis.* 1997;7:150–164.
4. Hall WD, Ferrario CM, Moore MA, et al. Hypertension-related morbidity and mortality in the southeastern United States. *Am J Med Sci.* 1997;313:195–209.
5. Howard G, Howard VJ, Katholi C, et al. Decline in US stroke mortality: an analysis of temporal patterns by sex, race, and geographic region. *Stroke.* 2001;32:2213–2220.
6. Lackland DT, Egan BM, Jones PJ. Impact of nativity and race on "stroke belt" mortality. *Hypertension.* 1999;34:57–62.
7. Lopes AAS, Port FK. The low birth weight hypothesis as a plausible explanation for the black/white differences in hypertension, non–insulin-dependent diabetes, and end-stage renal disease. *Am J Kidney Dis.* 1995;25:350–356.
8. National Center for Health Statistics. National Vital Statistics Report, Vol 48, No. 11, July 24, 2000. Available at: http://www.cdc.gov/nchs/fastats/stroke.htm. Accessed on October 21, 2002.
9. NHLBI Data Fact Sheet. *The Stroke Belt: Stroke Mortality by Race and Sex.* Washington, DC: U.S. Dept of Health and Human Services, Public Health Service; 1989.
10. Perry MH, Roccella EJ. Conference report on stroke mortality in the Southeastern United States. *Hypertension.* 1998;31:1206–1215.

Chapter B81

Cardiovascular Risk Factors and Hypertension

William B. Kannel, MD, MPH; Peter W. F. Wilson, MD

KEY POINTS

- Hypertension generally doubles the risk of cardiovascular diseases, of which coronary disease is the most common and lethal.
- Systolic and diastolic pressure are associated with a stepwise increase in cardiovascular events, even within the high-normal range.
- Elevated systolic pressure is strongly associated with cardiovascular disease even in the presence of normal diastolic pressure; high pulse pressure further enhances risk.
- Hypertension is usually accompanied by other risk factors, and the risk of cardiovascular disease varies with the total burden of risk factors.

See also Chapters A44, A45, A60, A67, A78, B82, B83, B97, C110, and C127

Hypertension is an established risk factor for all clinical manifestations of atherosclerosis. It is a common and powerful independent predisposing factor for development of coronary heart disease (CHD), stroke, peripheral arterial disease, and heart failure. The high prevalence of hypertension, its powerful impact on the incidence of cardiovascular disease (CVD), and the potential impact on control justify high priority efforts to detect and treat elevated blood pressure (BP).

Atherosclerotic Hazards

CVD sequelae imposed by hypertension occur at a 2- to 4-fold increased rate compared with normotensive persons of the

Table B81.1. Risk of Cardiovascular Events in Subjects with Hypertension: 36-Year Follow-Up in Framingham Heart Study Participants 35 to 64 Years Old

CARDIOVASCULAR EVENTS	AGE-ADJUSTED BIENNIAL RATE PER 1,000		AGE-ADJUSTED RISK RATIO[a]		EXCESS PER 1,000	
	MEN	WOMEN	MEN	WOMEN	MEN	WOMEN
Coronary disease	45	21	2.0[b]	2.2[b]	23	12
Stroke	12	6	3.8[b]	2.6[b]	9	4
Peripheral artery disease	10	7	2.0[b]	3.7[b]	5	5
Cardiac failure	14	8	4.0[b]	3.0[b]	10	4
Cardiovascular events	65	35	2.2[b]	2.5[b]	36	21

[a]Relative to nonhypertensives.
[b]$p < .001$.

same age. Although the risk ratio it imposes is greatest for heart failure and least for coronary disease, CHD is the most common hazard of hypertension because of its greater incidence in the general population (**Table B81.1**). The lower-than-expected efficacy of antihypertensive therapy for prevention of CHD in trials led to doubt about the etiologic role of hypertension in development of CHD. However, risk of all clinical manifestations of CHD is related to the severity of antecedent hypertension in population-based investigations. BP is critical in atherogenesis because atherosclerosis seldom occurs in low-pressure segments of the circulation such as the pulmonary arteries or veins. Also, animal experiments indicate that lipid-induced atherogenesis can be accelerated or retarded by raising or lowering the BP.

Elevated BP is related to development of CVD in a continuous graded fashion, with no indication of a critical value. Risk of CVD increases with each increment in BP, even within the high-normal range (**Figure B81.1**). As compared with normal BP, high-normal (130–139/85–89 mm Hg) pressure is associated with a 2.5- and 1.6-fold hazard of CVD in women and men, respectively. Stage 1 hypertension is a substantial contributor to atherosclerotic CVD, and because it is so much more prevalent than severe grades of hypertension, a large proportion of the CVD attributable to it derives from this seemingly innocuous level of BP.

Importance of Systolic Hypertension

Comparison of the impacts of systolic and diastolic BP components gives no indication of a greater influence of the diastolic pressure for any sequela of hypertension. Isolated systolic hypertension has been shown to be hazardous, particularly in the elderly (**Figure B81.2**). With increasing age, there is a gradual shift from diastolic to systolic BP and then to pulse pressure as dominant predictors of CHD. Only before age 50 years is diastolic pressure a stronger predictor. Systolic hypertension is a persistent risk factor, even taking arterial compliance into account. Treatment of elevated systolic BP, whether isolated or accompanied by elevated diastolic BP, greatly reduces the risk of CVD. Over-reliance on diastolic pressure to assess hypertensive risk is misleading, particularly in advanced age when the predominant type of hypertension is of the isolated systolic variety. After age 60, diastolic pressure is inversely related to CHD, and wide pulse pressure also predicts CHD. The relative importance of pulse pressure versus systolic BP as a predictor of clinical cardiovascular events is uncertain.

Risk Factor Clustering

Hypertension seldom occurs in isolation from other CVD risk factors. It tends to occur in association with other atherogenic risk factors that promote its occurrence and greatly influence its CVD impact. Hypertension appears to be metabolically linked to

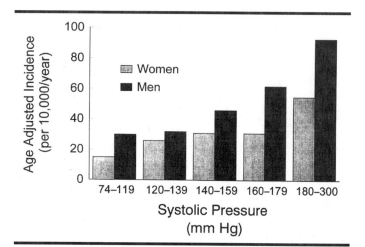

Figure B81.1. Risk of cardiovascular events by level of systolic blood pressure: 38-year follow-up for Framingham subjects 65 to 94 years old.

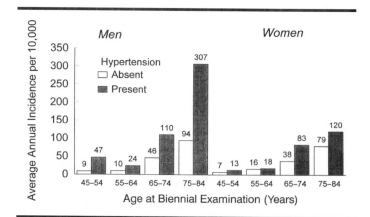

Figure B81.2. Risk of atherothrombotic brain infarction in isolated systolic hypertension: experience of Framingham men and women 45 to 84 years old over 24 years of follow-up. [Adapted from Kannel WB. Hypertension as a risk factor for cardiac events—epidemiologic results of long-term studies. *Cardiovasc Pharmacol.* 1993;21(Suppl 2):S27–S37.]

Table B81.2. Number of Other Risk Factors: Framingham Heart Study Offspring with Elevated Blood Pressure 18 to 65 Years Old

NUMBER OF RISK FACTORS	% WITH RISK FACTORS		OBSERVED/EXPECTED RATIO	
	MEN	WOMEN	MEN	WOMEN
0	24.4	19.5	0.74	0.59
1	29.1	28.1	0.71	0.69
≥2	46.5	52.4	1.8	2.01

dyslipidemia, glucose intolerance, abdominal obesity, hyperinsulinemia, and hyperuricemia, among others. Clustering of these risk factors with hypertension was investigated in the Framingham Study, and hypertension was found to occur in isolation <20% of the time. Clusters of 2 or 3 major risk factors with hypertension were found to occur approximately 50% of the time, a rate twice that expected by chance (**Table B81.2**). Approximately 63% of CHD occurring in hypertensive Framingham Study men had 2 or more additional risk factors. Hence, in evaluating patients with elevated BP, other atherogenic risk factors should be evaluated. This is important because the hypertensive risk of CVD varies widely depending on the burden of associated risk factors (**Figure B81.3**). The risk of coronary events in hypertensive Framingham Study participants increased with the degree of risk factor clustering, so that 39% of the coronary events in men with elevated BP were attributable to having 2 or more additional risk factors. The influence of risk factor clustering is particularly important in stage 1 hypertension, in which the average risk is modest, and many people must be treated to prevent 1 CVD event.

The same cluster of atherogenic risk factors that often accompanies hypertension also influences the hazard of developing a stroke, peripheral arterial disease, or heart failure. Atrial fibrilla-tion, CHD, and left ventricular hypertrophy (LVH) also play an important role in stroke risk. For heart failure risk, CHD, heart murmurs, cardiomegaly, low vital capacity, and rapid heart rate are additional factors.

A rapid resting heart rate is more common in persons with hypertension and also predisposes to its occurrence. Hypertension associated with a rapid resting heart rate has a higher CVD mortality. Rapid resting heart rate, low vital capacity, proteinuria, LVH, and silent myocardial infarction often signify organ damage in hypertension and escalate the risk of developing overt CVD by 2- to 3-fold in hypertensives.

Determinants of Clustering

Postulated causes of metabolic clustering of hypertension with dyslipidemia, glucose intolerance, hyperinsulinemia, obesity, LVH, and hyperuricemia include insulin resistance and sympathetic neurons overactivity. Abdominal obesity promotes this syndrome in hypertensive persons. In the Framingham Study, the tendency for these atherogenic traits to cluster with elevated BP increased in a stepwise fashion with the degree of obesity and the amount of weight gained on follow-up (**Table B81.3**). A 5-lb weight increase in hypertensives was associated with a 30% increment in atherogenic risk factor clustering.

Left Ventricular Hypertrophy

Hypertrophy of the left ventricle is no longer accepted as an incidental compensatory feature of hypertension and is now recognized as an ominous harbinger of CVD. Recent population-based investigation indicates that each 39 g increase in left ventricular mass/m^2 confers a 40% increase in CVD events. Risk of heart failure, myocardial infarction, and stroke increase when long-standing or severe hypertension induces LVH. It is a prominent feature of evolving heart failure, increasing the hypertension-imposed risk 2- to 3-fold. Approximately 20% of heart failure cases have antecedent electrocardiogram-LVH and 60% to 70% demonstrate LVH by echocardiogram, which is more sensitive.

Global Cardiovascular Risk

The impact of hypertension on CHD, atherothrombotic brain infarction, intermittent claudication, heart failure, and all CVD in Framingham Study participants ages 35 to 64 and 65 to 94 years is shown for men (**Figure B81.4**). Hypertension (BP ≥140/90 mm Hg) is associated with greater risk of all atherosclerotic vascular disease outcomes compared with persons with normal BP (<140/90 mm Hg). However, arterial pressure should not be considered in isolation, because age, sex, blood lipids, cigarette smoking, and diabetes also contribute to hypertensive CHD risk (Figure B81.3). In both sexes, CHD risk rises with the burden of other risk factors. Figure B81.3 shows the risks for hypothetic 55-year-old Framingham men and women with various combinations of cardiovascular risk factors. Persons with multiple risk factors typically experience the highest CHD rates. As shown in Figure B81.3, men or women with diabetes who smoke cigarettes, have LVH and a low HDL cholesterol in the presence of systolic pressure of 160 mm Hg have an estimated 10-year CHD risk that exceeds 55%. Predicted CHD rates for men are typically greater than those for women by 1.3 to 1.5 times when only a few risk factors are present, but the male to female difference is small when risk factor levels,

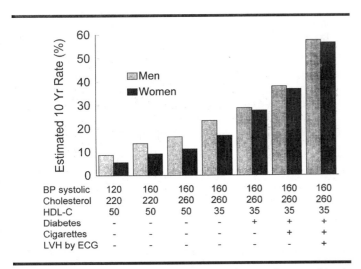

Figure B81.3. Estimated 10-year coronary heart disease risk in hypothetical 55-year-old adult according to levels of various factors. BP, blood pressure; ECG, electrocardiogram; HDL-C, HDL cholesterol; LVH, left ventricular hypertrophy.

Table B81.3. Risk Factor Clustering in the Framingham Study Offspring with Elevated Blood Pressure According to the Body Mass Index: Subjects 18 to 74 Years Old[a]

MEN		WOMEN	
BODY MASS INDEX	AVERAGE NUMBER OF RISK FACTORS	BODY MASS INDEX	AVERAGE NUMBER OF RISK FACTORS
<23.7	1.68 ± 0.91	<20.8	1.80 ± 0.87
23.7–25.5	1.85 ± 0.95	20.8–22.3	2.00 ± 1.02
25.6–27.2	2.06 ± 1.05	22.4–23.9	2.22 ± 1.06
27.3–29.5	2.28 ± 1.09	24.0–26.8	2.20 ± 0.99
≥29.5	2.35 ± 1.08	≥26.8	2.66 ± 1.09

[a]*Elevated blood pressure* was defined as systolic pressure ≥138 mm Hg (men) and ≥130 mm Hg (women). Other risk factors included the top quintiles for the factors total cholesterol, body mass index, triglycerides, and glucose and bottom quintile for high-density lipoprotein cholesterol.

including diabetes, smoking, and LVH by electrocardiogram, are all present.

Preventive Implications

Hypertension and dyslipidemia are the most common modifiable risk factors for atherosclerotic CVD. Treatment of these risk factors has been proven to reduce the risk of atherosclerotic disease. Aside from age, hypertension is the most common modifiable risk factor in high-risk dyslipidemic patients. Aggressive BP control is required. High-normal and normal BPs frequently progressed to hypertension in Framingham Study subjects. Over a period of 4 years, 37.5% of those younger than age 65 years developed hypertension and 49.5% of those older than age 65 years. Obesity and weight gain significantly contributed to progression to hypertension. A 5% weight gain increased the odds of progression 20% to 30%.

Goal blood pressure. Many hypertensive patients do not achieve Joint National Committee VI–recommended goals of <140/90 mm Hg for uncomplicated patients, and <130/85 mm Hg for hypertensive diabetics. Among diabetics, 81% are not at their Joint National Committee VI–recommended goal, and 64% of uncomplicated hypertensive patients are not at the recommended goal. Isolated systolic hypertension is the condition

least likely to be treated and least likely to be brought to the recommended goal.

Risk profiles. Optimal CVD protection from hypertension also requires more than simply lowering the BP. At the cellular level, CVD risk factors can promote vascular disease via the common pathway of endothelial dysfunction impaired by hypertension, dyslipidemia, and impaired glucose tolerance. The potential for development of CVD and the optimal choice for therapy are best evaluated by determining the multivariable risk of the hypertension, taking into account associated risk factors. This can be conveniently done for strokes and coronary disease using multivariable risk factor scoring profiles based on Framingham Study data that require only ordinary office procedures and simple laboratory tests. In this way, hypertensive persons can be efficiently targeted for cost-effective treatment using more optimal therapy likely to maximize the benefit. In particular, antihypertensive therapy should be tailored to take into account the often associated dyslipidemia, glucose intolerance, and any associated cardiovascular condition as well as the severity and type of BP elevation.

SUGGESTED READING

1. Franklin SS, Larson MG, Kahn BS, et al. Does the relation of blood pressure to coronary heart disease change with aging? The Framingham Heart Study. *Circulation.* 2001;103:1245–1249.
2. Kannel WB. Blood pressure as a cardiovascular risk factor: prevention and treatment. *JAMA.* 1996;275:1571–1576.
3. Kannel WB, Wolf PA, McGee DL, et al. Systolic blood pressure, arterial rigidity, and risk of stroke: the Framingham study. *JAMA.* 1981;245:1225–1229.
4. Reaven GM. Insulin resistance and compensatory hyperinsulinemia: role in hypertension, dyslipidemia, and coronary heart disease. *Am Heart J.* 1991;121:1283–1288.
5. The Sixth Report of the Joint National Committee on Prevention, Detection, Evaluation and Treatment of High Blood Pressure. *Arch Intern Med.* 1997;157:2413–2446.
6. Vasan RS, Larson MG, Leip EP, et al. Assessment of frequency of progression to hypertension in non-hypertensive subjects in the Framingham Heart Study. A cohort study. *Lancet.* 2001;358:1682–1686.
7. Vasan RS, Larson MG, Leip EP, et al. Impact of high-normal blood pressure on the risk of cardiovascular disease. *N Engl J Med.* 2001;345:1291–1297.
8. Verdecchia P, Carini G, Circo A, et al. Left ventricular mass and cardiovascular morbidity in essential hypertension: the MAVI Study. *J Am Coll Cardiol.* 2001;38:1829.
9. Wilson PWF, D'Agostino RB, Levy D, et al. Prediction of coronary heart disease using risk factor categories. *Circulation.* 1998;97:1837–1847.
10. Wolf PA, D'Agostino RB, Belanger AJ, Kannel WB. Probability of stroke: a risk profile from the Framingham Study. *Stroke.* 1991;22:312–318.

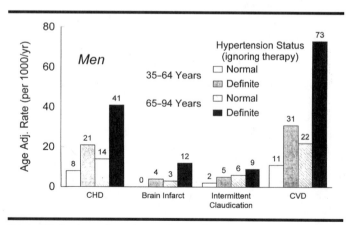

Figure B81.4. Age-adjusted annual rate of coronary heart disease (CHD) according to hypertension status in Framingham cohort men followed up for 30 years, with examinations and reclassification of blood pressure every 2 years. CVD, cardiovascular disease.

Cerebrovascular Risk

Philip A. Wolf, MD

KEY POINTS

- Hypertension is the most common and important risk factor for brain infarction and hemorrhage.

- Incidence of initial and recurrent stroke rises in proportion to increases in blood pressure. In the elderly, stroke risk is more strongly related to the level of systolic than diastolic blood pressure.

- Treatment of hypertension decreases stroke incidence. This is especially important in diabetics, in whom strict control of elevated blood pressure is the most effective stroke prevention measure available.

- It is estimated that control of hypertension may prevent nearly 50% of the approximately 500,000 annual initial stroke events in the United States.

See also Chapters A68, B80, B81, C125, C127, and C160

Death and disability from cardiovascular disease increase steadily with age. After the age of 65 years, cardiovascular disease accounts for nearly 50% of all deaths. Fully 20% of all cardiovascular disease deaths in the elderly are attributable to stroke. Although cerebrovascular disease is the third leading cause of death in the United States, stroke is 4 times more likely to produce disability than death. Also, stroke is the leading cause of neurologic disability in the elderly. The American Heart Association estimated that in 1998, 500,000 Americans sustained an initial stroke, 100,000 had a stroke recurrence, and 158,448 of these 2 groups combined died as a result of a stroke, corresponding to 1 death every 3.3 minutes. However, death data do not portray the toll in human suffering experienced by stroke survivors and their families, whose lives are irrevocably altered by this neurologic catastrophe. There are nearly 4 million stroke survivors in the United States, many of whom require chronic care.

Stroke is not limited to the elderly; nearly 20% of strokes occur in persons <60 years old, of whom more than one-third never work again. To many functionally independent persons, stroke represents a condition considered to be worse than death itself. To these stroke survivors, the loss of function and independence signals the end of worthwhile life.

Secular Trends in Stroke Incidence and Mortality

Since 1972, stroke death rates in the United States have fallen by approximately 60% and rates of death from coronary heart disease (CHD) by 46%, whereas noncardiovascular death rates have remained unchanged. Similar improvement in stroke and CHD mortality has occurred in other industrialized nations. The acceleration of a 1% annual decline in stroke death rates from 1915 to 1965 to 5% per year since then strongly highlights the role of modifiable environmental factors in stroke mortality. Stroke death rates have declined as part of the decrease in total death rates and in deaths from cardiovascular disease.

In some populations, the incidence of stroke has declined, with hemorrhage incidence declining more strikingly than that of cerebral infarctions. In other studies, no decline in incidence has occurred, although most studies have found a decrease in stroke severity. However, the age-adjusted death rate for stroke reached a nadir in 1992 to 1993 and is now rising for the first time since 1915 (**Figure B82.1**). With a growing number of elderly people, it is likely that the number of persons who will die of, or be disabled by, stroke will increase during the next century.

Etiology of Stroke

Unlike CHD, in which atherosclerosis of the arteries supplying the myocardium is the underlying disease process, stroke is a heterogeneous condition (see Chapter A68). Approximately 85% of strokes are owing to cerebral infarction, a consequence of interruption of the blood supply to the brain. The remainder are due to hemorrhage, half from intracerebral hemorrhage and half from subarachnoid hemorrhage. Hemorrhage is easy to distinguish from infarction by computed tomography scan of the brain, whereas it is often more difficult to determine the mechanism of infarction. With the exception of embolism from a cardiac source, most brain infarctions result from thrombotic occlusion of large and small arteries in the intracranial and extracranial circulation. Hypertension is the most common and potent risk factor for hemorrhage and ischemic stroke, and reduction of elevated blood pressure (BP) clearly prevents stroke regardless of infarct subtype.

Incidence of Stroke

In the general population sample at Framingham, Massachusetts, after 40 years of follow-up, stroke occurred in 718 persons, 312 in men and 406 in women. Incidence increased with age, approximately doubling in each successive decade after age 55 years (**Table B82.1**). Because the most common type, atherothrombotic brain infarction (ABI), may be considered to be analogous to myocardial infarction (MI), it is informative to compare

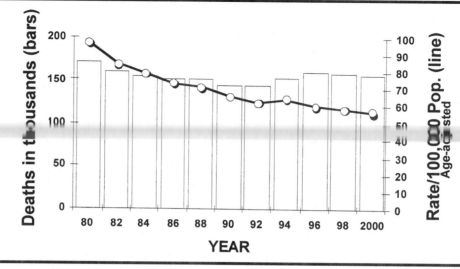

Figure B82.1. Mortality from stroke in the United States, 1980 to 2000. Pop., population. Data from Vital Statistics of United States, National Center for Health Statistics.

the incidence, by age and sex, of these 2 manifestations of cardiovascular disease (**Figure B82.2**). Although both increase with age, approximately doubling in successive decades, there are clear differences. Before the age of 65 years, MI has a striking male predominance; the male to female ratio is 4:1. The incidence of MI in women lags 20 years behind that of men; the rate of MI in women 65 to 74 years old approximates that of men 45 to 54 years old. ABI incidence is approximately 30% higher in men, and this ratio is quite constant across the adult age span, without the striking male predominance at younger ages seen for MI.

Among stroke subtypes, the most prevalent was ABI resulting from atherosclerosis and thrombosis without a cardiac source for embolism, accounting for 61% of cases (**Table B82.2**). ABI includes infarction resulting from large-vessel atherothrombosis, lacunar infarction, and infarct of undetermined cause. Stroke from cerebral embolus occurred in 24% of cases, chiefly from a left atrial clot in the presence of atrial fibrillation and from left ventricular thrombus after acute MI.

Stroke Risk Profile

At any level of BP, probability of stroke is strongly related to the presence and level of other risk factors. By using the Framingham Stroke Risk profile, a gender-specific model with points assigned

for age, systolic BP level, antihypertensive drug usage, cigarette smoking, diabetes, atrial fibrillation, and other cardiovascular disease, it is clear that the probability of stroke is strongly related to these associated risk factor abnormalities as well as level of BP.

Hypertension and the Risk of Stroke

The incidence of stroke rises progressively with increasing BP levels. Using the Joint National Committee VI classification of systolic BP, the incidence of stroke generally, and ABI in particular, was approximately 3 times greater in persons with stage 2 or 3 hypertension ($\geq$160 and $\geq$180 mm Hg systolic, respectively) and 50% higher in stage 1 hypertension (140 to 159 mm Hg systolic) than in persons with high-normal BP (130 to 139 mm Hg) and normotensives (<130 mm Hg systolic) (**Figure B82.3**). This was true in both sexes and in all age categories, including persons 75 to 84 years of age. Hypertension was a powerful and significant independent risk factor for incident ABI even after age and other pertinent risk factors had been taken into account.

Although the level of stroke risk rises progressively with level of BP, most initial strokes occurred in persons with stage 1 sys-

Table B82.1. **Annual Incidence of Completed Strokes in Men and Women Ages 35 to 94 Years**

AGE (YR)	MEN		WOMEN	
	NUMBER	RATE/1,000	NUMBER	RATE/1,000
35–44	3	0.37	3	0.30
45–54	25	1.61	20	1.04
55–64	60	3.13	60	2.41
65–74	127	8.07	115	5.07
75–84	126	14.29	199	12.65
85–94	28	15.25	112	22.25
Total	**369**	**5.34**[a]	**509**	**5.22**[a]

[a]Age adjusted, 35–94 years.
Data are from the Framingham Study: 50-year follow-up.

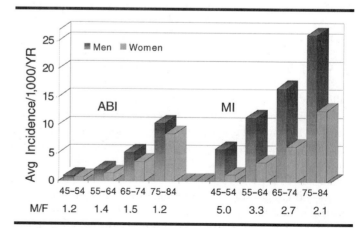

Figure B82.2. Atherothrombotic brain infarction (ABI) and myocardial infarction (MI) incidence. M/F, male/female. 50-Year follow-up, the Framingham Study.

Table B82.2. Frequency of Completed Stroke by Type in Men and Women 35 to 94 Years

COMPLETED STROKE	MEN	WOMEN	TOTAL	%
Atherothrombotic brain infarction	227	301	528	0.1
Cerebral embolus	87	131	218	24.8
Intracerebral hemor-rhage	31	42	73	8.3
Subarachnoid hemor-rhage	20	28	48	5.5
Other	4	7	11	1.3
Total	**369**	**509**	**878**	**100**

Data are from the Framingham Study: 50-year follow-up.

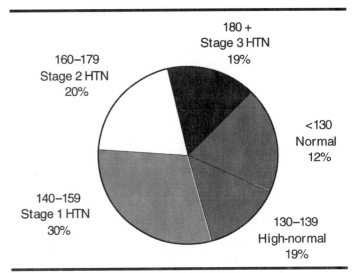

Figure B82.4. Percent of stroke by systolic blood pressure in subjects 45 to 64 years of age. The Framingham Study. HTN, hypertension.

tolic hypertension (systolic pressure, 140 to 159 mm Hg). This was true for strokes owing to hemorrhage as well as infarction (**Figure B82.4**). Approximately half the initial stroke events in Framingham occurred in subjects with high-normal (systolic pressure, 130 to 139 mm Hg) and stage 1 hypertension (**Figure B82.5**).

Traditionally, greater importance has been ascribed to the diastolic than the systolic pressure level. Although most clinical trials of hypertension treatment have classified subjects by the diastolic level, evidence for the ascendancy of diastolic BP over systolic BP is lacking; the opposite is probably true. With advancing age, systolic BP continues to rise into the 70s, whereas diastolic pressures decline after reaching a plateau in the early 50s. Systolic pressure level is clearly directly related to risk of stroke, particularly after age 65 years.

Isolated systolic hypertension. In the elderly, stage 2 and stage 3 isolated systolic hypertension, ≥160/<90 mm Hg, becomes highly prevalent, affecting approximately 25% of per-

sons older than 80 years. In Framingham, elderly subjects (65 to 84 years of age) with isolated systolic hypertension had twice the risk of stroke in men and 1.5 times increased risk in women.

Antecedent blood pressure and risk of stroke. Stroke risk predictions are generally based on measurement of current BP. Clearly, the duration of the BP level, the height of the pressure, and host factors contribute to cardiovascular risk. Using 50 years of BP data, it is evident that elevated midlife BP during the prior 10 years increases the relative risk of stroke by 1.68 (95% confidence interval, 1.25–2.25) per standard deviation increment in women and 1.92 (95% confidence interval, 1.39–2.66) per standard deviation increment in men at age 60 years. Similar increases in relative risk by elevated antecedent pressures were also seen at age 70. These data confirm clinical experience as well as prior prospective epidemiologic data that, at any level of pressure, persons with evidence of a large left ventricle by electrocardiograph or on echocardiography is at increased risk of stroke and other cardiovascular outcomes.

Treatment Trials for Stroke Prevention

Primary protection. Multiple clinical trials have shown that reduction of elevated BP in hypertensives in middle and advanced age with systolic as well as diastolic hypertension incontrovertibly reduces stroke incidence. Since the first VA trial in 1967, stroke and other hypertensive outcomes have been shown clearly to be reduced by drug treatment of patients with very elevated levels of BP (stages 2 and 3). Since then, a host of clinical trials have consistently demonstrated that stroke can be prevented in those with milder forms (stage 1 hypertension), regardless of age.

Isolated systolic hypertension is not as resistant to antihypertensive medications as had been previously thought and treatment does not precipitate stroke, syncope, or produce an excess of confusion, falls, or depression as had been feared. The Systolic Hypertension in the Elderly Program (SHEP) and the Systolic Hypertension in Europe Trial (Syst-Eur) trials demonstrate that reducing elevated systolic pressure significantly reduces stroke incidence.

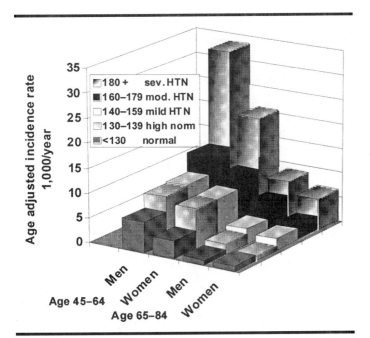

Figure B82.3. Incidence of stroke and systolic blood pressure level according to Joint National Committee VI categories. HTN, hypertension; sev., severe. 50-Year follow-up, the Framingham Study.

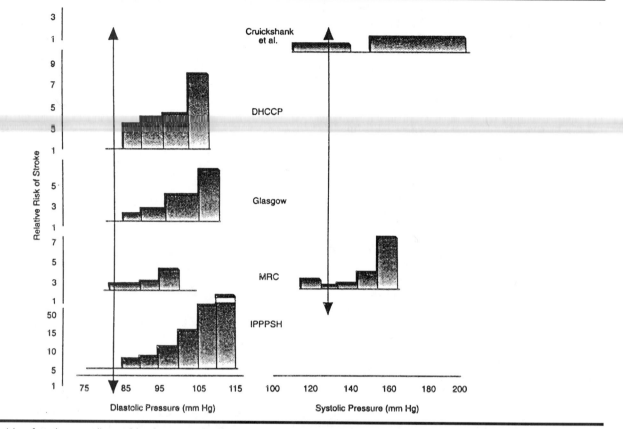

Figure B82.5. Relative risks of stroke according to blood pressure during treatment for hypertension in 8 studies and metaanalyses. Arrows indicate levels of treated systolic and diastolic blood pressure associated with lowest risks of stroke. DHCCP, Department of Health Hypertension Care Computing Project; IPPPSH, International Prospective Primary Prevention Study in Hypertension; MRC, Medical Research Council. (From Fletcher and Bulpitt, Massachusetts Medical Society; 1992, with permission.)

Secondary protection against recurrence. Data from a metaanalysis of 4 trials of BP-lowering drugs suggested that a BP reduction of approximately 6 to 8 mm Hg systolic and 3 to 4 mm Hg diastolic is associated with approximately 20% fewer recurrent strokes. In addition, BP reduction lowered stroke recurrence in the Post-Stroke Antihypertensive Study (PATS) using the diuretic indapamide. The combination of indapamide and the angiotensin-converting enzyme (ACE) inhibitor was tested in the Perindopril Protection against Recurrent Stroke Study (PROGRESS) trial; the average BP reduction of 9/4 mm Hg was associated with a 28% relative risk reduction of stroke recurrence. In the Heart Outcomes Prevention Evaluation (HOPE) trial, the ACE inhibitor ramipril reduced initial stroke incidence and stroke recurrence, but the mean BP reduction was modest; the contribution of BP reduction versus ACE-inhibition in the HOPE trial remains uncertain. The LIFE study showed that a regimen beginning with the angiotensin-receptor blocker losartan reduced strokes more effectively than one starting with atenolol, in spite of the fact that the degree of BP reduction was equivalent.

Optimal Blood Pressure

The optimal level to which elevated BP should be reduced for stroke prevention remains undefined, but it is clearly lower than has been thought previously. Fears that overzealous BP reduction would reduce cerebral blood flow in persons with cerebral atherosclerosis and precipitate stroke have not been borne out. Analyses of a large number of clinical trials suggest that systolic pressure should be reduced to <125 mm Hg and diastolic pressure to <85 mm Hg (Figure B82.5). However, this issue of target BP levels has yet to be resolved and remains under study. Because the bulk of the population has BP levels in the high-normal and stage 1 ranges, the major effort in stroke prevention must be focused here.

Preventive Implications

Of the estimated 50 million hypertensives in the United States, only 10.5 million have their BP controlled. It has been estimated that nearly 250,000 new strokes could be prevented each year by treatment of elevated BP alone.

Demonstration of the benefits of treatment in preventing stroke and of the potential to control hypertension suggests that considerable progress remains to be achieved.

SUGGESTED READING

1. Bosch J, Yusuf S, Pogue J, et al. on behalf of the HOPE Investigators. Use of ramipril in preventing stroke: double blind randomized trial. *BMJ.* 2002;324:1–5.
2. Fletcher AE, Bulpitt CJ. How far should blood pressure be lowered? *N Engl J Med.* 1992;326:251–254.
3. Kannel WB, Wolf PA, Verter J, McNamara PM. Epidemiologic assessment of the role of blood pressure in stroke. The Framingham study. *JAMA.* 1970;214:301–310.
4. Lindholm LH, Ibsen H, Dahlof B, et al. The LIFE Study Group. Cardiovascular morbidity and mortality in patients with diabetes in the Losartan

Intervention For Endpoint reduction in hypertension study (LIFE): a randomised trial against atenolol. *Lancet.* 2002;359:1004–1010.

5. Progress Collaborative Group. Randomised trial of a perindopril-based blood-pressure-lowering regimen among 6,105 individuals with previous stroke or transient ischaemic attack. *Lancet.* 2001;358:1033–1041.

6. Seshadri S, Wolf PA, Beiser A, et al. Elevated Midlife Blood Pressure Increases Stroke Risk in Elderly Persons: The Framingham Study. *Arch Int Med.* 2001;161:2343–2350.

7. SHEP Cooperative Research Group. Prevention of stroke by antihypertensive drug treatment in older persons with isolated systolic hypertension:

final results of the Systolic Hypertension in the Elderly Program (SHEP). *JAMA.* 1991;265:3255–3264.

8. Staessen JA, Fagard R, Thijs L, et al. for the Systolic Hypertension in Europe (Syst-Eur) Trial Investigators. Randomised double-blind comparison of placebo and active treatment for older patients with isolated systolic hypertension. *Lancet.* 1997;350:757–764.

9. Yusuf S, Sleight P, Pogue J, et al. Effects of an angiotensin-converting-enzyme inhibitor, ramipril, on cardiovascular events in high-risk patients. The Heart Outcomes Prevention Evaluation Study Investigators. *N Engl J Med.* 2000;342:145–153.

Chapter B83

Left Ventricular Hypertrophy Risk

Daniel Levy, MD

KEY POINTS

- Left ventricular hypertrophy, whether on the electrocardiogram or the echocardiogram, is associated with an increased risk of several cardiovascular disease outcomes.

- Aggressive hypertension treatment can promote reversal of left ventricular hypertrophy.

- Observational studies have suggested that reversal of left ventricular hypertrophy confers a reduction in risk for cardiovascular disease events.

- New clinical trials reveal that reversing left ventricular hypertrophy leads to a reduced risk of cardiovascular disease.

See also Chapters A60–A62, A78, B81, C115, C116, C155, and C156

Etiology and Diagnosis

Left ventricular hypertrophy (LVH) is the response of the heart to chronic pressure, volume overload, or both. The most common stimuli to cardiac hypertrophy are hypertension and valvular heart disease. Genetic factors determine the extent of the hypertrophic response to existing stimuli (see Chapter A78), and several mutations have been identified in kindreds with severe familial forms of LVH, which can occur even in the absence of hypertension. The diagnosis of LVH can be made in several ways, but most commonly it is identified on the electrocardiogram (ECG) on the basis of increased voltage and repolarization abnormalities, or on the echocardiogram by measuring LV wall thickness and internal chamber dimensions and calculating left ventricular mass (LVM).

Left ventricular hypertrophy on the electrocardiogram.

The first studies to document the cardiovascular disease (CVD) hazards associated with LVH were based on its appearance on the ECG. The ECG hallmarks of LVH are increased R-wave and S-wave voltage, reflecting left ventricular forces; a widened QRS complex; a leftward frontal plane axis shift; ST- and T-wave repolarization abnormalities; and P-wave abnormalities reflecting left atrial enlargement. Several reports from the Framingham Heart Study and elsewhere found that individuals with ECG LVH were at increased risk for coronary heart disease (CHD), stroke, congestive heart failure, and sudden death.

The CVD risks associated with LVH are greatest when increased QRS voltage is accompanied by repolarization abnormalities. More than 30 years ago, investigators reported that among more than 5,000 original participants in the Framingham Heart Study, the new development of LVH on the ECG (increased voltage with accompanying major repolarization abnormalities) carried a relative risk for developing CHD of 2.2 to 5.1 in men and 1.4 to 2.5 in women. A more recent investigation from Framingham examined the separate contributions of increased voltage and repolarization abnormalities to CVD risk in those with ECG LVH. That study was based on follow-up of 524 subjects who exhibited ECG LVH during nearly 40 years of observation. Among persons free of CVD at baseline, the relative risk for developing CVD, comparing subjects in the top quartile of Cornell ECG voltage (sum of R wave in augmented voltage unipolar left arm lead plus S wave in V_3) with those in the bottom quartile, was 3.08 [95% confidence interval (CI), 1.87 to 5.07] in men and 3.29 (95% CI, 1.78 to 6.09) in women. The presence of major repolarization abnormalities also identified individuals with LVH who were at increased risk for CVD.

LVH by ECG is associated with an increased risk of several CVD outcomes. **Table B83.1** summarizes the incidence rates for a variety of CVD outcomes as a function of ECG LVH status for men and women in 2 age groups. For all end points, the risks were substantially higher in those with ECG LVH than in those without it.

Table B83.1.   Two-Year Rates of Cardiovascular Disease Events per 1,000 Subjects Free of Designated Event at Baseline in Persons with and without Left Ventricular Hypertrophy (LVH) by Electrocardiogram[a]

	AGE-ADJUSTED BIENNIAL RATE/1,000 MEN				AGE-ADJUSTED BIENNIAL RATE/1,000 WOMEN			
	AGE 35–64 YR		AGE 65–94 YR		AGE 35–64 YR		AGE 65–94 YR	
	NO LVH	WITH LVH	NO LVH	WITH LVH	NO LVH	WITH LVH	NO LVH	WITH LVH
Cardiovascular disease	35	164[b]	83	234[b]	18	135[b]	57	235[b]
Coronary heart disease	27	79[b]	52	138[b]	12	55[b]	31	94[b]
Congestive heart failure	5	71[b]	21	77[b]	1	81[b]	15	160[b]
Stroke	5	29[b]	23	71[b]	3	20[b]	20	90[b]

[a]Based on 36-year follow-up of Framingham Heart Study subjects.
[b]$p < .0001$.

Left ventricular hypertrophy on the echocardiogram. The advent of echocardiography has provided a new and more sensitive tool for the detection of LVH. Whereas ECG LVH was present in only approximately 2% of subjects from the Framingham Heart Study, echocardiographic LVH was detected in approximately 15%. The echocardiographic diagnosis of LVH is based on the presence of increased LVM. LVH, whether considered as a dichotomous variable (i.e., LVH present vs. absent), and LVM examined as a continuous variable are both associated with increased risk for CHD, CVD, stroke, and sudden death.

Risks

General population. In a large sample of 3,220 subjects ≥40 years old from the Framingham Heart Study, 208 subjects developed new CVD events and 124 died during 4 years of follow-up. As shown in **Figure B83.1**, LVM predicted the incidence of CVD, and the association was continuous and graded. In multivariable models adjusting for age and traditional CVD risk factors [blood pressure (BP), antihypertensive treatment, lipids, diabetes, cigarette smoking, body mass index, and ECG LVH], in men a 50-g/m² increment in LVM

was associated with a relative risk of 1.49 (95% CI, 1.20 to 1.85) for CVD events. The corresponding relative risk in women was 1.57 (95% CI, 1.20 to 2.04). Increased levels of LVM were also associated with increased risk for CVD death and death from all causes. In a subsequent report from Framingham, an association of LVM with risk for stroke or transient ischemic attack was observed. This finding suggests that the target organ damage identified by echocardiography may be reflective of parallel damage throughout the cardiovascular system.

Hypertensives. The association of echocardiographic LVH with increased risk for CVD has also been observed in studies of hypertensive patients. In one study, 140 men with uncomplicated hypertension were followed up for a mean of 4.8 years, during which time there were 14 "hard" CVD events. The definition of LVH was an LVM index >125 g/m². The event rate was 4.6/100 patient-years among men with LVH versus 1.4/100 patient-years in those without LVH ($p < .01$). In a multivariable analysis adjusting for age, systolic BP, diastolic BP, and left ventricular fractional shortening, LVM index remained predictive of a CVD risk ($p = .026$) and was the most powerful predictor of events of all the variables examined.

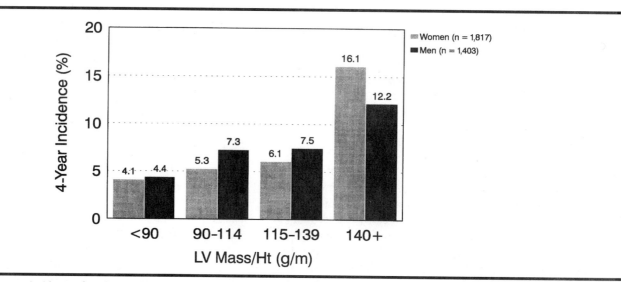

Figure B83.1.   Four-year incidence of cardiovascular disease events in Framingham Heart Study men and women who were free of cardiovascular disease at baseline as a function of echocardiographic left ventricular (LV) mass [adjusted for height (Ht)]. (From Levy D, Garrison RJ, Savage DD, et al. Prognostic implications of echocardiographically determined left ventricular mass in the Framingham Heart Study. *N Engl J Med.* 1990;322:1561–1566, with permission.)

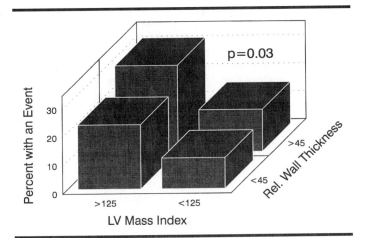

Figure B83.2. Incidence of cardiovascular disease events in hypertensive subjects according to baseline left ventricular (LV) geometry. Four mutually exclusive groups are defined on the basis of LV mass and relative (Rel.) wall thickness. (Koren MJ, Devereux RB, Casale PN, et al. Relation of left ventricular mass and geometry to morbidity and mortality in uncomplicated essential hypertension. *Ann Intern Med.* 1991;114:345–352, with permission.)

In another study, 280 patients with uncomplicated hypertension were followed up for an average of 10.2 years, during which time there were 40 incident CVD events. The authors looked at CVD outcome in relation to left ventricular geometry by separating subjects into 4 mutually exclusive groups on the basis of LVM and relative wall thickness (the ratio of 2-times posterior wall thickness to left ventricular end-diastolic dimension): normal geometry (LVM <125 g/m^2 and relative wall thickness <0.45), concentric remodeling (LVM <125 g/m^2 and relative wall thickness >0.45), eccentric LVH (LVM >125 g/m^2 and relative wall thickness <0.45), and concentric LVH (LVM >125 g/m^2 and relative wall thickness >0.45). Of the 4 geometric patterns, concentric LVH carried the greatest risk for the development of CVD (**Figure B83.2**). It remains to be determined whether concentric LVH contributes causally to the increased risk for CVD events or, as some have suggested, whether the increased risk is due to the increase in LVM that is also present in patients with this geometric pattern of hypertrophy.

Impact of Left Ventricular Hypertrophy and Coronary Artery Disease

A key question is whether the association of LVH with risk for CHD is attributable to the coexistence of subclinical coronary artery disease. In a study of 785 predominantly black subjects who underwent coronary angiography and echocardiography, there were 80 deaths during 4 years of follow-up. Echocardiographic LVH appeared to confer increased risk whether coronary artery disease was present or absent. Among patients with documented coronary artery disease, the relative risk for death from any cause among subjects with echocardiographic LVH was 2.14 (95% CI, 1.24 to 3.68) after adjustment for age, sex, and baseline hypertension. Similarly, among subjects without significant coronary artery disease, the adjusted relative risk for death was 4.14 (95% CI, 1.77 to 9.71) among subjects with echocardiographic LVH. In a subsequent study, echocardiographic LVH carried the greatest attributable risk for mortality of all risk factors studied; 37% of deaths were attributed to LVH. A possible explanation for

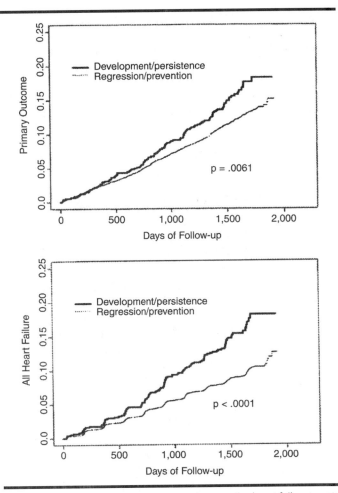

Figure B83.3. Primary outcome events and congestive heart failure events in the HOPE trial. [From Mathew J, Sleight P, Lonn E, et al. for the Heart Outcomes Prevention Evaluation (HOPE) Investigators. Reduction of cardiovascular risk by regression of electrocardiographic markers of left ventricular hypertrophy by the angiotensin-converting enzyme inhibitor ramipril. *Circulation.* 2001;104:1615–1621, with permission.]

the risk conferred by LVH in patients without epicardial (large-vessel) coronary disease is that it may be associated with malignant ventricular arrhythmias, microvascular coronary disease, and impaired coronary reserve.

Regression of Left Ventricular Hypertrophy

In hypertensive patients, aggressive BP control can prevent the development of LVH and reverse or regress it. Numerous clinical trials of antihypertensive drug therapy have documented the occurrence of regression of LVH in response to BP lowering. It remains unresolved whether, and to what extent, there are differential drug effects on reversing LVH.

In light of the association of LVH with risk for CVD, there has been great interest in studying the impact of LVH regression on CVD risk. A report from Framingham used serial ECGs to examine the implications of reversal of ECG LVH. In that study, subjects with a serial decline in ECG LVH voltage were at lower risk for CVD than were those with no serial change (men: odds ratio after adjustment for age and baseline voltage, 0.46; 95% CI, 0.26 to 0.84; women: odds ratio, 0.56; 95% CI, 0.30 to 1.04). The results of this investigation suggest that regression of LVH confers an improvement in risk for CVD. The benefits of LVH regression are also supported by studies of hypertensive patients undergoing repeat echocardiographic assessment of LVM; these reports similarly have suggested that regression of LVH is associated with a reduction in CVD risk.

Recently, the Heart Outcomes Prevention Evaluation (HOPE) trial examined whether treatment of high-risk patients with the angiotensin-converting inhibitor ramipril could prevent the development of LVH on ECG or promote its regression when compared with placebo in 8,281 eligible participants. The prevention or regression of LVH occurred more commonly in those receiving active therapy, whereas development or persistence of LVH were more frequent in those receiving placebo ($p = .008$). Prevention or regression of LVH was associated with a 25% reduction in CVD risk compared with the new development or persistence of LVH; of 7,539 patients with prevention/regression of LVH, 12% experienced a primary cardiovascular event (cardiovascular death, myocardial infarction, or stroke) compared with 16% of patients with development/persistence of LVH ($p = .006$). Risk of heart failure was especially reduced in those who experienced prevention/regression of LVH versus its development/persistence (9% vs. 15%; $p < .0001$). This placebo-controlled trial documented the feasibility of LVH regression and confirmed the benefits conferred by LVH regression (**Figure B83.3**).

SELECTED READING

1. Arnett DK. Genetic contributions to left ventricular hypertrophy. *Curr Hypertens Rep.* 2000;2:50–55.

2. Casale PN, Devereux RB, Milner M, et al. Value of echocardiographic measurement of left ventricular mass in predicting cardiovascular morbid events in hypertensive men. *Ann Intern Med.* 1986;105:173–178.
3. Gottdiener JS, Reda DJ, Massie BM, et al. for the Department of Veterans Affairs Cooperative Study Group on Antihypertensive Agents. Effect of single-drug therapy on reduction of left ventricular mass in mild to moderate hypertension: comparison of six antihypertensive agents. *Circulation.* 1997;95:2007–2014.
4. Koren MJ, Devereux RB, Casale PN, et al. Electrocardiographic left ventricular hypertrophy and risk of coronary heart disease: the Framingham Study. *Ann Intern Med.* 1970;72:813–822.
5. Koren MJ, Devereux RB, Casale PN, et al. Relation of left ventricular mass and geometry to morbidity and mortality in uncomplicated essential hypertension. *Ann Intern Med.* 1991;114:345–352.
6. Levy D, Garrison RJ, Savage DD, et al. Prognostic implications of echocardiographically determined left ventricular mass in the Framingham Heart Study. *N Engl J Med.* 1990;322:1561–1566.
7. Levy D, Salomon MS, D'Agostino RB, et al. Prognostic implications of baseline electrocardiographic features and their serial changes in subjects with left ventricular hypertrophy. *Circulation.* 1994;90:1786–1793.
8. Liao Y, Cooper RS, McGee DL, et al. The relative effects of left ventricular hypertrophy, coronary artery disease, and ventricular dysfunction on survival among black adults. *JAMA.* 1995;273:1592–1597.
9. Liebson PR, Grandits GA, Dianzumba S, et al. Comparison of five antihypertensive monotherapies and placebo for change in left ventricular mass in patients receiving nutritional-hygienic therapy in the Treatment of Mild Hypertension Study (TOMHS). *Circulation.* 1995;91:698–706.
10 Mathew J, Sleight P, Lonn E, et al. for the Heart Outcomes Prevention Evaluation (HOPE) Investigators. Reduction of cardiovascular risk by regression of electrocardiographic markers of left ventricular hypertrophy by the angiotensin-converting enzyme inhibitor ramipril. *Circulation.* 2001;104:1615–1621.

Chapter B84

Renal Risk

Michael J. Klag, MD, MPH

KEY POINTS

- Approximately 90% of persons with end-stage renal disease have a history of hypertension.

- The link between blood pressure and end-stage renal disease has been demonstrated in ecologic, case-control, and prospective cohort studies; renal risk is a continuum that begins with the lowest levels of blood pressure elevation.

- Renal risk is more closely related to systolic than diastolic blood pressure.

- Black men have a greater risk of developing end-stage renal disease at every level of blood pressure than do white men.

See also Chapters A49, A71, B81, B89, C124, and C159

In 1836, Bright first described the association of kidney disease, as evidenced by the presence of small kidneys and proteinuria and hypertension, manifested by left ventricular enlargement and stroke. Bright believed that kidney disease was the causal factor. In contrast, physicians later in the century argued that high blood pressure (BP) led to the development of kidney disease. This controversy persists to the present day, but both camps are probably correct. Renal disease elevates BP; approximately 90% of persons with end-stage renal disease (ESRD) have a history of hypertension. Elevated BP, however, also increases the rate of progression of renal insufficiency and may initiate renal damage. Thus, it is often difficult, both in clinical practice and research, to determine which comes first. Causal inferences are best made from clinical trials of BP lowering in which change in renal function is the outcome, but observational studies of the risk of renal disease associated with BP also add important information.

Impact of End-Stage Renal Disease

During the last 10 years, the substantial public health impact of renal disease has been recognized. The incidence of ESRD has increased every year since 1973, the first year from which such data are available. In 1994, almost 90,000 persons entered ESRD treatment programs in the United States. In 26% of these cases, the underlying cause of the ESRD was ascribed by the treating nephrologist to hypertension. This number underestimates the importance of the contribution of BP to the burden of ESRD, however, because the etiology of renal disease is multifactorial and higher BP contributes to the incidence of all forms of ESRD. The increasing incidence of ESRD coupled with improvements in patient survival have led to a large number of persons with prevalent ESRD each year. In 1999, for example, almost 400,000 persons received treatment for ESRD in the United States. The economic impact of ESRD is also profound. The cost to Medicare for direct care of patients with ESRD in 1999 was more than $11 billion. Although patient survival after initiation of renal replacement therapy is improving, it is still dismal. The most recent survival data indicate that only 38% of persons with ESRD are alive 5 years after beginning treatment, with the most common cause of death being cardiovascular disease. An increased risk of death from cardiovascular disease is also present in persons with milder forms or renal disease without ESRD.

Blood Pressure and End-Stage Renal Disease

The strong association between malignant hypertension and the development of renal failure was first recognized at the beginning of this century. Only relatively recently, however, has the risk of developing renal disease associated with less severe hypertension been determined.

Maryland study. A link between BP and ESRD has been demonstrated in ecologic, case-control, and prospective cohort studies. In an analysis of 26 geographic areas in Maryland, the incidence of hypertensive ESRD correlated closely with prevalence of hypertension, especially severe hypertension. During a 15-year follow-up of 11,912 male hypertensive veterans, pretreatment systolic BP associated with development of ESRD was more predictive of developing ESRD than was diastolic pressure. Greater decrease in BP with treatment, in an observational analysis, was associated with lower risk of incident ESRD.

Multiple risk factor intervention trial follow-up study. The risk of ESRD across a wide range of BP was determined in a prospective study of 332,544 men screened for the Multiple Risk Factor Intervention Trial (MRFIT). Between 1973 and 1975, 361,662 men aged 35 to 57 years in 18 U.S. cities were screened for entry into the trial, and 12,866 men entered the trial. Men with evidence of end-organ damage based on medical history or physical examination and a serum creatinine level ≥2.0 mg/dL (176 μmol/L) were excluded from the trial. Excluded from the analysis were 3 men already being treated for ESRD at time of screening and 29,115 men for whom information about systolic BP or income was not available, leaving 332,544 men for analysis.

Blood pressure follow-up. This large cohort was followed for 16 years; 814 cases of *all-cause ESRD*, defined as treatment for ESRD or death from renal failure, were identified. Use of all-cause ESRD as the primary outcome precludes misclassification

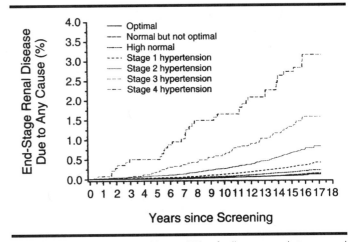

Figure B84.1. Cumulative incidence (%) of all-cause end-stage renal disease by Joint National Committee V categories of systolic and diastolic blood pressure in 332,544 men screened for the Multiple Risk Factor Intervention Trial. (From Klag MJ, Whelton PK, Randall BL, et al. Blood pressure and end-stage renal disease in men. *N Engl J Med.* 1996;334:13–18, with permission.)

of causes of ESRD. **Figure B84.1** shows cumulative incidence of all-cause ESRD during follow-up by BP assessed at baseline, grouped according to the 7 Joint National Committee V categories. The incidence of ESRD rose progressively with successively higher BP compared with men with optimal BP. In men with stage 4 hypertension (a category not used in the Joint National Committee VI), the highest BP group, the excess incidence was evident within the first 2 years of follow-up. Incidence curves for the other groups did not separate until later in follow-up. The early increase in ESRD incidence in men with the highest BP may reflect preexisting renal disease in this group. **Table B84.1** gives the number of men in each stratum of BP, the number of men who developed ESRD, age-adjusted incidence rates of ESRD, and multivariate-adjusted relative risk. Of the ESRD cases, 49% occurred at hypertension of stage 1 or higher. The consistency and strength of the association of BP categories with ESRD incidence are impressive. Men with high normal BP have a 2-fold increased risk of development ESRD compared with men with optimal BP. Stage 4 hypertension imparted a 22-times greater risk than optimal BP. In men who survived the first 10 years without ESRD, the relative risks of ESRD among those with stages 1, 2, 3, and 4 hypertension were 2.8, 5.0, 8.4, and 12.4, respectively, compared with men with optimal BP. The risk of ESRD associated with BP was strong, positive, and statistically significant overall in subgroups defined by age and other baseline covariates. However, positive associations were weaker among older men, men with diabetes, and black men.

Race. Black men had a greater risk of developing ESRD at every level of BP than did white men (**Figure B84.2**). The risk of ESRD associated with BP, however, was similar in the 2 groups. For every 16 mm Hg higher systolic BP at baseline, the multivariate-adjusted relative risk of ESRD was 1.54 in black men compared to 1.77 in white men. These relative risk estimates were statistically significantly different owing to the large numbers of men in the cohort, but the differences were not of clinical importance. Thus, the higher incidence of ESRD in black men compared with white men was not owing to a greater sen-

Table B84.1. Baseline Blood Pressure and All-Cause End-Stage Renal Disease (ESRD)

BLOOD PRESSURE CATEGORY[a]	MEN (N)	ALL-CAUSE ESRD (N)	AGE-ADJUSTED RATE/100,000 PERSON-YEARS[b]	ADJUSTED RELATIVE RISK[c] (95% CONFIDENCE INTERVAL)
Optimal	61,089	51	5.3	1.0
Normal, but not optimal	81,621	86	6.6	1.2 (0.8 to 1.7)
High normal	73,798	134	11.1	1.9[d] (1.4 to 2.7)
Hypertension				
Stage 1	85,684	275	21.0	3.1[d] (2.3 to 4.3)
Stage 2	23,739	158	45.9	6.0[d] (4.3 to 8.7)
Stage 3	5,464	73	96.1	11.2[d] (7.7 to 16.2)
Stage 4	1,429	37	187.1	22.1[d] (14.2 to 34.3)
Overall	332,544	814	15.6	—

[a]Classification of blood pressure is based on the higher of systolic or diastolic pressure according to Joint National Committee V standards: optimal, systolic <120 and diastolic <80 mm Hg; normal, not optimal, systolic 120 to 129 and diastolic <84 mm Hg or diastolic 80 to 84 and systolic <130 mm Hg; high normal, systolic 130 to 139 and diastolic <90 mm Hg or diastolic 85 to 89 and systolic <140 mm Hg; stage 1, systolic 140 to 159 and diastolic <100 mm Hg or diastolic 90 to 99 and systolic <160 mm Hg; stage 2, systolic 160 to 179 and diastolic <110 mm Hg or diastolic 100 to 109 and systolic <180 mm Hg; stage 3, systolic 180 to 209 and diastolic <120 mm Hg or diastolic 110 to 119 and systolic <210 mm Hg; stage 4, systolic ≥210 mm Hg or diastolic ≥120 mm Hg.
[b]Adjusted using the direct method for the age distribution of all men screened.
[c]Estimated using proportional hazards regression model stratified by clinic and adjusted for age, ethnicity, income, serum cholesterol, reported cigarettes per day, use of medication for diabetes, and previous myocardial infarction.
[d]$p < .001$.
From Klag MJ, Whelton PK, Randall BL, et al. Blood pressure and end-stage renal disease in men. *N Engl J Med*. 1996;334:13–18, with permission.

sitivity to the effects of BP in black men. Higher BP in the black men did explain a substantial portion of the excess ESRD risk seen in this group. Adjustment for systolic BP reduced the relative risk of all-cause ESRD in black men compared with white men from 3.20 to 2.56 (**Table B84.2**).

Systolic versus diastolic pressure. Systolic and diastolic BP imparted a similar magnitude of ESRD risk. With multivariate adjustment for the covariates listed in the footnotes to Table B84.1, for example, the relative risk of developing ESRD associated with 1 standard deviation higher BP at baseline was 1.7 [95% confidence interval (CI), 1.7 to 1.8] for systolic BP and 1.7 (95% CI, 1.6 to 1.8) for diastolic BP. However, when systolic and diastolic pressure were considered together in the same proportional hazards model with adjustment for all other vari-

ables, systolic BP (relative risk, 1.6; 95% CI, 1.5 to 1.7) had more predictive power than diastolic pressure (relative risk, 1.2; 95% CI, 1.1 to 1.2). Stratified analyses without use of statistic models also showed that the risk relationships were stronger and more consistent for systolic pressure than diastolic pressure when both were considered together. Risk associated with BP was similar for ESRD ascribed to hypertension compared with all-cause ESRD; 193 men developed hypertensive ESRD. After adjustment for the covariates listed in Table B84.1, the relative risk of this outcome associated with a 1 standard deviation higher BP was 2.0 (95% CI, 1.8 to 2.1) for systolic and 1.94 for diastolic (95% CI, 1.8 to 2.2). Higher BP in men with diabetes is also an important contributor to the risk of ESRD associated with diabetes mellitus. Adjustment for systolic BP reduced the relative risk of all-cause ESRD associated with diabetes by 18%, from 11.4 to 9.3, and the relative risk of diabetic ESRD by 15%, from 11.4 to 9.3.

Multiple Risk Factor Intervention Trial intervention group. The relationship between BP and all-cause ESRD was also investigated in the 12,866 men who were screened and who entered the trial. In this group, BP was unlikely to be elevated as a consequence of preexisting renal disease. The availability of serum creatinine measurements and dipstick assessment of urinary protein in these men at entry into the trial also permitted analysis of the relation of BP to incidence of ESRD, taking into account renal function at baseline. Among the men in the trial, an increase in systolic BP of 1 standard deviation (15.8 mm Hg) was associated with a 2-fold increased risk of ESRD, similar to the 1.8-fold increased risk seen in those not in the trial. Risk estimates associated with diastolic BP were also similar in men who entered the trial compared with those who did not. When serum creatinine and urinary protein excretion at time of entry into the trial were included as covariates in multivariate models, the relative risk of ESRD associated with BP was unchanged (2.0; 95% CI, 1.5 to 2.7 for systolic BP; and 2.5; 95% CI, 1.4 to 4.3 for diastolic BP). Moreover, when analysis was confined to the 7,817 men with a serum creatinine <1.2 mg/dL (106 μmol/L) and <1+ urinary protein excretion at entry, among

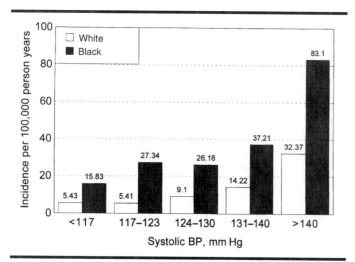

Figure B84.2. Age-adjusted 16-year incidence of all-cause end-stage renal disease by level of systolic blood pressure in 300,645 white men and 20,222 black men screened for the Multiple Risk Factor Intervention Trial. (From Klag MJ, Whelton PK, Randall BL, et al. End-stage renal disease in African-American and white men: 16-year MRFIT findings. *JAMA*. 1997;277:1293–1298, with permission.)

Table B84.2. Adjusted Relative Risk (95% Confidence Intervals) of Developing End-Stage Renal Disease (ESRD) for 20,222 Black Men Compared with 300,645 White Men Screened for Multiple Risk Factor Intervention Trial: Cox Proportional Hazards Analysis

| | RELATIVE RISK, BLACK COMPARED TO WHITE (95% CONFIDENCE INTERVAL) | | |
ADJUSTED FOR	ALL-CAUSE ESRD[a]	HYPERTENSIVE ESRD[b]	NONHYPERTENSIVE ESRD[c]
Age	3.20 (2.62, 3.91)	5.16 (3.64, 7.31)	2.61 (2.04, 3.35)
Age, systolic blood pressure[d]	2.56 (2.09, 3.13)	3.84 (2.68, 5.48)	2.14 (1.66, 2.75)
Age, serum cholesterol	3.25 (2.66, 3.98)	5.21 (3.68, 7.40)	2.65 (2.07, 3.40)
Age, cigarettes/d	3.26 (2.67, 3.98)	5.35 (3.77, 7.59)	2.64 (2.06, 3.39)
Age, median income	2.32 (1.82, 2.95)	2.83 (1.80, 4.45)	2.05 (1.53, 2.74)
Age, diabetes	2.73 (2.23, 3.34)	4.83 (3.40, 6.86)	2.16 (1.68, 2.78)
Age, previous myocardial infarction	3.20 (2.62, 3.91)	5.19 (3.66, 7.35)	2.61 (2.04, 3.35)
All of the above	1.87 (1.47, 2.39)	2.42 (1.52, 3.84)	1.63 (1.22, 2.18)

[a]Entry into ESRD registry or death from renal disease.
[b]Entry into ESRD registry with renal disease attributed to hypertension or death from hypertensive renal disease.
[c]Entry into ESRD registry with other than hypertensive renal disease or death from renal disease other than hypertension.
[d]Systolic blood pressure modeled as a continuous variable.

whom 19 men developed ESRD, the relative risk estimates were not significantly different from analyses including all 12,866 men (1.8; 95% CI, 1.2 to 2.7 for systolic BP; 1.7; 95% CI, 0.8 to 3.4 for diastolic BP). The similar relationships between BP and all-cause ESRD in the men who were included in the trial and those who were not, the independence of the association of baseline serum creatinine and urinary protein excretion in the men entering the trial, and the persistence of the association after 10 years of follow-up in the screened men argue against prevalent renal disease as an important contributor to the observed associations. The lack of information on renal function at baseline and during follow-up does mean, however, that we cannot say whether the strong association between BP and incidence of ESRD is owing to initiation of renal disease or accelerated progression of preexisting renal disease.

Blood Pressure and Moderate Renal Dysfunction (Hypercreatinemia)

Several studies have examined hypercreatinemia, an intermediate stage between normal renal function and ESRD, as an outcome. In an analysis of the 10,940 participants with hypertension in the Hypertension Detection and Follow-Up Program, the incidence of *clinically significant hypercreatinemia* (defined as a creatinine ≥2.0 mg/dL and at least 1.25 times the level at entry into the trial) during 5 years of follow-up was strongly related to diastolic BP at baseline. Incidence of renal insufficiency in the Stepped-Care group rose from 13.2 per 1,000/5 years in the 90 to 104 mm Hg BP stratum, to 34.4 in those with a BP of 105 to 114 mm Hg, and 63.7 per 1,000/5 years in the ≥115-mm Hg BP category. The relation of systolic BP to change in renal function was not studied. Smaller clinical observational studies of persons with hypertension have also demonstrated that higher BP is associated with decline in renal function. Such studies also suggest that control of high BP slows loss of renal function, consistent with results of clinical trials.

Overview

BP measured carefully on a single occasion is a strong independent risk factor for development of renal disease (either hypercreatinemia or ESRD). The increased risk associated with high BP is graded, continuous, and present throughout the entire distribution of BP above optimal. Risk estimates are graded for systolic and diastolic BP, but systolic BP is the stronger predictor of subsequent ESRD. Most of the risk estimates are based on BP measured on a single occasion, resulting in an underestimation of the strength of the real association of ESRD with BP owing to regression-dilution. Most observational data were generated before the widespread use of angiotensin-converting enzyme inhibitors, a class of antihypertensive drugs that appears to offer special renal protection. Widespread use of these drugs in the population may alter the relation between BP and ESRD observed in studies to date. The results of these studies also suggest that risk of renal disease associated with BP is present in individuals without clinical evidence of renal disease. Lastly, the presence of renal disease increases the risk of cardiovascular disease.

SUGGESTED READING

1. Brancati FL, Whelton PK, Randall BL, et al. Risk of end-stage renal disease in diabetes mellitus: a prospective cohort study of men screened for MRFIT. *JAMA.* 1997;278:2069–2074.
2. Klag MJ, Whelton PK, Randall BL, et al. Blood pressure and end-stage renal disease in men. *N Engl J Med.* 1996;334:13–18.
3. Klag MJ, Whelton PK, Randall BL, et al. End-stage renal disease in African-American and white men: 16-year MRFIT findings. *JAMA.* 1997;277:1293–1298.
4. Perneger TV, Nieto FJ, Whelton PK, et al. A prospective study of blood pressure and serum creatinine: results from the "Clue" Study and the ARIC Study. *JAMA.* 1993;269:488–493.
5. Perry HM Jr, Miller JP, Fornoff JR, et al. Early predictors of 15-year end-stage renal disease in hypertensive patients. *Hypertension.* 1995;25:587–594.
6. Shulman NB, Ford CE, Hall WD, et al. Prognostic value of serum creatinine and effect of treatment of hypertension on renal function: results from the Hypertension Detection and Follow-up Program. *Hypertension.* 1989;13:I-80–I-93.
7. U.S. Renal Data System. USRDS 1998 Annual Data Report. Bethesda, MD: The National Institutes of Health, National Institute of Diabetes and Digestive and Kidney Diseases; 1998.
8. Whittle JC, Whelton PK, Seidler AJ, Klag MJ. Does racial variation in risk factors explain black-white differences in the incidence of hypertensive end-stage renal disease? *Arch Intern Med.* 1991;151:1359–1364.

Chapter B85

Peripheral Arterial Disease and Hypertension

Michael H. Criqui, MD, MPH; Julie O. Denenberg, MA; Robert D. Langer, MD, MPH; Arnost Fronek, MD, PhD

KEY POINTS

- Cigarette smoking and diabetes appear to be the most important risk factors for peripheral arterial disease.

- The association of peripheral arterial disease with systolic blood pressure appears to be stronger than the association with diastolic blood pressure.

- Compared to individuals without peripheral arterial disease, the prevalence of hypertension is ≥50% higher in those with moderate peripheral arterial disease and nearly twice as high in those with severe peripheral arterial disease.

- Hypertension appears to be an important causal factor in the pathogenesis of peripheral arterial disease.

See also Chapters A67, B81, C122, and C157

It is generally accepted that the 3 most important modifiable risk factors for coronary heart disease are cigarette smoking, dyslipidemia, and elevated blood pressure. Other important risk factors for coronary heart disease include diabetes, obesity, and physical inactivity. Cigarette smoking and diabetes appear to be the most important risk factors for peripheral arterial disease (PAD). The prevalence of PAD also increases with age, and PAD is more common among men than women.

Diagnosis of Peripheral Arterial Disease

Intermittent claudication. Intermittent claudication (IC) is the classic symptom of PAD, consisting of ambulatory leg pain not present at rest and relieved by rest. By definition, this criterion excludes asymptomatic and presumably less extensive PAD. However, studies using IC as their PAD definition have produced somewhat conflicting results. Some studies showed no association; in other studies showing a positive association, the relationship was stronger for systolic blood pressure (SBP) than for diastolic blood pressure (DBP). Cross-sectional studies such as these could be biased by a number of factors. First, IC is an imprecise end point for PAD. Although IC reflects symptomatic and thus usually significant obstruction, surprisingly, nearly half of patients reporting IC in a population study had no demonstrable reduction in arterial flow on extensive noninvasive testing. Second, a bias could also be introduced by diet, lifestyle, or pharmaceutic interventions after the diagnosis of IC.

Ankle-brachial index. In general, an ankle pressure that is less than 90% of the brachial pressure is considered diagnostic for PAD. Studies using this criterion, or a more conservative criterion such as an ankle-brachial index (ABI) of <0.80 or even <0.75, have generally found an association with elevated blood pressure. In several studies, the association with SBP appeared stronger than the association with DBP. In the Cardiovascular Health Study, there was a gradation of effect, with an inverse relationship between ABI and either percent reported hypertension (SBP >160 mm Hg, DBP >95 mm Hg, or self-report of hypertension along with use of antihypertensive medications) and SBP. After adjustment for age and gender, as the ABI decreased, the number of persons reporting hypertension and the relative risk of hypertension increased significantly, as did the mean SBP. The trend was highly significant. DBP did not differ significantly with varying levels of ABI. In the Rotterdam Study, men and women with PAD (ABI <0.9) had a 60% greater prevalence of hypertension (≥160/95 mm Hg or use of antihypertensive medications) compared with men and women without PAD (ABI ≥0.9). Other studies have similarly shown an association between ABI and hypertension. However, these studies may have the usual limitations of cross-sectional studies, and the use of the ABI as the only criterion for PAD also limits specificity and sensitivity.

Combined assessment. A community-based study in an older population in the United States used several combined evaluations.

Lower-extremity pressure-flow evaluation. The ratios of systolic pressures at several levels of the lower extremity to the systolic brachial pressure, as well as flow velocity determination in the femoral and posterior tibial arteries, define PAD. In addition, a small proportion of cases who had had PAD surgery were included. Of the nonsurgical cases, only 20% had ambulatory leg pain, and overall approximately two-thirds of the cases were asymptomatic. This resulted in a broader spectrum of disease with many more mild cases of PAD than usually found in epidemiologic studies. In this study, the extensive use of noninvasive testing minimized the number of false-positive and false-negative cases.

Blood pressure and antihypertensive drugs. Moderate PAD cases had a somewhat higher SBP than normal individuals, but the difference was not statistically significant. Severe PAD cases had a significantly higher SBP than normals (11.7 mm Hg), but the increase in DBP (1.8 mm Hg) was not statistically significant (**Table B85.1**). This association was further explored by includ-

Table B85.1. Age-Adjusted Mean Levels of Blood Pressure by Peripheral Arterial Disease (PAD) Status

PAD STATUS	MEN	WOMEN	MEN AND WOMEN (SEX ADJUSTED)
Normal (N)	183	225	408
SBP	131.2	128.2	129.2
DBP	77.2	73.9	75.4
Moderate PAD (N)	22	27	49
SBP	138.9[a]	125.4	131.4
DBP	80.0	71.6	75.2
Severe PAD (N)	12	6	18
SBP	140.4[a]	141.9[a]	140.9[b]
DBP	78.2	74.8	77.2

DBP, diastolic blood pressure; SBP, systolic blood pressure.

[a] $p \leq .05$.

[b] $p \leq .01$, compared to normal group.

Table B85.3. Adjusted Odds Ratios[a] for Systolic Blood Pressure Greater Than 140 mm Hg with Presence of Isolated Arterial Lesions

	MALE		FEMALE	
	ODDS RATIO	95% CONFIDENCE INTERVAL	ODDS RATIO	95% CONFIDENCE INTERVAL
Aortoiliac	3.0	1.6–5.4	5.1	1.6–16.0
Femoropopliteal	2.3	1.3–4.3	2.4	1.2–4.9
Tibioperoneal	0.9	0.5–1.9	5.0	1.7–14.4

[a] Adjusted for age, current smoker, former smoker, diabetes, history of angina, ischemic heart disease, stroke, and congestive heart failure.

ing information on use of antihypertensive medication (**Table B85.2**). *Hypertension* is defined either liberally as an SBP ≥140 mm Hg or a DBP ≥90 mm Hg or use of hypertensive medications (HTN1), or more conservatively by changing the BP criteria to an SBP ≥160 mm Hg or a DBP ≥95 mm Hg or medication use (HTN2). By either definition, there is in both sexes a stepwise increase in the proportion of hypertensives from normals to persons with moderate PAD to people with severe PAD. For both sexes combined, with analyses adjusted for age and sex, individuals with moderate PAD had a 50% or greater prevalence of hypertension. Individuals with severe PAD had nearly twice the prevalence of hypertension as normals, and these findings are highly statistically significant. The results suggest a stronger relationship between hypertension and PAD when antihypertensive medication use is included in the hypertension definition.

Threshold pressures. In a study of subjects from a vascular laboratory, which used segmental pressures to assess PAD, an SBP >140 mm Hg was highly associated with PAD at all levels in the lower extremity in women, and in the 2 proximal levels in the

men (**Table B85.3**). In the San Luis Valley Diabetes Study, Hiatt, using the 2-vessel criteria (both the dorsalis pedis and the posterior tibial artery meeting ABI criteria), found that the odds ratio for hypertension increased with worsening PAD percentiles. At the fifth percentile, the hypertension odds ratio was 1.63; at the 2.5 percentile, it was 2.16; and at the first percentile, it was 3.12. All p values were <.05.

Angiography. When clinical or laboratory tests are coupled with angiography, the diagnosis of PAD is highly reliable, and most patients have disease severe enough to be symptomatic. Nonetheless, similar to studies in which PAD is defined as IC, the results are mixed, ranging from no association to strong associations. An Italian study found a statistically significant 5-fold increase in the prevalence of hypertension (SBP >160 mm Hg or DBP >95 mm Hg) among patients with PAD when compared with age- and gender-matched controls. In another study that matched PAD patients and controls on mean arterial pressure, PAD patients had increased systolic pressure and decreased diastolic pressure, and thus increased pulse pressure. Pulse pressure was inversely correlated with arterial compliance, owing to changes in viscoelastic properties of the arterial wall (see Chapter A60). In addition, unlike population-based epidemiologic studies, angiographic studies use selected clinical samples that may not be representative of the general population.

Incidence of Peripheral Arterial Disease

If blood pressure measurements are made before the development of the PAD, a more reliable incidence rate can be obtained. Carefully collected data in the Framingham Study showed a steep, near-linear gradient between the baseline level of SBP and the 26-year incidence of IC (**Figure B85.1**). For baseline DBP, the data suggest a threshold effect beginning at the fourth quintile (87 to 94 mm Hg) in women and the fifth quintile (≥95 mm Hg) in men. For the fifth quintile of SBP (≥180 mm Hg) compared to the first quintile of SBP (≤119 mm Hg), the relative risk in men was 2.7 and in women 5.2. Interestingly, the attributable (or excess) risk in men and women for the fifth versus the first quintile was the same in both men and women (8/1,000 biennial rate). The misclassification inherent in defining PAD by IC would suggest that these strong associations might be conservative.

Peripheral Arterial Disease Progression

Palumbo et al. have reported on the prospective progression of PAD as defined by the rate of change in the postexercise ABI

Table B85.2. Age- and Sex-Adjusted Percentages of Hypertensives by Peripheral Arterial Disease (PAD) Status Using 2 Different Definitions of Hypertension (HTN):

HTN1 = (HTN Drugs or SBP ≥140 or DBP ≥90)

HTN2 = (HTN Drugs or SBP ≥160 or DBP ≥95)

PAD STATUS	MEN	WOMEN	MEN AND WOMEN (SEX ADJUSTED)
Normal (N)	183	225	408
% HTN1	39.5	46.6	41.6
% HTN2	24.3	32.8	26.9
Moderate PAD (N)	22	27	49
% HTN1	65.4[a]	58.5	60.3[b]
% HTN2	54.2[b]	43.8	46.5[b]
Severe PAD (N)	12	6	18
% HTN1	74.5[a]	90.0[a]	81.2[c]
% HTN2	53.8[a]	61.8	55.7[a]

[a] $p \leq .05$.

[b] $p \leq .01$.

[c] $p \leq .001$, compared to normal group.

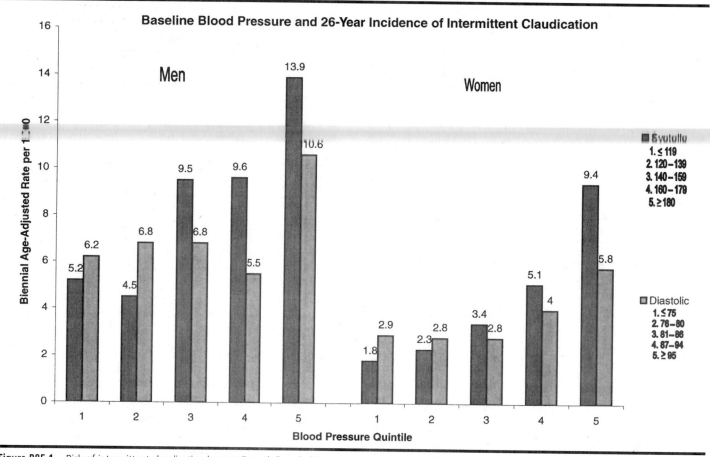

Figure B85.1.   Risk of intermittent claudication by systolic and diastolic blood pressure. Subjects aged 35 to 84 years. Trends significant at *p* <.001. Data from 26-year follow-up of the Framingham Study. (From Kannel WB, McGee DL. Update on some epidemiologic features of intermittent claudication: the Framingham Study. *J Am Geriatr Soc*. 1985;33:13–18, with permission.)

over 4 years, as well as the occurrence of clinical events, such as PAD surgery, including amputation. In multivariate analyses, SBP was independently and significantly predictive of PAD progression. Similar data exist in other studies.

Randomized Controlled Trials of Hypertension and Peripheral Arterial Disease

Limited data are available. In the Prevention of Atherosclerosis Complications with Ketanserin (PACK) study, nearly 4,000 patients with IC and an ABI ≤0.85 were randomized, and 46% had hypertension (SBP ≥160 mm Hg and/or DBP ≥95 mm Hg). Above-ankle amputations were reduced 47% (17 vs. 32) in the ketanserin group. Although this finding is consistent with a causal association between hypertension and PAD, it does not represent definitive proof because ketanserin, in addition to being an antihypertensive, also inhibits platelet aggregation and has favorable hemorheologic effects.

SUGGESTED READING

1. Criqui MH, Langer RD, Fronek A, et al. The epidemiology of large vessel and isolated small vessel peripheral arterial disease. In: Fowkes FGR, ed. *Epidemiology of Peripheral Vascular Disease*. London, UK: Springer-Verlag; 1991.

2. Fowkes FGR, Housley E, Riemersma RA, et al. Smoking, lipids, glucose intolerance, and blood pressure as risk factors for peripheral atherosclerosis compared with ischemic heart disease in the Edinburgh artery study. *Am J Epidemiol*. 1992;135:331–340.

3. Hiatt WR, Hoag S, Hamman RF. Effect of diagnostic criteria on the prevalence of peripheral arterial disease. The San Luis Valley Diabetes Study. *Circulation*. 1995;91:1472–1479.

4. Hirsch AT, Criqui MH, Treat-Jacobson D, et al. Peripheral arterial disease detection, awareness, and treatment in primary care. *JAMA*. 2001;286:1317–1324.

5. Kannel WB, McGee DC. Update on some epidemiologic features of intermittent claudication: the Framingham Study. *J Am Geriatr Soc*. 1985;33:13–18.

6. Meijer WT, Hoes AW, Rutgers D, et al. Peripheral arterial disease in the elderly: the Rotterdam Study. *Aerterioscler Thromb Vasc Biol*. 1998;118:185–192.

7. Newman AB, Siscovick DS, Manolio TA, et al. CHS Collaborative Research Group. Ankle-arm index as a marker of atherosclerosis in the Cardiovascular Health Study. *Circulation*. 1993;88:837–845.

8. Palumbo PJ, O'Fallon WM, Osmundson PJ, et al. Progression of peripheral occlusive arterial disease in diabetes mellitus. What factors are predictive? *Arch Intern Med*. 1991;151:717–721.

9. Prevention of Atherosclerotic Complications with Ketanserin Trial Group. Prevention of atherosclerotic complications: controlled trial of ketanserin. *BMJ*. 1989;298:424–430.

10. Strano A, Novo S, Avellone G, et al. Hypertension and other risk factors in peripheral arterial disease. *Clin Exp Hypertens*. 1993;15:71–89.

Chapter B86

Gender and Blood Pressure

David A. Calhoun, MD; Suzanne Oparil, MD

KEY POINTS

- There is a sexual dimorphism in blood pressure, such that men have higher systolic blood pressure levels than women during early adulthood years, whereas the opposite is true after the sixth decade of life. Diastolic blood pressure tends to be slightly higher in men than women regardless of age.

- The effects of hormone replacement therapy on blood pressure are not well defined. On an individual basis, the effect is likely modest, but warrants close monitoring.

- Women are more likely than men to be aware of their hypertension, to be treated with antihypertensive drugs, and to have their blood pressure controlled.

- Antihypertensive therapy induces similar blood pressure reductions in men and women. However, men experience larger reductions in total cardiovascular risk with successful treatment of high blood pressure.

See also Chapters A53, A57, B81, B102, C151, and C165

Age and Blood Pressure

Blood pressure (BP) manifests a sexually dimorphic pattern in humans with mean BP being generally higher in men than in women regardless of age. In a study of normotensive Danish men and women, ambulatory BP monitoring was used to assess 24-hour BP levels in healthy adults. In subjects aged 20 to 79 years, 24-hour mean systolic BP (SBP) increased progressively with age in men and women but was higher in men than women at all ages except for the oldest age group, 70 to 79 years (**Figure B86.1**). The largest difference was in the 30 to 39 year olds, in whom the mean SBP was approximately 16 mm Hg higher in men than women. There was no gender difference in 24-hour mean diastolic BP (DBP), which increased by approximately 10 mm Hg with aging in men and women.

Systolic blood pressure. In the overall population, mean SBP increases progressively throughout adult life in men and women (**Figure B86.2**). The Third National Health and Nutrition Examination Survey (NHANES III) found that mean SBP is higher in men than women during early adulthood, but the subsequent rate of rise in BP is steeper for women than men. As a result, in all 3 ethnic groups (non-Hispanic blacks, non-Hispanic whites, and Mexican-Americans), mean SBP in women is as high or higher than the corresponding values for men during and after the seventh decade of life.

Diastolic blood pressure. In the overall population, mean DBP increases progressively in men and women until approximately the fifth decade of life, after which it decreases progressively (Figure B86.2). The consequence is a widening pulse pressure in men and women after the age of 60 years. This widening pulse pressure is thought to be due to loss of aortic and other large vessel elasticity. Recent reports indicate that a wide pulse pressure predicts cardiovascular risk and that pulse pressure may be superior to SBP as a predictor of cardiovascular risk, especially in the elderly. Throughout adult life, men have a slightly higher average level of DBP than women (Figure B86.2). Black women have a higher mean DBP than white or Hispanic women. The same is true of men until the end of the fifth decade. Thereafter, mean DBP is similar in the 3 ethnic groups.

Prevalence of hypertension. The prevalence of hypertension increases progressively with age in men and women (**Figure B86.3**). By the age of 65, the majority of whites are hypertensive. Blacks tend to develop hypertension earlier than whites, such that the majority of black men and women are hypertensive by the age of 55. In early adulthood, hypertension is more common among men than women. However, after the fifth decade of life, the incidence of hypertension increases more rapidly in women than men, with the prevalence of hypertension in women equal to or exceeding that in men during the sixth decade of life. The highest prevalence rates of hypertension are observed in elderly black women, with hypertension occurring in more than 75% of women older than 75 years of age.

Gender and blood pressure awareness, treatment, and control. Overall and in each of the 3 ethnic groups studied in NHANES III, women are more likely to know that they have hypertension, are more likely to have it treated, and are more likely to have it controlled (**Figure B86.4**). In NHANES III, approximately 75% of hypertensive black and white women were aware of their high BP in contrast to just 65% of hypertensive men in these ethnic groups. In Hispanic hypertensives, 64% of women and 44% of men were aware that they had hypertension.

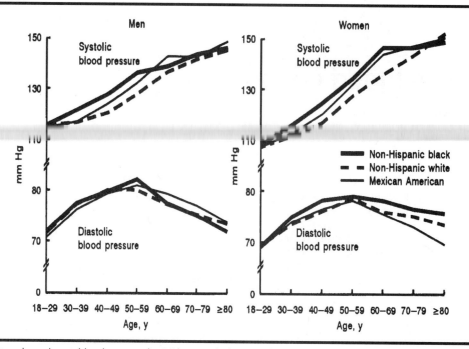

Figure B86.1. Effect of age and gender on blood pressure by 24-hour ambulatory technique in a Danish normotensive cohort. Data presented as mean ± standard error of mean. $p <.05$ compared with women of similar age. (From Wiinberg N, Hoegholm A, Christensen HR, et al. 24-h Ambulatory blood pressure in 352 normal Danish subjects, related to age and gender. *Am J Hypertens.* 1995;8:978–986, with permission.)

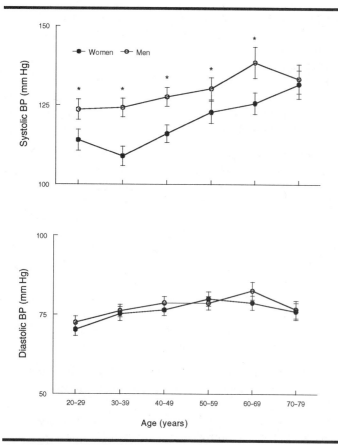

Figure B86.2. Mean systolic and diastolic blood pressures by age and race/ethnicity for men and women [Third National Health and Nutrition Examination Survey (NHANES III), 1988–1991]. (From Burt VL, Whelton P, Roccella EJ, et al. Prevalence of hypertension in the US adult population: results of the Third National Health and Nutrition Examination Survey, 1988–1991. *Hypertension.* 1995;25:305–313, with permission.)

Overall, 61% of hypertensive women but only 44% of men were being treated with antihypertensive medications. The higher antihypertensive treatment rates in women have been attributed to increased numbers of physician contacts because of visits for reproductive health and childcare, as well as a lower probability of employment outside the home. Finally, only 28% of women and 19% of men had their BP controlled (<140/90 mm Hg).

Menopause and Blood Pressure

The effect of menopause on BP is controversial.

Age versus menopause. Longitudinal studies such as Framingham have not documented a rise in BP with menopause. In contrast, cross-sectional studies have found significantly higher SBP and DBP in postmenopausal versus premenopausal women. In NHANES III, the rate of rise in SBP tends to be steeper in postmenopausal women compared to premenopausal women until the sixth decade, when the rate of increase tends to slow. Staessen et al. reported a 4-fold higher prevalence of hypertension in postmenopausal women than in premenopausal women (40% vs. 10%, $p <.001$). After adjustment for age and body mass index, postmenopausal women were still more than twice as likely to have hypertension as premenopausal women. In a recent prospective study of conventional and ambulatory BP levels in pre-, peri-, and postmenopausal women, the postmenopausal women had high SBP (4 to 5 mm Hg) compared to the pre- and perimenopausal controls. The increase in SBP per decade was 5 mm Hg greater in the peri- and postmenopausal women compared to the premenopausal group. Thus, there is disagreement between longitudinal and cross-sectional studies as to the effect of menopause on BP, but there is convincing evidence that at least part of the rise in BP (particularly SBP) seen later in life in women is owing to menopause. A menopause-

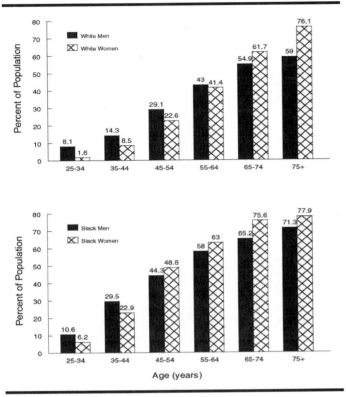

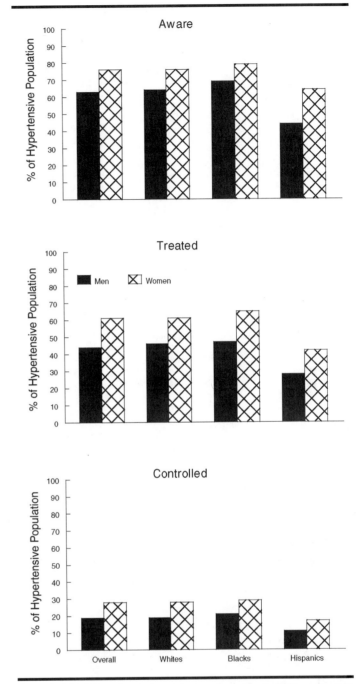

Figure B86.3. Prevalence of hypertension in the United States by age, gender, and race, 1988–1994. (From Wolz M, Cutler J, Roccella EJ, et al. Statement from the National High Blood Pressure Education Program: prevalence of hypertension. *Am J Hypertens*. 2000;13:103–104, with permission.)

related increase in BP has been attributed to a variety of factors, including estrogen withdrawal, overproduction of pituitary hormones, weight gain, or a combination of these and other yet undefined neurohumoral influences.

Postmenopausal Hormone Replacement Therapy and Blood Pressure

Clinical studies. Studies evaluating the effects of hormone replacement therapy (HRT) on BP have been inconsistent. The Baltimore Longitudinal Study on Aging (BLSA), the largest observational study to address this question, followed 226 normotensive postmenopausal women for an average of 5.7 years. Women receiving HRT (oral or transdermal estrogen and progestin) had a significantly smaller increase in SBP over time than nonusers. HRT users had a 1.6 mm Hg average increase in SBP, whereas nonusers had an average increase of 8.9 mm Hg. DBP was not affected by HRT.

Results of the Postmenopausal Estrogen/Progestin Intervention (PEPI) trial and Women's Health Initiative (WHI) contrast with those of BLSA. In the former, 596 normotensive, postmenopausal women, aged 45 to 64 years, were followed for an average of 3 years. HRT (conjugated equine estrogen and native or synthetic progestin) had no significant effect on SBP or DBP. In the WHI, cross-sectional analysis of almost 100,000 women aged 50 to 79 years indicated that current HRT use was associated with a 25% greater likelihood of having hypertension compared to past use or no prior use of HRT.

Figure B86.4. Rates of awareness, treatment, and control of hypertension by race and gender (age 18 years and older, NHANES III, phase 1, 1988–1991). The control rate represents the proportion of persons with hypertension who are controlled to <140/90 mm Hg. (From Burt VL, Whelton P, Roccella EJ, et al. Prevalence of hypertension in the US adult population: results of the Third National Health and Nutrition Examination Survey, 1988–1991. *Hypertension*. 1995;25:305–313, with permission.)

Smaller studies have used 24-hour ambulatory monitoring to evaluate the effects of HRT on BP in normotensive and hypertensive women. Although results are inconsistent overall, several of the studies suggest that HRT improves or restores the normal nighttime reduction ("dipping") in BP that may be diminished in postmenopausal women. Such an effect would tend to reduce total BP load and thereby reduce target organ damage.

Because of the existing contradictory results of published studies, even larger, prospective, randomized trials would be

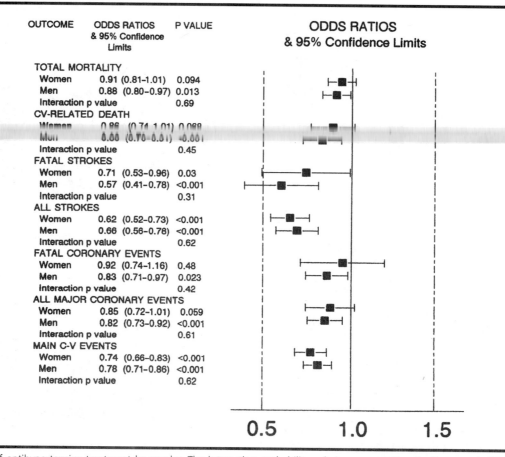

OUTCOME	ODDS RATIOS & 95% Confidence Limits	P VALUE
TOTAL MORTALITY		
Women	0.91 (0.81–1.01)	0.094
Men	0.88 (0.80–0.97)	0.013
Interaction p value		0.69
CV-RELATED DEATH		
Women	0.86 (0.74–1.01)	0.068
Men	0.88 (0.76–0.81)	<0.001
Interaction p value		0.45
FATAL STROKES		
Women	0.71 (0.53–0.96)	0.03
Men	0.57 (0.41–0.78)	<0.001
Interaction p value		0.31
ALL STROKES		
Women	0.62 (0.52–0.73)	<0.001
Men	0.66 (0.56–0.78)	<0.001
Interaction p value		0.62
FATAL CORONARY EVENTS		
Women	0.92 (0.74–1.16)	0.48
Men	0.83 (0.71–0.97)	0.023
Interaction p value		0.42
ALL MAJOR CORONARY EVENTS		
Women	0.85 (0.72–1.01)	0.059
Men	0.82 (0.73–0.92)	<0.001
Interaction p value		0.61
MAIN C-V EVENTS		
Women	0.74 (0.66–0.83)	<0.001
Men	0.78 (0.71–0.86)	<0.001
Interaction p value		0.62

Figure B86.5. Effects of antihypertensive treatment by gender. The interaction probability values represent the significance of difference in odds ratios between men and women. CV, cardiovascular. (From Gueyffier F, Boutitie F, Boissel J-P, et al. for the INDANA Investigators. Effect of antihypertensive drug treatment on cardiovascular outcomes in women and men: a meta-analysis of individual patient data from randomized, controlled trials. *Ann Intern Med.* 1997;126:761–767, with permission.)

needed to rigorously define the effects of HRT on BP. Overall, HRT-related change in BP is likely to be modest and should not preclude HRT use in normotensive or hypertensive women. At the same time, benefit in terms of BP reduction cannot be assumed, either individually or on a population basis. Thus, HRT should not be prescribed for any benefit on BP. It is recommended that all hypertensive women treated with HRT have their BP monitored closely at first and then at 6-month intervals.

Oral Contraceptives and Blood Pressure

Many women taking oral contraceptives experience a small but detectable increase in BP; a small percentage experience the onset of frank hypertension, which resolves with withdrawal of oral contraceptive therapy. This is true even with modern preparations that contain only 30 μg estrogen.

Clinical studies. The Nurses' Health Study found that current users of oral contraceptives had a significantly increased [relative risk (RR), 1.8; 95% confidence interval, 1.5–2.3] risk of hypertension compared with women who never used oral contraceptives. Of note, absolute risk was small: Only 41.5 cases of hypertension per 10,000 person-years could be attributed to oral contraceptive use. Risk decreased quickly with cessation of contraceptive use: Past users had only a slightly increased risk (RR, 1.2; 95% confidence interval, 1.0–1.4) compared with women who never used oral contraceptives. Controlled pro-

spective studies have demonstrated a return of BP to pretreatment levels within 3 months of discontinuing oral contraceptives, indicating that oral contraceptives' BP effect is relatively acute and readily reversible.

Mechanisms of disease. Oral contraceptives occasionally appear to precipitate accelerated, or malignant, hypertension. Genetic characteristics, such as family history of hypertension, as well as environmental characteristics, including preexisting pregnancy-induced hypertension, occult renal disease, obesity, middle age (>35 years), and duration of oral contraceptive use, increase susceptibility to oral contraceptive–induced hypertension. The mechanism of contraceptive-induced hypertension is unclear but appears to be related to the progestogenic, not the estrogenic, potency of the preparation. The risk of hypertension is greater among users of monophasic combination oral contraceptives than among users of biphasic or triphasic combinations, perhaps because the total dose of progestin delivered is greater with the monophasic preparation.

Outcomes of Antihypertensive Trials by Gender

Most of the large multicenter trials of antihypertensive therapy with "hard" end points have included slightly larger numbers of women than men, and none of these trials included enough women to analyze data from gender subgroups independently. Subgroup analyses from individual trials have yielded variable results regarding the risk/benefit ratio of pharmacologic treatment of hypertension in women, leading some to conclude that women derive less benefit than men from antihypertensive treatment. A subgroup metaanalysis of individual patient data according to gender based on 7 trials from the INDANA (Individual Data Analysis of Antihypertensive Intervention Trials) database was recently carried out to quantify treatment effect by sex and to determine whether there are gender differences in treatment effect. These trials included 20,802 women and 19,975 men recruited between 1972 and 1990 and treated with thiazide diuretics or β-blockers. In women, significant treatment benefits included reductions in strokes (total and fatal) and major cardiovascular events (**Figure B86.5**). In men, treatment benefits were significant for all 7 outcomes considered. In terms of RR, treatment benefits did not differ between the sexes. Absolute risk reduction, in contrast, is dependent on untreated risk, and untreated risk for stroke was similar in the 2 sexes; for coronary events, untreated risk was greater in men. Accordingly, absolute risk reduction for stroke attributed to treatment was similar in men and women; for coronary events, absolute risk reduction was greater in men. These results cannot be extrapolated to the newer classes of antihypertensive drugs without further research or analysis of results of recent clinical trials by gender. Because the risk of stroke is similar in both sexes, the sex of the patient should not play a role in decisions about whether to treat high BP.

Gender Considerations in Choice of Antihypertensive Drugs

Women generally respond to antihypertensive drugs similarly to men, but some special considerations may dictate treatment choices for women.

Angiotensin-converting enzyme inhibitors and AT_1-receptor blockers are contraindicated for women who are or intend to become pregnant because of the risk of fetal developmental abnormalities. Diuretics are particularly useful in women, particularly elderly women, because their use is associated with decreased risk of hip fracture. Increasing evidence suggests that antihypertensive drugs have gender-specific adverse effect profiles. In the Treatment of Mild Hypertension Study (TOMHS), women reported twice as many adverse effects as men. Biochemical responses to drugs may be gender dependent with women who are more likely to develop diuretic-induced hyponatremia and men who are more likely to develop gout. Hypokalemia is more common in women taking a diuretic. Angiotensin-converting enzyme inhibitor–induced cough is twice as common in women as in men, and women are more likely to complain of calcium channel blocker–related peripheral edema and minoxidil-induced hirsutism. The effect of antihypertensive therapy on sexual function is a major obstacle to successful therapy in men, and there is evidence that sexual dysfunction is a problem in hypertensive women as well. However, additional evaluation is needed in this area, as sexual dysfunction in women is seldom assessed in clinical trials.

SUGGESTED READING

1. Burt VL, Whelton P, Roccella EJ, et al. Prevalence of hypertension in the US adult population: results of the Third National Health and Nutrition Examination Survey, 1988–1991. *Hypertension*. 1995;25:305–313.
2. Chasan-Taber L, Willett WC, Manson JE, et al. Prospective study of oral contraceptives and hypertension among women in the United States. *Circulation*. 1996;94:483–489.
3. Gueyffier F, Boutitie F, Boissel J-P, et al. for the INDANA Investigators. Effect of antihypertensive drug treatment on cardiovascular outcomes in women and men: a meta-analysis of individual patient data from randomized, controlled trials. *Ann Intern Med*. 1997;126:761–767.
4. Klungel OH, de Boer A, Paes AH, et al. Sex differences in the pharmacological treatment of hypertension: a review of population-based studies. *J Hypertens*. 1997;15:591–600.
5. PEPI Trial Writing Group. Effects of estrogen or estrogen/progestin regimens on heart disease risk factors in postmenopausal women: the Postmenopausal Estrogen/Progestin Intervention (PEPI) trial. [Published correction appears in *JAMA*. 1995;274:1676.] *JAMA*. 1995;273:199–208.
6. Rosenthal T, Oparil S. Hypertension in women. *J Human Hypertens*. 2000;14:691–704.
7. Scuteri A, Bos AJ, Brant LJ, et al. Hormone replacement therapy and longitudinal changes in blood pressure in postmenopausal women. *Ann Intern Med*. 2001;135:229–238.
8. Wassertheil-Smolller S, Anderson G, Psaty BM, et al. Hypertension and its treatment in postmenopausal women: baseline data from the Women's Health Initiative. *Hypertension*. 2000;36:780–789.
9. Wiinberg N, Hoegholm A, Christensen HR, et al. 24-h Ambulatory blood pressure in 352 normal Danish subjects, related to age and gender. *Am J Hypertens*. 1995;8:978–986.
10. Wolz M, Cutler J, Roccella EJ, et al. Statement from the National High Blood Pressure Education Program: prevalence of hypertension. *Am J Hypertens*. 2000;13:103–104.

Blood Pressure in Children

Alan R. Sinaiko, MD

KEY POINTS

- Measurement of blood pressure is recommended yearly after the age of 3 years. The diagnosis of hypertension in children now uses the fifth Korotkoff sound to define diastolic blood pressure and also depends on height.

- Blood pressure is considerably lower in children than adults and increases steadily throughout the first 2 decades of life.

- Factors known to be associated with higher levels of blood pressure in children and adolescents include greater weight, greater height, and a family history of hypertension.

- There are no significant blood pressure differences between ethnic groups until late adolescence.

See also Chapters A54, A75, A78, B97, B103, and C166

Arterial hypertension has a relatively low prevalence in children compared with adults. Nonetheless, for some children, the problem is clinically significant, and guidelines on detection, evaluation, and treatment are of considerable importance in their care. Moreover, because the essential hypertensive adults of tomorrow will emerge in large part from the normotensive, seemingly healthy children of today, it is important from a preventive standpoint to consider hypertension as a risk factor in the pediatric age group, even before clinical manifestations of the disease become apparent.

Prevalence and Risks of Hypertension in Children

Prospective cohort data on the relationship between childhood blood pressure (BP) and cardiovascular risk are not yet available. Yet, there continue to be compelling reasons for developing the broadest base of information about BP in children and adolescents. First, the prevalence of essential hypertension in the U.S. adult population has been estimated to be 25%, or greater than 50 million Americans. Although the prevalence of clinical hypertension is of a far lesser magnitude in children than in adults, ample evidence supports the concept that the roots of essential hypertension extend back into childhood. Second, familial patterns for BP have been established from early infancy, and children with BP in the higher distributional percentiles are more likely to come from families with histories of hypertension. Third, although it is generally agreed that early essential hypertension poses little immediate risk to most children, evidence from preliminary studies in children and adolescents has shown cardiac ventricular and hemodynamic changes consistent with an adverse effect of mild hypertension before the third decade of life. Fourth, high BP is associated with the insulin resistance syndrome (hyperinsulinemia, dyslipidemia, obesity) before adulthood. Although BP is not significantly correlated with insulin resistance in childhood, it

appears that a significant relation develops during adolescence. Adolescents with high BP have a significantly greater clustering effect for the insulin resistance syndrome factors when compared to adolescents with low BP. Thus, elevation of BP during the first 2 decades is an early warning sign of overall cardiovascular risk.

Evolution of guidelines. From a historic standpoint, the initial orientation of health care providers to BP in children and adolescents was toward identification and pharmacologic treatment of secondary forms of hypertension, such as renal parenchymal disease and renal artery stenosis. However, the incorporation of BP measurement into the routine pediatric examination during the past 20 years and publication of national survey data on BP in children confirmed that elevations in BP during childhood are more common than previously recognized, particularly in adolescents (i.e., beginning with the second decade of life). The First Task Force on Blood Pressure Control in Children was convened in 1977 by the National Heart, Lung, and Blood Institute in response to the need to establish guidelines for the measurement and classification of BP and to develop recommendations for the treatment of childhood hypertension. The second Task Force report, published in 1987, revised and strengthened the norms for childhood BP; these were further strengthened by an update of the 1987 report, published in 1996.

Age and Blood Pressure

BP is considerably lower in children than adults and increases steadily throughout the first 2 decades of life.

Infants. The average systolic BP (SBP) at 1 day of age is approximately 70 mm Hg in full-term infants, and it increases to approximately 85 mm Hg by 1 month of age. BP increases at a greater rate in premature infants than full-term infants during the first year of life, and there is a significant inverse relation between birth weight and the risk of hypertension in adulthood.

Tracking during growth and development. During the preschool years, BP begins to follow a tracking pattern in which children tend to maintain specific levels of BP distribution relative to their peer group as they age. Tracking has been demonstrated using a number of statistical methods, including percentile and raw BP data, and may increase in significance when evaluating groups of subjects selected from the extremes of the BP distribution. Of particular importance is the documentation that BP tracking bridges the gap between childhood and early adulthood.

Other Risk Factors for Hypertension

A number of factors known to be associated with hypertension in adults also have been associated with higher levels of BP in children and adolescents. A direct relation between weight and BP has been documented as early as 5 years of age and is more prominent in the second decade. Height is independently related to BP at all ages. Sex and race do not have the same impact on BP in children as in adults. No significant differences have been found in comparisons of whites, blacks, Hispanics, and Southeast Asians until adolescence. Even then, the differences are small and have varied among epidemiologic studies. Reference standards for BP in children do not distinguish between ethnic groups, because the differences are not clinically relevant. BP in male children is slightly higher than in female children during the first decade of life. The difference between males and females begins to widen around the onset of puberty, and BP is significantly higher in males by the end of the teenage years.

Family history. Children from hypertensive families tend to have BPs that are higher than children from normotensive families, and the significant correlation of BP and cardiovascular risk factors between parents and their children is widely recognized. Siblings of children with high BP have significantly higher BP than siblings of children with low BP. The BP correlation is higher between mothers and their children than between fathers and their children, suggesting a direct prenatal influence.

Blood Pressure Measurement Techniques

There are some special features to the measurement and evaluation of BP in children. Measurement by usual auscultation methods is not feasible in infants and very young children because of practical problems with anxiety and cooperation. Therefore, automated devices are widely used in this age group, and these devices are generally reliable. Measurement of BP is recommended yearly after the age of 3 years.

Cuff size. Use of an appropriately sized BP cuff is necessary to ensure accurate measurement, and the current commercially marketed series of pediatric cuffs along with the regular and oversized adult arm and thigh cuffs provides a sufficiently broad range of sizes. In a busy clinical setting, correctness of cuff size can be determined by using the manufacturer's suggested markings on the cuff or selecting a cuff size with a width approximately two-thirds of the distance between the shoulder and

elbow. Choosing an inappropriate cuff size may falsely elevate the BP, in the case of a small cuff, or falsely reduce the BP, in the case of a large cuff. However, when choosing between 2 cuffs, both of which are close in size to the measured width of the arm, the larger cuff should be selected; it is uncommon for a slightly larger cuff to mask true hypertension, whereas it is more likely that use of a small cuff may lead to an elevated reading.

Korotkoff sounds. The 4th phase Korotkoff sound was traditionally used to designate diastolic BP (DBP) in children less than 13 years, and the 5th phase Korotkoff sound was used for DBP in children 13 years and older. With the addition of more childhood epidemiologic BP data and reanalysis of the database used to establish previous standards, the 1996 update of the Task Force report determined that the 5th phase Korotkoff sound is a reliable measure of DBP for children of all ages.

Ambulatory pressures. Ambulatory BP monitoring (ABPM) is being used in pediatrics, but its role in complementing or replacing the casual office measurement is not yet defined. Recent studies have shown that the frequency of "white coat" hypertension in children is inversely related to the degree of hypertension. Thus, ABPM does not provide much additional information in the child with moderate or severe hypertension. Although the frequency of white coat hypertension is greater in children with only minimal elevations of BP, ABPM is also of limited usefulness in planning therapy in these children. Because many are overweight, clinicians rarely treat these children with pharmacologic agents before attempting nonpharmacologic therapy. In contrast, ABPM has been a valuable addition in epidemiologic studies, drug trials, and other types of clinical BP research.

Current Definitions and Classification of High Blood Pressure

As with adults, there are no data to support the rigorous classification of BP as normotensive or hypertensive or to further delineate hypertensive categories. Nonetheless, it becomes a matter of practical necessity to have definitions and classifications of hypertension to determine when and how vigorously hypertension should be treated. Definitions of hypertension are, of necessity, based on clinical experience and consensus rather than on risk data and are determined on the basis of percentile BP distribution within the pediatric population as follows: (a) normal BP: SBP and DBP <90th percentile for age and sex; (b) high normal BP: average SBP or DBP (or both) between the 90th and 95th percentiles for age and sex; (c) high BP (hypertension): average SBP or DBP (or both) ≥95th percentile for age and sex, with measurements obtained on at least 3 occasions.

Nomograms. Tables used to classify hypertension in children were revised by the 1996 Task Force and take into account the documented effect of body size and differential rates of growth in children by relating BP to age and height. The average 95th percentile systolic and DBPs for boys and girls by height at selected ages are provided in **Table B87.1**. For any given age, BP norms increase as height rises. Use of these published norms should prevent mislabeling of tall nonoverweight children as hypertensive or missing a diagnosis of elevated BP in shorter or

Table B87.1. Systolic and Diastolic Blood Pressure Levels for the 95th Percentile for Boys and Girls 3 to 6 Years Old According to Height[a]

AGE, YR	SYSTOLIC BLOOD PRESSURE							
	HEIGHT PERCENTILES							
	BOYS				GIRLS			
	5TH	25TH	75TH	95TH	5TH	25TH	75TH	95TH
3	104	107	111	113	104	105	108	110
6	109	112	115	117	108	110	112	114
10	114	117	121	123	116	117	120	122
13	121	124	128	130	121	123	126	128
16	129	132	136	138	125	127	130	132
	DIASTOLIC BLOOD PRESSURE							
3	63	64	66	67	65	65	67	68
6	72	73	75	76	71	72	73	75
10	77	79	80	82	77	77	79	80
13	79	81	83	84	80	81	82	84
16	83	84	86	87	83	83	85	86

[a]Height percentile is determined from standard growth curves.
Reprinted from *N Engl J Med.* as adapted from the Update on the 1996 Task Force Report on High Blood Pressure in Children and Adolescents, with permission.

heavier children, as was the case when only the BP level was used for each age. Obese children are unlikely to have another cause for their high BP other than their excessive weight. If a child or adolescent has an average BP greater than the 95th percentile for age but is not tall or heavy, there is greater probability that the elevation is the result of some scientific pathologic process. In this case, the child needs further evaluations for secondary causes and special consideration for treatment.

Surveillance and Records

Except in cases of severe hypertension with evidence of target organ damage, identifying children with high BP requires multiple BP measurements on several visits. Specifically, if the BP is above the 90th percentile, the child is scheduled for repeat BP measurements over several visits. If the average BP is then below the 90th percentile, the child should return to continuing health care. If the average BP is between the 90th and 95th percentiles, the child has high normal BP and should remain under surveillance, with BP measurements at least every 6 months. If the average BP after several visits places the child in the 95th percentile or higher, the child should undergo a diagnostic evaluation and consideration should be given to therapy. If the child is obese, a trial of weight control may be attempted before proceeding to the evaluation and other therapeutic interventions.

Under optimal circumstances, children receive care from a continuing source, and good records are kept of their clinical progress. A record of the patient's BP should be maintained throughout the years and plotted against the BP/age percentile charts. In this way, the health care provider is able to determine whether the child is trending in a favorable or an unfavorable direction. Such trends provide guidance for determining how closely the child should be monitored.

SUGGESTED READING

1. Lurbe E, Redon J. Ambulatory blood pressure monitoring in children and adolescents: the future. *J Hypertens.* 2000;18:1351–1354.
2. National High Blood Pressure Education Program Working Group on Hypertension Control in Children and Adolescents. Update on the Task Force (1987) on High Blood Pressure in Children and Adolescents: A working group from the National High Blood Pressure Education Program. *Pediatrics.* 1996;98:649–658.
3. Proceedings from the Houston symposium on Ambulatory Blood Pressure Monitoring in the Pediatric Population. *Blood Pressure Monit.* 1999;4:105–205.
4. Sinaiko AR. Hypertension in children. *N Engl J Med.* 1996;335:1968–1973.
5. Sinaiko AR, Steinberger J, Moran A, et al. Relation of insulin resistance to blood pressure in children. *J Hypertens.* 2002;20:509–518.
6. Task Force on Blood Pressure Control in Children. Report of the Second Task Force on Blood Pressure Control in Children—1987. *Pediatrics.* 1987;79:1–25.

Ethnicity and Socioeconomic Status in Hypertension

John M. Flack, MD, MPH; Samar A. Nasser, MS, PA-C

KEY POINTS

- Epidemiologic data consistently show a higher age-adjusted incidence and prevalence of hypertension in blacks than in whites; age-adjusted hypertension burden is similar between whites and Hispanics.

- Aggregate comparisons of various ethnic groups on mean blood pressure levels and hypertension risk are confounded by differences in average age, geographic factors, socioeconomic status, and other lifestyle attributes.

- Blood pressure control rates are slightly higher in blacks than in whites and considerably higher in both these groups than in Hispanics; blood pressure control rates within each ethnic group are usually higher in women than in men.

- Blood pressure levels and overall cardiovascular disease burden are higher in lower socioeconomic status women of all 3 major ethnic groups.

See also Chapters B79, B80, B86, B89, B90, B100, B102, B108, C136, and C167

Increasing blood pressure (BP), particularly systolic BP (SBP) occurs commonly with advancing age in industrialized countries such as the United States, with the lifetime risk of hypertension for most Americans probably exceeding 70%. Despite improvements in the treatment and control of hypertension in recent years, ethnic disparities remain within the United States. There are persistent differences in health status experienced by ethnic minority and low socioeconomic status (SES) groups with an inverse relationship between SES and hypertension prevalence.

Ethnic Patterns and Age

Cross-sectional data from the first phase of the Third National Health and Nutrition Examination Survey (NHANES III) (**Figure B88.1**), which evaluated 9,901 participants (non-Hispanic whites, non-Hispanic blacks, and Mexican Americans), men and women, 18 years and older, from 1988 to 1991, indicated that 24% (or at least 43 million persons) of the noninstitutionalized adult U.S. population have hypertension (Figure B88.1). The overall prevalence of hypertension reported in the survey was slightly greater among men than among women (24.7% and 23.4%, respectively), and age-adjusted hypertension prevalence was higher in non-Hispanic blacks than in non-Hispanic whites and Mexican Americans (32.4%, 23.3%, and 22.6%, respectively). For both men and women, non-Hispanic blacks had the highest mean SBP until the end of the fifth decade. Between the sixth and seventh decades, Mexican-American men had the highest mean SBP level. Among women, non-Hispanic blacks had the highest mean SBP until the end of the sixth decade; thereafter, all 3 ethnic groups had similar mean levels of SBP. In comparison, mean diastolic BP (DBP) levels in men and women of all 3 ethnic groups gradually increased from early adulthood through the fifth decade but plateaued and subsequently declined with advancing age. Over the last 3 decades, the average BP differential for black and white adults has narrowed considerably.

Blacks. Blacks collectively have a higher prevalence of hypertension than whites, with severe hypertension (>180/110 mm Hg) being approximately 8.5 times more prevalent among blacks than whites. The excess rate of hypertension in blacks is greatest at younger ages, particularly in women, and declines progressively with advancing age. Mean BP levels are higher in black men than non-black men at all ages until 70 years of age. In women, mean BP levels are higher in blacks than non-blacks at all ages, although the differential narrows with advancing age. This ethnic differential in hypertension rates and premature hypertension onset probably results, in part, from a greater prevalence of obesity and lower levels of physical activity in blacks, particularly among women. Other factors possibly contributing to higher levels of hypertension in blacks include lower potassium and calcium intakes, lower levels of physical activity, greater exposure to psychosocial stressors, and, perhaps, greater salt sensitivity. The impact of genetic factors on interethnic hypertension differentials has not been elucidated and therefore remains speculative.

Hispanics. Hispanics, a rapidly growing heterogeneous group, are currently the second largest minority population in the United States. The Hispanic share of the population is projected to increase significantly over the 1995 to 2025 time frame, accounting for 44% of all the U.S. population growth (32 million Hispanics out of a total of 72 million persons added to the nation's population). Although the overall prevalence of hypertension among Mexican Americans was similar during 1982 to 1984 and 1988 to 1991, age- and sex-specific prevalences suggest a slight downward trend (except among men aged 40 to 49 years). Accordingly, this is a finding consistent with an overall decline in the prevalence of hypertension in the United States. Although the data for Hispanics do not indicate an excess population disease burden, socioeconomic factors likely place many Hispanics at significant disadvantage for optimal hypertension detection and management.

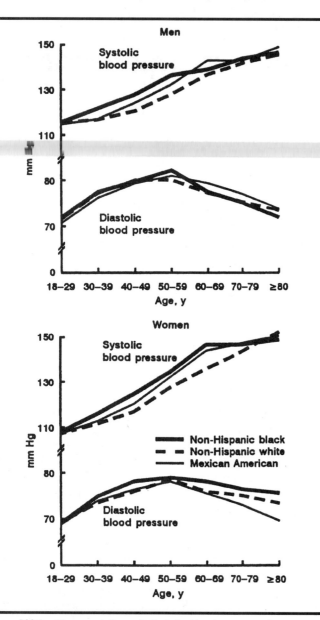

Figure B88.1. Mean systolic and diastolic blood pressures by age and race/ethnicity for men and women, U.S. population 18 years of age and older. (From Burt VL, Whelton P, Roccella, EJ, et al. Prevalence of hypertension in the US adult population. Results from the Third National Health and Nutrition Examination Survey, 1988–1991. *Hypertension.* 1995;25:305–313.)

Geography and Urbanization

Geographic location influences hypertension risk (see Chapters B79 and B80). A recent report from the Coronary Artery Risk Development in Young Adults (CARDIA) study on a cohort of more than 5,000 black and white men and women, aged 18 to 30 years, studied at 4 clinical centers located in different regions of the country, reported on hypertension prevalence and incidence over 7 years. There was no difference in hypertension prevalence at baseline. Nevertheless, over 7 years of follow-up, differences in hypertension incidence and prevalence emerged; at the 7-year follow-up visit, hypertension prevalence differed significantly by region (Birmingham, AL, 14%; Oakland, CA, 11.2%; Minneapolis, MN, 7%; and Chicago, IL, 6.6%). Also at the 7-year follow-up, hypertension prevalence in

black and white men was 9% to 5%, respectively, in Chicago and 25% to 14%, respectively, in Birmingham. Among women, elevated BP did not differ significantly by regional center, but hypertension prevalence was highest in black and white women in the Birmingham cohort. Regional dietary intake habits may contribute, at least in part, to these regional differences in hypertension. Accordingly, CARDIA participants in the Birmingham clinic had the highest level of dietary sodium intake, as well as the lowest consumption of potassium and magnesium, a trend that was present in both black and white participants. The Strong Heart Study (SHS) was a longitudinal study of cardiovascular disease (CVD) and its risk factors in 4,549 American Indians involving Arizona, southwestern Oklahoma, and regions of South and North Dakota. The SHS reported prevalence rates of hypertension in American Indians residing in Arizona and Oklahoma were similar to the rates for whites, but rates were lower for Indians living in the Dakotas.

Diet and Socioeconomic Status

SES indicators (e.g., education and income) function as surrogate markers of a constellation of lifestyle characteristics, including diet, physical activity, psychosocial and environmental stressors, social support, coping mechanisms, and health-seeking behaviors, as well as access to health-related information and medical care.

Salt intake and socioeconomic status. The Treatment of Mild Hypertension Study (TOMHS) was a multicenter, randomized, double-blind, placebo-controlled clinical trial evaluating the efficacy of different classes of antihypertensive agents in 902 men and women, aged 45 to 69 years, with stage I diastolic hypertension. Analyses of baseline TOMHS data showed discrepant levels of urinary Na^+ and $Na^+:K^+$ ratio in blacks and whites that correlated to socioeconomic differences. Higher levels of urinary Na^+ levels and $Na^+:K^+$ ($p < .001$ and $p < .05$, respectively) were documented for individuals of lower income and education attainment among blacks, but not among whites. The higher urinary Na^+ levels and $Na^+:K^+$ ratio in lower SES TOMHS blacks represent a pattern of dietary electrolyte intake that, if present in the black population at large, would be a contributing factor to the excessive incidence and prevalence of hypertension as well as pressure-related target-organ damage (e.g., stroke, left ventricular hypertrophy, and proteinuria).

Ethnicity and Socioeconomic Status

In 1998, Winkleby et al. reported data from NHANES III to determine whether differences among women in CVD risk factors by ethnicity could be attributed to differences in SES. The findings, based on a national sample of 1,762 black, 1,481 Mexican-American, and 2,023 white women, support the idea that multiple factors influence the risk of developing elevated BP. Winkleby et al. reported that black and Mexican-American women had steeper upward slopes of BP with advancing age than white women, resulting in progressively larger ethnic differences at older ages (the black-white difference of 4 mm Hg at ages 25 to 34 years increased to 11 mm Hg at ages 55 to 65 years). In addition, black and Hispanic women had a higher prevalence of CVD risk factors—BP, body mass index, physical inactivity, and diabetes—than white women even after adjustment for education.

Also, lower SES women from all 3 ethnic groups had significantly higher prevalences of smoking, physical inactivity, and higher non–high-density lipoprotein cholesterol and body mass index than higher SES women of the same ethnic group.

Confounder of ethnic associations. Aggregate comparisons of various ethnic groups on mean BP levels and hypertension risk are, to some degree, confounded by different average levels of SES indicators, such as income and education. Moreover, anthropometric measures, such as obesity, which correlate with low SES, especially in women, can also influence biologic systems that are involved in BP regulation and the expression of pressure-related target-organ damage. For example, obesity is a major anthropometric correlate of salt sensitivity in blacks and whites and is extremely prevalent among lower SES persons, particularly women. Cooper and co-workers reported data documenting positive association between obesity and both serum angiotensin-converting enzyme and angiotensinogen levels. This observation represents a potential mechanism through which obesity might contribute to elevated BP as well as to pressure-related target-organ damage. These data also highlight the complex interrelationships of ethnicity, SES, and body size with biologic mechanisms likely to be involved in BP regulation.

Psychosocial Factors and Socioeconomic Status

Psychosocial factors correlated with lower SES may also contribute to the excess risk of developing elevated BP and to the disparity of hypertension incidence of prevalence among blacks and whites. Strogatz and colleagues examined the relationship between social support and perceived stress with BP in a cross-sectional, community-based sample of 1,784 black men and women, aged 25 to 50 years, living in the southeastern United States. After adjustment for age, obesity, and waist to hip ratio, separate analyses of emotional support, instrumental support, and perceived stress, there was an inverse association of support and a direct association of stress with BP that was stronger for SBP than DBP. Differences in SBP associated with low support and high stress ranged from 3.6 to 5.2 mm Hg in women and 2.5 to 3.5 mm Hg in men. These data suggest that chronic stress, low SES, and low social support may contribute to the development of hypertension among blacks. An additional study by Krieger and Sidney examined the relationship between self-reported experience of racial discrimination and BP and the contribution of racial discrimination to explain black-white disparities in elevated BP. The results indicate that racial discrimination likely affects patterns of BP among the U.S. black population and black-white differences on BP. The study consisted of individuals who were enrolled in the CARDIA study and included 4,086 black and white women and men 25 to 37 years old. A self-administered questionnaire was used to elicit experiences of racial discrimination and unfair treatment. Both working class and professional blacks had SBP that ranged from 7 to 10 mm Hg higher if they did not challenge discriminatory or unfair treatment or if they reported that they never experienced discriminatory treatment in any of the 7 situations about which they were queried. These data suggest that internalizing discriminatory or unfair treatment leads to higher levels of SBP among blacks in the 25- to 37-year-old age range.

Education

Aggregate measures of an individual's attainment of durable goods appear to have a role in the relationship between education and BP. A recent study by Kaufman and colleagues suggests interactions between possession of material goods and level of education among populations of African origin in the United States, Africa, and the Caribbean. Unlike previously reported associations between education and hypertension in the United States, in this report, education was actually associated with a greater, not lesser, risk of hypertension among Caribbean women (odds ratio 1.69, confidence interval, 1.15–2.48). In the First National Health and Nutrition Examination Study (NHANES I) Epidemiologic Follow-up Study (NHEFS), Vargas and co-workers found that the incidence rate for hypertension was higher among persons with less than 12 years of education versus those with more than 12 years of education for all demographic groups.

Income

According to Winkleby et al., the rate of black and Mexican-American women with more than 12 years of education who were living in poverty was more than twice the rate observed in white women (18.9% and 18.6% vs. 7.1%), suggesting a different relationship between education and income among women of color. According to the U.S. Department of Health and Human Services from 1988 to 1994, the prevalence of hypertension was 26% to 27% for poor, near poor, and middle-income men, whereas for men with high family incomes, there was a lower prevalence of hypertension (22%). On the other hand, there was a significant income-related gradient in hypertension prevalence among women, which ranged from 31% for poor women to 19% for high-income women.

Ethnic Patterns of Blood Pressure Control

Over the past 2 decades, the number of Americans aware of their hypertensive condition has increased. Data from NHANES III indicated that overall hypertension awareness was greatest among non-Hispanic blacks (74%) and non-Hispanic whites (70%) compared with the younger Mexican-American population (54%). Aside from Hispanics exhibiting lower awareness of their hypertension than either non-Hispanic white or black adults, according to Sudano and colleagues, they also have a lower rate of antihypertensive medication use. According to Crespo and co-workers, Hispanic women are more aware of their hypertension than men, and the percentage of hypertensive women under treatment and with controlled BP was greater than among men. Nevertheless, BP is not adequately controlled in the large majority of hypertensives of any racial/ethnic group. Hypertension control rates (<140/90 mm Hg) are highest among non-Hispanic blacks and non-Hispanic whites, and lowest among Mexican Americans (25%, 24%, and 14%, respectively). Non-Hispanic black women have the highest levels of hypertension awareness, treatment, and control (79%, 65%, and 29%, respectively).

Poor BP control may be an important factor contributing to the high rate of pressure-related complications among blacks in the southeastern United States. Approximately one-half of adult U.S. blacks reside in 13 southeastern states. Thus, race/ethnic contrasts involving U.S. blacks is, to a degree, influenced by geography. Interestingly, the risk of stroke death among blacks varies by geographic region; rates are ~50% higher in blacks residing in the Southeast as compared to their white counterparts living in the same region. Accordingly, Svetkey and colleagues reported a cross-sectional population survey of 4,162 men and women, aged 65 years and older, who resided in mostly rural areas of North Carolina. Among treated hypertensives, women were 52% more likely than men to have adequate BP control (DBP ≤90 mm Hg), and blacks were 40% less likely than whites to have adequate BP control. This black/white difference is directly opposite of the previously mentioned national survey.

SUGGESTED READING

1. Bell AC, Adair LS, Popkin BM. Ethnic differences in the association between body mass index and hypertension. *Am J Epidemiol.* 2002;155: 346–353.
2. Flack JM, Neaton JD, Daniels B, Esunge P. Ethnicity and renal disease: lessons from the multiple Risk Factor Intervention trial and the Treatment of Mild Hypertension Study. *Am J Kidney Dis.* 1993;219:31–40.
3. Ganguli MC, Grimm RH Jr, Svendsen KH, et al. Higher education and income are related to a better Na:K ratio in blacks. Baseline results of the Treatment of Mild Hypertension Study (TOMHS) data. *Am J Hypertens.* 1997;10:979–984.
4. Kaufman JS, Tracy JA, Durazo-Arvizu RA, Cooper RS. Lifestyle, education, and prevalence of hypertension populations of African origin: results from the International Collaborative Study on Hypertension in Blacks. *Ann Epidemiol.* 1997;7:22–27.
5. Kiefe CI, Williams OD, Bild DE, et al. Regional disparities in the incidence of elevated blood pressure among young adults: the CARDIA study. *Circulation.* 1997;96:1082–1088.
6. Krieger N, Sidney S. Racial discrimination and blood pressure: the CARDIA study of young black and white adults. *Am J Public Health.* 1996;86:1370–1378.
7. Strogatz DS, Croft JB, James SA, et al. Social support, stress, and blocked pressure in black adults. *Epidemiology.* 1997;8:482–487.
8. U.S. Department of Health and Human Services. Health in America tied to income and education. 1998. Available at: http://www.cdc.gov/nchs/releases/98news/huspr98.htm. Accessed on October 29, 2002.
9. Vargas CM, Ingram DD, Gillum RF. Incidence of hypertension and educational attainment. *Am J Epidemiol.* 2000;152:272–278.
10. Winkleby MA, Kraemer HC, Ahn DK, Varady AN. Ethnic and socioeconomic differences in cardiovascular disease risk factors. *JAMA.* 1998;280:356–362.

Chapter B89

Hypertension in Blacks

Keith C. Ferdinand, MD

KEY POINTS

- Hypertension is more prevalent, begins earlier in life, and is of greater severity in blacks compared to non-blacks.

- Clinical trials have documented that blacks benefit from lifestyle modification and from appropriate pharmacologic therapy.

- Thiazide diuretics are useful as the first step of pharmacologic therapy in blacks with uncomplicated hypertension, but other agents can also be used effectively, especially when there are compelling indications such as coexisting cardiovascular or renal indications.

See also Chapters B79–B81, B84, B86, B88, B106, and C167

Blacks have one of the highest prevalence rates of hypertension in the world, with hypertension earlier in life, a higher prevalence of stage 3 hypertension, and greater risk for developing blood pressure (BP)–related target organ damage (heart failure, end-stage renal disease, fatal and nonfatal stroke, and overall heart disease). Hypertension is a predominant cause of the excess risk of morbidity and mortality from heart failure in this population.

Race as a Social Construct

Although medical researchers continue to use terms such as *race, racial groups, racial differences,* and *ethnic backgrounds,* the biologic basis for such classifications is uncertain. Race is best viewed as a social concept rather than a firm scientific construct. Furthermore, because of marked heterogeneity within groups, it is important not to consider race or ethnicity as a marker for individual responsiveness to antihypertensive therapies.

Etiologic factors in blacks. In blacks, elevated BP can be attributed to potentially modifiable lifestyle factors including increased body mass index, physical inactivity, inadequate potassium intake, and increased sodium intake. Whereas various biochemical and endocrine mechanisms have been hypothesized, a recent 7-population study of patients of West African decent, including African, Afro-Caribbean, and black populations, has highlighted the importance of lifestyle factors. Using standardized procedures, this study documented that elevated BP was more prevalent in the black population in comparison to the Afro-Caribbean and native African populations. The high prevalence of hypertension appeared to be related to increased body mass and a high ratio of sodium to potassium intake (as indicated by urinary electrolyte excretion).

Treatment Issues in Blacks

Lifestyle modification. Lifestyle modifications (population-based and individual) should particularly benefit blacks, in part because of the high prevalence of overweight, obesity, sedentary lifestyle, excess dietary sodium intake, and low potassium intake, along with excess consumption of alcohol. Much needs to be learned about the optimum strategy to accomplish the needed lifestyle modification. Potential settings include the traditional medical office for intensive counseling of high-risk patients, whereas population-based options include community centers such as senior centers and churches. Population-based programs should also include screening and referral of persons with elevated BP; in such persons, pharmacologic therapy in addition to lifestyle modification is typically warranted.

Clinical trials have documented the effects of lifestyle modifications in blacks. In phase 2 of the Trials of Hypertension Prevention, which included a large number of blacks, the weight loss intervention led to significant reductions in systolic and diastolic BP. As in previous trials, blacks tended to lose less weight than non-blacks. Still, BP reduction per kg of weight lost (0.45 mm Hg reduction in systolic BP and 0.35 mm Hg reduction in diastolic BP per kg lost) did not differ by race. Although large population surveys, including the International Study of Salt and Blood Pressure (INTERSALT), have not consistently demonstrated higher dietary sodium intake in blacks compared to whites, blacks often experience greater BP reductions from dietary changes such as lower sodium intake or increased potassium intake [Dietary Approaches to Stop Hypertension (DASH) diet]. In the initial DASH trial, the DASH diet, which is rich in fruits, vegetables, and low-fat dairy products and limits total and saturated fat, led to significantly greater BP reduction in blacks compared to whites (e.g., systolic BP reduction of 6.8 vs. 3.0). In the subsequent DASH-Sodium trial, which tested the effects of sodium reduction in 2 different diets, BP reductions from a lower sodium intake (~65 mmol/day) were consistently greater in blacks than whites.

Responses to drug therapy. Diuretics. In patients with uncomplicated hypertension, including blacks, the first step of pharmacologic therapy should usually be thiazide-type diuretics, which are efficacious in both blacks and whites. The addition of thiazide or loop diuretics increases the efficacy of angiotensin-converting enzyme (ACE) inhibitors, angiotensin receptor blockers (ARB), and β-adrenergic blockers. Use of diuretic therapy essentially removes any racial or ethnic differences in BP response when used in combination with agents.

The Antihypertensive Lipid Lowering in Heart Attack (ALLHAT) trial will report the cardiovascular effects of initial therapy with lisinopril, amlodipine, and chlorthalidone in a large cohort of 42,448 high-risk patients that includes 35% blacks. An interim analysis demonstrated reduced risk of combined cardiovascular events including heart failure with thiazide diuretics in comparison to doxazosin in the whole study population, including the black cohort. A recent study of the C825T polymorphism of the G protein β-subunit appears to identify those who respond better to diuretics. Systolic and diastolic BP reductions appear to be greater with diuretics among those with the TT versus CC homozygotes. Univariate analysis predicted a greater response to being black, female, higher pretreatment BP, age, lower waist to hip ratio, and lower renin-angiotensin-aldosterone activity.

Other agents. Calcium antagonists effectively lower BP in blacks, perhaps more so than monotherapy with ACE inhibitor, β-blockers, and ARBs. However, at present, none of the clinical outcome trials have enrolled sufficient numbers of blacks to assess the impact of ACE inhibitors and ARBs on cardiovascular morbidity and mortality in this population.

Monotherapy with agents that modulate the renin-angiotensin-aldosterone system appears to be less effective at reducing BP in blacks compared to whites. Still, ACE inhibitors, β-blockers and, potentially, ARBs remain attractive choices in blacks because of their potential benefits on higher rates of end-organ damage, specifically renal disease with or without diabetes, left ventricular hypertrophy, left ventricular systolic dysfunction, and heart failure. Still, as noted earlier, the addition of a diuretic or of sodium reduction greatly enhances the efficacy of ACE inhibitors in blacks. Also, BP lowering response can be achieved with higher doses of ACE inhibitors. This phenomenon was demonstrated in a recent trial with trandolapril in which black hypertensives appeared to require 2 to 4 times the dose of ACE inhibitor versus similar age- and sex-matched white hypertensives.

Outcome studies. Few trials have documented the effects of ACE inhibitors on clinical outcomes in blacks. The recently reported African-American Study of Kidney Disease (AASK) documented the effects of ramipril versus amlodipine on renal outcomes in hypertensive blacks with nephrosclerosis. Among participants with urinary protein/creatinine ratio greater than 0.22 (corresponding to approximately 300 mg/day of proteinuria), the ramipril group had a 36% slower mean decline in glomerular filtration rate over 3 years and 48% reduction in risk of clinical end points compared to the amlodipine group.

In hypertensives with heart failure, secondary analyses of some trials have suggested that treatment with ACE inhibitors may be less beneficial in blacks than in whites. The potential for inadequate dosing in these studies clouds the interpretation, however. In contrast, recent analyses have demonstrated equal benefits with the use of carvedilol.

Adverse effects. One potential barrier to the use of drug therapy with ACE inhibitor in blacks is the increased risk of angioedema, perhaps 2 to 5 times higher in blacks than U.S. whites. This side effect profile may lead to frequent discontinuation of ACE inhibitor therapy in blacks. Although angioedema is a rare complication, it may be higher in blacks perhaps because of a greater sensitivity to bradykinin. Accordingly, a recent American Diabetes Association position statement suggested that in hypertensive type 2 diabetic patients with microalbuminuria or clinical albuminuria, ARBs are the initial agents of choice. Yet these agents were studied primarily in white populations, and the benefits of ARBs for renal and cardiovascular protection have not yet been conclusively confirmed in blacks.

SUGGESTED READING

1. Agodoa L, Appel L, Barkis G, et al. Effects of ramipril versus amlodipine on renal outcomes on hypertensive nephrosclerosis. A randomized controlled trial. *JAMA* 2001;285:2719–2728.
2. ALLHAT Collaborative Research Group. Major Cardiovascular Events in Hypertensive Patients Randomized to Doxazosin Versus Chlorthalidone: The Antihypertensive and Lipid Lowering Treatment to Prevent Heart Attack Trial (ALLHAT). *JAMA.* 2000;283:1967–1975.
3. American Diabetes Association. Diabetic Nephropathy. *Diabetes Care.* 2002;25:S85–S89.
4. Clark L, Ferdinand K, Flack J, Gavin J III. Coronary heart disease in African Americans. *Heart Dis.* 2001;3:97–108.

5. Cooper R, Rotimi C. Hypertension in blacks. *Am J Hypertens.* 1997;10:804–812.

6. Ferdinand K. New approaches to pharmacologic treatment of hypertension. *The Cardiology Clinics: Annual of Drug Therapy.* 1999;3:63–80.

7. Papademetriou V. Selection of antihypertensive therapy in patients with hypertensive renal disease. [Editorial] *JAMA.* 2001; 285:2774–2776.

8. Schwartz RS. Racial profiling in medical research. [Editorial] *N Engl J Med.* 2001;344:1392–1393.

9. The Trials of Hypertension Prevention Collaborative Research Group. Effects of weight loss and sodium reduction intervention on blood pressure and hypertension incidence in overweight people with high-normal blood pressure. The Trials of Hypertension Prevention, Phase II. *Arch Intern Med.* 2001;134:1–11.

10. Turner ST, Schwartz GL, Chapman AB, Boerwinkle E. C825T polymorphism of the G protein β_3-subunit and antihypertensive response to a thiazide diuretic. *Hypertension.* 2001;37:739–743.

Chapter B90

Hypertension in Hispanic Americans

Carlos J. Crespo, PhD, MS; Ellen Smit, PhD; Mario R. Garcia Palmieri, MD

KEY POINTS

- Heart disease remains the leading cause of death in Hispanics.

- Hypertension among Hispanics varies by gender and by country of origin.

- Despite a greater prevalence of obesity and diabetes, the prevalence of hypertension in Hispanics is lower than that of the general population.

See also Chapters B79, B80, B88, B97, B102, B106, C164, and C167

Hispanics constitute approximately 13% of the general population of the United States. Hispanics are a heterogeneous group of subpopulations that share the common bond of the Spanish language, and each subgroup has racial, ethnic, and cultural characteristics that distinguish it from other Hispanic subgroups. The largest Hispanic subgroups in the United States are Mexican Americans, Puerto Ricans, and Cuban Americans, but persons with ethnic backgrounds from Central and South America and the Caribbean combined make a significant portion of the total Hispanic population. Social and economic disadvantages, compounded with language barriers, have made it very difficult for Hispanics to obtain comparable preventive and primary health care services.

Coronary Heart Disease in Hispanics

Heart disease continues to be the leading cause of death in Hispanics, but the decline in heart disease mortality rates observed in the general population in recent years has occurred to a much lesser extent among Hispanics. Also, progress in the percent reduction in the prevalence of hypertension observed in non-Hispanic whites and non-Hispanic blacks has not been observed in Mexican Americans. Coronary heart disease and other chronic diseases are expected to increase among Hispanics over the next 20 years as this population ages. Mean age of Hispanics is less than whites in the United States; the relative young age of Hispanics presents the opportunity to intervene with preventive measures to modify risk factors and prevent cardiovascular disease in this popula-tion. Mortality from coronary heart disease and stroke also differs according to Hispanic subgroup (**Figure B90.1**). Mexican Americans represent more than two-thirds of the Hispanic population, so estimates for all Hispanics are more representative of Mexican Americans than other subgroups. **Figures** B90.1 and **B90.2** show that Puerto Ricans living in the United States have age-adjusted coronary heart disease and stroke mortality rates that are higher than those observed for other Hispanics and the general population.

Hypertension in Hispanics

Hypertension among Hispanics varies by gender and by country of origin. Despite a greater prevalence of obesity and diabetes, the prevalence of hypertension in Hispanics is lower than that of the general population. Most of the literature report hypertension rates in Mexican Americans and Puerto Ricans, with limited data among Cuban Americans. The Hispanic Health and Nutrition Examination Survey (HHANES) was conducted between 1982 and 1984 by the National Center for Health Statistics, Centers for Disease Control and Prevention. HHANES sampled Mexican Americans in the southwest part of the United States, Puerto Ricans in the New York City metropolitan area, and Cuban Americans in Miami, Dade County, FL. **Tables B90.1** and **B90.2** show the prevalence status of hypertension and its respective awareness treatment and control levels. The observed disparities in awareness, treatment, and control of hypertension warrant attention and an educational campaign targeted to members of different gender and ethnic subgroups.

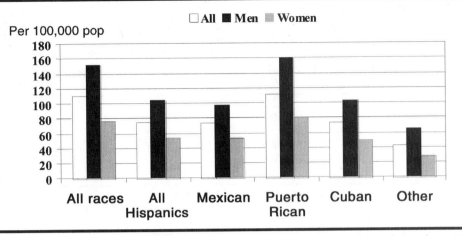

Figure B90.1. Mortality from coronary heart disease among Hispanics in the United States, 1994. pop, population. (From National Center for Health Statistics, Healthy People 2000 Progress Review. Personal Communication, June 24, 1997.)

The San Antonio Heart Study observed similar findings as HHANES. Despite higher frequency of obesity and type 2 diabetes mellitus in Mexican Americans, hypertension rates were lower than in non-Hispanic whites. Mexican-American men and women, however, suffered from poor control of their hypertension [systolic blood pressure (BP) ≥160 mm Hg or diastolic BP ≥95 mm Hg]. Findings from hypertension data in Mexican Americans from Starr County in Texas show different results. Starr County is on the border between Texas and Mexico, with approximately 97% of the residents reported being of Mexican descent. Prevalence of hypertension by age and gender were elevated in this population group compared with those in the general population. These differences, concluded the authors, are not simple functions of measurement protocols, but are likely to be caused by differences in population structure, employment, and socioeconomic status.

Social and Cultural Factors

The Mexico City Diabetes Study examined diabetes and cardiovascular disease in men and women, age 35 to 64 years, and provided comparative data on people of Mexican origin living in Mexico City and San Antonio, TX. After careful analysis of social and economic indicators in these 2 groups, hypertension in men of Mexican origin living in Mexico City and San Antonio has a biphasic curve related to modernization. This suggests that modernization affects health until a transition point is reached, after which modernization is beneficial to health. This biphasic pattern was not observed in women, however; modernization and education among women were consistently inversely associated with systolic and diastolic BP.

The San Luis Valley Diabetes Study found no differences in hypertension between nondiabetic rural Hispanics and non-Hispanic whites in Colorado. The risk of hypertension in diabetic Hispanics was somewhat lower than in non-Hispanic white diabetics. The Stanford Five-City Project reported hypertension results from 7,087 non-Hispanic white and 933 Hispanics, ages 25 to 74 years, from 5 separate cross-sectional surveys conducted biennially from 1979 to 1990. Significant differences were observed among the groups, with higher levels of hypertension (29%) reported among non-Hispanic whites

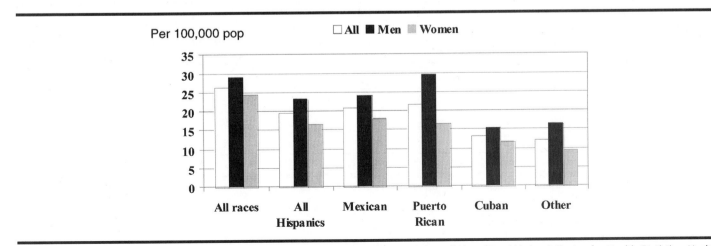

Figure B90.2. Mortality from stroke among Hispanics in the United States, 1994. pop, population. (From National Center for Health Statistics, Healthy People 2000 Progress Review. Personal Communication, June 24, 1997.)

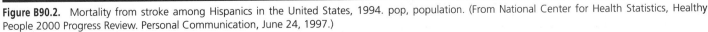

Table B90.1. Age-Adjusted Prevalence of Hypertension; Awareness, Treatment, and Control of Hypertension; and High Blood Pressure Distribution among Mexican Americans, Cuban Americans, and Puerto Ricans Ages 18 to 74 Years from the Hispanic Health and Nutrition Examination Survey

RACE/ETHNICITY	SEX	AGE (YR)	SAMPLE SIZE (N)	PREVALENCE[a] (%)	AWARE[b] (%)	TREATMENT[c] (%)	CONTROL[d] (%)	STAGE 1[e] (%)	STAGE 2–4[f] (%)
Mexican Americans	Men	35	1,554	22.7	40	16	8	15	6
	Women	37	1,964	19.2	76	55	34	11	3
Cuban Americans	Men	43	401	20.0	40	33	0	13	5
	Women	44	497	13.6	91	41	14	7	4
Puerto Ricans	Men	37	495	20.4	6	19	9	13	6
	Women	36	835	17.6	66	43	28	9	4

[a]Hypertension is defined as systolic or diastolic blood pressure greater than or equal to 140/90 or currently on antihypertensive medication.
[b]Aware is defined as hypertensives who have been told by a physician or health professional that they have high blood pressure or hypertension.
[c]Treatment is defined as hypertensives who are currently on antihypertensive medication.
[d]Control is defined as hypertensives who are currently treated and who have mean blood pressures less than 140/90 mm Hg.
[e]Stage 1 is defined as mean systolic blood pressure distribution between 140 to159 mm Hg or mean diastolic blood pressure between 90 and 99 mm Hg, regardless of medication.
[f]Stage 2 to 4 is defined as mean systolic blood pressure ≥160 mm Hg or diastolic blood pressure ≥100 mm Hg, regardless of medication.
Adapted from Crespo CJ, Loria CM, Burt VL. Hypertension and other cardiovascular disease risk factors among Mexican Americans, Cuban Americans, and Puerto Ricans from the Hispanic Health and Nutrition Examination Survey. *Public Health Rep.* 1996;111:7–10, with permission.

(22.9% among Hispanic men and women). Further adjustment of the data by matched pairs by sociodemographic factors showed no significant differences between the groups. The findings stressed the need to consider social and economic indicators when examining ethnic differences in BP.

Puerto Rico

The Puerto Rico Heart Health Program examined risk factors, morbidity, and mortality of coronary heart disease among Hispanics living on the island of Puerto Rico. Urban men had higher average BP than rural men and systolic BP showed increasing mean values with increasing education in the rural and urban areas. The mean value of systolic BP increased by approximately 8 mm Hg when comparing those with no educa-tion with those with a high school education or higher. This inverse relationship is not consistent with other findings from the United States. The implication is that the urban and more educated Puerto Rican men may have adopted lifestyles that were more conducive to increased systolic BP and other coronary heart disease risk factors than their less acculturated counterparts, a finding that concurs with the biphasic curve observed in the Mexico City Diabetes Study. Dark-skinned Puerto Rican men had a higher prevalence of definite and possible left ventricular hypertrophy (assessed by electrocardiogram) than light-skinned Puerto Rican men. Among persons younger than 45 years of age, the prevalence of hypertension in Puerto Rico is twice (8.1%) the rate observed in the United States (4.2%). Deaths caused by heart disease have also been

Table B90.2. Age-Adjusted Mean Body Mass Index and Prevalence of Overweight, Overweight among Hypertensives, High Serum Cholesterol, Smoking, and the Combination of Hypertension plus High Serum Cholesterol and Hypertension plus Smoking among Mexican Americans, Cuban Americans, and Mainland Puerto Ricans Ages 20 to 74 Years from the Hispanic Health and Nutrition Examination Survey

RACE/ETHNICITY GROUP	SEX	BODY MASS INDEX[a]	PREVALENCE OF OVER-WEIGHT[b] (%)	OVERWEIGHT BY HYPERTENSION YES[c] (%)	OVERWEIGHT BY HYPERTENSION NO[d] (%)	HIGH SERUM CHOLESTEROL[e] (%)	SMOKING[f] (%)	HYPERTENSION PLUS HIGH CHOLESTEROL[e] (%)	HYPERTENSION PLUS SMOKING[f] (%)
Mexican Americans	Men	26.1	30.6	48	26	18.5	43.4	5.6	9.2
	Women	27.0	41.8	63	40	19.4	23.8	7.0	3.3
Cuban Americans	Men	26.0	28.0	60	25	15.2	41.8	7.0	7.7
	Women	25.5	31.4	74	29	16.0	25.8	6.0	2.3
Puerto Ricans	Men	25.8	25.3	39	24	17.1	40.9	6.3	5.6
	Women	26.6	40.0	44	38	20.6	31.4	7.2	3.0

[a]Body mass index is defined as weight in kilograms divided by height in meters squared.
[b]Men are considered overweight if their body mass index is ≥27.8; women are considered overweight if their body mass index is ≥27.3.
[c]Percent of men and women with high blood pressure (systolic blood pressure or diastolic blood pressure≥140/90 mm Hg or currently taking antihypertensive medication) who are overweight.
[d]Percent of normotensives (not taking antihypertensive medication and systolic blood pressure and diastolic blood pressure <140/90 mm Hg) who are overweight.
[e]High serum cholesterol is defined as serum cholesterol levels ≥240 mg/dL.
[f]Smoking based on self-reported data of smoking 1 or more cigarettes a day.
Adapted from Crespo CJ, Loria CM, Burt VL. Hypertension and other cardiovascular disease risk factors among Mexican Americans, Cuban Americans, and Puerto Ricans from the Hispanic Health and Nutrition Examination Survey. *Public Health Rep.* 1996;111:7–10, with permission.

increasing in Puerto Rico by approximately 72% since 1960, whereas in the United States, mortality from coronary heart disease and stroke has been declining during the last 25 years. Concomitantly, end-stage renal disease in Puerto Rico is higher than any other Latin American country.

SUGGESTED READING

1. Crespo CJ, Loria CM, Burt VL. Hypertension and other cardiovascular disease risk factors among Mexican Americans, Cuban Americans, and Puerto Ricans from the Hispanic Health and Nutrition Examination Survey. *Public Health Rep.* 1996;111:7–10.
2. Garcia-Palmieri MR, Sorlie PD, Havlik RJ, et al. Urban-rural differences in 12 year coronary heart disease mortality: the Puerto Rico Heart Health Program. *J Clin Epidemiol.* 1988;41:285–292.
3. Haffner SM. Hypertension in the San Antonio Heart Study and the Mexico City Diabetes Study: clinical and metabolic correlates. *Public Health Rep.* 1996;111:11–14.
4. Hanis CL. Hypertension among Mexican Americans in Starr County, Texas. *Public Health Rep.* 1996;111:15–17.
5. Hazuda HP. Hypertension in the San Antonio Heart Study and the Mexico City Diabetes Study: sociocultural correlates. *Public Health Rep.* 1996; 111:18–21.
6. Rewers M, Shetterly SM, Hamman RF. Hypertension among rural Hispanics and non-Hispanic whites: the San Luis Valley Diabetes Study. *Public Health Rep.* 1996;111:27–29.
7. Sica DA, Cangiano JL. Hypertension and renal disease in Puerto Ricans. *Am J Med Sci.* 1999;318:369–373.
8. Sorlie PD, Garcia-Palmieri MR. Left ventricular hypertrophy among dark- and light-skinned Puerto Rican men: the Puerto Rico Heart Health Program. *Am Heart J.* 1988;111:777–783.
9. Sorlie PD, Garcia-Palmieri MR. Education status and coronary heart disease in Puerto Rico: the Puerto Rico Heart Health Program. *Int J Epidemiol.* 1990;19:59–65.
10. Winkleby MA, Kramer H, Lin J, et al. Sociodemographic influences on Hispanic-White differences in blood pressure. *Public Health Rep.* 1996;111:30–32.

Chapter B91

Hypertension in South Asians

Prakash C. Deedwania, MD; Rajeev Gupta, MD, FACC

KEY POINTS

- Hypertension is a major public health problem in the Indian subcontinent and among South Asians worldwide.
- In India, the prevalence of hypertension is lower in rural compared to urban populations.
- The prevalence of hypertension in emigrant South Asians residing in Western countries is high but may be similar to other populations in these countries.
- The prevalence of hypertension is increasing in South Asians in proportion to the degree of urbanization.

See also Chapters A78, B79, B92, and B97

Hypertension is a major public health problem in the Indian subcontinent and among South Asians worldwide. Although large population-based prospective studies have not been conducted, available data indicate that the prevalence of hypertension is increasing substantially in these populations.

India

The World Health Organization (WHO) reported that hypertension is an important public health problem in developing countries. This WHO report also emphasized that in adults aged 40 to 55 years, blood pressure (BP) levels were the highest among Indian men in comparison to those of 20 other developing countries. The International Clinical Epidemiology Network study using WHO criteria documented that the prevalence of hypertension was more than 20% among 6 of the 12 communities studied in different parts of Asia and Latin America.

Recent studies among Indians have shown a high prevalence of hypertension in urban and rural areas. Prevalence rates are almost similar to those in the United States. Trends of hypertension prevalence in Indian urban and rural populations, aged 20 to 70 years, from several epidemiologic studies are displayed in **Table B91.1**. Indian urban population studies in the mid-1950s reported hypertension prevalence of 1.2% to 4.0%. Subsequent studies that used the standardized WHO guidelines for the diagnosis of hypertension (known hypertension, systolic BP $\geq$160 or diastolic BP $\geq$95 mm Hg) show a steadily increasing trend in hypertension prevalence: 4.35% in Agra (1961), 6.43% in Rohtak (1975), 15.52% in Bombay (1980), 14.08% in Ludhiana (1985), 10.99% in Jaipur (1995), and 11.59% in Delhi (1997) **(Figure B91.1)**. The prevalence of hypertension defined by Joint National Committee V criteria also shows a steep increase from 6.2% (Delhi, 1959) to 30.9% (Jaipur, 1995), 44.0% (Mumbai, 1999), and 36% (Chennai, 2001).

Although the prevalence of hypertension is lower in rural compared to urban Indian populations, there has been a steady increase in hypertension over time in rural and urban regions: 0.52% in Bombay (1959), 1.99% in Delhi (1959), 3.57% in Haryana (1978), 5.41% in Delhi (1983), 5.59% in Rajasthan (1984),

Table B91.1. Indian Hypertension Prevalence Studies (Blood Pressure ≥160/95 mm Hg)

FIRST AUTHOR	YEAR PUBLISHED	AGE GROUP	PLACE	SAMPLE SIZE	PREVALENCE (% ± STANDARD ERROR)
			Urban		
Dotto BB	1949	18–50	Calcutta	2,500	1.24 ± 0.2
Dubey VD	1954	18–60	Kanpur	2,262	4.24 ± 0.4
Sathe RV	1959	20–80	Bombay	4,120	3.03 ± 0.3
Mathur KS	1963	20–80	Agra	1,634	4.35 ± 0.5
Malhotra SL	1971	30–58	Railways	4,333	0.34 ± 0.4
Gupta SP	1970	20–69	Rohtak	2,023	6.43 ± 0.5
Dalal PM	1980	20–80	Bombay	5,723	15.52 ± 0.5
Sharma BK	1985	20–75	Ludhiana	1,008	14.08 ± 1.1
Gupta R	1995	20–80	Jaipur	2,212	10.99 ± 0.7
Chadha SL	1998	25–69	Delhi	13,134	11.59 ± 1.0
			Rural		
Shah VV	1959	30–60	Bombay	5,996	0.52 ± 0.1
Padmavati S	1959	20–75	Delhi	1,052	1.99 ± 0.4
Gupta SP	1977	20–69	Haryana	2,045	3.57 ± 0.4
Wasir HS	1983	20–69	Delhi	905	5.41 ± 0.8
Baldwa VS	1984	21–60	Rajasthan	912	5.59 ± 0.8
Sharma BK	1985	20–75	Punjab	3,340	2.63 ± 0.3
Kumar V	1991	21–70	Rajasthan	6,840	3.83 ± 0.2
Joshi PP	1993	16–60	Maharashtra	448	4.02 ± 0.9
Jajoo UN	1993	20–69	Maharashtra	4,045	3.41 ± 0.3
Gupta R	1994	20–80	Rajasthan	3,148	7.08 ± 0.5
Chadha SL	1998	25–69	Delhi	1,732	3.58 ± 0.5

2.63% in Punjab (1985), 4.02% in Maharashtra (1993), 3.41% in Maharashtra (1993), 7.08% in Rajasthan (1994), and 3.58% in Delhi (1998). In South Indian urbanized rural subjects, hypertension prevalence has been reported to be as high as 17.8% (1993) and 12.46% (1994). Overall, there is a significant increase in hypertension prevalence in rural areas, although the rise is not as steep as in urban populations. This increasing trend remains after exclusion of Kerala studies that show a disproportionately high prevalence of hypertension (**Figure B91.2**). The increased prevalence of hypertension, along with the rising rates of diabetes and dyslipidemia, has dire public health consequences, including a potential epidemic of coronary artery disease in India.

Other South Asian Populations

Data from other South Asian countries are sparse. A study in Nepal in the early 1980s reported hypertension in 10% of urban subjects. In Bangladesh, a recent study reported hypertension in less than 5% of rural subjects.

Emigrant South Asians report a similar high prevalence of hypertension. In Britain, population prevalence studies have reported hypertension prevalence similar to whites. Bhatnagar et al. reported that mean systolic BP among emigrant South Asians as compared with Indian siblings was 146 ± 23 versus 132 ± 22 in men and 143 ± 28 versus 142 ± 23 in women. Williams analyzed various South Asian emigrant studies and commented that hypertension prevalence was not different in this group as compared with whites. Bhopal et al. compared hypertension prevalence rates in Indians, Pakistanis, and Bangladeshi living in Britain and reported that the hypertension was more common in Indians as compared to other South Asian groups. In the Study of Health Assessment and Risk in Ethnic Groups (SHARE) Study in Canada, prevalence of self-reported hypertension in South Asians was 12.5%. This was almost similar to Europeans (11.0%) but lower than that of the Chinese (15.9%).

Reasons for the Increasing Prevalence of Hypertension

Although the precise reasons for the increase in hypertension prevalence in South Asians are not established, several possibilities exist.

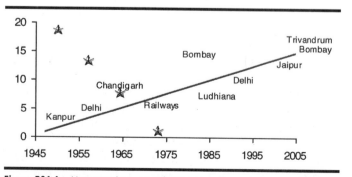

Figure B91.1. Hypertension prevalence in urban Indian populations. Hypertension diagnosis is based on known hypertensives or blood pressure >160 mm Hg systolic, >95 mm Hg diastolic, or both.

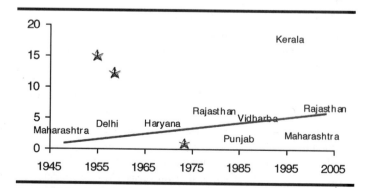

Figure B91.2. Hypertension prevalence trends in rural Indian populations.

Acculturation. Studies among unaccultured societies have shown lower BP levels that are not influenced by age. Among the so-called unaccultured and less-cultured Indian rural populations, there is only a small increase in prevalence in hypertension over time (Gupta et al., 1996). On the other hand, in urban populations that are exposed to acculturation and modernization, the hypertension prevalence rates have more than doubled in the last 30 years.

Gene-environmental interactions. Essential hypertension may be considered the result of interactions between genes and environment. The environmental effects are powerful and explain most of the BP differences between populations. Obesity, especially truncal obesity, is a powerful influence because of the associated insulin resistance that often leads to the cardiovascular dysmetabolic syndrome, which is often associated with hypertension. Other important environmental factors are excess alcohol intake, physical inactivity, high dietary intake of sodium, and deficiency of potassium.

Socioeconomic factors and urbanization. There is epidemiologic evidence that the population demographic changes in India have caused increased life expectancy, urbanization, development, and affluence. In 1901, only 11% of the population was living in an urban area; this proportion was 17.6% in 1951, 18.3% in 1961, 20.2% in 1971, 23.7% in 1981, and 26.1% in 1991. There is a strong, direct association between urbanization and the increased prevalence of hypertension. Affluence as measured by evaluation of per capita net domestic product, growth of production, and human development index has also increased sharply in India in recent years and correlates positively with the hypertension increase. Tobacco production, which is a surrogate for its consumption, is increasing at a very high rate in India. Per capita fat and oil consumption has also increased in the last 40 years. It was 5.79 kg per person per year in 1961, 5.85 in 1971, 6.48 in 1981, and 6.96 in 1987. Salt consumption was 10.7 g per person per day in 1971 and increased to 13.0 in 1981, 15.8 in 1991, and 16.9 in 1994. In this setting, it is reasonable to hypothesize that summation of these sociodemographic and lifestyle factors is accelerating the hypertension epidemic currently sweeping India and other parts of South Asia.

SUGGESTED READING

1. Anand SS, Yusuf S, Vuksan V, et al. Differences in risk factors, atherosclerosis and cardiovascular disease between ethnic groups in Canada: the Study of Health Assessment and Risk in Ethnic Groups (SHARE). *Lancet.* 2000;356:279–284.
2. Bhatnagar D, Anand IS, Durrington PN, et al. Coronary risk factors in people from the Indian subcontinent living in West London and their siblings in India. *Lancet.* 1995;345:405–409.
3. Bhopal R, Unwin N, White M, et al. Heterogeneity of coronary heart disease risk factors in Indian, Pakistani, Bangladeshi, and European origin population: cross sectional study. *BMJ.* 1999;319:215–220.
4. Deedwania P. The changing face of hypertension—is systolic blood pressure the final answer? *Arch Intern Med.* 2002;162:506–508.
5. Gupta R. Hypertension epidemiology in India: meta-analysis of fifty-year prevalence rates and blood pressure trends. *J Human Hypertens.* 1996;10:465–472.
6. Gupta R. Defining hypertension in the Indian population. *Natl Med J India.* 1997;10:139–143.
7. Nissinen A, Bothig S, Grenroth H, Lopez AD. Hypertension in developing countries. *World Health Statistics Q.* 1988;41:141–154.
8. Toshima H, Koga Y, Blackburn H, Keys A, eds. *Lessons for Science from the Seven Countries Study.* Tokyo: Springer-Verlag; 1994:63–175.
9. Williams B. Westernised Asians and cardiovascular disease: nature or nurture? *Lancet.* 1995;345:401–402.
10. Zaman MM, Rouf MA. Prevalence of hypertension in a Bangladeshi adult population. *J Human Hypertens.* 1999;13:547–549.

Chapter B92

Hypertension in East Asians and Native Hawaiians

Nathan D. Wong, PhD, MPH

KEY POINTS

- The prevalence of hypertension has increased in developing Asian nations, is high among Native Hawaiians, and varies dramatically among Asian ethnic subgroups.

- The prevalence of hypertension is lower in rural than urban Chinese, but rural Japanese demonstrate high prevalence rates of hypertension.

- In clinical trials, pharmacologic therapy effective in white populations is also effective in East Asian populations, but drug side effects such as cough or flushing may be greater among certain Asian ethnic subgroups.

See also Chapters A78, B79, B88, and B94

Hypertension has become increasingly prevalent in developing East Asian populations and among immigrant East Asian and Pacific Islander populations living in the United States (**Table B92.1**). Hypertension is a major contributor to cardiovascular disease morbidity and mortality, which may even be higher among some Asian immigrants to the United States than among their white counterparts.

China

Between 1982 and 1994, among 9 regions of China (N = 2,000 to 4,000 in each center), the prevalence of hypertension among those aged 35 to 59 years increased from 17.8% to 25.5% in men and 17.7% to 24.0% in women, with slight decreases more recently in 1998 (24% in men and 22% in women). Hypertension is less common among those living in southern China, particularly in rural areas, where dietary and exercise patterns are substantially different from those in northern or urban areas. Among those living in the United States, 1 study of 346 elderly Chinese immigrants aged 60 years and above showed a prevalence rate of hypertension of 29.7% for men and 33.5% for women. Others studies report lower prevalence rates but also a poor level of awareness and knowledge of hypertension.

Japan

Among native Japanese, a recent national survey of 12 rural communities (N = 11,302 subjects; mean age, 55 years) revealed a prevalence of hypertension of 37% for men and 33% for women. Only 7% of those hypertensive, however, were controlled to a systolic blood pressure (BP) <140 mm Hg systolic and diastolic BP <90 mm Hg. In Japanese aged 60 years and older, an overall prevalence of hypertension of 53% has been reported, with more than one-third of these having isolated systolic hypertension. Among Japanese Americans, systolic and diastolic BP have been shown to be the most important independent predictors of total, cardiovascular, and coronary heart

disease and stroke mortality. In the Honolulu Heart Study, the prevalence of hypertension increased among men from 53% in those aged 60 to 64 years to 67% among those aged 75 to 81 years. Those who had isolated systolic hypertension, isolated diastolic hypertension, and systolic/diastolic hypertension at baseline were 4.8, 1.4, and 4.3 times more likely to experience a stroke over the next 20 years compared to normotensive subjects. Among second- and third-generation Japanese aged 34 to 75 years living in King County, Washington, 41.5% of men and 33.8% of women were hypertensive; three-fourths were aware of their hypertension, more than half were on treatment, and, of those treated, more than 40% were controlled.

Korea

In a large metaanalysis, hypertension was a strong risk factor in Koreans for ischemic, hemorrhagic, and overall stroke (odds ratios of 3.3 to 6.6). A Korean national BP survey among 21,242 persons older than 30 years of age showed 20% with hypertension, but only 25% aware, 16% treated, and 5% controlled. Among more than 100,000 Korean workers, aged 35 to 59 years, the prevalence of hypertension was 28.9% in men and 15.9% in women.

Native Hawaiians

Relevant data in Native Hawaiians is limited to 1 survey conducted among those aged 20 to 59 years in the Molokai Heart Study. Hypertension prevalence rates ranged from 6% in men and 8% in women, ages 20 to 24, to 37% of men and 41% of women, ages 45 to 54. In addition to hypertension, other aspects of the metabolic syndrome, including abdominal obesity and glucose intolerance/diabetes, are common among Native Hawaiians.

Benefits of Hypertension Control

Ethnic differences in response to antihypertensive agents have long been recognized, but only recently have data become

Table B92.1. Prevalence Rates of Hypertension among East Asians and Native Hawaiians

	PREVALENCE (%) IN MEN	PREVALENCE (%) IN WOMEN	REFERENCE
Chinese, aged 35–54 yr	24	22	Chinese Academy of Medical Sciences 2001
Chinese Americans, aged 60 yr and above	29.7	33.5	Choi 1990
Japanese, mean age 55 yr	37	33	Asai 2001
Japanese Americans, men aged 60–81 yr	53 (60–64 y), 67 (75–81 y)	—	Curb 1996
Japanese Americans, aged 34–75 yr	41.5	33.8	Fujimoto 1996 [*Public Health Rep.* 1996;111(Suppl 2):56–58]
Korean, aged 35–59 yr	28.9	15.9	Jee 1998
Korean, aged 18–92 yr	41.5	24.5	Jo 2001
Native Hawaiians, aged 20–54 yr	6 (20–24 y), 37 (45–54 y)	8 (20–24 yr), 41 (50–54 yr)	Curb 1996

available in East Asian populations. Comparative efficacy and tolerability data are still lacking for Native Hawaiian and Pacific Islander populations. The Systolic Hypertension in China trial was conducted in 1,253 older patients with isolated systolic hypertension, assigned to active therapy (nitrendipine with addition of captopril or hydrochlorothiazide, if needed) and 1,141 patients assigned to placebo. Active therapy reduced total strokes by 38%, all-cause mortality by 39%, and cardiovascular mortality by 39%, relative to placebo. Among 7,443 Japanese patients treated and followed for 5 years, a reduced cardiovascular event risk was seen with the use of diuretics and β-blockers, but an increased risk was noted with calcium antagonists.

Specific Treatment Issues

A review of hypertension management in 200 Asian patients and 196 white patients revealed that medication changes, dose reductions, and side effects were all more common in the Asian patients. Among 6,289 Japanese patients receiving antihypertensive treatment, calcium antagonists were most often prescribed, followed by angiotensin-converting enzyme inhibitors, β-blockers, and diuretics. Hypertension control was similar regardless of class of agent. Among Chinese patients (in Hong Kong and Taiwan), similar effectiveness and tolerability of commonly used medications (amlodipine, atenolol, felodipine, and isradipine) have been observed, with some reports of higher side effect rates in those taking felodipine. Studies of angiotensin-converting enzyme inhibitors in Chinese subjects show similar efficacy to whites, but Chinese subjects appear to experience more cough from this class of medications. Flushing is also more common.

There is some evidence that Chinese and other Asian-based herbal therapeutic approaches may reduce BP. Among 50 well-matched patients with mild to moderate hypertension, reductions in BP were greater among those assigned to the Western therapy, including dihydrochlorothiazide and atenolol, but those assigned to the Chinese mixtures of 9 herbs still showed modest control of BP from a mean systolic/ diastolic BP of 168/96 mm Hg to 146/81 mm Hg.

SUGGESTED READING

1. Asai Y, Ishikawa S, Kayaba K, et al. Prevalence, awareness, treatment, and control of hypertension in Japanese rural communities. *Nippon Koshu Eisei Zasshi*. 2001;48:827–836.
2. Cardiovascular Institute of the Chinese Academy of Medical Sciences, unpublished data, 2001.
3. Choi E. The prevalence of cardiovascular risk factors among elderly Chinese Americans. *Arch Intern Med*. 1990;150:413–418.
4. Curb JD, Aluli NE, Huang BJ. Hypertension in elderly Japanese Americans and adult native Hawaiians. *Public Health Rep*. 1996;111:53–55.
5. Hui KK, Pasic J. Outcome of hypertension management in Asian Americans. *Arch Intern Med*. 1997;157:1345–1348.
6. Jee SH, Appel LJ, Suh I, et al. Prevalence of cardiovascular risk factors in South Korean adults: results from the Korea Medical Insurance Corporation (KMIC) Study. *Ann Epidemiol*. 1998;8:1–2.
7. Jo I, Ahn Y, Lee J, et al. Prevalence, awareness, treatment, control and risk factors of hypertension in Korea: the Ansan study. *J Hypertens*. 2001;19:1523–1532.
8. Liu L, Wang JG, Gong L, et al. Comparison of active treatment and placebo in older Chinese patients with isolated systolic hypertension. Systolic Hypertension in China (SYST-China) Collaborative Group. *J Hypertens*. 1998;16:1823–1829.
9. Uchiyama M, Kondo T, Tsuzuki Y, et al. Difference in occurrence of cardiovascular events according to class of antihypertensive agent, based on a follow-up study of Japanese hypertension patients. *Jpn Heart J*. 2001;42:585–595.
10. Wong ND, Ming S, Zhou HY, Black HR. A Comparison of Chinese traditional and Western medical approaches for the treatment of mild hypertension. *Yale J Biol Med*. 1991;64:79–87.

Chapter B93

Dietary Patterns and Blood Pressure

Frank M. Sacks, MD

KEY POINTS

- Populations eating mainly vegetarian diets have lower blood pressure levels and lesser blood pressure rises with age than those eating omnivorous diets.

- The Dietary Approaches to Stop Hypertension diet, which emphasizes fruits, vegetables, low-fat dairy products, whole grains, poultry, fish, and nuts, with only small amounts of red meat, sweets, and sugar-containing beverages, lowers blood pressure; combining the Dietary Approaches to Stop Hypertension diet with lower sodium intake lowers blood pressure further.

- High fruit and vegetable consumption is also associated with decreased stroke and ischemic heart disease.

- Fish oil (omega fatty acid) has a mild blood pressure–lowering effect.

See also Chapters A44–A47, A65, A76, B81, B87, B94–B97, B103, C127, C129, C135, C151, C152, C162–C164, C166, and C167

There are striking differences in the blood pressures (BPs) of populations worldwide. BP is higher and rises more steeply with age in industrialized than in nonindustrialized societies. A predominantly vegetarian dietary pattern is often present in those cultures that have generally low BP. In industrialized countries, vegetarians have lower average BP levels than do comparable nearby nonvegetarian populations.

Epidemiologic Surveys

The lowest average BPs in an industrialized country have been found in strict vegetarians in Massachusetts ("macrobiotics") who consume almost no animal products of any kind (**Figure B93.1**). Their diet is very plentiful in whole grains, green leafy vegetables, squash, and root vegetables. The entire BP distribution of the vegetarians is shifted to lower levels than nonvegetarians who reside in the same area. This indicates that diet could have a population-wide effect on BP.

Less rigorous dietary restriction is also associated with lower BP; a dietary pattern high in potassium and polyunsaturated fats and low in starch, saturated fat, and cholesterol was inversely associated with BP in a large population of U.S. men. Prospective studies in the United States, one in women (Nurses' Health Study) and the other in men (Health Professionals Follow-Up Study), found that a high intake of fruits and vegetables was associated with lower BP and less change in BP with age. In a representative population sample of the United States [National Health and Nutrition Examination Survey (NHANES) Follow-Up Study], fruit and vegetable intake 3 times a day or more was associated with reductions in stroke and ischemic heart disease mortality of 25% to 40%.

Dietary Approaches to Stop Hypertension Study

DASH (Dietary Approaches to Stop Hypertension) was a multicenter trial that tested 2 dietary patterns compared with a control dietary pattern that was typical of what many Americans eat. One diet, now termed the *DASH diet*, emphasized fruits, vegetables, and low-fat dairy products, included whole grains, poultry, fish and nuts, and contained only small amounts of red meat, sweets, and sugar-containing beverages, with decreased amounts of total fat, saturated fat, and cholesterol. The other diet, termed the *fruits-and-vegetables diet*, emphasized fruits and vegetables and included nuts and reduced amounts of sweets and sugar-containing beverages; it was otherwise similar in other nutrients to the control dietary pattern. All food for the experimental diets was provided to the participants. The experimental diets were eaten for 8 weeks. The dietary patterns were constructed with commonly consumed food items, so that the results could be conveniently implemented in dietary recommendations to the general public.

The study population consisted of 459 healthy men and women, mean age 44 years, with systolic BP <160 mm Hg and diastolic BP 80 to 95 mm Hg. The BPs of the population would be classified as either stage 1 hypertension, high-normal, or normal but above optimal. Blacks composed 60% of the population. In the initial DASH trial, sodium intakes were the same in all diets and participants maintained their prestudy body weights during the trial. The DASH diet significantly reduced BP by 5.5 mm Hg systolic and 3.0 mm Hg diastolic, according to measurements made in the clinics, and by 4.5 mm Hg systolic and 2.7 mm Hg diastolic as measured by 24-hour ambulatory monitoring (**Figure B93.2**). In contrast, the fruits-and-vegetables diet reduced BP by approximately half this amount, −2.8/−1.1 mm Hg for clinic readings and −3.1/−2.1 mm Hg for ambulatory readings. The effects of the dietary patterns were similar in men and women. The BP reductions in black participants were greater than those in whites, and the diets were more effective in hypertensives than in those with high-normal or normal BP. In hypertensives, who composed 29% of the group, the reductions

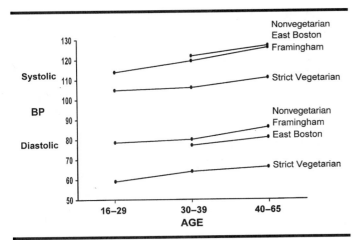

Figure B93.1. Blood pressure (BP) in a strict vegetarian population in Boston and in nonvegetarian populations in East Boston and Framingham, Massachusetts. (Adapted from Sacks FM, Kass EH. Low blood pressure in vegetarians: effects of specific foods and nutrients. *Am J Clin Nutr.* 1988; 48:795–800.)

in BP were −11.4/−5.5 mm Hg for the DASH diet and −7.2/−2.8 mm Hg for the fruits-and-vegetables diet. The therapeutic effects of the DASH diet in the hypertensives approached the magnitude of pharmacologic treatment with a single drug.

Explaining the Dietary Approaches to Stop Hypertension Diet Effect

Potassium and other nutrients. If we compare the BP lowering caused by the fruits-and-vegetables diet with that caused by the DASH diet, it may be surmised that the high intake of fruits and vegetables, including nuts and reduced amounts of sweets and sugar-containing beverages was responsible for approximately 50% of the effect of the DASH diet. Fruits and vegetables are high in potassium, magnesium, fiber, and many other nutrients. Of

these, potassium is the most well-established for lowering BP, particularly in hypertensives, persons with low potassium intake, and in blacks. The DASH population had these characteristics associated with potassium-sensitive BP, and the magnitude of BP lowering in the fruits-and-vegetables group is similar to that in potassium trials in such populations. Thus, a plausible explanation is that raising potassium intake by fruits and vegetables from a low intake, 1,700 mg (44 mmol), to a high level, 4,100 mg (105 mmol), reduced BP. It is also possible that reduced amounts of sweets and sugar-containing beverages contributed to the BP lowering.

Limitations to interpretation. The DASH study was not designed to determine which additional foods or nutrients are responsible for the overall BP-lowering effect. Compared with the fruits-and-vegetables diet, the DASH diet had more low-fat dairy products, vegetables, poultry, fish, calcium, magnesium, potassium, protein, and cereal grains and was lower in saturated, monounsaturated, and total fat, as well as cholesterol, red meat, sweets, and high-carbohydrate snacks. Overall, trials that tested certain of these nutrients individually (e.g., fat, fiber, calcium, or magnesium) have not found effects on BP that could account for the effects of the DASH combination diet. However, it could be that very small hypotensive effects of several nutrients, too small to be detected in a clinical trial or in a metaanalysis (e.g., 0.5 to 1.0 mm Hg), could combine to reduce BP. Alternative explanations include the possibility that a nutrient in the DASH diet that has BP-lowering properties has not yet been identified or that the DASH dietary pattern itself has a unique effect.

Combining the Dietary Approaches to Stop Hypertension Diet and Low Sodium

The combined effects on BP of lower sodium intake and the DASH diet are greater than either alone and are substantial. The DASH diet lowers BP even when sodium intake is low, and sodium reduction lowers BP even without the DASH diet.

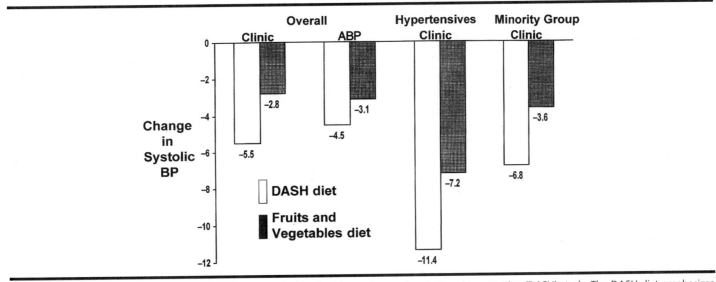

Figure B93.2. Effect of dietary patterns on blood pressure (BP) in the Dietary Approaches to Stop Hypertension (DASH) study. The DASH diet emphasizes fruits, vegetables, and low-fat dairy products; it includes whole grains, poultry, fish, and nuts and contains only small amounts of red meat, sweets, and sugar-containing beverages. The DASH diet contains decreased amounts of total and saturated fat and cholesterol. The fruits-and-vegetables diet was high in fruits and vegetables, included nuts, and reduced amounts of sweets and sugar-containing beverages but was similar in other nutrients to the control dietary pattern resembling average intake in the United States. ABP, ambulatory blood pressure.

However, the combined effects are not as much as estimated from strict additivity of DASH and low sodium, perhaps caused by lower sodium attenuating the hypotensive effects of potassium in the DASH diet, or by the high potassium or calcium content of the DASH diet attenuating the effects of lower sodium. Nevertheless, the combination of both interventions of the DASH-Sodium Trial achieved the greatest effect on BP, and therefore both merit recommendation, not just one or the other.

Fish Oil

From a physiologic viewpoint, it is attractive to propose that fish oil lowers BP. Fish oil has highly unsaturated fatty acids that stimulate the synthesis of vasodilating prostaglandins, inhibit platelet aggregation, and limit the release of vasoconstrictors. Fish oil is often prescribed as capsules that contain 1 mL of purified oil or as crude cod liver oil. Large doses of fish oil (e.g., 30 to 45 mL daily) clearly lower BP levels in hypertensive patients. However, intervention trials of moderate, more practical amounts of fish oil have been inconsistent. Metaanalyses of these trials found a small hypotensive effect (−3.0/−1.5 mm Hg) of 10 to 15 mL of fish oil, particularly in hypertensive patients. A smaller dose (e.g., 6 capsules daily) had no effect in hypertensive and normotensive persons. The unpleasant taste of the fish oil and belching interfere with compliance. Therefore, fish oil is not considered a practical therapy for hypertension.

Dietary Protein and Carbohydrate Content

Vegetarians have relatively low protein intake, although in almost all cases it is above the recommended dietary allowance. In Japan, in contrast, a high protein intake is associated with a low incidence of hypertension. High protein for lowering BP has not been adequately tested in a clinical trial. Carbohydrate, when substituted for fat, has not lowered BP in most trials. However, the type of carbohydrate has not been studied adequately. It is possible that a complex or unrefined carbohydrate that produces a low glucose and insulin response affects BP differently than does sugar or refined carbohydrate (e.g., white bread) or that dietary fiber could be involved.

Applications to Public Health and Clinical Practice

If the population shifted to a DASH type of diet, and more so if sodium intake is reduced, the BP distribution would shift to lower levels, thereby reducing the incidence of cardiovascular disease. For clinicians, the BP reductions demonstrate an alternative to medications as initial therapy for stage 1 hypertension. The Sixth Joint National Committee on the Prevention, Detection, Evaluation, and Treatment of Hypertension endorsed the results of DASH and recommended the DASH diet with low sodium for the population and clinical practice.

SUGGESTED READING

1. Appel LJ, Moore TJ, Obarzanek E, et al. A clinical trial of the effects of dietary patterns on blood pressure: DASH collaborative research group. *N Engl J Med*. 1997;336:1117–1124.
2. Ascherio A, Hennekens CH, Willett WC, et al. Prospective study of nutritional factors, blood pressure, and hypertension among US women. *Hypertension*. 1996;27:1065–1072.
3. Ascherio A, Rimm EB, Giovannucci EL, et al. A prospective study of nutritional factors and hypertension among US men. *Circulation*. 1992;86:1475–1484.
4. Bazzano KA, He J, Ogden LG, et al. Fruit and vegetable intake and risk of cardiovascular disease in US adults: the First National Health and Nutrition Examination Survey epidemiologic follow-up study. *Am J Clin Nutr*. 2002;76:93–99.
5. Morris MC, Sacks FM, Rosner B. Does fish oil lower blood pressure: a meta-analysis of controlled trials. *Circulation*. 1993;88:523–533.
6. Sacks FM, Kass EH. Low blood pressure in vegetarians: effects of specific foods and nutrients. *Am J Clin Nutr*. 1988;48:795–800.
7. Sacks FM, Svetkey LP, Vollmer WM, et al. Effects on blood pressure of reduced dietary sodium and the Dietary Approaches to Stop Hypertension (DASH) diet. *N Engl J Med*. 2001;344:3–10.
8. Stamler J, Caggiula A, Grandits GA, et al. for the MRFIT Research Group. Relationship to blood pressure of combinations of dietary macronutrients: findings of the Multiple Risk Factor Intervention Trial (MRFIT). *Circulation*. 1996;94:2417–2423.

Salt and Blood Pressure

Paul Elliott, PhD, FRCP, FFPHM, FMedSci

KEY POINTS

- Evidence of an adverse effect of high sodium intake on blood pressure comes from animal experimental studies, anthropology, clinical observations, controlled clinical trials, and epidemiologic studies both within and across populations.

- Within-population analyses from the International Co-Operative Study of Salt and Blood Pressure yield estimates of systolic and diastolic blood pressure lower by 3 to 6 mm Hg and 0 to 3 mm Hg, respectively, for each lower daily sodium intake; the Dietary Approaches to Stop Hypertension–Sodium feeding trial found that lower versus higher sodium (77 mmol sodium difference) reduced systolic blood pressure and diastolic blood pressure by 6.7 and 3.5 mm Hg, respectively.

- At the population level, downward shifts in blood pressure of this order are estimated to have sizable effects on mortality from cardiovascular diseases; for the individual patient, lowered sodium intake may help lower blood pressure and reduce or obviate the need for antihypertensive drugs.

- Most sodium consumed in the diet is added as sodium chloride (common salt) in food processing and manufacturing; cooperation of the food industry is required to help lower sodium consumption in the population.

See also Chapters A37, A41, A46, A47, A76, B89, B93, B102, C127, C129, C139, and C152

There is considerable evidence relating sodium (or salt) intake to blood pressure (BP).

Animal Studies

Various animal models of salt-induced hypertension in dogs, chickens, and rats have been used to study the relationship of sodium and hypertension. Several strains of rat develop hypertension and have strokes when fed high doses of salt. In the spontaneously hypertensive rat, salt restriction attenuates the severity of hypertension. Increased potassium (K) intake, meanwhile, offsets to some extent the adverse effects of a high-salt diet. More recently, a controlled study of added salt in chimpanzees unequivocally showed that salt intake causes a large rise in BP among the species phylogenetically closest to humans. In the wild, the chimpanzee consumes a diet high in fruits and vegetables, high in K and low in salt. When up to 15 g of salt per day were added to the diets of the experimental group of chimpanzees over a 20-month period, systolic BP (SBP) and diastolic BP (DBP) rose 33 mm Hg and 10 mm Hg, respectively, with rapid reversal to baseline values once the added salt was removed.

Anthropology and Early Clinical Observations

The addition of salt to the human diet is a relatively recent phenomenon, dating back only some 6,000 to 8,000 years ago, around the same time that agriculture and animal husbandry developed. Humans evolved on a low-salt diet of no more than 20 to 40 mmol sodium per day, and became (and remain) adapted to the physiologic conservation of the limited salt naturally present in foods and not for excretion of a sodium load some 10 to 20 times higher than the physiologic need (8 to 10 mmol/day). Current consumption of sodium in the United Kingdom, United States and other western countries averages around 140 to 150 mmol/day (8 to 9 g/day salt).

Although sodium reduction was advocated in the treatment of hypertension early in the twentieth century, it was not until the 1940s that it gained favor when Kempner's low-sodium rice diet proved to be an effective treatment of malignant hypertension. The introduction of diuretic therapy, which promotes sodium as well as water loss, revolutionized the management of hypertension and added support to the concept that sodium was important in the development and control of high BP. Subsequently, a number of controlled trials showed that lowered sodium intake could reduce, or even obviate, the need for antihypertensive medication among people who had been treated for high BP.

Epidemiologic Studies

Salt and blood pressure. Epidemiologic evidence for a positive association between salt and BP comes from cross- and within-population studies. A positive cross-population association of salt and hypertension was first described by Dahl in 1960, and subsequently by other authors, although based on published data from different studies and subject to varying degrees of possible bias and confounding. By contrast, up until the 1980s, the within-population (individual) level studies were largely considered to be negative, but methodologic problems—especially large day-to-day variation in sodium intake—caused estimates of association to be biased downward ("regression dilution"). Many studies were too small to find any effect. However, in an overview by Elliott of 14 studies (16 populations) that reported BP and 24-hour urinary sodium excretion data (excluding INTERSALT), a highly significant positive association of sodium with SBP and DBP was found, larger among women than men.

Table B94.1. International Study of Salt and Blood Pressure (INTERSALT), Pooled Within-Population Regression Estimates of Blood Pressure Difference per 100 mmol/Day Sodium Excretion, without and with Correction for Reliability

RELIABILITY CORRECTED[b]	ESTIMATED DIFFERENCE IN SBP (MM HG)			ESTIMATED DIFFERENCE IN DBP (MM HG)		
	SAMPLE-AGE-SEX ADJUSTED	MULTIPLE ADJUSTMENT[a]		SAMPLE-AGE-SEX ADJUSTED	MULTIPLE ADJUSTMENT[a]	
		WITH BMI	WITHOUT BMI		WITH BMI	WITHOUT BMI
Men and women (N = 10,074)						
No	1.8 (0.2)	1.0 (0.3)	2.1 (0.3)	0.7 (0.2)	0.04 (0.2)	0.9 (0.2)
Yes	4.3 (0.8)	3.1 (0.9)	6.0 (1.1)	1.8 (0.5)	0.1 (0.6)	2.5 (0.7)
Men (N = 5,042)						
No	1.2 (0.3)	0.6 (0.3)	1.5 (0.3)	0.6 (0.2)	−0.08 (0.3)	0.8 (0.3)
Yes	3.2 (0.9)	1.8 (1.2)	4.6 (1.2)	1.5 (0.6)	−0.2 (0.9)	2.3 (0.9)
Women (N = 5,032)						
No	2.2 (0.4)	1.3 (0.4)	2.6 (0.4)	0.9 (0.3)	0.09 (0.3)	0.9 (0.3)
Yes	5.7 (1.2)	4.0 (1.4)	7.5 (1.5)	2.3 (0.7)	0.3 (0.9)	2.8 (0.9)

BMI, body mass index; DBP diastolic blood pressure; SBP, systolic blood pressure.
[a]Adjusted for sample, age, sex, 24-hour urinary potassium excretion, alcohol intake.
[b]Multivariate correction for reliability (regression dilution bias); standard error estimated approximately by bootstrap sampling.

The INTERSALT study is the most extensive epidemiologic investigation yet published on the relation of sodium to BP. It included over 10,000 men and women 20 to 59 years of age from 52 population samples in 32 countries. Both cross- and within-population analyses were reported. In the cross-population analyses, a highly significant relationship of sodium with upward slope of BP with age was found across the 52 population samples, such that mean BP rise with age over a 30-year period (e.g., 25 to 55 years) was estimated to be less for SBP/DBP by 10/6 mm Hg for sodium intake lower by 100 mmol/day; adjusted median SBP/DBP was estimated to be lower by 4.5/2.3 mm Hg for sodium intake lower by 100 mmol/day.

Results for the within-population analyses, both uncorrected and corrected for reliability, are shown in **Table B94.1**. The coefficients in the table are pooled from sample-specific multiple regression analyses, weighting each individual coefficient by the inverse of its variance. Data are shown both sample-age-sex adjusted and multiple adjusted, with and without body mass index (BMI) in the model. (This is because inclusion of BMI may represent overadjustment: Sodium and BMI are positively correlated, and at least some of the BMI/BP relationship may be operating through association with sodium.) Whereas sodium is poorly estimated, BMI is well-estimated and therefore tends to dominate in the regression models. Table B94.1 shows that in the sample-age-sex models and in the multiple-adjusted models excluding BMI, sodium is highly significant and positively associated with SBP and DBP. With BMI in the model, sodium remains significantly associated with SBP for men and women combined and in women only. As with the overview of other epidemiologic studies noted in the first paragraph of this section, associations tended to be larger in women than in men, and also at older ages (not shown). Overall, in men and women combined, 100 mmol lower sodium intake was associated with SBP and DBP lower by 3 to 6 mm Hg and 0 to 3 mm Hg, respectively, after correction for reliability.

Salt and mortality. A few studies have investigated the association of sodium intake and subsequent mortality, although most were flawed methodologically. In 2001, a Finnish group reported up to 14-years mortality follow-up of over 1,400 men and women from whom 24-hour urinary sodium excretion was obtained in the 1980s. There was a significant positive association between urinary sodium excretion and subsequent coronary heart disease, cardiovascular disease, and all-cause mortality, with multiple adjusted hazard ratios (men and women combined) of 1.56 (95% confidence interval, 1.15–2.12), 1.36 (1.05–1.76), and 1.22 (1.02–1.47) per 100 mmol of sodium, respectively.

Controlled Clinical Trials

Controlled clinical trials of reduced sodium intake on BP have been summarized in various metaanalyses published since the mid 1990s. Three metaanalyses showed that lower sodium intake resulted in lower BP among hypertensive and normotensive individuals. One of these, published in 1998, found a mean decrease in SBP/DBP of 4.5/2.3 mm Hg among hypertensive people and 1.6/0.4 mm Hg, among normotensive people for reductions in mean sodium intake of 129 mmol/day and 165 mmol/day, respectively. Interpretation of the metaanalyses is not straightforward because the quality of the trials is variable. The adherence of participants to counseling for salt-intake reduction is different (leading to underestimation of true effects on BP), and some of these metaanalyses include many short-duration trials with large fluctuations in sodium intakes. Well-conducted trials of longer duration (4 weeks or more) tend to show larger effects.

Two high-quality trials have investigated different levels of sodium intake on BP. MacGregor and colleagues used the double-blind randomized cross-over design and either placebo or salt tablets to provide 3 sodium intake levels. Comparing the lowest sodium group (49 mmol/day) to the highest (190 mmol/day), SBP/DBP was lower by 16/9 mm Hg in the lowest sodium group.

The second study, the DASH-Sodium trial, was a feeding trial with all food supplied to participants to achieve high adherence. Its design also provided for 3 levels of sodium [higher (141 mmol/day), intermediate (106 mmol/day), lower (64 mmol/day)], as verified by 24-hour urine collections. The effects of sodium reduction were tested in 2 diets. The DASH

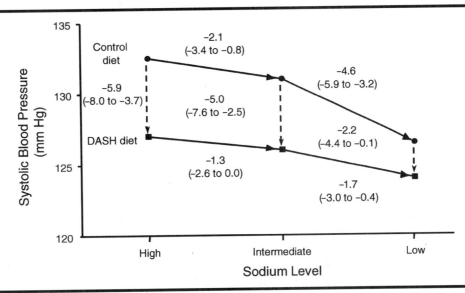

Figure B94.1. DASH-Sodium Trial: Effect of DASH diet and 3 different levels of sodium intake on systolic blood pressure. [Re-drawn from Sacks FM, Svetkey LP, Vollmer WM, et al. for the DASH-Sodium Collaborative Research Group. Effects on blood pressure of reduced dietary sodium and the Dietary Approaches to Stop Hypertension (DASH) diet. *N Engl J Med.* 2001;344:3–10, with permission.]

diet is rich in fruits, vegetables, and low-fat dairy products and reduced in saturated and total fats; this diet had already been shown to lower BP independently of sodium (see Chapter B93). **Figure B94.1** displays results for SBP. Among participants assigned to the control diet, lower versus higher sodium (i.e., 77 mmol/day lower sodium) reduced SBP by 6.7 mm Hg, whereas in participants randomized to the DASH diet, SBP reduction was 3.0 mm Hg. The combined effect of the DASH diet with lower sodium compared to the control diet with higher sodium was a reduction in SBP of 8.9 mm Hg. Significant reductions were also found for DBP. Crucially, for nonhypertensive participants assigned to the control diet, lower versus higher sodium produced a 5.6 mm Hg fall in SBP (7 mm Hg in blacks, 4 mm Hg in other groups). Further, the effect of salt reduction on BP was greater for lower versus intermediate than for intermediate versus higher sodium.

One further trial, concerning sodium reduction in newborns, merits discussion here. This trial was conducted in The Netherlands in the early 1980s before no-added-salt baby formula was widely available. With reduction in sodium intake by approximately two-thirds, SBP at 6 months was significantly lower than in the "usual" (high) sodium group by 2.1 mm Hg. At follow-up 15 years later, the reduced sodium group continued to have lower BP than the usual sodium group, despite no further intervention since infancy.

SUGGESTED READING

1. Chobanian AV, Hill M. National Heart, Lung, and Blood Institute Workshop on sodium and blood pressure. A critical review of current scientific evidence. *Hypertension.* 2000;35:858–863.
2. Denton D, Weisinger R, Mundy NI, et al. The effect of increased salt intake on blood pressure in chimpanzees. *Nat Med.* 1995;1:1009–1016.
3. Elliott P. The INTERSALT study: an addition to the evidence on salt and blood pressure, and some implications. *J Hum Hypertens.* 1989;3:289–298.
4. Elliott P. Observational studies of salt and blood pressure. *Hypertension.* 1991;17: I-3–I-8.
5. INTERSALT Cooperative Group. INTERSALT: an international study of electrolyte excretion and blood pressure. Results for 24-hour urinary sodium and potassium excretion. *BMJ.* 1988;297:319–328.
6. MacGregor GA, Markandu ND, Sagnella GA, et al. Double-blind study of three sodium intakes and long-term effects of sodium restriction in essential hypertension. *Lancet.* 1989;2:1244–1247.
7. National Research Council, Committee on Diet and Health, Food and Nutrition Board, Commission on Life Sciences. *Diet and health: implications for reducing chronic disease.* Washington, DC: National Academy Press; 1989:413–430.
8. Sacks FM, Svetkey LP, Vollmer WM, et al. for the DASH-Sodium Collaborative Research Group. Effects on blood pressure of reduced dietary sodium and the Dietary Approaches to Stop Hypertension (DASH) diet. *N Engl J Med.* 2001;344:3–10.
9. Stamler J. The INTERSALT Study: background, methods, findings, and implications. *Am J Clin Nutr.* 1997;65:626S–642S.
10. Tuomilehto J, Jousilahti P, Rastenyte D, et al. Urinary sodium excretion and cardiovascular mortality in Finland: a prospective study. *Lancet.* 2001;357:848–851.

Potassium and Blood Pressure

Paul K. Whelton, MD, MS

KEY POINTS

- Many studies suggest that potassium intake is inversely related to systolic and diastolic blood pressure; potassium deficiency may play a special role in the high incidence and prevalence of hypertension in blacks.

- Increased potassium intake reduces systolic and diastolic blood pressure; this effect is more pronounced in hypertensives compared to normotensives, in blacks compared to whites, and in those consuming a high intake of sodium.

- Increased potassium intake in combination with weight loss, sodium restriction, moderation in alcohol consumption, and increased physical activity may provide the optimal means for prevention and treatment of hypertension.

- Increased potassium intake may reduce the risk of stroke independent of its effects on blood pressure.

See also Chapters A26, B93, B94, B103, C129, C139, and C140

Evidence from a variety of sources, including interpopulation and migrant studies, suggests that diet and physical inactivity play an important role in the genesis of age-related increases in blood pressure (BP) and in the occurrence of hypertension. Weight gain, alcohol consumption, excessive intake of sodium and insufficient dietary potassium are leading possibilities as dietary causes of hypertension. Interest in the potassium-BP relationship dates back to the early part of the twentieth century, when increased potassium intake was advocated as a treatment for hypertension. Recent publications, including numerous cross-sectional studies in economically developed and developing countries, and metaanalyses of clinical trial results have rekindled interest in the role of increasing potassium intake as a means to prevent and treat hypertension.

Epidemiology

Cross-sectional studies conducted in the United States, Japan, England, Scotland, Sweden, Belgium, St. Lucia, Kenya, Zaire, and China have identified an inverse relationship between BP and various measures of serum, urine, total body, and dietary potassium. The most precise estimates come from the International Study of Salt and Blood Pressure (INTERSALT), a cross-sectional investigation conducted in 10,079 men and women aged 20 to 59 years from 52 populations around the world. In this study, a 50 mmol/day higher level of urinary potassium excretion was associated with a 3.4 [95% confidence interval (CI), 1.5 to 5.2] mm Hg lower level of systolic and 1.9 (95% CI, 0.7 to 3.0) mm Hg lower level of diastolic BP after adjustment for the potentially confounding influences of age, sex, body mass index, alcohol consumption, and urinary sodium excretion and correction for regression dilution bias. Epidemiologic studies are also consistent with the suggestion that potassium deficiency may play a special role in the strikingly high incidence and prevalence of hypertension in blacks and the elderly.

Isolated populations with a low prevalence of hypertension and a blunted age-related increase in BP almost uniformly consume a diet that is relatively high in potassium and low in sodium content (**Table B95.1**). Potassium intake is often lower in economically developed countries than in isolated rural societies because commercially prepared foods are an important part of the diet, and potassium is frequently removed during the manufacturing process. Migration studies have identified a relationship between progressive diminution in potassium intake and increasing levels of BP and hypertension. Typically, these changes have been noted in a setting in which there is a concurrent increase in sodium, calorie, and alcohol consumption and a decrease in physical activity. It has been hard to separate the independent contribution of each of these changes to the concurrent change in BP. It is conceivable that they all play a role in the age-related increase in BP that is so common in the United States and most other societies.

Clinical Trials

A critically important question is whether the inverse association between potassium intake and BP is causal or merely reflects the presence of a confounding relationship between potassium and another variable. Clinical trials provide the most satisfactory study design for resolution of this question. Potassium was widely advocated as a means to lower BP during the 1920s and 1930s. The rice/fruit diet of Kempner, which received considerable attention during the 1950s, was characterized by a relatively high content of potassium and a low sodium to potassium ratio. Kempner's diet, however, also resulted in weight loss and a variety of metabolic changes. During the 1960s and 1970s, a series of animal experiments were conducted that suggested potassium administration could blunt the rise in BP after sodium loading in a variety of salt-sensitive rat models. Similar findings have been reported in humans who were exposed to extremely high and extremely low intakes of dietary sodium. The first controlled trial

Table B95.1. Urinary Excretion of Potassium and Sodium/Potassium Ratio in 7 Low Blood Pressure Populations

POPULATION	URINARY POTASSIUM, MMOL/24 HR	URINARY SODIUM/ POTASSIUM RATIO
Yanomamo Indians, Brazil	152	0.01
Kung bushmen, Botswana	70–103	0.28–0.44
Xingu Indians, Brazil	78–96	0.19–0.20
Asaro Valley, Papua New Guinea	62–79	0.53–0.70
Luo tribesmen, Kenya	32–35	1.9

Data from He J, Whelton PK. Potassium, blood pressure, and cardiovascular disease: an epidemiologic perspective. *Cardiol Rev.* 1997;5:255–260.

Table B95.3. Reduction of Blood Pressure from Potassium

Mechanism of action
　Direct natriuretic effect
　　Suppression of the renin-angiotensin and sympathetic nervous systems
　　Effect on kallikreins and eicosanoids
　　Improvement of baroreceptor function
　　Antagonism of the effects of natriuretic hormone
　　Direct arterial vasodilatation

of the efficacy of increased potassium intake in essential hypertension, however, was not reported until 1981. Since that time, a large number of randomized, controlled trials as well as many uncontrolled experimental studies have reported on the effect of increased and decreased potassium intake on BP in hypertensive and normotensive persons.

Whelton et al. identified 33 randomized, controlled trials (2,565 participants) in which the effects of an increased intake of potassium on BP were evaluated. Of these, 21 trials (2,565 participants) were conducted in hypertensive and 12 in normotensive (1,005 participants) persons. In all but 2 trials, the dose of potassium prescribed in the active intervention arm was >60 mmol per day. The weighted mean net change in urinary potassium excretion for the intervention versus control group was 53 mmol per 24 hours in the 31 trials in which such information was available. Overall, increased potassium intake was associated with a significant reduction in mean (95% CI) systolic and diastolic BP of 4.4 (2.5–6.4) and 2.5 (0.7–4.2) mm Hg, respectively (**Table B95.2**). After exclusion of 1 trial in which there was an extreme effect on systolic (–41 mm Hg) and diastolic (–17 mm Hg) BP, the overall mean (95% CI) reduction was 3.1 (1.9–4.3) for systolic and 2.0 (0.5–3.4) for diastolic BP. Subgroup analysis suggested that the treatment effect was enhanced in hypertensives, blacks, and those consuming a high intake of sodium. In trials in which the participants were consuming a diet high in sodium content, there was a

significant ($p < .001$) dose-response relationship between 24-hour urinary potassium excretion and treatment effect size.

In a subsequent trial, conducted in China, potassium supplementation resulted in a 5.0 mm Hg (95% CI, 2.1–7.9 mm Hg) reduction in systolic BP. Using randomized, cross-over design trials, Krishna et al. have demonstrated that short-term potassium depletion produces an increase in BP in hypertensive and normotensive persons.

Two randomized controlled trials have explored the efficacy of increased potassium intake in reducing the need for antihypertensive drug therapy in patients with well-controlled hypertension. In a dietary modification trial, an increased intake of potassium significantly reduced the need for antihypertensive drug therapy. In contrast, in a large and rigorously controlled trial of potassium chloride pill supplementation, Grimm et al. were unable to identify any apparent effect of potassium supplementation on BP. That the participants in this study were concurrently counseled to reduce salt intake may have blunted the effect of the potassium supplements.

Clinical trials have shown that consumption of a diet that is rich in fruits, vegetables, and low-fat dairy foods and with a reduced saturated and total fat content [Dietary Approaches to Stop Hypertension (DASH) diet] results in a substantial lowering of BP in hypertensive and normotensive persons. The high intake of dietary potassium in the DASH diet may contribute to its efficacy in lowering BP (see Chapter B93).

Mechanism of Action

Various mechanisms have been proposed to explain the purported influence of potassium on BP (**Table B95.3**). Many studies have demonstrated short-term changes in sodium

Table B95.2. Pooled Estimates of Change in Blood Pressure (BP) after Potassium Supplementation in 33 Randomized Controlled Clinical Trials

TRIALS IN ANALYSIS	SYSTOLIC BP MEAN CHANGE	SYSTOLIC BP 95% CONFIDENCE INTERVAL	DIASTOLIC BP MEAN CHANGE	DIASTOLIC BP 95% CONFIDENCE INTERVAL
All trials (N = 33)	–4.4	–2.53, –6.36	–2.5	–0.74, –4.16
Obel trial excluded (N = 32)	–3.1	–1.91, –4.31	–2.0	–0.52, –3.42
Hypertensive trials[a] (N = 20)	–4.4	–2.2, –6.6	–2.5	–0.1, –4.9
Normotensive trials (N = 12)	–1.8	–0.6, –2.9	–1.0	0.0, –2.1
Trials in blacks[a] (N = 6)	–5.6	–2.4, –8.7	–3.0	–0.7, –5.3
Trials in whites (N = 25)	–2.0	–0.9, –3.0	–1.1	–0.1, –2.1
Urinary Na, mmol/d[b]				
<140 (N = 10)	–1.2	0.0, –2.4	0.1	1.1, –1.0
140–164 (N = 10)	–2.1	–0.3, –4.0	–1.4	0.0, –2.8
≥165 (N = 10)	–7.3	–4.6, –10.1	–4.7	–1.1, –8.3

[a]Excludes outlier trial by Obel AO.
[b]Urinary sodium excretion during follow-up.
Adapted from Whelton PK, He J, Cutler JA, et al. Effects of oral potassium on blood pressure: meta-analysis of randomized controlled clinical trials. *JAMA.* 1997;277:1624–1632.

Table B95.4. Hazard Ratio and Corresponding 95% Confidence Interval of Stroke Associated with a Low Dietary Intake of Potassium during 19 Years of Follow-Up of 9,805 Male and Female Participants in the National Health and Examination Survey I Epidemiologic Follow-Up Study

ADJUSTMENT MODEL	HAZARD RATIO (95% CONFIDENCE INTERVAL)	P VALUE
Age-, energy-adjusted	1.37 (1.20–1.54)	<.0001
Age-, race-, sex-, energy-adjusted	1.26 (1.11–1.45)	.0007
Multivariate[a]	1.28 (1.11–1.47)	.0001

[a]Additionally adjusted for systolic blood pressure, serum cholesterol, body mass index, history of diabetes, physical activity, education level, regular alcohol consumption, current cigarette smoking, vitamin supplement use, saturated fat intake, cholesterol intake, sodium intake, calcium intake, dietary fiber, vitamin C intake, and vitamin A intake (N = 9,244).

Adapted from Bazzano LA, He J, Ogden LG, et al. Dietary potassium intake and risk of stroke in US men and women. National Health and Nutrition Examination Survey I Epidemiologic Follow-Up Study. *Stroke.* 2001;32:1473–1480.

excretion, but it remains unclear whether any long-term effects on BP can be ascribed to a decrease in intravascular volume resulting from this initial and transient natriuresis.

Effects on Stroke and Heart Disease

In addition to its hypotensive effects, increased potassium intake may have independent vasculoprotective properties. In a series of animal models, including spontaneously hypertensive and Dahl salt-sensitive rats, Tobian reported that the addition of potassium chloride or potassium citrate markedly reduced the probability of death from a stroke. An inverse relationship between 24-hour dietary potassium intake at baseline and subsequent stroke-associated morbidity and mortality has been noted in several population-based cohort studies. In the most generalizable and statistically powerful investigation, Bazzano et al. studied 9,805 U.S. men and women who had participated in the First National Health and Nutrition Examination Survey (NHANES I) who were followed for more than an average of 19

years, yielding 927 stroke and 1,847 coronary heart disease events (**Table B95.4**). After adjustment for a broad array of potential cardiovascular disease risk factors, those who had consumed a low potassium diet at baseline (first quartile, <34.6 mmol/day) experienced a 28% higher (95% CI, 11% to 47%) risk of stroke compared to the remainder of the cohort. Recognizing the limitations of observational studies in answering therapeutic questions, the accumulated experience from prospective analyses suggests that a high potassium diet reduces the risk of stroke. Evidence from a number of epidemiologic studies suggests that stroke mortality is inversely related to intake of vegetables and fruits. Although this evidence is indirect, these reports are consistent with a vasculoprotective effect from increased potassium intake.

SUGGESTED READING

1. Appel LA, Moore TJ, Obarzanek E, et al. for the DASH Collaborative Research Group. A clinical trial of the effects of dietary patterns on blood pressure. *N Engl J Med.* 1997;336:1117–1124.
2. Bazzano LA, He J, Ogden LG, et al. Dietary potassium intake and risk of stroke in US men and women. National Health and Nutrition Examination Survey I Epidemiologic Follow-up Study. *Stroke.* 2001;32:1473–1480.
3. Gu D, He J, Wu X, et al. Effect of potassium supplementation on blood pressure in Chinese: a randomized, placebo-controlled trial. *J Hypertens.* 2001;19:1325–1331.
4. INTERSALT Cooperative Research Group. INTERSALT: an international study of electrolyte excretion and blood pressure: results for 24-hour urinary sodium and potassium excretion. *BMJ.* 1988;297:319–328.
5. Johnston SC. Potassium, stroke, and the bounds of epidemiological studies. *Stroke.* 2001;32:1479–1480.
6. Joshipura KJ, Ascherio A, Manson MJ, et al. Fruit and vegetable intake in relation to risk of ischemic stroke. *JAMA.* 1999;282:1233–1239.
7. Klag MJ, He J, Coresh J, et al. The contribution of urinary cations to the blood pressure differences associated with migration. *Am J Epidemiol.* 1995;142:295–303.
8. National High Blood Pressure Education Program Working Group. Report on primary prevention of hypertension. *Arch Intern Med.* 1993;153:186–208.
9. The sixth report of the Joint National Committee on prevention, detection, evaluation, and treatment of high blood pressure. *Arch Intern Med.* 1997;157:2413–2446.
10. Whelton PK, He J, Cutler JA, et al. Effects of oral potassium on blood pressure: meta-analysis of randomized controlled clinical trials. *JAMA.* 1997;277:1624–1632.

Calcium, Magnesium, Heavy Metals, and Blood Pressure

Lawrence J. Appel, MD, MPH

KEY POINTS

- In observational studies, an increased intake of calcium and magnesium is often associated with lower blood pressure.

- In clinical trials, the effects of calcium and magnesium supplements on blood pressure are small and inconsistent; overall, available data do not support use of these pill supplements as a means to lower blood pressure.

- Chronic exposure to lead may raise blood pressure, but the relationship is weak.

See also Chapters A47, B93, and C129

In addition to weight, salt, potassium, and alcohol, other aspects of nutrition may affect blood pressure (BP) and account in part for the high prevalence of hypertension in most societies. Calcium and magnesium are two such nutrients.

CALCIUM

Overview of Basic Physiology and Nutrition

The adult body contains approximately 1,200 g of calcium, of which 99% is present in the skeleton. The remaining 1%, found in intracellular space, cell membranes, and extracellular fluids, affects numerous body functions, including nerve conduction, muscle contraction, blood clotting, and membrane permeability. Blood levels are tightly regulated within narrow limits through the effects of several hormones (vitamin D, parathyroid hormone, calcitonin, estrogen, testosterone, and perhaps others). These hormones control calcium absorption and excretion, as well as bone metabolism.

Absorption and metabolism. Calcium absorption occurs through active transport and passive diffusion across the intestinal mucosa. Active transport, which accounts for the absorption of calcium at low to moderate levels, is dependent on vitamin D. Passive diffusion becomes more important at higher levels of calcium intake. Fractional absorption depends on several factors including age (greater in infants and during puberty), pregnancy status (greater during the last 2 trimesters), and race (greater in blacks).

Calcium is lost through the body in feces, urine, and sweat. Urinary calcium excretion is typically 100 to 250 mg per day and varies as a function of the filtered load and the efficiency of reabsorption, which is regulated by parathyroid hormone levels. Increased intake of sodium, protein, and caffeine may increase calcium excretion. Other than a direct association between sodium intake and nephrolithiasis, the clinical relevance of these effects is unclear.

United States intake levels. According to the U.S. Department of Agriculture 1994 Continuing Survey of Food Intakes, the median dietary intake of calcium is less in women than in men and tends to decrease throughout adult ages (857 mg/day in men 31 to 50 years old and 708 mg/day in men >70 years old, 606 and 571 mg/day in women at corresponding ages). Also, in both sexes and across all age groups, blacks consume less calcium than whites. In terms of food sources, 73% of calcium in the food supply is from milk, 9% from fruits and vegetables, 5% from grain products, and the remaining 12% from all other sources. Milk products contain <300 mg of calcium per serving (e.g., 8 oz of milk, 1.5 oz of cheddar cheese). Other calcium-rich foods include kale, calcium-fortified orange juice, and broccoli. Use of calcium supplements is high among adult women (25% in 1986) and is probably rising as a result of efforts to prevent osteoporosis through increased calcium intake. In nutrition guidelines issued by the Institute of Medicine, an adequate intake of calcium for adults (men and women) is 1 g per day at 19 to 50 years of age and 1.2 g per day at older ages. Few people meet this guideline. For instance, among persons ≥70 years old, <1% of women and <5% of men meet this dietary guideline.

Clinical Studies of Calcium and Blood Pressure

Epidemiology. Reports from ecologic studies of an inverse association between drinking water hardness and mortality from atherosclerotic diseases stimulated interest in the roles of calcium and magnesium intake on BP. Evidence of an effect of calcium on BP comes from a variety of sources including animal studies, observational studies, clinical trials, and metaanalyses of observational studies and controlled trials. In a metaanalysis of 23 observational studies, Cappuccio et al. documented an inverse association between BP and dietary calcium intake (as measured by 24-hour dietary recalls or food frequency questionnaires). However, the size of the effect was relatively small, and there was evidence of publication bias and of heterogeneity across studies.

Clinical trials. Two metaanalyses of randomized trials have documented that calcium supplementation significantly

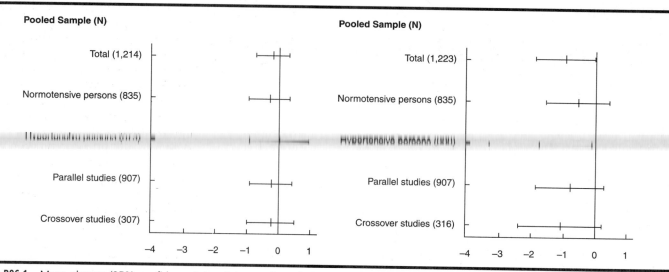

Figure B96.1. Mean change (95% confidence interval) in systolic and diastolic blood pressure, overall and by subgroups, from a metaanalysis of 22 randomized trials. (From Allender PS, Cutler JA, Follmann D, et al. Dietary calcium and blood pressure: a meta-analysis of randomized clinical trials. *Ann Intern Med.* 1996;124:825–831.)

reduced systolic BP (by 0.89 mm Hg in one analysis and 1.27 mm Hg in the other) but not diastolic BP (**Figure B96.1**). Typical calcium doses in the trials were 1.0 to 1.5 g per day. The unimpressive results of pill supplementation trials in the setting of inverse relationships in observational studies have several possible explanations. First, calcium may have an effect but only in combination with a high intake of other nutrients. However, in 1 trial of combinations of cation supplements (calcium, magnesium, and potassium) in hypertensive patients, none of the combinations reduced BP. Alternatively, some nutrients closely associated with calcium (e.g., protein, phosphorus, vitamin D, or an unknown nutrient) may be responsible for the BP-lowering effect attributed to calcium. One small trial demonstrated that milk consumption in the context of a low-calcium diet reduced systolic BP. The Dietary Approaches to Stop Hypertension (DASH) diet lowers BP. This low-fat diet is rich in fruits, vegetables, and dairy products (i.e., high in calcium).

Potential response heterogeneity. One issue still unanswered is whether certain subgroups of the population are particularly sensitive to the effects of calcium. Such groups may include pregnant women at risk for preeclampsia and persons with a low dietary intake of calcium or sodium. In the large and well-controlled Trials of Hypertension Prevention, calcium supplementation did not reduce BP overall in the trial but may have reduced diastolic BP in white women, particularly those with low urinary sodium excretion, calcium excretion, or low body mass index. In contrast, in another trial conducted in 300 female nurses with low dietary intakes of calcium, magnesium, and potassium, calcium supplementation did not lower BP. Likewise, in 1 trial of 4,589 pregnant women, calcium supplements had no effect on hypertension, BP, or preeclampsia. Surprisingly, the effects of calcium supplementation on BP in blacks has not been well studied, although they consume much less calcium than their white counterparts. Although the effects of calcium supplementation on BP have been small and inconsistent, clinical trials have demonstrated that calcium supplementation in combination with vitamin D can reduce the risk of bone fractures in older persons.

MAGNESIUM

Overview of Basic Physiology and Nutrition

The adult body contains <25 g of magnesium, of which 40% is in soft tissues, 60% in the skeleton, and only 1% in extracellular fluids. Magnesium is a cofactor in >300 enzyme systems and is required for aerobic and anaerobic energy production, glycolysis, membrane function, and DNA and RNA synthesis. It has been called *nature's physiologic calcium channel blocker.* In magnesium depletion states, intracellular calcium rises and leads to contraction of smooth muscle and skeletal muscle along with a rise in BP. Such findings raise the possibility that magnesium may be involved in BP homeostasis in healthy populations.

Absorption and metabolism. The mechanisms controlling blood levels and intestinal absorption of magnesium are poorly understood. The kidney has a predominant role in magnesium homeostasis, reabsorbing most filtered magnesium, particularly in magnesium deficiency states. As with calcium, fractional absorption is inversely proportional to the amount of magnesium ingested.

United States intake levels. According to data from the 1994 Continuing Survey of Food Intake, the median dietary intake of magnesium is nearly 330 mg per day in adult men and <230 mg per day in women. Magnesium intake decreases to a minor extent with age. Approximately 45% of dietary magnesium comes from fruits, vegetables, grains, and nuts and <30% from milk, meat, and eggs. According to recent guidelines, the recommended dietary allowance of magnesium is 420 mg for adult men (>30 years old) and 320 mg for adult women.

Clinical Studies of Magnesium and Blood Pressure

The body of evidence implicating magnesium as a major determinant of BP is inconsistent.

Epidemiologic studies. In observational studies, often cross-sectional in design, a common finding is an inverse association of dietary magnesium with BP. This relationship was seen in cross-sectional analyses of 15,248 participants in the Atherosclerosis Risk in Communities study, in which hypertensive participants also had lower serum magnesium levels than did normotensives. In 1 prospective observational study, dietary magnesium intake was inversely related to systolic and diastolic BP and change in BP; however, these relationships did not persist after adjustment for fiber.

Clinical trials. Evidence from clinical trials has been inconsistent. In phase 1 of the Trials of Hypertension Prevention, supplemental magnesium had no effect on BP in 461 persons with high normal BP. Magnesium in combination with either potassium or calcium had no effect on BP in a trial of 125 hypertensives. Most recently, in a trial of 300 female nurses with low dietary intake of magnesium, potassium, and calcium, magnesium had no effect on BP. In contrast, in a crossover, dose-response trial of only 17 hypertensive patients, oral magnesium resulted in a significant dose-dependent reduction in BP. In a metaanalysis of 20 clinical trials, there were nonsignificant reductions in systolic and diastolic BP of 0.6 and 0.8 mm Hg, respectively. A dose-dependent effect of magnesium was present for systolic but not diastolic BP. Overall, it appears that magnesium supplementation in nondeficient general populations has little impact on BP. However, as mentioned previously, the DASH diet that is rich in magnesium (>400 mg/day) and other nutrients substantially lowered systolic and diastolic BP.

HEAVY METALS

Heavy metals such as lead and mercury may have direct and indirect effects on BP, the latter mediated through renal toxicity. Humans are exposed to lead from environmental sources, including lead from gasoline, soldered cans, paint, dust, and soil. National survey data suggest lead exposure has decreased, at least between 1976 and 1991. In the human body, most lead (more than 95%) is stored in calcified tissues, predominantly bone. The turnover of lead in bone is extremely slow.

Toxic levels of lead can lead to cardiovascular-renal disease. However, from a public health perspective, the most relevant issue is whether chronic exposure to nontoxic levels affects health. A large number of observational studies, often population-based surveys, have correlated blood lead with BP. Many but not all studies adjusted for potential confounders, including alcohol intake, body mass index, and use of antihypertensive medication. In a metaanalysis of 31 observational studies with 58,518 participants, there was a weak, statistically significant, direct association of blood lead with BP; specifically, a 2-fold rise in blood lead was associated with a 1.0 mm Hg increase in systolic BP and a 0.6 mm Hg increase in diastolic BP.

In children, toxic exposure to elemental mercury can simulate pheochromocytoma, with its markedly high BP and tachycardia. The most common type of toxic exposure is mercury spillage from a thermometer or sphygmomanometer. At room temperature, mercury vaporizes easily. The vapors can then be inhaled and subsequently absorbed through alveolar membranes. Fortunately, cases of acute toxicity are uncommon.

SUGGESTED READING

1. Allender PS, Cutler JA, Follmann D, et al. Dietary calcium and blood pressure: a meta-analysis of randomized clinical trials. *Ann Intern Med.* 1996;124:825–831.
2. Appel LJ, Moore TJ, Obarzanek E, et al. for the DASH Collaborative Research Group. A clinical trial of the effects of dietary patterns on blood pressure. *N Engl J Med.* 1997;336:1117–1124.
3. Cappuccio FP, Elliott P, Allender PS, et al. Epidemiologic association between dietary calcium intake and blood pressure: a meta-analysis of published data. *Am J Epidemiol.* 1995;142:935–945.
4. Institute of Medicine. *Dietary Reference Intakes: Calcium, Phosphorus, Magnesium, Vitamin D, and Fluoride.* Washington, DC: National Academy Press; 1997.
5. Jee SH, Guallar E, Singh VK, et al. The effect of magnesium supplementation on blood pressure: a meta-analysis of randomized clinical trials. *Am J Hypertens.* 2002;15:691–696.
6. Levine RJ, Hauth JC, Curet LB, et al. Trial of calcium to prevent preeclampsia. *N Engl J Med.* 1997;337:69–76.
7. Nawrot TS, Thijis L, Den Hond EM, et al. An epidemiological re-appraisal of the association between blood pressure and blood lead: a meta-analysis. *J Hum Hypertens.* 2002;16:123–131.
8. Sacks FM, Willett WC, Smith A, et al. Effect on blood pressure of potassium, calcium, and magnesium in women with low habitual intake. *Hypertension.* 1998;31:131–138.
9. Torres AD, Rai AN, Hardiek ML. Mercury intoxication and arterial hypertension: report of two patients and review of the literature. *Pediatrics.* 2000;105:E34. Available at: http://www.pediatrics.org/cgi/content/full/105/3/e34. Accessed on October 28, 2002.
10. Yamamoto ME, Applegate WB, Klag MJ, et al. Lack of blood pressure effect with calcium and magnesium supplementation in adults with high-normal blood pressure: results from Phase I of the Trials of Hypertension Prevention (TOHP). *Ann Epidemiol.* 1995;5:96–107.

Obesity, Body Fat Distribution, and Insulin Resistance: Clinical Relevance

Steven M. Haffner, MD

KEY POINTS

- Obesity is widely recognized as a risk factor for the development of hypertension; an association between abdominal or visceral fat and blood pressure has been shown to be independent of obesity.

- An adverse body fat distribution is associated with insulin resistance, which may be an important cause of hypertension.

- Persons who develop hypertension at an early age have an increased frequency of lipid disorders (familial dyslipidemic hypertension); many of these people have increased glucose and insulin concentrations.

- Diuretics and β-blockers tend to exacerbate glucose intolerance, whereas α-blockers, angiotensin-converting enzyme inhibitors, and angiotensin blockers tend to have favorable effects.

See also Chapters A44, A45, A76, B87, B93, B98, B103, C127–C129, C152, C162, and C166

Obesity in clinical and epidemiologic studies is most often assessed by body mass index (BMI: weight in kg divided by the square of height in meters). Obesity is widely recognized as a risk factor for the development of hypertension. In the follow-up study of the First National Health and Nutrition Examination Survey (NHANES I), overall adiposity measured by BMI strongly predicted the incidence of hypertension in blacks and whites and weight loss has been shown to be associated with decreases in blood pressure (BP) in many studies. These relationships are evident in many ethnic groups.

Body Fat Distribution

Recently, the pattern of body fat distribution has been recognized as a major risk factor, with upper-body obesity being associated with dyslipidemia, type 2 diabetes, and hypertension.

Assessment techniques. The most common clinical and epidemiologic assessments of body fat distribution have been made from measures of central or upper-body adiposity, such as subscapular skinfolds, the ratio of subscapular to triceps skinfolds, or the ratio of waist to hip circumferences (WHR). Unfortunately, there is no agreement on landmarks for the measurement of circumferences. Often, waist circumference is measured at the umbilicus or, alternatively, at the minimum diameter between the thorax and the hips. Hip circumference can be measured at the maximum diameter of the hips or, alternatively, at the level of the greater trochanter. There are also no internationally recognized standards as to what constitutes upper-body adiposity, although some authors have suggested a WHR >0.95 in men and a WHR >0.85 in women. The WHR and ratio of skinfolds are related to the general degree of adiposity. Central adiposity, as assessed by skinfolds, has been related to BP cross-sectionally in whites, blacks, and Hispanics. Waist to hip circumferences have also been related to BP in Hispanics and whites. The association between body fat distribution and BP has been shown to be independent of obesity in a number of studies.

Visceral fat. Recently, interest has focused on the possible role of visceral fat (measured by computerized tomography) as compared to the less metabolically active central subcutaneous fat. The ratio of visceral fat to subcutaneous fat is more closely correlated with the risk of type 2 diabetes than are assessments of fat distribution using circumferences or skinfolds. Fewer data are available on the possible role of visceral fat in hypertension, although a recent report has suggested very high correlations between visceral and retroperitoneal adipose tissue mass and BP in normoglycemic humans. Waist circumference may even be a better indicator of visceral fat than WHR.

Insulin Resistance and the Pathogenesis of Hypertension

The mechanisms by which obesity and body fat distribution lead to an increased risk of hypertension are not well understood. An adverse body fat distribution has been associated with insulin resistance, which may be an important cause of hypertension. The clustering of cardiovascular risk factors, including dyslipidemia, diabetes, hypertension, obesity, and central adiposity, has long been recognized. Many studies have shown that lean, normoglycemic untreated hypertensive subjects are more insulin-resistant than comparable normotensive subjects. Furthermore, subjects who develop hypertension at an early age have an increased frequency of lipid disorders (familial dyslipidemic hypertension); a subset of these patients have increased glucose and insulin concentrations. Insulin resistance may underlie this cluster of atherogenic changes. Multiple mechanisms have been proposed to explain a possible relationship between insulin resistance and hypertension, including increased sympathetic nervous system activity, proliferation of vascular smooth muscle cells, altered cation transport, and increased sodium retention.

Race effects. The association between insulin and hypertension is still controversial, in part because of inconsistent evidence. One reason for the discrepancy between studies is the possibility that the etiology of hypertension is different among ethnic groups. One cross-sectional study suggested a relationship between insulin resistance and BP in whites but not in blacks or Pima Indians, whereas another found a definite association between insulin resistance and mild hypertension in young, lean black men. A relationship between insulin resistance and hypertension has been shown in lean type 1 diabetic subjects but not in obese type 2 diabetic subjects. Because the blacks in the later report were much leaner than those in the former study (BMI, 24 vs. 31 kg/m^2, respectively), the discrepancy of whether insulin resistance is associated with hypertension may have been due to differences in adiposity. Studies using the hyperinsulinemic euglycemic clamp showed that decreased insulin sensitivity is directly associated with BP in a large number of nonobese nondiabetic Europeans.

Insulin effects. Other studies have disputed some of the proposed mechanisms that might underlie the relationship of insulin resistance and hypertension. Short-term insulin infusions (2 hours) raise catecholamines but not BP in normotensive men. Similarly, short-term infusion leading to vasodilation rather than vasoconstriction has also been shown in humans and in dogs. However, the effect of chronic hyperinsulinemia (i.e., lasting months or years) is not known. Ecologic data also do not support a strong relationship between insulin and BP. Pima Indians and Mexican Americans have high rates of type 2 diabetes, hyperinsulinemia, and insulin resistance and yet have a lower prevalence of hypertension. Certain antihypertensive agents have been reported to increase insulin resistance and induce dyslipidemia. Many studies have avoided this problem by studying hypertensive subjects not currently on medications. However, another potential problem with cross-sectional studies is that the clustering of risk factors (including insulin resistance) could result from compensatory mechanisms that induce secondary metabolic changes such as increased catecholamines.

Risk Factor Clustering

A prospective study examined the role of obesity, body fat distribution, and insulin concentrations in relation to the development of hypertension in 1,440 nonhypertensive Mexican-American and non-Hispanic white subjects over 8 years. Obesity, glucose intolerance, and fasting insulin were each significantly related to the incidence of hypertension in univariate analyses. Subjects in the highest category of BMI ($\geq$30 kg/m^2) had an increased incidence of hypertension relative to subjects with lower BMIs [13.8% vs. 6.3%, respectively; relative risk (RR) = 2.00; p <.001]. Similarly, subjects in the highest third of insulin concentrations (>95 pmol/L) had an increased incidence of hypertension relative to subjects with lower insulin concentrations (13.4% vs. 6.9%, respectively; RR = 1.93; p = .001). Sub-

jects with type 2 diabetes had an increased incidence of hypertension relative to subjects with normal glucose tolerance (17.1% vs. 7.8%, respectively; RR = 2.18; p = .04). None of the interactions of ethnicity with BMI, insulin, and glucose tolerance status were statistically significant (p >.50), suggesting that the effects of BMI, insulinemia, and glucose intolerance category on hypertension incidence were similar in both ethnic groups. In nondiabetic populations, subjects had dyslipidemia (increased triglyceride and decreased high-density lipoprotein cholesterol levels) before the onset of hypertension. This observation supports the general concept of the clustering of the cardiovascular risk factors with hypertensive subjects, as has been proposed in the familial dyslipidemia hypertension syndrome; furthermore, the lipid disorder may precede the development of hypertension. Because the relative impact of insulin resistance may be greater in lean than in obese subjects, the incidence of hypertension was examined stratified simultaneously by BMI and fasting insulin concentrations. In nonobese subjects (BMI <25 kg/m^2), the incidence of hypertension increased with baseline fasting insulin concentrations in a stepwise fashion. This relation was not consistently observed in more obese subjects. In lean subjects, the incidence of hypertension for those in the highest third of insulin concentration compared with those in the lowest two-thirds was 10.1% versus 4.5%, respectively (RR = 2.24; p = .0032), in subjects with BMI between 25 and 30 kg/m^2, and the incidence in the corresponding insulin categories was 11.5% versus 15.0%, respectively (RR = 0.70; p = not significant). Thus, the effect of fasting insulin on the incidence of hypertension decreased with increasing obesity.

Antihypertensive Agents and Glucose Intolerance

A number of studies have suggested that thiazides and β-blockers might worsen glucose tolerance and insulin resistance. In contrast, calcium antagonists (with the possible exception of nifedipine) are believed not to affect insulin sensitivity, and certain angiotensin-converting enzyme inhibitors, angiotensin blockers, and α-blockers tend to improve insulin sensitivity. Antihypertensive agents that worsen insulin sensitivity might be expected to increase the risk of diabetes because hyperinsulinemia and insulin resistance are strongly related to the incidence of type 2 diabetes. This is important because hypertensive persons appear to be at increased risk of diabetes, as evidenced by the clustering of diabetes and hypertension.

In a longitudinal study of Swedish women, it was observed that hypertensive women taking diuretics have a significant 3.4-fold–higher risk of developing diabetes than untreated hypertensive women. Relative to hypertensive subjects not on therapy, the risk of developing diabetes was even higher in hypertensive subjects taking β-blockers and hypertensive subjects taking both thiazides and β-blockers. In a 10-year follow-up study, 12.7% of hypertensive men developed diabetes, as opposed to 3.6% of nonhypertensive men (p <.001). Others have found that whereas the use of antihypertensive agents is associated with an increased risk of diabetes, the risk of diabetes with thiazide diuretics is not different from that with other antihypertensive agents.

In another prospective study, subjects who were hypertensive at baseline had a higher 8-year incidence of type 2 diabetes (8.9% vs.

4.9%, $p = .041$) and impaired glucose tolerance (25.2% vs. 10.0%, $p < .001$) than subjects who were normotensive at baseline. After adjustment for age, sex, ethnicity, obesity, body fat distribution, fasting glucose, and insulin, this excess was present only for impaired glucose intolerance. Thus, the excess risk of type 2 diabetes in hypertensive patients can be explained by their greater age, obesity, more unfavorable body fat distribution, and hyperinsulinemia, whereas their excess risk of impaired glucose intolerance is independent of these factors. The odds of developing type 2 diabetes for hypertensive subjects on β-blockers and thiazides versus other hypertensives were not greater than with other agents, contrary to the Swedish studies. In the Heart Outcomes Prevention Evaluation (HOPE) trial, ramipril, an angiotensin-converting enzyme inhibitor, was associated with a decreased risk of developing type 2 diabetes. A similar reduced incidence of new type 2 diabetes was observed in the Losartan Intervention for Endpoint (LIFE) trial in which a regimen beginning with an adrenergic receptor binder (losartan) was compared to a β-blocker (atenolol).

SUGGESTED READING

1. Blair D, Habicht JP, Sims EA, et al. Evidence for an increased risk for hypertension with centrally located body fat and the effect of race and sex on this risk. *Am J Epidemiol.* 1984;119:526–540.

2. Ferrannini E, Natali A, Capaldo B, et al. Insulin resistance, hyperinsulinemia, and blood pressure. *Hypertension.* 1997;30:1144–1149.
3. Haffner SM, Ferrannini E, Hazuda HP, Stern MP. Clustering of cardiovascular risk factors in confirmed prehypertensive individuals. *Hypertension.* 1992;20:38–45.
4. Hunt SC, Wu LL, Hopkins PN, et al. Apolipoprotein, low density lipoprotein subfraction, and insulin associations with familial combined hyperlipidemia: study of Utah patients with familial dyslipidemic hypertension. *Arteriosclerosis.* 1989;9:335–344.
5. Litholl HOL. Effect of antihypertensive drugs on insulin glucose and lipid metabolism. *Diabetes Care.* 1991;14:203–209.
6. Lorenzo C, Serrano-Rios M, Martinez-Larrad MT, et al. Prevalence of Hypertension in Hispanic and non-Hispanic white populations. *Hypertension.* 2002;39:203–208.
7. Morales PA, Mitchell BD, Valdez RA, et al. Incidence of NIDDM and impaired glucose tolerance in hypertensive subjects: the San Antonio Heart Study. *Diabetes.* 1993;42:154–161.
8. Pouliot MC, Després JP, Lemieux S, et al. Waist circumference and abdominal sagittal diameter: best simple anthropometric indexes of abdominal visceral adipose tissue accumulation and related cardiovascular risk in men and women. *Am J Cardiol.* 1994;73:460–468.
9. Saad MF, Lillioja S, Nyomba BL, et al. Racial differences in the relation between blood pressure and insulin resistance. *N Engl J Med.* 1991;324:733–739.
10. Yusuf S, Sleight P, Pogue J, et al. Effects of an angiotensin-converting-enzyme inhibitor, ramipril, on cardiovascular events in high-risk patients. The Heart Outcomes Prevention Evaluation Study Investigators. *N Engl J Med.* 2000;342:145–153.

Chapter B98

Physical Activity and Blood Pressure

Denise G. Simons-Morton, MD, PhD

KEY POINTS

- Numerous epidemiologic studies, both cross-sectional and longitudinal, have observed inverse relationships between amount of physical activity and blood pressure level.

- Clinical trials demonstrate that physical activity significantly decreases systolic blood pressure in all population groups and diastolic blood pressure in all but those with isolated systolic hypertension.

- At least 120 minutes per week of aerobic activity of moderate intensity (e.g., brisk walking) appears to be needed for a clinically relevant BP effect.

See also Chapters B87, B97, B103, C117, C127, C129, C130, C162, and C166

Physical activity has an important influence on blood pressure (BP) as well as on overall cardiovascular disease (CVD) risk. Physical activity (a behavior that results in energy expenditure) and cardiorespiratory fitness (a physiologic attribute of the body's ability to use oxygen that is increased by physical activity) are inversely associated with BP level and hypertension incidence. Randomized trials have demonstrated that increasing physical activity can lower BP. A substantial body of evidence strongly supports the assertion that a physically active lifestyle can delay or prevent the development of hypertension and thus the need for antihypertensive medication.

Benefits of Physical Activity

In addition to effects on BP and cardiorespiratory fitness, physical activity provides other benefits that reduce risk of CVD, including favorable effects on blood lipids, body weight, and blood glucose levels. Physical activity and cardiorespiratory fitness are inversely associated with CVD incidence and mortality as well as with total mortality. In addition, physical activity has favorable effects on other conditions, such as osteoporosis, risk of some cancers, depression, and physical functioning in the elderly. Physical activity also increases the general sense of well-being. Therefore, physical activity should be promoted for a variety of benefits, of which a favorable effect on BP is only 1.

Table B98.1. Exercise Prescription to Control Blood Pressure and to Develop and Maintain Cardiorespiratory Fitness

PARAMETER	DESCRIPTION
Mode of activity	Large-muscle activity that is rhythmic and aerobic (e.g., walking, running, cycling)
Frequency	3–5 d per week
Duration	20–60 min
Intensity	60–90% of maximum heart rate (50–85% of maximum oxygen uptake)

Source: American College of Sports Medicine.

Physical Inactivity and Hypertension

Observational evidence. Prospective studies have found that the incidence of hypertension is higher in those with lower activity levels or lower levels of cardiorespiratory fitness. The associations generally have held when age, sex, smoking, weight, body mass index, blood lipids, or other potentially confounding factors are controlled. Although the evidence from observational studies is strong for an inverse relationship between physical activity level and BP, these studies are limited by the inability to ensure that all other factors that affect BP are the same between active and nonactive groups.

Clinical trials. More than 50 controlled trials have been conducted that have examined the effects on BP of physical activity or exercise regimens. Most of the physical activity regimens tested have been *aerobic exercise*, defined as rhythmic exercise that involves large muscle movements (running, walking, cycling, or swimming) and causes increases in heart and respiration rates (which results in increased oxygen consumption). The exercise regimens tested in most studies have used a frequency, intensity, and duration based on the American College of Sports Medicine (ACSM) exercise prescription for improving cardiorespiratory fitness (**Table B98.1**). Some studies have examined the effects of dynamic resistance exercise (weight training) and more moderate intensities of activity, such as walking.

Metaanalyses. At least 8 quantitative metaanalyses have been conducted to examine the effects of exercise on BP in controlled trials. These results have included effects of aerobic exercise on BP overall (54 trials), in normotensive and hypertensive individuals (approximately 15 and 25 trials, respectively), in women (10 studies), and in adults ≥50 years old (7 studies) (**Figure B98.1**). In addition, other metaanalyses have examined the effects on BP of resistance (weight) training (11 studies) and walking (16 studies). All have concluded that physical activity significantly decreases systolic and diastolic BP in all population groups analyzed and by all types of exercise examined, except for diastolic BP reduction in older adults, which was not significant. Effects are greater in those hypertensive individuals who routinely perform more minutes of training. The BP-lowering effects of exercise are independent of weight changes.

Types of Exercise and Duration

At least 120 minutes of exercise of moderate intensity appears to be needed for a clinically relevant BP effect (reduction of approximately 5.0/2.5 mm Hg) (Figure B98.1). Although some

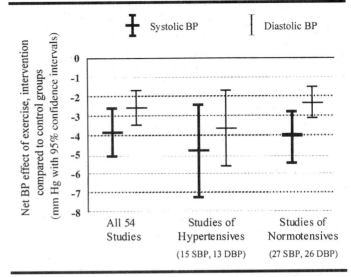

Figure B98.1. Results of a metaanalysis of 54 controlled trials published through September 2001 that tested effects of aerobic exercise on blood pressure (BP). DBP, diastolic blood pressure; SBP, systolic blood pressure. (Based on data reported by Whelton SP, Chin A, Zin Z, He J. Effect of aerobic exercise on blood pressure: a meta-analysis of randomized controlled trials. *Ann Intern Med.* 2002;136:493–503.)

reviewers have concluded that moderate-intensity activity has BP-lowering effects as great as or greater than those of vigorous-intensity activity (running), few studies have directly compared the effects on BP of differing exercise intensities. Making comparisons across studies is problematic because of differences in populations, exercise protocols, length of follow-up, and other characteristics. One randomized trial compared the effects of incorporating physical activity into daily activities (walking up stairs instead of taking the elevator or being more active in home and yard endeavors) with a more traditional exercise regimen based on the ACSM prescription for cardiorespiratory fitness. Both interventions lowered BP, with no significant difference between groups, although the traditional exercise group experienced increased cardiovascular fitness. One metaanalysis found that BP reductions at lower levels of training intensity were proportional to the minutes of training.

Although more evidence is needed about the relative biologic effects of moderate- and vigorous-intensity activity, behavioral intervention studies provide evidence that people may be more able to achieve moderate- than vigorous-intensity activity. The implication is that initial changes in activity levels in sedentary or irregularly active people should employ moderate-intensity activities, such as brisk walking.

National Recommendations

Consensus statements. The National High Blood Pressure Education Program recommends physical activity as an adjunctive treatment for patients with stage 2 and stage 3 hypertension and in those with stage 1 or high-normal BP who are diabetic or have demonstrable target-organ damage. It should be used as a first-line intervention for patients with high-normal and stage 1 hypertension who are free of target-organ damage and as a population-wide behavior for preventing the increase in BP that occurs with age. Numerous organizations recommend that physicians and other health care providers should counsel their patients to be physically active. For controlling BP, the ACSM recommends the exercise regimen used for developing and maintaining cardiorespiratory fitness (Table B98.1). More recently, the focus has been on health in general rather than on cardiorespiratory fitness. The ACSM and the Centers for Disease Control and Prevention, as well as the Surgeon General's Report on Physical Activity and Health, recommend a minimum of 30 minutes of moderate-intensity physical activity on most days. These recommendations also state that additional activity, which can be achieved by increasing frequency, duration, intensity, or a combination of these, can result in additional health benefits.

Activity requirements. An intensity of 50% to 69% of maximum heart rate is considered to be moderate, and an intensity of ≥70% of maximum heart rate is considered to be vigorous. Moderate-intensity activity for most people is comparable to a brisk walking pace of 3 to 4 miles per hour, and vigorous-intensity activity is comparable to jogging or running. Maximum heart rate can be estimated by subtracting age from the constant 220. All of the recommendations focus on aerobic exercise as the primary activity. Some of the recommendations include weight training as part of an overall fitness regimen, but none recommend weight training as a sole mode of exercise. The role of weight training in hypertension treatment or prevention needs further study, but it is recommended for overall fitness (see Chapter C130).

SUGGESTED READING

1. American College of Sports Medicine. Position stand: physical activity, physical fitness, and hypertension. *Med Sci Sports Exerc*. 1993;25:i–x.
2. American College of Sports Medicine. Position stand: the recommended quantity and quality of exercise for developing and maintaining cardiorespiratory and muscular fitness, and flexibility in healthy adults. *Med Sci Sports Exerc*. 1998;30:975–991.
3. Fletcher GF, Blair SN, Blumenthal J, et al. Statement on exercise: benefits and recommendations for physical activity programs for all Americans: a statement for health professionals by the Committee on Exercise and Cardiac Rehabilitation of the Council on Clinical Cardiology, American Heart Association. *Circulation*. 1992;86:340–344.
4. Kelley GA, Kelley KA, Tran ZV. Aerobic exercise and resting blood pressure: a meta-analytic review of randomized, controlled trials. *Prev Cardiol*. 2001;4:73–80.
5. Kelley GA, Kelley KS. Progressive resistance exercise and resting blood pressure: a meta-analysis of randomized controlled trials. *Hypertension*. 2000;35:838–843.
6. NIH Consensus Development Panel on Physical Activity and Cardiovascular Health. Physical activity and cardiovascular health. *JAMA*. 1996;276:241–246.
7. Pate RR, Pratt M, Blair SN, et al. Physical activity and public health: a recommendation from the Centers for Disease Control and Prevention and the American College of Sports Medicine. *JAMA*. 1995;273:402–407.
8. U.S. Department of Health and Human Services. *Physical Activity and Health: A Report of the Surgeon General*. Atlanta, GA: U.S. Department of Health and Human Services, Centers for Disease Control and Prevention, National Center for Chronic Disease Prevention and Health Promotion; 1996.
9. Whelton SP, Chin A, Zin Z, He J. Effect of aerobic exercise on blood pressure: a meta-analysis of randomized controlled trials. *Ann Intern Med*. 2002;136:493–503.

Chapter B99

Alcohol Use and Blood Pressure

William C. Cushman, MD

KEY POINTS

- Many epidemiologic studies have shown a direct relationship between alcohol intake and hypertension, especially above an average intake of 2 drinks per day.

- Reduction in alcohol intake is associated with lowering of blood pressure in at least 15 randomized controlled trials: Each reduction by 1 drink per day lowers systolic and diastolic blood pressure approximately 1 mm Hg.

- Although regular alcohol intake is associated with lower risk for atherothrombotic cardiovascular events, excessive intake increases the risk of many medical and psychosocial problems, including hypertension.

- For persons with hypertension who drink excessively, average maximum alcohol intakes of 1 drink per day in women and 2 drinks per day in men are reasonable goals if drinking is not otherwise contraindicated.

See also Chapters A56, B97, and C129

Regular alcohol consumption can produce positive psychosocial effects and some beneficial effects on health, especially reduced atherothrombotic events and death. However, excessive alcohol intake causes many serious adverse psychosocial and health consequences. One of the harmful effects of excess alcohol intake is its impact on blood pressure (BP). Hemodynamic effects of alcohol have been reported at least since the middle of the nineteenth century. The first population-based study of alcohol use and prevalence of hypertension was reported in 1915 by a French surgeon, Lian, who found a linear

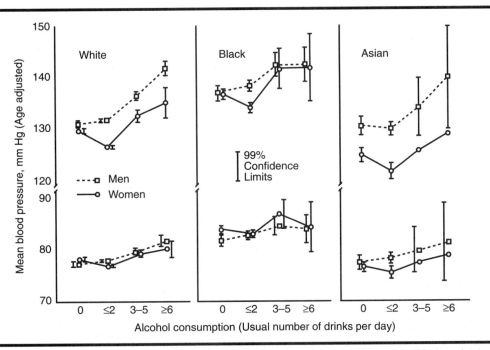

Figure B99.1. Mean systolic blood pressures (*upper half*) and mean diastolic blood pressures (*lower half*) for white, black, and Asian men and women with known drinking habits. Small circles represent data based on fewer than 30 persons. (From Klatsky AL, Friedman GD, Siegelaub AB, Gerard M. Alcohol consumption and blood pressure. *N Engl J Med.* 1977;296:1194–1200, with permission.)

relationship between the amount of wine regularly ingested by French troops on the western front and the prevalence of hypertension. Most studies on the relationship between alcohol intake and BP, however, have been reported in the past several decades.

Epidemiology

Amount and type of alcohol. A standard drink in the United States is usually defined as 14 g of alcohol (ethanol). This amount of alcohol is in 12 oz of beer, 5 oz of table wine, or 1.5 oz of 80 proof (40% alcohol) distilled spirits. Some studies suggest that one type of alcoholic beverage, such as beer or liquor, is more strongly associated with BP than other types of beverages, such as wine. However, when all studies are taken together, it appears that the relationship between alcohol and BP is primarily dependent on the amount of alcohol ingested, rather than the type of beverage.

Epidemiologic associations. The relationship between the amount of alcohol consumed and BP is robust. Cross-sectional epidemiologic studies from many cultures have shown progressively higher BP levels or a higher prevalence of hypertension with increasing levels of alcohol intake. Alcohol intake also predicts future BP elevation and development of hypertension in prospective observational studies.

Above an average intake of 2 drinks per day, the higher the alcohol intake is, the higher the BP. This relationship is usually still present even when taking into account other factors, such as age, weight (or body mass index), sodium and potassium intake, cigarette smoking, and education. Alcohol has been found to increase BP in whites, blacks, and Asians (**Figure B99.1**). Sometimes a J-shaped relationship is found, that is, the lowest BP levels are seen with low levels of alcohol intake compared with no drinking or drinking 3 or more drinks per day. Although low levels of alcohol intake are occasionally associated with higher BP levels than no drinking, most often there is no BP difference on average between nondrinkers and those drinking no more than 2 drinks per day. However, even when BP is reported to be different between these 2 groups, the difference is small. In the Atherosclerosis Risk in Communities (ARIC) study, it was estimated that in subjects drinking ≥30 g per day of alcohol, 1 in 5 cases of hypertension could be attributed to the consumption of alcohol.

Patterns of blood pressure elevation. Studies of both the pattern of alcohol consumption and the temporal relationship of alcohol with BP suggest that there may be an acute BP elevation from the alcohol withdrawal syndrome in episodic and predominantly weekend drinkers and a direct pressor effect in regular daily drinkers. Sustained heavy drinking, however, may cause less reversible hypertensive effects, with evidence suggestive of residual chronic pressor effects of alcohol in heavy drinkers and alcoholics even after subjects have become abstinent.

Drug resistance. Alcohol intake has also been associated with resistance to antihypertensive therapy. Some of the apparent resistance may be from poor medication adherence in heavy drinkers, but some resistance is also clearly from true interference with the BP-lowering effects of medications.

Randomized Controlled Trials

Randomized controlled trials provide strong support of a direct causal link between chronic alcohol consumption and raised BP. They also provide a strong basis for public health and individual recommendations to reduce alcohol intake, if above 2 drinks per day, as part of a program to prevent or treat hypertension.

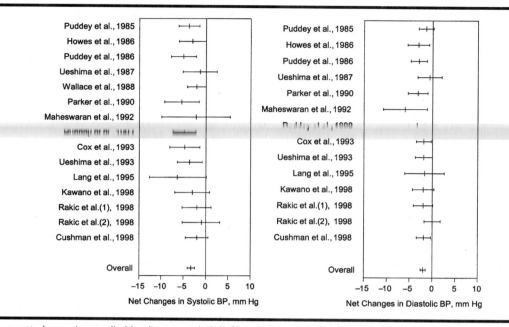

Figure B99.2. Average net change in systolic blood pressure (BP) (*left*) and diastolic BP (*right*) and corresponding 95% confidence intervals related to alcohol reduction intervention in 15 randomized controlled trials. (From Xin X, He J, Frontini MG, et al. Effects of alcohol reduction on blood pressure: a meta-analysis of randomized controlled trials. *Hypertension.* 2001;38:1112–1117, with permission.)

At least 15 randomized controlled trials have examined the effect of a reduction in alcohol intake on BP (**Figure B99.2**). Most trials demonstrate a significant reduction in systolic BP, diastolic BP, or both. Figure B99.2 displays results from a meta-analysis of these 15 studies that included 2,234 participants. Alcohol reduction was associated with a significant reduction in mean (95% confidence interval) systolic and diastolic BP of 3.3 mm Hg (2.5–4.1 mm Hg) and 2.0 mm Hg (1.5–2.6 mm Hg), respectively. A dose-response relationship was observed between mean percentage of alcohol reduction and mean BP reduction. Effects of intervention were enhanced in those with higher baseline BP. Although the majority of these studies included relatively few subjects, were of short duration, and were not designed as effectiveness trials, the results are consistent with the epidemiologic evidence on the relationship of alcohol with BP. The authors of this metaanalysis concluded that "alcohol reduction should be recommended as an important component of lifestyle modification for the prevention and treatment of hypertension among heavy drinkers."

Prevention and Treatment of Hypertension Study. The largest and longest of the randomized controlled trials was the Prevention and Treatment of Hypertension Study (PATHS). The primary objectives of this U.S. National Institutes of Health and Veterans Affairs Cooperative Studies Program trial were to determine whether alcohol could be reduced for at least 6 months and whether BP was lowered by sustained reductions in alcohol intake in 641 moderate to heavy drinkers with diastolic BP 80 to 99 mm Hg. Anyone with evidence of alcoholism, complications of excess alcohol intake, or significant cardiovascular or psychiatric diseases was excluded. Although differences in alcohol intake between randomized groups were highly significant over the 3 to 24 months of follow-up, the difference only averaged 1.3 drinks per day rather than the anticipated 2.0 drinks per day that was projected. This shortfall resulted in part because the control group lowered alcohol intake more than anticipated. The average difference in BP reduction was 0.9/0.6 mm Hg. Although not statistically different, this BP difference is consistent with the approximately 1 mm Hg change in BP for each drink per day change in alcohol intake seen in controlled studies with larger alcohol intake differences. In most other controlled trials of alcohol reduction and BP, baseline levels of alcohol intake were higher and differences in alcohol intake larger than in PATHS.

Other trials. Short-term intervention trials have consistently demonstrated a decline in BP within 1 to 2 weeks of alcohol restriction with further gradual declines in BP after 4 to 6 weeks. In an 18-week study, in which alcohol restriction (by 4–5 standard drinks per day) was combined with caloric restriction (reducing weight by 7.5 kg), the 2 interventions had an additive effect, that is, reducing BP by approximately 10 mm Hg. The 5 studies from Perth, Australia, in normotensive and hypertensive participants are probably the best from which to estimate the expected change in BP with a change in alcohol intake. The investigators typically recruited middle-aged heavy-drinking men and randomized them to continue their usual intake of beer or to drink low-alcohol beer, usually in a crossover design. In these studies, the difference in alcohol intake in the randomized groups averaged 3 to 4 drinks per day: This resulted in 3.8 to 5.4/1.4 to 3.3 mm Hg average difference in BP, although most of the participants in these trials did not have hypertension or were normotensive on therapy. In the first 2 studies, a 3.0 drink per day net reduction in alcohol intake produced a 4.4/2.2 mm Hg average reduction in BP. Across all studies, for every 1 drink per day difference in reduction in alcohol intake, systolic or diastolic BP was reduced approximately 1 mm Hg. In aggregate, the randomized controlled trials provide strong evidence that among persons who drink 3 or more drinks per day, a reduction in alcohol intake can effectively lower BP.

Table B99.1. Suggested Mediators of Direct Effects of Alcohol on Blood Pressure

Stimulation of the sympathetic nervous system, endothelin, renin-angiotensin-aldosterone system, insulin (or insulin resistance), and corticotropin or cortisol

Inhibition of vascular relaxing substances (nitric oxide)

Calcium depletion

Magnesium depletion

Increased intracellular calcium or other electrolytes in vascular smooth muscle

Increased acetaldehyde

Potential Mechanisms of Effect on Blood Pressure

Several mechanisms have been proposed for the relationship between alcohol and elevated BP. An immediate effect of alcohol ingestion is vasodilation in some vascular beds. Sustained intake accompanied by high blood alcohol levels, however, results in short-term elevation of BP. In addition, BP levels usually correlate best with alcohol intake within the previous 24 hours, and BP levels fall within hours to days after cessation or reduction in intake. Therefore, it seems likely that the effect of alcohol on BP is not mediated by long-term structural alterations, but by neural, hormonal, or other reversible physiologic changes. Some evidence, however, also supports a chronic state of alcohol withdrawal in frequent heavy drinkers as the hypertensive effect of alcohol, but there is much evidence in favor of a direct effect of alcohol on BP. There are several suggested mediators for the direct effect of alcohol on BP (**Table B99.1**). There appears to be more evidence to support the role of the sympathetic nervous system or cellular transport and electrolytes, or both, than the other mechanisms suggested, but this remains an open question.

Cardiovascular Protective Effects of Alcohol Intake

Low to moderate levels of alcohol intake are associated with a lower incidence of atherosclerotic cardiovascular events, including myocardial infarction, atherothrombotic stroke, and peripheral and renal vascular disease, compared with no alcohol ingestion. These beneficial epidemiologic observations of alcohol may be related to increases in high-density lipoprotein and apolipoproteins A_1 and A_2, antioxidant effects, decreases in fibrinogen, and reduced ability of platelet aggregation. However, higher intake levels are associated with increased risk of hypertension, cardiomyopathy and other cardiac complications, hemorrhagic and thrombotic strokes, certain kinds of cancer, hepatitis, cirrhosis, pancreatitis, gastritis, suicides, accidents, violence, and alcohol abuse and dependence. Because of these adverse risks, most medical authorities and consensus guidelines do not encourage initiation of alcohol consumption to reduce cardiovascular disease risk. However, for those who choose to drink and have no contraindications, low levels of drinking can be considered prudent.

Clinical Recommendations

All hypertensive patients should be asked about recent drinking, including quantity and frequency of drinking. Those who drink should be given appropriate screening for alcohol dependence. Effective interventions, such as the cognitive-behavioral technique used in the PATHS trial, have been developed to reduce alcohol consumption in nondependent heavy drinkers. Referral to alcohol treatment specialists is necessary in many cases, if there is evidence of alcohol dependence or more serious health consequences of drinking, but primary care physicians and other health care providers should routinely discuss alcohol consumption with their patients and recommend limitation of excessive intake whenever present.

Because of the association between heavy drinking and hypertension, other detrimental health and psychosocial effects, and the potential benefits of alcohol consumption, the current public health recommendation in the United States for those who drink is that average alcohol intake should not exceed 2 drinks per day in men and 1 drink per day in women, because women are generally smaller and have markedly reduced gastric alcohol dehydrogenase compared with men. Many persons should not drink at all, for example, pregnant women and anyone with a history of or who appears to be at risk of a drinking problem or serious medical complications from alcohol. For those who are not in a high-risk category and who drink within the limits outlined above, the risk of developing hypertension is probably not increased and beneficial effects of alcohol may predominate. Persons drinking more than 1 to 2 drinks per day should be encouraged to reduce their intake and thereby reduce BP as well as the risk of developing hypertension and of other alcohol-related problems.

The reductions in BP seen from reducing alcohol intake in randomized controlled trials is comparable to or quantitatively greater than the differences found for most other effective lifestyle interventions. In the Trials of Hypertension Prevention, Phase I (TOHP-I), weight reduction was most effective in reducing BP (2.9/2.3 mm Hg), although sodium reduction also significantly reduced BP (1.7/0.9 mm Hg) and was comparable to the results of alcohol intervention in PATHS. Exercise has also produced reductions in BP at least of this magnitude. Therefore, reduction in alcohol intake should be considered along with weight reduction, limitation of sodium intake, and exercise as the primary lifestyle changes to encourage in patients with or at risk for hypertension. If alcohol intake exceeds an average of 1 to 2 drinks per day, then reduction in alcohol consumption should be included in the initial management plan.

SUGGESTED READING

1. Cushman WC, Cutler JA, Hanna E, et al. for the PATHS Group. The Prevention and Treatment of Hypertension Study (PATHS): effects of an alcohol treatment program on blood pressure. *Arch Intern Med.* 1998;152:1197–1207.

2. Di Castelnuovo A, Rotondo S, Iacoviello L, et al. Meta-analysis of wine and beer consumption in relation to vascular risk. *Circulation.* 2002;105:2836–2844.

3. MacMahon S. Alcohol consumption and hypertension. *Hypertension.* 1987;9:111–121.

4. Marmot MG, Elliott P, Shipley MJ, et al. Alcohol and blood pressure: the INTERSALT study. *BMJ.* 1994;308:1263–1267.

5. *Nutrition and Your Health: Dietary Guidelines for Americans*, 4th ed. Washington, DC: U.S. Department of Agriculture, U.S. Department of Health and Human Services; 1995:40–41.

6. Puddey IB, Beilin LJ, Vandongen R, et al. Evidence for a direct effect of alcohol consumption on blood pressure in normotensive men: a randomized controlled trial. *Hypertension.* 1985;7:707–713.

7. Suh I, Shaten BJ, Cutler JA, Kuller LH. Alcohol use and mortality from coronary heart disease: the role of high-density lipoprotein cholesterol: the Multiple Risk Factor Intervention Trial Research Group. *Ann Intern Med.* 1992;116:881–887.
8. Thun MJ, Peto R, Lopez AD, et al. Alcohol consumption and mortality among middle-aged and elderly US adults. *N Engl J Med.* 1997;337:1705–1714.
9. Xin X, He J, Frontini MG, et al. Effects of alcohol reduction on blood pressure: a meta-analysis of randomized controlled trials. *Hypertension.* 2001;38:1112–1117.

Chapter B100

Stress and Blood Pressure

Norman K. Hollenberg, MD, PhD

KEY POINTS

- Stress is an important environmental factor contributing to acute and chronic elevation of blood pressure.

- Stress is difficult to quantify, but stressful situations can be identified or induced and effects on blood pressure observed.

- Treatment of stress or its psychological consequences is an important adjunct to successful management of hypertension.

See also Chapters A40, A43, A56, B88, B101, C112, C113, and C129

Hypertension is a complex process in which a genetic component, representing 30% to 50% of the total pathogenesis of hypertension, is acted on by environmental factors to result in a sustained increase in blood pressure (BP). Although we know a great deal about factors that regulate BP, we know substantially less about the pathogenesis of essential hypertension.

What Is Stress?

Environmental factors can be divided into 2 major categories: those relating to what we eat and drink and those relating to what is broadly described as *stress*. The general community and the medical community use the word *stress* in a number of ways. A cardiovascular stress test, for example, employs exercise or the infusion of a vasoactive agent in search of evidence of ischemic heart disease. In this chapter, the word *stress* is applied to a psychosocial situation that provokes a negative response, emotional and circulatory. The assessment of stress arising spontaneously in daily life is difficult, both in identifying whether a stimulus is stressful, and if it is, how stressful. One person's source of stress might be another person's exhilarating challenge. Another important consideration involves whether stress is viewed as a primary cause of hypertension, a BP modifier, or a BP amplifier. Although the role stress might play in BP regulation is clearly important, it is remarkable how few studies have addressed the issue.

Clinical anecdotes. Anecdotes can be very dramatic. A young woman, a recently married nurse, was admitted to the hospital with a BP of 260/140 mm Hg. Her BP had been recorded as normal several times in the preceding 2 years. While on vacation at a local lake, she heard her husband approach the dock in a motorboat. She was prompted to go down to the dock by his failure to appear and the sound of the motor boat engine racing

in the harbor. There, she found her husband's headless body floating in the blood-tinged bay and his head looking up at her from the bottom of the boat; he had been decapitated by a tree branch while approaching the dock. Her BP was managed as though she had a pheochromocytoma. After several days, BP medication was weaned, and she was normotensive, remaining so for at least the next 2 years.

A second less dramatic example was provided by woman in her early 30s who migrated to Boston from Cuba. In Boston, she became the leader of a strong anti-Castro movement. Her BP was strikingly labile, but at its nadir, she was always hypertensive. During a renal arteriogram obtained to rule out a renal vascular source of hypertension, we recorded beat-to-beat BPs from the arterial catheter. After a stable 15 minutes, I mentioned Fidel Castro's name to her and asked her opinion. Within 5 heartbeats, her BP had increased from 135/85 mm Hg to 240/120 mm Hg, and renal blood flow fell by half. Plasma norepinephrine doubled within 10 minutes, and plasma epinephrine was increased 5-fold. We concluded that in her basal state she had relatively mild essential hypertension, with an enormous amplification induced by sympathetic nervous system activation, consequent to stress. Her basic medical management had involved treatment with a diuretic and a β-adrenergic blocking agent along with treatment for her anxiety, which removed many if not all of the peaks.

Research Approaches

As stress is so elusive, what strategies can we use to identify its contribution to hypertension? There are 3 approaches available. Perhaps the most engaging, although anecdotal in nature, is individual clinical experience. Second, controlled experiments in animals can explore the influence of acute stress on BP in individual animals or the influence of chronic stress on

BP in a group of animals. Finally, in humans, either laboratory studies of BP in the individual or epidemiologic studies in groups of subjects can be performed. Evidence from each of these sources provides information that suggests that stress does influence BP in groups and can play an important role in BP regulation in individuals.

Animal Studies

Similar studies have been performed in primates, trained to sit tethered in a chair with recording of arterial BP from an implanted catheter, in response to various provocations. As in the case of the patients described in the section Clinical Anecdotes, the primates could be easily provoked into pressor responses. In another approach, rats have been housed in population cages, in which overcrowding is a source of stress; such conditions raised BP in the group as a whole. Social interaction in mice housed in population cages revealed the interesting and somewhat surprising fact that pecking order (i.e., social status) influences BP. Subordinates have lower BPs than dominant animals, and the highest BPs are found in subdominants that are attempting to take over the dominant role.

Human Studies

In humans, a number of models have been examined, and, in general, each has provided evidence for a contribution of stress to BP levels.

Socioeconomic status. As one example, the contribution of stress to the BP level found in blacks was examined in several neighborhoods, which were labeled as stressful or nonstressful according to the population's socioeconomic status, income, home ownership, and educational level. The highest BP levels were seen in black men under the age of 40 living in high-stress neighborhoods. Conversely, ethnicity played no role in low-stress neighborhoods, in which black and white men had essentially identical BP levels. In other studies, where the degree of "blackness" was estimated by a reflectometer, BP levels were influenced by degree of blackness as a surrogate for socioeconomic status.

Job stress. As an alternative approach to examining the effect of chronic stress, a series of studies on BP levels associated with job stress have been performed. Stressful jobs are those which make great demands but provide little control. Although many blue collar jobs share this feature, air traffic controllers, who are not blue collar by any criterion, also show substantial job stress. Increased job stress is associated with a higher average BP level, increased frequency of hypertension, and substantially greater levels of anxiety and depression.

Low-stress environments. As an alternative, one can examine the influence of a stress-free, or at least low-stress, environment on BP. Perhaps the best known and most persuasive study is an observational examination of nuns living in a secluded order in Italy. The nuns were compared with a noncloistered control group both at entry and after 30 years of cloistered life. BP level in the nuns and controls at the beginning of the study were essentially identical. After 30 years of living in the protected environment provided by a cloister, the nuns failed to show the usual increase in BP associated with aging and had

significantly lower average BP; systolic BP had risen by approximately 30 mm Hg in the controls. As a confirmation of the reduction in stress, renal catecholamine excretion was also lower in the nuns.

Migration studies. Kuna Indians residing in their traditional isolated islands off the Caribbean coast of Panama show no BP rise with age and little hypertension. With migration to the city and adoption of an urban life, the Kuna experience all of the sequelae of modern western urban life, including a rise in BP with age and a substantial prevalence of hypertension.

Exaggerated Vasoreactivity

Are there individuals who are especially responsive to stressful situations? Despite a substantial number of studies, we still do not have a clear answer to this question (see Chapter A43). In a major epidemiologic study, Julius and coworkers found in Tecumseh, Michigan, that exaggerated vascular reactivity did not predict future BP levels in a prospective epidemiologic study.

In a smaller physiologic study, the authors found that hypertensives' response to the stress associated with performing a nonverbal intelligence quotient test (Raven's progressive matrices) was too weak to raise BP directly but that renal vasoconstriction and activation of the renin-angiotensin-aldosterone system (RAAS) were evident. Normotensive individuals free of a family history of hypertension showed no RAAS activation at all, whereas normotensive offspring of hypertensives showed RAAS activation and renal vasoconstriction approximately 50% of the time—approximately halfway between the normotensive and hypertensive participants. This physiologic response pattern could predispose to sodium retention and thus to a rise in BP.

Other recent studies suggest that medications such as angiotensin-converting enzyme inhibitors have a much greater effect on basal or resting BP than on acute stress-induced BP elevations. These reactive responses appear to be less exaggerated in individuals with higher levels of perceived social support and in individuals with a sense of environmental control.

Anxiety and Depression

Another subset of patients in whom stress responses may be altered are those who are hypertensive but also are chronically anxious, depressed, or both (see Chapter A56). Both impose a substantial clinical burden on the patient. In the case of depression, the patient has little interest in prolonging his or her life, which is perceived as a burden. To suggest antihypertensive medications, which do not give short-term relief of symptoms but will extend life, must be considered absurd by such patients. Until the depression is adequately managed, antihypertensive therapy may be futile.

In patients with substantial anxiety, the problem is different. BP may not be fully controlled until the anxiety is controlled. The management of anxiety, and especially the anger that often accompanies it, goes beyond the scope of this chapter, but there are several points that should be made. First, either drugs or brief supportive psychotherapy (approximately 12 weeks) can help, but the combination is much more effective. In this regard, the practice of benzodiazepine use on an as-needed basis may be counterproductive—analogous to suggesting that a patient drop into a bar for a drink when he or she feels anxious. The best advice, I believe, is to use techniques that allow affected individuals to cope with their anxiety and anger. There are specific techniques for anger management, if that is a major element in the clinical story, and for anxiety. In both cases, daily medications can be effective adjuncts to supportive psychotherapy. The regimen is often effective after approximately 12 weeks.

SUGGESTED READING

1. Dressler WW. Social support, lifestyle incongruity, and arterial blood pressure in a southern black community. *Psychosom Med.* 1991;53:608–620.
2. Harburg E, Erfurt JC, Chape C, et al. Socioecological stressor areas and black-white blood pressure: Detroit. *J Chronic Dis.* 1973;26:595–611.
3. Henry JP, Liu J, Meehan WP. Psychosocial stress and experimental hypertension. In: Laragh JH, Brenner BM, eds. *Hypertension: Pathophysiology, Diagnosis, and Management*, 2nd ed. Vol 1. New York, NY: Raven Press; 1995:905–921.
4. Hollenberg NK, Martinez G, McCullough M, et al. Aging, acculturation, salt intake and hypertension in the Kuna of Panama. *Hypertension.* 1997;29:171–176.
5. Hollenberg NK, Williams GH, Adams DF. Essential hypertension: abnormal renal vascular and endocrine responses to a mild psychological stimulus. *Hypertension.* 1981;3:11–17.
6. Julius S, Jones K, Schork N, et al. Independence of pressure reactivity from pressure levels in Tecumseh, Michigan. *Hypertension.* 1991;17: III12–21.
7. Oparil S, Chen Y-F, Berecek KH, et al. The role of the central nervous system in hypertension. In: Laragh JH, Brenner BM, eds. *Hypertension: Pathophysiology, Diagnosis, and Management*, 2nd ed. Vol 1. New York, NY: Raven Press; 1995:713–740.
8. Pickering TG, Devereux RB, James GD, et al. Environmental influences on blood pressure and the role of job strain. *J Hypertens Suppl.* 1996;14:S179–186.
9. Rostrup M, Kjeldsen S, Eide JK. Awareness of hypertension increases blood pressure and sympathetic responses to cold pressor test. *Am J Hypertens.* 1990;3:912–917.
10. Timio M. Blood pressure trend and psychosocial factors: the case of the nuns in a secluded order. *Acta Physiol Scand Suppl.* 1997;640:137–139.

Chapter B101

White Coat Hypertension

Thomas G. Pickering, MD, PhD

KEY POINTS

- *White coat hypertension* is generally defined as a persistently elevated clinic pressure in combination with a normal ambulatory pressure in a hypertensive not on treatment.

- The prevalence of white coat hypertension increases with age and varies according to the definition used and the population studied, but is approximately 20% of stage 1 hypertensives.

- White coat hypertension is relatively benign; target organ damage is less frequent in white coat hypertension than in sustained hypertension, but in some studies, target organ damage is more prevalent in white coat hypertension patients than in normotensive patients.

- Antihypertensive medication in white coat hypertension patients usually decreases clinic pressure, with little or no change in ambulatory blood pressure; thus drug treatment may not confer substantial benefit.

See also Chapters A43, B88, B89, B100, C109, C112, C128, and C152

White coat hypertension (WCH) is the most commonly used term to describe patients whose blood pressure (BP) is high only in a medical setting. The term should be reserved for those not on treatment. *Office resistance* is probably a better description for those on treatment whose blood pressure is high in the office but normotensive in other settings. The concept of WCH has been widely adopted in the lay press as well as professional publications. Alternatives that have been proposed are *isolated office hypertension* and *isolated clinic hypertension*. WCH should be distinguished from the *white coat effect*, which is a measure of the pressor response to the clinic visit and is generally defined as the difference between the average clinic BP and the daytime ambulatory pressure. The white coat effect is present to a greater or lesser degree in most hypertensive patients and is greatest in patients with the highest clinic pressures, perhaps because hypertension is identified primarily on the basis of an elevated clinic pressure. Accordingly, there may be a selection bias in the diagnosis of hypertension favoring individuals who tend to show a large white coat effect. In normotensive subjects and some hypertensives, the white coat effect may be absent or even reversed (i.e., the clinic pressure is lower than the daytime pressure).

Definition

WCH is not a discreet entity, so any definition is arbitrary. The most commonly used definition is a persistently elevated clinic or office BP together with a normal ambulatory pressure. The most widely used criterion has been a clinic pressure greater than 140/90 mm Hg together with a daytime ambulatory pressure below 135/85 mm Hg. As shown in **Figure B101.1**, this method of classification identifies 4 groups of indi-

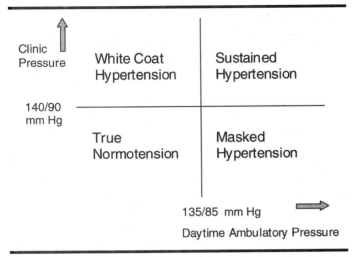

Figure B101.1. Classification of hypertension status according to clinic and ambulatory blood pressure criteria.

viduals: those who are hypertensive by both criteria (true hypertension), normotensive by both (true normotension), hypertensive only by clinic criteria (WCH), and hypertensive only by ambulatory criteria (masked hypertension).

It should be emphasized that WCH cannot be defined on the basis of a single clinic visit, especially the first visit. Many individuals have a relatively high BP when first seen, but BP tends to fall with repeated visits. A related question is whether WCH can be diagnosed by home BP monitoring, without the use of ambulatory BP monitoring. Although a high home BP excludes the diagnosis of WCH, normal home pressures (<135/85 mm Hg) do not establish the diagnosis because the pressure might be high under other conditions, especially at work.

Prevalence

The prevalence of WCH depends on the definition and on demographic features of the population being surveyed, including whether it is a random sample or referred clinic population. Most studies have suggested that WCH occurs in 20% or more of the hypertensive population. Factors associated with WCH are female sex, increasing age, less severe hypertension by clinic measurement, and less frequent clinic visits and measurements. In 1 study in a population of newly diagnosed hypertensives referred for evaluation, 25.8% were classified as white coat hypertensives after the first visit (when an ambulatory BP monitoring was also performed); after the fifth visit, the prevalence was 13.6% (17.7% became clinically normotensive). Because of the magnitude of the white coat effect, WCH should always be considered in the evaluation of elderly patients. The increase of BP that characterizes the white coat effect is not necessarily accompanied by any increase of heart rate.

Natural History and Progression

At least 3 studies have included repeat ambulatory monitoring but have given very different estimates of how many patients make the transition from WCH to true hypertension, ranging from 12.5% to 75.0%. The apparent transition of a patient from white coat to true hypertension could have several explanations. The one that has been most widely advocated is that WCH represents a prehypertensive state, but an equally plausible explana-

tion is that the transition is nothing more than regression to the mean. Because WCH is defined by a relatively high clinic pressure and a relatively low ambulatory pressure, it is to be expected that some patients will have a lower clinic pressure and higher ambulatory pressure on repeat testing. Evidence in support of this comes from the Hypertension and Ambulatory Recording Venetia Study (HARVEST), in which patients with mild hypertension had ambulatory monitoring repeated after 3 months. Of 90 patients initially diagnosed with WCH, only 38 had the same diagnosis 3 months later; the other 52 showed higher ambulatory BPs, such that they were subsequently diagnosed as having true hypertension. Thus, all patients with a diagnosis of WCH must be followed indefinitely with both clinic and home or ambulatory readings.

Metabolic and Biochemical Characteristics of White Coat Hypertension

Some studies have claimed that WCH is associated with metabolic changes that would put white coat hypertensives at higher cardiovascular risk than normotensives, such as high plasma triglycerides, insulin, and insulin to glucose ratios, and low high-density lipoprotein cholesterol. These changes are associated with central obesity. However, the majority of studies show that there is no specific metabolic or obesity-related abnormality associated with WCH.

Target Organ Damage

The extent to which WCH patients exhibit target organ damage is of interest for 2 reasons. First, absence of target organ damage supports the hypothesis that WCH is characterized only by an elevation of BP only in the physician's office. Second, it would imply a benign prognosis. Although the bulk of studies have supported this view, the data have not been consistent, in some cases perhaps because of failure to match groups for demographic confounders. Some studies have showed increased left ventricular mass in WCH, but in these studies, the average daytime pressure has been significantly higher in white coat hypertensives than in normotensives. In general, left ventricular mass in WCH is closer to that found in true normotensives than true hypertensives.

Other measures of target organ damage have also been investigated, but less extensively. In studies using carotid ultrasonography, white coat hypertensives generally have less intimal-medial thickness and less atherosclerotic plaque than true hypertensives. Another index of target organ damage is microalbuminuria, which has been found to be an independent predictor of morbidity. Hoegholm et al. compared microalbuminuria in normotensives, white coat hypertensives, and true hypertensives. Defining WCH as a daytime ambulatory level of <136/90 mm Hg identified a group of patients whose prevalence of target organ damage was no higher than in normotensives. There is no correlation between the magnitude of the white coat effect and left ventricular mass, which is consistent with the idea that chronic BP burden is more important than increased BP reactivity in determining target organ damage.

Morbidity and Mortality

Several prospective studies have provided data consistent with the hypothesis that WCH is associated with a relatively low risk of morbidity, intermediate between truly normotensive and truly hypertensive subjects. Those subjects whose daytime ambulatory pressures are low in relation to their clinic pressure are at lower risk of morbidity. A study of a group of 1,187 normotensive and hypertensive individuals followed for 3 years identified a subgroup of patients with WCH (daytime BP of 131/86 mm Hg in women and 136/87 in men as the upper limit of normal ambulatory pressure). The WCH group experienced an event rate (0.49 per 100 patient-years) that was similar to the rate (0.47) in the normotensives and much lower than hypertensive dippers who constituted the majority (1.79) and in hypertensive nondippers (4.99). In another study of 479 hypertensive patients originally studied with intraarterial monitoring and followed for an average of 9 years (24-hour average of 140/90 mm Hg used to separate WCH from true hypertension), the event rate in WCH was lower than in the true hypertensives (1.32 vs. 2.56 events per 100 patient-years). A substudy of the Systolic Hypertension in Europe (SYST-Eur) trial of treatment of isolated systolic hypertension in the elderly found that patients with WCH were at lower risk of strokes than patients with true hypertension. In a cohort of 958 elderly Japanese patients, most of whom had isolated systolic hypertension and who were followed for an average of 42 months, the relative risk for stroke was 5.5 times higher in the true hypertensives than in white coat hypertensives, with no difference in events between the WCH and normotensive groups. Other prognostic studies, although not defining a distinct group of white coat hypertensives, have concluded that ambulatory BP monitoring gives a better predictor of risk than clinic BP.

Management

The most controversial issue in the management of WCH is whether antihypertensive drug treatment should be prescribed. Most experts favor the view that there is less need to start white coat hypertensives on antihypertensive medication than patients with true hypertension. The principal rationale for this approach to medications is that WCH appears to have a more benign prognosis than true hypertension and that WCH confers only slightly higher risk than true normotension. Several studies have analyzed the effects of antihypertensive medica-

tions in patients with true hypertension and WCH. For example, doxazosin, a long-acting α-blocker, lowered clinic BP to the same extent in both groups, but lowered the ambulatory pressure only in those with true hypertension. Other studies have obtained virtually identical results with calcium antagonists. In WCH, therefore, the white coat effect was reduced by drug treatment. However, there are also reports that angiotensin-converting enzyme inhibitors may lower ambulatory pressure, although clinic pressure is still affected to a greater extent. In the majority of patients with true hypertension, treatment reduces but does not eliminate the white coat effect.

SUGGESTED READING

1. Fagard RH, Staessen JA, Thijs L, et al. Response to antihypertensive therapy in older patients with sustained and nonsustained systolic hypertension. Systolic Hypertension in Europe (Syst-Eur) Trial Investigators. *Circulation.* 2000;102:1139–1144.
2. Fogari R, Corradi L, Zoppi A, et al. Repeated office blood pressure controls reduce the prevalence of white-coat hypertension and detect a group of white-coat normotensive patients. *Blood Press Monit.* 1996;1:51–54.
3. Hoegholm A, Kristensen KS, Bang LE, Nielsen JW. White coat hypertension and target organ involvement: the impact of different cut-off levels on albuminuria and left ventricular mass and geometry. *J Hum Hypertens.* 1998;12:433–439.
4. Kario K, Shimada K, Schwartz JE, et al. Silent and clinically overt stroke in older Japanese subjects with white-coat and sustained hypertension. *J Am Coll Cardiol.* 2001;38:238–245.
5. Palatini P, Dorigatti F, Roman E, et al. White-coat hypertension: a selection bias? Harvest Study Investigators. Hypertension and Ambulatory Recording Venetia Study. *J Hypertens.* 1998;16:977–984.
6. Perloff D, Sokolow M. Ambulatory blood pressure: mortality and morbidity. *J Hypertens Suppl.* 1991;9:S31–S33.
7. Pickering TG, Levenstein M, Walmsley P. Differential effects of doxazosin on clinic and ambulatory pressure according to age, gender, and presence of white coat hypertension. Results of the HALT Study. Hypertension and Lipid Trial Study Group. [See comments.] *Am J Hypertens.* 1994;7:848–852.
8. Verdecchia P. Prognostic value of ambulatory blood pressure: current evidence and clinical implications. *Hypertension.* 2000;35(3):844–851.
9. Verdecchia P, Porcellati C, Schillaci G, et al. Ambulatory blood pressure. An independent predictor of prognosis in essential hypertension. [Published erratum appears in *Hypertension.* 1995;25:462.] [See comments.] *Hypertension.* 1994;24:793–801.
10. White WB, Daragjati C, Mansoor GA, McCabe EJ. The management and follow-up of patients with white-coat hypertension. *Blood Press Monit.* 1996;1:S33–S36.

Chapter B102

Trends in Blood Pressure Control and Mortality

Thomas J. Thom, BA; Edward J. Roccella, PhD, MPH

KEY POINTS

- Approximately 50 million Americans have hypertension, but national surveys show that among persons 18 to 74 years of age, average systolic blood pressures have decreased since the 1960s.

- More hypertensive persons are aware of their condition, are being treated, and have their blood pressure under control since the 1971 to 1974 survey, but preliminary data suggest that improvement in the 1990s was seen only in men.

- Stroke mortality has declined markedly since 1972, resulting in the United States having one of the lowest death rates from stroke in the world; this decline has continued after a period of flattening in the mid-1990s.

See also Chapters B79–B81, B86, B87, B103, B104, B108, C126, and C127

An estimated 50 million Americans have hypertension, one of the major risk factors for stroke, coronary heart disease (CHD), heart failure, and other cardiovascular and renal diseases. The effectiveness of detection, treatment, and control of hypertension plays a major role in the primary and secondary prevention of these diseases. For stroke and heart failure, the relationship between blood pressure (BP) and risk is stronger than the relationship between BP and CHD. The marked acceleration of the downward trend in age-adjusted stroke mortality in the United States after 1972 coincided with the formation of the National High Blood Pressure Education Program, a major national health education effort of the National Heart, Lung, and Blood Institute of the National Institutes of Health to detect, treat, and control hypertension.

Definitions and Data Source

Data from the 1960–1962 National Health Examination Survey, from the National Health and Nutrition Examination Survey (NHANES) studies (1971–1974, NHANES I; 1976–1980, NHANES II; 1988–1994, NHANES III), from 1999 to 2000 (preliminary NHANES IV), and from national vital (mortality) statistics from the National Center for Health Statistics are the primary sources of data. *Hypertension* is defined as a systolic BP of ≥140 mm Hg, a diastolic pressure ≥90 mm Hg, or the use of antihypertensive medication. To examine long-term trends, the formerly accepted definition of 160 mm Hg for systolic and 95 mm Hg for diastolic BP or on treatment has been used. In the health interviews, respondents were asked whether a physician had ever told them that they had hypertension or whether they were taking antihypertensive medication. On the basis of the 2 interview questions plus actual BP measurements, awareness of hypertension diagnosis, treatment, and control status can be ascertained. Mortality data for stroke (cerebrovascular diseases), CHD, and major cardiovascular diseases are based on tabulation of U.S. death certificates as coded by the International Classification of Diseases of the World Health Organization.

Trends

Average blood pressure and prevalence of hypertension.

National surveys show that among persons 18 to 74 years of age, average systolic and diastolic BPs have decreased since the 1960s (**Table B102.1**). Decreases were observed in men and women and in the white and black populations. Declines were greater among older age groups than among younger age groups. Mean systolic and diastolic pressures were significantly higher in the black than in the white population, and mean BPs were higher in men than women overall. Men had higher mean BPs than women at younger ages, but later in life the reverse was true. The prevalence of hypertension for persons 20 to 74 years of age was essentially unchanged during the 1960s and 1970s for white and black men and women, but data from NHANES III indicate a substantial decline in prevalence (**Table B102.2**). Preliminary data from the most recent

Table B102.1. Average Blood Pressure in Persons 18 to 74 Years of Age by Sex and Race, United States, 1960–1962 to 1988–1994 National Health Examination Surveys[a]

	WHITE		BLACK	
	MEN	**WOMEN**	**MEN**	**WOMEN**
Systolic blood pressure, mm Hg				
1960–1962	130	127	135	137
1971–1974	133	129	138	136
1976–1980	129	121	130	127
1988–1994	123	116	127	122
Diastolic blood pressure, mm Hg				
1960–1962	78	77	83	83
1971–1974	85	81	89	86
1976–1980	82	77	84	81
1988–1994	75	69	77	71

[a]Values are age-adjusted. Blood pressures are based on 1, 2, or (usually) 3 seated measurements on 1 occasion.

Table B102.2. Percent Prevalence of Hypertension[a] in Persons 20 to 74 Years of Age by Sex and Race, United States, 1960–1962 to 1988– 1994 National Health Examination Surveys

	WHITE		BLACK	
	MEN	WOMEN	MEN	WOMEN
1960–1962	39.3	31.7	48.1	50.8
1971–1974	41.7	32.4	51.8	50.3
1976–1980	43.5	32.3	48.7	47.5
1988–1994	24.3	19.3	34.9	33.8

[a]Either systolic blood pressure ≥140 mm Hg or diastolic ≥90 mm Hg or taking antihypertensive medication. Values are age-adjusted.

NHANES show a modest although not statistically significant increase in prevalence in men and women from the 1988–1994 lows, but it is still considerably lower than in 1976–1980.

Hypertension awareness, treatment, and control. For persons ages 18 to 74 years, **Figure B102.1** shows the marked improvement since 1971 to 1974 in the proportion of individuals with hypertension who are aware of their condition, are being treated, and have their BP under control. For these analyses, hypertension was defined by a BP >160/95 mm Hg or the use of antihypertensive medication to include older data. Comparable percentages (numbers inside the bars in Figure B102.1) are available only for the 1976–1980 and 1988–1994 periods for the BP threshold >140 mm Hg systolic or >90 mm Hg diastolic or those taking antihypertensive medication.

During the NHANES III survey, which was conducted in 2 phases (1988–1991 and 1991–1994), there were small declines in awareness (73% to 68%), therapy (55% to 54%), and control (29% to 27%) of hypertension based on 140/90 mm Hg cut

points in persons 18 to 74 years of age. Preliminary data from the NHANES IV (1999–2000) show improvement from 1988 to 1994 in awareness, treatment, and control in men but no change in women.

These survey data collected over 4 separate periods document the progress made during the 3 decades of national and community hypertension control efforts. These programs have alerted the public to the dangers of uncontrolled hypertension and its sequelae and have successfully encouraged the public to visit their physicians, have their BPs measured, follow their doctors' advice, and stay on therapy. Of concern is the recent report by the Surgeon General that 61 percent of Americans are overweight; accordingly, further improvements in hypertension control may be slower than in previous decades.

Evidence is mounting that treatment of those with isolated systolic hypertension and of persons with high-normal BP levels is highly beneficial. An estimated 34 million Americans have high-normal BP levels, and approximately half of the population of hypertensives (approximately 25 million) has isolated systolic hypertension. Hypertension remains the major population-attributable risk factor for heart failure, the prevalence of which is approaching 5 million.

Mortality. Stroke is the third leading cause of death in the United States, accounting for >160,000 deaths each year. **Figure B102.2** shows that the age-adjusted death rates for stroke declined at a modest rate (28% overall) during the 22 years from 1950 to 1972. After that year, there was a sharp acceleration in the rate of decline, followed by a flat trend from 1992 to 1996, and resumption of the decline from 1996 to 2000. Between 1972 and 1992, the decline was 58%. The annual decline was <2% per year before 1972 and as much as 6% per year thereafter. Acceleration of the rate of decline occurred in all age, race, and sex groups. Figure B102.2 also shows the reduction in mortality from CHD

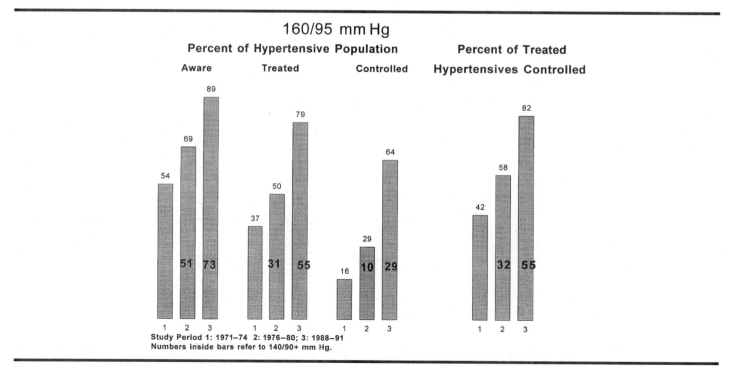

Figure B102.1. Hypertension awareness, treatment, and control rates reported in the National Health and Nutrition Examination Survey; age 18 to 74 years.

Age-Adjusted Death Rate/100,000 Pop.

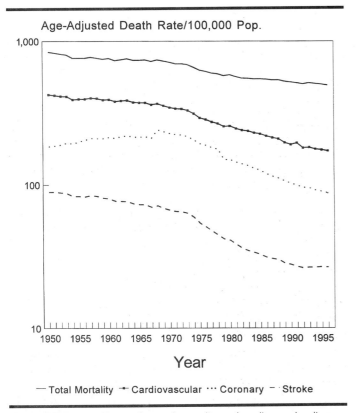

Figure B102.2. Death rates for total mortality and cardiovascular diseases in the United States, 1950 to 1995. Rates adjusted to U.S. population, 1940. No correction made for changes caused by revision in the International Classification of Diseases.

and demonstrates that the trend for total cardiovascular disease improved considerably more than did the trend for all causes of death combined.

Evidence of declining trends in incidence and immediate or long-term survival after stroke is not available on a national scale. Hospital discharge statistics for broad age groups show very modest increases in rates of hospitalization for stroke between 1970 and 1985, followed by modest declines to 2000. They also show steady and significant increases in the percentage of stroke and CHD patients discharged alive from hospitals and decreases in the length of stay since 1970. These statistics, however, are an incomplete measure of incidence and case-fatality, and they are affected by repeat admissions and changes in hospital admission practices.

In addition, community-based studies conducted during the 1970s and 1980s (the Minnesota Heart Survey, the Honolulu Heart Program, the Framingham Study, and the study in Rochester, MN) also report substantial declines in stroke incidence and rates of hospitalizations for stroke as well as improved survival.

Role of Education

In 1972, a large national effort, the National High Blood Pressure Education Program, designed to educate the public, health professionals, and hypertensive patients about the health risks posed by hypertension and the health benefits of its detection, treatment, and control, commenced. This program also developed a national infrastructure that supported and disseminated BP management guidelines, including the 6 periodic reports of the Joint National Committee on Detection, Evaluation, and Treatment of High Blood Pressure. The program has also produced numerous clinical advisories. It is widely believed that part of the mortality decline for stroke and CHD was the result of the massive and successful national campaign to detect, treat, and control hypertension. Simultaneous reductions in the prevalence of smoking and high blood cholesterol and improvements in the treatment of cardiovascular diseases undoubtedly contributed to the decline in cardiovascular mortality. It should be noted that many countries have also adopted U.S. guidelines and procedures for national efforts to control BP and have experienced long-term declines in stroke mortality and, in some cases, acceleration of the rate of decline over the past 20 years.

The sharp and accelerated rate of decline in stroke mortality that began after 1972 still continues. As a result, the United States has one of the lowest death rates from stroke in the world. Many factors contributed to the decline in mortality from stroke and from CHD. These include the introduction of well-tolerated oral antihypertensive drugs and heightened efforts to treat hypertension with these agents and with changes in lifestyle as both adjunctive and definitive care. Improvements in the management of acute stroke (see Chapter A68) and acute coronary disease also contribute. Clinicians have become motivated to manage hypertension more effectively when clinical trial evidence demonstrated reductions in the risks of nonfatal and fatal cardiovascular diseases from lowering BP.

SUGGESTED READING

1. Brown CD, Higgins M, Donato KA, et al. Body mass index and the prevalence of hypertension and dyslipidemia. *Obes Res.* 2000;8:605–619.
2. Burt VL, Cutler JA, Higgins M, et al. Trends in prevalence, awareness, treatment, and control of hypertension in the adult US population: data from the Health Examination Surveys, 1960 to 1991. [Published correction appears in *Hypertension.* 1996;27:1192.] *Hypertension.* 1995;26:60–69.
3. Himmelmann A, Hedner T, Hansson L, et al. Isolated systolic hypertension: an important cardiovascular risk factor. *Blood Press.* 1998;7:197–207.
4. Hyman DJ, Pavlik VN. Characteristics of patients with uncontrolled hypertension in the United States. *N Engl J Med.* 2001;345:479–486.
5. Lenfant C, Roccella EJ. Trends in hypertension control in the United States. *Chest.* 1984;86:459–462.
6. National Heart, Lung, and Blood Institute. Morbidity and Mortality Chartbook on Cardiovascular, Lung, and Blood Diseases. Bethesda, MD: U.S. Dept. of Health and Human Services, Public Health Service, National Institutes of Health; 2002.
7. Proceedings of the National Heart, Lung, and Blood Institute Conference on the Decline in Stroke Mortality, Bethesda, Maryland, November 30–December 1, 1992. *Ann Epidemiol.* 1993;3:453–575.
8. The Sixth Report of the Joint National Committee on Prevention, Detection, Evaluation, and Treatment of High Blood Pressure. Bethesda, MD: National Institutes of Health; 1997. NIH publication 98B4080.
9. U.S. Health, 2001 with Urban and Rural Health Chartbook. Hyattsville, MD: National Center for Health Statistics; 2001:1201.
10. Vasan RS, Larson MG, Leip EP, et al. Impact of high-normal blood pressure on the risk of cardiovascular disease. *N Engl J Med.* 2001;345:1291–1297.

Prevention of Hypertension

Jeffrey A. Cutler, MD, MPH; Jeremiah Stamler, MD

KEY POINTS

- Epidemiologic and clinical trial evidence supports the potential for hypertension prevention through weight control, increased physical activity, moderation of sodium and alcohol intake, increased potassium intake, and a dietary pattern rich in fruits, vegetables, and low-fat meat, fish, and dairy products.

- Both targeted (individual) and population-wide (public health) strategies are important approaches to hypertension prevention.

See also Chapters B81, B93–B99, B102, B104, B105, B108, C126, C129, and C152

Strategic Challenge

In the United States, the prevalence of hypertension in adults is estimated at approximately 1 in 5, or 50 million persons. Each year, there are approximately 1 million new cases. Tens of millions of others have blood pressure (BP) levels above optimal, although not hypertensive (**Figure B103.1**), and these persons are at increased risk of cardiovascular and renal diseases. As large as this BP problem is overall, it is even more severe among those of lower socioeconomic status, regardless of race and ethnicity.

Public Health Strategies

High-risk approach. Until the 1990s, the approach to coping with this mass BP problem was primarily a "high-risk" strategy: detect, evaluate, and treat people with hypertension. This emphasis has accomplished much; it ended therapeutic nihilism in regard to hypertension and has resulted in control of hypertension for millions of Americans. It is a reasonable inference that this effort has been one of the most important factors contributing to the decades-long substantial declines in mortality rates from coronary heart disease and stroke and consequent increases in life expectancy for adult men and women.

But this high-risk strategy has serious limitations. It is late (i.e., defensive rather than proactive), and it relies primarily on drug treatment, with its mix of favorable and unfavorable effects and costs. In addition, millions of Americans with hypertension are treated inadequately or not at all, and tens of millions of other people with nonhypertensive BP elevations are neglected despite their increased cardiovascular-renal risk. Above all, this high-risk strategy is never-ending; it offers no possibility of terminating the epidemic of high BP. Only the primary prevention of this major risk factor offers this possibility.

A pivotal fact is that adverse BP levels result from the rise in systolic and diastolic pressure experienced by most people during the decades from youth through middle age, with a continuing rise in systolic pressure through later years (**Figure B103.2**). Lifelong maintenance of favorable BP levels common among young adults would end high BP as a mass problem. Recent research advances make this strategic goal possible.

Prevention of Age-Related Blood Pressure Increases

Evidence is now clear on the relationship to BP of lifestyle, particularly suboptimal nutritional habits that are common in the population. These include caloric imbalance with consequent obesity, habitual high salt (NaCl) intake, inadequate potassium intake, excess alcohol consumption, and sedentary habits. By the early 1990s, extensive data on these traits served as a scientific foundation for the first international and U.S. expert group reports on the prevention of high BP. During the mid-1990s, new findings from observational studies and randomized trials, and animal experiments suggested other dietary factors in hypertension.

Observational studies of dietary factors and blood pressure of individuals

International Study of Salt and Blood Pressure. The International Study of Salt and Blood Pressure (INTERSALT) involved >10,000 men and women 20 to 59 years old, sampled at 52 centers in 32 countries. It tested both cross-population (ecologic) ($N = 52$) and within-population ($N > 10,000$) prior hypotheses. To deal with the methodologic problem in assessing individual intake, it had a large sample size and one carefully collected 24-hour urine per person. Its cross-population and within-population analyses gave concordant results. They substantiated independent relationships of sodium and potassium excretion (direct and inverse, respectively) and the direct associations of body mass index and alcohol intake with BP levels, hypertension prevalence, and slope of BP on age. INTERSALT also found an inverse relation between years of education and BP of individuals, with higher intake of sodium and alcohol and higher body mass among the less educated, as well as lower potassium intake. These dietary factors accounted significantly for higher BP levels of less educated persons.

Dietary protein and other factors. Subsequent analyses from INTERSALT, based on measurement of urinary nitrogen excretion as a marker of dietary protein, provided evidence for an inverse association of total protein intake with BP. Additional support for this intriguing relationship has come from other observational studies, including analyses of data collected over

Average DBP mm Hg	Average SBP mm Hg			
	< 120	120–129	130–139	≥ 140
< 80	Optimal†	Normal	High Normal	High
80–84	Normal	Normal	High Normal	High
85–89	High Normal	High Normal	High Normal	High
≥ 90	High	High	High	High

Figure B103.1. Systolic blood pressure (SBP) and diastolic blood pressure (DBP) criteria for classification of blood pressure (BP) as optimal, normal (not optimal), high-normal, and high for adults age 18 years or older. The recommendation is to classify on the basis of average BP for an individual from ≥2 readings at each of ≥2 visits after an initial screening, with the individual not taking drugs and not acutely ill. Optimal BP, with regard to cardiovascular risk, is SBP <120 mm Hg and DBP <80 mm Hg; however, unusually low readings should be evaluated for clinical significance. When systolic and diastolic BPs fall into different categories, the higher category should be selected to classify the individual's BP status (e.g., 138/82 should be classified as high-normal BP). (From the *Fifth Report of the Joint National Committee on Detection, Evaluation, and Treatment of High Blood Pressure.* National High Blood Pressure Education Program, National Institutes of Health, National Heart, Lung, and Blood Institute. Bethesda, MD: The Institute, 1995. NIH publication 93-1088, with permission.)

6 years from 11,342 middle-aged men in the Multiple Risk Factor Intervention Trial (MRFIT). The MRFIT results support the concept that multiple dietary factors influence BP independently and additively, including direct associations with overweight and with saturated fat, cholesterol, sodium, and alcohol intake, and inverse associations with potassium and protein intake. This concept receives further support from the International Population Study on Macronutrients and Blood Pressure (INTERMAP), involving 4,680 men and women ages 40 to 59 from 17 population samples in China, Japan, the United Kingdom and the United States (2,195 Americans of diverse ethnicities). Nutrients were assessed by 4 standardized in-depth dietary recalls and two 24-hour urine collections; 8 standardized BP measurements were made at 4 visits over 2 to 4 weeks. For U.S. participants, significant direct associations to systolic BP were found for body mass, alcohol intake and 24-hour sodium excretion, as expected, and in addition, with total fat, saturated fat, monounsaturated fat, and Keys dietary lipid score. There were significant inverse associations to systolic BP for vegetable protein, total carbohydrate, fiber, vitamins A, C, and B_6, β-carotene, thiamin, riboflavin, folacin, magnesium,

and iron. For several of these nutrients, intakes were less favorable for less educated individuals, and these factors considered together accounted significantly for the higher systolic BP levels of less educated persons (for both sexes and for blacks, Hispanic Americans, and white Americans). Multiple dietary variables also accounted significantly for the higher average BP of blacks compared to others.

Other studies. In the Chicago Western Electric Study of 1,714 middle-aged men examined annually for 9 years, usual dietary intake during the previous month was assessed by in-depth interview at years 0 and 1. Baseline dietary cholesterol, alcohol intake, and Keys dietary lipid score were directly related to BP change over time; dietary vegetable protein and antioxidant intake (vitamin C and β-carotene) were inversely related. Change in weight over the years was also directly related to BP change. (Sodium and potassium intake were not measured.)

Two large cohort studies of health professionals, conducted entirely by questionnaire, relied on self-report of usual postbaseline BP or diagnosis of incident hypertension. Usual intake of foods and nutrients was determined at baseline by food frequency questionnaire. Several of the expected variables—weight (body mass index) and alcohol intake—were found to be strong BP predictors. Dietary potassium, magnesium, and fiber were inversely related to BP change over time and incidence of high BP. Sodium intake was not, but salt intake is particularly difficult to measure accurately by questionnaire, and those health professionals with originally higher intake and high-normal BPs may have reduced dietary salt, with resultant confounding of the analysis.

These findings from epidemiologic studies on the relationship of several dietary variables to BP and BP change, along with previous reports on inverse relationships of vegetarian diets with BP and hypertension, gave impetus to the conduct of the Dietary Approaches to Stop Hypertension (DASH) trials (see the section Dietary Approaches to Stop Hypertension diet and Chapter B93).

Dietary. Randomized trials in adults and children with high-normal BPs have reported findings on the effects of nutritional and other lifestyle changes on BP levels and hypertension incidence.

Primary Prevention of Hypertension study. The 5-year Primary Prevention of Hypertension (PPH) study found that multifactor intervention (weight loss, reduction of sodium and alcohol intake, increased physical activity) significantly lowered average follow-up BP by 1 to 2 mm Hg and hypertension incidence by 54% (8.8% vs. 19.2% for intervention and control participants, respectively). This outcome was attributable to modest weight loss (average of approximately 3 kg) and, to a lesser extent, sodium reduction (approximately 20% on average).

Hypertension Prevention Trial study. The Hypertension Prevention Trial (HPT) studied sodium reduction and weight loss both separately and combined and tested increased dietary potassium as well. Again, weight loss lowered BP throughout the 3 years of the trial, with waning effect as weight was partially regained. Nevertheless, the data trended toward 27% lower incidence of hypertension. Low-order sodium reduction (10% at 3 years) did not significantly lower mean BP, although incidence of hypertension was apparently reduced. Combined intervention encoun-

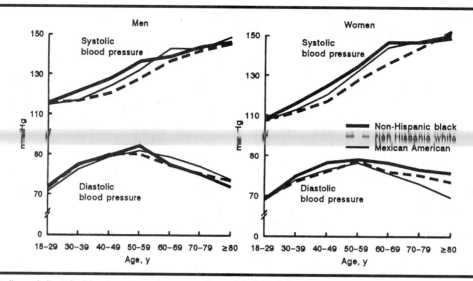

Figure B103.2.   Mean systolic and diastolic blood pressures by age and race/ethnicity for men and women, U.S. population ≥18 years old. (From Burt VL, Whelton P, Roccella EJ, et al. Prevalence of hypertension in the US adult population: results from the Third National Health and Nutrition Examination Survey, 1998–1991. *Hypertension*. 1995;25:305–313, with permission.)

tered diminished effectiveness in producing weight reduction, with BP results no better than with single interventions. Only modest sustained increase (8%) in potassium intake was achieved, with minimal BP effect.

Trials of Hypertension Prevention studies. The Trials of Hypertension Prevention (TOHP) phase I tested a broad range of interventions aimed at factors thought to be related to BP levels. In addition to counseling overweight participants for weight reduction (with inclusion of an exercise component) or sodium reduction, a third lifestyle approach (stress management) was evaluated; also, 4 nutritional supplements (calcium carbonate, magnesium diglycine, potassium chloride, and fish oil) were tested in placebo-controlled, double-blind designs. During the first 6 months of intervention, only weight loss and sodium reduction produced significant BP reductions, by 2 to 4 mm Hg systolic and 1 to 3 mm Hg diastolic BP. By design, lifestyle groups were also followed for 18 months to assess maintenance of behavioral change. During this period, weight and sodium reduction each demonstrated tendencies to decrease hypertension incidence, by 51% and 24%, respectively. Stress management showed no such trend.

TOHP phase II, a longer trial, further evaluated weight loss and sodium reduction, singly and in combination. The most important additional finding of TOHP-II was that each of the interventions lowered incidence of hypertension significantly, by approximately 20% over 3 to 4 years. In addition, during the initial 6-month follow-up period, at the height of intervention adherence, effects of weight loss and sodium reduction on hypertension incidence were additive.

Trial of Nonpharmacological Intervention in the Elderly study. A combination of weight loss and salt reduction was more effective than either one alone (although weight loss and sodium reduction were individually effective) in the 2.5-year Trial of Nonpharmacological Intervention in the Elderly (TONE), which studied hypertensive participants age 60 to 79 years.

Newborns. Among newborn infants, consumption of formula with decreased sodium content resulted in lower systolic BP at

6 months. Of potentially great significance, reexamination of 35% of these infants after 15 years showed maintenance of a 3.6/2.2 mm Hg advantage in BP levels for the group assigned to the reduced sodium formula, despite little evidence of difference in current sodium intake or any other BP determinants at follow-up.

Moving from Clinical Studies to Public Policy

Participants in clinical trials are volunteers and thus are apt to be more highly motivated toward lifestyle change. They also enjoy socioeconomic circumstances more conducive to modifying behavior than other social groups. To achieve broad public health benefits, efficacious methods to prevent hypertension must be shown to be effective in broadly representative populations. Reducing dietary salt should be one approach that is particularly amenable to a population approach, because more than 85% of dietary sodium comes from processed foods. Two community-intervention salt-reduction trials have been completed in Europe using "quasi experimental" designs (1 intervention, 1 control community).

Portuguese salt trial. In the Portuguese salt trial, 2 rural communities were compared, with random samples of residents 15 to 69 years old examined before intervention, then annually for 2 years. The health education program in the intervention community was facilitated by the fact that 50% of the very high salt consumption (360 mmol/day sodium) came from salt that was added in cooking at home, and another 33% was derived from 1 food item, salt-dried codfish. There was also a focus on reducing salt used in commercial bread baking. Results of this trial showed sodium excretion to be 42% lower in the intervention community at 1 year, and there were significant reductions of mean BPs of 4 to 5 mm Hg at years 1 and 2.

Belgian salt trial. In contrast, the Belgian salt trial was much less successful in its intervention; there were no net changes in sodium excretion or BP for men, sodium changes for women were modest (20%), and net mean BP reductions (2.9 mm Hg systolic and 1.6 mm Hg diastolic BP) were not significant. In contrast to the Portuguese trial, the same individuals were not examined at baseline and follow-up, leading to less precise estimation of BP change.

Other population interventions. Another community intervention experiment studied adolescents at 2 boarding schools. In a crossover design with each phase lasting 1 academic year, sodium intake was reduced 15% to 20% by changes in food purchasing and preparation, with a significant effect on systolic and diastolic BP of approximately 2 mm Hg. This study is encouraging because of simplicity of intervention and because prevention is theoretically most attractive when begun in childhood. Positive results also have been reported from a 3-year community trial in urban north China, which found significant reductions of systolic BP (5 mm Hg in men and 6 mm Hg in women 15 to 64 years old) associated with net reductions in sodium intake of only 14% in men and 6% in women.

Current Recommendations and Future Directions

National and international guidelines. Consistent recommendations for preventive medicine and public health have emerged from the World Health Organization/International Society of Hypertension Guidelines Committee and the U.S. Working Group Report on the Primary Prevention of Hypertension. The reports emphasize (a) weight control and increased physical activity, (b) no more than moderate alcohol intake [daily average of ≤2 drinks (i.e., no more than 1 oz or 26 g of ethanol)] for men and half these amounts for women, (c) limitation of dietary sodium to ≤2.4 g per day (equivalent to 6 g of sodium chloride), and (d) increased dietary potassium.

Regarding reduction of psychosocial stress, more study is required, and no specific roles for supplementing calcium or magnesium intake were noted.

Dietary Approaches to Stop Hypertension diet. The 1997 Sixth Report of the Joint National Committee on Prevention, Detection, Evaluation, and Treatment of High Blood Pressure gave special emphasis to the landmark DASH trial. In this 8-week outpatient feeding trial, DASH found that a diet rich in fruits, vegetables, and fat-free and low-fat dairy foods, with reduced total and saturated fat, dietary cholesterol, and sugars, plus modestly increased protein, lowered BP in adults by 5.5/3.0 mm Hg. Body weight and sodium intake were maintained at constant levels in all participants, who consumed little or no alcohol. Also, in nonhypertensives evaluated separately, the diet reduced BP by 3.5/2.1 mm Hg. In a second feeding trial (DASH-Sodium), the same investigators reproduced the foregoing results at each of 3 levels of sodium intake, showed that lowered salt intake had independent stepwise effects on BP, and further documented

that the greatest BP-lowering (e.g., by 7.1 mm Hg systolic in the nonhypertensive subgroup) was with the combination of the DASH diet and sodium intake reduced to approximately 65 mmol (approximately 3.8 g salt) per 24 hours.

Thus, the results of DASH and DASH-Sodium add to the extensive evidence on established lifestyle causes of rise in BP with age and resultant high incidence of hypertension. This evidence leads to the reasonable inference that most of the knowledge is in hand for the primary prevention of high BP. While ongoing or needed research pursues such issues as (a) the full potential of combined lifestyle approaches, (b) the effects in special population groups, (c) better methods for estimation of food and nutrient intake, and (d) potential for incorporation of hypertension prevention into primary medical care, it is possible to apply existing knowledge in pursuit of making the rise in BP with age rare and optimal BP levels common in all population subgroups, thereby ending the epidemic.

SUGGESTED READING

1. Ellison RC, Capper AL, Stephenson WP, et al. Effects on blood pressure of a decrease in sodium use in institutional food preparation: the Exeter-Andover project. *J Clin Epidemiol.* 1989;42:201–208.
2. Forte JG, Miguel JM, Miguel MJ, et al. Salt and blood pressure: a community trial. *J Hum Hypertens.* 1989;3:179–184.
3. Geleijnse JM, Hofman A, Witteman JC, et al. Long-term effects of neonatal sodium restriction on blood pressure. [Published erratum appears in *Hypertension.* 1997;29:1211.] *Hypertension.* 1996;29:913–917.
4. The Hypertension Prevention Trial Research Group. The Hypertension Prevention Trial: three-year effects of dietary changes on blood pressure. *Arch Intern Med.* 1990;150:153–162.
5. Stamler J, Caggiula A, Grandits GA, et al. Relationship to blood pressure of combinations of dietary macronutrients: findings of the Multiple Risk Factor Intervention Trial (MRFIT). *Circulation.* 1996;94:2417–2423.
6. Stamler J, Liu K, Ruth KJ, et al. Eight-year blood pressure change in middle-aged men: relationship to multiple nutrients. *Hypertension.* 2002;39:1000–1006.
7. Stamler J, Stamler R, Neaton JD. Blood pressure, systolic and diastolic, and cardiovascular risks: US population data. *Arch Intern Med.* 1993;153:598–615.
8. Stamler R, Stamler J, Gosch FC, et al. Primary prevention of hypertension by nutritional-hygienic means: final report of a randomized, controlled trial. [Published erratum appears in *JAMA.* 1989;262:3132.] *JAMA.* 1989;262:1801–1807.
9. The Trials of Hypertension Prevention Collaborative Research Group. The effects of nonpharmacologic interventions on blood pressure of persons with high normal levels: results of the Trials of Hypertension Prevention, phase I. [Published erratum appears in *JAMA.* 1992;267:2330.] *JAMA.* 1992;267:1213–1220.
10. The Trials of Hypertension Prevention Collaborative Research Group. Effects of weight loss and sodium reduction intervention on blood pressure and hypertension incidence in overweight people with high-normal blood pressure: the Trials of Hypertension Prevention, phase II. *Arch Intern Med.* 1997;157:657–667.
11. Whelton PK, He J, Appel LJ, et al. Primary prevention of hypertension: clinical and public health advisory from The National High Blood Pressure Education Program. *JAMA.* 2002;288:1882–1888.

Community-Based Management Programs

Brent M. Egan, MD; Daniel T. Lackland, PhD

KEY POINTS

- The risk of cardiovascular disease is likely to rise over the next 20 years given the increasing age and weight of the U.S. population and the growing numbers of high-risk ethnic groups.

- The *community*, defined as places and groups in which people learn, work, worship, and play, can be approached to implement cost-effective lifestyle and health care delivery system changes.

- Reliance of U.S. health care policy on treatment of an ever-increasing proportion of high-risk patients is costly and perhaps ineffective by itself.

- Strategies for implementing evidence-based guidelines in primary care settings can improve the efficacy of the high-risk strategy and reinforce lifestyle change.

See also Chapters B79, B80, B88, B89, B103, B105, C129, and C134–C136

In the United States, truly impressive declines in cardiovascular disease (CVD) have occurred (see Chapter B102). From the 1960s through the mid-1990s, age-adjusted death rates for heart disease and stroke in the United States fell by more than 50%, but relative disparities persist.

Rationale for Community Programs: Failure to Reach Goals

Despite these advances, the population at risk for CVD remains too large. Approximately 60% of adults have a total cholesterol >200 mg per dL. Moreover, one-third of patients with coronary heart disease have a total cholesterol <200 mg per dL. Many of them have low high-density lipoprotein, high triglycerides, and dense low-density lipoprotein cholesterol. More than half of individuals older than 50 years of age have hypertension according to Joint National Committee (JNC) VI Hypertension Guidelines, and 16% have diabetes. Only a minority of patients at risk are treated to evidence-based goals. Despite long-standing evidence that treatment of hypertension reduces cardiovascular morbidity and mortality, only 1 in 4 patients has a blood pressure (BP) <140/90 mm Hg. With the more stringent goal of <130/85 mm Hg for JNC risk group C, control rates are even lower. Control rates of hypercholesterolemia and diabetes are typically no better and often worse than corresponding rates for high BP. Low control rates reflect provider and system barriers. Adequate evidence-based interventions are often not prescribed, and patient variables, such as adherence to appropriate therapy, are often suboptimal. Despite decades of efforts to generate and disseminate treatment guidelines to providers and a plethora of studies to enhance patient adherence, the gap between potential and realized medical benefits remains wide.

Potential Target Populations

Elderly. The median age of the U.S. population is rising rapidly. In the next 20 years, the number of Americans ≥60 years old is projected to grow by more than 30 million, whereas the population from 30 to 49 years old is expected to decline. Cardiovascular risk and disease advance sharply with increasing age, whereas control rates, for hypertension in particular, decline. The major demographic changes are projected to place an extraordinary demand on financial and health care resources, including nursing homes.

Young. Cardiovascular risk among young Americans is rising even more rapidly than in older adults. The increasing risk among youth largely reflects the burgeoning obesity epidemic. More than half of diabetes in children and teenagers in many areas is now type 2 (non–insulin dependent). The proportions of obesity and sedentary lifestyles are increasing in children.

Obesity. More than 60% of U.S. adults are now overweight or obese, reflecting a major increase during the 1990s. Compared to normal weight individuals, overweight and obese subjects who are currently without cardiovascular risk factors are at 2- to 4-fold greater risk for developing hypertension and CVD and 10 to 60 times more likely to develop diabetes mellitus in the next 10 years. The health risks of obesity are greater over longer periods of time. Consequently, the impact of the obesity epidemic in this country is likely to become more fully manifest in the next 20 years with devastating effects on public and individual health and finances.

Racial and regional disparities. Individuals living in the southeast United States are 50% more likely to experience CVD (see Chapter B80). Given long-term trends, including lower birth weights, greater proportions of high-risk minorities, and preferential relocation of retirees, the Southeast disparities are likely to persist and grow. Moreover, blacks are twice as likely to die from a stroke and 5 times more likely to die from end-stage renal disease than whites, especially in the Southeast. The Hypertension Detection and Follow-Up Program showed >20 years ago that a systematic approach to treating high BP reduced the racial disparity in stroke mortality from >2:1 to 4:3 and also reduced the racial differential in total mortality. Despite the evidence, large ethnic disparities persist. Socioeconomic factors other than race appear to contribute significantly to health disparities (see Chapter B85). Evidence suggests that insurance and access to health care account for less than half of observed health disparities between ethnic groups.

Public Health Strategies for Risk Reduction

The numerous problems currently encountered suggest that public health strategies should be reevaluated.

Targeted high-risk strategy. The traditional Western approach to chronic disease prevention is to identify those at highest risk and implement an intensive strategy aimed at improving outcome for the individual. Given the time and resource intensity of this approach, the high-risk strategic approach works best when the proportion of the population meeting the diagnostic criteria for intervention is relatively small (i.e., ±5% of the total). A BP of ≥180/110 mm Hg or total cholesterol ≥280 mg per dL, roughly define the upper 5%. Initial clinical trials for hypertension and hypercholesterolemia focused on these high-risk patients. Later trials demonstrated that treatment benefits extend well beyond the upper 5% to 10% of the distribution. These studies suggest that 50% or more of adults will probably benefit from a high-risk approach to CVD prevention. Nevertheless, attempts to apply the high-risk strategy on a mass basis have proven costly and of limited efficacy. Continued reliance on this model given the demographic changes cited may be intrinsically inefficient.

Mass strategy. Cardiovascular risk and disease are virtually absent in unacculturated peoples. However, these people develop CVD with acculturation. These observations strongly implicate a crucial role for lifestyle in the pathogenesis of CVD. The relationship between cardiovascular risk and disease is continuous. When a population is at high risk, small reductions in risk factor levels of the population (e.g., 2–3 mm Hg BP) can equal or exceed the life-saving potential of intensive treatment of a substantial number of high-risk individuals. This is especially true when considering the actual benefits of the high-risk approach, which includes provider, patient, and system failures. The mass strategy has suffered from perceptions that people are unwilling to change lifestyle sufficiently to obtain benefit and that genetic factors predominate in determining disease. Both notions minimize the role of individual responsibility for health outcomes. However, lifestyle changes have probably accounted for more than half of the 30% age-adjusted reduction of coronary heart disease in the United States from 1968 to 1976 and for a >50% reduction of CVD among the intervention group in the Oslo Diet and Heart Study. Lifestyle may account for up to 10 years of interindividual differences in longevity.

Lifestyle changes are probably easier to initiate and sustain when embraced by the community and supported by policy and insurance and tax law changes. For example, evidence that cigarette smoking is deleterious and that smoking cessation is beneficial has been reinforced by relevant public health messages, policy changes to limit smoking locations, and punitive taxes and court decisions. Incentives in insurance policies have not been explored adequately.

Community-Based Interventions

The traditional notion of community as a local neighborhood of people that care for each other has not disappeared entirely. However, as our society and family structure become more fluid, human relationships in the local neighborhood are being replaced by interactions in the places people learn, work, worship, and enjoy leisure time together. A growing body of studies documents that health care interventions in schools, worksites, and places of worship can have substantial and sustained beneficial impact on health behaviors and risk factors. Moreover, each of these locations addresses important issues raised earlier.

Principles of prevention in community health models. Three basic components define our overall strategy to any of the community-based interventions as outlined in **Table B104.1.** The first and overall objective is to translate research into practice by extending the academic mission to the community. The second aim is to implement a successful intervention model. The third objective is to provide centralized data management for monitoring progress and providing reports to community leaders. This model allows for a dynamic structure that can be owned and modified by the community to best meet local needs.

School programs. School programs inside and outside the classroom can reach youth, raise awareness, and establish healthy lifestyle patterns early in life. Successful interventions in our nation's schools have tremendous potential for progressively reducing the burden of CVD risk over the long term. A primary area for improvement would be school lunch programs that provide far too much fat and caloric intake.

Worksite programs. Health promotion in the workplace, especially programs that combine education with healthy lifestyle change and risk factor monitoring are highly cost-effective (see Chapter B105). Moreover, the worksite is an ideal place to reach young adults and men who are less likely to receive crucial preventive services.

Faith-based programs. Health programs centered at sites of worship represent an excellent forum for risk factor screening and lifestyle interventions. In minority communities especially, the site of worship is often the heart of the community. Many individuals who do not access primary health care services can be reached at their site of worship with health messages and can be assisted in making important and sustained lifestyle changes.

Table B104.1. Model for Community Intervention

Translate research into practice by extending the academic mission of patient care, education, and health services research to the community.

Enhance and enlist local experts and leaders, then implement a proven model for intervention through the community leaders.

Provide administrative support for coordinating services together with ongoing monitoring of the intervention and relevant feedback to community leaders.

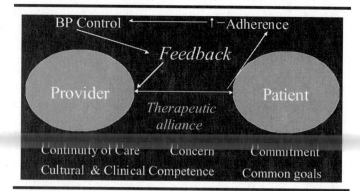

Figure B104.1. The importance of feedback in blood pressure control. Continuity of primary care with an effective therapeutic alliance between the patient and provider emerges as a critical component of chronic risk factor control. Relevant feedback to the provider appears to enhance the therapeutic alliance, improve adherence, and facilitate risk factor control. BP, blood pressure.

Provider-Based Programs

Primary care providers. In controlling risk factors for chronic disease, a regular source of primary health care is paramount. The therapeutic alliance between the patient and his or her provider is critical in obtaining and adhering to appropriate therapy (**Figure B104.1**). The managed care program at the University of Pennsylvania School of Medicine nearly tripled hypertension control in 1 year from 19% to 53% with monitoring of BP control rates and comparative feedback to providers. This model has been adapted to the predominantly fee-for-service paradigm in rural and suburban South Carolina. With some 70 providers and 7,000 hypertensive patients in the program thus far, control rates at <140/90 mm Hg are in excess of 50%.

Pharmacies. The pharmacist can improve patient adherence with BP medications by providing information and monitoring. Effective strategies to improve communication between the patient's provider and pharmacist would probably be beneficial but are usually lacking.

SUGGESTED READING

1. Egan BM, Lackland DT. Strategies of prevention and the importance of public health and community programs. *Ethn Dis.* 1998;8:143–154.
2. Egan BM, Lackland DT, Basile JN. American Society of Hypertension Regional Chapters: leveraging the impact of the clinical hypertension specialist in the local community. *Am J Hypertens.* 2002;15:372–379.
3. Jones D, Basile J, Cushman W, et al. Managing hypertension in the southeastern United States: applying the JNC VI guidelines. *Am J Med Sci.* 1999;318:357–364.
4. Lackland DT, Egan BM. The dominant role of systolic hypertension as a vascular risk factor: evidence from the Southeast. *Am J Med Sci.* 1999;318:365–368.
5. Oexmann MJ, Ascanio R, Egan BM. Preventing cardiovascular disease: efficacy of a church-based intervention on cardiovascular risk reduction. *Ethn Dis.* 2001;11:817–822.

Chapter B105

Workplace Management of Hypertension

Michael H. Alderman, MD

KEY POINTS

- Providing diagnostic and therapeutic services in the occupational setting has proved acceptable, effective, and highly efficient.

- Medical cost savings over an 8-year period have more than paid for the Worksite Hypertension Treatment program.

- Isolated screening at the workplace or in other nonmedical settings may not be beneficial.

See also Chapters B102, B104, B108, C131, C132, and C134–C136

Millions of workers have high blood pressure (BP), so the ability to efficiently reach such large numbers of hypertensive patients in their working environment is an attractive opportunity to improve health. Employers' efforts, through their own medical departments, have included screening and case finding as well as the actual provision of diagnostic and therapeutic services in the workplace.

Problems of Isolated Screening

During the early years of the National High Blood Pressure Program, on-site screening was popular. Frequently provided by outside vendors or volunteers, these efforts were too often isolated activities. BP was measured and, on the basis of the numbers, employees were advised to seek further medical care. Although many hypertensives were appropriately identified, problems were also created. Measuring techniques were often unreliable or the diagnosis was based on single recordings that often resulted in misleading or incorrect information. All too often, the result was disaffection of community physicians, coupled with frustration and confusion among patients. This well-meaning exercise actually produced occasional adverse effects through the "labeling" phenomenon, in which inappropriately identified "hypertensive" persons experienced measurable adverse physiologic, economic, and even physical consequences.

Although most Americans have had their BPs recorded within the past 2 years, roughly one-third of those with *hypertension* (defined at a single encounter as >140/90 mm Hg) are not aware of their current status. Clearly, the first step toward BP control is improved identification. But screening by itself, in or out of the workplace, is probably not the optimal solution.

Rationale for the Worksite Program

An alternative approach is to provide all diagnostic and therapeutic services in the occupational setting. Experience has proved this approach to be acceptable, effective, and highly efficient. This initiative was stimulated by the observation that treatment in medical clinics of the urban teaching hospital centers or in most private practice settings failed to retain more than half of patients in continuing care for 1 year. Only approximately half of all the remaining cases achieved BP control—findings disturbingly reminiscent of current control rates in the general population among treated patients.

The premise tested by the creation of the worksite management program was that the main impediments to achieving effective long-term BP control in conventional therapeutic settings were essentially structural. The first step in closing the gap in hypertension control was to bring care directly to patients to overcome the barriers imposed by having patients come to therapists. An equally important element of the program was to provide care according to a protocol that assured standardized practice for each patient, in general following the strategies from clinical trials.

Principles of the Program

The model program was established in New York City in 1973 for the employees of Bloomingdale's and Gimbel's department stores. The guiding principles of the program were (a) provision of all services at the workplace; (b) adherence to a formal diagnostic and therapeutic protocol; (c) a team approach to treatment, in which nurses were the primary caregivers and physicians played a supervisory, educational, and consultative role; (d) no out-of-pocket patient expenses; (e) convenience in care, which included visits on-site or nearby and delivery of medications; and (f) use of the cohesive resources of the union structure to enhance participation, persistence, and adherence to treatment.

Screening. The program began with screening 75% of employees at the stores. Initially, qualifying individuals had BPs >160/95 mm Hg on 3 separate occasions, each of which involved 3 measurements, with the average of the final 2 recorded pressures. Approximately two-thirds of those screened opted to remain in the on-site treatment program, a remarkably high acceptance given that it was an experimental program that depended on nurses for most direct care and that these employees were eligible for conventional health care financed by union insurance. This initial success was probably owing to the overt support by the union leadership, articulated in meetings at which advocates presented the program.

Patient evaluation strategies. Entrants were evaluated in facilities provided by the union, thus assuring members of a supportive environment. The nurse obtained initial history and performed laboratory studies including blood, urine, and electrocardiogram. Testing was parsimonious and limited to

"action measures" that helped to determine appropriate drug therapy, assessed potential treatment toxicity, or established overall cardiovascular disease risk. Blood tests included serum creatinine, fasting blood glucose, potassium, uric acid, and thyroid function. Urine was assessed for protein qualitatively, and an electrocardiogram was performed. The culmination of the 4- to 6-week intake process was an examination and review of all previously obtained data by the supervising physician. At that visit, protocol-based therapy was begun.

Drug therapy. Initial drug selection was largely guided by the recommendations of the Joint National Committee reports (JNC I through VI) that have varied over the past 25 years. More recently, plasma renin activity was added to further measure cardiovascular risk and guide drug selection. In general, lacking contraindications or specific indications, low-renin patients (<30%) were begun on therapy with a diuretic. High-renin subjects (<18%) were begun with β-blockers, angiotensin-converting enzyme inhibitors, or angiotensin II receptor blockers. Demographic factors as well as coincident disease have influenced the selection of initial therapy. Medications have been provided through a union-sponsored central delivery system and mailed directly to the patient's home.

Follow-up. All subsequent visits, dictated by patient need, have been with the nurse. These generally total 4 to 6 per year, after an initial year of somewhat more frequent attendance. Each patient had an annual revisit to the physician, who remained available for consultation as dictated by patient need.

Recordkeeping. Over the years, what began as a system of paper encounter forms has evolved into an electronic management system that includes all patient data and is used for scheduling, patient visits, laboratory tests, and consultations. This facilitates oversight and ensures that deviations from protocol can be noted and, when necessary, investigated.

Program Evaluation

Several medical care elements of the program are believed to be keys to its success. These include the following: (a) systematic care delivered according to a protocol that is appropriately revised as new information or experience is gained; (b) provision of most direct patient care by a physician-supervised, specially trained hypertension nurse-expert; and (c) constant oversight of all patient data by the supervising physician.

Over the 25 years of program existence, patterns of drug treatment have varied widely, in response to emerging pharmacologic innovation and to changing JNC recommendations. However, despite dramatic shifts in patterns of first-drug use, all measures of BP response, including BP control, adverse effects, persistence in treatment, visits, change in medication, and use of laboratory, have been constant. In other words, vastly different medication use patterns have had no discernible short-term effects.

More recently, the growing recognition of the ability to maximize cardiovascular disease prevention by comprehensive attention to all cardiovascular risk factors has led to a broadening of intervention patterns. The program has lost its initial "one size fits all" character and has evolved to an approach that uses the capacity to stratify patients according to absolute cardiovascular risk while tailoring therapy according to need and opportunity for benefit. For example, BP targets are lower and are pursued more aggressively in patients at higher risk.

BP control has been achieved and maintained by roughly 70% of patients with attrition from all causes <10%. Participants, when compared with those receiving conventional treatment, have enjoyed a 40% reduction in cardiovascular events and reduced absenteeism from work. Medical cost savings over an 8-year period have more than paid for the program. A formal prospective comparison of several worksite-based approaches to care has indicated that the full on-site model was most effective in achieving BP control.

SUGGESTED READING

1. Alderman MH. Blood pressure management: individualized treatment based on absolute risk and the potential for benefit. *Ann Intern Med.* 1993;119:329–335.
2. Alderman MH, Cohen H, Madhavan S. Distribution and determinants of cardiovascular events during twenty years of successful antihypertensive treatment. *J Hypertens.* 1998;16:761–769.
3. Alderman MH, Davis TK. Blood pressure control programs on and off the worksite. *J Occup Med.* 1980;22:167–170.
4. Alderman MH, Lamport B. Labeling of hypertensives: a review of the data. *J Clin Epidemiol.* 1990;43:195–200.
5. Alderman MH, Madhavan S, Cohen H. Antihypertensive drug therapy: the effect of JNC criteria on prescribing patterns and patient status through the first year. [Published correction appears in *Am J Hypertens.* 1996;9:840.] *Am J Hypertens.* 1996;9:413–418.
6. Alderman MH, Madhavan S, Davis TK. Reduction of cardiovascular disease events by worksite hypertension treatment. *Hypertension.* 1983;5 (Suppl III):III-138–III-143.
7. Alderman MH, Schoenbaum EE. Detection and treatment of hypertension at the worksite. *N Engl J Med.* 1975;293:65–68.
8. Foote A, Erfurt JC. Hypertension control at the worksite: comparison of screening and referral alone, referral and follow-up, and on-site treatment. *N Engl J Med.* 1983;308:809–813.
9. Sixth report of the Joint National Committee on prevention, detection, evaluation, and treatment of high blood pressure (JNC VI). *Arch Intern Med.* 1997;157:2413–2446.
10. Stockwell DH, Madhavan S, Cohen H, et al. The determinants of hypertension awareness, treatment, and control in an insured population. *Am J Public Health.* 1994;84:1768–1774.

Chapter B106

Antihypertensive Treatment Trials: Morbidity and Mortality Data

Bruce M. Psaty, MD, PhD; Curt D. Furberg, MD, PhD

KEY POINTS

- Control of elevated systolic or diastolic blood pressure reduces the risk of stroke, myocardial infarction, heart failure, and death.

- High-risk patients, such as the elderly, are prime candidates for antihypertensive therapy.

- Diuretics in low doses are economical and safe, especially in the elderly, and are effective at preventing heart attacks, strokes, and heart failure.

- β-blockers and angiotensin-converting enzyme inhibitors are effective in treating established heart failure and myocardial infarction, and calcium antagonists are useful in treating angina and preventing stroke.

See also Chapters B102, B107, B108, C126, C127, C138, C139, C141, C144–C146, C151, and C152

Pharmacologic treatment is initiated to prevent the major-disease complications of untreated hypertension. Therapeutic strategies are based on randomized trials of antihypertensive therapy. In most of these trials, cardiovascular morbidity and mortality are the primary outcomes.

Clinical Trial Design Principles

The preferred design to evaluate a pharmacologic therapy is the randomized controlled clinical trial.

Randomization. On average, randomization produces groups that are similar at baseline with respect to their expected response to therapy, their propensity for compliance, and their risk for the outcome(s) of interest. With randomization, the study becomes an unbiased test of the therapy. Complete follow-up of subjects, careful ascertainment of events, and blinded classification of outcomes ensure the validity of the comparison between the treatment and the control groups. Even if some participants are noncompliant with therapy or cross over to the other therapy, the analysis should generally follow the intention-to-treat principle, which compares the treatment and the control groups exactly as they were initially randomized.

Outcomes and end points. Randomized controlled clinical trials can assess a given therapy in terms of a variety of outcomes. For antihypertensive therapy, examples include physiologic measures such as level of blood pressure (BP), measures of subclinical disease such as angiographically assessed coronary atherosclerosis, or major disease end points such as stroke and myocardial infarction. In the absence of evidence from trials that include major disease end points, it is common to consider evidence concerning other intermediate or surrogate end points. The underlying assumption is that the effect of the therapy on BP, for instance, is an adequate surrogate for its effect on major disease end points. In practice, this assumption has not always turned out to be true. In one randomized clinical trial of patients with coronary disease, nifedipine suppressed the development of new coronary lesions but unexpectedly and significantly increased total mortality. Thus, randomized trials that specify major disease end points as their primary outcomes are most likely to provide the best evidence regarding the key health benefits or risks associated with specific forms of antihypertensive therapy.

Adverse effects. Randomized trials are also important to evaluate adverse drug reactions, including symptoms that may influence quality of life or general well-being. Because high BP is asymptomatic or associated with only low-level symptoms, it is important that treatment have as few side effects as possible.

A comparison of side effects among various drugs is of interest when the drugs are equally effective in preventing the major disease end points associated with hypertension.

Early Randomized Trial Results

Design issues. Once the early Veterans' Administration studies had shown a benefit from treating participants with diastolic BPs >115 mm Hg, it was no longer ethical to randomize subjects with high diastolic pressures to receive a placebo. The Hypertension Detection and Follow-up Program (HDFP) and Medical Research Council (MRC) investigators addressed the placebo issue in different ways (Table B106.1). In the HDFP trial, researchers recruited subjects with elevated levels of diastolic BP and randomized them to either diuretic-based stepped care or referred (usual) care. Referred-care participants had an opportunity to be evaluated by their own physicians for some form of therapy, whereas the stepped-care group received systematic care. Conversely, the MRC investigators limited eligibility to those with lower levels of BP, and participants were randomized to one of two active drugs or matching placebos. In both studies, the intervention reduced mean diastolic BP by about 5 mm Hg more than control groups. These initial choices affected other

Table B106.1. **Two Major Randomized Trials of the Treatment of Hypertension: The Hypertension Detection and Follow-up Program (HDFP) and the Medical Research Council (MRC) Trials**

	HDFP (1979)	MRC (1985)
Sampling centers, N = 14,176	Population-based	General practice clinic
Eligibility		
Age (yr)	30–69	35–64
Blood pressure (BP)		
Systolic, mm Hg	—	<200
Diastolic, mm Hg	>90	90–109
Subjects excluded	Bedfast and institutionalized	Those with secondary or treated hypertension, heart failure, angina, recent myocardial infarction, diabetes, gout, asthma
Subject		
Screened, N	178,009	515,000
Randomized, N	10,940	17,354
Blinding	Neither subjects nor physicians	Subjects only
Treatment	Offered free standardized program of stepped-care antihypertensive therapy	Thiazide diuretic (bendrofluazide) or β-blocker (propranolol)
Control	Referred to personal sources of medical care	Matching thiazide placebo or matching β-blocker placebo
Target diastolic BP	<90 mm Hg if entry DBP >100 mm Hg; 10 mm Hg reduction if entry DBP was 90–99 mm Hg	<90 mm Hg
Trial duration (yr)	5.0	5.5
Primary end point	Total mortality	Fatal and nonfatal stroke

RESULTS	STEPPED CARE	REFERRED CARE	ACTIVE	PLACEBO
Baseline diastolic BP, mm Hg	101.1	101.2	98.5	98.0
Subjects with diastolic BP at or below target at the end of trial (%)	64.9	43.6	74.1	46.3
Total mortality				
Randomized	5,485	5,455	8,700	8,654
Deaths, N	349	419	248	253
Cumulative mortality (%)	6.4	7.7	2.9	2.9
Relative risk (95% CI)	0.83 (0.72–0.95)		0.98 (0.82–1.16)	
Total strokes				
Events, N	102	158	60	109
Cumulative incidence (%)	1.9	2.9	0.7	1.3
Relative risk (95% CI)	0.64 (0.50–0.82)		0.55 (0.40–0.75)	

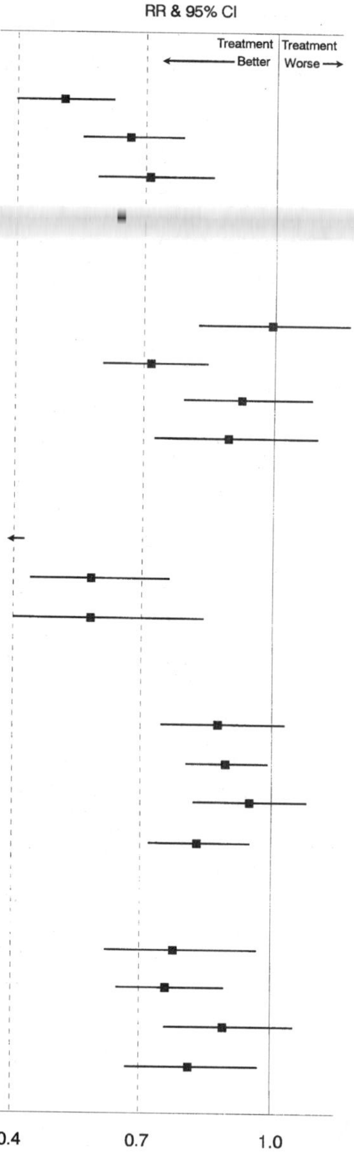

Figure B106.1. Metaanalysis of randomized, controlled clinical trials in hypertension according to first-line treatment strategy. For these comparisons, the numbers of participants randomized to active therapy and control were 7,768 and 12,075 for high-dose diuretic therapy, 4,305 and 5,116 for low-dose diuretic therapy, and 6,736 and 12,147 for β-blocker therapy. Because the MRC trials included 2 active arms, the control group is included twice in these totals, once for a diuretic comparison and again for a β-blocker comparison. The total numbers of participants randomized to active therapy and control therapy were 24,294 and 23,926, respectively. CI, confidence interval; HDFP, Hypertension Detection and Follow-up Program Study (5,484 in stepped care and 5,455 in referred care); Trials, number of trials with at least 1 end point of interest; RR, relative risk. (Reprinted with permission from JAMA.)

aspects of the design. In the HDFP, the referral of participants to their personal sources of medical care as the "control" therapy precluded the possibility of blinding. To avoid any potential bias in ascertaining morbid events, the investigators defined total mortality as the outcome of primary interest. In the MRC trial, the use of a matching placebo allowed blinding, and the investigators defined their primary end point as fatal or nonfatal stroke.

Results. Table B106.1 also summarizes the primary results of the HDFP and MRC trials. The typical measure of the intervention effect is the *relative risk* (RR), which is the event rate in the intervention group divided by the event rate in the control group. In the HDFP study, the RR of total mortality was 0.83 [(349/5,485)/

(419/5,455)]. Values <1.0 indicate a benefit from therapy and values >1.0 indicate an adverse effect from therapy. The 95% confidence interval (CI) uses the observed data to estimate the likely range of the true underlying RR. A 95% CI that excludes 1.0 corresponds to a value of $p < .05$. On occasion, the benefits of therapy are expressed in terms of the *RR reduction*, which is calculated as 1 minus the RR. An alternative measure is the number requiring treatment to prevent one event or number needed to treat, which is calculated as 1 divided by the difference in event rates between the treatment and comparison groups. In the HDFP trial, stepped care was associated with a RR reduction of 17% for total mortality $(1–0.83) \times 100$; 76 hypertensive subjects received stepped care for 5 years to prevent 1 death $[1/(0.077–0.064)]$. Benefit may be under-

Table B106.2. Estimates of Treatment Effect by Sex[a]

OUTCOME	WOMEN		MEN	
	ODDS RATIO	95% CONFIDENCE INTERVAL	ODDS RATIO	95% CONFIDENCE INTERVAL
Total mortality	0.91	0.81–1.01	0.88	0.81–1.01
Cardiovascular disease–related death	0.86	0.74–1.01	0.80	0.70–0.91
Fatal strokes	0.71	0.53–0.96	0.57	0.41–0.78
All strokes	0.62	0.52–0.73	0.66	0.56–0.78
Fatal coronary events	0.92	0.74–1.16	0.83	0.71–0.97
All major coronary events	0.85	0.72–1.01	0.82	0.73–0.92
Main cardiovascular disease events	0.74	0.66–0.83	0.78	0.71–0.86

[a]None of the differences in the odds ratios between men and women were statistically significant (all interaction p values ≥.31).
Adapted from Gueyffier F, Boutitie F, Boissel JP, et al. Effect of antihypertensive drug treatment on cardiovascular outcomes in women and men: a metaanalysis of individual patient data from randomized, controlled trials. The INDANA investigators. *Ann Intern Med*. 1997;126:761–767.

estimated in clinical trials when a high proportion of the comparison group (e.g., the placebo group in the MRC trial) receives drug treatment or when patients assigned to active treatment drop out.

Metaanalyses of Placebo-Controlled Treatment Trials

In 1986, the term *metaanalysis* first appeared in the Medline database of the National Library of Medicine. In the same year, MacMahon and colleagues published the first metaanalysis of the randomized trials to estimate the overall effect of the treatment of hypertension on morbidity and mortality. The technique of metaanalysis is now commonly used to combine data from studies to gain statistical power. As new trials have been completed, additional metaanalyses have been published.

Effects on blood pressure. Compared with control groups, active treatment generally produces a long-term difference of 5 to 6 mm Hg in diastolic BP. The reduction in stroke incidence is quite close to the estimate of 35% to 40% derived from the association of BP with event rates in epidemiologic studies. For coronary heart disease, the risk reduction of 8% to 14% is less than the 20% to 25% predicted from the epidemiologic studies.

Outcomes. In a metaanalysis of placebo-controlled trials, the findings of 18 trials were synthesized according to the first-line treatment strategy (**Figure B106.1**). Compared with the control group, β-blocker therapy was effective in preventing stroke (RR, 0.71; 95% CI, 0.59 to 0.86) and heart failure (RR, 0.58; 95% CI, 0.40 to 0.84). The findings were similar for high-dose diuretic therapy (for stroke: RR, 0.49; 95% CI, 0.39–0.62, and for heart failure: RR, 0.17; 95% CI, 0.07–0.41). Low-dose diuretic therapy prevented not only stroke (RR, 0.66; 95% CI, 0.55–0.78) and heart failure (RR, 0.58; 95% CI, 0.44–0.76) but also coronary disease (RR, 0.72; 95% CI, 0.61–0.85) and total mortality (RR, 0.90; 95% CI, 0.81–0.99). These data indicate clearly that the use of low-dose diuretic therapy is especially effective in preventing many of the major disease complications of untreated high BP. Another recent metaanalysis of the treatment trials suggests that the benefits of treatment are similar in men and women (**Table B106.2**).

Metaanalyses of Active-Control Treatment Trials

The use of a placebo or untreated control group in a clinical trial answers the question of treatment efficacy. The generation of trials that evaluated diuretics and β-blockers has documented the importance of BP lowering (Figure B106.1), and it is no longer ethical to randomize participants to placebo in large long-term trials. The current generation of clinical trials is active-control, which is not only ethical, but also important in documenting the relative benefit of one drug versus another.

In the current generation of active-control trials, calcium-antagonists and angiotensin-converting enzyme (ACE) inhibitors have figured prominently. In a metaanalysis of 9 active-control randomized clinical trials that assessed major-disease end points, calcium antagonists were compared to other forms of antihypertensive therapy in 27,743 patients (**Table B106.3**). Compared with other forms of antihypertensive therapy, calcium antagonists were associated with significantly higher risks of myocardial infarction [odds ratio (OR), 1.26; 95% CI, 1.11–1.43], heart failure (OR 1.25; 95% CI, 1.07–1.46) and major cardiovascular events (OR, 1.10; 95% CI, 1.02–1.18). Although the treatment regimens did not differ in stroke mortality or total mortality, the risk of stroke was slightly but not significantly lower with calcium antagonists (OR, 0.90; 95% CI, 0.80–1.02). According to currently available evidence, diuretics, β-blockers, and ACE inhibitors are more effective in preventing major-disease complications than calcium antagonists.

Antihypertensive Lipid-Lowering Treatment to Prevent Heart Attack Trial.
Table B106.4 summarizes the Antihypertensive Lipid-Lowering Treatment to Prevent Heart Attack Trial (ALLHAT), a 6-year, double-blind, active-control randomized trial evaluating low-dose chlorthalidone (N = 15,255), amlodipine (N = 9,048), lisinopril (N = 9,054), and doxazosin (N = 9,061). The doxazosin arm was terminated prematurely because of an increased incidence of cardiovascular events (25%) and a 2-fold increase in heart failure incidence. On combined fatal and nonfatal coronary artery disease, there was particularly an increase in heart failure episodes. At the trial's completion, systolic BP was slightly lower in those on low-dose chlorthalidone than in those on amlodipine (0.8 mm Hg) or lisinopril (2.0 mm Hg). After an average of 4.9 years, there were no significant differences for the primary outcome. Risk of heart failure was significantly higher in those randomized to amlodipine (RR, 1.38; 95% CI, 1.25–1.52). Among those randomized to lisinopril, risks were higher for stroke (RR, 1.15; 95% CI, 1.02–1.30), heart failure (RR, 1.19; 95% CI, 1.07–

Table B106.3. Metaanalysis of 9 Trials That Compared Calcium Antagonists with Other Antihypertensive Agents[a]

OUTCOME	EVENTS	ODDS RATIO	95% CONFIDENCE INTERVAL
Myocardial infarction	1,050	1.26	1.11–1.43
Stroke	1,227	0.90	0.80–1.02
Heart failure	717	1.25	1.07–1.46
Major cardiovascular events	2,409	1.10	1.07–1.18
Total mortality	2,078	1.03	0.94–1.13

Events, total number of events in both arms of the trials.
[a]There were 12,699 subjects randomized to calcium antagonists and 15,044 randomized to other antihypertensive therapies. Odds ratio >1.0 suggests that other agents are more favorable than calcium antagonists.
Adapted from Pahor M, Psaty BM, Alderman MH, et al. Health outcomes associated with calcium antagonists compared with other first-line antihypertensive therapies: a meta-analysis of randomised controlled trials. *Lancet.* 2000;356:1949–1954.

1.31), and combined cardiovascular disease (RR, 1.10; 95% CI, 1.05–1.16). Low doses of thiazide diuretics are superior in preventing one or more major forms of cardiovascular disease. Because they are at least equally effective and less expensive than other drug therapies, the authors suggested that low-dose diuretics should be first-line antihypertensive drugs.

Overview: Value of Diuretic Therapy

The first generation of randomized trials that examined major disease end points as an outcome generally used diuretics (with or without β-blockers) as first-line therapy for high BP and found significant reductions in incidence of stroke and heart failure. Low-dose diuretic therapy also reduces the incidence of coronary disease and total mortality (Figure B106.1). These outcomes are consistent across a number of metaanalyses, and the health benefits of the treatment of hypertension are similar in men and women (Table B106.2).

The second generation of clinical trials comparing one active treatment to another found diuretics, β-blockers, and ACE inhibitors have been more effective in preventing major disease complications, such as myocardial infarction and heart failure, than

calcium antagonists. ALLHAT results confirm that thiazide diuretics are at least as effective as ACE inhibitors, calcium antagonists, or α-blockers in preventing heart attack, heart failure, and stroke. ALLHAT did not test the important question of whether an ACE inhibitor–diuretic combination was superior to combinations of β-blocker with diuretic or calcium antagonist with diuretic.

SUGGESTED READING

1. The ALLHAT Officers and Coordinator for the ALLHAT Collaborative Research Group. Major cardiovascular events in hypertensive patients randomized to doxazosin vs chlorthalidone: The Antihypertensive and Lipid-Lowering Treatment to Prevent Heart Attack Trial (ALLHAT). *JAMA.* 2000;283:1967–1975.
2. Gueyffier F, Boutitie F, Boissel JP, et al. Effect of antihypertensive drug treatment on cardiovascular outcomes in women and men: a metaanalysis of individual patient data from randomized, controlled trials. The INDANA Investigators. *Ann Intern Med.* 1997;126:761–767.
3. Hypertension Detection and Follow-up Program Cooperative Group. The effect of treatment on mild hypertension: Results of the Hypertension Detection and Follow-up Program. *N Engl J Med.* 1982;307:976–980.
4. MacMahon SW, Cutler JA, Furberg CD, Payne GH. The effects of drug treatment for hypertension on morbidity and mortality from cardiovascular disease: a review of randomized controlled trials. *Prog Cardiovasc Dis.* 1986;29:99–118.
5. Medical Research Council Working Party. MRC trial of treatment of mild hypertension: principal results. *BMJ.* 1985;291:97–104.
6. Pahor M, Psaty BM, Alderman MH, et al. Health outcomes associated with calcium antagonists compared with other first-line antihypertensive therapies: a metaanalysis of randomised controlled trials. *Lancet.* 2000;356:1949–1954.
7. Psaty BM, Heckbert SR, Koepsell TD, et al. The risk of myocardial infarction associated with antihypertensive drug therapies. *JAMA.* 1995;274:620–625.
8. Psaty BM, Smith NL, Siscovick DS, et al. Health outcomes associated with antihypertensive therapies used as first-line agents: a systematic review and metaanalysis. *JAMA.* 1997;277:739–745.
9. Psaty BM, Weiss NS, Furberg CD, et al. Surrogate end points, health outcomes, and the drug approval process for the treatment of risk factors for cardiovascular disease. *JAMA.* 1999;282:786–790.
10. SHEP Cooperative Research Group. Prevention of stroke by antihypertensive drug treatment in older persons with isolated systolic hypertension: final results of the Systolic Hypertension in the Elderly Program (SHEP). *JAMA.* 1991;265:3255–3264.
11. The Collaborative Research Group. Major outcomes in high-risk hypertensive patients randomized to angiotensin-converting enzyme inhibitor or calcium-channel blocker vs diuretic: The Antihypertensive and Lipid-Lowering Treatment to Prevent Heart Attack Trial (ALLHAT). *JAMA.* 2002;288:2981–2997.

Table B106.4. Primary Results of the Antihypertensive and Lipid-Lowering Treatment to Prevent Heart Attack Trial (ALLHAT): Chlorthalidone as the Reference Group

OUTCOME	CHLORTHALIDONE		AMLODIPINE		LISINOPRIL	
	N	RATE	RR[a]	95% CI	RR[a]	95% CI
CHD	1,362	11.5	0.98	0.90–1.07	0.99	0.91–1.08
Combined CHD	2,451	19.9	1.00	0.94–1.07	1.05	0.98–1.11
Stroke	675	5.6	0.93	0.82–1.06	1.15	1.02–1.30
Combined CVD	3,941	30.9	1.04	0.99–1.09	1.10	1.05–1.16
Heart failure	870	7.7	1.38	1.25–1.52	1.19	1.07–1.31
Angina	1,567	12.1	1.02	0.94–1.10	1.11	1.03–1.20
Coronary revascularization	1,113	9.2	1.09	1.00–1.20	1.10	1.00–1.21
Total mortality	2,203	17.3	0.96	0.89–1.02	1.00	0.94–1.08

Angina, hospitalized angina; CHD, fatal coronary heart disease and nonfatal myocardial infarction; CI, confidence interval; combined CHD, CHD plus coronary revascularization and hospitalized angina; combined CVD, combined CHD plus heart failure and peripheral arterial disease; N, number of events in chlorthalidone group; rate, 6-year event rate per 100 persons; RR, relative risk.
[a]RR <1.0 indicates alternative therapy is better than chlorthalidone, the reference group.

Antihypertensive Treatment Trials: Quality of Life

Richard H. Grimm, Jr, MD, PhD; Carrie L. Hildebrant, MA

KEY POINTS

- *Quality of life* is defined as the patient's ability to function well in daily living, including psychological and physical well-being, social and leisure activity, and satisfaction with life.

- In 2 recent clinical trials, the Hypertension Optimal Treatment study and the Treatment of Mild Hypertension Study, better control of blood pressure was associated with enhanced quality of life.

See also Chapters B106, C127, C131, and C136

Historically, the treatment of hypertension with drugs was thought to diminish quality of life owing to side effects and adverse events. However, in the past several years, major clinical trials have shown an improvement in quality of life when blood pressure (BP) control is achieved with drugs or lifestyle modifications.

Quality of Life: Definition and Measurement

Quality of life is generally thought to be the patient's ability to function well in daily living, including psychological and physical well-being, social and leisure activity, and satisfaction with life. It has also been suggested that quality of life is the measure of the gap between patient expectations and achievements. A wide variety of instruments is used to measure quality of life. Most quality-of-life instruments are questionnaire-based. These range from the Sickness Impact Profile, which comprises 136 questions, to the Battery-of-Scales Quality-of-Life Questionnaire, which has 22 questions. One of the most common questionnaires is the Short Form 36, which consists of 36 questions. Seven domains have been identified as relevant to hypertensive patients: general health, psychological well-being, sleep disturbance, social function, sexual function, cognitive function, and symptom bother.

Clinical Trials

Dietary Approaches to Stop Hypertension studies. The Dietary Approaches to Stop Hypertension (DASH) trial (see Chapter B93) examined the effects of 3 dietary patterns on BP and quality of life. The combination diet, also termed the *DASH diet* (rich in fruits, vegetables, and low-fat dairy products and reduced in saturated and total fat) significantly reduced BP compared to the control diet. Another diet that was rich in fruits and vegetables but otherwise similar to the control diet also significantly reduced BP. None of the intervention diets included sodium reduction or weight loss. Quality of life was measured with the Short Form 36 questionnaire and showed improvement in all 3 treatment groups. When the subscales were summed into a total score, quality of life improved 4.0% in the control diet group, 5.0% in the fruits and vegetables diet group, and 5.9% in the DASH diet group.

Salt restriction studies. Two trials of nonpharmacologic therapies, the Trials of Hypertension Prevention (TOHP) and the Trial of Nonpharmacological Interventions in the Elderly (TONE), tested the effects of sodium reduction and weight loss. In each case, decreased BP was associated with improved quality of life.

Treatment of Mild Hypertension Study. The Treatment of Mild Hypertension Study (TOMHS) compared medical therapies but also included a nonpharmacologic component to reduce weight and dietary sodium and alcohol intake and to increase physical activity. Quality of life was measured based on a 35-item questionnaire and included 7 indexes: general health, energy or fatigue, mental health, general functioning, satisfaction with physical abilities, social functioning, and social contacts.

Weight loss. Almost all measures of quality of life improved significantly with greater weight loss. Overall, greater weight loss, increased physical activity, and improved BP control were each associated with improvements in quality of life.

Drug comparisons. In TOMHS, quality of life improved in all active drug groups compared to placebo (**Table B107.1**). The most significant improvement among drugs was with the diuretic, chlorthalidone, and the β-blocker acebutolol.

Adverse Drug Effects and Placebos

All drug treatments have the potential to produce bothersome side effects. An adverse effect by convention in drug development studies is considered to be a symptom or complaint that occurs in a patient taking a drug, but the symptom is not necessarily causally related to the drug. In placebo-controlled studies, incidence rates of adverse effects in patients on placebo are frequently the same or sometimes greater than in active drug-treated patients as has been seen in comparisons of angiotensin-receptor blockers to placebos.

Certain hypertension treatment drugs have known common side effects. For instance, in the Swedish Trial in Old Patients with Hypertension (STOP-2), calcium antagonists resulted in ankle edema in 25.5% of patients, and angiotensin-converting enzyme inhibitors caused dry cough in 30% of patients.

Table B107.1. Mean Change from Baseline in Quality-of-Life Indices Averaged over All Follow-Up Visits for All Active Drugs Combined (plus Lifestyle) and Placebo (plus Lifestyle) in the Treatment of Mild Hypertension Study (TOMHS)

QUALITY-OF-LIFE INDEX	ALL ACTIVE (N = 653)		PLACEBO (N = 230)		p VALUE
	MEAN	SE	MEAN	SE	ACTIVE VS. PLACEBO
General health	1.26	0.16	0.98	0.25	.10
Energy or fatigue	0.95	0.1	0.67	0.17	.03
Mental health	3.14	0.22	1.17	0.41	.01
General functioning	−0.03	0.06	−0.32	0.1	.01
Satisfaction with physical abilities	0.38	0.03	0.25	0.05	.07
Social functioning	0.12	0.03	−0.12	0.06	.004
Social contacts	0.09	0.06	0.15	0.11	.75
Global quality-of-life statistic	450.10	5.65	420.31	9.39	.007

From Grimm RH Jr, Prineas RJ, Roel J, Grandits G. The Treatment of Mild Hypertension (TOMHS): design and additional analyses. In: Black HR: *Clinical Trials in Hypertension*. New York, NY: Marcel Dekker; 2001, with permission.

The Hypertension Optimal Treatment (HOT) study tested the impact on cardiovascular events of 3 different levels of diastolic BP control (<80 mm Hg, <85 mm Hg, and <90 mm Hg) in patients with mild to moderate diastolic hypertension. In this trial, diastolic BP could be reduced to below 90 mm Hg in almost 90% of patients and to below 80 mm Hg in nearly 60% of patients when treated with structured, stepped-care therapy in a general practice setting. There was a low incidence of side effects among all 3 treatment groups, indicating that antihypertensive drugs, used in combination, can achieve target BP with minimal side effects.

SUGGESTED READING

1. Bulpitt CJ, Fletcher AE. Quality of life evaluation of antihypertensive drugs. *Pharmaco Economics*. 1992;2:95–102.
2. Fletcher A. Quality of life in the management of hypertension. *Clin Exp Hypertens*. 1999;21:961–972.
3. Grimm RH Jr, Grandits GA, Cutler JA, et al. for the TOMHS Research Group. Relationships of quality of life measures to long-term lifestyle and drug treatment in the Treatment of Mild Hypertension Study (TOMHS). *Arch Intern Med*. 1997;157:638–648.
4. Hansson L, Lindholm LH, Ekbom T, et al. Randomised trial of old and new antihypertensive drugs in elderly patients: cardiovascular mortality and morbidity in the Swedish Trial in Old Patients with Hypertension-2 Study. *Lancet*. 1999;354:1751–1756.
5. Hansson L. The Hypertension Optimal Treatment study and the importance of lowering blood pressure. *J Hypertens Suppl*. 1999;17:S9–S13.
6. McInnes G. Integrated approaches to management of hypertension: promoting treatment acceptance. *Am Heart J*. 1999;138:S252–S255.
7. Nunes MI. Quality of life in the elderly hypertensive. *J Cardiovasc Risk*. 2001;8:265–269.
8. Plaisted C, Lin P-H, Ard J, et al. The effects of dietary patterns on quality of life: a substudy of the Dietary Approaches to Stop Hypertension trial. *J Am Diet Assoc*. 1999;99:S84–S89.
9. Roel JP, Hildebrant CL, Grimm RH Jr. Quality-of-life with nonpharmacologic treatment of hypertension. *Curr Hypertens Rep*. 2001;3:466–472.
10. Testa M. Methods and applications of quality-of-life measurement during antihypertensive therapy. *Curr Hypertens Rep*. 2000;2:598–615.

Economic Considerations in Hypertension Management

William J. Elliott, MD, PhD

KEY POINTS

- Cost-effectiveness calculations compute the cost per year of life saved, balancing the overall cost of treatment against its effectiveness in avoiding expensive adverse clinical outcomes.

- Cost-utility analyses incorporate quality-of-life data and adjust for disabilities from side effects of treatment and nonfatal adverse outcomes.

- Beneficial cost-effectiveness ratios occur in patients at high risk of cardiovascular disease (e.g., diabetics or older patients with higher initial blood pressures).

- The cost-benefit ratio for treating hypertension may be improved by accurately diagnosing hypertension, assessing absolute risk for cardiovascular events, selecting treatments that minimize the total cost of care (while not adversely affecting quality of life), enhancing medication adherence, and avoiding unnecessary office visits or laboratory testing.

See also Chapters B81, B101, B106, C127, C128, C131, and C136

Calculations of Economic Aspects of Hypertension Therapy

Cost-effectiveness. Cost-effectiveness calculations are a formalized method of comparing the cost of an intervention with the (discounted) benefits that presumably accrue to a population to whom it is administered. The impact of treatment on public health recommendations has been limited by regional and temporal variations in the cost of medicines and medical services, accurate data on the prevalence of drug use, and the paucity of morbidity and mortality data with specific medications. Economic considerations for hypertension treatment are becoming more important and widely appreciated, both nationally [in Joint National Committee (JNC) guidelines] and locally (by managed care organizations). The cost-effectiveness ratio is the cost per year of extended life and depends on several factors (**Table B108.1**). Cost-utility analyses have units of cost per quality-adjusted life-year saved and adjust downward the value of each year of extended life, using quality-of-life data for discomfort or disability owing to either side effects of treatment or nonfatal adverse events. Early cost-effectiveness calculations were based on theoretic and computer models (e.g., Coronary Heart Disease Policy Model, Framingham Heart Study). More recently, data from large outcome studies in actual patients have provided "real-world" estimates of costs and benefits. The most accurate results from a large single-country experience come from Sweden, where the government pays for nearly all of the medical care. Therefore, solid data on costs and morbid events are available; results are summarized in **Table B108.2**.

Effect of risk. Table B108.2 shows, as have previous studies, that higher-risk patients [older people with higher initial blood pressures (BPs)] have more beneficial cost-effectiveness ratios, and that there are some subgroups for whom antihypertensive

drug therapy actually saves money in the long term. Similar money-saving ratios also exist in secondary prevention (for people who have survived an initial myocardial infarction or stroke) and in very-high-risk hypertensives (e.g., diabetics).

Improving the Cost-Effectiveness of Hypertension Therapy

Giving antihypertensive drugs to everyone with elevated BP costs money, overall. Nonetheless, there are several simple steps that can be easily incorporated into medical practice that should improve the cost-effectiveness ratio of hypertension treatment. These include the following: (a) accurate diagnosis and classification of hypertension, (b) baseline risk assessment to determine whether costly medications should be prescribed, (c) choosing drug therapy that leads to the lowest overall cost, (d) maximizing patients' adherence to medications, and (e) reducing unnecessary office visits and laboratory testing.

Accurate diagnosis of hypertension. Approximately 20% of individuals with elevated BPs in the medical office setting have white coat hypertension (see Chapter B101) and probably

---

Table B108.1. Major Determinants of the Cost-Effectiveness Ratio

The absolute risk for cardiovascular events for a given patient (which depends on age, blood pressure stage, and concomitant diseases and comorbidities)

The efficacy of treatment in reducing the future risk of expensive adverse clinical events (e.g., stroke, myocardial infarction, heart failure, dialysis, or renal transplantation)

The (discounted) future cost of these adverse events

The total cost of treatment

Table B108.2. **Cost for 1 Additional Year of Life for Swedish Hypertensives Treated with Diuretics or β-Blockers, Converted into 1992 U.S. Dollars**

DIASTOLIC BP (MM HG)	AGE <45 YR		AGE 45–69 YR		AGE ≥70 YR	
	MEN ($)	WOMEN ($)	MEN ($)	WOMEN ($)	MEN ($)	WOMEN ($)
90–94	118,375	313,250	8,500	26,875	3,125	2,625
95–99	97,500	236,750	4,250	16,625	1,750	875
100–104	79,500	173,500	8,500	7,375	375	Saves[a]
≥105	55,000	93,250	Saves[a]	Saves[a]	Saves[a]	Saves[a]

[a]For this subgroup, antihypertensive drug therapy *saves* money.
Adapted from Jönsson BG. Cost-benefit of treating hypertension. *J Hypertens Suppl.* 1994;12:S65–75, with permission.

do not benefit from drug therapy to the same extent as people with sustained hypertension. Ambulatory BP monitoring is effective in documenting white coat hypertension, so selective use of ambulatory BP monitoring could lead to an overall reduction in costs. This procedure has recently been approved for reimbursement by federal authorities in the United States. However, home BP monitoring and multiple office visits to document the presence of sustained hypertension are still more commonly recommended to avoid "wasting" treatment on patients who are at low cardiovascular risk.

Risk stratification before therapy. Risk stratification before prescribing drug therapy has been widely recommended by JNC and other guideline committees. For patients with low baseline risk (without other risk factors, target organ damage, or cardiovascular disease), even with BPs as high as 159/99 mm Hg, JNC VI recommended a year of lifestyle modifications before initiating drug therapy. This should improve the cost-effectiveness ratio, because it delays starting costly drug therapy for patients with a very low risk of cardiovascular events. At the other extreme, drug therapy should be intensified for patients with diabetes or chronic renal impairment until the BP is below 130/85 mm Hg. Antihypertensive drug therapy saved lives and money in the United Kingdom Prospective Diabetes Study. Compared to the usual target of 140/90 mm Hg, the lower BP goal is also cost saving (because of reductions in expensive hypertension-related morbidity) in American diabetics over age 60, as long as the marginal annual cost of such treatment does not exceed $414.

Cost of lifestyle modifications. Lifestyle modifications are still routinely recommended for all hypertensives, although their efficacy in reducing cardiovascular events has never been proven. The Treatment of Mild Hypertension Study showed a slightly but significantly lower rate of cardiovascular events in hypertensive individuals randomized to receive drugs in addition to an excellent program of lifestyle modifications. Lifestyle modification programs are often expensive to implement and maintain, and long-term adherence among the general population to a low-salt diet, weight control, and physical activity is likely to be lower than adherence to antihypertensive drug therapy. Public health programs directed toward lifestyle modifications are, however, relatively cost-effective, because the cost of public service advertisements is low and the potential for lower BPs across large exposed populations is substantial.

Limiting costs of medicines. Lower-cost medications are easily recommended over higher-cost drugs with the same efficacy in reducing BP, but the cost of antihypertensive drugs is a com-

plex subject. The American Heart Association estimates that medications accounted for the largest single portion (32.8%) of the total cost of care for hypertension in 2002 in the United States. The annualized increase in drug expenditures for hypertension since 1995 is 22%, 50% higher than overall spending on hypertension (14.1%) and approximately 4.4 times higher than the rate of inflation. Pricing of medications is variable, particularly at the retail pharmacy. Generic medications, with lower average wholesale prices than their branded counterparts, have a markup up to 10 times more than the traditional 7% for branded drugs, so retail costs may be quite similar.

Pharmacy benefits managers have implemented many strategies that reduce pharmaceutical expenditures. Although some of these are beneficial, worsened BP control and increased morbid events have been found in several studies. Some "innovations" (e.g., monthly bidding for an exclusive contract to use a single angiotensin-converting enzyme inhibitor in a large health maintenance organization) reduce the pharmacy budget but incur more office visits and lead to a higher total cost of care. Patient and physician satisfaction also are negatively affected. One large clinic in Omaha demonstrated no significant differences in total cost of the first year of treatment across 5 different classes of first time antihypertensive drugs, after adjusting for the cost of other needed medications, office visits, laboratory studies, and evaluation of adverse experiences. When more than 1 medication is needed to control BP, some pharmacy programs vigorously pursue prescribing economically advantageous fixed-dose combination products that often cost less than 2 separate prescriptions for the individual components.

A low-dose diuretic has most often been suggested (on economic grounds) to be the best initial choice for an antihypertensive drug in an otherwise uncomplicated patient. More expensive drugs (e.g., ramipril) can be justified if the absolute risk for costly events (e.g., dialysis) is extremely high, because such drugs then save money overall. The better long-term tolerability of some of the newer medications (e.g., angiotensin II receptor antagonists) carries greater weight in cost-utility analyses. These incorporate not only the costs of "extra" visits to health care providers for evaluation of perceived side effects but also the subjective annoyance caused by some antihypertensive drugs in some patients.

Enhanced medication adherence. Long-term adherence to a medication (sometimes called *persistence*) is seldom considered when performing cost-effectiveness calculations but may be the most important factor in everyday medical practice. Patients who are prescribed antihypertensive medications but who do not take them properly clearly incur the costs attendant to obtaining such therapy but derive no benefit: an infinite cost to benefit ratio. Simple procedures to enhance adherence include educating the patient about the disease and the medication, prescribing once-daily pills that do not adversely affect quality of life, and minimizing out-of-pocket costs.

Reducing health care provider–associated costs.

Current American Heart Association estimates of $47.2 billion spent on hypertension treatment in the United States suggest that 27% goes for indirect costs (transportation, time off work, and lost productivity), 18% goes to health care providers, and 18% goes to hospital and nursing home services. If patients were able to monitor home BPs and receive health care advice by telephone or Internet rather than making costly office visits, costs could be reduced. Similarly, laboratory testing can often be minimized by choosing effective doses of drug therapy with few adverse metabolic effects.

The discussion about how to improve the cost-effectiveness of hypertension treatment is expected to intensify in the next several years as studies are completed that compare the effectiveness of newer and somewhat more expensive drug classes with the traditional (and generically available) diuretics and β-blockers. Cost-effectiveness analyses are likely to guide how policy makers incorporate these clinical trial results into "critical pathways" for hypertension treatment.

SUGGESTED READING

1. Elliott WJ, Weir DR, Black HR. Cost-effectiveness of the lower treatment goal (of JNC VI) in hypertensive diabetics. *Arch Intern Med.* 2000;160:1277–1283.
2. Hilleman DE, Mohiuddin SM, Lucas BD Jr, et al. Cost-minimization analysis of initial antihypertensive therapy in patients with mild-to-moderate essential diastolic hypertension. *Clin Ther.* 1994;16:88–102.
3. Johannesson M. The cost-effectiveness of hypertension treatment in Sweden. *Pharmacoeconomics.* 1995;7:242–250.
4. Jönsson BG. Cost-benefit of treating hypertension. *J Hypertens Suppl.* 1994;12:S65–75.
5. Mar J, Rodriguez-Artalejo F. Which is more important for the efficiency of hypertension treatment: hypertension stage, type of drug, or therapeutic compliance? *J Hypertension.* 2001;19:149–155.
6. Neaton JD, Grimm RH Jr, Prineas RJ, et al. Treatment of Mild Hypertension Study: final results. *JAMA.* 1993;270:713-724.
7. Raikou M, Gray A, Briggs A, et al. Cost-effectiveness analysis of improved blood pressure control in hypertensive patients with type 2 diabetes: UKPDS 40. U.K. Prospective Diabetes Study Group. *BMJ.* 1998;317:720–726.
8. Schadlich PK, Brecht JG, Brunetti M, et al. Cost-effectiveness of ramipril in patients with non-diabetic nephropathy and hypertension: economic evaluation of Ramipril Efficacy In Nephropathy (REIN) Study for Germany from the perspective of statutory health insurance. *Pharmacoeconomics.* 2001;19:497–512.
9. Swales JD. The costs of not treating hypertension. *Blood Press.* 1999;8:198–199.
10. Yarows SA, Khoury S, Sowers JR. Cost effectiveness of 24-hour ambulatory blood pressure monitoring in evaluation and treatment of essential hypertension. *Am J Hypertens.* 1994;7:464–468.

Part C. CLINICAL MANAGEMENT

Section 1. *General Diagnostic Aspects*

Chapter C109

Blood Pressure Measurement

Carlene M. Grim, MSN, SpDN; Clarence E. Grim, MS, MD

KEY POINTS

- Hypertension detection, referral, and treatment guidelines are based on measurements by trained observers using the mercury sphygmomanometer, following standard techniques recommended by the American Heart Association.

- Indirect blood pressure measurement is one of the most frequent and, in many cases, most poorly performed health care procedures.

- Clinicians should encourage the use of the mercury sphygmomanometer until aneroid and automated devices are better validated.

- Validation and calibration of aneroid and automated devices is often neglected; a program of regular maintenance and calibration of all instruments should be the standard of care in all settings.

See also Chapters B101, C110, C112, C128, C133, C135, and C136

Indirect Blood Pressure Measurement

Indirect blood pressure (BP) measurement is safe, painless, and provides reliable information when performed accurately. Virtually all the epidemiologic data used to determine hypertension detection, referral, and treatment guidelines are based on BPs obtained by the American Heart Association (AHA) standardized indirect measurement method. Health professionals base crucial clinical decisions on these measurements; therefore, the proven benefits of treating high BP can be accomplished only when BP measurement is performed accurately. Accurate BP measurement requires the ability to hear, interpret, and record Korotkoff sounds; and operate the equipment properly. Failure to practice correct technique and the use of inaccurate equipment are the major reasons for inaccurate BP determinations.

Selecting and Caring for Blood Pressure Measurement Equipment

The manometer is a mercury or an aneroid instrument calibrated to the nearest 2 mm Hg. The mercury manometer is read at the top edge (the meniscus) of the mercury column. It is the most accurate measurement device available and is considered the "gold standard" for all blood pressure measurements. The aneroid manometer consists of a metal bellows that expands as the pressure in the cuff increases and is read at the point indicated by a needle on its dial. Accuracy of the mercury manometer is assessed by noting whether the mercury meniscus rests at zero. The aneroid manometer is fragile and easily damaged. Users cannot be certain that it is accurate even when the needle is positioned at zero. Therefore, it is necessary to use a Y connector to compare the aneroid device to an accurate mercury manometer at least every 6 months (**Figure C109.1**). Calibration is required when the readings differ from the standard mercury manometer by ≥3 mm Hg. All practice settings should have a regular (at least every 6 months) calibration program in place. The stethoscope head should have a low-frequency detector (bell) for listening to the low-pitched sounds. Earpieces should fit comfortably forward in the direction of the ear canal and block out external noise. For best sound transmission, the tubing should be thick and no longer than 15 in.

Automated Blood Pressure Measurement Devices

Before using any automated BP instrument, the observer must document the accuracy of its pressure-registering system by using a Y tube to connect and compare the automated BP instrument to an accurate mercury device. Next, simultaneous digital and mercury readings on the patient should be compared. The use of automated devices is discouraged in most clinical settings because they are often difficult to calibrate, fail to give accurate readings on many individuals, and do not eliminate human error.

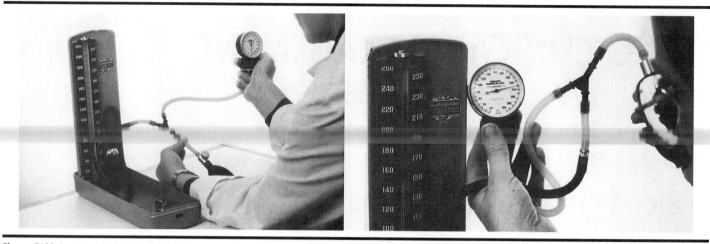

Figure C109.1.   Aneroid instrument being tested by inserting a Y-tube connector or stopcock to create a communicating system with one pressure source, allowing simultaneous pressure application to both instruments. (Courtesy of Shared Care Research and Education Consulting, Inc., Torrance, CA.)

Steps Needed to Obtain Accurate and Reliable Readings

Step 1: environment.   The setting should be private and quiet, with a comfortable room temperature. To get the best estimate of the patient's usual BP, environmental factors that may cause BP variation or interfere with hearing Korotkoff sounds must be controlled. The manometer must be positioned so the observer can view it at eye level. Viewing the manometer above or below the observer's eye level results in inaccurate readings. The room should have a straight-backed chair to seat the patient next to a table or desk with feet flat on the floor. A seat for the BP observer should be provided along with an adjustable surface to support the arm at heart level during standing measurements. The height of the table should be such that the midpoint of the cuff is in place on the patient's right arm (or the arm that is known to produce the higher BP reading) and is supported at heart level. It is important to avoid errors induced by differences in hydrostatic pressure between the point of artery compression by the cuff and the heart. If the center of the cuff on the arm or leg is above the heart level, the reading will be falsely low by 0.8 mm Hg for each 1 cm above the heart level. If below heart level, it will be falsely high by a similar amount. Supporting the back in the seated position and the arm in any position avoids increases in BP due to isometric muscle contraction.

Step 2: preparation and rest period.   Inquire about biologic factors that may affect the reading at this time, including the time and dose of medications. If not wearing short, loose sleeves, patients should bare their arm(s). To get the best estimate of the patient's usual BP, biologic factors that may cause BP variation such as pain, stress, full urinary bladder, and recent meal should be minimized. Recent ingestion of prescription, over-the-counter or street drugs, caffeine, and nicotine can affect BP readings. Clothing interferes with cuff placement, pressure, and sound transmission. Proper preparation avoids elevated readings due to anxiety about the procedure. Repeated readings increase accuracy. Instruct patients to sit up straight with legs uncrossed, back resting against the chair, and feet flat on the floor, and to remain silent until after BP readings. Allow a 5-minute rest period before the first reading. The lack of back

and foot support, such as occurs when the patient is seated on an examination table, causes BP elevation averaging 5 mm Hg diastolic. Talking or active listening during measurement causes BP elevation.

Step 3: proper cuff (bladder) size.   To get an accurate reading, the width of the cuff bladder should encircle at least 40% of the arm circumference; the length of the cuff bladder should encircle at least 80% of the arm circumference. At the first visit, measure circumference at the midpoint of the upper arm, between the olecranon and acromion processes. Chart the arm circumference for future reference. Arms >53 cm in circumference should have the BP measured with a cuff of the appropriate size on the forearm. When arm circumference measurement is not practical, as during screening situations, it is acceptable to estimate the proper cuff size by comparing the bladder width and length to arm circumference. When BP is not measured in both arms, the reading should be taken in the right arm unless it is known that BP in the left arm is higher. Note the appropriate cuff and bladder size on each chart. Using a bladder that is too narrow or short for the limb is a common error that is serious because it yields false high readings. Diseases that cause BP differences between the arms are much more likely to cause a falsely low BP in the left arm.

Step 4: cuff placement.   Locate the patient's brachial artery at the midpoint of the upper arm by palpating between the biceps and triceps muscles on its inner surface. Wrap the cuff smoothly and snugly around the arm with its bladder center directly over the palpated artery and the lower edge of the cuff 2.5 cm above the antecubital fossa. This technique avoids false high readings that occur when cuff pressure is not equally distributed over the artery and avoids errors that result from extra sounds when the stethoscope comes in contact with the cuff or tubing.

Step 5: determine the maximum inflation level

(1) Before listening for the BP, determine the inflation level necessary to obtain an accurate systolic reading, the maximum inflation level (MIL). To do this, locate the radial pulse and note the heart rate and rhythm. When the heart rate is irregu-

lar, systolic BP may vary beat to beat, and additional readings are needed to get the best estimate of the systolic BP.

(2) Continue feeling the pulse and rapidly inflate the cuff to 60 mm Hg and then by 10-mm increments until the pulse is no longer palpable. This is the first estimate of the palpated pressure. Stop inflating the cuff.

(3) Begin deflation at 2 mm Hg per second. Note the pressure at which the pulse reappears. This is the palpated systolic pressure and is usually within 10 mm Hg of the level at which the pulse disappeared.

(4) Immediately release all pressure. Add 30 mm Hg to the palpated systolic reading to determine the MIL. This maneuver determines the minimum pressure needed to get an accurate systolic BP on a patient, decreases patient discomfort, and avoids errors that result from failure to inflate above systolic BP reading, including an inaccurately low systolic BP reading, which occurs when the observer begins listening during an auscultatory gap.

Step 6: stethoscope placement. Position the stethoscope earpieces pointing forward in your ears. Sound is not transmitted well when the eartips fail to point into the ear canal. Find the point at which the brachial artery pulse is the strongest, usually just above the antecubital fossa on the inner aspect of the arm. Using light pressure, position the chestpiece over this point with all edges gently touching the skin surface. The stethoscope bell or a low-frequency detector is recommended. The loudest sounds can be heard over this pulse and errors owing to difficulty hearing and interpreting Korotkoff sounds are minimized along with errors from too much stethoscope pressure that may cause artery occlusion and distortion of BP sounds. Do not allow the stethoscope head to touch the cuff or tubing because extraneous sounds mask and confuse Korotkoff sounds.

Step 7: inflation and deflation. Rapidly inflate the cuff to the MIL. If sounds are heard immediately, completely release all pressure and repeat step 5 to repeat the palpated pressure. Rapid inflation to the correct MIL ensures listening above systolic BP. Slow inflation traps venous blood in the arm and may result in pain and diminished or distorted sounds. Release the air from the cuff so that the mercury falls at a rate of 2 mm Hg per second until Korotkoff sounds are heard. Continue deflation at the rate of 2 mm Hg per beat. If unable to hear sounds clearly, quickly release all pressure and check position of eartips and stethoscope. Repeat the procedure. Slow deflation is necessary to allow the observer to hear the systolic and diastolic pressures at the point of onset. A reading can be no more accurate than the rate of deflation (i.e., a deflation rate of 10 mm Hg/second results in a pressure accurate to only 10 mm Hg, and if 1 beat is missed, to only 20 mm Hg).

Step 8: systolic blood pressure. Read to the nearest 2 mm Hg mark. Remember the systolic pressure at the onset of Korotkoff phase 1, the first of at least 2 regular "tapping" sounds (**Table C109.1**). Forgetting the reading is a very common source of errors of 8 to 10 mm Hg, especially in the presence of a wide pulse pressure (difference between the systolic and diastolic pressures). When the reading falls between two 2 mm Hg marks, round to the higher of the 2. Concentrate and remember the

Table C109.1. Phases of the Korotkoff Sounds[a]

Phase 1
   The pressure level at which the first faint, consistent tapping sounds are heard. The sounds gradually increase in intensity as the cuff is deflated. The first of at least 2 of these sounds is defined as the *systolic pressure*.
Phase 2
   The time during cuff deflation when a murmur of swishing sounds are heard.
Phase 3
   The period during which sounds are crisper and increase in intensity.
Phase 4
   The time when a distinct, abrupt, muffling of sound (usually of a soft blowing quality) is heard. This is defined as the *diastolic pressure* in anyone in whom sounds continue to zero.
Phase 5
   The pressure level when the last regular blood pressure sound is heard and after which all sound disappears. This is defined as the *diastolic pressure* unless sounds are heard to zero.

[a]To avoid error, the observer must be prepared to recognize 2 normal Korotkoff sound variations associated with BP readings. The auscultatory gap is a period of silence occurring during Korotkoff phases 1 and 2. This disappearance of sound is temporary and is usually short, but the gap can occur over a period of 40 mm Hg. It seems to be associated with higher BP readings. An absent Korotkoff phase 5 occurs when sounds are heard to zero. When this is the case, phase 4 should be recorded along with phase 5. In this case, phase 4 is the best reference for diastolic pressure.

reading by silently repeating the systolic number with every heartbeat until you confirm disappearance. Observers must learn to rule out sound artifacts. Single sounds inconsistent with heart rate are insignificant artifacts unless the pulse was irregular during palpation. In the case of arrhythmia, additional readings are needed to get the best estimate of the systolic BP.

Step 9: diastolic blood pressure. Remember the point at which the last regular Korotkoff sound is heard. (Korotkoff sounds are designated as K1 through K5.) Immediately record systolic and diastolic BPs. When the sounds continue to very low diastolic levels or zero, remember the reading at the onset of K4, the point at which sounds begin to muffle, as well as the last sound heard. The onset of K5 (disappearance) is more reliably interpreted when observers listen for the last sound heard. The absence of K5 occurs often in children, during pregnancy, and in other high-cardiac-output states. In these cases, the onset of K4 is the most accurate diastolic indicator. If the diastolic BP is heard above 90 mm Hg, listen for an additional 40 mm Hg. Otherwise, listen for 10 to 20 mm Hg below the last sound to confirm disappearance to avoid inaccurately high diastolic BP owing to failure to listen until sounds reappear after a period of silence (auscultatory gap).

Step 10: recording. Immediately record the reading, the arm used, the position of the patient, and the cuff size used to avoid recall artifact. Record the reading as K1/K5. If K4 is recorded, write the 3 numbers as K1/K4/K5. If sounds do not cease, record K5 as 0. Standardized recording methods are necessary to correctly interpret and compare readings by different observers. When phase 5 is absent, Korotkoff phase 4 is the best indication of diastolic pressure.

Step 11: repeat the reading. Make certain all air is out of the cuff and wait 1 to 2 minutes, then repeat steps 6 through 10.

BP normally changes from minute to minute, especially during clinical measurements. The average of 2 or more BP readings in a single arm is more reliable and a better indicator of usual readings than is a single reading or 1 reading in each arm.

Step 12: repeat the process. Repeat the measurements in the other arm during initial workup and standing or supine as dictated by the patient's situation. Postural changes in BP are measured after 1 and 3 minutes of standing. Note the arm with the higher reading for future comparisons. BP can differ by >10 mm Hg between arms. The higher pressure more accurately reflects intraarterial pressure.

Special Techniques and Populations

Absence of Korotkoff phase 5. When cardiac output is high, as in some children, in thyrotoxicosis, during fever, and in pregnant women, K5 is often absent. In this event, Korotkoff sounds are heard until the mercury column falls to zero. BP should be recorded as 3 numbers (K5/K4/0).

Blood pressure measurement in children. The principles of measurement are the same in newborns, infants, and children. A most important consideration is the selection of a cuff that is appropriate for the arm circumference, as described above.

Blood pressure measurement in the elderly. In the elderly, the brachial arteries occasionally become very thickened and stiff. When this happens, the indirect cuff pressure may overestimate intraarterial pressure, because higher cuff pressure is required to compress such a rigid vessel. The presence of a radial artery that is still palpable after the cuff is inflated above the systolic BP should be a warning of this error. If the artery feels excessively thick when rolled back and forth under the finger, the BP reading measured with indirect techniques may be falsely high. Recheck the pressure by palpation in the forearm. If the palpated systolic pressure differs by >15 mm Hg, then a direct arterial punc-

ture may be needed to be certain of the true pressure, although this is rare.

Very large, cone-shaped, and muscular arms. If the patient's arm is >41 cm in circumference or if it is shaped so that a cuff does not fit on it well, then accurate pressure measurement may be impossible. In this case, palpated and auscultated readings should be attempted, with a cuff of the appropriate size, in the upper arm and forearm. If these differ by >15 mm Hg, then a better estimate of true pressure is the palpated systolic pressure with the cuff on the forearm.

SUGGESTED READING

1. Bailey RH, Knaus VL, Bauer JH. Aneroid sphygmomanometers: an assessment of accuracy at a university hospital and clinics. *Arch Intern Med.* 1991;151:1409–1412.
2. Grim CM, Grim CE. A curriculum for the training and certification of blood pressure measurement for health care providers. *Can J Cardiol.* 1005;11:38H–42H.
3. Hayes MV. Managing mercury: simple, effective methods for cleaning up small spills. *Med Waste.* 1993;1:3–7.
4. Jones DW, Frohlich ED, Grim CM, et al. Mercury sphygmomanometers should not be abandoned: an advisory statement from the Council for High Blood Pressure Research, American Heart Association. *Hypertension.* 2001;37:185–186.
5. Nash CA. How do you test a digital sphygmomanometer? *Am J Nurs.* 1992;92:66–69.
6. National High Blood Pressure Education Program Working Group Update on the 1987 Task Force Report on High Blood Pressure in Children and Adolescents: a working group report from the National High Blood Pressure Education Program. *Pediatrics.* 1996;90:649–658.
7. O'Brien E, Waeber B, Gianfranco, P, et al. Blood pressure measuring devices: recommendations of the European Society of Hypertension. *BMJ.* 2001;322:531–536.
8. Perloff D, Grim CM, Flack J, et al. Human blood pressure determination by sphygmomanometry. *Circulation.* 1993;88:2460–2470.
9. Prisant LM, Alpert BS, Robbins CB, et al. American national standard for nonautomated sphygmomanometers: summary report. *Am J Hypertens.* 1995;8:210–213.
10. Sixth Report of the Joint National Committee on Prevention, Detection, Evaluation, and Treatment of High Blood Pressure (JNC VI). *Arch Intern Med.* 1997;157:2413–2446.

Chapter C110

Initial Workup of the Hypertensive Patient

Ray W. Gifford, Jr, MD, MS; Marvin Moser, MD

KEY POINTS

- A history, physical examination, basic serum chemistries that include a lipid profile and fasting triglycerides, urinalysis, and an electrocardiograph are recommended for the initial evaluation of a hypertensive patient.

- Goals of initial evaluation are (a) estimation of the severity of the hypertension, including the presence or absence of target organ disease; (b) evaluation of other cardiovascular risk factors; and (c) evaluation for secondary hypertension. Repeat visits are often necessary to be certain that hypertension is sustained.

- An echocardiogram, 24-hour ambulatory blood pressure monitoring, and renin determinations are not recommended unless there are specific indications for these procedures.

- Particular attention should be paid to systolic blood pressure, which more closely predicts morbidity and mortality than diastolic pressure.

See also Chapters A72, B81, B101, C109, C111–C115, C120–C125, C128, and C173

The initial diagnostic evaluation of the hypertensive patient has 4 major objectives: (a) to define the severity of the hypertension including presence or absence of target organ disease, (b) to determine the presence or absence of other risk factors for cardiovascular disease, (c) to search for clues of secondary causes for hypertension, and (d) to confirm that hypertension is sustained, by repeating measurements in the office and at home.

Sixth Joint National Committee on the Prevention, Detection, Evaluation, and Treatment of High Blood Pressure Recommendations

The Sixth Joint National Committee on the Prevention, Detection, Evaluation, and Treatment of High Blood Pressure (JNC VI) recommends a careful history, a complete physical examination, several basic laboratory tests, and an electrocardiogram (ECG) for the pretreatment evaluation. It is recognized from epidemiologic studies that hypertension in conjunction with any one of several other cardiovascular risk factors, such as a history of cigarette smoking, elevated serum lipid levels, diabetes mellitus, heavy alcohol consumption, and obesity, puts a patient at greater risk than when hypertension is the only risk factor. The presence of target organ involvement, such as left ventricular hypertrophy (LVH), indicates that treatment should be undertaken more readily than in subjects without evidence of target organ involvement. Although a low percentage (<1%) of all cases of hypertension in the general population is secondary to an identifiable and possibly curable cause, patients with these diseases should be identified, if possible, because they may be cured by specific treatment.

Establishing the Diagnosis of Hypertension

The initial step in the evaluation of a patient with newly discovered hypertension is to decide whether he or she actually has a sustained blood pressure (BP) elevation. Before a diagnosis of hypertension is established, BP should be measured on at least 2 occasions after the original determination unless initial levels are >180/110 mm Hg (stage 3 hypertension), in which case the diagnosis is considered established, and therapy should be initiated promptly. Follow-up readings are often lower than the first reading, and fewer people would be categorized as hypertensive if these subsequent pressures are considered. Individuals with initially elevated BPs who become normotensive on further evaluation should not be ignored, however, because they have a tendency to develop more consistently elevated BPs in the future. They should be carefully followed up at regular intervals of between 6 months and 1 year. Careful attention should be paid to measurement techniques to ensure that BP readings are accurate.

Systolic Blood Pressure Level and Risk

Risk increases as pressure rises: The higher the level of BP, the greater the incidence of cardiovascular complications at all ages and in both genders. Recent data from more than 300,000 men screened for the Multiple Risk Factor Intervention Trial (MRFIT) determined that an elevation of systolic BP may be a more reliable and important prognostic factor than an elevated diastolic BP, at least in men. For example, a systolic BP of 150 to 159 mm Hg suggests a greater risk for cardiovascular events than a diastolic BP of 95 to 100 mm Hg. This finding confirms data from Framingham and other studies, which include women, but the misperception persists that the diastolic BP is of more importance than systolic BP as a predictor of events. An exception is in individuals <50 years of age, in whom diastolic pressure is a reliable risk predictor. An increased pulse pressure (systolic minus diastolic), which reflects decreased arterial compliance in older persons, may be an even better index of cardiovascular risk.

White Coat Hypertension?

Routine use of ambulatory BP monitoring to diagnose *white coat hypertension*, defined as persistently elevated BPs in a doctor's office with normal BPs at home or at work, was not recommended in JNC VI. This opinion and recommendation were based on the following:

(1) All of the major epidemiologic studies have based their estimations of risk on casual BPs taken on 1 or 2 occasions in a doctor's office or clinic, not on home or work-site pressures. If the office BP is high, the risk of a future cardiovascular event is increased compared with someone with a normal casual BP.

(2) In all of the long-term clinical trials, patients were treated on the basis of BPs measured in a clinic or doctor's office. The lower the office BP, the better the outcome.

(3) Recent data from the Tecumseh study have established that patients with slightly elevated BPs in doctors' offices but with normal pressures at home are different physiologically from those who are normotensive (<135/85 mm Hg) at home and in a medical office; peripheral resistance is increased, and changes in left ventricular diastolic function and in certain metabolic parameters such as insulin resistance, levels of serum cholesterol, and serum glucose, have already occurred. Other studies have shown that patients with white coat hypertension have a slightly greater tendency to develop LVH, coronary disease, and stroke than patients who have normal BPs at home and in the physician's office. However, other experts in the field have found that the degree of target organ damage and the overall morbidity and mortality in white coat hypertensives are closer to levels observed in normotensives than those seen in sustained hypertensives (see Chapter B101). Ambulatory BP monitoring has been approved for reimbursement by Medicare. Further studies are necessary to establish clear policy in this area.

Clues for Secondary Hypertension

If an elevated BP is discovered, efforts should be made to rule out, if possible, the presence of secondary hypertension (**Table C110.1**). Although a number of very rare causes exist, most fall into a few diagnostic groups. Every case of accelerated

---

Table C110.1. Some Symptoms or Findings That May Suggest Further Studies for Identifiable Causes of Hypertension

---

Obesity, unusual truncal distribution of fat and abdominal striae, and excessive body or facial hair (Cushing's syndrome)

Anxiety, tremor, headaches, sweating, rapid pulse, recent weight loss (pheochromocytoma)

Skin lesions (pheochromocytoma is sometimes associated with von Recklinghausen's disease; pigmented striae are consistent with Cushing's syndrome)

Muscle weakness, cramps (primary aldosteronism)

Periods of impaired consciousness (cerebrovascular disease or hypersomnolence owing to sleep apnea that may be associated with hypertension)

Snoring (obstructive sleep apnea)

Absent or diminished femoral pulses (coarctation of aorta)

Periumbilical holosystolic bruit with or without diastolic component (renovascular disease)

---

or malignant hypertension should be evaluated for secondary hypertension after the BP is lowered.

Chronic renal insufficiency. Chronic renal insufficiency can usually be ruled out by the absence of proteinuria and the presence of a normal serum creatinine level.

Renovascular hypertension. Renovascular hypertension should be suspected if there is (a) new-onset hypertension in a patient older than 55 to 60 years of age, particularly in smokers; (b) definite hypertension in a child <10 to 12 years of age; (c) sudden increase in BP in patients who were previously controlled by medication; (d) failure of triple-drug therapy (employing adequate doses and usually including a diuretic); and (e) a periumbilical bruit with radiation to the flanks, especially in younger women. This bruit is characteristically holosystolic and high-pitched with a short diastolic component.

Adrenal steroid excess. Primary aldosteronism should be suspected if the serum potassium level is consistently <3.5 mEq per L in the absence of diuretic therapy or <3.0 mEq per L on a diuretic. Cushing's syndrome, a rare form of hypertension, should be suspected in a person with abdominal obesity, purple abdominal striae, and abnormal blood chemistries.

Aortic coarctation. Coarctation of the aorta can be identified by the presence of a short, rough systolic murmur in the second left interspace, the palpation or auscultation of bruits over the back, the absence of or marked decrease in the amplitude of the femoral pulses or BPs in the legs, a chest radiograph demonstrating notching of the posterior ribs, or an imaging test.

Pheochromocytoma. Pheochromocytoma should be suspected when there is a history of palpitations, sweating, headaches, weight loss, and the presence of orthostatic hypotension.

Specific Aspects of the History

Family history. To determine the urgency of treatment, it is often helpful to establish whether there is a strong family history of hypertension, stroke, or coronary disease, especially if any of these events have occurred in close relatives <60 years old. The history should specifically include information regarding symptoms and any prior cardiovascular disease (e.g., stroke, myocardial infarction, angina, congestive heart failure). The presence of early coronary artery disease is another cardiovascular disease risk factor.

General symptomatology. Although stages 1 and 2 hypertension (BPs of 140–159/90–99 and 160–179/100–109 mm Hg, respectively) are generally asymptomatic, data demonstrating improvement in general well-being when BP is lowered with antihypertensive agents suggest that hypertensive individuals may not be as free of symptoms as has been commonly believed.

Nonprescription medications and nonsteroidal antiinflammatory drugs. A history of the use of other medications (prescribed or over-the-counter) should be obtained because these medications may cause an elevation of pressure or aggravate existing hypertension. Among drugs that may increase BP are high-dose estrogens, adrenal steroids, nonsteroidal antiinflammatory drugs, nasal decongestants, appetite suppressants, cyclosporine, and tricyclic antidepressants. The number of patients, however, who experience an elevated BP from these agents is small. If BP is well controlled in treated subjects, there is little reason to interdict the use of any of these medications, including the cyclooxygenase-2 inhibitors for arthritis, if they are indicated for medical reasons and prescribed in usual doses. In some patients, however, cyclooxygenase-2 inhibitors clearly raise BP.

Alcohol and street drugs. Chronic alcohol use predisposes to hypertension by unknown mechanisms. This type of hypertension can be quite refractory to drug therapy. Use of stimulants such as amphetamines or cocaine can cause marked BP elevations. Withdrawal of alcohol, opiates, and other street drugs is also associated with acute BP increases.

Sleep history. Sleep apnea is commonly associated with hypertension. It should be suspected in obese individuals with disrupted sleep patterns. Snoring is a frequent finding but is more reliably reported by the sleep partner (or other family member) than by the affected individual. Daytime somnolence and fatigue are also common in this condition.

Physical Examination

Blood pressure. On the first visit, it is useful to measure BP in both arms using standard technique (see Chapter C109). These readings should be similar, although if there is a time lapse between the 2 measurements, there may be a difference of approximately 5 to 10 mm Hg. If the difference between arms is much more than 15 to 20 mm Hg of systolic BP, an atherosclerotic plaque may be present in the circulation supplying the arm with the lower pressure. Always use the BP measured in the arm with the highest reading to monitor therapy.

Funduscopic examination. Funduscopic examination is not very helpful in the majority of subjects with stage 1 or 2 hypertension, but the presence of significant arteriolosclerosis or arteriovenous nicking indicates that BP has been elevated for a considerable length of time or has been higher at other times in the past. Flame-shaped hemorrhages, exudates, or papilledema with an elevated BP suggest severe target organ damage and a poor prognosis unless therapy is instituted quickly (see Chapter A72 and figures on back cover).

Cardiac examination. Physical examination of the heart includes an evaluation of rate and rhythm. Ectopic beats are not uncommon in persons with hypertension, especially if LVH is present. Atrial fibrillation is not a common finding unless there are other complicating factors. Physical signs of cardiomegaly may be present, with a forceful apical impulse and palpation of cardiac dullness to the left of the midclavicular line. An accentuated aortic second sound is frequently present, especially if the diastolic BP is >100 mm Hg. A fourth heart sound is common in adults with hypertension and atrial enlargement, but a third heart sound suggests decreased ventricular function. Specific valvular murmurs are not usually related to hypertension, but marked elevations of systolic and diastolic pressures may cause dilatation of the aortic ring and an aortic diastolic murmur which occasionally is heard on this basis (see Chapter C115).

Table C110.2. Initial Laboratory Evaluation Test

Urinalysis
Serum creatinine[a]
Serum potassium[a]
Serum glucose elevation[a]
Uric acid[a]
Serum total cholesterol with high-density lipoprotein, low-density lipoprotein, and triglycerides[a]
Serum calcium[a]
Electrocardiogram

[a]An automated blood chemistry may be less expensive than individual determinations.

Peripheral pulses. Examination of the peripheral pulses helps to rule out peripheral arterial disease and to confirm the diagnosis of aortic coarctation. The carotid arteries should be palpated and auscultated for the presence of bruits, which might indicate narrowing or plaques (see Chapter C125).

Abdomen. During examination of the abdomen, special efforts should be made to listen for a periumbilical bruit (renovascular disease) and to palpate for a spongy mass that might suggest polycystic kidneys. Active, forceful pulsations along the aorta might be a normal finding in young, thin people but might suggest an abdominal aortic aneurysm in older individuals. Palpation of the abdomen, especially laterally, may trigger a typical attack in individuals with a pheochromocytoma.

Laboratory Evaluation

The JNC VI report stressed that the laboratory evaluation of hypertensive patients need not be extensive or costly (**Table C110.2**). If proteinuria is absent, renal parenchymal disease as a cause of the hypertension is rarely found, but renovascular disease may present with a normal urinalysis. White and red blood cells with proteinuria or casts suggest the presence of accelerated or malignant hypertension or chronic renal parenchymal disease. Certain blood chemistries are suggested as baseline data (Table C110.2). An automated blood chemistry is recommended to include those tests to provide baseline information for the treatment of hypertension as well as other risk factors, such as diabetes and hyperlipidemia. A complete blood cell count is also advised.

An ECG is suggested to determine the presence or absence of arrhythmias, myocardial ischemia, LVH, or a combination of all or some of these factors. The presence of heart block would indicate caution in the use of a β-blocker or one of the nondihydropyridine calcium antagonists. Although an echocardiogram is a more sensitive index of LVH than an ECG, a full echocardiogram is expensive, and the information other than ventricular mass is probably not of great importance for the average hypertensive patient. Echocardiogram, chest radiograph, intravenous pyelogram, and plasma renin activity are not recommended as routine procedures in the evaluation of the hypertensive patient. These tests are relatively insensitive indicators of secondary hypertension and should be reserved for use in individuals in whom there is a high suspicion of a specific disease.

SUGGESTED READING

1. Executive Summary of the third report of the National Cholesterol Education Program (NCEP) Expert Panel on Detection, Evaluation, and Treat-

ment of High Blood Cholesterol in Adults (Adult Treatment Panel III). *JAMA*. 2001;285:2486–2497.

2. Gifford RW Jr, Kirkendall W, O'Connor DT, et al. Office evaluation of hypertension: a statement for health professionals by a writing group of the Council for High Blood Pressure Research, American Heart Association. *Circulation*. 1989;79:721–731.

3. Guidelines Subcommittee. 1999 World Health Organization–International Society of Hypertension Guidelines for the Management of Hypertension. *J Hypertens*. 1999;17:151–183.

4. Julius S, Mejia A, Jones K, et al. "White coat" versus "sustained" borderline hypertension in Tecumseh, Michigan. *Hypertension*. 1990;16:617–623.

5. The Sixth Report of the Joint National Committee on Prevention, Detection, Evaluation, and Treatment of High Blood Pressure. *Arch Intern Med*. 1997;157:2413–2446.

6. Stamler J, Stamler R, Neaton JD. Blood pressure, systolic and diastolic, and cardiovascular risks. U.S. Population Data. *Arch Intern Med*. 1993;153:598–615.

Chapter C111

Evaluation of Electrolyte Abnormalities

John W. Graves, MD

KEY POINTS

- Disturbances in sodium in the hypertensive patient suggest underlying diseases such as hyperaldosteronism, renal failure, thyroid and parathyroid disorders, renal failure, and heart failure.

- Disturbances in potassium are seen in diabetics, the elderly, renal failure, hyperaldosteronism, renovascular hypertension, and Cushing's disease.

- Hyponatremia and hyperkalemia may influence choices of antihypertensive drugs.

See also Chapters A50, A52, C110, C159, C170, and C171

Evaluation of the patient with hypertension is aimed at identifying secondary causes of hypertension, assessing evidence of target organ involvement and uncovering additional factors that may influence choice of antihypertensive treatment. A thorough history and physical examination is complemented by a list of suggested laboratory tests. Those recommended by the Sixth Report of the Joint National Committee on Prevention, Detection, Evaluation, and Treatment of High Blood Pressure (JNC VI) include urinalysis, complete blood cell count, serum sodium, serum potassium, serum creatinine, fasting blood glucose, and total and high-density lipoprotein cholesterol measurements. The prevalence of secondary hypertension is too low to justify extensive diagnostic testing in all hypertensives. The serum sodium and serum potassium values at the time of diagnosis can aid the clinician in 2 ways: They may heighten suspicion of the presence of secondary forms of hypertension and they may be helpful in decisions about initiation of hypertension drug therapy.

SODIUM AND HYPERTENSION

Hypernatremia

The presence of hypernatremia (**Table C111.1**), particularly when accompanied by hypokalemia, should alert the physician to the possibility of primary hyperaldosteronism. Subsequent measurement of plasma renin activity and plasma aldosterone levels and 24-hour urinary excretion of sodium and aldoster-

one after 3 days of a high salt diet can confirm the presence of primary hyperaldosteronism. Hypernatremia in primary hyperaldosteronism has been shown to be due to a resetting of the osmostat "to the right"; there is a normal response to water loading and to dehydration but at a higher than normal serum sodium or serum osmolality.

Hyponatremia

Hypertension. Hyponatremia (Table C111.1) at initial diagnosis of hypertension may be evidence of hypertensive target organ damage from hypertensive heart or renal disease. When the glomerular filtration rate falls below 30 mL per minute, patients with acute or chronic renal failure manifest difficulties with water handling and develop hyponatremia. In a patient with renal failure, the onset of hypertension aids in deciding the cause of renal failure. In glomerular and vascular disease of the kidney, hypertension occurs early in the course of renal disease. In interstitial renal disease, hypertension and hyponatremia usually are seen when renal insufficiency is far advanced. The hyponatremic-hypertensive syndrome has been reported with acute renal ischemia in malignant hypertension and also in the presence of chronic renal artery stenosis. Hypertensive hypertrophic cardiomyopathy may lead to congestive heart failure and a decrease in effective arterial blood volume. In congestive heart failure, antidiuretic hormone is released as a result, the kidney is unable to excrete dilute urine, free water is reabsorbed, and hyponatremia may result.

Table C111.1. Sodium Electrolyte Disorders and Their Associated Diseases

ELECTROLYTE DISORDER	ASSOCIATED DISEASE
Hypernatremia	Hyperaldosteronism
Hyponatremia	Acute and chronic renal failure
	Acute renal ischemia syndrome
	Malignant hypertension
	Renovascular hypertension
	Hypertensive heart disease
	Endocrine disease
	Hyperparathyroidism
	Hypothyroidism
	Syndrome of inappropriate secretion
	of antidiuretic hormone and
	hypertension
	Increased intracranial pressure
	Medications (e.g., amitriptyline)

Table C111.3. Electrolyte Disorders and Impact on Initial Antihypertensive Therapy

DISORDER	DRUGS TO AVOID	DRUGS TO USE
Hyponatremia	Diuretics	ACE inhibitors
		Angiotensin II blockers
Hypokalemia	Diuretics	ACE inhibitors
		Angiotensin II blockers
		β-blockers
		Potassium-sparing diuretics
Hyperkalemia	ACE inhibitors	Diuretics
	Angiotensin II blockers	
	β-blockers	
	Potassium-sparing	
	diuretics	

ACE, angiotensin-converting enzyme.

Endocrine conditions. Primary hyperparathyroidism may be associated with the development of hypertension when far-advanced bone disease has developed. Hyponatremia may also occur with hypercalcemia. The advent of multichannel chemistry analyzers in clinical medicine has made early diagnosis of primary hyperparathyroidism common, before significant hypercalcemia and hyponatremia develop. A second endocrine disease that may present with hyponatremia and hypertension is hypothyroidism. Thyroid hormone is required for normal handling of water in the distal tubule. Deficiencies of thyroid hormone may lead to hyponatremia and hypertension.

Medications. Some medications may cause hypertension and hyponatremia; for example, amitriptyline can cause acute elevations of the blood pressure and hyponatremia owing to release of antidiuretic hormone. Increased intracranial pressure from brain tumors, brain abscess, meningitis, subdural hematoma, or other diseases may cause release of antidiuretic hormone as well as acute, often severe elevations of blood pressure and hyponatremia.

POTASSIUM AND HYPERTENSION

Potassium and hyper/hypokalemia are discussed in **Table C111.2.**

Hyperkalemia

Hyperkalemia is a common occurrence in acute and chronic renal insufficiency. Hyperkalemia is usually caused by more

Table C111.2. Potassium Electrolyte Disorders and Their Associated Diseases

ELECTROLYTE DISORDER	ASSOCIATED DISEASE
Hyperkalemia	Acute and chronic renal failure
	Immunosuppressive drugs (cyclosporin, tacrolimus)
Hypokalemia	Hyperaldosteronism
	Renovascular hypertension
	Pheochromocytoma
	Cushing's syndrome
	Liddle's syndrome

than a single defect in potassium homeostasis. Thus, hyperkalemia is more common in diabetics and the elderly in whom low aldosterone levels are coupled with renal failure. Hyperkalemia is often seen in the renal transplant patient, including those with good graft function. It may be associated with immunosuppressive medications such as cyclosporin and tacrolimus, which interfere with potassium metabolism.

Hypokalemia

The presence of hypokalemia is perhaps the most helpful clue to secondary hypertension from the screening blood tests. Diseases that stimulate the renin-angiotensin-aldosterone system often present with hypokalemia and hypertension. Primary hyperaldosteronism may present not only with hypokalemia but also hypernatremia. More valuable clues are present in the history and physical examination. The hypokalemic hypertensive patient with a history of smoking, episodes of flash pulmonary edema, other manifestations of vascular disease such as claudication, an abdominal bruit, or the abrupt onset of hypertension should have diagnostic tests for renovascular hypertension. Palpitations, weight loss, hypokalemia, and paroxysms of hypertension should lead to testing for pheochromocytoma. Hypertension is, however, a late manifestation of Cushing's disease, so diagnosis should not be difficult. Liddle's syndrome, which mimics primary aldosteronism (owing to a specific mutation in the epithelial Na+ channel) and other conditions of mineralocorticoid excess result in hypertension in the setting of hypokalemic metabolic alkalosis. Liddle's syndrome may be differentiated clinically by the failure of hypokalemia and hypertension to respond to the mineralocorticoid receptor blocker spironolactone.

ELECTROLYTES AND HYPERTENSION THERAPY

Disorders of serum potassium can have a significant impact on choices of antihypertensive therapy. The presence of hyperkalemia sometimes limits the use of antihypertensive drugs that can increase potassium, such as potassium-sparing diuretics (spironolactone, amiloride, and triamterene), angiotensin-converting enzyme inhibitors, angiotensin II blockers, and β-blockers. Use of these agents in proteinuric renal disease or congestive heart failure requires monitoring of serum potassium. Diuretics may worsen preexisting hypokalemia or hyponatremia. Angiotensin-converting enzyme inhibitors and angiotensin II blockers may help normalize serum potassium and serum sodium. Potassium-sparing agents such as spironolactone, amiloride, and triamterene can cause profound hyponatremia, especially in the elderly. Electrolytes and hypertension are discussed in **Table C111.3**.

SUGGESTED READING

1. Agarwal M, Lynn KL, Mark ToT, Nicholls MG. Hyponatremic-hypertensive syndrome with renal ischemia: an under-recognized disorder. *Hypertension*. 1999;33:1020–1024.
2. Cohen JJ. Disorders of potassium balance. *Hosp Pract*. 1979;14:119–128.
3. Friedler RM, Koffler A, Kurokawa K. Hyponatremia and hypernatremia. *Clin Nephrol*. 1977;7:163–172.
4. Gregoire JJ. Adjustment of the osmostat in primary aldosteronism. *Mayo Clin Proc*. 1994;69:1108–1110.
5. Pacak K, Linehan WM, Eisenhofer G, et al. Recent advances in genetics, diagnosis, localization, and treatment of pheochromocytoma. *Ann Intern Med*. 2001;134(4):315–329.
6. Palmer BF, Alpern RJ. Liddle's syndrome. *Am J Med*. 1998;104:301–309.
7. Safian RD, Textor SC. Renal artery stenosis. *N Engl J Med*. 2001;344:431–442.
8. Young WF, Hogan MJ, Klee GG, et al. Primary aldosteronism: diagnosis and management. *Mayo Clin Proc*. 1990;65:96–110.

Chapter C112

Ambulatory and Home Blood Pressure Monitoring

William B. White, MD

KEY POINTS

- An important advantage of self-monitoring of blood pressure is that multiple readings at different times of the day may be taken and recorded and blood pressure patterns can be observed.

- A useful feature of self-monitoring of blood pressure is that it usually avoids the pressor response (white coat effect) seen in 15% to 20% of stage 1 or 2 hypertensive patients in the doctor's office; average home-office blood pressure differences typically are in the range of 5 mm Hg.

- Out-of-office blood pressures correlate better with left ventricular hypertrophy, hypertensive cerebrovascular disease, renal disease, retinopathy, and alterations in vascular compliance.

- Ambulatory blood pressure monitoring may be useful in separating those who truly require antihypertensive drug therapy from those who can be managed by lifestyle modification.

See also Chapters B101, B104, B105, C109, C113, C128, C133, and C152

Blood pressure (BP) monitoring outside of the medical care environment is an increasingly important part of clinical hypertension assessment and management. There are 2 main forms of out-of-office BP monitoring: (a) self- or home monitoring, usually performed by the patient with a portable semiautomatic device or aneroid manometer plus stethoscope and (b) ambulatory BP monitoring, which uses automatic detection and recording devices for repeated determinations during an extended time period, typically 24 hours. Both techniques have been shown to enhance substantially the clinician's understanding of BP behavior in patients and to aid in diagnosis and therapeutic decision making.

Self- or Home Monitoring of Blood Pressure

There are several advantages of self-monitoring or home measurement of BP (**Table C112.1**). One important advantage is that patients may take and record multiple BP readings during different times of the day. These values can be reviewed by the physician as adjunct information to the office pressures for therapeutic decision making. A second useful feature is that self-monitoring or home measurement of BP may avoid the pressor response (white coat effect) seen in approximately 15 to 20% of stage 1 and 2 hypertensive patients in the doctor's office.

Techniques for self-monitoring. Several types of BP monitors are available for use at home, including aneroid (dial-type) manometers, semiautomatic electronic sphygmomanometers [generally using an oscillometric method of BP measurement (see Recorders)], and mercury column sphygmomanometers. Electronic devices are most convenient and have become the devices of choice for home or self-monitoring during the past few years. Before they are used in practice by patients, they should be independently validated according to a rigorous standard, such as the American Association for Medical Instrumentation guidelines. Aneroid manometers with a stethoscope are relatively simple to use and generally are the most economic type of self-monitoring units available. However, in older patients lacking manual dexterity, or when hearing loss is an

Table C112.1. Usefulness of Self- or Home-Bound Blood Pressure Monitoring

Distinguishes sustained hypertension from white coat hypertension
Assesses response to antihypertensive therapy
Improves patient adherence to treatment
Potentially reduces management costs

Note: Only validated electronic devices or aneroid sphygmomanometers are recommended with appropriately sized cuffs and bladders.

issue, an electronic device may be preferable to a nonautomated sphygmomanometer. In rare patients or those with arrhythmias, oscillometric devices may not sense accurately. Clinical calibration against a mercury column sphygmomanometer or other validated non-mercury pressure meter should be performed on a regular basis. Patients are usually fairly accurate when transcribing their own pressures, but may tend to underreport high BP levels. They also tend to measure BP at home while relaxed, rather than during work or other stressful situations. For the diagnosis of hypertension based on an average of home BPs, 135/85 mm Hg is comparable to an office average of 140/90 mm Hg.

Self-monitored blood pressures in hypertension management. Although the theoretic advantages of self-monitoring are obvious, there are no definitive prognostic data comparing the prediction of cardiovascular risk by home BP versus doctor's office BP.

Diagnosis. Several cross-sectional studies have shown that self-monitored BPs correlate better with echocardiographically determined left ventricular mass than clinic pressures. One population study based in Japan has suggested that home BP is a better predictor of cardiovascular risk than office BP in older patients. The self-monitored BP has the potential for reducing the bias and error in assessing the "true" pressure in a patient. Because BP variation is quite large in some people, single readings may give a false impression. Bias may be quite large if a small number of readings in the doctor's office are used. In some studies, the self-monitored pressure has been shown to be similar to the attenuated BP seen with repeated measurements over time (i.e., weeks and months) in the clinic. Self-monitored BP may be more representative of the 24-hour BP. In a study recently performed in Scotland, not only was the reproducibility of the self-measurement twice as good as the clinic BP, it agreed with the results of an ambulatory recording in 81% of the patients.

Therapeutic decisions. Monitored BPs can be useful in therapeutic decision making. After antihypertensive therapy has been initiated, self-monitoring is an excellent way to evaluate the effectiveness of the therapy and to avoid multiple doctor or nurse visits. Furthermore, the relationship between time of dosing of antihypertensive therapy and BP levels may be easier to assess with self-monitoring patients. As a final attribute, adherence to therapy and BP control have been shown to improve when patients (even previously noncompliant ones) self-monitor their BP.

Clinical trials. Self-monitoring has been used in clinical trials of antihypertensive therapy. The rationale for use of self-BP in clinical trials includes the improved precision of the measurement compared to clinic measurements, an absence of the white coat effect, little to no placebo effect, and greater reproducibility compared to the measurements made by physicians or nurses in the clinic setting. Staessen and co-workers have compared conventional clinic and automated self-BP in the THOP (Treatment of Hypertension According to Home or Office Blood Pressure) clinical trial and showed that differences between the 2 were nearly the same as the differences between ambulatory and clinic BP. Thus, it is possible that self-BP is a reasonable surrogate for daytime ambulatory BP monitoring.

Ambulatory Monitoring

Recorders. Over the past 20 years, noninvasive automatic devices have been developed for hypertension management and clinical research. Ambulatory BP monitors have become much more practical to use in patient care as the devices are quite small (less than 1 lb in most instances), simple to apply by a nurse or technician, and precise. Fully automatic, programmable recorders are capable of 100 to 200 BP and pulse measurements from an energy source of 2 to 4 small batteries. The devices measure BP by oscillometry (most commonly) or auscultation of Korotkoff sounds. Oscillometric measurement depends on the detection of pulsatile oscillations from the brachial artery into the BP cuff. The amplitude of the oscillations is related to a standard form of BP (usually mercury column measurements by auscultation), and an algorithm is then developed. The oscillometric methodology is fairly accurate in patients with midrange BPs who hold their arms still during cuff inflation and deflation. Oscillometric BP determination is less accurate in older patients or those with extremely low or high pressures. Auscultatory measurements mimic those of clinicians and use a microphone for detection of the Korotkoff sounds. Auscultatory devices are also subject to noise artifact when the patient has excessive arm motion during the actual BP measurement.

Ambulatory blood pressure versus office or clinic measurements. The clinical use of ambulatory BP recordings requires a frame of reference for the values derived. Usually,

Table C112.2. Values of Clinic and Ambulatory Blood Pressures (BPs) in Normal and Untreated Hypertensive Patients (Based on Clinic Pressures)

	NORMOTENSIVES	HYPERTENSIVES
Clinic systolic BP	120 ± 9	151 ± 10
Clinic diastolic BP	79 ± 6	101 ± 6
24-h systolic BP	113 ± 9	139 ± 12
24-h diastolic BP	72 ± 5	87 ± 8
Awake systolic BP	118 ± 9	149 ± 12
Awake diastolic BP	76 ± 5	93 ± 9
Sleep systolic BP	98 ± 9	117 ± 9
Sleep diastolic BP	60 ± 5	77 ± 7

From White WB, Morganroth J. Usefulness of ambulatory blood pressure monitoring in assessing antihypertensive therapy. *Am J Cardiol.* 1989;63:94–98, with permission.

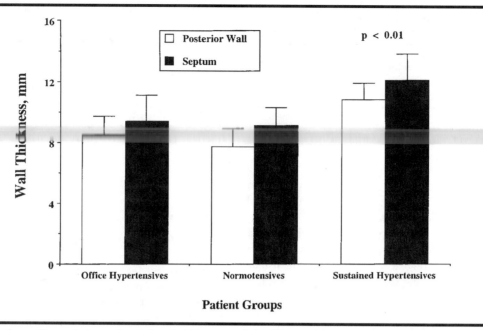

Figure C112.1. This figure shows the posterior and septal wall thicknesses of the left ventricle in 3 groups of patients stratified according to their ambulatory blood pressure (BP) monitoring results. Office hypertensive patients had an office BP >140/90 mm Hg and an awake BP <130/80 mm Hg; normotensives had an office BP <140/90 mm Hg and an awake BP <130/80 mm Hg; sustained hypertensives had an office BP and awake BP >140/90 mm Hg. The wall thicknesses were significantly greater in the sustained hypertensive patients (*p* <.01) compared with the 2 other groups. (From White WB, Schulman P, McCabe EJ, Dey HM. Average daily blood pressure, not office blood pressure, determines cardiac function in patients with hypertension. *JAMA.* 1989; 261:873–877, with permission.)

physicians set the recorders to measure 50 to 100 BPs in 24 hours. There is a reproducible diurnal/nocturnal pattern to BP during a 24-hour period of measurement in approximately 80% of patients. Typically, the pressure is highest while awake (especially during work) and lowest during sleep. The data are expressed as 24-hour mean BP and often as the values during wakefulness and sleep. BP during sleep is quite low compared to the office or clinic pressure, whereas BP during wakefulness is similar to the values obtained in the office (**Table C112.2**).

These differences must be kept in mind when interpreting ambulatory BP recordings. Based on several new outcome studies comparing ambulatory versus clinic BP in patients with hypertension, most consensus groups have defined a 24-hour BP >135/85 mm Hg as abnormal.

Ambulatory blood pressure and hypertensive disease. The majority of cross-sectional studies published to date have shown that ambulatory BP is superior to office BP in predicting target

Table C112.3. Studies Demonstrating That the Relations for Ambulatory Blood Pressure (ABP) with Hypertensive Outcomes Is Superior to Clinic Blood Pressure (CBP)

AUTHOR (YR)	TYPE OF STUDY	N	KEY FINDING(S)
Staessen (1997)	Clinical trial	419	Ambulatory blood pressure monitoring (ABPM) superior to CBP for determining antihypertensive requirements.
Staessen (1999)	Clinical trial	808	In elderly, ambulatory systolic blood pressure (SBP) is independent predictor of risk.
Redon (1998)	Cohort study	86	ABPM is useful in stratifying risk in patients with refractory hypertension. Measured by CBP.
Ohkubo (1997)	Cohort study	1,542	Ambulatory SBP was related to the risk of mortality whereas CBP was not.
Verdecchia (1997)	Case series	1,522	The white coat effect was not associated with cardiovascular outcome.
Imai (1997)	Cohort study	1,192	ABPM group showed decreased survival in the highest quintile of SBP and in the highest and lowest quintiles of diastolic BP.
Lemne (1995)	Cross-sectional	161	Casual BP levels correlated poorly with the degree of left ventricular (LV) hypertrophy in borderline hypertension; ambulatory BP correlates much more closely with LV wall dimensions.
Boley (1997)	Cross-sectional	280	In hypertensive, unmedicated adults, ambulatory BPs during waking hours and at home are related to LV and arterial function.
Lantelme (2000)	Cross-sectional	88	True white coat effect and its estimation are not equivalent. In addition, the white coat effect had no impact on target organ involvement.
Lin (1995)	Cross-sectional	171	The severity of hypertensive complications was more closely related to mean ambulatory SBP than mean ambulatory diastolic CBP.
Musialik (1998)	Cross-sectional	30	Nocturnal mean arterial pressure correlated with LV mass in elderly hypertensives and a dependency of nocturnal BP load with LV mass.
Palatini (1997)	Cohort	1,095	ABPM was useful in identifying those patients with white coat hypertension.

Table C112.4. Clinical Diagnoses or Problems in Which Noninvasive Ambulatory Blood Pressure Monitoring May Be Useful

Office or white coat hypertension
Borderline hypertension with or without target organ involvement
Evaluation of patients refractory to antihypertensive therapy
Episodic hypertension
Hypotensive symptoms associated with antihypertensive medications
Autonomic dysfunction/nocturnal hypertension
Exclusion of placebo reactors when determining efficacy of antihypertensive drug therapy in controlled clinical trials

Adapted from National High Blood Pressure Education Program Working Group report on ambulatory blood pressure monitoring. *Arch Intern Med.* 1990;150:2270–2280.

organ involvement (**Table C112.3**). The most striking evidence has come from assessment of the relations among office pressure, ambulatory BP, and indices of left ventricular hypertrophy (**Figure C112.1**). Ambulatory BP is superior to office BP in predicting hypertensive cerebrovascular disease, retinopathy, renal abnormalities, and alterations in vascular compliance. Certain studies using intraarterial BP measurements (hence beat-to-beat BP values are obtained) show that variability of BP may be a predictor of morbidity in hypertension. Older patients and those with severe hypertension might be among those with excessive BP variability. Numerous studies have shown that ambulatory BP is an independent predictor of cardiovascular risk (Table C112.3). Most of these studies have also demonstrated that a loss of nocturnal decline in BP (so-called nondippers) conveys excessive risk for stroke and myocardial infarction.

Clinical usefulness

Diagnosis. Several subsets of hypertensive diagnoses have been elucidated as a result of ambulatory BP monitoring (**Table C112.4**). Clinical problems seen most often by practicing physicians that are appropriate for ambulatory BP monitoring include the assessment of possible white coat hypertension, borderline hypertension (with and without evidence for target organ damage), and evaluation of refractory hypertension in patients on complex antihypertensive regimens. A number of well-performed studies in these areas show that patients might benefit clinically when the ambulatory BP is known in addition to the measurements made in the medical care environment.

Evaluation of therapy. It is not uncommon that refractory patients (regardless of age) on antihypertensive drugs have a pressor response in the medical care environment that brings them into hypertensive ranges although their out-of-office values remain normal. Conversely, it is not unusual to perform ambulatory BP monitoring in a hypertensive patient with reasonably good office pressures and find that BP levels are not normal late in the dosing period of the medication (**Figure C112.2**).

Problem areas. Ambulatory BP monitoring is usually well tolerated by patients, especially as the technology has improved. A few problems do exist, however. An important minority of patients do not sleep well with the recorders and tend to have somewhat higher BP values. Those who remain in bed have much lower values than those who get out of bed and move about. Cuffs can also rotate and different arm positions can change BP significantly. Rarely, patients may develop erythema, ecchymoses, petechiae, or superficial phlebitis in the area distal to cuff placement. These soft tissue injuries are typically mild and self-limiting.

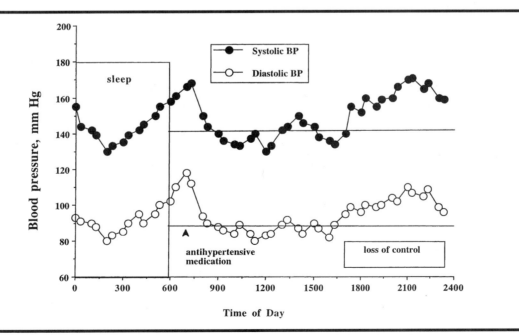

Figure C112.2. Twenty-four–hour profile obtained by noninvasive ambulatory blood pressure (BP) monitoring in a stage 3 hypertensive patient. After antihypertensive medication, the BP is relatively well controlled. At approximately 5 PM (1700 hours), BP control is lost as the antihypertensive effect of the medication is attenuated. The early morning BP is also high before drug administration. The patient's office BP was 135 to 140/85 mm Hg on 3 long-acting medications. However, self-monitoring showed BPs to be variably high and low, leading to this ambulatory BP study.

Cost and coverage considerations. The cost to the patient of self-monitoring using a nonautomated recording device is relatively low (approximately $50–$150 for the instrumentation and $20–$60 for the training session by a nurse), and the data that it yields are helpful in hypertension management. To set up ambulatory BP monitoring may cost the provider many thousands of dollars for 2 adequate recorders and the software for data analysis and reports. The patient charges range from $60 for short daytime studies to $75 to $300 for 24-hour studies. Although more costly than self-monitoring, ambulatory BP monitoring is still useful because it may lead to identifying those who truly require antihypertensive therapy as well as those who may be best managed with nonpharmacologic therapy. During 2001, the Center for Medicare and Medicaid Services independently evaluated the U.S. national insurance coverage policy for ambulatory BP monitoring and approved a national policy that pays for the study when it is used in the diagnosis of white coat hypertension. Other potential diagnoses, such as episodic hypertension, refractory hypertension, and evaluation of antihypertensive therapy, are not covered in the policy.

SUGGESTED READING

1. Mansoor GA, White WB. Ambulatory blood pressure is a useful clinical tool in nephrology. *Am J Kidney Dis.* 1997;30:591–605.
2. National High Blood Pressure Education Coordinating Committee. National High Blood Pressure Education Program Working Group Report on Ambulatory Blood Pressure Monitoring. *Arch Intern Med.* 1990;150:2270–2280.
3. Pickering TG, Kaplan NM, Krakoff L, et al. American Society of Hypertension Expert Panel: conclusions and recommendations on the clinical use of home (self) and ambulatory blood pressure monitoring. *Am J Hypertens.* 1996;9:1–11.
4. Soghikian K, Casper SM, Fireman BH, et al. Home blood pressure monitoring: effect on use of medical services and medical costs. *Med Care.* 1992;30:855–865.
5. Staessen JA, Bienaszewski L, O'Brien E, et al. An epidemiological approach to ambulatory blood pressure monitoring: the Belgian population study. *Blood Press Monit.* 1996;1:13–26.
6. Staessen JA, Celis H, Den Hond E, et al. Comparison of conventional and automated blood pressure measurements: interim analysis of the THOP trial. *Blood Press Monit.* 2002;7:61–62.
7. Tsuji I, Imai Y, Nagai K, et al. Proposal of reference values for home blood pressure measurement: prognostic criteria based on a prospective observation of the general population in Ohasama, Japan. *Am J Hypertens.* 1997;10:409–418.
8. White WB, Daragjati C, Mansoor GA, McCabe EJ. The management and follow up of patients with white-coat hypertension. *Blood Press Monit.* 1996;1:S33–S36.

Chapter C113

Diurnal and Other Cyclic Variations of Blood Pressure

Joseph L. Izzo, Jr, MD; Thomas G. Pickering, MD, PhD

KEY POINTS

- There are regular variations in blood pressure, the most important of which is the diurnal (circadian or daily) rhythm; blood pressure is generally highest on arising from sleep, with a gradual fall throughout the day; normally, sleep blood pressures are the lowest recorded.

- Blunting or reversal of day-night blood pressure patterns occurs in several conditions, including obstructive sleep apnea, autonomic dysfunction (most commonly with diabetes), hypertension caused by excess adrenal steroids, cardiac transplantation, and in certain subpopulations of essential hypertensives, such as blacks.

- Because there are atypical diurnal rhythms, blood pressure should optimally be taken at different times of the day; with normal diurnal rhythm, therapeutic decisions should be made on the basis of morning BPs.

- Seasonal cycles lead to wintertime vasoconstriction; winter blood pressures tend to be slightly higher than summer blood pressures.

See also Chapters A34–A38, A40, A50, A55, B100, B101, B105, C112, C127, C152, C161, C167, C170, C172, and C174

Cyclic variation of blood pressure (BP) in reproducible patterns is a consistent feature of BP regulation in the vast majority of people, regardless of overall BP level. Diurnal variation is clearly the most prominent cycle, but shorter and longer cycles are also present.

Pathophysiology of Diurnal Blood Pressure Variation

Over the 24-hour cycle, there are regular variations in BP (**Figure C113.1**). The onset of sleep is associated with a significant BP decrease of 10% to 20%. BP levels during sleep are generally associated with the stage of sleep, with the lowest levels occurring during stage IV (deep) sleep. Embedded within the 24-hour diurnal variation are ultradian rhythms with 90-minute periodicity, similar to "sleep cycles." Ultradian rhythms are more apparent in animals than humans, probably because ultradian rhythms are masked by stronger environmental stress responses in humans.

Hemodynamic and neuroendocrine changes. In the predawn hours, BP begins to increase steadily back toward conscious levels; this change is driven by the increased nocturnal

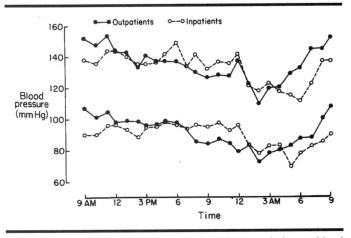

Figure C113.1. Usual diurnal pattern of 24-hour ambulatory blood pressure (BP) recordings. Automated ambulatory BP recordings are similar whether performed at home or in hospitalized subjects. Typically, first-morning BPs are the highest of the day. BP tends to fall in the afternoon and evening and is dramatically lower during sleep. Before awakening, BP begins to rise again, concomitant with increases in blood volume and neurohumoral activation. This pattern is absent in nondippers (see text).

blood volume and the prearousal increase in activity of the sympathetic nervous and renin-angiotensin systems. Waking and assumption of the upright posture immediately after waking cause substantial additional sympathetic nervous activation. Consequently, for the vast majority of people, first morning BPs are among the highest of the day. In hypertensives, cardiac output and systemic resistance are inappropriately high at this time. It is also well known that the peak incidence of myocardial infarction and stroke coincide with the morning peak in BP.

Impact of activity levels. Whether there is an intrinsic diurnal variation in BP or whether the observed patterns is simply the summation of stimulated versus resting BPs has been debated. Clearly, levels of arousal and activity and the overall degree of environmental stimulation together exert the major influence over the circadian BP changes.

Abnormal Day-Night Blood Pressure Variation (Dippers and Nondippers)

The increasing use of ambulatory BP monitoring (see Chapter C112) has uncovered different patterns of diurnal variation. One of the most common variations involves blunting or reversal of sleep-waking BP patterns. People with this condition have been characterized as nondippers, as compared to those who experience a normal degree of BP dipping during sleep.

Pathophysiology. The pathophysiologic mechanisms for reversal of day-night BP patterns have not been systematically identified, but may fall into 2 separate groups. Excessive nocturnal activation of the sympathetic nervous system occurs in obstructive sleep apnea owing to intermittent hypoxemic episodes. In other types of nondippers, it appears that there is an exaggerated BP response to the blood volume expansion that occurs as plasma is redistributed into the vascular space overnight.

Clinical conditions associated with day-night blood pressure reversal. Blunted or reversed diurnal variation is useful in identifying subpopulations of people with essential hyper-

tension and can be a valuable diagnostic clue to the presence of certain forms of secondary hypertension.

Adrenal steroid or catecholamine excess. Syndromes of excess mineralocorticoids (primary aldosteronism or licorice intoxication) or excess glucocorticoids (Cushing's syndrome or high-dose corticosteroids) often manifest the nondipping pattern. Certain patients with pheochromocytomas exhibit the same pattern. In steroid- or catecholamine-induced hypertension, the diurnal abnormality resolves with successful treatment of the underlying condition.

Autonomic dysfunction. The central role of the sympathetic nervous system in controlling diurnal BP rhythms is demonstrated by the pattern of nondipping seen in people with autonomic dysfunction, in whom baroreflexes are not fully functional. This pattern is seen most commonly in long-standing diabetes and is often associated with fixed high heart rate, diminished heart rate variability, and postural hypotension. The largest group of such patients is that of advanced diabetics, especially those with superimposed chronic renal failure.

Diabetes. The nondipping pattern is characteristic of early diabetes, and predicts the onset of albuminuria. Early diabetics tend to have marked increases in cardiac output and are likely to be sensitive to increased cardiac preload caused by centralization of blood volume and subsequent plasma volume expansion during recumbency.

Renal disease. Impaired renal function from any cause is associated with nondipping. As with diabetics, these individuals tend to have high blood volume and preload-dependent high cardiac output. It has been proposed that nondipping status may accelerate the decline of renal function, perhaps by sustaining glomerular capillary hyperperfusion and hypertension.

Cardiac transplant recipients. Disordered cardiopulmonary baroreflex function is relatively frequent in cardiac transplant recipients, who may have excessive sympathetic activation and a degree of volume sensitivity. Antirejection drugs (corticosteroids and cyclosporin) further exacerbate the problem.

Accelerated hypertension and preeclampsia/toxemia. Preeclampsia and toxemia are hemodynamically characterized by marked activation of the sympathetic and renin-angiotensin systems and excessive systemic vasoconstriction. It seems likely that exquisite volume sensitivity in these conditions is the basis for blunting or reversal of normal day-night BP variation in response to overnight blood volume expansion.

Obstructive sleep apnea. The frequent periods of hypoxia in this condition cause marked sympathetic activation, usually accompanied by increases in heart rate and BP (see Chapter A55). Treatment with airway pressurization and supplemental oxygen can restore normal diurnal patterns and lower daytime BP as well (see Chapter C172).

Black race. The nondipper pattern is relatively more common in blacks than whites, even in adolescence. This finding is not invariable, however, and may be caused by environmental rather than genetic influences.

Seasonal Hemodynamic and Blood Pressure Variations

The large reproducible hemodynamic changes that accompany seasonal adaptation in higher latitudes are largely unrecognized because of the internal compensation that typically occurs.

Winter months are associated with decreases in blood volume of approximately 1 L and corresponding decreases in stroke volume and cardiac output of 10% to 15% compared to summer. BP does not change substantially in normotensives because systemic vascular resistance increases by the same 10% to 15%. The wintertime vasoconstriction is driven by increased sympathetic nervous and renin-angiotensin system activation. In hypertensives, however, there is a small trend to higher winter BPs; in the MRC (Medical Research Council) Trial, a 3 to 4 mm Hg BP increase in systolic BP was found during the winter months.

Impact of Cyclic Variation on Hypertension Management

Initiation and modification of drug therapy.
All major clinical studies in hypertension have employed morning BP recordings. Differences between morning and afternoon readings are quite commonly 5 mm Hg, thus the decision to treat may very well depend on the time of day at which BPs are consistently measured. Similarly, decisions to titrate or combine medications can easily be affected by diurnal rhythms. Thus, to be consistent, clinical decisions regarding treatment should also be made on the basis of morning BP readings.

Evening medication dosing.
Several experts have recommended that evening dosing of once-a-day BP drugs is preferable to morning dosing in the majority of hypertensives. The rationale for this recommendation is the finding that the peak daily incidence of stroke and myocardial infarction coincides with the morning peak in BP. By administering BP drugs in the evening, it has been assumed that peak drug effects effectively blunt the morning BP peak. A few clinical trials have tested this point but are not yet conclusive.

Seasonal blood pressure changes.
In the Medical Research Council studies, BP was higher in the winter by a few mm Hg. This corresponds to a wintertime increase in sympathetic and systemic resistance and a decrease in blood volume and cardiac output. The potential impact of seasonal hemodynamic changes on BP management has not been tested in clinical studies. Anecdotally, patients withdrawn from BP medications during the summer experience a longer period of lower pressures and a slower return to hypertensive pressures than those withdrawn from medications during the winter.

SUGGESTED READING

1. Giles TD. Factors affecting circadian variability. *Blood Press Monit.* 2000;5:S3–S7.
2. Izzo JL Jr, Larrabee PS, Sander E, Lillis LM. Hemodynamics of seasonal adaptation. *Am J Hypertens.* 1990;3:405–407.
3. Neutel JM, Smith DH. The circadian pattern of blood pressure: cardiovascular risk and therapeutic opportunities. *Curr Opin Nephrol Hypertens.* 1997;6:250–256.
4. Parati G. Blood pressure reduction at night: sleep and beyond. *J Hypertens.* 2000;18:1725–1729.
5. Pickering TG. What is the 'normal' 24 h, awake, and asleep blood pressure? *Blood Press Monit.* 1999;4:S3–S7.
6. Pickering TG, Kario K. Nocturnal non-dipping: what does it augur? *Curr Opin Nephrol Hypertens.* 2001;10:611–616.
7. Scarpelli PT, Gallo M, Chiari G. Chronobiology of blood pressure. *J Nephrol.* 2000;13:197–204.
8. Sica DA. What are the influences of salt, potassium, the sympathetic nervous system, and the renin-angiotensin system on the circadian variation in blood pressure? *Blood Press Monit.* 1999;4:S9–S16.
9. Smolensky MH, Haus E. Circadian rhythms and clinical medicine with applications to hypertension. *Am J Hypertens.* 2001;14:280S–290S.
10. White WB. Cardiovascular risk and therapeutic intervention for the early morning surge in blood pressure and heart rate. *Blood Press Monit.* 2001;6:63–72.

Genetic Profiling in Hypertension

Haralambos Gavras, MD

KEY POINTS

- Essential hypertension is a polygenic multifactorial disorder attributed to interplay of multiple causative or modifier genes with the environment, limiting at this time the usefulness of genetic profiling in individual patients.

- Essential hypertension is associated with genetic variants or polymorphisms in several candidate genes, but the findings are inconsistent in different racial or ethnic groups.

- Rare hypertensive disorders with distinct phenotypes and mendelian inheritance owing to a single abnormal gene have been described.

- It is anticipated that in the future, genotyping may provide novel diagnostic and prognostic information, as well as permit pharmacogenetic applications.

See also Chapters A75–A78

The absence of a bimodal distribution of blood pressure (BP) that separates the population into clear-cut normal and abnormal groups indicates that hypertension is a polygenic or "complex" trait. The hypertensive phenotype thus does not follow the classic mendelian rules of dominant or recessive inheritance attributable to a single gene locus. Approximately 30% to 50% of the variation in BP between individuals is attributed to genetic factors (see Chapter A78).

Candidate Genes

Genes encoding for various hormones, hormone precursors, enzymes, receptors, or other biologic principles relevant to the pathophysiology of BP regulation are reasonable candidates for analysis. Such "candidate genes" include those encoding for various components of the renin-angiotensin-aldosterone system, the kallikrein-kinin system, the cation-transport systems regulating flux across cell membranes, the sympathetic system, vasoactive autacoids, and neurotransmitters. Genetic variants or polymorphisms in these genes have been proposed to confer susceptibility to hypertension or to specific target organ complications, such as cardiac hypertrophy, coronary disease, renal failure, and stroke.

Racial Interactions

Several linkage and association studies have implicated a number of candidate gene variants in the etiology of essential hypertension, but the results differ, depending on the ethnic and racial background of the population studied. Examples include variants of the angiotensinogen gene (see Chapters A75 and A76) that are associated with hypertension in French and North American but not in British or Mexican-American subjects. An association between the SA gene and hypertension has been found in Japanese hypertensives but not white hypertensives. A renin gene restriction fragment length polymorphism

has been associated with hypertension in blacks but not in whites. α_2-Adrenoceptor or β_2-adrenoceptor variants have been associated with hypertension in selected racial groups. In some cases, when an association was found between a gene polymorphism and hypertension (e.g., the angiotensin II receptor AT_1 gene), no linkage could be demonstrated by sibpair analysis.

Monogenic Forms of Hypertension

Within the large population with essential hypertension, there are rare families with particular phenotypic characteristics and quasi-Mendelian inheritance of hypertension, suggesting a single abnormal gene (see Chapter A77). Such hypertensive syndromes include glucocorticoid-remediable aldosteronism, the syndrome of apparent mineralocorticoid excess, Liddle's syndrome (pseudoaldosteronism), Gordon's syndrome (pseudohypoaldosteronism), and a syndrome characterized by severe hypertension, short stature, and brachydactyly. Some of these syndromes are associated with specific hypertensive complications. For example, subjects affected by the syndrome of glucocorticoid-remediable aldosteronism, which was found to be due to a chimeric gene involving the aldosterone synthase and 11β-hydroxylase genes, appear to be particularly prone to hemorrhagic strokes. Members of the brachydactyly/hypertension kindred are also prone to neurovascular malformation and early strokes.

Current Status of Genetic Profiling in Hypertension

Genetic profiling is not yet part of the routine diagnostic workup of the hypertensive patient. Exceptions are the rare cases of secondary hypertension in which clinical data, family history, and biochemical profiling point to anatomic or functional aberrations, such as abnormal production of hormones or abnormal receptor responses. Other rare sporadic or familial hypertensive disorders with distinct clinical and biochemical characteristics are also likely to be discovered in the future and found to be caused by specific gene mutations. In such cases, genotyping may confirm the diagnosis and dictate specific treatment strategies for the affected individual or may help identify other family members at risk.

For the vast majority of hypertensives (i.e., those who remain classified as having essential hypertension), genetic profiling at this time is not useful as a guide to diagnosis or treatment. Furthermore, polymorphisms in some of the candidate genes associated with hypertension in one population appear to be common variants unrelated to hypertension in other populations of different ethnic ancestry and genetic background. It is likely that new developments in the molecular genetics of hypertension, further study of homogeneous hypertensive populations subgrouped by intermediate phenotypic characteristics, advances in genome-wide scanning and gene mapping technology (see Chapter A74), and further development of high-throughput methods and microarray techniques for mutation analysis will eventually provide the means for identifying and localizing aberrant genes in a more efficient and practical manner. However, the diagnostic value of genotyping for a polygenic and multifactorial disorder such as hypertension is diminished by the interplay of multiple causative or modifier genes with the environment, so that most molecular variants have a limited effect at the individual level.

Therapeutic Implications

With the exception of the rare monogenic mendelian disorders, it is difficult at this point to contemplate gene treatment as a therapeutic option for hypertension. However, it is possible that discovery of specific genotypes potentially linked to defined pathogenic mechanisms might lead to selective application of preventive or therapeutic measures in appropriate subgroups of the hypertensive population. Traits related to an individual's susceptibility to specific medication side effects or predisposition to exaggerated target organ damage may be identifiable (see Chapter A78). Such strategies might replace the current indiscriminate application of expensive and not innocuous lifelong pharmaco-

therapy to all hypertensives on an empiric basis and might improve the success rates and cost-effectiveness of treatment in reducing cardiac and renal complications.

Pharmacogenetics is a discipline still in its infancy. Already, there is information about single gene polymorphisms of drug metabolizing enzymes that affect pharmacokinetic differences among individuals. Ongoing research may identify additional genes affecting pharmacodynamic responses. Although the prospect that genotyping used as a guide for the choice of antihypertensive therapy seems to be in the distant future and may never become practical or cost-effective for the average patient, it may well become a useful tool for selected patients with particularly resistant and difficult to treat hypertension.

SUGGESTED READING

1. Corvol P, Persu A, Gimenez-Roqueplo AP, Jeunemaitre X. Seven lessons from two candidate genes in human essential hypertension: angiotensinogen and epithelial sodium channel. *Hypertension.* 1999;33:1324–1331.
2. Lifton RP, Dluhy RG, Powers M, et al. A chimaeric 11β-hydroxylase/aldosterone synthase gene causes glucocorticoid-remediable aldosteronism and human hypertension. *Nature.* 1992;355:262–265.
3. Litchfield WR, Weiss RJ, Coolidge CR, et al. Glucocorticoid-remediable aldosteronism is associated with hemorrhagic stroke. [Abstract.] *Hypertension.* 1997;30:479.
4. Mansfield TA, Simon DB, Farfel Z, et al. Linkage of familial hyperkalemia and hypertension, pseudohypoaldosteronism type II, to 1q3–42 and 17p11–q21. [Abstract.] *Hypertension.* 1997;30:475.
5. Mune T, Rogerson FM, Nikkilä H, et al. Human hypertension caused by mutations in the kidney isozyme of 11β-hydroxysteroid dehydrogenase. *Nat Genet.* 1995;10:394–399.
6. Naraghi R, Schuster H, Toka HR, et al. Neurovascular compression at the ventrolateral medulla in autosomal dominant hypertension and brachydactyly. *Stroke.* 1997;28:1749–1754.
7. Schuster H, Wienker TE, Bähring S, et al. Severe autosomal dominant hypertension and brachydactyly in a unique Turkish kindred maps to human chromosome 12. *Nat Genet.* 1996;13:98–100.
8. Shimkets RA, Warnock DG, Bositis CM, et al. Liddle's syndrome: heritable human hypertension caused by mutations in the β subunit of the epithelial sodium channel. *Cell.* 1994;79:407–414.
9. Timberlake DS, O'Connor DT, Parmer RJ. Molecular genetics of essential hypertension: recent results and emerging strategies. *Curr Opin Nephrol Hypertens.* 2001;10:71–79.
10. Turner ST, Schwartz GL, Chapman AB, et al. Antihypertensive pharmacogenetics: getting the right drug into the right patient. *J Hypertens.* 2001;19:1–11.

Chapter C115

Basic Cardiac Evaluation: Physical Examination, Electrocardiogram, and Chest Radiograph

Clarence Shub, MD

KEY POINTS

- Hypertensive heart disease can be detected by clinical examination, electrocardiogram, and cardiac imaging.

- Left ventricular hypertrophy is a manifestation of "target organ damage" and implies an adverse prognosis and the need for aggressive therapy in the hypertensive patient.

- Electrocardiogram remains the traditional and standard method for detecting left ventricular hypertrophy despite its relative lack of sensitivity.

See also Chapters A61, C110, C116, C117, C121, and C155

Because the heart is one of the major target organs adversely affected by high blood pressure, a careful and thorough evaluation of cardiac structure and function is an obligatory part of the examination of the hypertensive patient.

Physical Examination

The presence of abnormalities on the cardiac and vascular physical examination contributes significantly to the cardiac assessment of the hypertensive patient and to cardiovascular risk stratification as recommended by the Sixth Report of the Joint National Committee on Prevention, Detection, Evaluation, and Treatment of High Blood Pressure (JNC VI). The presence of "target organ" damage or clinical cardiovascular diseases [e.g., the detection of left ventricular hypertrophy (LVH) or peripheral vascular disease] prompts more aggressive antihypertensive therapy and risk factor modification.

Palpation. One of the most important physical signs of LVH is a localized, sustained, and forceful apical impulse. This is best appreciated with the patient in the left lateral decubitus position, but it may be more difficult to elicit in obese patients and in those with chronic obstructive pulmonary disease. If the apical impulse in the supine position is laterally displaced, left ventricular (LV) dilatation should be suspected. In patients with hypertensive heart disease, LV dilatation is frequently associated with impaired ventricular function.

Auscultation

Heart sounds. A loud first heart sound (S_1) and brisk carotid upstroke in a hypertensive patient suggest a hyperdynamic circulatory state. The second heart sound (S_2) is usually narrowly split, and the aortic component may be accentuated. Although paradoxic splitting of S_2 may occur, it is uncommon and, in the absence of left bundle-branch block, suggests LV systolic dysfunction. A third heart sound (S_3) is unusual except when LV systolic failure occurs. In almost all patients, a fourth sound (S_4) develops before the S_3 is heard; when the S_3 is heard, the S_4 is almost always present. The incidence of an S_4 in hypertensive patients has been estimated to be between 50% and 70%, especially in the presence of LVH and in older patients. An S_4 is the auscultatory counterpart of a vigorous atrial contraction into a relatively noncompliant left ventricle. An S_4 may be associated with a palpable presystolic impulse or A wave. The S_4 is best appreciated when the patient is in the left lateral decubitus position and the bell of the stethoscope is gently placed directly on the point of maximal apical impulse. Because of the difficulty in routine clinical assessment of an S_4, the presence of a palpable A wave appears to be more specific for the pathophysiologic mechanisms described above. An aortic systolic ejection sound (or click) is occasionally heard in hypertensive patients and appears to be related to forceful expansion of a dilated aortic root.

Systolic murmurs. A systolic murmur can frequently be heard in older hypertensive patients. This murmur is usually ejection in type, early in timing, and of low intensity (grade 1 or 2). It most often represents aortic outflow turbulence related to a sclerotic aortic valve. This murmur can be heard at both the apex and the base, but, occasionally, the murmur is localized to the apex alone and can be confused with mitral regurgitation. Some hypertensive patients with systolic murmurs may have LV outflow tract obstruction, a condition that has been referred to as *hypertensive hypertrophic cardiomyopathy*. Such patients often have a small LV cavity with hypertrophied walls and normal or hyperdynamic systolic function. Recognition of this disorder is important, because it may worsen with the administration of certain antihypertensive drugs, especially diuretics or direct-acting vasodilators. Bedside hemodynamic maneuvers, such as the Valsalva maneuver, that accentuate the systolic murmur may provide an important clue to the presence of LV outflow tract obstruction.

Diastolic murmurs. An early diastolic murmur of aortic regurgitation, which may be variable in intensity and duration, may occasionally be found in hypertensive patients. Unless there is a separate anatomic defect of the aortic valve, the aortic regurgitation represents a "functional" abnormality secondary to dilatation of the aortic ring. This abnormality is more common in older hypertensive patients and may lessen in severity or even disappear as BP is lowered.

Peripheral pulses. Examination of the carotid, femoral, and extremity arterial pulses is also important (see Chapter C125). Reduced volume of the femoral pulses or a delay in femoral pulse timing (especially in a young patient) compared with simultaneous palpation of the radial pulse suggests the possibility of coarctation of the aorta. The presence of femoral or carotid bruits and reduced arterial pulses in the lower extremities suggests vascular obstructive disease, which, in older patients, is most commonly due to atherosclerosis. This process of vascular damage is enhanced and accelerated in the presence of systemic hypertension.

Electrocardiogram

Standard electrocardiography is a specific but poorly sensitive tool for the diagnosis of LVH. Compared with the chest radiograph, the routine scalar electrocardiogram (ECG) is more sensitive in detecting LVH in hypertensive patients. In the late stages of hypertensive heart disease, typical signs of LVH are almost always seen on the ECG. Thus, when a patient presents with heart failure that is attributed to hypertension, in addition to other target organ involvement, he or she almost always has some evidence of LVH on the ECG; if not, other causes for heart failure should be considered. The ECG is the traditional and standard method for detecting LVH. However, it detects only 20% to 50% of instances of autopsy-proven LVH in patient populations and <10% of echocardiographic LVH in the general population. Despite this relative insensitivity, ECG LVH is a strong predictor of cardiovascular morbidity and mortality. The cost-effectiveness of the ECG may be questioned when detection of hypertensive LVH is the only goal and its prognostic value appears to be less than that of echocardiography. However, it does provide important information when other clinical abnormalities (e.g., myocardial ischemia or infarction, arrhythmias, or conduction defects) are sought.

Voltage criteria. Various ECG diagnostic criteria for diagnosing LVH exist [e.g., the scoring system recommended by Estes; the Sokolow-Lyon criteria; the criteria of McPhie (sum of tallest precordial R and S waves >45 mm); the sum of 12-lead QRS voltages; and the Minnesota code]. Conventional ECG criteria correlate with echocardiographic LV mass index (see Chapter C116) but do not predict specific geometric patterns very well (**Figure C115.1**). ECG evidence of left atrial enlargement may occur in the early stages of hypertension, is associated with LV diastolic dysfunction, and may precede abnormalities in the QRS complex. Improved diagnostic sensi-

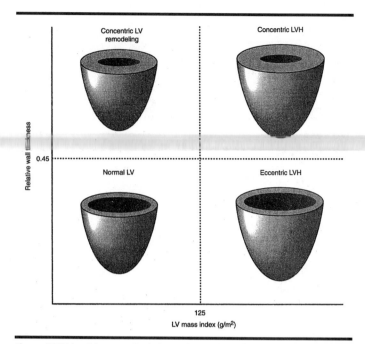

Figure C115.1. Diagram depicting relation between left ventricular (LV) mass index and relative wall thickness. An increase in LV mass index (defined as >125 g/m^2) denotes development of left ventricular hypertrophy (LVH). If relative wall thickness (ratio of wall thickness/LV cavity radius) does not increase proportionately, chamber volume is increased and a more volume-dependent "eccentric" LVH occurs. However, if there is an increase in relative wall thickness along with LV mass index, a more "concentric" pressure-dependent LVH occurs. Conversely, if LV mass index does not increase but selective wall thickness increases, the more recently described "remodeling" phenomenon occurs. (Adapted with permission from Frohlich ED, Apsten C, Chobanian AV, et al. The heart in hypertension. *N Engl J Med.* 1992;327:998–1008.)

tivity with excellent specificity, especially in obese patients, is provided by sex-specific Cornell voltage criteria ($S_{V3} + R_{V1} \geq 20$ mm in women or ≥ 28 mm in men). Combining various ECG criteria improves sensitivity. With regard to QRS amplitudes, considerable overlap exists in normal and hypertensive patients. Factors such as age, sex, race, and body weight affect the QRS amplitude and may influence the predictive value of QRS criteria for the diagnosis of LVH. In the presence of left bundle-branch block, LVH is difficult to diagnose. Thus, when precordial QRS voltages alone are used as criteria for LVH, significant numbers of false-positive and false-negative results may occur.

Vectorcardiography. Vectorcardiographic analysis increases diagnostic sensitivity. The vectorcardiographic forces are shifted posteriorly and to the left. This is manifested in the scalar ECG as an increased R wave in leads I, aVL, V_5, and V_6. As anterior forces decrease (diminished R waves in precordial leads V_1 through V_3), the pattern of anterior infarction may be simulated. Left axis deviation in the frontal plane may occur. Hypertensive patients with ECG-LVH are more likely to have impaired LV performance and greater LV mass.

Strain pattern. With increasing severity of hypertension, T-wave amplitude decreases, and T-wave inversion may occur, especially in ECG leads I, aVL, V_5, and V_6. The addition of J-point and ST-segment depression constitutes the pattern that has been called *LV strain*. Relative subendocardial ischemia may be responsible for these repolarization abnormalities. The ECG diagnosis of LVH is considerably strengthened in the presence of increased QRS voltages combined with typical repolarization abnormalities (LV strain). The LV strain pattern correlates with increased echocardiographic LV mass—especially when there is concomitant coronary artery disease.

QRS duration and Cornell product. The QRS duration has been reported to widen with increasing severity of hypertension, and the finding of ventricular conduction delay on the ECG has been correlated with certain histologic abnormalities (e.g., myocardial fibrosis). Inclusion of conduction abnormalities with voltage criteria further improves specificity. LVH can be reliably diagnosed with the Cornell voltage product, calculated as (R wave in aVL + S wave in V_3) × QRS duration ≥2,440. The ECG abnormalities may improve or even revert to normal with successful antihypertensive therapy (decreased QRS voltages and resolution of ST-T–wave abnormalities).

QT changes. The QT interval may be prolonged in patients with LVH, and QT dispersion (difference between maximal and minimal corrected QT intervals) has been reported to be increased in elderly hypertensives and is associated with LVH and ventricular arrhythmias.

24-Hour Ambulatory Electrocardiogram Monitoring

Clinical investigations using 24-hour ambulatory ECG monitoring have shown a greater incidence of ventricular arrhythmias in hypertensive patients with LVH. Ventricular arrhythmias appear to worsen as the hypertrophy progresses, and LVH patients have an increased risk of sudden cardiac death. Atrial fibrillation, especially in the elderly, and other supraventricular tachycardias are more common in patients with hypertension than in the general population. Although it is not indicated for asymptomatic patients, 24-hour ambulatory ECG monitoring can be useful in assessing atrial and ventricular arrhythmias in patients with palpitations, near syncope, or syncope.

Chest Radiograph

The chest radiograph of patients with uncomplicated hypertension usually is normal, although occasionally an abnormal cardiac contour suggesting LV enlargement or LVH may be found. However, one cannot rely on the routine chest radiograph to diagnose LVH. Subtle dilation of the ascending aortic shadow can be found in many patients with hypertension and no evidence of cardiac disease. In young patients and sometimes in adults, the presence of aortic coarctation as a cause of hypertension can be suspected on the chest radiograph.

SUGGESTED READING

1. Bulatov VA, Stenehjem A, Os I. Left ventricular mass assessed by electrocardiography and albumin excretion rate as a continuum in untreated essential hypertension. *J Hypertens.* 2001;19:1473–1478.
2. Okin PM, Devereux RB, Nieminen MS, et al. Relationship of the electrocardiographic strain pattern to left ventricular structure and function in hypertensive patients: The LIFE study. *J Am Coll Cardiol.* 2001;38:514–520.
3. Chapman N, Mayet J, Ozkor M, et al. Ethnic and gender differences in electrocardiographic QT length and QT dispersion in hypertensive subjects. *J Hum Hypertens.* 2000;14:403–405.
4. Ciaroni S, Cuenoud L, Bloch A. Clinical study to investigate the predictive parameters for the onset of atrial fibrillation in patients with essential hypertension. *Am Heart J.* 2000;139:814–819.
5. Gryglewska B, Grodzicki T, Czarnecka D, et al. QT dispersion and hypertensive heart disease in the elderly. *J Hypertens.* 2000;18:461–464.
6. Wachtell K, Rokkedal J, Bella JN, et al. Effect of electrocardiographic left ventricular hypertrophy on left ventricular systolic function in systemic hypertension (The LIFE Study). Losartan Intervention For Endpoint. *Am J Cardiol.* 2001;87:54–60.
7. Verdecchia P, Dovellini EV, Gorini M, et al. Comparison of electrocardiographic criteria for diagnosis of left ventricular hypertrophy in hypertension: the MAVI study. *Ital Heart J.* 2000;1:207–215.
8. Terpstra WF, May JF, Smit AJ, et al. Silent ST depression and cardiovascular end-organ damage in newly found, older hypertensives. *Hypertension.* 2001;37:1083–1088.
9. Enstrom I, Burtscher IM, Eskilsson J, et al. Organ damage in treated middle-aged hypertensives compared to normotensives: results from a cross-sectional study in general practice. *Blood Press.* 2000;9:28–33.

Cardiac Imaging Techniques

Clarence Shub, MD

KEY POINTS

- Determination of left ventricular mass by echocardiography is the most commonly used noninvasive clinical method of diagnosing left ventricular hypertrophy.

- Radionuclide angiography can be used to assess the dynamic changes in the left ventricular blood pool but cannot directly evaluate the myocardium or the great vessels.

- Magnetic resonance imaging is a precise method to image the heart and great vessels, generally without need for contrast.

- Choice of imaging modality depends on clinical presentation, availability, and local expertise.

See also Chapters A61, C110, C115, C118, C121, and C155

Proper evaluation of the heart in hypertension often requires the use of imaging procedures.

Echocardiography

Overall, echocardiography is probably the most useful cardiac imaging technique for patients with hypertension and its complications.

Patterns of left ventricular hypertrophy. The type of overload to which the heart is subjected determines not only the specific chamber (or chambers) involved but also the pattern of left ventricular hypertrophy (LVH) (see Figure C115.1). In concentric hypertrophy, the ratio of ventricular wall thickness to radius (relative wall thickness) is increased to >0.45. The ratio is decreased in eccentric hypertrophy. Eccentric hypertrophy should not be confused with the term *asymmetric hypertrophy*, in which a portion of the ventricle, usually the ventricular septum, is thicker than the other wall segments. *Eccentric* (or volume-overload) *hypertrophy* refers to a ventricle with an expanded cavitary volume in proportion to wall thickness, whereas *concentric hypertrophy* refers to a ventricle with thick walls relative to cavity volume. These specific geometric patterns appear to have prognostic implications.

Left ventricular mass determination. Increased ventricular septal and posterior wall thicknesses and left ventricular (LV) internal dimensions indicate LVH and LV chamber dilation, respectively. These parameters are more sensitive for detection of LVH when used to determine LV muscle mass, which has been shown to impart an adverse prognosis. LV muscle mass is calculated by use of standard M-mode echocardiographic measurements of the LV in necropsy-validated formulas. LV mass is directly related to body size and should be indexed to body surface area or body height with use of sex-specific normative values. In addition, age appears to have a small but significant independent effect on LV mass in women

but not in men. In comparison with autopsy-validated LVH, echocardiography has a specificity of 97%. Its sensitivity is 57% for mild, 92% for moderate, and 100% for severe LVH. In contrast, the sensitivity for the Romhilt-Estes electrocardiographic point score for LVH is only 7% in the general population and 54% in autopsied patients with relatively severe LVH. Thus, echo is more sensitive and specific (but also more expensive) than standard electrocardiogram criteria. LV dimensions, mass, and ejection fraction (EF) can also be measured by 2-dimensional echocardiography, a technique that provides more complete global and regional information than M-mode echocardiography. Recent studies have shown that 3-dimensional echocardiography is more accurate and reproducible than M-mode or 2-dimensional echocardiography in the diagnosis of LVH. However, technical and feasibility issues need to be overcome before this modality becomes available for clinical purposes.

Left ventricular hypertrophy criteria. Partition values for detection of LVH by M-mode echocardiography, derived from apparently normal subjects in the primarily white Framingham population, were an LV mass index in men >131 g/m^2 and in women >100 g/m^2. The upper-normal limits derived in a racially mixed normotensive population were >134 g/m^2 and 110 g/m^2, respectively. In obese subjects, identification of LVH is enhanced without loss of prognostic power by indexing LV mass to height. LV mass is best viewed as a continuous variable, and current partition values should ultimately be replaced by upper-normal limits that identify subjects with a more adverse prognosis. Echocardiographic LV mass is elevated in 20% to 50% of patients with stage 1 hypertension and up to 90% of hospitalized patients with stage 2 to 3 hypertension. Echocardiography and, in selected circumstances, comprehensive echocardiography and Doppler assessment, would appear to be appropriate in the situations listed in **Table C116.1**. Limited, or focused, echocardiography has been proposed as a less costly screening method to

Table C116.1. Indications for Use of Echocardiography, Comprehensive Echocardiography, and Doppler Assessment

Possible cardiac involvement requires further confirmation (e.g., electro-cardiography diagnosis of left ventricular hypertrophy based on volt-age criteria alone).[a]
Patient has a coexisting cardiac condition (e.g., valvular heart disease).
A child or adolescent has mild hypertension.[a]
Etiology and significance of systolic murmurs need better definition.
Hypertension occurs during exercise, but resting pressures are normal.[a]
Dyspnea of unknown etiology (differentiate systolic vs. diastolic dys-function and assess pulmonary artery pressures by Doppler).

[a]Limited or focused echocardiography to assess left ventricular hypertrophy only may be appropriate under these circumstances.

detect LVH in hypertensive patients. Its clinical role in hypertensive patients needs to be further defined.

Other diagnostic uses. Hypertensive hypertrophic cardiomyopathy can be readily diagnosed by combined 2-dimensional and Doppler echocardiography. Echocardiography also allows imaging of the aorta, which can be useful in the evaluation of suspected aortic coarctation. Transesophageal echocardiography is especially valuable for the rapid diagnosis of aortic dissection.

Ventricular function. LV systolic function can be assessed by calculating systolic fractional shortening by M-mode echocardiography or EF or by 2-dimensional echocardiography. The latter is preferable if LV shape or pattern of wall motion is abnormal. Standard measurements of cardiac function in hypertensive patients show that EF is preserved but that diastolic filling, as assessed by radionuclide angiography (RNA) or Doppler echocardiography, is often impaired. Studies using Doppler echocardiography have shown a high prevalence (<30% to 45%) of impaired diastolic function in hypertensive patients, especially in older patients, even in the absence of sys-

tolic dysfunction or LVH. These diastolic abnormalities reflect impaired ventricular relaxation but may also represent impaired chamber compliance owing to LVH, deposition of increased or altered collagen tissue, and abnormalities of contractile proteins or intracellular calcium flux.

Doppler Echocardiography

Doppler echocardiography allows separation of diastolic dysfunction into different patterns of LV filling abnormalities (e.g., delayed relaxation or restrictive filling patterns). Restrictive filling patterns reflect a more severe diastolic abnormality and are more likely to be associated with clinical symptoms, (e.g., dyspnea). The compliance curve of the stiff and poorly compliant ventricle is shifted to the left and is steeper than normal in patients with LVH. This implies that for an equivalent increase in diastolic volume, the diastolic pressure increases more in the hypertrophic than in the normal ventricle.

Radionuclide Angiography

RNA is a widely available and extensively used, validated method to assess cardiac size and function, especially dynamic changes in LV chamber volumes during the cardiac cycle. Because RNA examines the blood pool and not the myocardium directly, LV muscle mass cannot be quantified.

Ejection fraction. By registering externally the dynamic changes in the ventricular "blood pool," RNA examines relative changes in total LV chamber blood pool "counts" during the cardiac cycle. No assumptions regarding LV geometry are needed to quantify EF (as are necessary with echocardiography). As a result, RNA remains a very accurate clinical method to determine LV EF, although imaging is suboptimal in very obese subjects.

Volume curves. By defining dynamic changes in the left ventricle during the cardiac cycle, the dynamics of contraction and relaxation can be defined (**Figure C116.1**). Radionuclide LV

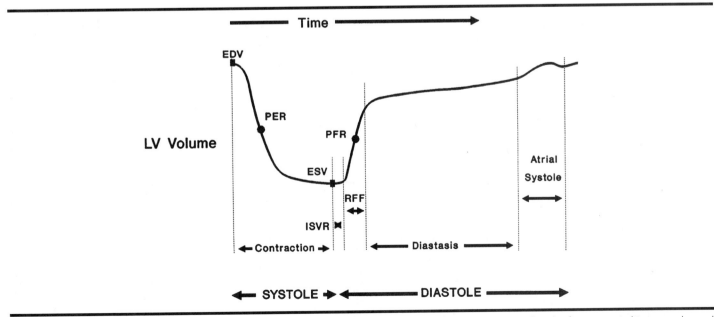

Figure C116.1. Dynamics of left ventricular (LV) volume and function as may be assessed by radionuclide angiography, ultrafast computed tomography, and magnetic resonance imaging. Ejection fraction can be determined directly from the end-diastolic volume (EDV) and end-systolic volume (ESV). ISVR, isovolumetric relaxation phase; PER, peak systolic emptying rate; PFR, peak (early) diastolic filling rate; RFF, rapid (early) diastolic filling phase.

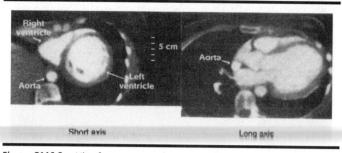

Figure C116.2. Ultrafast computed tomography scans at end diastole in the cardiac short-axis (transverse cardiac) and horizontal long-axis planes from the mid left ventricle in a patient with congestive heart failure. Note that this well-known complication of hypertension results in a dilated left ventricle that has poor contractile performance. Similar images can be obtained with magnetic resonance imaging.

"volume" curves can be analyzed to determine relative rates of systolic contraction (peak emptying rate) and early diastolic relaxation (peak filling rate). Abnormalities of early diastolic filling are frequently observed in patients with hypertension before there is evidence of systolic dysfunction.

Electron Beam (Ultrafast) Computed Tomography

Electron beam computed tomography (EBCT), also known as *ultrafast computed tomography* (CT) and *cine CT*, uses an electron beam and stationary target/detector pairing to replace the physical rotation of the x-ray source/detector pair required by conventional CT. Ultrafast CT can acquire tomographic images very rapidly. The methods for image display and analysis of cardiac (50-microsecond) images are derived from 2-dimensional echocardiography to quantify regional myocardial motion, EF, and chamber volumes (**Figure C116.2**) and from RNA to define the dynamics of LV volumes during the cardiac cycle. Unlike RNA and magnetic resonance imaging (MRI), imaging by EBCT is "triggered" (as opposed to "gated") by the patient's electrocardiogram. Thus, dynamic imaging from the entire heart can be completed in seconds. EBCT, like echocardiography and MRI, defines the cardiac chambers and myocardium and can also be used to define great-vessel anatomy in hypertensive patients. Because of the speed at which imaging can be done, EBCT, if available, is extremely useful in assessing diseases of the aorta in severely ill patients and (because no sedation is necessary) in children.

Table C116.3. Advantages and Disadvantages of Radionuclide Angiography, Computed Tomography, and Magnetic Resonance Imaging in Assessing Patients with Hypertension

IMAGING MODALITY	ADVANTAGES	DISADVANTAGES
Radionuclide angiography	Widely available in major medical centers	Radiation, limitations in large patients
Conventional computed tomography	Widely available in major medical centers	Radiation, contrast media
Ultrafast computed tomography	Highly versatile and precise	Availability to only a few major medical centers, radiation, contrast
Magnetic resonance imaging	Versatile, precise, no radiation	Limited availability,[a] contrast,[b] prolonged imaging

[a]Although magnetic resonance imaging is widely available, at present there are limited facilities that can perform dynamic cardiac studies.
[b]See section Magnetic Resonance Imaging.

Magnetic Resonance Imaging

MRI provides exquisite tomographic images of the heart and great vessels that can be displayed from virtually any plane or orientation. There is no radiation exposure to the patient. There is also no need for contrast injection, and patients can be imaged with any level of renal excretory function. MRI is useful to image the cardiac chambers or great vessels. Specific cine techniques (or magnetic resonance angiography) have been developed to allow quantification of EF, LV volumes, and LV muscle mass. Cine MRI can be used to assess the effects of drug therapy on cardiac remodeling (i.e., regression of LVH, left atrial size, and improvement in diastolic function) over time. MRI is used extensively to define aortic dissection and coarctation and to follow such patients after surgical or pharmacologic therapy. The major disadvantages to MRI are the necessity of prolonged times for completion of the entire study (15 minutes to 1 hour) and the fact that the subject needs to remain still during image acquisition. Patients with claustrophobia or pacemakers or who are acutely ill cannot be imaged effectively with MRI. Although the method is safe for patients who have prosthetic (natural or metallic) valve replacements, MRI is contraindicated in patients who have metal plates anywhere in the body or metallic hip replacements. Although MRI technology is widely available, its application to

Table C116.2. Comparison of Radionuclide Angiography, Computed Tomography, and Magnetic Resonance Imaging Methods to Define Cardiac Function and Great Vessel Anatomy

IMAGING MODALITY	EJECTION FRACTION	LEFT VENTRICULAR MASS	LEFT VENTRICULAR VOLUME	DIASTOLIC FUNCTION	REGIONAL WALL MOTION (CONTRACTION) ABNORMALITIES	GREAT VESSEL ANATOMY
Radionuclide angiography	Yes	No	Yes	Yes	Yes	No
Conventional computed tomography	No	No	No	No	No	Yes
Ultrafast computed tomography	Yes	Yes	Yes	Yes	Yes	Yes
Magnetic resonance imaging	Yes	Yes	Yes	Yes	Yes	Yes

cardiac imaging is not, mainly because of the need for additional software for analysis and proper image sequencing and limited experience in cardiac MRI.

Comparison of Imaging Modalities

Echocardiography, RNA, EBCT, and MRI can be used effectively to diagnose or quantify cardiovascular manifestations of hypertension (**Table C116.2**). Their relative uses depend heavily on availability and the degree of local expertise with each technique. Each has a role in defining specific complications of hypertension, such as diastolic dysfunction, reduced EF, heart failure, aortic aneurysm, and dissection, or concomitant cardiac disease (e.g., valve abnormality). In addition, each has distinct advantages and disadvantages in clinical practice (**Table C116.3**). The clinician must choose which method to apply to a specific patient, largely guided by individual clinical circumstances, the objectives of the study, relative costs of the various techniques, and the expertise of the local or referral laboratory or imaging center. Mere availability of a particular technique to image the heart and great vessels does not absolve the clinician of first establishing the necessity and objectives of the study.

SUGGESTED READING

1. Celentano A, Palmieri V, Esposito ND, et al. Inappropriate left ventricular mass in normotensive and hypertensive patients. *Am J Cardiol.* 2001;87:361–363, A10.
2. Cuspidi C, Lonati L, Macca G, et al. Cardiovascular risk stratification in hypertensive patients: impact of echocardiography and carotid ultrasonography. *J Hypertens.* 2001;19:375–380.
3. Gopal AS, Keller AM, Shen Z, et al. Three-dimensional echocardiography: in vitro and in vivo validation of left ventricular mass and comparison with conventional echocardiographic methods. *J Am Coll Cardiol.* 1994;24:504–513.
4. Hamouda MS, Kassem HK, Salama M, et al. Evaluation of coronary flow reserve in hypertensive patients by dipyridamole transesophageal Doppler echocardiography. *Am J Cardiol.* 2000;86:305–308.
5. Hoffmann U, Globits S, Stefenelli T, et al. The effects of ACE inhibitor therapy on left ventricular myocardial mass and diastolic filling in previously untreated hypertensive patients: a Cine MRI study. *J Magn Reson Imaging.* 2001;14:16–22.
6. Linss G. Noninvasive investigations of systolic and diastolic heart function in arterial hypertension: from calibrated and differentiated apexcardiography to echocardiography. *J Cardiol.* 2001;37:65–69.
7. Mineoi K, Shigematsu Y, Ochi T, Hiwada K. Left ventricular mass and atrial volume determined by cine magnetic resonance imaging in essential hypertension. *Am J Hypertens.* 2000;13:1103–1109.
8. Okin PM, Devereux RB, Jern S, et al. Baseline characteristics in relation to electrocardiographic left ventricular hypertrophy in hypertensive patients: the Losartan intervention for endpoint reduction (LIFE) in hypertension study. The Life Study Investigators. *Hypertension.* 2000;36:766–773.
9. Park SH, Shub C, Nobrega TP, et al. Two-dimensional echocardiographic calculation of left ventricular mass as recommended by the American Society of Echocardiography: correlation with autopsy and M-mode echocardiography. *J Am Soc Echocardiogr.* 1996;9:119–128.
10. Resnick LM, Militianu D, Cunnings AJ, et al. Pulse waveform analysis of arterial compliance: relation to other techniques, age, and metabolic variables. *Am J Hypertens.* 2000;13:1243–1249.
11. Rusconi C, Sabatini T, Faggiano P, et al. Prevalence of isolated left ventricular diastolic dysfunction in hypertension as assessed by combined transmitral and pulmonary vein flow Doppler study. *Am J Cardiol.* 2001;87:357–360, A10.
12. Verdecchia P, Carini G, Circo A, et al. Left ventricular mass and cardiovascular morbidity in essential hypertension: The MAVI Study. *J Am Coll Cardiol.* 2001;38:1829–1835.

Chapter C117

Exercise Stress Testing

Michael F. Wilson, MD; Mofid N. Khalil-Ibrahim, MD, PhD

KEY POINTS

- Exercise stress testing provides useful information for cardiac diagnosis, prognosis, and management.

- An exaggerated blood pressure response to exercise stress testing is due in part to impaired vasodilation.

- Subjects who exhibit this exaggerated blood pressure response have increased risk of target organ damage.

- Added prognostic value is provided by stress myocardial perfusion imaging.

See also Chapters B98, C115, C116, C118, and C130

Traditionally, blood pressure (BP) has been measured in a semiactivated state (sitting position in a medical office). It is well known that exercise and other stressors increase BP (see Chapter A43), but the diagnostic and prognostic value of stress testing has not been fully investigated.

Cardiovascular Responses to Exercise

Exercise stimulates the sympathetic nervous system, which in turn alters hemodynamics.

Blood pressure responses. With exercise, there is an increase in metabolic demand for oxygen, and the cardiac output (CO) responds through an increase primarily in heart rate (HR) but also in stroke volume (SV). CO is the product of HR and SV ($CO = HR \times SV$). Normally, systemic vascular resistance decreases with exercise, but the increase of CO is greater. Therefore, mean arterial blood pressure increases according to the relationship systemic vascular resistance $\times$ CO = mean arterial blood pressure. With exercise, the normal pattern is for sys-

Table C117.1. Indications for Stress Testing

Diagnosis
  Chest pain syndrome
  Screening for latent heart disease
  Evaluation of dysrhythmias
Prognosis and severity of disease
  Functional capacity and exercise prescription
  After myocardial infarction
  Before noncardiac surgery
Management
  Evaluating effects of medical and surgical treatment
  Stimulus to change lifestyle
Myocardial viability

tolic BP (SBP) to increase and diastolic blood pressure (DBP) to decrease. The widened pulse pressure thus reflects the increase in SV.

Heart rate responses. HR is a useful and practical index to record the level of stress placed on the heart. The maximum HR level in beats per minute is a function of age (HR = 220 – age in years). Myocardial work, oxygen consumption, coronary blood flow, CO, and HR all increase proportionally. Optimum stress testing requires an HR ≥85% of age-predicted maximum. Physical conditioning decreases the HR response to a given workload, as do some cardiac medications, such as β-blockers.

Rate-pressure product. Rate-pressure product (RPP = HR × SBP) is recorded as a clinical measure of myocardial work, oxygen consumption. A value of ≥25,000 (beats per minute × mm Hg) at peak exercise is considered to be an adequate response for stress testing purposes. See **Table C117.1** for indications for exercising or pharmacologic stress testing. If ≥85% of optimum

HR and adequate RPP is reached and the exercise tolerance test is normal [negative by electrocardiographic (ECG) criteria with no defects in myocardial perfusion imaging], there is a high probability that clinically significant coronary artery disease is not present. However, the sensitivity is substantially lower if the HR and RPP maximal responses are less than optimal.

Exaggerated Pressure Responses to Exercise

In normotensive individuals, an exercise SBP >220 mm Hg or DBP >100 mm Hg is considered abnormal. Only a small percentage of the population exhibits an exaggerated BP response to exercise, but several subgroups are at risk for this pattern. Normotensive individuals with a parental history of hypertension are at greater risk for developing hypertension and more frequently display the exaggerated BP pattern. Borderline hypertensives and those with treated hypertension (with an adequate resting BP) may also display an exaggerated pressure response to exercise or mental stress. Some investigators have suggested that this pattern is associated with higher cardiovascular disease risk (see Chapter A43). Hemodynamic measurements demonstrate vasodilatory impairment in those with exaggerated BP responses to exercise (**Figure C117.1**). This blunted vasodilation is manifest even at submaximal exercise and is associated with a trend toward a reduced CO response. It has been proposed that individuals with endothelial dysfunction (see Chapter A66) may respond in this fashion.

Treadmill Protocols

Stress testing (exercise tolerance testing) is commonly performed by use of a programmed treadmill ECG evaluation. The treadmill ECG protocol developed by Bruce is generally recognized as the standard. This protocol begins at 1.7 miles per

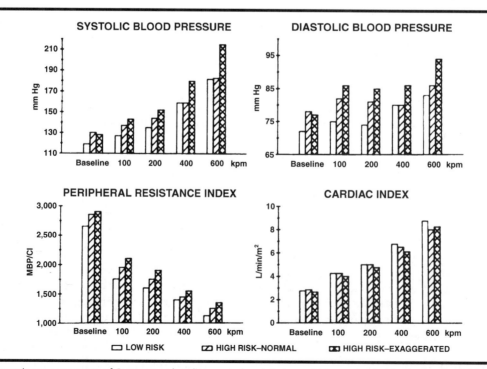

Figure C117.1. Hemodynamic measurements of 3 groups at baseline control and during mild to moderate bicycle exercise (100 to 600 kpm). CI, cardiac index; MBP, mean blood pressure. (From Wilson MF, Sung BH, Pincomb GA, Lovallo WR. Exaggerated pressure response to exercise in men at risk for systemic hypertension. *Am J Cardiol.* 1990;66:731–736, with permission.)

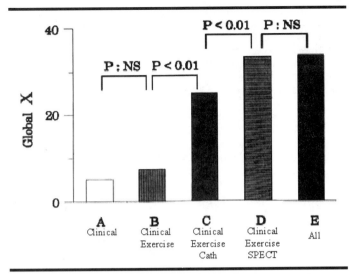

Figure C117.2. Incremental prognostic power of clinical, imaging, catheterization, and single-photon emission computed tomographic (SPECT) imaging. NS, not significant. [From Iskandrian AS, Chae SC, Heo J, et al. Independent and incremental prognostic value of exercise single-photon emission computed tomographic (SPECT) thallium imaging in coronary artery disease. *J Am Coll Cardiol*. 1993;22:665–670, with permission.]

hour and a 10% grade, then increases both speed and grade at 3-minute intervals to symptom-limited exercise capacity. Others believe that treadmill speed should be held constant while the grade is increased gradually (Balke test) or that speed and grade should be increased separately (Naughton test) to produce a linear progression of workload.

Imaging Methods

Bike exercise ergometry is a valuable method for stress testing (**Figure C117.2**) that is especially useful in conjunction with radionuclide ventriculography. Both the first-pass and the multigated acquisition techniques measure ventricular contractile (ejection fraction) response to exercise. However, myocardial perfusion imaging in conjunction with treadmill stress testing or with a vasodilating agent (dipyridamole or adenosine) has largely replaced exercise ventriculography in many institutions. The multigated acquisition scan at rest remains valuable to assess resting ventricular function through accurate ejection fraction and regional wall motion measurements. Nuclear cardiology myocardial perfusion imaging with exercise or pharmacologic stress has increased sensitivity and specificity compared with exercise ECG testing and also increased precision in prognosis and management decisions. Abstinence from caffeine is important 10 to 12 hours before stress MPI and from food 3 to 4 hours. Caffeine increases BP response with exercise and blocks pharmacologic response. Other imaging techniques are discussed in Chapter C116.

Contraindications for Stress Testing

There are both absolute and relative contraindications to stress testing (**Table C117.2**).

Absolute contraindications. Patients with left main coronary artery disease or left main equivalent [i.e., those with

Table C117.2. **Contraindications to Stress Testing**

Acute myocardial infarction
Acute myocarditis or pericarditis
Rapid ventricular or atrial arrhythmias
Severe aortic stenosis, hypertrophic obstructive cardiomyopathy
Second- or third-degree heart block without pacemaker
Stage 3 elevated blood pressure ≥180/110 mm Hg
Unstable progressive angina
Severe illness from infection or other processes (e.g., hyperthyroidism, severe anemia, or liver, renal, pulmonary, or cardiac failure)

high-grade obstruction (≥80% diameter narrowing) in all proximal branches of the left main coronary artery] should not undergo stress testing. The danger is that a large mass of myocardium is at risk for ischemia, myocardial infarction, arrhythmia, and sudden cardiac death secondary to ventricular fibrillation.

Relative contraindications. **Severe hypertension.** Because of the danger of further aggravating an unstable and progressive hypertensive state, hypertension should usually be brought under control before the exercise stress test. However, stress testing in the presence of stage 1 or 2 hypertension (SBP <180 mm Hg) does not present significant additional risk. Sometimes the SBP and DBP are modestly elevated in the stress testing milieu before exercise, even when the BP was previously normal with or without medication. This is considered a variant of white coat hypertension secondary to augmented sympathoadrenal activity.

Aortic stenosis. Patients with clinical signs of critical aortic stenosis and angina should not undergo a stress test. These patients should usually be referred directly to the cardiac catheterization laboratory for evaluation of the aortic valve and the coronary arteries. In adults with evidence of moderate aortic stenosis, stress testing has some increased risk but may be quite useful, especially when accompanied by myocardial perfusion imaging. In children, stress testing in the presence of aortic stenosis has been useful and safe.

Unstable angina syndrome. A progressive increase in the intensity, frequency, duration, or new onset of exertional angina or angina at rest heralds the potential to develop into an acute myocardial infarction. Stress testing could aggravate this situation by increasing platelet aggregability and triggering the coagulation cascade through augmented sympathoadrenal and neurohumoral pathways. However, after appropriate therapy to control unstable angina, it is sometimes useful to perform a stress test, especially in association with myocardial perfusion imaging, to assist in management and follow-up (**Figure C117.3**).

Compensated heart failure. Patients who have heart failure with dependent edema and pulmonary rales by auscultation should not undergo exercise stress testing until these signs have responded to therapy. Conversely, careful exercise tolerance testing that monitors symptoms, HR, and BP responses relating to workload (and measures of oxygen consumption and carbon dioxide elimination when available) is useful for determining the appropriate rehabilitation exercise schedule. The Naughton stress test and the Borg scale of perceived effort are commonly used.

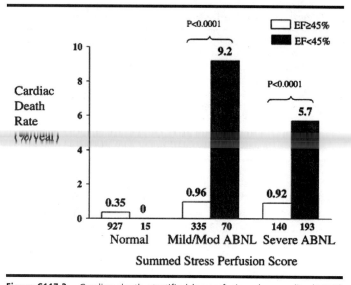

Figure C117.3. Cardiac death stratified by perfusion abnormality (ABNL) and ejection fraction (EF). Mod, moderate. (From Sharir T, Germano G, Kavanagh PB, et al. Incremental prognostic value of poststress left ventricular ejection fraction and volume by gated myocardial perfusion single photon emission computed tomography. *Circulation.* 1999; 100:1035–1042, with permission.)

SUGGESTED READING

1. Beller GA. New directions in myocardial perfusion imaging. *Clin Cardiol.* 1993;16:86–94.

2. Borer JS, Brensike JF, Redwood DR, et al. Limitations of the electrocardiographic response to exercise in predicting coronary artery disease. *N Engl J Med.* 1975;293:367–371.

3. Bruce RA, Kusumi F, Hosmer D. Maximal oxygen intake and nomographic assessment of functional aerobic impairment in cardiovascular disease. *Am Heart J.* 1973;85:546–562.

4. Ellestad MH. Cardiovascular limits to exercise. In: Ellestad MH, ed. *Stress Testing: Principles and Practice.* 3rd ed. Philadelphia, PA: FA Davis; 1975:177–195.

5. Esquivel L, Pollock SG, Beller GA, et al. Effect of the degree of effort on the sensitivity of the exercise thallium 201 stress test in symptomatic coronary artery disease. *Am J Cardiol.* 1989;63:160–165.

6. Iskandrian AS, Chae SC, Heo J, et al. Independent and incremental prognostic value of exercise single-photon emission computed tomographic (SPECT) thallium imaging in coronary artery disease. *J Am Coll Cardiol.* 1993;22:665–670.

7. Machecourt J, Longere P, Fagret D, et al. Prognostic value of thallium-201 single-photon emission computed tomographic myocardial perfusion imaging according to extent of myocardial defect: study in 1,926 patients with follow-up at 33 months. *J Am Coll Cardiol.* 1994;23:1096–1106.

8. Pollock SG, Abbott RD, Boucher CA, et al. Independent and incremental prognostic value of tests performed in hierarchical order to evaluate patients with suspected coronary artery disease: validation of models based on these tests. *Circulation.* 1992;85:237–248.

9. Sharir T, Germano G, Kavanagh PB, et al. Incremental prognostic value of post–stress left ventricular ejection fraction and volume by gated myocardial perfusion single photon emission computed tomography. *Circulation.* 1999;100:1035–1042.

10. Wilson MF, Sung BH, Pincomb GA, Lovallo WR. Exaggerated pressure response to exercise in men at risk for systemic hypertension. *Am J Cardiol.* 1990;66:731–736.

Hemodynamic Profiles in Essential and Secondary Hypertension

Robert C. Davidson, MD; Suhail Ahmad, MD

KEY POINTS

- Hypertension results from an altered hemodynamic relationship between cardiac output and total peripheral resistance, either or both of which may be elevated.

- Antihypertensive agents can be characterized by their relative abilities to lower either cardiac output or total peripheral resistance.

- Use of an antihypertensive agent appropriate for the underlying hemodynamic abnormality is generally more effective and is associated with less untoward effects than random selection of drugs.

- High cardiac output occurs most commonly in borderline hypertension, diabetes, and renal failure; in secondary hypertension, high cardiac output occurs in renal artery stenosis with a single kidney, in chronic renal failure, and in pheochromocytoma.

See also Chapters A38, A40, A48–A51, A59, and A60

Hypertension is recognized as a disturbed relationship between cardiac output (CO) and vascular resistance. The value of hemodynamic profiling in management, however, remains controversial but many experts have suggested that knowledge of hemodynamics aids in the management of hypertension.

Physiology

Systemic blood flow (CO) is dependent on the difference between mean arterial pressure (MAP) and right atrial pressure (RAP), expressed as $CO = MAP - RAP/TPR$ (where TPR is total peripheral resistance). Because RAP is small, the formula $MAP = CO \times TPR$ is generally used. There is always a compensatory relationship between flow and resistance; reducing CO increases TPR and vice versa. Thus in hypertension either TPR or CO is increased, with or without a concomitant decrease in the other. In a sense, there is inappropriate CO and inappropriate TPR. Factors affecting CO and TPR are shown in **Figure C118.1**. [Cardiac index (CI) normal = 2.5 to 3.5 L/min/m^2 and total peripheral index normal is <2,400 dyne/cm^{-5}.]

Methods for Measuring Hemodynamics

CO can be measured by invasive or noninvasive techniques.

Noninvasive methods. Invasive methods provide measurements in various positions and during exercise but are not practical for most clinical settings. Relatively precise estimates of CO can be derived from echocardiography/Doppler methods that measure aortic root diameter by echo, and the velocity of blood and cardiac ejection time by Doppler; stroke volume is calculated from these parameters. Other acceptable methods include gas rebreathing techniques. Pulse contour analysis is generally unreliable. Impedance cardiography can be used to determine stroke volume but it is more suitable for comparing changes within an individual than comparing between individuals. Impedance methods can also be used to determine thoracic fluid volume, which has been proposed as a guide to therapy.

Estimating hemodynamics without measuring cardiac output. Clinical observation and judgment can often be used to estimate CO or TPR. For example, rapid heart rate, bounding pulse, and hyperdynamic circulation suggest hyperadrenergic activity and increased CO. Poorly controlled hypertension in a patient who is taking multiple vasodilating agents also suggests high CO. On the other hand, bradycardia, a quiet heart, cold extremities, and the use of β-blockers suggest a low CO. If clinical observations and the hemodynamic action of antihypertensive drugs are kept in mind when instituting or changing drug therapy, successful management of hypertension is more readily attained than by randomly prescribing drugs. For example, a calcium antagonist would be a logical complement to a β-blocker. Clinical judgment or direct measurement of the hemodynamics, when matched with the action of antihypertensive drugs, often result in more successful treatment.

Aging and Hemodynamics in Essential Hypertension

In longitudinal 20-year studies in hypertensive men, Lund-Johansen has reported the hemodynamics both in the resting state and with exercise. He found that hypertension starts at varying ages either with a high CO and rapid heart rate or with a high TPR. With aging, TPR increases and blood pressure (BP) continues to rise. With exercise, but not at rest, stroke index is abnormally low in early hypertension, and decreases further with time. Low stroke index may reflect reduced compliance of the left ventricle. In Eich's studies, the initial cardiac index was high in 15 of 41 patients younger than 50 years of age, whereas only 1 of 7 older

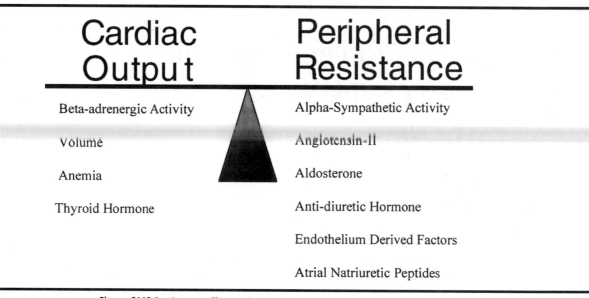

Figure C118.1. Factors affecting hemodynamics and blood pressure.

than age 50 years had a high cardiac index. After 50 months, all patients had higher BPs, with lower cardiac indices, and higher vascular resistances. In another longitudinal study in younger subjects (average age, 32.6 years), Julius et al. reported that approximately one-third with borderline hypertension had an increased CO and heart rate. When hypertension became sustained, CO normalized and vascular resistance increased. In the elderly, hypertension is characterized by progressive lowering of CO and increasing vascular resistance. Messerli et al. compared 30 patients older than 65 years of age with 30 younger than 42 years of age with similar mean arterial pressures and found that the older group had a lower CO and higher TPR.

Hemodynamic Subgroups in Essential Hypertension

Hyperdynamic hypertension. One specific subgroup has been defined with very high CO: hyperdynamic hypertension. The prevalence rate of this condition is not precisely known (probably a few %), partly because a clear definition has not been established. A high incidence of high CO hypertension has been said to occur in borderline (nonsustained) hypertension (see Chapter C152).

Obesity and diabetes. Most obese people have increased CO, although they may also have increased vascular resistance. Similarly, early diabetes is often associated with a hyperdynamic circulatory state. These individuals respond favorably to diuretics, angiotensin-converting enzyme inhibitors, angiotensin-receptor blockers, and β-blockers.

Race. In general, total peripheral resistance is higher in blacks than whites, but the overlap is broad. Blacks respond well to the vasodilator effects of thiazides and calcium antagonists (see Chapter C167).

Secondary Hypertension

Renovascular hypertension. Renal artery stenosis is usually caused by atherosclerosis or fibromuscular dysplasia. Whether the disease is unilateral or bilateral determines the hemodynamics of the accompanying hypertension. In unilateral renal artery disease, high levels of renin and angiotensin II increase central sympathetic activity and cause high peripheral vascular resistance (see Chapter A48). In bilateral renal artery stenosis, both kidneys conserve sodium, blood volume is expanded, and CO is high, which may trigger flash pulmonary edema. High CO hypertension also is caused by renal artery stenosis in a single kidney.

Primary aldosteronism. Tarazi et al. found a positive correlation between CO and blood volume in hyperaldosteronism. However, somewhat unexpectedly, the BP was better correlated with vascular resistance than CO. In addition to the mechanical effects of high BP, aldosterone can damage the vasculature (see Chapter A50). In addition, aldosterone also directly affects vascular tone. Wehling et al. reported that intravenous aldosterone acutely increased BP and vascular resistance and lowered CO within 3 to 10 minutes (nongenomic effect). Aldosterone antagonists (spironolactone and eplerenone) may be effective by preventing vascular injury and lowering vascular tone and resistance.

Chronic renal failure and dialysis. In renal parenchymal disease and renal failure, multiple factors influence hemodynamics and BP (see Chapter A49). The most important factor is sodium retention and volume excess but the sympathetic nervous system, renin-angiotensin-aldosterone system, and other hormones and autocoids are also elevated. Anemia and hyperparathyroidism are also often present. Thus, the hemodynamics of renal failure can be complex and vary with severity of the disease and presence of associated complications. Studies in nonuremic renal disease have shown that hypertension is basically maintained by elevated TPR and CO is usually in normal ranges. However, longitudinal studies involving renal insufficiency patients without anemia suggest that increased CO is seen first, then TPR increases. In untreated anemic dialysis patients, CO is also increased. However, after the correction of anemia by blood transfusion or erythropoietin, BP increases as a result of increased TPR.

Table C118.1. Hemodynamic Effects of Antihypertensive Drug Classes

REDUCE CO	BALANCED EFFECT (REDUCE CO AND TPR)	REDUCE TPR
β-blockers	Angiotensin-converting enzyme inhibitors	Direct arterial dilators (hydralazine, minoxidil)
Thiazide diuretics (acute)	Angiotensin receptor blockers	Calcium antagonists
	α-Blockers	Thiazide diuretics (chronic)

CO, cardiac output; TPR, total peripheral resistance.

Pheochromocytoma. Pheochromocytoma causes episodic or sustained hypertension, usually with increased TPR (see Chapter A51). Characteristic orthostatic hypotension is caused by decreased blood volume (probably due to pressure-diuresis). Downregulation of α-receptors may also occur, further exacerbating the problem. Drugs with α-blocking action, including labetalol, are the mainstay of treatment before surgical removal of the tumor; volume expansion may also be required.

Antihypertensive Drug Effects

Antihypertensive agents can be conveniently divided in 3 categories based on their action to lower CO, TPR, or both as outlined in **Table C118.1**. Because hypertension is a state of altered hemodynamics, drug selection ultimately must be appropriate for the underlying hemodynamic abnormality. In some cases, combination therapy may be required for optimal effect.

SUGGESTED READING

1. Brod J, Bahlmann J, Cachovan M, Pretschner P. Development of hypertension in renal disease. *Clin Sci*. 1983;64:141–152.
2. Eich RH, Cuddy RP, Smulyan H, Lyons RH. Hemodynamics in labile hypertension. A follow-up study. *Circulation*. 1966;34:299–307.
3. Huntsman LL, Stewart DK, Barnes SR, et al. Noninvasive Doppler determination of cardiac output in man. Clinical validation. *Circulation*. 1983; 67:593–602.
4. Julius S, Krause L, Schork NJ, et al. Hyperkinetic borderline hypertension in Tecumseh, Michigan. *J Hypertens*. 1991;9:77–84.
5. Lund-Johansen P. Hemodynamics in essential hypertension. In: Swales JD. *Textbook of Hypertension*, Oxford: Blackwell Scientific Publications, 1994;61–76.
6. Messerli FH, Sundgaard-Riise K, Ventura HO, et al. Essential hypertension in the elderly: haemodynamics, intravascular volume, plasma renin activity, and circulating catecholamine levels. *Lancet*. 1983;2:983–986.
7. Rajagopalan S, Pitt B. Aldosterone antagonists in the treatment of hypertension and target organ damage. *Curr Hypertens Rep*. 2001;3:240–248.
8. Tarazi RC, Ibrahim MM, Bravo EL, et al. Hemodynamic characteristics of primary aldosteronism. *N Engl J Med*. 1973;289:1330–1335.
9. Wehling M, Spes CH, Win N, et al. Rapid cardiovascular action of aldosterone in man. *J Clin Endocrinol Metab*. 1998;83:3517–3522.

Chapter C119

Evaluation of Arterial Stiffness

Gary F. Mitchell, MD; Joseph L. Izzo, Jr, MD

KEY POINTS

- Systolic hypertension is largely attributable to exaggerated age-related increases in aortic and conduit arterial stiffness, an independent cardiovascular risk factor.

- Arterial stiffness, the inverse of "compliance," is a nonuniform property that primarily affects the aorta and central arteries but not peripheral arteries (such as the brachial artery).

- Functional assessment of arterial stiffness requires measurement of the amplitudes of the pulsatile pressure wave and the corresponding pulsatile flow wave (which determine characteristic impedance) and the propagation velocity of the pressure wave as it travels along the vessel.

- All of the currently available techniques to estimate arterial stiffness have significant limitations to widespread clinical use.

See also Chapters A59, A60, B81, C120, C122, and C151

There has been a major paradigm shift in hypertension that has changed our focus from diastolic to systolic hypertension. Isolated systolic hypertension is usually associated with increased stiffness of the aorta and central conduit arteries, which leads to increased systolic blood pressure (BP), decreased diastolic BP, and wide pulse pressure (PP) (see Chapter A60). The overriding importance of systolic hypertension has prompted the development of new techniques to assess arterial stiffness.

Structure-Function Relationships at Different Levels of the Arterial Tree

Three distinct levels of the arterial tree can be identified on a combined functional-anatomic basis: central arteries,

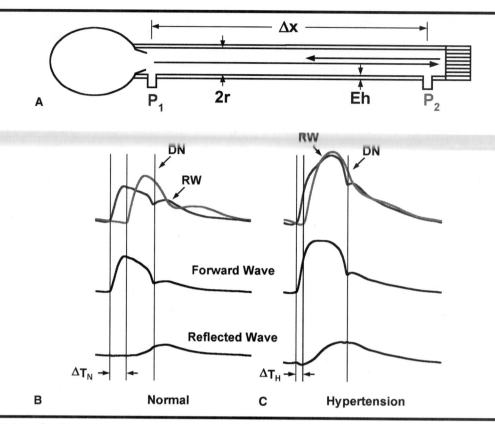

Figure C119.1.　An overview of pulsatile hemodynamics. **A:** The conduits are modeled as an elastic tube terminated by the peripheral resistance. The ventricle ejects blood into the low impedance aorta, which isolates the heart from the high impedance resistance vessels. This sets up a forward wave whose amplitude is determined by characteristic impedance of the aorta and peak flow. This wave travels down the aorta at a velocity [pulse wave velocity (PWV) = $\Delta X/\Delta T$] that depends on wall stiffness (Eh) and internal radius (r) (see text). When this forward wave meets changing impedance distally, a partial reflection occurs, and this reflected wave travels back to the heart. **B:** In normotensive patients, balance between PWV, heart rate, and body length results in a ΔT_N that is approximately one-half of the systolic ejection period. Thus, the reflected wave (RW) returns in diastole ($2 \times \Delta T_N$) and enhances diastolic perfusion of coronary and cerebral circulations. **C:** In a hypertensive patient with stiff conduits, PWV and characteristic impedance are elevated, resulting in a larger forward wave that travels down the aorta too fast ($\Delta T_H < \Delta T_N$). The RW returns prematurely, before the dicrotic notch (DN), and further augments central systolic pressure, thereby increasing load on heart and central vessels. Normal amplification of the waveform as it propagates distally (pulse pressure at $P_1 < P_2$) is lost ($P_1 \approx P_2$).

peripheral arteries, and arterioles. In all cases, structural and functional characteristics of the arterial wall are important in the maintenance of appropriate organ blood flow and function.

Central arteries. The large central arteries (aorta and its proximal branches) are often called *central conduit arteries*, but this terminology is not ideal because it implies that the central arteries are only pipes that allow the passage of blood to the periphery. In reality, the central arteries function as the "third chamber" of the cardiac pumping system, converting highly pulsatile aortic flow into more continuous flow in distal organs. The principal pathogenetic abnormality in systolic hypertension is stiffening of these vessels.

Peripheral arteries. Some investigators consider the second- and third-order arteries (distal carotids, coronaries, brachial, etc.) to be "peripheral conduit arteries." These relatively thick-walled muscular arteries must be differentiated from the thin-walled central arteries because they often respond in opposite fashion than the central arteries. In hypertensives, aortic stiffening occurs prematurely whereas brachial arteries remain normal or demonstrate less age-

related stiffening. Decreased stiffness of peripheral arteries may be an important obligatory offload mechanism if central arteries become too stiff.

Arterioles. Arteriolar changes are important because arteriolar constriction directly increases systemic resistance, diastolic pressure, and mean arterial pressure. Arteriolar vasoconstriction also contributes indirectly to systolic hypertension because it elevates mean arterial pressure and also because the constricted arterioles are major sites of wave reflection. Reflected pressure waves cause late augmentation of central systolic pressure (see Chapter A60). In addition, adaptive changes in vessels with diameters less than 1 mm may be important in modulating pressure transmission and flow distribution in the capillary beds.

Applied Pathophysiology

Functional assessment principles. Clinical assessment of arterial wall properties is complex and requires an understanding of several basic principles (**Figure C119.1**). Characteristic impedance (Z_c) is important because it determines the amplitude of the initial pressure wave produced by the flow wave. Pulse wave velocity (PWV) is important because of its impact on reflected pulse waves, another important phenomenon in the peripheral circulation. These related variables (Z_c and PWV) are each dependent on an interplay between wall stiffness, wall thickness, and vessel geometry according to the following relationship:

$$Y \propto \sqrt{\frac{Eh}{r^x}}$$

where Y is either PWV or Z_c, Eh is the elastance–wall thickness product (see Arterial stiffness and elastic modulus) and r is radius, which is raised to some power x (for PWV, x = 1, whereas for Z_c, x = 5). Thus, PWV and Z_c differ dramatically in their relative dependence on geometry and do not necessarily change in parallel in various disease states or with changes in BP. For example, smooth muscle contraction can dramatically increase Z_c via the reduction in radius although having only a modest effect on PWV.

Arterial stiffness and elastic modulus. The intrinsic stiffness of the vessel wall can be described by Young's elastic modulus (E, the slope of the stress-strain relationship of the vessel wall), in which higher values mean stiffer arteries. The effective stiffness of the wall is determined by the product Eh, where h is wall thickness. The vessel wall is composed of a heterogeneous mixture of materials with varying elastic properties. The Maxwell model describes the parallel load-bearing contributions of each of the 3 major wall components (collagen, elastin, and smooth muscle). With respect to vessel geometry, collagen is loaded by forces that elongate arteries, elastin is loaded by elongation and circumferential stretch, and smooth muscle is loaded circumferentially. Muscle and elastin, the predominant load-bearing elements in normal vessels at physiologic distending pressures, have a much lower elastic modulus than collagen. As distending pressure (particularly systolic) increases, progressively more load is borne by collagen, which leads to a nonlinear increase in wall stiffness. As a result, elastic modulus and most other indices of conduit vessel stiffness must be interpreted in the context of ambient mean arterial pressure. Clinically, Eh is somewhat difficult to measure directly because it requires simultaneous measurement of arterial pressure, diameter, and wall thickness.

Pulse wave velocity. Aging and hypertension strongly affect PWV, which is directly proportional to the stiffness of the arterial wall (see Chapter A60). PWV has been shown to provide important prognostic information in patients with hypertension. Regional assessment of PWV is necessary because central and peripheral conduits behave differently in various disease states including hypertension. These divergent changes in central and peripheral conduit stiffness may be missed if global parameters, such as total of "whole-body" arterial compliance, are used to describe conduit vessel properties. PWV is assessed via the calculation of the time required for a given pressure waveform to travel from a proximal to a distal site over a known distance (distance between sites/transit time, Figure C119.1). Transit time is readily assessed noninvasively using arterial tonometry of the carotid, brachial, radial, or femoral arteries (**Figure C119.2**). The foot of the waveform is used to assess transit time because the peak is affected by reflected pressure waves.

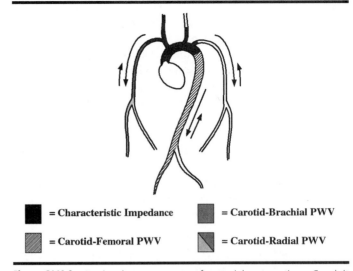

= Characteristic Impedance
= Carotid-Brachial PWV
= Carotid-Femoral PWV
= Carotid-Radial PWV

Figure C119.2. Regional assessment of arterial properties. Conduit properties are not uniform and should be assessed in different regions of the body. Central conduit stiffness is assessed using characteristic impedance and carotid-femoral pulse wave velocity (PWV). Peripheral (muscular) conduit stiffness may be assessed using carotid-brachial and carotid-radial PWV.

There are at least 3 important limitations of PWV measurements. First, the distance between recording sites must be sufficiently large to allow for accurate assessment of the time delay. Second, the transit distance often spans vessel segments with varied properties (Figure C119.2). Third, true transit distance often cannot be measured directly. By convention, carotid-femoral transit distance is estimated by measuring from suprasternal notch to the carotid artery and subtracting this distance from the suprasternal notch-to-femoral distance, which creates a "blind spot" for carotid-femoral PWV in the proximal aorta. This is an important limitation because this segment of the aorta supplies nearly half of the buffering capacity of the arterial system.

Pulse wave reflection. As the forward-traveling pressure wave encounters areas of impedance mismatch in the peripheral circulation (branch points, areas of turbulence, areas of arterial diameter change, etc.), a partial reflection of the pressure waveform occurs (Figures C119.1 and C119.2). The transition from large, low-impedance central arteries to higher impedance peripheral arteries and resistance vessels also affects PWV and wave reflection. Normally the primary reflected wave returns to the central aorta in diastole and augments coronary and cerebral perfusion (Figure C119.1). However, if PWV is elevated, the reflected wave arrives back in the central aorta during systole rather than diastole and adds to pulsatile load on the heart and central vessels (see Chapter A60).

In theory, the central aortic pressure waveform can be reconstructed from a peripheral arterial waveform through the use of a mathematic transfer function. Commercial devices (SphygmoCor, AtCor Medical, West Ryde, Australia) have been marketed that use noninvasive acquisition of the peripheral (usually radial arterial) waveform to calculate the timing and amplitude of wave reflections, assessed by finding the first (primary) and second (reflected wave) peaks on the reconstructed central pressure waveform. The degree of augmentation of systolic pressure is quantitated as the increment between the first and second systolic peaks, and a systolic augmentation index (augmentation pressure/total PP) can be calculated.

The transfer function, which is a mathematic description of the changes in waveform shape that occur as the wave travels distally (Figure C119.1), is assumed to be equal to a population-derived mean or "generalized" transfer function that is assumed to be constant between patients and after interventions. Recent studies suggest that the waveforms reconstructed from a transfer function lack sufficient fidelity to allow for analysis of waveform landmarks, including the timing of wave reflection or augmentation index, and that gender-specific transfer functions may be required. These limitations aside, a central pressure waveform can be assessed more directly by performing carotid artery tonometry, which does not require analysis by transfer function.

Characteristic impedance of the aorta.

Characteristic impedance of the proximal aorta at the point of coupling of heart and arteries (ventricular-vascular coupling, see Chapter A59) is the major determinant of pulsatile load in humans and is the pulsatile equivalent of resistance. *Characteristic aortic impedance* (Z_c) is the change in pressure as it related to the corresponding change in flow in early systole, before the return of the reflected pressure wave (Figure C119.1).

Z_c is assessed noninvasively by using Doppler flow and calibrated carotid tonometry. The carotid waveform is carefully calibrated from the brachial waveform and cuff BP, assuming the same mean and diastolic pressures in the carotid and brachial arteries. This technically demanding approach requires a trained technician and an echo machine and depends on several independent components, each with its own potential sources of error. Properly obtained pressure and flow waveforms provide a robust assessment of Z_c, steady-flow hemodynamics, and amplitude and timing of reflected waves and provide insight into the relationship between pulsatile load and ventricular ejection; this approach, however, is more applicable to research than clinical practice at present.

Other Compliance-Related Variables

Historically, principles of engineering and fluid mechanics have been applied to description of arterial wall characteristics. Other concepts have been advanced to use more readily available clinical data. Each concept has major limitations.

Compliance.

Compliance is the most familiar term in the field. Arterial compliance relates to the "give" in the arterial wall [change in luminal volume (dV), diameter, or area] caused by a corresponding change in distending pressure (dP) (dV/dP, usually in mL/mm Hg). The use of local compliance as a measure of arterial properties is limited because compliance characteristics are not uniform across the entire arterial system. Similarly, whole-body compliance is only a hypothetical concept. Waveforms travel through the arterial system at a finite velocity (Figure C119.1), so the heart normally does not "see" total arterial compliance during systole because the advancing pressure wave has not yet distributed to the entire arterial system.

Distensibility.

Distensibility is the compliance adjusted for the initial volume (V) (dV/VdP, in 1/mm Hg). As with compliance, relatively little information about intact functional arterial properties is afforded by this measure. Many studies have suffered from a common flaw of measuring dP and dV at different sites (e.g., combining brachial PP and carotid dV) which is invalid because PP differs at various sites in the arterial system.

Pulse pressure.

Clinically, wide PP is associated with systolic hypertension and increased conduit arterial stiffness but is a late manifestation of a complex process. Changes in PP include contributions from reflected waves and therefore are affected by systemic hemodynamics and distal vasoconstriction. For the vast majority of hypertensives, especially those older than age 50 years, wide PP is a reasonable surrogate for increased central arterial stiffness. However, wide PP may also accompany states in which cardiac peak flow or stroke volume is high (hyperdynamic hypertension, aortic insufficiency, thyrotoxicosis, vitamin deficiency, arteriovenous malformations, anemia, etc.).

Stroke volume to pulse pressure ratio.

To adjust for the effect of cardiac stroke volume on PP, it is possible to relate a given PP to the corresponding change in stroke volume (expressed in arbitrary units) as a measure of whole-body compliance. Although potentially preferable to using PP alone, this ratio assumes that the peripheral circulation is a single compartment, which is physiologically incorrect and fails to account for arterial runoff from the aorta during systole. Thus, as with PP alone, changes in peripheral resistance, PWV, wave reflection, and ejection pattern can alter stroke volume to PP ratio.

Diastolic pulse contour analysis (Windkessel model).

In theory, the diastolic waveform yields important information about arterial elastic properties that can be unlocked by decomposing the waveform into 2 main components: proximal (C_1) and distal (C_2) arterial compliance. This model represents an idealized waveform as a 4-element electrical Windkessel model, in which the main slope of the diastolic decay function is assumed to be related to the proximal (aortic) compliance (C_1). The presence of a superimposed decaying sinusoid function represents the damping (or compliance) of the distal arterial tree (C_2).

This approach suffers from several technical and theoretical limitations that have been described in detail by several groups. First, the model-based parameters C_1 and C_2 have unclear physiologic significance. C_2, which is intrinsically interdependent with systemic vascular resistance, recently has been claimed to be a surrogate measure for endothelial dysfunction because maneuvers that increase vascular nitric oxide tend to increase C_2. However, convincing proof of this hypothesis remains lacking. A more important issue is that the model fails to account for wave reflections, which significantly affect the calculation of model parameters. Other questions arise from the lack of correlation between whole-body compliance values derived from the arm versus the leg, the high percentage of uninterpretable (negative) values in hypertensive patients, and the lack of correlation between C_1 or C_2 and other measures of arterial stiffness. Given the numerous theoretical and technical limitations, the Windkessel model has unclear value in clinical practice or research.

Brachial plethysmography.

Several systems are available that estimate local brachial artery compliance by using a specially calibrated automated BP cuff as a plethysmograph. Theoretically, this approach allows for an assessment of local compliance across a wide range of effective transmural pressures (the difference between cuff pressure and mean arterial pressure), but there are important technical limitations. The algorithms usually depend on equal pressure transmission along the full length of the pneumatic cuff, but the pressure is actually nonuniform. Furthermore, the volume change occurring with each pressure pulse represents a combination of vessel filling from a collapsed state (which is not related to compliance) and the quantitatively much smaller vessel distension (which is the desired compliance-related volume change). As a result of these limitations, the diameter calculations using this technique are artifactually high. More importantly, the applicability of brachial compliance data to hypertension and cardiovascular disease is unclear because changes in central arterial stiffness and brachial arterial stiffness are not uniform.

Arterial imaging. Vessel wall tracking and simple image-based (ultrasound or magnetic resonance imaging) assessment of systolic and diastolic diameter have been used to assess local arterial stiffness. Pulsatile vessel diameter is obtained and coupled with simultaneous PP to derive the pressure-diameter relationship of the vessel and the corresponding effective elastic modulus (Eh). This approach has been applied in a research setting but is difficult to apply clinically because of the training required and the high cost of the imaging device. An important limitation of the approach is that the pressure waveform must be obtained from the same site as the diameter waveform because pulse pressure can differ considerably at various sites in the arterial system.

SUGGESTED READING

1. Domanski MJ, Davis BR, Pfeffer MA, et al. Isolated systolic hypertension: prognostic information provided by pulse pressure. *Hypertension.* 1999;34:375–380.
2. Domanski MJ, Norman J, Wolz M, et al. Cardiovascular risk assessment using pulse pressure in the First National Health and Nutrition Examination Survey (NHANES I). *Hypertension.* 2001;38:793–797.
3. Izzo JL, Manning TS, Shykoff BE. Office blood pressures, arterial compliance characteristics, and estimated cardiac load. *Hypertension.* 2001;38:1467–1470.
4. Laurent S, Boutouyrie P, Asmar R, et al. Aortic stiffness is an independent predictor of all-cause and cardiovascular mortality in hypertensive patients. *Hypertension.* 2001;37:1236–1241.
5. Manning TS, Shykoff BE, Izzo JL Jr. Validity and reliability of diastolic pulse contour analysis (Windkessel model) in humans. *Hypertension.* 2002;39:963–968.
6. Mitchell GF, Izzo Jr JL, Lacourcière Y, et al. Omapatrilat reduces pulse pressure and proximal aortic stiffness in patients with systolic hypertension: results of the conduit hemodynamics of omapatrilat international research study. *Circulation.* 2002;105:2955–2961.
7. Mitchell GF, Pfeffer MA, Finn PV, Pfeffer JM. Equipotent antihypertensive agents variously affect pulsatile hemodynamics and regression of cardiac hypertrophy in spontaneously hypertensive rats. *Circulation.* 1996;94:2923–2929.
8. O'Rourke MF, Staessen JA, Vlachopoulos C, et al. Clinical applications of arterial stiffness; definitions and reference values. *Am J Hypertens.* 2002;15:426–444.
9. Rietzschel ER, Boeykens E, De Buyzere ML, et al. A comparison between systolic and diastolic pulse contour analysis in the evaluation of arterial stiffness. *Hypertension.* 2001;37:e15–e22. See also Cohn JN, Rietzschel ER. Techniques for studying arterial elastic properties. *Hypertension.* 2002;39:e20 (Letter).

Chapter C120

Evaluation of Aortocarotid Baroreflexes

Addison A. Taylor, MD, PhD

KEY POINTS

- Hypertension leads to baroreceptor resetting, blunted baroreflex control of the blood pressure, and increased blood pressure variability.

- Autonomic failure is associated with wide fluctuations in blood pressure, usually manifest as supine hypertension and orthostatic hypotension.

- Exaggerated baroreflex responses in the carotid sinus hypersensitivity syndrome can cause bradycardia, excessive vasodilation, or syncope.

- Pathophysiologically based diagnosis of autonomic dysfunction in patients with hypertension or orthostatic hypotension and syncope can improve therapeutic management.

See also Chapters A34–A37, A41, A60, C128, C151, and C161

The autonomic nervous system, through its sympathetic and parasympathetic divisions, modulates rapid adaptation of the cardiovascular system to changing conditions. This system is intimately involved in the maintenance of normal blood pressure (BP) during posture or temperature changes, metabolic alterations, or other environmental stresses. This precise regulation is achieved through a series of highly differentiated but closely integrated reflex arcs, including the aortocarotid, or high-pressure, and cardiopulmonary, or low-pressure, baroreflex arcs.

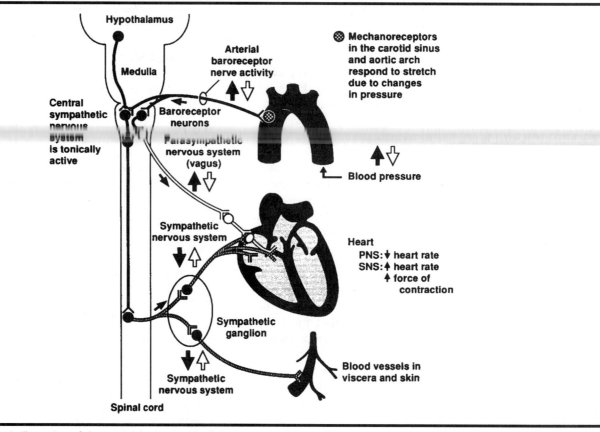

Figure C120.1. Schematic illustration of the essential components of the aortocarotid baroreflex arc. Autonomic neural responses to an increase in blood pressure (BP) are indicated by the upward pointing black arrows and autonomic neural responses to a decrease in BP by the downward pointing white arrows. PNS, parasympathetic nervous system; SNS, sympathetic nervous system.

Applied Pathophysiology

Components of baroreflex arcs. In its simplest form, the aortocarotid baroreflex arc consists of 3 basic components as illustrated in **Figure C120.1.** Sensory nerves located in the heart and in vascular tissue transmit afferent signals through the vagus and the glossopharyngeal cranial nerves and through the sympathetic nerves to the central nervous system. Internuncial neurons located in the brain stem integrate signals from the afferent sensory nerves and from the hypothalamus and higher cortical centers to modulate the activity of the autonomic efferent neurons. Efferent nerve tracts are divided into sympathetic and parasympathetic fibers, and each efferent tract consists of a 2-neuron chain.

The cell body of the first neuron in the sympathetic neuronal chain is located in the brain stem, and its axon terminates in the thoracic spinal sympathetic ganglion. The cell body of the second neuron in this chain is located in the sympathetic ganglion and terminates in a vascular structure such as the myocardium or blood vessel wall. In contrast, the first neuron in the parasympathetic chain extends from the brain stem to the vascular structure and synapses with a very short second neuron that is located entirely within that structure. Norepinephrine is the primary neurotransmitter released by the second neuron of the sympathetic chain, whereas acetylcholine is released by the second neuron of the parasympathetic chain.

Physiologic effects. The aortocarotid or arterial baroreflexes, also termed the *high-pressure baroreflexes*, derive their name

from the anatomic location of their afferent fibers. The sensory nerve fibers from the carotid arteries and aortic arch that comprise the afferent limb of this baroreflex are coupled to mechanoreceptors in the wall of the arteries that are sensitive to changes in stretch or transmural pressure. Chemoreceptor cells sensitive to carbon dioxide and, to a lesser extent, oxygen are also present in this region.

The aortocarotid baroreflex exhibits tonic activity under resting conditions. As illustrated by the black arrows in Figure C120.1, a rise in BP increases aortocarotid baroreceptor nerve activity. This heightened baroreceptor nerve firing stimulates parasympathetic nerve activity, resulting in a reduction in heart rate and cardiac output, and reduces sympathetic nerve activity, causing vasodilation and decreased cardiac contractility. These compensatory hemodynamic changes tend to return the elevated BP toward its previous value. As illustrated by the white arrows in Figure C120.1, the opposite effects are produced by a reduction in BP.

Several factors modulate the cardiovascular response to baroreflex activation. These include origin and strength of the activating stimulus, the "set point" of the reflex, neuronal input from the hypothalamus and higher cortical centers, and input from brain stem centers that modulate other autonomic functions such as respiration or gastrointestinal motility. Conditions influencing the heart and conduit arteries and the embedded stretch receptors such as arteriosclerosis can also lead to impaired baroreflex control. The modulatory influence of neurohumoral and vasoactive substances (catecholamines,

Table C120.1. Physiologic and Pharmacologic Maneuvers That Modulate Autonomic Cardiovascular Reflexes in Humans

AORTOCAROTID BAROREFLEXES	
ACTIVATE	**DEACTIVATE**
Neck pressure	Neck suction
Phenylephrine	Nitroglycerin
Angiotensin II	Amyl nitrite
Valsalva, phase IV	Nitroprusside

angiotensin, prostanoids, gonadal hormones, neuropeptides, etc.), and interactions of aortocarotid with cardiopulmonary baroreflex and chemoreflex arcs further modulate function of this complex system.

Assessment of Baroreflex Function

A variety of physiologic and pharmacologic maneuvers can be used to characterize the cardiovascular responses to autonomic reflex activation in normal subjects and to evaluate the integrity of the autonomic cardiovascular reflexes in patients with specific cardiovascular diseases. Some of the maneuvers and their effects on baroreflexes are summarized in **Table C120.1**.

Bedside assessment. Baroreceptor sensitivity is usually defined as a change in the R-R interval (reciprocal of the heart rate) on the electrocardiogram plotted as a function of the change in BP during the preceding cardiac cycle. Although a quantitative assessment of baroreceptor sensitivity requires continuous monitoring of the electrocardiogram and beat-to-beat BP, a qualitative assessment of baroreflex arc integrity can be obtained at the bedside by measuring the change in heart rate from baseline during Valsalva's maneuver for 15 seconds. The heart rate typically increases 10 to 30 beats per minute by the end of the 15-second Valsalva maneuver in normal individuals.

Laboratory assessment of autonomic function. BP and heart rate are the usual hemodynamic parameters monitored at the bedside to assess the effects of autonomic reflex activation, but a more comprehensive evaluation is obtained if 1 or more of the following hemodynamic measurements are also included: cardiac output, cardiac contractility, venous capacitance, peripheral and central venous pressure, and limb (forearm or leg) blood flow. Direct measurements of peripheral muscle sympathetic nerve firing rates in the arm or leg using microneurographic techniques provide a useful adjunct to these cardiovascular measures but are limited in their capacity to assess regional differences in sympathetic neural activity in specific vascular beds. In addition, these techniques are not widely available. Power spectral analysis of heart rate variability or arterial pressure signals provides an indirect assessment of changes in autonomic function, but there is controversy about which components of cardiovascular autonomic function are represented by low- versus high-frequency power spectra. Assessment of systemic and regional norepinephrine spillover rates, plasma norepinephrine and epinephrine concentrations, plasma renin activity, plasma angiotensin II concentrations, plasma arginine vasopressin, plasma atrial natriuretic peptides,

and measurements of adrenergic receptor number or affinity on circulating leukocytes or platelets offer additional, although indirect, information about the neurohormonal consequences of autonomic reflex activation.

Tilt-testing and other maneuvers. Changes in arterial high-pressure baroreceptor activity can be induced by any physiologic or pharmacologic maneuver that produces an abrupt increase or decrease in BP (Table C120.1). For example, the transient hypotension that occurs with standing or passive tilt results in a reflex increase in heart rate, whereas the post-Valsalva increase in BP causes reflex slowing. Substances such as α-adrenergic agonists or angiotensin II that increase BP produce reflex slowing of the heart rate, whereas agents such as sodium nitroprusside or hydralazine that lower BP directly by relaxing vascular smooth muscle augment sympathetic efferent nerve activity, heart rate, and cardiac contractility. The magnitude of the BP change in response to vasodilators and vasoconstrictors is inversely proportional to the degree of baroreceptor blunting. Maneuvers such as neck suction or neck pressure that alter the transmural pressure or stretch in the carotid sinus can also be used to activate or deactivate arterial baroreceptor reflexes (Table C120.1).

Age-adjustment. Because baroreceptor sensitivity decreases with age, the baroreceptor response obtained in a patient with suspected autonomic abnormalities should be compared with the response obtained in normal subjects of comparable age.

Clinical Syndromes of Baroreflex Dysfunction

Aortocarotid baroreflex abnormalities have been documented in a wide variety of clinical conditions in which autonomic neuronal control of BP is altered. Some of the more common conditions are summarized in **Table C120.2**. Optimal therapy in each of these conditions depends on the underlying pathophysiologic abnormality.

Impaired baroreflex function
Symptoms. Many of these conditions, most notably idiopathic orthostatic hypotension, multiple-system atrophy, and diabetes mellitus, are characterized by orthostatic lightheadedness, weakness, or syncope owing to interruption of the high-pressure baroreflex arc by the underlying disease. Palpitations and tachycardia may also occur, with or without accompanying BP change as in the postural orthostatic tachycardia syndrome.
Laboratory abnormalities. If the disease affects primarily the postganglionic nerve, as in diabetes mellitus or amyloidosis, supine resting plasma norepinephrine concentrations are reduced and do not increase with standing, a stimulus that usually results in an increase in plasma norepinephrine of 50% to 100% above the supine value. The patients also demonstrate increased pressor sensitivity to α-adrenergic agonists (phenylephrine) owing to vascular α-receptor upregulation. When the disease affects primarily the preganglionic sympathetic nerve, as in multiple-system atrophy, supine values for plasma norepinephrine are normal, but there is no increase with standing because the aortocarotid baroreflex arc is interrupted within the central nervous system. Because there is normal basal release of norepinephrine from the intact postganglionic nerve, sensitivity of vascular α-receptors to α-agonists is not altered.

Table C120.2. Selected Clinical Conditions Associated with Autonomic Dysfunction

Cardiovascular conditions	Environmental	Primary/unknown
Hypertension	Microgravity (space)	Carotid sinus hypersensitivity
Congestive heart failure	Prolonged bed rest	Idiopathic orthostatic hypotension
Myocardial infarction	Genetic diseases	Baroreceptor failure
Mitral valve prolapse	Familial dysautonomia	Psychiatric diseases
Drugs/toxins	Dopamine β-hydroxylase deficiency	Panic disorder
α-Adrenergic agonists	Neoplastic disorders	Agoraphobia
β-Adrenergic agonists	Spinal meningiomas	Trauma
Cocaine	Brain stem meningiomas	Spinal cord transection
Amphetamines	Systemic mastocytosis	Neurocardiogenic syncope
Endotoxin shock	Neurologic diseases	
Certain snake venoms	Friedreich's ataxia	
Cigarette smoking	Guillain-Barré syndrome	
Endocrine/metabolic diseases	Parkinson's disease	
Diabetes mellitus	Central nervous system demyelinating diseases	
Hyperthyroidism	Syringomyelia	
Fabry's disease	Multiple system atrophy	
	Familial dysautonomia	

Therapeutic implications. Identification of the site of baroreflex dysfunction has therapeutic implications. For example, orthostatic hypotension in patients with preganglionic disease often improves with a high-tyramine diet. Monoamine oxidase inhibitors can increase norepinephrine release from the normal postganglionic nerve and decrease its metabolism in the synaptic cleft in patients with preganglionic disease. On the other hand, patients with diseases involving the postganglionic nerve may respond to α-agonists such as phenylpropylamine, clonidine, and midodrine. All patients, regardless of the site of baroreflex dysfunction, require fluid volume expansion with a high-salt diet, often combined with the mineralocorticoid hormone, fludrocortisone.

Carotid sinus hypersensitivity
Clinical findings. Orthostatic lightheadedness, weakness, or syncope may also occur in patients with exaggerated activity of the aortocarotid baroreflex. Carotid sinus hypersensitivity is characterized by hypotension and syncope or near-syncope owing to mechanical deformation of the carotid sinus located at the bifurcation of the common carotid artery. Symptoms may be produced by lateral rotation or hyperextension of the neck or by wearing garments with tight-fitting collars that impinge on the carotid arteries. This condition has also been observed in patients with tumors of the neck that impinge on the carotid artery or encircle the glossopharyngeal or vagus nerves and in patients with extensive scarring in the neck secondary to radical neck dissection or prior radiation. In the majority of these patients, however, there is no obvious cause for the condition, although it tends to occur more frequently in the elderly. The diagnosis is established by demonstrating that massage of 1 carotid sinus for 5 to 10 seconds produces a fall of more than 50 mm Hg in the BP or a sinus pause of >3 seconds accompanied by near-syncopal or syncopal symptoms.
Subtypes and therapeutic implications. Three different types of carotid sinus syndrome have been noted and form the basis of the classification of this syndrome: (a) cardioinhibitory type (bradycardia only), (b) vasodepressor type (hypotension without bradycardia), and (c) mixed cardioinhibitory plus vasodepressor type. In patients who meet the criteria for cardioinhibitory carotid sinus

syndrome, it is essential to repeat the carotid sinus massage after insertion of a temporary transvenous pacemaker to maintain the heart rate. This excludes the possibility of a vasodepressor component that was undetected during the initial evaluation. If no significant vasodepressor component is demonstrated during carotid sinus massage with cardiac pacing, a permanent cardiac pacemaker of the dual chamber type usually prevents further symptoms. In the newest pacemakers, a rate-drop algorithm is incorporated into the firmware that activates the pacemaker impulse in response to a predetermined reduction in heart rate. A patient who has a significant vasodepressor component should be managed medically with elastic support garments, α-agonists, and with fluid expansion in a fashion similar to that described above for orthostatic hypotension. Should these options fail, surgical interruption of the carotid sinus reflex by stripping the adventitia from the carotid artery or by transection of the glossopharyngeal nerve as it enters the brain can be considered; this procedure has been reported to prevent symptoms in a small series of patients.

SUGGESTED READING

1. Akselrod S, Oz O, Greenberg M, et al. Autonomic response to change of posture among normal and mild-hypertensive adults: investigation by time-dependent spectral analysis. *J Auton Nerv Syst*. 1997;64:33–43.
2. Bannister R. *Autonomic Failure: A Textbook of Clinical Disorders of the Autonomic Nervous System*. 3rd ed. New York, NY: Oxford University Press; 1992.
3. Brignole M, Oddone D, Cogorno S, et al. Long-term outcome in symptomatic carotid sinus hypersensitivity. *Am Heart J*. 1992;123:687–692.
4. Farquhar WB, Taylor JA, Darling SE, et al. Abnormal baroreflex responses in patients with idiopathic orthostatic intolerance. *Circulation*. 2000;102:3086–3091.
5. Grubb BP, Olshansky B. *Syncope: Mechanisms and Management*. Armonk, NY: Futura Publishing; 1997.
6. Jordan J, Biaggioni I. How to diagnose, how to treat: diagnosis and treatment of supine hypertension in autonomic failure patients with orthostatic hypotension. *J Clin Hypertens (Greenwich)*. 2002;4:139–145.
7. Jordan J, Tank J, Shannon JR, et al. Baroreflex buffering and susceptibility to vasoactive drugs. *Circulation*. 2002;105:1459–1464.
8. Parati G, Di Rienzo M, Mancia G. How to measure baroreflex sensitivity: from the cardiovascular laboratory to daily life. *J Hypertens*. 2000;18:7–19.
9. Robertson D, Hollister AS, Biaggioni I, et al. The diagnosis and treatment of baroreflex failure. *N Engl J Med*. 1993;329:1449–1455.
10. Smit AA, Timmers HJ, Wieling W, et al. Long-term effects of carotid sinus denervation on arterial BP in humans. *Circulation*. 2002;105:1329–1335.

Chapter C121

Evaluation of the Failing Heart

Jay N. Cohn, MD

KEY POINTS

- Symptoms and signs of early heart failure can be very subtle and are best detected by careful history and examination for signs of sodium retention or exercise intolerance.

- Heart failure must be distinguished from depression, deconditioning, pulmonary diseases, venous diseases, and miscellaneous edema states.

- Left ventricular dysfunction and structural remodeling are assessed by physical examination and imaging, especially by detection of a sustained and diffuse apical impulse and by echocardiographic evidence of left ventricular dilation, increased wall thickness, or reduced wall motion.

See also Chapters A59–A62, A66, A67, A78, B81, B83, C115, C116, C155, and C156

Major Pathogenetic Factors in Heart Failure

Heart failure commonly develops in patients with a history of hypertension. It also dramatically increases in prevalence with increasing age. The pathogenesis of heart failure in the hypertensive individual is multifactorial. Three major factors must be considered in the patient presenting with signs and symptoms: increased afterload, aging influences, and the presence of coronary artery disease. Occasionally other etiologies exist.

Systolic hypertension (increased afterload). A chronic increase in systolic blood pressure (BP), both at rest and during daily activity, imposes a load on the left ventricle that results in myocyte hypertrophy, interstitial collagen growth, and relative coronary insufficiency. Impaired diastolic relaxation is usually the first manifestation of left ventricular (LV) dysfunction, but impaired contraction (systolic dysfunction) also may occur.

Aging. Aging interacts with hypertension in several ways to increase ventricular load and decrease ventricular performance (see Chapters A59–A62); it is associated with myocyte loss, hypertrophy of surviving myocytes, and interstitial growth. The resulting diastolic and systolic dysfunction in older individuals may be indistinguishable from those complicating systolic hypertension.

Coronary artery disease. Coronary insufficiency, myocardial ischemia, and myocardial infarction are complications of obstructive coronary atherosclerosis that may be accelerated in hypertensive individuals. Regional wall motion abnormalities from these coronary syndromes commonly contribute to systolic dysfunction.

Other causes. Valvular, idiopathic, postviral, infiltrative, toxic, and other rare causes of heart failure exist and can be recognized by characteristic patterns.

Diagnosis

Heart failure must be distinguished from other clinical conditions (e.g., depression, deconditioning, pulmonary disease, venous insufficiency) and miscellaneous edema states, including that induced by vasodilator drugs.

Symptoms. Heart failure is a symptomatic disease, but a long course of asymptomatic LV dysfunction usually precedes overt heart failure. Early diagnosis can be hampered by the fact that symptoms may be quite subtle, often depending on the activity level of the individual patient. Fatigue, orthopnea, nocturnal dyspnea, nocturia, and pedal edema are common early manifestations.

Clinical signs

Jugular veins. The most sensitive guide to volume overload is an elevated jugular venous pressure (JVP), either at rest or in response to right upper quadrant abdominal pressure (positive hepatojugular reflux), passive leg raising, or exercise. Detecting the top of the deep venous pulsation in the neck is facilitated by positioning the patient in a partially upright position. A resting JVP level more than 10 cm above the right atrium or a sustained increase in response to these maneuvers suggests heart failure. Because the JVP only indirectly assesses LV function, this assessment cannot distinguish right ventricular dysfunction (e.g., cor pulmonale) from LV dysfunction.

Cardiac examination. The presence of LV structural change can often be detected by physical examination. With the patient lying in the left lateral position, palpation of the LV apex can detect LV hypertrophy (a sustained outward thrust rather than a short tap) and LV dilation (a heave that covers an area of the chest larger than a 50-cent piece).

Auscultation of the heart can reveal murmurs of aortic valve or, more commonly, mitral valve dysfunction. Mitral regurgitation is a common finding with a dilated left ventricle, but severe mitral regurgitation also may contribute to progressive LV remodeling. Aortic insufficiency may be detected in the presence of a high diastolic pressure and may disappear with BP control. A fourth heart sound (S_4) is common in heart failure, particularly when hypertension is an important contributor, and is usually indicative of increased atrial pressure and increased ventricular stiffness, with or without chamber dilation. A third heart sound (S_3) suggests more severe LV dysfunction, usually with ventricular dilation.

Pulmonary examination. Lung sounds vary in heart failure. The presence of fine rales is usually a sign of increased lung water and high left atrial pressure. The presence of decreased breath sounds or dullness to percussion at the lung bases may indicate pleural effusion and increased right atrial pressure.

Extremities. Dependent edema is a common finding in heart failure. Edema also may occur in patients with venous insufficiency, decreased serum albumin concentration, or renal failure and in response to vasodilator drugs (in particular, calcium antagonists).

Electrocardiogram and arrhythmias.

The electrocardiogram is usually, but not always, abnormal in heart failure. Commonly, there are voltage criteria for LV hypertrophy, widened QRS complex, ST-T abnormalities, localized loss of voltage (see Chapter A61), or Q waves.

Atrial and ventricular arrhythmias are common in patients with LV dysfunction. They are best viewed as manifestations of the structural disease rather than abnormalities requiring specific antiarrhythmic therapy. Adequate management of dilated cardiomyopathy often causes marked improvement in the frequency of atrial and ventricular arrhythmias. However, recent data suggesting the benefit on life expectancy of implanted defibrillators may encourage Holter monitoring to detect nonsustained ventricular tachycardia, especially when accompanied by presyncopal symptoms.

Echocardiogram.

Echocardiography is essential for quantitating wall thickness, chamber size, systolic emptying [ejection fraction (EF)], and regional wall motion abnormalities. The clinical syndrome of heart failure is always accompanied by LV dysfunction, which can be manifested by a spectrum of abnormalities from pure diastolic dysfunction (impairment of filling) to a dilated, remodeled ventricle with reduced wall motion. Doppler examination can provide an assessment of diastolic filling characteristics by the relationship between filling in early and late diastole (see Chapters C116 and C165).

Biochemical tests.

A blood sample for assay of B-type natriuretic peptide (BNP), a test available in many medical facilities, may help to distinguish heart failure from other conditions (see Chapter A15). A level above 100 pg per mL is usually indicative of LV dysfunction, which can confirm that symptoms are likely due to heart failure.

Systolic versus Diastolic Dysfunction

Echo distinction between diastolic dysfunction and so-called systolic dysfunction (dilated, remodeled ventricle) is somewhat subjective. All patients with elevated cardiac filling pressure have an element of diastolic dysfunction. When the left ventricle is not enlarged (diastolic transverse diameter <2.7 cm/m^2 body surface area) and EF nearly normal (>45%), the syndrome is often called *pure diastolic dysfunction* or *heart failure with preserved systolic function* (see Chapter C155). The distinction is of considerable importance because most clinical trial data have been collected in patients with EF ≤35%. In the latter group, therapy to prevent progressive LV remodeling (angiotensin-converting enzyme inhibitors, β-blockers) is essential. In those patients with predominant diastolic dysfunction, treatment to normalize hemodynamics takes precedence.

Overall Strategy

In planning the workup and therapeutic strategy for patients presenting with heart failure, the physician must attempt to determine the relative contribution of hypertension, aging, and coronary artery disease to the development of the syndrome. When elevated BP is paramount, aggressive pressure control may be an adequate approach. When myocardial ischemia or infarction is suspected, studies of myocardial perfusion or coronary anatomy may be required. Therapeutic goals in heart failure depend on the nature and severity of the underlying condition. The goals in managing patients with high risk for heart failure is early recognition and aggressive therapy to prevent progression. Early recognition before the development of advanced symptoms provides the possibility of effective preventive strategies that can result in normal lifestyle and normal life expectancy. The hypertensive individual is at particular risk and should be screened at regular intervals for early markers of symptoms or signs of LV dysfunction. Symptomatic heart failure is a progressive disease with a poor overall prognosis for quality of life and life expectancy. Effective therapy of advanced symptomatic disease relieves symptoms and substantially prolongs life (see Chapter C156). Most of the therapy currently used to treat the failing heart results in a lowering of BP. Although BP reduction is not the sole benefit of these drugs, it is clear that the dysfunctional left ventricle performs best when there is a low impedance to ejection. Thus, both in preventing heart failure and in treating it, BP control must be aggressively pursued.

SUGGESTED READING

1. Cohn JN. Vasodilator therapy for heart failure: the influence of impedance on left ventricular performance. *Circulation.* 1973;48:5–8.
2. Cohn JN. Jugular venous pressure monitoring: a lost art? *J Card Fail.* 1997;3:71–73.
3. Cohn JN. Pathophysiology and clinical recognition of heart failure. In: Willerson JT, Cohn JN, eds. *Cardiovascular Medicine.* 2nd ed. New York, NY: Churchill Livingstone; 2000:1147–1164.
4. Kannel WB, Castelli WP, McNamara PM. Role of blood pressure in the development of congestive heart failure. The Framingham Study. *N Engl J Med.* 1972;287:781–787.
5. Maisel A. B-Type natriuretic peptide levels: a potential "white count" for congestive heart failure. *J Card Fail.* 2001;7:183–193.
6. Wong M, Johnson G, Shabetai R, et al., for the V-HeFT VA Cooperative Studies Group. Echocardiographic variables as prognostic indicators and therapeutic monitors in chronic congestive heart failure: Veterans Affairs Cooperative Studies V-HeFT I and II. *Circulation.* 1993;87:VI-65–70.

Evaluation of the Peripheral Circulation

Jeffrey W. Olin, DO

KEY POINTS

- Evaluation of the entire vascular system is important because of the increased prevalence of peripheral arterial disease in patients with hypertension.

- The primary symptom of peripheral arterial disease is intermittent claudication, but many patients have atypical leg symptoms or no symptoms at all.

- Evaluation of the peripheral circulation includes functional testing (ankle-brachial index, pulse volume recordings) and imaging (duplex ultrasound, computed tomography angiography, magnetic resonance angiography, arteriography).

- Blood pressure should be measured in both arms to detect the presence of innominate or subclavian artery stenosis due to atherosclerosis.

See also Chapters A65–A68, B81, B85, C110, C119, C157, and C158

Evaluation of the peripheral circulation is extremely important in the hypertensive patient because hypertension is a potent risk factor for the development of peripheral arterial disease (PAD), carotid atherosclerosis, and aneurysmal disease. The Framingham Study showed a significant relationship between systolic and diastolic blood pressure (BP) levels and the 26-year incidence of intermittent claudication.

Signs and Symptoms

Cold hands and feet are poor clues to the presence of arterial insufficiency because they also occur in patients who are extremely anxious, have overactivity of the sympathetic nervous system, or have vasospastic disease. Some patients have a condition called *vasomotor instability* that prevents the blood vessel from reacting normally to exogenous stimuli such as differences in ambient temperature. There are several clues in a patient's history that suggest the presence of carotid atherosclerosis, PAD, or aneurysmal disease.

Transient ischemia. A history of transient ischemic attacks (focal neurologic deficit that resolves within 24 hours), including amaurosis fugax (monocular blindness), aphasia, dysphagia, hemiparesis, hemiplegia, focal sensory abnormalities, and stroke suggests the presence of cardiac disease, aortic arch atherosclerosis, or carotid artery atherosclerosis.

Claudication. The primary symptom of PAD is intermittent claudication, which is characterized as discomfort, pain, cramping, tightness, heaviness, or tiredness in 1 or more muscle groups in the lower extremities. Most commonly, it occurs in the calf as a result of superficial femoral artery obstruction. However, thigh, hip, or buttock claudication may occur in patients with aortoiliac occlusive disease. As a general rule, the discomfort is brought on by exercise (usually walking) and is quickly relieved within 2 to 5 minutes after the individual stops

walking. Intermittent claudication can usually be differentiated from pseudoclaudication (neurogenic claudication) caused by lumbar canal stenosis or disc disease on the basis of the history and physical examination (**Table C122.1**). In recent years, it has been recognized that some patients with PAD [identified by a low ankle-brachial index (ABI)] have atypical leg symptoms or no symptoms at all. This has led some investigators to suggest that ABI be measured in all patients >70 years old or in patients between 50 and 69 years of age with a history of smoking or diabetes.

Advanced vascular disease. When vascular disease becomes advanced, the patient may experience pain at rest, indicating that critical limb ischemia is present. It is not uncommon for individuals with rest pain to hang their leg over the side of the bed or sleep sitting in a chair so that gravity can improve the circulation to the lower extremity and thus relieve the nocturnal pain. This may lead to significant edema, which may falsely lead the clinician to suspect venous or lymphatic disease.

Physical Examination of the Circulation

Blood pressure measurements. At the initial physical examination, BP should be measured in both arms. If the BPs are different, the higher value should be used for subsequent BP readings. A discrepancy in BP readings between arms is usually indicative of innominate or subclavian artery stenosis (commonly owing to atherosclerosis but may also occur secondary to radiation-induced vascular disease, fibromuscular dysplasia, or inflammatory vascular diseases such as Takayasu's arteritis or giant cell arteritis) on the side of the lower BP. Occasionally, bilateral subclavian artery stenosis occurs. Under these circumstances, the BP is higher in the legs than in the arms.

Table C122.1. Differentiating (Vascular) Claudication from Pseudoclaudication

	CLAUDICATION	PSEUDOCLAUDICATION
Character of discomfort	Discomfort, pain, cramping, tightness, heaviness, tiredness, numbness.	Same or tingling, weakness, or clumsiness.
Location of discomfort	Buttock, hip, thigh, calf, foot.	Same.
Exercise induced	Always.	May or may not be.
Distance to claudication	Same each time.	Highly variable.
Occurs with standing	No.	Yes or no.
Relief	Stop walking. Discomfort usually disappears in 2–5 min	Often must sit, lean, or change body positions. Discomfort may take up to 15–20 min to disappear.

Adapted from Krajewski LP, Olin JW. Atherosclerosis of the aorta and lower extremities. In: Young JR, Graor RA, Olin JW, Bartholomew JR, eds. *Peripheral Vascular Diseases*. St. Louis, MO: Mosby Year Book; 1991:183.

Neck examination

Palpation. The carotid arteries should be palpated in every hypertensive patient. The carotid artery should be palpated low in the neck, at the level of the thyroid gland anterior to the sternocleidomastoid muscle. The carotid bifurcation (located at the angle of the jaw) should be avoided because palpation of this area may cause significant bradycardia or asystole in patients who have a hypersensitive carotid sinus; palpation at the carotid bifurcation may also cause dislodgment of atheromatous material, producing a transient ischemic attack or a stroke. A fullness in the carotid pulsation in the elderly is most commonly due to a tortuous (kinked) carotid artery. Carotid artery aneurysms are quite uncommon. The subclavian artery pulse should be palpated in the supraclavicular fossa with the thumb while the fingers are placed behind the neck. The character of the pulsation as well as the presence or absence of an aneurysm should be noted. Next, the superficial temporal artery should be palpated. A decrease in the arterial pulsation may indicate stenosis of the common or external carotid artery.

Auscultation. After careful palpation, one should listen in the cervical and supraclavicular regions for the presence of bruits. Bruits can be heard best with the bell of the stethoscope with the patient in the sitting position. The location and quality of the bruit should be described and characterized as being a systolic bruit or a combined systolic and diastolic bruit. It is important to listen over the base of the heart to be certain that the bruit is not a transmitted murmur from the aortic or pulmonary valve. A bruit that is heard during both systole and diastole indicates that there may be severe bilateral carotid artery disease. In fact, the artery on the contralateral side to the systolic/diastolic bruit is often more severely stenotic than the index vessel or is totally occluded (**Figure C122.1**). Other conditions that cause a systolic/diastolic bruit include arteriovenous malformation, arteriovenous fistula, and a venous hum. A venous hum is usually heard at the base of the neck and can easily be detected by its disappearance on light compression of the external jugular vein.

Upper extremities. The axillary, brachial, radial, and ulnar pulses should be palpated. If there is evidence of ischemia of the hands or fingers or if there is any reason to believe that the arteries distal to the wrist are diseased, an Allen test should be performed. The patient is asked to make a tight fist, which causes most of the blood to empty from the hands and fingers. The examiners' thumbs then swipe over the thenar and hypothenar eminences to occlude the radial and ulnar arteries. When the patient opens his or her hand, it should be blanched.

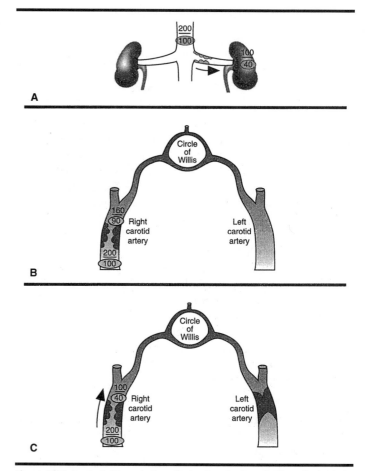

Figure C122.1. Systolic and diastolic bruits. **A:** Systolic/diastolic bruit in the renal artery. During systole, blood moves through a narrow arterial segment, turbulence is produced, and a bruit is heard. If the stenosis is severe enough, there is a significant pressure gradient during diastole as well (i.e., 100 vs. 40 mm Hg), blood continues to flow in a forward direction (*arrow*), and a systolic/diastolic bruit is heard. **B:** The right carotid artery is severely narrowed, turbulence is produced, and a systolic bruit is heard. Because the left carotid artery is patent, there is crossover flow from the left carotid through the circle of Willis maintaining pressure up in the distal right carotid artery. No forward flow occurs during diastole, and no diastolic bruit is heard. **C:** The left carotid artery is occluded, and there is no crossover from the left cerebral hemisphere. Pressure in the distal right carotid artery is very low, there is a substantial diastolic pressure gradient (*circled numbers*), blood flows forward (*arrow*) during diastole, and a systolic/diastolic bruit is heard, indicating severe stenosis or occlusion of the contralateral carotid artery.

When the radial or ulnar artery is released, prompt return of color to the hand indicates that the artery is open distal to the wrist. The maneuver is then repeated releasing the second artery. A positive test is failure of the hand to return to normal color promptly on release of the occluded artery.

Chest examination. The chest should be examined because occasionally a large aneurysm in the ascending aorta may be visualized or palpated as a pulsation high in the chest near the suprasternal notch. The bruit of aortic coarctation is best heard over the left subscapular area in most cases.

Abdominal examination. An attempt should be made to palpate the abdominal aorta during the physical examination. Infrarenal abdominal aortic aneurysms are not uncommon in the elderly hypertensive patient. By palpating the lateral border and the medial border of the aorta at the same time, the examiner can assess the size of the aorta. Gently rolling the aorta back and forth under the fingertips can help differentiate an aneurysm from a tortuous aorta. Careful auscultation of the abdomen for the presence of bruits (systolic, systolic/diastolic) in the epigastric region may reveal stenosis of the celiac artery, superior mesenteric artery, or renal arteries. A short systolic bruit is often heard in thin individuals and is generally not a cause of concern (Figure C122.1A).

Lower extremities. Pulses in the lower extremities should be graded as normal, diminished, or absent. The femoral pulse should be palpated just below the inguinal ligament, with firm, constant pressure applied to feel the pulse, which is deep in most individuals. The size of the femoral artery should be noted, and an aneurysm should be considered if it is large. The amplitude and timing of the pulse should be compared with those of the radial artery, which may be diminished and delayed in coarctation of the aorta. The popliteal pulse should be palpated in every individual. This pulse is often the most difficult for physicians to detect. Normally, the pulse can be found directly under the lateral aspect of the patella with the knee flexed <10 degrees. Firm pressure must be applied to allow the fingers to go deep into the popliteal space. The artery should be palpated with the pads of the fingers and not the fingertips. Popliteal artery aneurysms occur in 20% of patients with abdominal aortic aneurysms. The major complication of a popliteal aneurysm is thrombosis; when thrombosis occurs, the limb may become acutely ischemic, leading to limb loss in up to 50% of individuals. Next, the posterior tibial, dorsalis pedis, and peroneal pulses should be palpated. The posterior tibial pulse can be felt posterior to the medial malleolus. The dorsalis pedis pulse is usually located over the second metatarsal bones. The dorsalis pedis pulse may not be detected in some normal individuals because the anterior tibial artery dives deep at the level of the ankle. If the dorsalis pedis pulse cannot be detected, one should attempt to find the anterior tibial artery. If neither can be felt, the peroneal artery can often be detected in the lateral aspect of the ankle.

Advanced Diagnostic Studies

Carotid imaging. If carotid artery atherosclerosis is suspected, a duplex ultrasound examination of the carotid arteries is warranted. The indications for carotid duplex ultrasound are

---

Table C122.2. Indications for Carotid Ultrasonography

Asymptomatic cervical bruit
Amaurosis fugax
Hemispheric transient ischemic attack
Stroke in a potential candidate for carotid endarterectomy or stent
Follow-up of a known stenosis (>20%) in asymptomatic individuals
Follow-up after carotid endarterectomy or stent
Intraoperative assessment of carotid endarterectomy
Unexplained neck pain (to evaluate for carotid dissection)

---

listed in **Table C122.2.** Carotid ultrasonography can determine the degree of stenosis of the common carotid artery, the external carotid artery, and the internal carotid artery. The intracranial portion of the internal carotid artery cannot be adequately visualized with this technique. Although arteriography has been required in the past if carotid endarterectomy was to be performed, most centers now perform carotid endarterectomy on the basis of the results of carotid ultrasound alone. Therefore, it is very important to be certain that the vascular laboratory is accredited and that appropriate quality control measures are followed.

Abdominal imaging. An ultrasound, spiral computed tomography scan, or magnetic resonance angiogram can confirm the presence of an abdominal aortic aneurysm and give an accurate assessment of its size and location. An ultrasound examination is useful in determining the size of the femoral or popliteal arteries if aneurysms are suspected. Often, the vascular surgeon operates on the basis of a computed tomography scan or magnetic resonance angiogram. Aortic stent grafting has replaced open aortic aneurysm reconstruction in many patients, therefore an angiogram is obtained at the time of the stent graft placement.

Peripheral arterial disease detection. If the patient has intermittent claudication, ischemic rest pain, or digital ulcerations, the circulation can be assessed noninvasively with Doppler BPs and pulse volume recordings (pulse waveform analysis). **Ankle-brachial index.** The least expensive way to screen for the presence of PAD is to measure the ABI. An ABI can easily be performed in any physician's office to accurately predict the severity of PAD and the risk of future cardiovascular events. With a hand-held Doppler (5–10 MHz), the systolic BP should be measured in both arms, followed by the systolic BP in the right and left posterior tibial and dorsalis pedis arteries. A sample worksheet for measuring the ABI is shown in **Figure C122.2.** Recent data have shown that 29% of primary care patients >70 years old or between the ages of 50 and 69 years (with at least a 10–pack year history of smoking or the presence of diabetes) have PAD documented by measuring the ABI. More than 50% of patients identified with PAD on the basis of an abnormal ABI do not have typical claudication or leg pain at rest but nondescript leg pain, reduced ambulation, and a reduced quality of life. It has clearly been shown that the lower the ABI, the greater the risk of a cardiovascular death (myocardial infarction, stroke, vascular death). Patients with an ABI <0.40 and critical limb ischemia have a mortality of 25% per year. A useful algorithm for the evaluation of patients is shown in **Figure C122.3.** Patients with calcified blood vessels and a falsely elevated ABI should have a toe-brachial index measured.

Patient Name: _____

Date: _____   Patient Number: _____

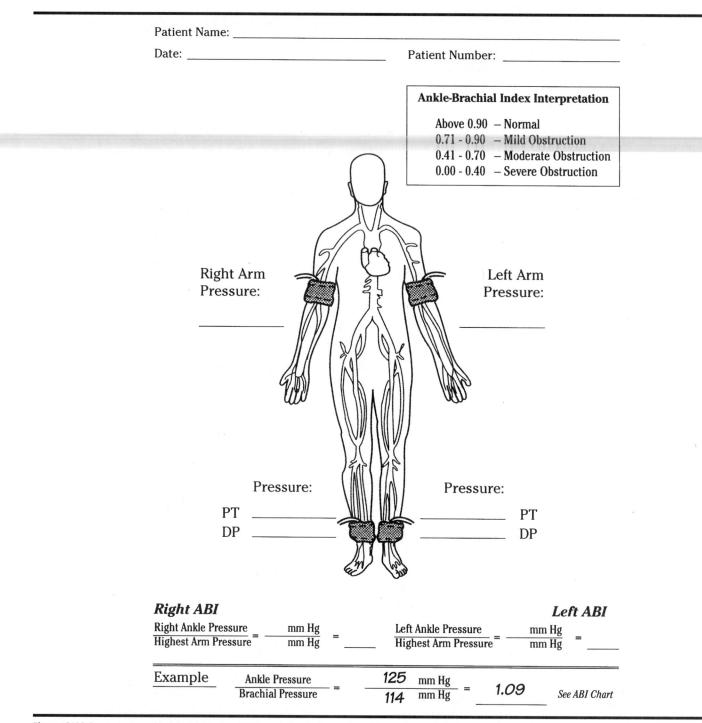

Ankle-Brachial Index Interpretation

Above 0.90 – Normal
0.71 - 0.90 – Mild Obstruction
0.41 - 0.70 – Moderate Obstruction
0.00 - 0.40 – Severe Obstruction

Right Arm
Pressure:

Left Arm
Pressure:

_____

_____

Pressure:

Pressure:

PT _____

_____ PT

DP _____

_____ DP

Right ABI

$$\frac{\text{Right Ankle Pressure}}{\text{Highest Arm Pressure}} = \frac{\text{mm Hg}}{\text{mm Hg}} = \underline{\quad}$$

Left ABI

$$\frac{\text{Left Ankle Pressure}}{\text{Highest Arm Pressure}} = \frac{\text{mm Hg}}{\text{mm Hg}} = \underline{\quad}$$

Example $\dfrac{\text{Ankle Pressure}}{\text{Brachial Pressure}} = \dfrac{125 \text{ mm Hg}}{114 \text{ mm Hg}} = 1.09$ *See ABI Chart*

Figure C122.2.   Sample ankle-brachial index (ABI) worksheet. (Reproduced from the Society for Vascular Medicine and Biology, *Peripheral arterial disease: marker of cardiovascular risk*, with permission.)

Segmental pressures and waveforms. Segmental pressures can be measured by placing BP cuffs at the high thigh, calf, ankle, transmetatarsal region, and toe. Pressures and pulse volume waveforms are obtained at each level, and an ABI is obtained by comparing BPs in the ankle and in the arm. After this examination is performed in the resting position, the patient exercises on a treadmill, and repeat BPs and pulse waveforms are obtained. Segmental pressure measurements help determine the location of the arterial obstruction or predict the level at which an amputation should occur. Although most patients with significant PAD demonstrate a decrease in the arterial pulsation, some have normal arterial pulses at rest. Therefore, it is important to perform pulse volume recordings and Doppler BPs not only at rest but after the patient has walked on a treadmill until symptoms are reproduced. When arterial obstruction is present, the pressures in the ankles decrease after exercise.

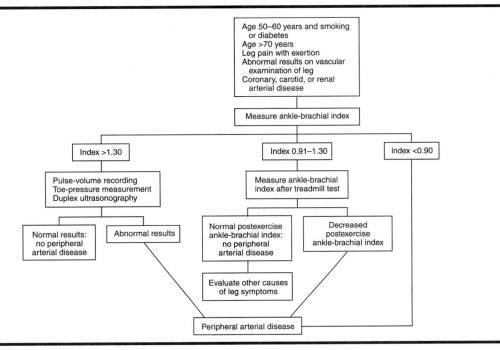

Figure C122.3. Evaluation algorithm for arterial disease.

Studies in advanced disease. In severe arterial insufficiency (rest pain, ischemic ulcerations, or gangrene) or disabling claudication, the patient may require a magnetic resonance arteriogram or a digital subtraction arteriogram to determine whether revascularization (endovascular or surgical) is feasible.

SUGGESTED READING

1. Hiatt WR. Medical treatment of peripheral arterial disease and claudication. *N Engl J Med*. 2001;344:1608–1621.
2. Hirsch AT, Criqui MH, Treat-Jacobson D, et al. Peripheral arterial disease detection, awareness, and treatment in primary care. *JAMA*. 2001;286:1317–1324.
3. Kannel WB, McGee DL. Update on some epidemiologic features of intermittent claudication: the Framingham Study. *J Am Geriatr Soc*. 1985;33:13–18.
4. Sumner DS. Volume plethysmography in vascular disease. In: Bernstein EF, ed. *Vascular Diagnosis*. 4th ed. St. Louis, MO: Mosby; 1993:181–193.
5. Thompson RW, Geraghty PJ, Lee JK. Abdominal aortic aneurysms: basic mechanisms and clinical implications. *Curr Probl Surg*. 2002;39:110–230.
6. Dormandy JA, Rutherford RB. Management of peripheral arterial disease (PAD). TASC Working Group. TransAtlantic Inter-Society Consensus (TASC). *J Vasc Surg*. 2000;31:S1–S296.
7. Yao JST. Pressure measurement in the extremity. In: Bernstein EF, ed. *Vascular Diagnosis*. 4th ed. St. Louis, MO: Mosby; 1993:169–175.
8. Young JR. Physical examination. In: Young JR, Olin JW, Bartholomew JR, eds. *Peripheral Vascular Diseases*. 2nd ed. St. Louis, MO: CV Mosby Co; 1996:18–32.

Chapter C123

Evaluation of Renovascular Disease

Stephen C. Textor, MD

KEY POINTS

- Evaluation of renovascular hypertension is undertaken to determine the potential benefits versus risks of renal revascularization; potential hazards and expense of diagnosis and intervention must be weighed against the likelihood of progressive vascular occlusion and compromised renal function.

- Magnetic resonance angiography provides nontoxic intravascular imaging and estimation of renal functional mass, whereas duplex ultrasonography provides an inexpensive means of following vascular lesions in serial fashion.

- Introduction of effective medical therapy, noninvasive imaging, and endovascular stent procedures make evaluation of renovascular disease a rapidly evolving field.

See also Chapters A41, A48, A58, A71, B84, C110, C111, C118, C128, C133, and C168

Recognition that reduced renal perfusion pressures can produce elevated blood pressure (BP) regularly leads to efforts directed at identification and correction of renal perfusion defects. Among older individuals with treatment-resistant hypertension, renovascular disease remains common. Recent advances in imaging, medical therapy (including agents capable of blocking the renin-angiotensin system), and endovascular techniques have combined to make this a rapidly changing clinical field.

Prevalence

Occurrence of renovascular disease may be increasing because declining mortality rates from coronary and cerebrovascular disease have increased the population available to develop atherosclerotic renal vascular disease. Some degree of renal artery stenosis may be found in 20% to 45% of patients with atherosclerotic disease of the coronary or peripheral vascular beds. Many instances of renal artery stenosis are of only minor hemodynamic significance because a 70% stenosis is usually necessary to cause hemodynamic compromise.

Definition and Applied Pathophysiology

True renovascular hypertension refers to the syndrome of elevated arterial BPs produced by reduced renal perfusion. Practically, this is best defined as a BP reduction after successful renal revascularization. Arterial hypertension due to renal artery stenosis results from 2 major mechanisms (see Chapter A48). The first is activation of renal pressor mechanisms, including activation of the renin-angiotensin system, which evokes a rise in systemic arterial hypertension sufficient to restore perfusion of the kidney. This pattern is characteristically seen in unilateral (Goldblatt) stenosis. The second mechanism that raises BP is reduced salt and water exaction, which characterizes bilateral renal artery stenosis or stenosis of the renal artery of a solitary kidney.

Goals of Evaluation

Studies to evaluate renovascular disease are typically directed toward 1 or more of the following: (a) establishing a causal role and hemodynamic significance of a lesion, (b) estimating the likelihood of benefit from renal revascularization, and (c) establishing whether "critical" renal artery stenosis poses the risk of progressive renal injury, often designated *ischemic nephropathy*. Advances in medical therapy have made "resistant hypertension" less pressing as the sole motivation for investigation and revascularization of renal artery stenosis. Concern about progressive vascular occlusion and loss of the kidneys is now the major rationale for diagnosing renovascular hypertension and initiating intervention. This analysis remains difficult, however, and there are no specific tests of renal viability. Hence, the clinician must consider from the beginning precisely what goals may be achieved by undertaking diagnostic evaluation of the renal circulation. Often this centers on examining the role of renal artery lesions in producing a spectrum of manifestations as identified in **Figure C123.1**.

Clinical Clues in Renovascular Disease

Demographics. Fibromuscular disease of the renal arteries can appear at any age but has a strong predilection for young women. Atherosclerotic disease has become the predominant renal artery lesion in Western countries and increases in frequency with advancing age. Most atherosclerotic disease is superimposed on essential hypertension, which accounts in part for the low rate of true "cure" with successful renal revascularization. The effectiveness of recent antihypertensive therapy and constraints on the cost of diagnostic testing contribute to the fact that many patients with renal artery stenosis and true renovascular hypertension remain undetected. When BP can be controlled with a simple regimen and renal function remains stable, there is little impetus to pursue correctable causes of hypertension. As a result, much renovascular disease

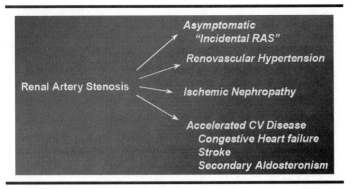

Figure C123.1. Issues in renovascular disease. CV, cardiovascular; RAS, renin-angiotensin system.

is identified during evaluation of recognizable syndromes as identified in **Table C123.1**.

"Functional" renal failure with angiotensin-converting enzyme inhibition. Introduction of agents that block the renin-angiotensin system has changed the presentation of renovascular disease and the implications of testing. Maintenance of glomerular filtration depends on the efferent arteriolar constrictive actions of angiotensin II during glomerular hypoperfusion. In this setting, blocking the generation or actions of angiotensin II has the potential to reduce filtration pressure, producing "*functional* acute renal insufficiency." Use of angiotensin-converting enzyme (ACE) inhibitors in proteinuric glomerular diseases and heart failure has inadvertently identified individuals at risk for unsuspected renovascular disease. Corollaries to this observation are 2-fold: (a) the clinician must be attuned to the possibility of unsuspected renal artery disease when encountering deteriorating renal function or "flash pulmonary edema," with circulatory congestion out of proportion to left ventricular systolic function, or (b) the clinician must give consideration to the possibility of progressive atherosclerotic occlusive disease if stenotic lesions are not corrected.

Imaging Studies

Renal artery lesions are commonly identified during noninvasive imaging procedures. In many instances, these procedures are undertaken primarily to exclude unilateral or bilateral renal artery disease.

Captopril renography. This test is widely used to rule out high-grade renal artery disease. Administration of captopril (or other ACE inhibitors) magnifies the functional difference between kidneys related to accumulation of radionuclide not removed by glomerular filtration in the affected kidney. The

Table C123.1. Syndromes of Renovascular Disease

Paroxysmal hypertension
Treatment-resistant hypertension
Bilateral disease/solitary functioning kidney
    Progressive renal failure in treated hypertension
    Renal failure limiting antihypertensive therapy
    Pulmonary vascular congestion ("flash" pulmonary edema)
    End-stage renal disease

renogram does not provide direct imaging of the renal vessels themselves and must be considered an indirect assessment of renal blood supply. When performed carefully in patients with near-normal renal function, several series indicate that a normal captopril renogram excludes renal artery stenosis with a very high negative predictive value. When renal function is poor (creatinine levels ≥ 2.0 mg/dL), the likelihood of false-positive scans rises, and the renogram is less reliable.

Doppler ultrasound of the renal arteries. In most institutions, Doppler study of the renal arteries is among the least expensive tests available, and it can measure gradients serially to track progression of stenosis. When carefully performed and identification of the renal arteries is unequivocal, Doppler studies can produce highly reliable estimates of renal artery flow velocity. A rise in velocity (to more than 200 cm/second or to a value higher than the aortic velocities with renal-aortic ratio ≥ 3.5) is considered predictive of stenosis (more than 60% luminal narrowing). Positive studies are nearly always confirmed at angiography, but the rates of false-negative studies are significant, particularly when obesity makes location of the renal vessels difficult. Examination of the Doppler waveforms distal to the main renal artery segments within the kidney can establish disturbances in waveforms (designated *parvus* and *tardus*) that indicate more proximal functional obstruction. The drawbacks of Doppler ultrasound include the fact that no functional assessment of the kidney itself is available, that it can be technically demanding and time consuming, and that some individuals are not technically suitable for study. Accessory renal arteries cannot be identified reliably by this method.

Gadolinium-contrast magnetic resonance angiography. Gadolinium-contrast magnetic resonance angiography provides imaging of the main renal arteries and some estimate of renal function, as assessed by clearance of the contrast agent. Although expensive, this method offers the most complete noninvasive imaging of the renal vasculature with a nonnephrotoxic agent. The latter feature makes it the method of choice for patients with impaired renal function. It is limited by cost and availability; because it offers clear images of only the proximal renal artery segments, it may miss distal lesions or accessory vessels.

Contrast arteriography. Contrast arteriography remains the gold standard for evaluation and identification of renal artery lesions and is now most commonly performed at the time of planned endovascular intervention (balloon angioplasty or stent deployment). It is also performed at the time of imaging of the aorta before planned surgical procedures that may involve aortic and renal artery repair. The hazards of arteriography include atheroembolic disease and contrast nephrotoxicity, particularly in older subjects with preexisting renal insufficiency or diabetes.

Assessment of Renal Artery Disease

Assessment of the functional significance of renal artery stenosis remains a challenge to clinicians. "Side-to-side" comparisons have been proposed to (a) establish whether hemodynamically significant lesions impair blood flow or activate release of renin and (b) establish whether correction of the vascular lesion is likely to produce improvement in blood flow or renal function.

Table C123.2. Functional Studies of Renal Artery Stenosis

Plasma renin activity
Captopril-stimulated renin activity
Renal vein renin activity
Intravenous pyelography
Radionuclide imaging with iodine-125 or diethylenetriamine pentaacetic acid for glomerular filtration
Captopril renography with technetium mercaptotriglycylglycine
Radionuclide imaging with technetium for renal blood flow

Comparative (side-to-side) tests. Table C123.2 lists several of these additional study techniques, including radionuclide renography, measurement of renal vein renin levels, intravenous pyelography, and functional testing of split renal function. These tests have the drawback of requiring comparison of a stenotic kidney with a presumed normal "contralateral" kidney, which is often actually abnormal. Such comparisons cannot be made if a solitary functioning kidney is present as in a renal transplant donor or recipient. Such tests may have value under specific circumstances of identifying a salvageable or culpable kidney, but are not widely applied as "screening" studies. To date, no absolute standards for interpretation have emerged.

Renin activation. Tests of activation of the renin-angiotensin system have been proposed to identify pressor lesions in the kidney. These tests have the drawback of being sensitive to the effects of basal conditions including sodium intake, drugs that affect renin release (including β-blockers, diuretics, sympatholytic agents, ACE inhibitors, and angiotensin receptor blockers) and kidney function. In clinical practice, these have limited predictive value and are not used commonly.

Renin lateralization. Renal vein renin determinations are illustrative: Several studies indicate that lateralization of renal vein measurements provides strong positive predictive benefit (more than 90%) from renal revascularization regarding improved BP control. However, failure to find a lateralizing measurement is also commonly associated with clinical benefit (50–60%). As a result, such measurements are of limited value in planning intervention.

Kidney size. Recent studies have been directed to identify kidneys not likely to respond to restoration of blood flow. It is generally recognized that small kidneys (less than 8 cm in length) are not likely to demonstrate restoration of function after revascularization.

Flow parameters. Assessment of poststenotic renal blood flow and vascular resistance within the kidney (e.g., measurement of "resistive index" by Doppler ultrasound) provides a guide to the potential salvageability of the kidney and the likelihood of BP response. Finding low distal resistance is reassuring, whereas a high parenchymal resistance argues against recovery of renal function. In practice, these guidelines are rarely absolute.

Renal function. Assessment of kidney function and proteinuria is important. Serum creatinine levels above 3.0 mg per dL indicate advanced renal insufficiency and predict a low probability of recovery of renal function after surgical or endovascular repair.

Proteinuria. The presence of proteinuria, particularly in subjects with diabetes, raises the possibility of other glomerular disease, which would not be expected to benefit directly from renal revascularization. Renovascular lesions producing hypertension have, however, been associated with nephrotic range proteinuria that has reverted to normal after renal revascularization, ACE inhibition, or nephrectomy. Hence, the presence of proteinuria itself is not a contraindication to revascularization.

Diabetes. Although not specifically studied in a randomized trial, revascularization is less effective in diabetics based on clinical experience. This trend may result from the presence of macro- and microvascular disease in diabetics.

Ischemic Renal Failure

Natural history. Atherosclerotic renal artery stenosis is recognized as a potentially progressive disorder leading to ischemic renal failure. Published reports of serial angiograms indicate that 30% to 50% of such lesions worsen during follow-up. Prospective series suggest that progression to higher ultrasound velocities occurs in 31% of lesions overall and 49% of lesions that are more than 60% stenotic. Remarkably, few lesions (3%) progressed to total occlusion in this series. Progression of the lesion thus does not usually translate into worsening hypertension or renal dysfunction. Several series of "incidental" renal artery lesions followed without revascularization indicate that true clinical progression is probably 10% to 15% over 3 to 5 years.

Impact on therapeutic decisions. These rates of progression are of clinical importance for several reasons. Because the majority of renal artery lesions do not worsen rapidly, the burden of comorbid risk and the hazards of vascular study and intervention (including complications of the procedure and restenosis) often outweigh the risk of intervention in a given patient. Thus, intense diagnostic evaluation and commitment to vascular repair are not always appropriate. Remarkably, renal function and BP outcomes in reported series of patients subjected to stenting or surgery do not differ greatly in bilateral or unilateral disease. However, the presence of bilateral disease is an independent predictor of cardiovascular mortality. Clinicians managing patients with renovascular hypertension therefore face a number of vexing challenges. Decisions regarding the extent of diagnostic evaluation must be predicated on a clear understanding of how the results will affect therapeutic recommendations and outcomes. Implicitly, the decision to initiate diagnostic evaluation implies that (a) the likelihood of renovascular hypertension is high and (b) the need for vascular intervention is justifiable (the diagnosis of bilateral disease will affect management or high-grade renal artery stenosis jeopardizes renal function). Because none of the available tests yields absolute answers to any of these critical questions, referral of patients to specialized centers with extensive clinical experience may be justifiable.

SUGGESTED READING

1. Caps MT, Perissinotto C, Zierler RE, et al. Prospective study of atherosclerotic disease progression in the renal artery. *Circulation*. 1998;98:2866–2872.

2. Caps MT, Zierler RE, Polissar NL, et al. Risk of atrophy in kidneys with atherosclerotic renal artery stenosis. *Kidney Int.* 1998;53:735–742.

3. Chabova V, Schirger A, Stanson AW, et al. Outcomes of atherosclerotic renal artery stenosis managed without revascularization. *Mayo Clin Proc.* 2000;75:437–444.

4. Conlon PJ, Little MA, Pieper K, Mark DB. Severity of renal vascular disease predicts mortality in patients undergoing coronary angiography. *Kidney Int.* 2001;60:1490–1497.

5. Grim CE, Weinberger MH. Diagnosis of renovascular hypertension: the case for renin assays. In: Narins RG, ed: *Controversies in Nephrology and Hypertension*. New York, NY: Churchill Livingstone; 1984:109–122.

6. Radermacher J, Chavan A, Bleck J, et al. Use of Doppler ultrasonography to predict the outcome of therapy for renal-artery stenosis. *N Engl J Med.* 2001;344:410–417.

7. Rieumont MJ, Kaufman JA, Geller SC, et al. Evaluation of renal artery stenosis with dynamic gadolinium-enhanced MR angiography. *AJR Am J Roentgenol.* 1997;169:39–44.

8. Safian RD, Textor SC. Medical progress: renal artery stenosis. *N Engl J Med.* 2001;344:431–442.

9. van Jaarsveld BC, Krijnen P, Derkx FHM, et al. The place of renal scintigraphy in the diagnosis of renal artery stenosis. *Arch Intern Med.* 1997;157:1226–1234.

Chapter C124

Evaluation of Renal Parenchymal Disease

Michael A. Moore, MD

KEY POINTS

• Clinical presentation of glomerular, renal cystic, or renal interstitial disease in hypertensive patients virtually always includes an abnormal urinalysis or renal insufficiency.

• Evaluation of hypertensive patients for renal parenchymal diseases should include a urinalysis, blood urea nitrogen or serum creatinine, and a renal sonogram.

• Glomerular disease presents as 1 of 5 clinical syndromes: isolated proteinuria, isolated hematuria, nephrotic syndrome, nephritic syndrome, or renal insufficiency.

• Percutaneous renal biopsy should be performed only when the information will contribute to the treatment of the patient.

See also Chapters A37, A49, A71, A78, B84, C110, C111, C113, C118, C159, and C174

Renal parenchymal diseases (RPDs) (cystic renal disease, glomerular disease, interstitial nephritis, nephrosclerosis, and end-stage kidney disease) usually cause hypertension and are almost always associated with impaired renal function and an abnormal urinalysis.

Evaluation of the Hypertensive Patient for Renal Parenchymal Diseases

Evaluation for RPD includes a history and physical examination seeking appropriate clues (**Table C124.1**). Laboratory studies include a urinalysis, renal sonogram, blood urea nitrogen (BUN), serum creatinine, electrolytes and albumin, spot urine albumin to creatinine ratio (A/C), and occasionally a 24-hour creatinine clearance or renal biopsy (**Figure C124.1**).

Proteinuria detection methods. Standard urinary reagent dipsticks detect albumin (not globulin) when it is present at concentrations >150 mg%. Urine should also be tested for total protein with sulfosalicylic acid (1 part sulfosalicylic acid to 9 parts urine), which precipitates all proteins including light chains in dysproteinemic states. Proteinuria should be quantified with a spot A/C from a randomly voided urine or a 24-hour urinary protein collection. The A/C correlates closely with a 24-hour urine albumin (normal A/C <0.2; 1.0 to 3.5 ratio correlates with 1.0 to 3.5 g/24 hours) and has the advantage of avoiding urine collection inaccuracies and unpleasantness. The amount of albuminuria also strongly predicts the risk of end-stage renal disease and cardiovascular disease.

Microalbuminuria. Proteinuria begins as microalbuminuria (30–299 mg/24 hours); concentrations of albumin below 150 mg per dL are not detected by standard urinary dipsticks and require radioimmunoassay methods. In nondiabetic patients, *significant proteinuria* is defined as >150 mg per 24 hours. Annual screening for microalbuminuria is important in all type 2 and postpubertal type 1 diabetic patients.

Implications of proteinuria. Except for the orthostatic variety, proteinuria is always of clinical concern. Orthostatic proteinuria, which has a benign prognosis, is present if protein is absent from the first voided (overnight) urine but is present in subsequent urine during the day. Orthostatic proteinuria has a good prognosis. RPDs cause variable amounts of proteinuria. Patients with persistent proteinuria (not orthostatic) should be screened for diabetes mellitus, connective tissue diseases, dysproteinemic conditions, and hypocomplementemia.

Table C124.1. **Clinical Clues for Renal Parenchymal Disease from the Medical History**

Recurrent urinary tract infections, particularly in young patients, suggest congenital bladder abnormalities or "reflux nephropathy."

A history of excessive proprietary analgesics use or use of any potential nephrotoxin (Table C124.3).

Previous renal failure. (Locate any previous renal function studies, such as blood urea nitrogen, serum creatinine, or urinalysis.)

A history of ingestion of moonshine or illicit alcohol suggests potential lead exposure.

Diabetic retinopathy establishes the diagnosis of diabetic nephropathy in a diabetic patient with proteinuria.

An abdominal bruit, particularly diastolic, suggests renal artery disease or an arteriovenous malformation.

Proteinuria always indicates glomerular disease.

Red cell casts always indicate glomerular inflammation.

A urine negative for protein by dipstick (albumin) but positive for protein by sulfosalicylic acid (any protein) suggests the presence of light chains with dysproteinemia.

CLINICAL CLUES FOR RENAL PARENCHYMAL DISEASE FROM THE PHYSICAL EXAMINATION

Periorbital edema	Expanded extracellular fluid volume
Lower back and leg edema	Expanded extracellular fluid volume
Rales	Expanded extracellular fluid volume
Pallor	Anemia of chronic renal failure
Systolic murmur	Functional flow murmur
Diastolic murmur	Precedes pericarditis
Pericardial rub	Uremic pericarditis
Decreased tactile sense	Uremic neuropathy
Loss of muscle mass	Uremic myopathy

Microscopic examination of urine. Cells and cellular casts are hallmarks of glomerular disease. When protein condenses in renal tubules, a cast of the internal shape of the tubule is created. These waxy or hyaline protein casts are always seen in patients with proteinuria but can also be seen in a normal urinalysis. Red blood cell (RBC) casts represent blood and protein derived from the glomerulus and are always indicative of glomerulonephritis. White blood cell casts or mixed cellular casts may also be present. A careful microscopic analysis is therefore considered to be a "poor man's renal biopsy."

Ultrasonography. Ultrasound examinations are useful to compare renal size, identify cysts, and screen for obstructive uropathy. Small dense "echogenic" kidneys on ultrasound also indicate diffuse RPD. Exceptions to the inverse correlation between cortical thickness and parenchymal disease are diabetes and amyloidosis, in which renal size is often increased.

Renal biopsy. Percutaneous renal biopsy should be performed only when the information will contribute to the treatment of the patient (i.e., alter therapy or provide critical prognostic information). Some treatable glomerular diseases, such as diabetes mellitus, lupus, dysproteinemias, and antinuclear cytoplasmic antibody glomerulonephritis, can be diagnosed from blood studies. Common specific indications for renal biopsy are (a) to establish a diagnosis in patients with idiopathic nephrotic syndrome or non-postinfectious glomerulonephritis, (b) to establish the severity or prognosis of an RPD such as lupus nephritis, or (c) to determine the etiology of acute renal failure. Renal biopsy is also done in potential renal transplant recipients to determine the primary RPD. Certain RPDs [membranoproliferative glomerulonephritis, focal glomerulosclerosis, immunoglobulin A (IgA) nephropathy, diabetic nephropathy, and oxalosis] can recur in the transplanted kidney. It is important to have an experienced renal pathologist for accurate interpretation. Open renal biopsy may be required in the severely obese, in noncooperative patients, and in patients with a solitary kidney.

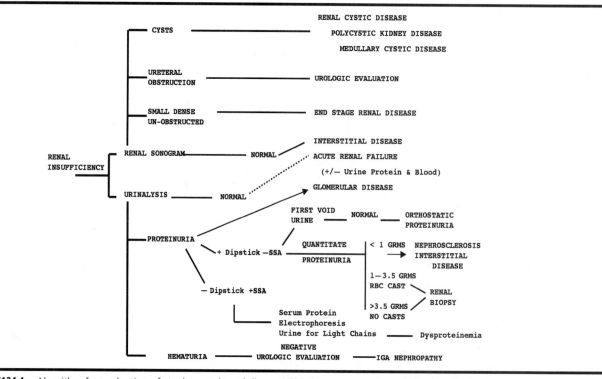

Figure C124.1. Algorithm for evaluation of renal parenchymal disease. GRMS, grams; RBC, red blood cell; SSA, sulfosalicylic acid.

Table C124.2. Calculation of Creatinine Clearance

Formula for creatinine clearance
[Urine creatinine (mg/dL) × urine volume (mL)]/[plasma creatinine (mg/dL) × collection time (min)]
Formula for estimating creatinine clearance

Men	[(140 − age) × weight (kg)]/[72 × serum creatinine (mg/dL)]
Women	[(140 − age) × weight (kg)]/[72 × serum creatinine (mg/dL)] × 0.85

Recognizing and Defining Renal Insufficiency

Chemistries. Renal insufficiency can be recognized by measurement of BUN, serum creatinine, or creatinine clearance (**Table C124.2**). BUN is the least precise measurement; blood in the intestinal tract raises BUN but not the serum creatinine; overhydration, decreased dietary protein, or malnutrition lowers BUN. Creatinine is somewhat more reliable and is inversely related to glomerular filtration rate (GFR). It is a byproduct of daily muscle metabolism, and a fixed amount related to muscle mass is eliminated daily by the kidney.

Creatinine clearance. Creatinine clearance approximates the GFR and should be done if a more precise level of kidney function is needed. Because creatinine is also secreted by the renal tubules, the creatinine clearance overestimates the actual GFR with the discrepancy increasing as renal function decreases. A timed collection (3–24 hours) is used. The creatinine clearance can be estimated by several methods; the one most commonly used is shown in Table C124.2. Creatinine clearance calculations remain inaccurate because of widespread difficulties in precise collection of 24-hour urine samples.

There is an inverse relationship between the serum creatinine and creatinine clearance in which an initial relatively large fall in creatinine clearance is reflected in only a small change in serum creatinine (**Figure C124.2**). In an average-sized patient <60 years of age, a serum creatinine level of ≥1.6 mg% usually reflects a 40% loss of GFR. In patients >60 years of age with a smaller muscle mass and, hence, a lower normal serum creatinine, a serum creatinine level of ≥1.4 mg% may reflect a similar loss of renal function.

Imaging studies. Radiocontrast agents cleared by glomerular filtration (e.g., diethylenetriamine pentaacetic acid) can be used to calculate GFR and, when imaged, yield information on renal size and inhomogeneities as well as abnormalities in renal perfusion (see Chapter C123).

Glomerular Diseases

Glomerular disease presents as 1 of 5 clinical syndromes, including isolated proteinuria, idiopathic hematuria, nephrotic syndrome, nephritic syndrome, or occasionally, end-stage renal disease.

Isolated proteinuria. These patients typically have <3.5 g (nonnephrotic range) of nonorthostatic proteinuria per day with no hematuria. All proteinuric patients should have annual urinary protein measurements to determine if the glomerular disease is progressing. Renal biopsy may be necessary.

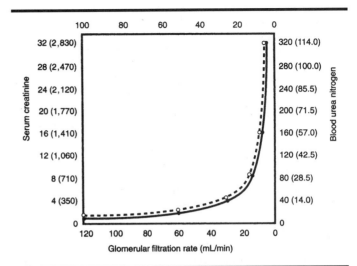

Figure C124.2. Percent of normal glomerular filtration rate. Relation among serum creatinine, blood urea nitrogen, and glomerular filtration rate. Dashed line, blood urea nitrogen, mg/dL (mmol/L); solid line, serum creatinine, mg/dL (μmol/L). (Adapted from Kassirer JP. Clinical evaluation of kidney function-glomerular function. *N Engl J Med.* 1971;285:385–389, with permission.)

Idiopathic hematuria. Hematuria usually requires urologic evaluation. If no urologic disease is found and kidney function is normal, IgA nephropathy is probably present. Approximately half of IgA patients develop renal insufficiency, especially those with coexistent hypertension. If kidney function is decreased or if proteinuria is also present, further workup may be necessary, including a renal biopsy.

Nephrotic syndrome. Proteinuria >3.5 g per day is nephrotic range proteinuria. Serum albumin can be low (<3.5 g/dL), which produces edema. Approximately one-fourth of nephrotic patients have secondary elevated serum cholesterol. Renal biopsy is usually done in patients with idiopathic nephrotic syndrome, but many centers first treat nephrotic adults and children with 6 to 8 weeks of corticosteroids, reserving renal biopsy for those with corticosteroid-resistant proteinuria. Hypertension in these individuals may result from progressive renal disease or corticosteroid therapy.

Nephritic syndrome. Patients with the nephritic syndrome have proteinuria to a lesser degree than those with the nephrotic syndrome (<3.5 g/day), variable amounts of hematuria, and RBC casts in the urine. RBC casts are pathognomonic of the nephritic syndrome and indicate glomerular arteritis. Serum complement should be measured because a low level of 1 or more components of the complement system is characteristic of several types of glomerulonephritis. Renal biopsy should be considered early in the course of nephritic patients who do not have postinfectious glomerulonephritis because treatment information can be obtained.

End-Stage Kidney Disease

End-stage kidney disease is diagnosed by azotemia, elevated serum phosphorus (>5.5 mg/dL), anemia, urinalysis with variable amounts of proteinuria, broad urinary casts, and small dense unobstructed kidneys on renal sonogram. By the time of

Table C124.3. **Drugs Associated with Chronic Interstitial Nephritis**

Lithium	Lead (moonshine whiskey)
Analgesics	Cisplatinum
Cyclosporine	Penicillamine
Gold	Pentamidine
Amphotericin	

diagnosis, serum creatinine is generally higher than 5 mg per dL. Hypertension is present in more than 85% of these patients, and the need for renal replacement therapy (dialysis or transplantation) is usually imminent.

Interstitial renal disease. Chronic interstitial disease presents with renal insufficiency (often nonoliguric), a history of exposure to a known cause of interstitial disease, and an essentially normal urinalysis (**Table C124.3**). Chronic interstitial disease typically has <1 g per day of proteinuria, a reduced maximum urinary concentrating capacity, and minimal urinary cellular elements. The finding of eosinophils in the urine, although uncommon even in proven cases of interstitial nephritis, is pathognomonic for "allergic" or drug-induced interstitial disease.

Renal Cystic Diseases

Simple, thin, smooth-walled renal cysts containing fluid under tension have been associated with reversible hypertension after cyst decompression or removal. Typically, the cysts are asymptomatic and develop as individuals age. Medullary cystic disease in children usually presents with renal insufficiency. Polycystic disease can present in adults as back pain, hematuria, hypertension, or renal insufficiency. Polycystic disease is usually an autosomal dominant inherited condition, but it can occur in an autosomal recessive pattern and generations can be skipped. Cystic renal disease is usually diagnosed with renal sonography. Hypertension is a common feature in medullary and polycystic diseases.

Nephrosclerosis

Nephrosclerosis is usually associated with chronic hypertension and worsens with advancing age. The hallmark lesion is thickening and hyalinosis of the afferent renal arterioles. Nephrosclerotic patients usually have some degree of renal insufficiency, a history of hypertension, <2 g per day proteinuria, and an otherwise unremarkable urinalysis. Renal sonography often demonstrates symmetric normal to small kidneys and a uniform increase in echogenicity.

SUGGESTED READING

1. American Diabetes Association. Diabetic nephropathy. *Diabetes Care.* 2002;25:S85–S89.
2. Bakris GL, Williams M, Dworkin L, et al. Preserving renal function in adults with hypertension and diabetes. National Kidney Foundation Hypertension and Diabetes Executive Committee Working Group. *Am J Kidney Dis.* 1999;33:1004–1010.
3. Ginsberg JM, Chang BS, Matarese RA, Garella S. Use of single voided urine samples to estimate quantitative proteinuria. *N Engl J Med.* 1983;309:1543–1546.
4. Jennette JC, Falk RJ. Glomerular clinicopathologic syndromes. In: Greenberg A, ed. *Primer on Kidney Disease.* 3rd ed. San Diego, CA: Academic Press; 2001.
5. National High Blood Pressure Education Program Working Group. 1995 update of the working group reports on chronic renal failure and renovascular hypertension. *Arch Intern Med.* 1996;156:1938–1947.

Chapter C125

Neurologic Evaluation in Hypertension

Irene Meissner, MD, FRCPC; Stephen J. Phillips, MBBS, FRCPC

KEY POINTS

- Neurovascular evaluation is indicated in all hypertensive patients with focal or global cerebral dysfunction or with painless monocular vision loss.

- In stroke, the clinical assessment is directed at localization, differentiation of infarct from hemorrhage, and determination of cause.

- Computerized tomography and magnetic resonance imaging can be used to confirm localization and stroke type.

- Vascular imaging is a priority in patients with carotid-territory transient ischemic attack or minor ischemic stroke.

See also Chapters A68–A70, A72, B81, C122, and C160

Among the principal aims of antihypertensive treatment is prevention of neurovascular complications such as hypertensive encephalopathy, transient retinal ischemia, retinal infarction, anterior ischemic optic neuropathy, transient focal cerebral ischemia, cerebral infarction, and intracerebral hemorrhage. Neurovascular evaluation is indicated if the hypertensive patient presents with clinical features of acute global cerebral dysfunction, acute painless monocular vision loss, or acute focal cerebral dysfunction. In each of these situations, precise diagnosis is necessary to optimize subsequent management of the patient. The most important part of the evaluation is a careful history and neurologic examination.

Hypertensive Encephalopathy

Diagnosis. Although there is some disagreement as to how to diagnose and classify hypertensive encephalopathy, there is usually a marked elevation of blood pressure (BP), typically ≈250/150 mm Hg, plus neurologic target organ damage characterized by severe headache, impaired consciousness (confusion, drowsiness, stupor, or coma), nausea and vomiting, vision disturbances, fleeting focal neurologic symptoms and signs, seizures, or retinopathy (papilledema, hemorrhages, and exudates). Rarely are all of these features present in the same patient, but usually 3 or more are noted.

Neurologic investigation. Computed tomography (CT) of the brain should be performed to exclude subarachnoid hemorrhage, cerebral infarction, and intracerebral hemorrhage. A magnetic resonance image (MRI) may show diffuse or multifocal cerebral edema or small focal ischemic infarcts. Neither is necessary for the emergency management of the patient, however, and appropriate treatment should not be delayed to obtain these tests.

Retinal Ischemia

The retina and optic nerve head are supplied by branches of the internal carotid artery. Thromboembolic disease of the eye is an important cause of vision impairment and an indicator of increased risk of cerebral and myocardial infarction (see Chapter A72).

Clinical syndromes

Amaurosis fugax. Transient monocular blindness (amaurosis fugax) is the sudden loss ("like a curtain coming down" or "graying out") of vision in 1 eye, lasting minutes. This is highly correlated with carotid occlusive disease in patients >50 years old but is usually owing to migraine in younger patients.

Retinal artery occlusion. Retinal artery occlusion causes sudden, painless, permanent monocular vision loss associated with ophthalmoscopic evidence of retinal infarction. In cases of central retinal artery occlusion, the vision loss is complete, there is an afferent pupillary defect, and the entire retina (excluding the macula) loses its transparency and appears milky white. The macula remains red because its choroidal blood supply is preserved. In cases of branch retinal artery occlusion, the vision loss is incomplete, pupil reactions are usually normal, and only a segment of the retina is infarcted.

Optic nerve disease. Anterior ischemic optic neuropathy (infarction of the optic nerve head) is sudden, painless, permanent, monocular vision loss accompanied by a nerve fiber bundle–type (arcuate) visual field defect, an afferent pupillary defect, and edema of the optic disc. The underlying lesion has been described as a lacunar infarct of the optic nerve head. Giant cell arteritis, lupus, or polyarteritis nodosa must be excluded by appropriate blood tests; for suspected giant cell arteritis, a temporal artery biopsy may be required.

Neurologic investigation

Brain imaging. A CT scan of the brain is useful to look for coexisting silent cerebral infarct(s). The presence of such a lesion indicates that the patient is at higher risk of subsequent cerebral reinfarction than a patient who has had an isolated retinal ischemic event.

Vascular imaging. The technique used depends on the clinical situation and the availability of resources and expertise. If the patient presents with a history of several recent episodes of amaurosis fugax and has an ipsilateral neck bruit, the probability of finding severe carotid occlusive disease is high. Although the most definitive procedure to evaluate the extracranial and intracranial circulation remains cerebral angiography, magnetic resonance angiography is a widely used technique to provide high-resolution images without the risks of catheter angiography. However, as with carotid ultrasound, it is limited in its ability to distinguish carotid occlusion from preocclusive stenosis and in defining intracranial stenoses and collateral supply, factors important in the surgical decision-making process. In other clinical situations, it is appropriate to first perform a noninvasive study, usually duplex ultrasound. If a technically adequate study shows a <50% diameter stenosis in the appropriate carotid artery, angiography usually need not be performed. Advances in the technique of duplex carotid ultrasound allow for the quantification of plaque noninvasively by the accurate measurement of arterial intimal medial thickness. Wall thickening as assessed by intimal medial thickness measurements has been demonstrated during sustained hypertension and may have significant implications as a marker of progression of cardiovascular disease and its response to antihypertensive therapy.

Transient Focal Cerebral Ischemia

A transient focal cerebral ischemic attack (TIA) is an episode of focal cerebral dysfunction of sudden onset and offset, of presumed vascular cause, that usually lasts for a few minutes and always <24 hours.

Diagnosis and implications. Diagnosis is often made on the basis of the patient's history and careful exclusion of other causes of transient focal cerebral dysfunction such as migraine or epilepsy. TIA is an indicator of increased risk of myocardial as well as cerebral infarction. The symptoms of an attack are variable and depend on the vascular territory involved (**Table C125.1**). Management of the patient also depends on the vascular territory involved, because surgical treatment may be indicated in patients with carotid-territory TIA but not vertebrobasilar-territory TIA. Carotid endarterectomy (CEA) substantially reduces the risk of stroke in patients who present with a carotid-territory TIA and an ipsilateral internal carotid artery diameter stenosis of ≥70%. Therefore, vascular imaging is a priority in patients with carotid-territory TIA. Percutaneous transluminal angioplasty and stenting have been explored as alternatives to CEA in select patients considered at high risk for surgery. To date, the indications for carotid stenting, as well as its efficacy and durability remain undefined. Multiple clinical trials are currently under way.

Imaging. Brain imaging may be unrevealing in patients with TIA; CT scan or MRI shows evidence of acute cerebral infarction in only a small proportion of patients who present with early resolution of symptoms. Patients in whom the CT scan shows white-matter rarefaction (leukoariosis) commonly have

Table C125.1. Differentiation of the Involved Vascular Territory in Patients with Transient Focal Cerebral Ischemic Attack or Stroke

VASCULAR TERRITORY	CLINICAL FEATURE
Carotid	1. Unilateral motor or sensory abnormalities (or both) 2. Aphasia 3. Combination of 1 and 2 4. Homonymous hemianopsia plus 1 or 2 5. Dysarthria with unilateral motor or sensory abnormalities
Vertebro-basilar	1. Bilateral motor or sensory abnormalities 2. Bilateral limb or gait ataxia 3. Bilateral homonymous hemianopsia 4. Any combination of 1 through 3 5. Dysarthria plus any combination of 1, 2, 3, 9, and 10 6. Homonymous hemianopsia alone 7. Homonymous hemianopsia plus any combination of 1, 2, 9, and 10 8. Unilateral motor or sensory abnormalities plus any combination of 2, 3, 9, and 10 9. Vertigo plus any combination of 1 through 8 10. Diplopia plus any combination of 1 through 9

chronic hypertension and a higher risk of subsequent stroke. A large study showed patients with these periventricular white-matter lucencies to have a less favorable outcome after CEA than those without this finding.

Cerebral Infarction and Intracerebral Hemorrhage

Cerebral infarction and intracerebral hemorrhage are considered together because they cannot be distinguished reliably on clinical grounds. They present as *stroke* (i.e., the sudden onset of a persistent focal neurologic deficit), by definition lasting >24 hours unless death occurs. The clinical picture depends on the part of the brain involved and the size of the infarct or hematoma. Diagnosis is a 3-step process: (a) localization, (b) differentiation of infarction from hemorrhage, and (c) determination of the cause of the stroke (see Chapter A69).

Localization. Clinical evaluation and a brain imaging study allow localization of the lesion in the majority of patients. Localization is important for the following 3 reasons. First, it may indicate the need for urgent intervention such as surgical decompression of the posterior fossa in cerebellar infarction or hemorrhage (clinical features of a cerebellar stroke are shown in **Table C125.2**). Second, it may indicate a potential for specific treatment, such as carotid revascularization, aimed at reducing the risk of stroke recurrence. Revascularization is not usually indicated for patients with vertebrobasilar-territory infarcts. Third, it helps predict the functional difficulties likely to be encountered by the patient, which is important for planning rehabilitation treatment. CT is the most useful brain imaging study because it is relatively fast, inexpensive, and accessible. The disadvantages of CT are that it may not show an infarct in the brain stem or any infarct within the first few hours of a stroke. However, determining whether an initial CT scan demonstrates hemorrhage, early edema, or subtle acute changes of infarction is crucial to the decision regarding the use

Table C125.2. Presenting Clinical Features of Cerebellar Stroke

Symptoms
 Dizziness or vertigo
 Nausea or vomiting
 Slurred speech
 Loss of balance
Signs
 Dysarthria
 Small pupils
 Ocular movement disorder
 Facial weakness or sensory loss
 Truncal, limb, or gait ataxia

of intravenous thrombolytic therapy. If localization is critical and the CT scan unhelpful, an MRI is indicated.

Differentiation of infarction from hemorrhage. For acute stroke, differentiation of infarction from hemorrhage is best achieved by CT. If the stroke occurred more than a few weeks before the diagnostic study, distinction can be made only by MRI. In the setting of acute stroke, intracerebral hemorrhage should be excluded by CT if the neurologic condition of the patient is deteriorating. In this setting, CT should be performed before thrombolytic or anticoagulant therapy is administered. Early CT is indicated also if a cerebellar stroke is suspected. In other situations, it is advantageous to delay the CT scan until ~48 hours after stroke onset because if the underlying lesion is an infarct, it is more likely to be visible at this time than in the first few hours. If the lesion is a hematoma, the characteristic CT signs will still be present.

Determining etiology

Intracerebral hemorrhage. The clinical evaluation and CT scan may be sufficient to diagnose the likely cause of the stroke and guide subsequent management. For example, cerebral amyloid angiopathy would be the most likely cause of a hemorrhage located superficially in the cerebral hemisphere of an 85-year-old patient. Such a patient could be spared cerebral angiography, might not require neurosurgical intervention, and should not be treated with antithrombotic drugs. Hemorrhages located in the basal ganglia, thalamus, pons, and cerebellum are usually owing to hypertension-induced rupture of small-diameter penetrating end arteries. If the patient is young or does not have a history of hypertension, an alternative explanation should be considered (**Table C125.3**) and the appropriate investigations performed.

Cerebral infarction. Ischemic strokes are due to (a) thrombotic or embolic occlusion of precerebral or cerebral arteries or (b) hemodynamic compromise with relative or absolute hypotension. Emboli may arise from the heart or from arterial lesions between the heart and the brain. Rarely, emboli may arise from the venous side of the circulation and gain access to the arterial circulation via a pulmonary arteriovenous fistula or an atrial septal defect. Therefore, determining the etiology of a cerebral infarct involves investigation of the heart, the precerebral and cerebral arteries, and the blood.

Factors affecting management decisions. The nature and extent of investigation should be guided by the patient's age, family history, timing of symptom onset, the severity of the

Table C125.3. Nonhypertensive Causes of Spontaneous Intracerebral Hemorrhage

Arteriovenous malformation
Intraparenchymal rupture of a saccular or mycotic aneurysm
Neoplasm
    Primary (e.g., glioblastoma multiforme)
    Secondary (e.g., bronchogenic carcinoma, renal cell carcinoma,
    melanoma, or choriocarcinoma)
Cerebral amyloid angiopathy
Bleeding diathesis
Anticoagulant therapy
Thrombolytic therapy
Sympathomimetic drugs (e.g., cocaine)

stroke, and the presence or absence of comorbid factors. There is a paucity of data concerning the effects of treatment on subtypes of cerebral infarction, and there is no consensus on the scope of evaluation. Young patients tend to be more extensively investigated than older patients because there is a greater likelihood of finding an unusual cause. A strong family history of stroke is suggestive of a hereditary disorder. Certain comorbid factors may point to the cause of the stroke. For example, a recent large transmural anterior myocardial infarction makes a cardioembolic mechanism likely. The recent U.S. Food and Drug Administration approval of tissue plasminogen activator as an intravenously administered thrombolytic agent for acute stroke has led to a more proactive approach to acute stroke management. Careful control of BP in the acute care setting, early timing of treatment after the onset of stroke symptoms, and minimal acute change or negative CT scan appear to be critical factors in the safe and efficacious administration of tissue plasminogen activator.

Hypertension and Dementia

The general consensus is that high BP has a negative impact on cognitive function. Trials are ongoing to assess the effect of drug action versus BP level on cognitive outcome measures (see Chapter A70).

SUGGESTED READING

1. Brown RD Jr, Evans BA, Wiebers DO, et al. Transient ischemic attack and minor ischemic stroke: an algorithm for evaluation and treatment. Mayo Clinic Division of Cerebrovascular Diseases. *Mayo Clin Proc.* 1994;69:1027–1039.
2. Elias MF, Wolf PA, D'Agostino RB, et al. Untreated blood pressure level is inversely related to cognitive functioning: the Framingham Study. *Am J Epidemiol.* 1993;138:353–364.
3. Forette F, Seux ML, Staessen JA, et al. Prevention of dementia in a randomised double blind placebo controlled systolic hypertension in Europe (Syst-Eur) trial. *Lancet.* 1998;352:1347–1351.
4. Jordan WD, Alcocer, F, Wirthlin D, et al. High risk carotid endarterectomy: challenges for carotid stent protocols. *J Vasc Surg.* 2002;35:16–22.
5. Kappelle LJ, Eliasziw M, Fox AJ, et al. Importance of intracranial atherosclerotic disease in patients with symptomatic stenosis of the internal carotid artery: the North American Symptomatic Carotid Endarterectomy Trial. *Stroke.* 1999;30:282–286.
6. Landi G. Clinical diagnosis of transient ischaemic attacks. *Lancet.* 1992;339:402–405.
7. Mayberg MR, Wilson SE, Yatsu F, et al. Carotid endarterectomy and prevention of cerebral ischemia in symptomatic carotid stenosis. *JAMA.* 1991;266:3289–3294.
8. Practice advisory: thrombolytic therapy for acute ischemic stroke—summary statement. Report of the Quality Standards Subcommittee of the American Academy of Neurology. *Neurology.* 1996;47:835–839.

Section 3. *Principles of Management*

Chapter C126

Interpretation and Evaluation of Clinical Guidelines

Edward J. Roccella, PhD, MPH; Norman M. Kaplan, MD

KEY POINTS

- Clinical guidelines are designed to assist clinicians in making decisions for their patients.

- Legitimate differences may exist among clinical guidelines based on uncertainties of data interpretation from clinical trials and on different needs of populations.

- Guidelines should include sufficient information for the reader to determine their validity and use.

See also Chapters B79, B80, B88, B102, B104–B108, and C127–C136

The past 3 decades have seen the unprecedented production of scientific information generated in the form of longitudinal and cross-sectional clinical studies and trials. Subsets of study populations have been analyzed or merged into metaanalyses yielding even more information. The abundant and rapid access to information has overwhelmed busy clinicians with published reports and editorials and a multitude of postgraduate educational programs all designed to promulgate the latest information. The diffusion of knowledge has occurred at an unequal rate, and patterns of practice continue to vary widely.

Purposes of Clinical Guidelines

In an effort to help the busy clinician digest rapidly produced and abundant information, clinical guidelines have been developed by a variety of governmental, professional, and voluntary bodies. Clinical guidelines present a cost-effective way to synthesize and filter study conclusions and provide credibility and clarity to the evidence that can then improve the effectiveness and efficiency of treatment. Changes in health care delivery systems throughout the world have created demands for evidence of the effectiveness and efficiency of treatments. Clinical guidelines are also intended to reduce variations in treatment patterns and to assist standard-setting groups such as the National Committee on Quality Assurance, large health care delivery bodies (such as managed care organizations), and the Department of Veterans Affairs.

Historical Aspects

The most well established practice guidelines in hypertension management are the reports of the Joint National Committee on the Prevention, Detection, Evaluation, and Treatment of High Blood Pressure issued by the National High Blood Pressure Education Program of the National Heart, Lung, and Blood Institute of the National Institutes of Health. Recommendations have evolved over the 7 reports issued between 1973 and 2003 in an attempt to improve blood pressure (BP) control rates and update overall management. The World Health Organization has also issued periodic reports aimed at the same goals. In addition, over the past 2 decades, dozens of practice guidelines for hypertension management have been issued by governmental, professional, and insurance-based expert groups around the world. Each group has approached the problem in a slightly different way based on the different needs of their constituents. Because of these heterogeneities, it has not been possible to formulate a single practice guideline that has been universally acceptable. The proliferation of guidelines, however, has added a measurable degree of confusion that remains a significant barrier to their acceptance.

Why Do Guidelines Differ?

The proliferation of guidelines has occurred in part because the science base that has been derived from clinical trials is sufficiently broad that different conclusions have been drawn from the results. There have been hundreds of clinical trials published in the last 3 decades. Most have been small trials that have insufficient statistical power unless they are aggregated in metaanalyses. There are also many assumptions within the process of metaanalysis that bias the overall results, particularly when inadequately designed clinical trials are included. Moreover, metaanalyses can be influenced by many intrinsic biases, most notably interpretation bias and selection bias intrinsic to criteria for inclusion or exclusion in particular studies. Guideline differences often reflect the choices and rankings of various forms of evidence used in supporting the benefits of therapy versus the costs to individual patients and to the general population. Guideline differences may also reflect both cultural attitudes regarding approaches to medical care and limits of available resources.

Limitations of Clinical Trials

Randomized clinical trials (RCTs) are widely viewed as the highest level of evidence available. However, clinical trials are based on several assumptions that can introduce bias. Some of the major sources of bias include selection and exclusion criteria, in which high- or low-risk populations are excluded. Use of inadequate sample sizes or short observation periods also influences interpretation. In addition, there is sometimes a failure to differentiate relative risk from absolute risk.

Underestimation of treatment benefits in randomized trials. RCTs may also underestimate potential benefits of therapy. Most RCTs do not include a true placebo and thus underestimate the beneficial effect of the therapy. RCTs may not represent true clinical practice because some patients, typically those at higher risk, are routinely excluded from the trial (e.g., patients with a recent stroke or myocardial infarction). Thus, the study cohort may be at lower risk than a general practice population, and the benefits of therapy would be proportionally underrepresented. RCTs also tend to focus primarily on a primary end point and a few secondary end points and not necessarily on all possible benefits of therapy. Short observation periods also contribute to underestimation of benefit. For example, consider the data on stage 1 hypertension and heart failure in the Framingham study (**Figure C126.1**). If decisions to treat are based on differences at the 5-year follow-up between those with stage 1 hypertension and normal BP, the benefit of treatment appears to be relatively small, and it could be concluded that treatment should not be initiated in stage 1 hypertension. At the 10-year mark, the difference between the treated and the untreated groups becomes quite large and clearly supports the conclusion that patients should be treated soon after diagnosis. Overall, the clinician must ask whether 5-year survival is an adequate health indicator in younger or middle-aged hypertensive patients or should the clinician consider the longer-term benefits of reducing morbidity and improving the quality of life more important? Guidelines should help clinicians answer these questions based at the crossroads where evidence-based medicine meets cost-effectiveness analysis. A guideline should not attempt to rigidly make clinical decisions for physicians and patients.

Clinical perspective: absolute versus relative risks and number-needed-to-treat. In considering the evidence to develop clinical policy, absolute rather than relative changes are often used. This is because the absolute benefit derived from treating hypertension depends on the absolute risk. Those at greater risk, such as older patients or those with preexisting coronary disease, receive the greatest immediate benefits from treatment. The inverse of absolute risk reduction is the number of patients needed to be treated during some time interval, usually 5 years, to prevent an event. It is clinically instructive to know that to prevent 1 stroke in younger women, 400 would need to be treated, whereas to prevent 1 stroke in older men, only 40 would require treatment. Thus, one might conclude that it may be more cost effective to treat the older patient. Because age and previous cardiovascular disease are the most powerful predictors of risk, the conclusion could be that, because treatment is more beneficial to those at greater risk, it should be recommended only in older people or in those who

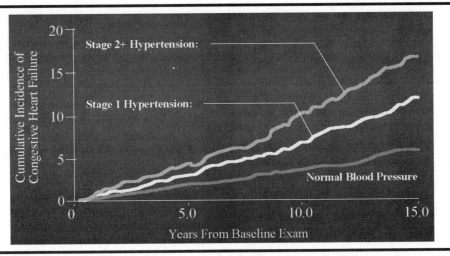

Figure C126.1. Cumulative incidence (in percent) of congestive heart failure in normotensive individuals and individuals with stages 1 and 2 hypertension as a function of time (in years) from baseline examination. Data from the Framingham Heart Study and National Heart, Lung, and Blood Institute, 1996.

have already experienced a cardiovascular event but this would deny therapy to many who would benefit. Thus, absolute and relative risk should be used to make clinical decisions.

Characteristics of Good Guidelines

Clinicians should be familiar with several key characteristics that define the quality of an individual guideline.

Methods. A clear description of the methods used to develop the guidelines is essential. Those who compose clinical guidelines use a range of methods, from highly quantitative analysis to group consensus to craft their recommendations. Although each has its place in guideline development, knowledge of the methods used to formulate guidelines helps the reader judge the credibility of the report and their applicability to clinical practice.

Strength versus applicability of evidence. Recommendations should be based on the best available scientific evidence, but the applicability of the evidence should also be considered. Most guidelines begin with a careful review of the literature; some attempt to grade the quality of published evidence. Although this practice seems to be attractive, grading is accompanied by a number of formidable challenges. For example, a small tightly controlled double-blind cross-over placebo trial conducted in an academic center typically receives a higher evidence grade than a larger trial conducted in an office-based setting, where a new therapeutic approach may be compared to usual care. But which study is more relevant to the clinician? Some guidelines classify the evidence used to make clinical recommendations, but the classification scheme may not adequately compare the differences between the types of available evidence.

Discussion of shortcomings. Guidelines that classify evidence should, if at all possible, describe the strength and limitations of the evidence. This information helps physicians to make more informed decisions for their patients. Regardless, the methods used to link the evidence to the guideline recommendation should be described.

Other considerations. Appropriate decisions about health care should rely on more than good literature reviews. Careful assessment of the needs of people using health services must remain a paramount consideration. Optimally, guidelines should use some method to gauge patient preferences. Finally, guidelines should be considered for their potential benefits and for their potential adverse effects.

If sufficient trial evidence is not available, the guideline should clearly acknowledge the information deficit. It still may be important to outline a therapeutic algorithm, but the guideline authors should then indicate the basis for the treatment recommendations.

Guidelines can be useful tools but are, as their name implies, only a guide. Each clinician must decide with his or her patient the best approach for managing hypertension.

SUGGESTED READING

1. Antman EM, Lau J, Kupelnick B, et al. A comparison of results of meta-analyses of randomized control trials and recommendations of clinical experts. *JAMA.* 1992;268:240–248.
2. Bero L, Rennie D. The Cochrane Collaboration. Preparing, maintaining, and disseminating systematic reviews of the effects of health care. *JAMA.* 1995;274:1935–1938.
3. Heffner J. Translating guidelines into practice: implementation and physician behavior change. *Chest.* 2000;118:1S–72S.
4. Lenfant C. NHLBI Clinical guidelines—another look. *Circulation.* 1995;91:617–618.
5. Levy D, Larson MG, Vasan RS, et al. The progression from hypertension to congestive heart failure. *JAMA.* 1996;275:1557–1562.
6. The National Committee on Quality Assurance Web site. Available at: http://www.ncqa.org/index.htm. Accessed January 15, 2003.
7. Selker HP. Criteria for adoption in practice of medical practice guidelines. *Am J Cardiol.* 1993;71:339–340.
8. Sixth Report of the Joint National Committee on Detection, Evaluation and Treatment of High Blood Pressure (JNC VI). *Arch Intern Med.* 1997;157:2413–2446.
9. United States National Library of Medicine Web site. Available at: http://www.nlm.nih.gov. Accessed January 15, 2003.
10. 1999 World Health Organization. International Society of Hypertension Guidelines for management of hypertension. *J Hypertens.* 1999;17:151–183.

Chapter C127

Approach to the Management of Hypertension

Joseph L. Izzo, Jr, MD; Henry R. Black, MD

KEY POINTS

- The ultimate goal of antihypertensive therapy is to reduce cardiovascular morbidity and mortality; lifestyle modification and aggressive management of other risk factors should be part of all treatment regimens for any individual whose systolic blood pressure is >120 mm Hg; in general, "lower is better."

- Thiazide diuretics are preferred as first-line drug therapy for medium-risk individuals with systolic blood pressure >140 mm Hg.

- Alternative first-line agents (e.g., angiotensin-converting enzyme inhibitors, β-blockers, calcium antagonists, angiotensin receptor blockers) are those proven to reduce morbidity and mortality; they may be chosen for concomitant treatment of hypertension and another coexisting condition or if thiazides are contraindicated.

- High-risk individuals (with systolic blood pressure ≥160 mm Hg, or with diabetes or target organ damage) should be treated initially with 2-drug combinations (usually diuretic and alternative first-line agent).

- In hypertensives who are not controlled on 2-drug combinations, other agents (e.g., sympatholytics, arterial vasodilators, α-blockers) can be added and titrated.

See also Chapters B81–B85, B101–C112, C126, C128–C138, C151, and C152

Hypertension is the major antecedent of adverse cardiovascular disease (CVD) events and is still the most common reason why adults see a health care provider. This chapter is intended to provide a streamlined, evidence-based, comprehensive, risk-stratified approach to the management of hypertension.

Risk Factors and Cardiovascular Disease

Blood pressure and cardiovascular disease risk. Blood pressure (BP) is a continuous risk factor for CVD events (see Chapter B80); thus, any choice of a particular threshold value to define hypertension is arbitrary. In the past, *hypertension* has been defined as a systolic BP value ≥140 mm Hg or a diastolic BP of ≥90 mm Hg based on actuarial observations indicating that above these levels, CVD death rates were at least doubled compared to BP levels below 120/80 mm Hg. Recently, a metaanalysis of 61 long-term clinical trials reconfirmed the same risk relationship in treated individuals: Trial participants with BPs below 120/80 mm Hg had half the CVD event rates of those with BPs above 140/90 mm Hg.

Importance of systolic blood pressure. It is now clear that systolic BP is more robust as a risk indicator and more important as a therapeutic target than diastolic BP, especially in those older than age 50 years, in whom systolic hypertension predominates (see Chapters A60 and C151). In hypertensives younger than age 50 years, diastolic BP may still be useful, but for the population at large, the greater impact and prevalence of systolic hypertension must be recognized.

Amplification of blood pressure–related risks by other cardiovascular disease risk factors. Age, male gender, postmenopausal status, diabetes mellitus or insulin resistance, left ventricular hypertrophy, and dyslipidemia are independent factors that interact to increase CVD risk and amplify the impact of BP on CVD risk (see Chapter B81). Thus, the greater the number of cardiovascular risk factors, the greater the likelihood that any increase in BP over 120/80 mm Hg will contribute to premature CVD and death. Thus, the greater the risk, the greater the need to achieve fastidious BP control. In the United Kingdom Prospective Diabetes Trial (UKPDS), for each 10-mm Hg lowering of systolic BP, CVD morbidity and mortality was reduced by 17%, including values lower than 120 mm Hg. Similar findings that "lower is better" have been derived from studies of diabetic and nondiabetic nephropathy; the exception is the African-American Study of Kidney Disease (AASK), a small trial that did not find an advantage of aggressive BP control in a mixed group of renal diseases.

Risk Stratification

The strategic approach to hypertension begins with an assessment of CVD risk. Therapeutic choices are based on the pattern of conditions present in the individual patient.

Target organ damage. The highest risk individuals are those with diabetes or preexisting target organ damage, especially renal failure, coronary artery disease (angina pectoris or prior myocardial infarction), left ventricular hypertrophy, heart failure, or peripheral vascular disease (**Table C127.1**).

Other cardiovascular disease risk factors. Each patient should be assessed for the presence of traditional risk factors (e.g., dyslipidemia, glucose intolerance or diabetes mellitus, cigarette smoking, obesity, sedentary lifestyle, family history of

Table C127.1. Hypertensive Target Organ Damage

Angina
Myocardial infarction
Left ventricular hypertrophy
Heart failure
Stroke
Transient ischemic attack
Chronic renal disease
Peripheral arterial disease

CVD). Although these conditions do not necessarily directly affect the therapeutic approach to hypertension, other risk factors should be viewed as additional mandates for aggressive BP control, and each modifiable risk factor should be managed aggressively on its own.

Lifestyle Modification: The Cornerstone of Therapy

The impact of the multiplicative nature of risk factors is that high-risk individuals with BP levels higher than 120/80 mm Hg should be treated more aggressively and with all the tools available. Because "therapy" does not necessarily mean drugs, lifestyle modifications are indicated for all individuals, especially those that help lower BP, cholesterol, and glucose values to their optimal ranges. Other studies suggest the added benefit of weight control (to a body mass index of 25 kg/m^2 or less), increased physical activity (at least 3 occasions per week of at least 30 minutes each), decreased salt intake (below 60–100 mmol/day), increased potassium intake (more than 60 mmol per day), elimination of excessive alcohol intake (1–2 oz/day, recommended), and aspirin therapy in at-risk individuals (see Chapters C129 and C130). As a population goal, if everyone with a systolic BP higher than 120 mm Hg followed lifestyle modification, complications of hypertension would be prevented in a major segment of the population. Even if drug therapy is used, lifestyle modifications should be continued to optimize drug effects and minimize doses and numbers of agents needed.

Risk-Based Antihypertensive Drug Therapy

The goal of antihypertensive therapy should be to lower systolic BP; in general, the lower the better. The ultimate target is the attainment of a systolic BP of 120 mm Hg or less. A comprehensive algorithm is provided in **Table C127.2**.

Low risk (systolic blood pressure <140 mm Hg without diabetes or target organ damage). Strict interpretation of the observational and metaanalytical data leads to the conclusion that anyone with a systolic BP ≥120 mm Hg is a potential candidate for therapy with lifestyle modification or drugs. Use of the 120 mm Hg systolic threshold for drug therapy is not practical because at least half of the adult population would be treated with medication, and no study, to date, has demonstrated that the benefits of treating all hypertensives to this goal outweigh the risks. Nevertheless, no prospective trial has proven that treating patients with systolic BPs below 140 mm Hg increases risk (i.e., no J-curve has been proven).

Moderate risk (systolic blood pressure ≥140 mm Hg without diabetes or target organ damage). Pharmacologic therapy should be used in addition to lifestyle modification when systolic BP is persistently ≥140 mm Hg. In general, a single drug, usually a low-dose thiazide diuretic, is preferred as initial therapy as suggested by the Antihypertensive and Lipid-Lowering Treatment to Prevent Heart Attack Trial (ALLHAT) study. If a thiazide cannot be used, an alternative first-line agent [angiotensin-converting enzyme (ACE) inhibitor, β-blocker, calcium antagonist, or angiotensin receptor blocker (ARB)] can be considered. These agents have undergone extensive study in hypertension and target organ damage (TOD) and have proven benefits in these conditions (**Table C127.3**). A justification for initial therapy with an alternative first-line agent is the simultaneous management of hypertension and a coexisting condition (e.g., β-blocker for migraine, calcium antagonist or β-blocker for angina, ARB for diabetic nephropathy, ACE inhibitor for nephrotic range proteinuria). Most individuals in this group eventually require ≥2 drugs, 1 of which should be a diuretic.

Table C127.2. Algorithm for the Management of Essential Hypertension[a]

| SYSTOLIC BLOOD PRESSURE (MM HG) | LIFESTYLE MODIFICATION[b] | RISK-STRATIFIED DRUG CHOICES | |
		NO DIABETES OR TARGET ORGAN DAMAGE[c]	DIABETES OR TARGET ORGAN DAMAGE[c]
120–139	Yes	No initial change in prescription	Condition-specific first-line alternative (see Table C127.3)[d]
140–159	Yes	Initial diuretic monotherapy **preferred** (first-line alternatives[e]: β-blocker, angiotensin-converting enzyme inhibitor, angiotensin receptor blocker, or calcium antagonist)	Initial monotherapy or 2-drug combinations (diuretic + condition-specific first-line alternative[d]); other drugs[f] as needed[g]
≥160	Yes	Initial monotherapy or 2-drug combinations (diuretic + first-line alternative[e]); other drugs[f] as needed[g]	

[a]Based on results of the Antihypertensive and Lipid-Lowering Treatment to Prevent Heart Attack Trial (ALLHAT) and other clinical trials in hypertensive target organ damage (see Table C127.3).
[b]Weight reduction, exercise, smoking cessation, salt restriction, alcohol restriction, and increased dietary potassium.
[c]Target organ damage as defined in Table C127.1.
[d]Drug choices should be modified according to specific trial results (see Table C127.3). Recommendations of the American Diabetes Association suggest that an appropriate treatment threshold in diabetics is 130 mm Hg systolic.
[e]First-line alternatives determined by clinical trial evidence are β-blockers, angiotensin-converting enzyme inhibitors, calcium antagonists, and angiotensin receptor blockers (see Table C127.1).
[f]Other drugs include central sympatholytics, arterial dilators, and α-blockers.
[g]For people with brittle hypertension (frail, elderly), single-drug may be preferred; ultimately, most will require 2 or more drugs.

Table C127.3. Large Controlled Studies Demonstrating Benefits of Alternative[a] First-Line Drugs in Diabetes and Various Forms of Target Organ Damage (versus Placebo or β-Blocker[b])

CONDITION	β-BLOCKERS	ANGIOTENSIN-CONVERTING ENZYME INHIBITORS	CALCIUM ANTAGONISTS	ANGIOTENSIN RECEPTOR BLOCKERS
Post myocardial infarction	BHAT	SAVE		
High coronary disease risk		HOPE		
Left ventricular hypertrophy				LIFE[b]
Heart failure	MERIT-HF, COPERNICUS	SOLVD, SAVE, AIRE, TRACE		ELITE I and II, Val-HEFT
Diabetes		MicroHOPE		
Diabetic nephropathy		Collaborative Group Study		RENAAL, IDNT, IRMA-2
Nondiabetic nephropathy		REIN, AASK[b]		
Stroke/transient ischemic attack		PROGRESS[c]	Syst-EUR	LIFE[b]
Cognitive impairment			Syst-EUR	

[a]Drug classes preferred in 2-drug combinations with thiazide diuretics or as first-line agents in thiazide-intolerant individuals (β-blockers, angiotensin-converting enzyme inhibitors, calcium antagonists, angiotensin receptor blockers).
[b]Comparison versus β-blocker.
[c]Low-dose angiotensin-converting enzyme inhibitor effective only in combination with diuretic.

High risk

Systolic blood pressure >160 mm Hg without diabetes or target organ damage. Two-drug combinations (diuretic + an alternative first-line agent) may be prescribed initially in this group because most people require at least 2 days to achieve control. In general, diuretic-based combinations should first use alternative first-line agents (β-blockers, ACE inhibitors, calcium antagonists, ARBs) before including other "second-line" drugs (sympatholytics, arterial vasodilators, α-blockers).
Systolic blood pressure <140 mm Hg with diabetes or target organ damage. In addition to lifestyle modification, alternate first-line agents, with or without diuretic, should be considered even when systolic BP is <140 mm Hg. In the setting of high CVD risk (e.g., diabetes, renal disease, coronary artery disease, cerebrovascular disease, left ventricular hypertrophy, or heart failure), the choice of agents should be "condition-specific" (Table C127.3). Recommendations from several professional societies, including the American Diabetes Association and the National Kidney Foundation/American Society of Nephrology working group, identify 130 mm Hg systolic as a drug treatment threshold in diabetics.

Highest risk (systolic blood pressure ≥140 mm Hg with diabetes or target organ damage). These individuals with classic hypertension and diabetes or TOD constitute the highest risk group and are most likely to benefit from BP reduction (they have the lowest number-needed-to-treat to prevent CVD events). One- or 2-drug therapy is indicated initially (diuretic and alternative first-line agent), but the vast majority of these individuals require additions and titrations of 3 or more drugs to reach target BPs of 120 mm Hg systolic or less. Based on the amount of available evidence (Table C127.3), ACE inhibitors and ARBs are probably the best choices for initial combination with a diuretic in most high-risk patients.

Other Concerns in Treatment: Whom, When, How, and How Far?

Nonsustained ("borderline") and white coat hypertension.
A substantial number of patients have BP elevations that are not sustained when rechecked. This includes so-called white coat hypertensives and those who have exaggerated elevations of BP in response to exercise or stress (see Chapters A43 and C152). These patients cannot be consistently classified as hypertensive, but many studies suggest that their cardiovascular risk is above that of sustained normotensives. No study has yet demonstrated the benefit of pharmacologic therapy in such individuals, but they are ideal candidates for aggressive lifestyle modification and careful follow-up.

Refractory hypertension.
Overall BP control (using the definition <140/90 mm Hg) can be achieved in at least 70% of the population based on the experience in ALLHAT, Controlled ONset Verapamil INvestigation of Cardiovascular Endpoints (CONVINCE) trial, and other trials. Diuretic therapy was an important feature of both studies. Nevertheless, certain individuals may be unable to be controlled at this level, even with a diuretic. If there is a failure of 3-drug combinations that is not explained by the lack of diuretic or patient nonadherence, the individual is said to have *refractory hypertension* (see Chapter C128). Perhaps the most common reason for true refractory hypertension is long-standing systolic hypertension in elderly people with severe central arteriosclerosis (see Chapters A60 and C151). Nonsteroidal antiinflammatory agents tend to blunt the antihypertensive effects of ACE inhibitors, ARBs, β-blockers, and diuretics (see Chapter C150). Although the addition of a fourth or fifth drug may reduce BP to goal, the individual physician must decide how aggressive to be with agents that are not as well tolerated.

Coexisting conditions and adverse effects, and other drugs.
Certain coexisting conditions that are common in hypertensive patients may influence drug choices. Patients with a history of asthma, for example, should not usually be given a β-blocker, whereas an individual with recurrent gout should usually not receive a thiazide diuretic. Adverse effects can also limit adherence; some occur more commonly in certain demographic groups. For example, ACE inhibitors are more likely to cause angioedema in blacks than in whites. Across individual patients, the acceptance of adverse effects is highly variable; nuisance side effects such as peripheral edema may be particularly annoying to some patients but not bothersome to others. The potential for drug–drug interactions can influence the choice of initial therapy. For example, immunosuppressives can be potentiated by diltiazem.

Pathophysiologic variation and patient profiling. Although the average efficacy of certain drugs is different in various patient subgroups (e.g., less effectiveness of ACE inhibitors and ARBs in blacks), there is considerable interindividual variation in these response patterns that are not sufficiently predictive in a given individual to support a specific therapeutic recommendation. Thus, the key issue is not so much which drug to choose first but which one(s) to add to optimize BP control.

Adherence and persistence with therapy. The barriers to long-term successful management of hypertension are formidable and must be addressed to achieve long-term adherence. **System-related barriers.** Physician and provider attitudes are major determinants of overall control rates, but even when the caregivers are committed to reaching goal BP, other barriers, such as limited patient contact time, inadequate reimbursement for services, suboptimal recordkeeping, and complex formularies, continue to act as barriers to successful control (see Chapter C136). In general, the provider should be familiar with the local barriers and should work to minimize them.

Patient-related barriers. The commitment of the patient to continue therapy remains critical. Several strategies are somewhat effective to improve adherence: fewer doses, fewer pills, fewer side effects, and matching the time of dosing to activities of daily living (e.g., morning teeth brushing or morning coffee) do work. Most authorities agree that patients are more likely to take their medication if the dosage schedule is simple (once or, at most, twice per day). All classes of antihypertensives have once-a-day preparations.

Cost. Although the price of drugs would appear to be a major problem for adherence, most studies have shown that cost is less of an issue than others. If, however, the patient for whom a particular regimen is prescribed cannot afford to buy it, then price becomes the most important factor. The clinician should not hesitate to ask about insurance status, the patient's drug plan and whether he or she will be able to pay for the pills.

SUGGESTED READING

1. Adler AI, Stratton IM, Neil HA, et al. Association of systolic blood pressure with macrovascular and microvascular complications of type 2 diabetes (UKPDS 36): prospective observational study. *BMJ.* 2000;321:412–419.
2. Cushman WC, Ford CE, Cutler JA, et al. Success and predictors of blood pressure control in diverse North American settings: The Antihypertensive and Lipid-Lowering treatment to prevent Heart Attack Trial (ALLHAT). *J Clin Hypertens.* 2002;4:393–404.
3. Furberg CD, Wright JR, Davis BR, et al. Major outcomes in high-risk hypertensive patients randomized to angiotensin-converting enzyme inhibitor or calcium channel blocker vs diuretic: The Antihypertensive and Lipid-Lowering treatment to prevent Heart Attack Trial (ALLHAT). *JAMA.* 2002;288:2981–2997.
4. Hebert LA, Kusek JW, Greene T, et al. Effects of blood pressure control on progressive renal disease in blacks and whites. Modification of Diet in Renal Disease Study Group. *Hypertension.* 1997;30:428–435.
5. Izzo JL Jr, Moser M. Clinical impact of renin-angiotensin system blockade: angiotensin-converting enzyme inhibitors vs. angiotensin receptor antagonists. *J Clin Hypertens.* 2002;4:11–19.
6. Lewington S, Clarke R, Qizilbash N, et al. Age-specific relevance of usual blood pressure to vascular mortality: a meta-analysis of individual data for one million adults in 61 prospective studies. *Lancet.* 2002;360:1903–1913.
7. Lindholm LH, Ibsen H, Dahlof B, et al. Cardiovascular morbidity and mortality in patients with diabetes in the Losartan Intervention For Endpoint reduction in hypertension study (LIFE): a randomized trial against atenolol. *Lancet.* 2002;359:1004–1010.
8. Schrier RW, Estacio RO, Esler A, Mehler P. Effects of aggressive blood pressure control in normotensive type 2 diabetic patients on albuminuria, retinopathy and strokes. *Kidney Int.* 2002;61:1086–1097.
9. Singer GM, Izhar M, Black HR. Goal-oriented hypertension management: translating clinical trials to practice. *Hypertension.* 2002;40:464–469.
10. Vasan RS, Larson MG, Leip EP, et al. Impact of high-normal blood pressure on the risk of cardiovascular disease. *N Engl J Med.* 2001;345:1291–1297.
11. Wright JT, Bakris G, Greene T, et al. Effect of blood pressure lowering and antihypertensive drug class on progression of hypertensive kidney disease. *JAMA.* 2002;288:2421–2431.

Chapter C128

Refractory Hypertension

Norman M. Kaplan, MD; Joseph L. Izzo, Jr, MD

KEY POINTS

- *Refractory hypertension* is defined as out-of-the-office blood pressure values persistently higher than 140/90 mm Hg for most hypertensive patients (or higher than 130/80 mm Hg for those with diabetes or renal insufficiency) despite a prescribed regimen of 3 or more medications from different classes, 1 of which should be a diuretic.

- Refractory hypertension is present in approximately 10% of patients seen by primary care providers and more than 30% of patients referred to hypertension specialists.

- Refractory hypertension falls into 2 broad categories: apparent resistance (e.g., medication doses too low or patient nonadherence) or true resistance (e.g., volume overload or secondary hypertension).

- Causes of refractory hypertension can be identified by history, physical examination, and appropriate laboratory testing.

See also Chapters A43, B97, B99, C109, C112, C131, C133, C136–C138, C140, C147, C150, C159, C161, C167, C168, C170, C173

Refractory Hypertension Definition

Refractory or *resistant hypertension* is defined as the persistence of out-of-the-office blood pressures (BPs) above the appropriate goal of therapy: above 140/90 mm Hg for most hypertensive patients, above 130/80 for those with diabetes or renal insufficiency, or above 140 mm Hg for those with isolated systolic hypertension. It is generally accepted that individuals labeled as having refractory hypertension will have been given prescriptions for 3 or more antihypertensive drugs from different classes, 1 of which is a diuretic.

General Approach to Management

Refractory or resistant hypertension can be arbitrarily divided into 2 broad categories: apparent resistance or true resistance (**Table C128.1**). The prevalence of apparent resistance is considerably higher than that of true resistance. Within these general categories is a long list of possible specific causes that can be identified by appropriate history, physical exam, and limited laboratory testing. Once the individual cause is identified, it can almost always be corrected, reducing the prevalence of actual resistant hypertensives to a small percentage of cases. If resistance persists, referral to a hypertension specialist is a logical next step (see Chapter C133).

APPARENT RESISTANCE

Patient nonadherence (see Chapter C131) and inadequate dosing (see Chapter C137) are the most common reasons for apparent resistance.

Cuff-Related Artifacts

Cuff too small. A common error is the use of a cuff that is too small for the arm. In general, the cuff should be large enough so that the bladder circles at least around 75% of the upper arm's circumference and extends at least two-thirds of its length (see Chapter C109).

Pseudohypertension. A rare cause of refractory hypertension is pseudohypertension, which can occur if there is severe arteriosclerosis or calcification of the brachial and radial arteries. Pseudohypertension has been said to be identifiable by the presence of Osler's sign (a palpable brachial artery even when cuff BP exceeds systolic), but this sign is unreliable because it is found in many elderly patients with normal BPs. The presence of pseudohypertension is usually suspected when hypotensive symptoms arise after therapies that seemingly do not lower BP very much. Oscillometric readings may be closer to intraarterial levels, but direct invasive measurements may be needed to confirm the presence of this condition.

Nonadherence to Therapy

A common cause of apparent resistance is patient nonadherence (see Chapter C131). There are several reasons for these patterns, including side effects of medications, lack of consistent and continuous primary care, inconvenient or chaotic dosing schedules, misunderstanding of instructions, memory defects from organic brain syndrome, personality disorders, social and cultural barriers, and medication cost. Various modalities can be used to reduce patient adherence problems, but strong physician motivation is very important (see Chapter C136).

Prescription Errors

Perhaps the most common reason for apparent lack of control is inadequate antihypertensive drug doses or failure to titrate medications to reach goal (see Chapters C136 and C137). The Antihypertensive and Lipid-Lowering Treatment to Prevent Heart Attack Trial (ALLHAT) study proved that community physicians could at least double their control rates (to approximately 68%) by following a titration algorithm. Closely related is the failure to use optimal combinations of drugs (see Chapter C138).

Table C128.1. Causes of Refractory (Resistant) Hypertension

Apparent drug resistance
  Cuff-related artifact
    Cuff too small
    Pseudohypertension (peripheral arterial calcification, rare)
  Nonadherence to therapy
    Side effects to therapy
    Lack of consistent and continuous primary care
    Inconvenient or chaotic dosing schedules
    Instructions not understood
    Organic brain syndrome with memory deficit
    Personality disorders
    Sociocultural barriers
    Cost
  Prescription errors
    Doses too low
    Suboptimal combinations
True drug resistance
  Exaggerated blood pressure reactivity or variability
    White coat hypertension
    Baroreflex failure
  Physiologic resistance (volume overload)
    Excess sodium intake
    Activation of blood pressure homeostatic mechanisms by vasodilators
    Fluid retention from reduced renal perfusion pressure
    Inadequate diuretic therapy
  Drug effects and interactions
    Nonsteroidal antiinflammatory drugs
    Sympathomimetics (nasal decongestants, appetite suppressants)
    Cocaine, amphetamines, and other street drugs
    Caffeine
    Oral contraceptives
    Adrenal steroids
    Natural licorice (also in chewing tobacco)
    Cyclosporine, tacrolimus
    Erythropoietin
  Associated conditions
    Smoking
    Obesity
    Metabolic syndrome (insulin resistance)
    Excess alcohol intake
    Anxiety-induced hyperventilation or panic attacks
    Chronic pain syndromes
    Intense vasoconstriction (arteritis)
  Genetic variation
    Racial/genetic differences in drug efficacy
    Rapid drug inactivation (hydralazine)
  Secondary forms of hypertension
    Renal impairment with volume overload
    Renal artery stenosis
    Pheochromocytoma
    Hyperaldosteronism
    Hypercortisolism (Cushing's syndrome)
    Sleep apnea

TRUE RESISTANCE

Among those with true resistance, the most common causes are inadequate diuretic therapy and the presence of factors that interfere with the efficacy of antihypertensive drugs.

Exaggerated Blood Pressure Reactivity or Variability

White coat hypertension. BP at rest does not predict the response an individual may manifest during physical or emotional stress (see Chapter A43). Importantly, these stress responses are not

fully treatable with standard antihypertensive drugs; thus, office readings remain high although home BPs may be normal. Approximately one-fourth to one-third of patients with office BP >140/90 mm Hg do not have hypertension on ambulatory monitoring (average awake BP is <135/85 mm Hg), a phenomenon commonly called the *white coat effect* or *white coat hypertension* (WCH) (see Chapter C112). WCH individuals often manifest a pattern of exaggerated sensitivity to antihypertensive drugs, which lower the "nonstressed" BPs and may cause hypotensive symptoms. WCH patients commonly self-discontinue their medications and may become difficult to manage. Therefore, several experts have recommended that out-of-the-office measurements (usually with automated ambulatory BP monitors) be obtained before additional testing or therapies are ordered. The exception to the recommendation for ambulatory BP is the presence of significant or progressive target organ damage, which mandates intensive drug therapy, regardless of whether out-of-the-office readings are below 140/90 mm Hg.

Baroreflex failure. Severe BP instability (increased lability) with very high and very low BPs occurs in individuals with impaired baroreflex function. This condition can be very difficult to treat (see Chapter C161).

Nonadherence to Therapy

Patients, physicians, and drugs may be responsible for nonadherence. Although patients are often responsible for not taking their prescribed therapies, the failure of their physicians to prescribe adequate therapy is likely as common, because twice as many patients are taking their medications than the number who are adequately controlled. As documented in a 2-year survey of physicians' behavior by Berlowitz et al., doses of drugs were increased only 26% of the time despite clear documentation on the patients' charts of inadequate control. Physician nonadherence to general principles of therapy may also be reflected in inconvenient and chaotic dosing schedules—for example, some drugs given once a day, others 2, 3, or 4 times a day, often at different times. With currently available formulations of agents in every class of antihypertensive drugs, there is no reason why more than 1 dose per day is needed (with the exceptions of labetalol and hydralazine). Medications may cause side effects that previously asymptomatic patients are unwilling to tolerate. Fortunately, most of these can be either circumvented (e.g., by substitution of an angiotensin II receptor blocker if an angiotensin-converting enzyme (ACE) inhibitor induces cough).

Drug-Related Causes

The most common of these interactions is the interference by nonsteroidal antiinflammatory drugs (NSAIDs) with the antihypertensive efficacy of all classes of antihypertensives except calcium antagonists (see Chapter C150). Even a single 300-mg tablet of aspirin can disrupt diuretic or ACE inhibitor effectiveness. Unfortunately, the newer cyclooxygenase-2–specific NSAIDs are as likely to interfere with antihypertensive medication effects as the first-generation NSAIDs. Such interference can often be circumvented with large doses of acetaminophen, but if a NSAID is required, larger doses of antihypertensive drugs usually can correct the problem. There is a long list of agents that can raise BP (see Chapter C173). Some have obvious pressor effects, such as sympathomimetic agents. Others raise BP by more subtle mechanisms, as with the mineralocorticoid excess caused by licorice-containing herbal remedies or chewing tobacco.

Physiologic Resistance (Pseudotolerance) and Volume Overload

In most series of truly resistant hypertensives, volume overload is the most common cause of hypertension. Arising from multiple interacting factors, the usual scenario is that there is an initial fall in BP caused by a vasodilator (especially minoxidil, see Chapters C137 and C147), which activates the mechanisms that "defend" arterial pressure (the sympathetic nervous and renin-angiotensin systems), which in turn cause sodium and water retention and volume overload. Marked volume expansion is seen unless adrenergic inhibitors and large doses of potent diuretics are also given. Any drug that lowers BP also reduces renal perfusion pressure and lowers glomerular filtration, a second mechanism that promotes volume overload.

A common culprit in the perpetuated volume overload state is the use of 1 daily dose of furosemide. The 3- to 4-hour natriuresis that follows each dose shrinks intravascular volume only until the next meal, when the activated renin system typically triggers sodium retention, often of a sufficient magnitude so as to replace all of the sodium excreted during the brief interval of natriuresis. In those with good renal function, a morning dose of the more long-acting hydrochlorothiazide (usually 12.5–25.0 mg) may avoid this antinatriuretic cycle. In those with impaired renal function, a morning dose of metolazone is usually effective, starting with 2.5 mg and increasing to 10.0 mg if needed. The case of longer acting loop active diuretics, such as torsemide, may also be effective. Dietary sodium reduction is also usually needed to enhance diuretic efficacy.

Associated Conditions

Patients who smoke, gain weight, or drink too much alcohol tend to have higher BPs (see Chapters B97 and B99) and are also less sensitive to antihypertensive drugs. Correction of these adverse lifestyle habits may allow patients with resistant hypertension to become more responsive to their regimen. The pressor effect of each cigarette cannot be recognized by BP readings taken in the clinic because the pressor effect wears off within 30 minutes, long after the patient put out his or her last cigarette. Only by out-of-the-office readings taken while the patient smokes can this pressor effect be recognized and used to further motivate the patient to quit smoking. Weight gain raises BP, the effect possibly mediated by concomitant insulin resistance and often with a contribution from obstructive sleep apnea. Too much alcohol (usually more than 3 usual-sized portions a day) can raise BP and is sometimes not recognized. Anxiety can interfere with therapy; patients who are appropriately concerned over the inability to have their hypertension controlled are often given more and more medication with little additional effect. These individuals often complain of dizziness, headache, paresthesias, fatigue, tachycardia, or atypical chest pain, which they commonly attribute to side effects of medications or even to other serious conditions such as migraine, transient ischemic attacks, or coronary disease, further adding to the patient's anxiety. The syndrome can sometimes be diagnosed by voluntarily hyperventilating, which sometimes reproduces the symptoms and can avoid unnecessary diagnostic procedures. For some individuals, all that is needed is an explanation of the syndrome and instructions to rebreathe into a no. 6 paper sack at the first appearance of symptoms.

Genetic Variation

The polygenic syndrome of essential hypertension encompasses a wide spectrum of hemodynamic and neuroendocrine variations. One of the most widely recognized variation is in plasma renin activity, which partly determines the degree of individual responsiveness to β-blockers, ACE inhibitors, and angiotensin receptor blockers. Genetic variations in the ACE gene have relatively little effect on ACE inhibitor efficacy. Increasingly recognized is the association of variants in the angiotensinogen gene with salt sensitivity. Thus, the variation in drug effectiveness across the population has a modest genetic component, but genetic profiling is not currently recommended (see Chapter C114). Genetically determined variation in drug metabolism can occur, such as rapid acetylation (metabolism) of hydralazine in affected individuals, but for the common classes of agents used today, no significant genetic differences in metabolism have been described.

Secondary Hypertension

The presence of any one of a large number of identifiable conditions may lead to resistant hypertension. Progressive renal insufficiency is the most common and is easily recognized (see Chapter C159). Renovascular disease should be suspected in those patients with previously controlled hypertension that suddenly goes out of control, particularly if atherosclerosis is evident in other target organs (see Chapter C168). In the last few years, it has been suggested that there is a higher prevalence of primary aldosteronism than was previously noted. Many of these patients are normokalemic but usually have an elevated plasma ratio of aldosterone to renin activity. A few of these patients have been found to have an aldosterone-producing adenoma (which should usually be removed), but most have bilateral adrenal hyperplasia, for which operative intervention is not indicated. Rather than subject all normokalemic resistant patients to an evaluation for primary aldosteronism, an evaluation that may be costly, modestly risky, and still inconclusive, a trial of aldosterone antagonist may be considered (see Chapters C140 and C170).

SUGGESTED READING

1. Berlowitz DR, Ash AS, Hickey EC, et al. Inadequate management of blood pressure in a hypertensive population. *N Engl J Med.* 1998;339:1957–1963.
2. Brown MA, Buddle ML, Martin A. Is resistant hypertension really resistant? *Am J Hypertens.* 2001;14:1263–1269.
3. Davies SJ, Ghahramani P, Jackson PR, et al. Panic disorder, anxiety and depression in resistant hypertension: a case-control study. *J Hypertens.* 1997;15:1077–1082.
4. Harris CJ, Brater DC. Renal effects of cyclooxygenase-2 selective inhibitors. *Curr Opin Nephrol Hypertens.* 2001;10:603–610.
5. Hyman DJ, Pavlik VN. Characteristics of patients with uncontrolled hypertension in the United States. *N Engl J Med.* 2001;345:479–488.
6. Kaplan NM. Anxiety-induced hyperventilation: a common cause of symptoms in patients with hypertension. *Arch Intern Med.* 1997;157:945–948.
7. Knight EL, Bohn RL, Wang PS, et al. Predictors of uncontrolled hypertension in ambulatory patients. *Hypertension.* 2001;38:809–814.
8. Logan AG, Perlikowski SM, Mente A, et al. High prevalence of unrecognized sleep apnea in drug-resistant hypertension. *J Hypertens.* 2001;19:2271–2277.
9. Nuesch R, Schroeder K, Dieterle T, et al. Relation between insufficient response to antihypertensive treatment and poor compliance with treatment: a prospective case-control study. *BMJ.* 2001;323:142–146.
10. Redon J, Campos C, Narciso ML, et al. Prognostic value of ambulatory blood pressure monitoring in refractory hypertension. *Hypertension.* 1998;31:712–718.

Chapter C129

Lifestyle Modifications

Theodore A. Kotchen, MD; Jane Morley Kotchen, MD, MPH

KEY POINTS

- Cardiovascular disease risk factors typically cluster within individuals; lifestyle modifications should address the overall risk of cardiovascular disease.

- Strategies to decrease cardiovascular disease risk should include the following: prevention and treatment of obesity; appropriate amounts of aerobic physical activity; avoidance of diets high in sodium chloride, total fat, and/or cholesterol; meeting recommended dietary intakes for potassium, calcium, and magnesium; limiting alcohol consumption; and avoiding cigarette smoking.

- Adoption of lifestyles targeted to reduce cardiovascular disease risk has a favorable impact on cardiovascular disease morbidity and mortality.

- Developing strategies for the successful implementation of recommended lifestyle modifications remains a challenge.

See also Chapters A11, A41, A43–A47, A53, A65, A76, B81, B87–B89, B93–B100, B102–B104, C127, C130, C136, C152, C162–C164, C166, and C167

Recommendations for lifestyle modifications should be included in a therapeutic plan for hypertensive patients based on convincing evidence from observational studies and clinical trials.

Risk Factor Clustering

Cardiovascular disease (CVD) risk factors tend to cluster within individuals. In the Framingham cohort, at baseline, clustering of 3 or more risk factors occurred at twice the rate predicted by chance. Adolescents and adults with higher levels of blood pressure (BP) tend to have higher serum concentrations of total cholesterol, triglycerides, glucose, apolipoprotein B, and lower high-density lipoprotein cholesterol values. Hypertensive individuals have an increased prevalence of dyslipidemia and glucose intolerance. Data from the National Health and Nutrition Examination Survey II (NHANES II) show that 40% of adults <55 years of age with BPs >140/90 mm Hg have serum cholesterol concentrations >240 mg/dL, whereas cholesterol was elevated to this level in only approximately 20% of normotensive age-matched control subjects. Likewise, of those individuals with blood cholesterol levels >240 mg/dL, approximately 46% had BPs >140/90 mm Hg. This clustering of risk factors within individuals is in part heritable, and resistance to insulin-stimulated glucose uptake may be the common link between hypertension and dyslipidemia.

Epidemiologic observations, including data from the Framingham Study, clearly document the additive risk associated with an increasing number of risk factors. Observations from autopsy studies also document a strong relation between CVD risk factors and atherosclerosis in young people. The severity of asymptomatic coronary and aortic atherosclerosis is related to the number of premortem cardiovascular risk factors. Conversely, according to a recent report of cohort studies conducted in 366,599 young and middle-aged men and women, persons with a low CVD risk profile (serum cholesterol <200 mg/dL, BP <120/80 mm Hg, and no

cigarette smoking) have a 72% to 85% lower mortality rate from CVD compared to those with 1 or more of these 3 risk factors. The recognition that CVD risk factors cluster within individuals dictates that any regimen for the prevention and treatment of hypertension should address overall CVD risk and not simply BP alone.

Impact of Lifestyle Interventions on Cardiovascular Risk Factors

BP is affected by body weight and diet composition. **Table C129.1** lists specific dietary factors that may have an impact on both the prevalence of hypertension and level of BP.

Hypertension. In short-term trials in both hypertensive and normotensive individuals, even modest weight loss (5%) can lead to a reduction in BP and an increase in insulin sensitivity. With a reduction in mean body weight of 9.2 kg, BP reductions of 6.3/3.1 mm Hg have been observed. Regular aerobic physical activity facilitates weight loss, decreases BP, and reduces the overall risk of CVD and all-cause mortality.

In short-term studies in hypertensives, reduction of alcohol consumption has been associated with a reduction of 4 to 8 mm Hg in systolic BP and a lesser reduction of diastolic BP. BP in normotensives may also decrease in response to reduced alcohol consumption.

As reviewed in several metaanalyses, the lowering of BP by limiting sodium chloride (NaCl) intake to 75 to 125 mEq/day results in systolic and diastolic BP reductions of 4 to 6 mm Hg and 2 to 4 mm Hg, respectively, in hypertensive individuals and lesser reductions in nonhypertensives. Many of the trials included in these analyses were of short duration, and the full impact of NaCl reduction on BP may not have been realized, because this effect may increase over time. Moderate reduction of NaCl intake and weight loss, alone and in combination, have

Table C129.1. Dietary Factors That May Influence Blood Pressure

DECREASE BLOOD PRESSURE	INCREASE BLOOD PRESSURE
Potassium (2.7 g/day = 69 mEq/day)	Sodium chloride (8.3 g/day = 140 mEq/day)
Calcium (767 mg/day)	Alcohol (8.8 g/day)
Magnesium (283 mg/day)	Cholesterol (298 mg/day)
Protein (79 g/day)	Saturated fat (26.3 g/day)
	Carbohydrate (254 g/day)

Note: Numbers in parentheses refer to average daily consumption by U.S. adults, as determined from the Third National Health and Nutrition Examination Survey (NHANES III) survey.

been shown to reduce BP and attenuate the development of hypertension in adults with high-normal BP.

Results of 2 metaanalyses of clinical trials have shown that oral potassium supplements (60–120 mEq/day) lower both systolic and diastolic BPs; the magnitude of the effect is greater in hypertensives (4.4/2.5 mm Hg) than nonhypertensives (1.8/1.0 mm Hg) and increases with the duration of the trial. Calcium supplementation may result in small but statistically significant reduction of systolic (1 to 2 mm Hg), but not diastolic BP.

Persons consuming vegetarian diets tend to have lower BPs than do nonvegetarians. The DASH (Dietary Approaches to Stop Hypertension) Trial convincingly demonstrated that over an 8-week period, a diet high in fruits, vegetables, and low-fat dairy products lowered BP in individuals with high normal BPs or mild hypertension. Reduction of NaCl intake below 100 mEq/day augmented the effect of this diet on BP. Fruits and vegetables in this diet provide an enriched source of potassium, magnesium, and fiber, and dairy products and are an important source of calcium. The DASH diet also lowered plasma concentrations of homocysteine, another risk factor for coronary artery disease (see Chapter B93).

Multiple risk factors. In a randomized, prospective clinical trial, the impact of a controlled meal plan that met the nutritional guidelines of the National Academy of Sciences was recently evaluated in men and women with essential hypertension, dyslipidemia, type 2 diabetes, or any combination of these diseases. Over a 10-week follow-up period, compared to participants consuming a self-selected diet, the intervention diet resulted in improvements in multiple risk factors, including hypertension, dyslipidemia, hyperinsulinemia, and excessive body weight.

Diabetes. The Diabetes Prevention Program Research Group recently conducted a large, randomized clinical trial involving U.S. adults who were at high risk for developing type 2 diabetes. Nondiabetic individuals with elevated fasting and post-load plasma glucose concentrations were randomized to placebo, metformin, or a lifestyle modification program with the goals of at least a 7% reduction in body weight and 150 minutes of physical activity per week. Over an average follow-up of 2.8 years, the lifestyle intervention reduced the incidence of diabetes by 58%; metformin reduced diabetes incidence by 31%. Similar beneficial results of the effect of diet and exercise on diabetes prevention have also been observed in other populations.

Impact of Lifestyle Interventions on Overt Cardiovascular Disease

Observational evidence consistently demonstrates a lower incidence of coronary heart disease among groups with the highest intake of fruits, vegetables, and grains. An increased intake of fish oil may also reduce the risk of coronary heart disease and stroke.

Several prospective studies confirm these observations. In a cohort of 44,875 men 40 to 75 years of age, a diet high in vegetables, fruit, legumes, whole grains, fish, and poultry and low in red meat, processed meat, high-fat dairy products, and refined grains reduced the risk of coronary heart disease over 8 years (relative risk, 0.70; $p < .0009$). Similarly, in a cohort of 42,254 women, with a median follow-up of 5.6 years, participants reporting dietary patterns that included fruits, vegetables, whole grains, low-fat dairy products, and lean meats had a lower risk of all-cause mortality (relative risk, 0.69; $p < .001$), as well as lower risk of mortality from cancer, coronary heart disease, and stroke.

Results of the Nurses' Health Study further document the beneficial impact of healthy lifestyles, including diet, on prevention of coronary heart disease. In that study, 84,129 middle-aged women were followed over 14 years. The incidence of coronary events among those women who did not smoke, were not overweight, maintained a "healthful diet," exercised moderately to vigorously for half an hour a day, and consumed alcohol moderately was 80% lower than in the remainder of the population. Subjects were considered to consume a healthful diet if they scored in the highest 40% of the cohort on a composite measure based on a diet low in trans fat and glycemic load; high in cereal fiber, marine omega-3 fatty acids, and folate; and with a high ratio of polyunsaturated to saturated fat. Several prospective studies, including the Nurses' Health Study, have reported that low daily intakes of calcium, potassium, and magnesium are each associated with an increased risk of ischemic stroke in both men and women; diets rich in potassium, magnesium, and cereal fiber are associated with a reduced stroke risk.

Lifestyle Recommendations for Blood Pressure Control and Cardiovascular Health

Implementation of lifestyles that most favorably impact BP has implications for the prevention and treatment of hypertension and for population-based strategies to shift the overall distribution of risk downward. Even if lifestyle modification does not produce a sufficient reduction of BP to avoid drug therapy, the number of medications or dosages required for BP control may be reduced.

Obesity and physical activity. Prevention and treatment of obesity are important for reducing BP and CVD risk (see Chapters B97 and C162). Physical activity or planned exercise should be an important component of any weight loss plan to prevent hypertension or reduce BP (see Chapters B98 and C130). It is likely that CVD mortality can be best reduced by motivating the sedentary segment of the U.S. population to perform some level of physical activity on at least a weekly basis. Further reductions in mortality may be achieved by encouraging people who are occasionally physically active to become active on a more regular basis. Sedentary individuals with normal BP have a 20% to 30% increased risk of developing hypertension compared with their more active peers.

For most people, BP can be lowered with 30 minutes of moderately intense physical activity, such as brisk walking, 6 to 7 days a week (see Chapter C130). In instances when less time is available, then less frequent, more intense workouts are needed, such as running for 20 to 30 minutes 3 to 4 days a week. In either instance, if an exercise program is sufficiently well maintained, the long-term impact on BP can be substantial.

Salt intake. Any population-based guideline for an upper limit of dietary salt intake is arbitrary. Recommendations for reduction in salt intake should be both safe and palatable. For the general population, the American Heart Association recommends that the average daily consumption of salt in adults not exceed 6 g (approximately 1 tsp table salt). There is no evidence that lowering salt consumption to this level poses any health risk, and this recommendation is consistent with guidelines of a number of other agencies both in the United States and abroad. Lower salt intakes may be recommended for certain hypertensive individuals, but the true risk to benefit ratio of rigorous salt restriction is unclear.

Potassium and other minerals. Adequate amounts of calcium, potassium, and magnesium should be included within the overall diet. Except in patients who take a diuretic and may require a potassium supplement, fruits and vegetables are the best source of potassium. Although calcium supplementation is not recommended as a means of controlling BP, calcium intake should be optimized to prevent osteoporosis.

Alcohol. Alcohol intake has little direct effect on BP unless it is consumed chronically in large amounts (see Chapter B99). Nevertheless, for general health reasons, The Sixth Report of the Joint National Committee on Prevention, Detection, Evaluation, and Treatment of High Blood Pressure (JNC VI) suggested that alcohol intake should be restricted to ≤1 oz of ethanol per day in men and 0.5 oz per day in women to optimize hypertension prevention efforts.

Stress. Emotional stress can raise BP acutely (see Chapter A43). Chronic exposure to environmental and occupational stress may also be associated with higher levels of BP (see Chapter B100). It has been suggested that psychosocial stress contributes to the increased prevalence of hypertension among inner-city blacks (see Chapter B88). However, controlled trials of relaxation therapies have not documented a consistent effect on BP. At present, there is no compelling rationale for the use of relaxation therapies for the prevention or treatment of hypertension.

Dietary guidelines. Expert panels periodically publish guidelines for the prevention and management of hypertension, obesity, hyperlipidemia, and diabetes. The most recent Amerian Heart Association (AHA) dietary guidelines for reducing cardiovascular disease risk in the general population are presented in **Table C129.2**. More stringent guidelines are recommended for high-risk indiviudals.

Antioxidants. AHA guidelines do not recommend additional antioxidant or plant sterol supplementation beyond that in the

Table C129.2. Summary of American Heart Association Dietary Guidelines

Maintain a healthy body weight by avoiding excess total energy intake and engaging in a regular pattern of physical activity.
Restrict total fat to <30% of total energy consumption, limit dietary saturated fat to <10% of energy, and cholesterol to <300 mg/day.
Consume at least 2 fish servings/week (particularly fatty fish).
Consume a diet with a high content of vegetables and fruits (5 or more servings/day), and low-fat dairy products.
Limit sodium chloride intake to <6 g/day.
For those who drink, limit alcohol (no more than 2 drinks/day for men and 1 drink/day for women).
Consume a variety of grain products, including whole grains (6 or more servings/day).

diet for either the primary or secondary prevention of CVD. Fruits, vegetables, and whole grains are ordinarily rich in antioxidants, plant sterols, and fiber (see Chapter A65).

Prevention and Implementation Strategies

For the primary prevention of CVD, it is important that healthy lifestyles be established at a young age. Recommendations should be comprehensive and address physical activity, nutrition, and smoking. Effective strategies will require a multifaceted approach for dealing with the population as a whole, targeted subgroups, and individuals with CVD risk factors and/or clinically evident CVD. Recommendations must also be practical if they are to be achieved, and dietary guidelines should be presented to the public in terms of overall diet and food choices. To facilitate change, different and culturally sensitive approaches may be targeted to special populations, such as children, the elderly, and minorities. Preliminary steps to the successful adoption of dietary change include assessment of the individual's readiness to make dietary change, current eating patterns and dietary intake, and the extent of family or social support. Development of strategies that are based on an understanding of the process of behavioral change may further assist in motivating people to make enduring lifestyle changes (see Chapter C162). In the future, genetic studies may identify those individuals who are most likely to benefit from a specific lifestyle intervention. For example, recent preliminary evidence suggests that the M235T variant of the angiotensinogen gene may have a modest influence on the BP pressure response to dietary NaCl reduction and weight loss.

SUGGESTED READING

1. AHA Dietary Guidelines. Revision 2000: a statement for healthcare professionals from the Nutrition Committee of the American Heart Association. *Circulation.* 2000;102:2284–2299.
2. Kotchen TA, Kotchen JM. Nutrition and cardiovascular health. In: *Nutritional Aspects and Clinical Management of Chronic Disorders and Diseases.* F. Bonner, ed. CRC Press 2002, 23–44.
3. Kotchen TA, McCarron DA. Dietary electrolytes and blood pressure: a statement for healthcare professionals from the American Heart Association Nutrition Committee. *Circulation.* 1998;98:613–617.
4. Appel LJ, Moore TJ, Obarzanek E, et al. A clinical trial of the effects of dietary patterns on blood pressure. *N Engl J Med.* 1997;336:1117–1124.
5. Sacks FM, Svetkey LP, Vollmer WM, et al. Effects on blood pressure of

reduced dietary sodium and the dietary approaches to stop hypertension (DASH) diet. *N Engl J Med.* 2001;344:3–10.

6. McCarron DA, Oparil S, Chait A, et al. Nutritional management of cardiovascular risk factors—a randomized clinical trial. *Arch Intern Med.* 1997;157:169–177.

7. Kand TK, Schatzkin AM, Graubard BI, et al. A prospective study of diet quality and mortality in women. *JAMA.* 2000;283:2109–2115.

8. Stampfer MJ, Hu FB, Manson JE, et al. Primary prevention of coronary heart disease in women through diet and lifestyle. *N Engl J Med.* 2000;343:16–22.

9. Hu FB, Rimm EB, Stampfer MJ, et al. Prospective study of major dietary patterns and risk of coronary heart disease in men. *Am J Clin Nutr.* 2000;72:912–921.

10. Diabetes Prevention Program Research Group. Reduction in the incidence of type 2 diabetes with lifestyle intervention or metformin. *N Engl J Med.* 2002;346:393–403.

11. Whelton PK, He J, Appel LJ, et al. Primary prevention of hypertension: clinical and public health advisory from the National High Blood Pressure Education Program. *JAMA.* 2002;288:1882–1888.

Chapter C130

Exercise Therapy

Denise G. Simons-Morton, MD, PhD

KEY POINTS

- Moderate physical activity should be recommended to the vast majority of sedentary individuals and patients with hypertension.

- Patient interventions to increase physical activity should include advice about recommended physical activity regimens, counseling that includes behavioral strategies, and follow-up contacts.

- At least 120 minutes per week of aerobic activity of moderate intensity (e.g., brisk walking) appears to be needed for a clinically relevant blood pressure effect.

- Screening examination and testing are recommended for individuals with cardiovascular symptoms or disease, older individuals, and those with 2 or more cardiovascular disease risk factors who wish to engage in vigorous exercise.

See also Chapters B97, B98, B100, B103, C117, C127, C129, C135, and C136

Physical activity is a key component of healthy behavior. Low levels of physical activity contribute substantially to obesity, hypertension, and premature cardiovascular disease (CVD) (see Chapter A98).

Physical Activity Advice and Counseling

To prevent or treat hypertension, patients should be advised to engage in moderate to vigorous aerobic activity on a regular basis, at least 3 times per week for vigorous activity and 5 times per week for moderate-intensity activity.

Physician endorsement. A physician's advice to increase physical activity can be a strong motivator to patients, although it should be accompanied by education about the recommended physical activity regimens as well as by counseling that employs behavioral approaches. Selecting an enjoyable activity, identifying and overcoming barriers, setting realistic goals, providing positive reinforcement, and enhancing social support are important components.

Behavioral counseling. Advice by a physician followed by behavioral counseling by other members of the health care team is a reasonable approach. The Activity Counseling Trial compared physician advice to patient education and counseling in primary care patients and found a significant increase in cardiorespiratory fitness over 2 years in women. This effect was achieved with approximately 3 hours of total contact time over 2 years (one 45-minute counseling session followed by monthly mailed printed material and written feedback), which was provided by an onsite health educator after physician endorsement.

Goals and reinforcement. The goal of vigorous activity 3 days a week or 30 minutes daily of moderate-intensity activity is a long-term (not short-term) goal to be discussed in physical activity counseling. The ultimate goal is the incorporation of regular moderate-to-vigorous physical activity as a permanent lifestyle behavior. Relapses to sedentary patterns should be considered temporary setbacks, not failures. Achievements should be reinforced, and short-term goals should be selected that are realistic. Follow-up visits should incorporate attention to physical activity, either by the physician or by other medical staff, because it is known from behavioral intervention studies that after follow-up intervention ceases, health behaviors begin to degrade.

Activity intensity and monitoring. Intensity of activity can be determined in a variety of ways.
Heart rate monitoring. The traditional method is self-monitoring of heart rate during exercise. To use this method, patients must be taught how to take a pulse (radial or carotid) or how to use a heart rate monitor. To identify the heart rate range that corresponds to an exercise prescription for moderate-to-vigorous activity (60–90% of maximum heart rate), one can estimate

Table C130.1. Recommendations for Medical Examination and Exercise Testing before Exercise Participation, by Patient Characteristics

| | APPARENTLY HEALTHY | | ≥2 CARDIOVASCULAR DISEASE RISK FACTORS | | |
EXERCISE INTENSITY	YOUNGER[a]	OLDER	NO SYMPTOMS	SYMPTOM(S)	KNOWN DISEASE[b]
Moderate	Not necessary	Not necessary	Not necessary	Recommended	Recommended
Vigorous	Not necessary	Recommended	Recommended	Recommended	Recommended

[a]≤40 years for men, ≤50 years for women.
[b]Persons with known cardiac, pulmonary, or metabolic disease.
From American College of Sports Medicine, with permission.

maximum heart rate by subtracting age from the constant 220 and then multiplying by 60% and by 90% to obtain the lower and upper values for the range, respectively. Thus, for a 50-year-old person, the target heart rate range during exercise is from 102 to 153 beats per minute (bpm), calculated as follows:

Lower limit: $(220-50) \times 0.60 = 102$ bpm
Upper limit: $(220-50) \times 0.90 = 153$ bpm

Less vigorous activity is also beneficial and may be preferred by some patients. A lower limit of the target heart rate range could be 50% of maximum, which for a 50 year old is 85 bpm. A heart rate anywhere within the heart rate range during activity is acceptable for achieving health benefits and improving fitness, but more intensive activity increases fitness to a greater degree. Individuals who are not used to physical activity should start at the lower end of the range, which will be more comfortable and safer. With increasing experience and fitness, values higher in the range can be targeted.

Perceived exertion scales. An alternative to heart rate monitoring is to achieve a relative perceived exertion of "moderate to very hard." Perceived exertion or heart rate monitoring is preferred to providing an absolute pace in an exercise prescription, such as walking 4 miles per hour, because an individual's age and physical condition affect the actual and perceived intensity of the activity. The phrase *brisk walking* should adequately convey a moderate intensity to most patients.

Specific Recommendations before Exercise

Safety issues. For safety and behavioral reasons, sedentary patients should start out slowly at a more moderate intensity and shorter duration than the ultimate goal. They could, for example, start with 10-minute walks 2 times a week and gradually increase over several weeks or months to 30 minutes of moderate-to-vigorous-intensity activity 3 or more times a week.

Hypertension. Although a person with hypertension may have a greater BP increase during exercise than a person without hypertension, there is evidence that the benefits of exercise outweigh the risks in hypertensives. General recommendations for screening before one engages in an exercise program have been provided by the American College of Sports Medicine (**Table C130.1**).

High-risk individuals. For people who wish to engage in moderate-intensity activity, no medical screening is needed unless the person has CVD symptoms or known disease. For older people or people with 2 or more CVD risk factors (older age, family history of early heart disease, cigarette smoking,

hypercholesterolemia, diabetes mellitus, hypertension) but no symptoms, screening is recommended only if they wish to engage in vigorous exercise. People with CVD symptoms or known CVD need a medical history and examination and, if not contraindicated, an exercise test no matter what intensity of activity they wish to engage in. The goals of an exercise test are to determine what intensity of exercise is safe and to determine whether exercise under supervision is necessary. In addition, the exercise test can determine the individual's maximum heart rate, which is much more accurate than using the constant 220 and which can be used to develop an individualized exercise prescription.

Contraindications to exercise. The goals of the medical history and examination are to determine whether there are any contraindications to exercise testing and to identify any medical conditions that would be contraindications to exercise. Absolute contraindications include acute ischemia, arrhythmias, and acute infections. Relative contraindications depend on the physician's clinical judgment. Diastolic BP >115 mm Hg or systolic BP >200 mm Hg are considered relative contraindications. Other relative contraindications include valvular heart disease, advanced stages of congestive heart failure, ventricular aneurysm, electrolyte abnormalities, and some chronic infectious diseases.

Exercise and antihypertensive medications. Use of antihypertensive medication is not a contraindication to exercise participation of moderate or vigorous intensity. β-Blockers diminish the heart rate response to exercise, so for patients taking β-blockers, a perceived exertion of "moderate to very hard" is a preferable recommendation to a target heart rate range. An individual on antihypertensive medication who begins a physical activity regimen may be able to maintain BP control on a lower level of medication, or possibly without medication, as long as the physical activity is continued.

SUGGESTED READING

1. American College of Sports Medicine. Position stand: physical activity, physical fitness, and hypertension. *Med Sci Sports Exerc.* 1993;25:i–x.
2. American College of Sports Medicine. *ACSM's Guidelines for Exercise Testing and Prescription.* 5th ed. Philadelphia, PA: Williams & Wilkins; 1995.
3. American College of Sports Medicine. Position stand: the recommended quantity and quality of exercise for developing and maintaining cardiorespiratory and muscular fitness, and flexibility in healthy adults. *Med Sci Sports Exerc.* 1998;30:975–991.
4. Fletcher GF, Blair SN, Blumenthal J, et al. Statement on exercise: benefits and recommendations for physical activity programs for all Americans: a statement for health professionals by the Committee on Exercise and Cardiac Rehabilitation of the Council on Clinical Cardiology, American Heart Association. *Circulation.* 1992;86:340–344.

Chapter C131

Adherence to Antihypertensive Therapy

Martha N. Hill, RN, PhD; Nancy Houston Miller, RN

KEY POINTS

- Adherence (or compliance) is not an end in itself, but a means to improved care and outcomes.

- The extent to which patients are able to adhere to treatment recommendations is a major issue in blood pressure control and depends on many factors.

- Patients, providers, and health care organizations taking action can prevent, monitor, and address adherence problems by using effective strategies.

See also Chapters B88, B102, B104, B105, B108, C112, C127, C128, and C134–C138

Nonadherence, or patients not carrying out recommended therapy, is an important, costly, and pervasive problem that contributes to low rates of hypertension control worldwide. If patients are unable or unwilling to adhere to lifestyle or medication recommendations, blood pressure (BP) control is unlikely and health may be adversely affected by complications such as stroke, heart failure, and end-stage renal disease. Patient nonadherence is also important because abrupt stopping or restarting increases the risk of rebound or first-dose effects.

Definitions

Adherence (compliance) is the extent to which the patient's behavior (in terms of taking medication, following a diet, or executing other lifestyle changes) coincides with the clinical prescription. Today, the terms *adherence* and *compliance* are commonly used interchangeably. Some prefer adherence because compliance connotes a paternalistic rather than collaborative relationship between provider and patient. More precise definitions vary according to the specificity of the recommended therapeutic behavior and the ability to measure the recommended behavior. For example, taking medication correctly at least 80% of the time is the most common definition of *medication compliance*. Taking the incorrect dose, taking a dose at the wrong time, forgetting to take a dose, or stopping a medication too early are forms of medication noncompliance. Underdosing in different patterns, particularly 2- to 3-day drug holidays or omissions, is the most common form of medication nonadherence. The frequency and length of missed doses affects BP variously depending on the medication. Medication nonadherence may begin with not having a prescription filled or refilled on schedule. In addition, missed appointments, continuation of unhealthy habits such as smoking tobacco, sedentary lifestyle and a diet high in calories, fat, and sodium also are prevalent and are important forms of nonadherence.

Measurement. Measurement of nonadherence is problematic. Information can be collected by physical examination, interview, self-administered questionnaires, electronic monitoring, and pharmacy records. Objective changes in BP, heart rate, and body weight may indicate adherence with recommendations. For example, a decrease in heart rate may indicate adherence with β-blocker therapy or increased physical activity. Compliance must be assessed carefully because worsening health status or other factors may also be responsible for such observed changes. Asking patients to self-report their degree of adherence is fraught with recall bias and the impulse to tell the provider what the patient thinks the provider wishes to hear. Counting returned unused medication can be unreliable because medications may be shared or put into other containers. Thus, adherence should be assessed with multiple methods.

Factors Associated with Adherence

Although it is important for the patient to know the consequences of untreated hypertension and the benefits of therapy, such knowledge is not sufficient to assure adherence.

Positive factors. Seeing a doctor regularly, having other health conditions, fear of complications of hypertension, a desire to control BP, and being on a simple medication regimen are factors associated with higher rates of adherence. In addition, the frequency of BP monitoring at home and in the office is strongly associated with improved medication taking and BP control. Social support from family members and friends, employment, and health insurance also have been shown to be determinants of adherence and BP control.

Negative factors. The reasons for nonadherence are numerous. Problems with adherence are seen in patients of all ages, diseases, and severity of illness. Generally, adherence decreases over time particularly in chronic conditions. Education, socioeconomic status, and gender do not predict nonadherence. Nonhealthy behaviors, such as smoking, excessive alcohol intake, and sedentary lifestyle, are predictive of nonadherence. Moreover, nonadherence varies within and between recommended behaviors to control BP. Patients' actual and perceived

Table C131.1. Successful Approaches of Cardiovascular Disease Prevention Strategies

Signed agreements
Behavioral skill training
Self-monitoring; telephone or mail contact, or both
Spouse support
Self-efficacy enhancement
Contingency contracting
Exercise prescriptions
External cognitive aids
Persuasive communication
Nurse-managed clinics
Work- or school-based programs

Table C131.2. Preventing, Monitoring, and Addressing Problems of Adherence

Educate about conditions and treatment.
    Assess patient's understanding and acceptance of the diagnosis and expectations of being in care.
    Discuss patient's concerns and clarify misunderstandings.
    Inform patient of BP level.
    Agree with a patient on a goal BP.
    Inform patient about recommended treatment and provide specific written information.
    Elicit concerns and questions and provide opportunities for patient to state specific behaviors to carry out treatment recommendations.
    Emphasize need to continue treatment, that patient cannot tell if BP is elevated, and that control does not mean cure.
Individualize the regimen.
    Include the patient in decision making.
    Simplify the regimen.
    Incorporate treatment into patient's daily lifestyle.
    Set, with the patient, realistic short-term objectives for specific components of the treatment plan.
    Encourage discussion of side effects and concerns.
    Encourage self-monitoring.
    Minimize cost of therapy.
    Indicate that you will ask about adherence at the next visit.
    If weight loss is established as a treatment goal, discourage quick weight loss regimens, fasting, or unscientific methods, because these are associated with weight cycling, which may increase cardiovascular morbidity and mortality.
Provide reinforcement.
    Provide feedback regarding BP level.
    Ask about behaviors to achieve BP control.
    Give positive feedback for behavioral and BP improvement.
    Hold exit interviews to clarify regimen.
    Make appointment for next visit before patient leaves office.
    Use appointment reminders and contact patients to confirm appointments.
    Schedule more frequent visits to counsel nonadherent patients.
    Contact and follow-up patients who miss appointments.
    Consider clinician-patient contract.
Promote social support.
    Educate family members to be part of the BP control process and provide daily reinforcement.
    Suggest small-group activities to enhance mutual support and motivation.
Collaborate with other professionals.
    Draw on complementary skills and knowledge of nurses, pharmacists, dietitians, optometrists, dentists, and physicians' assistants.
    Refer patients for more intensive counseling.

BP, blood pressure.
From *The fifth report of the Joint National Committee on Detection, Evaluation, and Treatment of High Blood Pressure/National High Blood Pressure Education Program, National Institutes of Health, National Heart, Lung, and Blood Institute.* Bethesda, MD: The Institute; 1995. NIH Publication 95-1088, with permission.

barriers to BP control influence adherence behaviors. Health care providers need to consider patients' beliefs, attitudes, perceptions, and prior experiences as well as their goals, values, and motivation. It is important to assess the reasons why patients do not follow advice. Factors in the social environment often create other priorities in daily life. Additional frequently cited reasons for not filling prescriptions or not taking medication as prescribed include a belief that their BP is normal or their hypertension controlled, concern about side effects, not believing medication is beneficial, and cost.

Effective Strategies to Improve Compliance

Successful interventions that enhance compliance and lead to improved patient outcomes are primarily behavioral. Patient knowledge is necessary but insufficient if appropriate action does not follow. Effective communication and trust between the patient and the health care provider are of paramount importance.

Multidisciplinary approach. The classic hypertension care and control clinical trials, such as Multiple Risk Factor Intervention Trial (MRFIT), Hypertension Detection and Follow-up Program (HDFP), Systolic Hypertension in the Elderly Program (SHEP), and Treatment of Mild Hypertension Study (TOMHS), demonstrated that extensive and continuous interventions provided by multidisciplinary teams improved adherence. These and other studies designed to meet patient, provider, and organizational needs and minimize barriers to BP control have been effective in a variety of clinical and community settings. Programs in which multidisciplinary teams address patients' beliefs and concerns, provide follow-up and feedback, and free medication, if needed, are the most successful. In these and other studies, BP control within weeks of initiation of treatment was significantly associated with control at later periods of time. Programs that focus on improving prioritized behaviors necessary for BP control can significantly improve adherence to antihypertensive therapy. Effective interventions include a variety of cognitive, educational, and behavioral strategies. Successful approaches are listed in **Table C131.1.** A multidisciplinary team approach to hypertension care and control permits flexibility in matching patients' needs with the competencies of staff with different, yet complimentary, skills and interests (see Chapter C134). Nonphysician health professionals, particularly nurses, pharmacists, and health educators have demonstrated effective,

safe, and well-received interventions that improve compliance and BP control. Nurse-supervised outreach workers, nurse case managers, and nurse practitioners, in collaboration with physicians and other health professionals in a variety of settings, have effectively improved the outcomes of patients with hypertension. Involving family, friends, community resources, and other health professionals can help change life-style habits and maintain these changes over time.

Long-term strategies. Successful BP control requires the initiation of appropriate therapies, achievement of the goal

Table C131.3. Actions to Increase Compliance with Prevention and Treatment Recommendations

ACTIONS BY PATIENTS	SPECIFIC STRATEGIES
Patients must engage in essential prevention and treatment behaviors.	
Decide to control risk factors	Understand rationale, importance of commitment
Negotiate goals with provider	Develop communication skills
Develop skills for adapting and maintaining recommended behaviors	Use reminder systems
Monitor progress toward goals	Use self-monitoring skills
Resolve problems that block achievement of goals	Develop problem-solving skills, use social support networks
Patients must communicate with provider about prevention and treatment services	Define own needs on basis of experience
	Validate rationale for continuing to follow recommendations

ACTIONS BY PROVIDERS	SPECIFIC STRATEGIES
Providers must foster effective communication with patients.	
Provide clear, direct messages about importance of a behavior or therapy	Provide verbal and written instruction, including rationale for treatments
	Develop skills in communication/counseling
Include patients in decisions about prevention and treatment goals and related strategies	Use tailoring and contracting strategies
	Negotiate goals and a plan
	Anticipate barriers to compliance and discuss solutions
Incorporate behavioral strategies into counseling	Use active listening
	Develop multicomponent strategies (i.e., cognitive and behavioral)
Providers must document and respond to patients' progress toward goals.	
Create an evidence-based practice	Determine methods of evaluating outcomes
Assess patient's compliance at each visit	Use self-report or electronic data
Develop reminder systems to ensure identification and follow-up of patient status	Use telephone follow-up

ACTIONS BY HEALTH CARE ORGANIZATIONS	SPECIFIC STRATEGIES
Develop an environment that supports prevention and treatment interventions	Develop training in behavioral science, office set-up for all personnel
	Use preappointment reminders
	Use telephone follow-up
	Schedule evening/weekend office hours
	Provide group and individual counseling for patients and families
Provide tracking and reporting systems	Develop computer-based systems (electronic medical records)
Provide education and training for providers	Require continuing education courses in communication, behavioral counseling
Provide adequate reimbursement for allocation of time for all health care professionals	Develop incentives tied to desired patient and provider outcomes
Health care organizations must adopt systems to rapidly and efficiently incorporate innovations into medical practice.	Incorporate nursing case management
	Implement pharmacy patient profile and recall review systems
	Use electronic transmission storage of patient's self-monitored data
	Obtain patient data on lifestyle behavior before visit
	Provide continuous quality improvement training

BP, and persistence of effective therapies overtime. From a behavioral perspective, to achieve long-term BP control patients must enter into and remain in care, make and maintain lifestyle changes, and for most, take medication. Achieving and maintaining goal BP levels over time also requires continuous educational and behavioral strategies so that patients have the knowledge, skills, motivation, and resources to carry out treatment recommendations with minimal relapses. Successful adherence requires that patients know what steps to take and develop skills in problem identification and problem solving to address barriers as well as in memory enhancement. Strategies to help patients develop these skills need to be adapted so that they are culturally salient and feasible for staff to implement.

Combinations. A combination of strategies is more likely to maximize long-term adherence by preventing, recognizing, and responding to adherence problems. The effective strategies in **Table C131.2** appeared in the Report of the Fifth Joint National Committee on Detection, Evaluation, and Treatment of High Blood Pressure. These evidence-based strategies are clustered under the following approaches: educate the patient and the family about high BP and its treatment, individualize the regimen, provide feedback to the patient, promote social support, and collaborate with other professionals.

Medication regimen simplification. Simplifying the regimen with once (or at most twice) daily dosing significantly improves adherence, although it does not resolve all problems with medication adherence.

Blood pressure monitoring. Self-monitoring BP levels at home or the work site increases patient involvement and provides much more frequent feedback on the basic relationship between adherence and BP levels than do physician office visits every 3 to 6 months.

Behavioral links and reminders. The pairing of adherence behavior with daily habits—for example, linking pill taking with brushing teeth or shaving—avoids missed medication doses. Reminders by telephone, mail, or electronic aids enhance memory and appropriate behavior. Compliance packaging, such as blister packaging, help patients remember when to take their medication and notice if they have forgotten. One of the most successful strategies in many practices is the use of "pill boxes" with individual bins for each day of the week. Multiple dose pill boxes are also available.

Multilevel Approach to Improve Care Delivery

A multilevel approach is needed with patients, providers, and health care organizations taking action to increase compliance. The delivery of care needs to be organized to address potential and real problems with adherence at all levels simultaneously. **Table C131.3** presents the actions and strategies encouraged by the American Heart Association for patients, providers, and health care organizations to increase compliance with prevention and treatment recommendations. It is important to work with individual patients to assure that they understand what is necessary to achieve treatment goals and that they participate in treatment decisions. Joint problem solving to prevent or minimize barriers to care and treatment is valuable. Provider responsiveness to patient concerns as well as reinforcement and support are also necessary. Provision of reminders, outreach, and follow-up services are beneficial. The use of 1 pharmacy to fill prescriptions improves surveillance, counseling, identification of drug–drug interactions, and monitoring of timely refilling of prescriptions. Integrated systems approaches with continuous quality improvement enhance the training and practice of providers and patient outcomes.

SUGGESTED READING

1. Burke LE, Dunbar-Jacob JE, Hill MN. Compliance with cardiovascular disease prevention strategies: a review of the research. *Ann Behav Med.* 1998;19:239–263.
2. Chalmers J, Chusid P, Cohn JN, et al. Working Group: practice guidelines for primary care physicians. *J Hypertens.* 1999;17:151–183.
3. The Fifth Joint National Committee on Detection, Evaluation, and Treatment of High Blood Pressure (JNC V). *Arch Intern Med.* 1993;153:154–183.
4. Hill MN, Miller NM. Compliance enhancement: a call for multidisciplinary team approaches. (Editorial) *Circulation.* 1996;93:4–6.
5. Miller NM, Hill MN, Kotke T, Ockene IS. The multilevel compliance challenge: recommendations for a call to action. *Circulation.* 1997;95:1085–1090.
6. Roter DL, Hall JA, Merisca R, et al. Effectiveness of interventions to improve patient compliance: a meta-analysis. *Med Care.* 1998;36:1136–1161.
7. Sackett DL, Haynes RB, eds. *Compliance with Therapeutic Regimens.* Baltimore, MD: The Johns Hopkins University Press; 1976.
8. Svensson S, Kjellgren KI, Ahlner J, Saljo R. Reasons for adherence with antihypertensive medication. *Int J Cardiol.* 2000;76:157–163.
9. Working Group on Health Education and High Blood Pressure Control, National High Blood Pressure Education Program. *The Physician's Guide: Improving Adherence among Hypertensive Patients.* Bethesda, MD: US Department of Health and Human Services, National Heart Lung, and Blood Institute; 1987.

Chapter C132

Hypertension Recordkeeping and Electronic Management Systems

Mary K. Goldstein, MD, MS; Brian B. Hoffman, MD

KEY POINTS

- Flowsheets and patient summary of hypertension-related clinical information facilitate treatment of hypertensive patients.

- Graphic displays can communicate quantitative information rapidly.

- Guideline-based decision support systems, individualized for the patient being seen, are being developed that can be presented to clinicians at the time of medical decision making in outpatient clinics.

See also Chapters B105, C127, C131, and C136

Rationale for Improved Recordkeeping Systems

Despite comprehensive, evidence-based, national guidelines for management of hypertension [e.g., Sixth Report of the Joint National Committee on Prevention, Detection, Evaluation, and Treatment of High Blood Pressure (JNC VI)], clinical management of hypertension often falls short of concordance with guideline goals for adequate control of blood pressure (BP) and optimal choices of drugs. To manage hypertension effectively over time, physicians and other health care professionals need rapid access to accurate medical record information about the patient's previous BPs and antihypertensive regimens. Such information can be difficult for the physician to extract from clinic charts unless they are structured to collect and display this specific information.

The increasing availability of electronic medical records offers an opportunity for improving the display of relevant clinical information. Electronic medical records, viewed at the time of clinic visits, can be used to present guideline-based recommendations about management of hypertension to physicians and other health care providers when medical decisions are actually being made.

Traditional Data Organization: A Barrier to Blood Pressure Control

Medical information in traditional clinical charts is often so extensive that it overwhelms the physician's capacity to evaluate it in the time available for most clinic visits. Prioritization of information value also does not occur. Presentation of information in graphic format can vastly improve the recipient's perception of important patterns. An early example of the power of graphic display of information is the famous dot map of Dr. John Snow, the physician who identified the Broad Street Water pump as the source of the cholera epidemic in London in 1854 by plotting the location of deaths. Clinical information intended to help physicians provide care for hypertensives may most effectively take the form of flowsheets and summaries.

Improved Information Systems

Flowsheets. Flowsheets aimed at providing important information for the management of hypertension, on paper or in electronic format, should present BPs and doses of antihypertensive medications over time. Flowsheets should provide detail in a time frame relevant to the clinical setting: For example, intensive care unit flowsheets may show minute-to-minute changes in BP, whereas outpatient primary hypertension flowsheets typically show more isolated values over weeks, months, and years. Flowsheets and graphs have been used routinely in paper charts for outpatients in many clinical domains, for example, growth charts and immunization records for children, fundal height and other parameters in prenatal care, and hematologic and renal parameters together with drug doses in chemotherapy protocols. Despite the fact that these are easy to maintain, hypertension flowsheets have not been widely used.

Patient summaries. Periodic summaries from a paper chart aid in making the particular clinical decision at hand. However, summaries from paper charts are extremely labor intensive. In contrast, an electronic record lends itself readily to automating the rapid extraction and display of patient data important to a particular clinical domain. Patient summaries from the electronic patient data may be presented in text format or, with the more recent wide availability of graphic user interfaces, in user-friendly visual displays.

Graphic displays. Many electronic medical record systems include graphing capabilities for display of single parameters. For example, the Computerized Patient Record System-

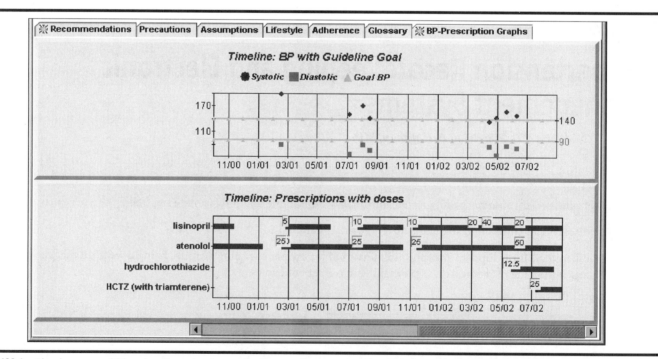

Figure C132.1. Blood pressures (BP) and antihypertensive medications on the same time line. This figure shows 1 tab, the BP-Prescription Graphs tab, from a hypertension advisory program, Automated Treatment of Hypertension Evaluator and Advisor (ATHENA) Decision Support System, built using EON technology for developing decision support systems for guideline-based care. This tab displays a time line with the patient's BP measurements (*top graph*) and antihypertensive drugs, including drug dose (*bottom graph*), on the same time line. The patient's goal BP (in this case 140/90) is shown as a gray line on the top graph so that it is readily apparent when the blood pressure is higher than the target pressure. The drug display shows how many days of prescription drug the patient had available; gaps in the line are a clue to the possibility of the patient not refilling prescriptions in a timely manner. In this case, the patient's prescription for hydrochlorothiazide (HCTZ) was changed to a prescription for combination HCTZ/triamterene, with the newer prescription entered (appropriately) before the patient had run out of the previous one.

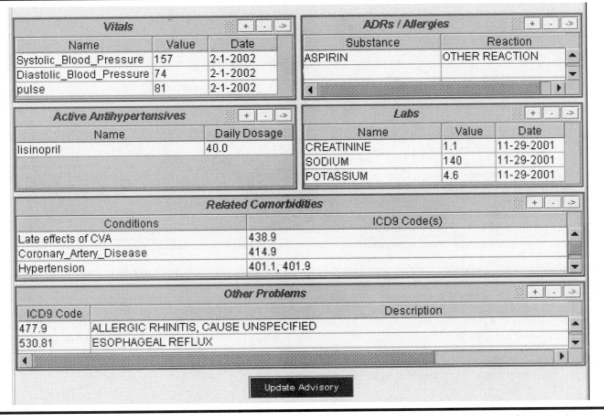

Figure C132.2. Summary of patient's hypertension-related information. The most recent patient data relevant to treatment of hypertension are pulled from various locations in the electronic medical record and summarized in this window. Information in the window can be changed, using the + and – buttons. For example, new diagnoses can be added to the list from a drop-down menu, or present diagnoses can be deleted. Recommendations made by the program can be updated with the new information by clicking the Update Advisory button at the bottom of the screen. The recommendations of the program (for a different patient) are shown in Figure C132.3. ADRs, adverse drug reactions; CVA, cardiovascular accident.

Graphical User Interface used nationally by the Department of Veterans Affairs in its hospitals and clinics includes a feature to display graphs of a single parameter in each instance for a time window selected by the user. This feature can be used to display every BP entered into the patient's electronic record.

The ability to display a graph of a patient's BPs over time is quite useful. It is also clinically advantageous to know what antihypertensive drugs, and at what doses, the patient was taking at the time these BP measurements were made. **Figure C132.1** shows a graphic display of BPs and antihypertensive drugs on the same time line. **Figures** C132.1 to **C132.3** are from Automated Treatment of Hypertension Evaluator and Advisor Decision Support System (ATHENA DSS), an automated hypertension advisory system built using EON technology for developing decision-support systems for guideline-based care. The graph shows the target BPs for adequate control, individualized to take into account comorbidities such as diabetes. The dose of each antihypertensive drug is shown at the time the drug was introduced or changed. Gaps in availability of the drug—for example, due to the patient not refilling the prescription on time—suggest the need to ask the patient about barriers to medical refill or other potential medication adherence difficulties.

Summary of hypertension-related information. The electronic medical records can be organized to present a summary of the patient's relevant clinical information (Figure C132.2). The summary shows the most recent vital signs, any known allergies or adverse reactions to drugs, the most recent relevant laboratory tests, a list of active antihypertensive medications, the diagnoses relevant to choice of antihypertensive medication, and other diagnoses.

Management decision support for hypertension management. The electronic medical record may be combined with hypertension guidelines to generate recommendations for management of each patient. A detailed description of the hypertension knowledge base for this program is beyond the scope of this chapter. These recommendations may be displayed visually. Figure C132.3 shows one such display. In this case, the recommendations are shown with icons indicating the clinical significance of each recommendation (e.g., a compelling indication per JNC VI). Additional information triggered by the patient data is available by clicking the Info button next to the recommendation. The clinician can also provide feedback about the recommendation from a checklist of options by clicking the Feedback button.

Testing of Records Systems

Automation provides many opportunities to improve medical care and patient safety through alerts, reminders, and other such systems. Studies of accidents, particularly in the

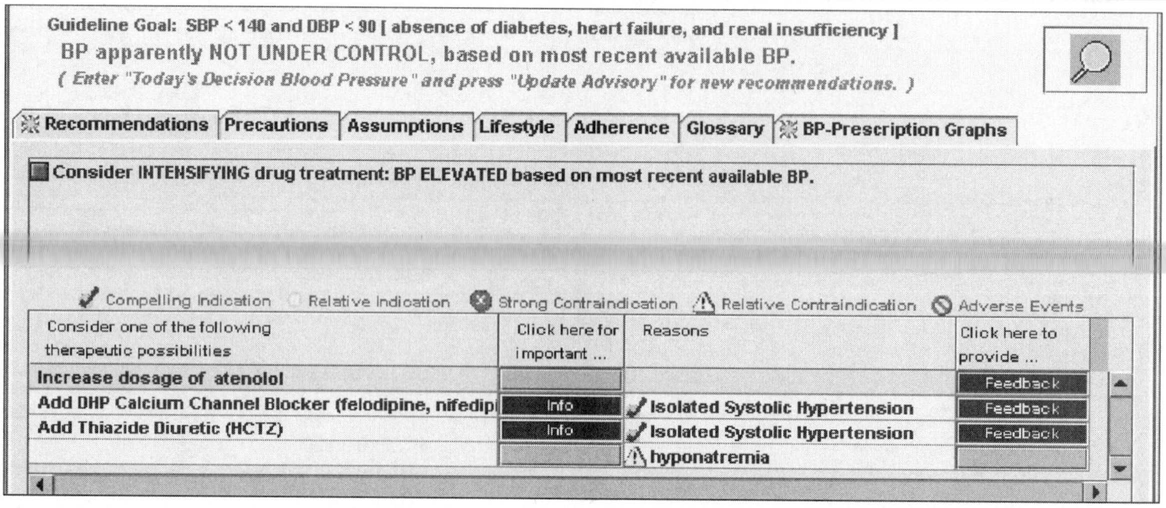

Figure C132.3. Display of guideline-based recommendations. The figure shows the mid-portion of screen displayed in a pop-up window in the electronic medical record. It includes goal blood pressure (BP) (<140/90); because this patient is above target, the information is displayed in red letters. A series of tabs give options for the clinician to select; the current screen shows the Recommendations tab, which is the default display when the window pops up. Because the BP is not adequately controlled, the primary recommendation is to intensify drug treatment.

The table shows recommended changes to drug treatment. Recognizing that drug choices must be individualized for the patient and that guideline-based recommendations may not apply to each individual patient, clinicians are asked to consider the possibilities. The first column in the table shows the specific drug recommendations for this patient, including an increase in the dose of a currently used drug, in this case atenolol, or the addition of a new drug. A variety of options are afforded in the boxes that prompt the user to make choices derived from guidelines and policies. DBP, diastolic blood pressure; DHP, dihydropyridine; HCTZ, hydrochlorothiazide; SBP, systolic blood pressure.

airline industry, have shown that the introduction of automated systems can also affect human problem solving in ways that can lead to unanticipated problems. New automated systems should be thoroughly tested in simulated clinical environments before they are deployed, and the systems should be monitored after deployment to detect and correct any problems that arise.

Health Insurance Portability and Accountability Act

The Health Insurance Portability and Accountability Act (HIPAA) of 1996, Public Law 104-191, specifies a number of regulations that include standard transaction and code sets and the national provider identifier; security standards; and a privacy rule that goes into effect in April 2003. A description of HIPAA is beyond the scope of this chapter. Physicians and health care systems should be aware of important security and privacy provisions of HIPAA. Further information is available from many sources, including the following Centers for Medicare and Medicaid Services Web site: http://cms.hhs.gov/hipaa/hipaa1/content/more.asp and the following Department of Health and Human Services Web site: http://www.hhs.gov/ocr/hipaa/assist.html.

SUGGESTED READING

1. EON Project at Stanford Medical Informatics. Available at: http://semi-web.stanford.edu/projects/eon/. Accessed on November 11, 2002.
2. Goldstein MK, Hoffman BB, Coleman RW, et al. Implementing clinical practice guidelines while taking account of changing evidence: ATHENA DSS. An easily modifiable decision-support system for managing hypertension in primary care. *Proc AMIA Symp.* 2000:300–304.
3. Goldstein MK, Hoffman BB, Coleman RW, et al. Patient safety in guideline-based decision support for hypertension management: ATHENA DSS. *Proc AMIA Symp.* 2001:214–218.
4. Kolodner RM, ed. *Computerizing Large Integrated Health Networks: The VA Success.* Computers in Health Care, ed. Hannah KJ, Ball MJ, eds. Springer: New York, NY; 1997.
5. McDonald CJ. Protocol-based computer reminders, the quality of care and the non-perfectibility of man. *N Engl J Med.* 1976;295:1351–1355.
6. National High Blood Pressure Education Program. *The Sixth Report of the Joint National Committee on Prevention, Detection, Evaluation, and Treatment of High Blood Pressure.* Washington, DC: National Institutes of Health; 1997.
7. Shankar RD, Martins SB, Tu SW, et al. Building an explanation function for a hypertension decision-support system. *Medinfo.* 2001;10:538–542.
8. Tang PC, McDonald CJ. Computer-Based Patient-Record Systems. In: *Medical Informatics: Computer Applications in Health Care and Biomedicine.* Shortliffe EH, Perreault LE, eds. New York, NY: Springer; 2001.
9. Tu SW, Musen MA. A flexible approach to guideline modeling. *Proc AMIA Symp.* 1999:420–424.
10. Tufte ER. *The Visual Display of Quantitative Information.* Cheshire, CN: Graphics Press; 1983.

Hypertension Consultations and Specialists

Lawrence R. Krakoff, MD

KEY POINTS

- Management of hypertension is complex; a large number of patients harbor a spectrum of disorders varying from the simple to the highly complicated.

- Specialists have been identified to provide expertise for management of hypertension; specialist expertise may occur as consultations for individual patients or for management of groups and populations.

See also Chapters B102–B105, B108, C111, C112, and C126–C128

Optimal management of the large fraction of the population with hypertension requires a multicomponent health care system. Most hypertensives are managed by primary care providers such as internists, family practitioners, pediatricians, and nurse practitioners. Using current diagnostic criteria for hypertension, most patients have stage 1 hypertension (140–159/90–94 mm Hg) before treatment. In general, these individuals have increased prevalence of other risk factors but are relatively free of target organ damage and can be effectively managed in a primary care environment.

Hypertension Specialists

A small fraction of the hypertensive population has secondary hypertension or unusual medical conditions not routinely encountered by primary care practitioners. Patients who are difficult to control or those with complex medical problems require the expertise of specialists trained and qualified to act as consultants. The role of experts in management of hypertension has been recognized in recent guidelines and by the American Society of Hypertension, which has developed the American Society of Hypertension Specialists Program. This program has designated nearly 800 physicians practicing in the United States or Canada as *Specialists in Clinical Hypertension* as of September 2002.

Hypertension Consultations

The problems that lead to consultations by hypertension specialists are shown in **Table C133.1**.

Blood pressure measurement issues. Several consultation issues raise the question "What is this patient's usual or average pressure?" as the basis for management decisions. This question may arise during the initial or early assessment of an untreated patient, in which the diagnosis of white coat hypertension is suspected. The same question is related to the patient who appears to be unresponsive to treatment with several antihypertensive drugs (refractory hypertension). For these situations, appropriate use of supplemental blood pressure (BP) measurements (ambulatory BP recording, recorded or telemetered home BP) may be needed. Hypertension consultants should be familiar with these techniques and their interpreta-

tion, as the normal ranges for these techniques may be lower than for clinic BPs.

Secondary and complicated hypertension. Problems related to secondary hypertension listed in Table C133.1 may require expertise from those with competence in nephrology, endocrinology, cardiology, or clinical pharmacology. Older patients with multiple risk factors may have advanced atherosclerotic disease

Table C133.1. Problems of Patient Care That May Require a "Hypertension Specialist" and Some of the Skills and Knowledge Base That Will Be Needed to Deal with These Problems

PROBLEMS	SKILLS OR SPECIAL KNOWLEDGE REQUIRED
White coat hypertension—suspected difference between clinic and outside pressures	Methods and interpretation of ambulatory blood pressures, home recordings
Refractory hypertension—apparent failure to respond to medications	Causes and management of complex drug regimens, awareness of issues related to out-of-clinic blood pressure assessment and compliance
Multiple adverse reactions to antihypertensive medication	Clinical pharmacology and individual barriers to adherence, including patient's perceptions
Secondary hypertension—renal diseases	Causes and diagnostic methods for renal hypertension
Secondary hypertension—adrenal or steroid abnormalities	Causes and diagnostic methods for adrenal steroid disorders and related syndromes
Secondary hypertension—other conditions	Awareness of unusual drug reactions, congenital and acquired syndromes
Complex vascular disease—carotid stenosis, peripheral artery disease, aortic aneurysm	Familiarity and experience in management of cerebrovascular disease, atherosclerosis syndromes, rare disorders (Takayasu's disease, fibromuscular dysplasias, etc.)
Other medical conditions requiring complex multi-drug treatment	Comprehensive skills for such disorders as depression, chronic lung disease, syndromes in the elderly

Table C133.2. Problems of Hypertension Care in Populations and Groups That May Require "Hypertension Experts"

PROBLEMS	SKILLS OR SPECIAL KNOWLEDGE REQUIRED
Screening groups or populations	Methods of unbiased measurement, epidemiology, guidelines for classification of hypertension
Quality assessment for care	Knowledge of current guidelines, strategies for review, data management, and interventions that may improve local practices
New care systems	Knowledge of alternate strategies to conventional office- or clinic-based care, awareness of worksite, rural health care, special systems
Cost-effective care for systems with limited resources	Medical economics, cost-effective analysis, including pharmacy and formulary review, results of clinical trials

in several arteries requiring experience with complex and complicated conditions. Some experience in geriatrics and psychiatry may assist in the management of patients with such disorders as dementia, panic disorder, and depression.

Groups and Population Issues: A New Role for Hypertension Specialists

Health policy issues. The magnitude of the need to detect and treat hypertension in societies with Western lifestyles has been recognized in the past. However, recent trends indicate that hypertension has become an even greater challenge for those countries that have large older populations. The lifetime risk of developing hypertension in suburban towns of the United States is now >85%. The design and results of many clinical trials have implications for how large groups of hypertensives and those at high risk of cardiovascular disease are best managed from the perspectives of optimal treatment and cost-effective care. Published trials include studies of drug treatment for established hypertension and high cardiovascular risk, but also document recent strategies relevant to preventing hypertension through lifestyle interventions (changes in diet and exercise patterns). Those with expert knowledge of cardiovascular epidemiology, prevention of hypertension, interpretation of relevant clinical trials, medical economics, and population

interventions can be of particular value to those responsible for health care policies and funding.

Practice guidelines. National and international committees have already written guidelines for management of hypertension. However, adaptation of these guidelines to local areas and specific health care systems requires experts with knowledge of clinical hypertension and the specific characteristics of their own communities. Hypertension experts may assist in finding strategies for overcoming barriers to optimal management through quality and process improvement and may participate in the development of care or surveillance systems outside of the offices and clinics that have been traditional sites of management. For example, management of hypertension at worksites has become an attractive supplemental system that may be suitable for expansion (see Chapter B105). Some of the issues that require expertise for groups and populations are shown in **Table C133.2.**

SUGGESTED READING

1. Berlowitz DR, Ash AS, Hickey EC, et al. Inadequate management of blood pressure in a hypertensive population. *N Engl J Med.* 1999;339:1957–1963.
2. Burt VL, Cutler JA, Higgins M, et al. Trends in the prevalence, awareness, treatment, and control of hypertension in the adult US population. Data from the health examination surveys, 1960–1991. *Hypertension.* 1995;26:60–69.
3. Guidelines Subcommittee. 1999 World Health Organization-International Society of Hypertension Guidelines for the Management of Hypertension. *J Hypertens.* 1999;17:151–183.
4. Krakoff LR. Hypertension specialists: ready or not, here we come. *Am J Hypertens.* 1999;12:242–243.
5. Meissner I, Whisnant JP, Sheps SG, et al. Detection and control of high blood pressure in the community: do we need a wake-up call? *Hypertension.* 1999;34:466–471.
6. Oliveria SA, Lapuerta P, McCarthy BD, et al. Physician-related barriers to the effective management of uncontrolled hypertension. *Arch Intern Med.* 2002;162:413–420.
7. Redon J, Campos C, Rodicio JL, et al. Prognostic value of ambulatory blood pressure monitoring in refractory hypertension: a prospective study. *Hypertension.* 2001;31:712–718.
8. Rogers MAM, Small D, Buchan DA, et al. Home monitoring service improves mean arterial pressure in patients with essential hypertension. *Ann Intern Med.* 2001;134:1024–1032.
9. The Sixth Report of the Joint National Committee on Prevention, Detection, Evaluation, and Treatment of High Blood Pressure. *Arch Intern Med.* 1997;157:2413–2445.
10. St. Peter RF, Reed MC, Kemper P, Blumenthal D. Changes in the scope of care provided by primary care physicians. *N Engl J Med.* 1999;341:1980–1985.

Nonphysician Providers and the Management of Hypertension

Nancy Houston Miller, RN; Martha N. Hill, RN, PhD

KEY POINTS

- Optimal treatment of hypertension requires a multidisciplinary team approach that integrates physician and nonphysician providers.

- Nonphysician providers (nurses, pharmacists, community health workers, health educators, social workers, and exercise physiologists) can effectively identify, educate, and monitor patients with hypertension.

- Advanced practice nonphysician providers (nurse practitioners, clinical nurse specialists, physician assistants, and clinical pharmacists) are trained and licensed to manage hypertension.

See also Chapters B104, B105, B108, C129, C131, C132, C135, and C136

Due to its prevalence and asymptomatic nature, hypertension control presents a public health challenge that requires the expertise of multiple health professionals in addition to physicians.

History of Multidisciplinary Hypertension Management

For more than 30 years, in clinical trials and practice settings, education to improve hypertension control by nonphysician health care providers has improved patient outcomes. Nonphysician providers such as nurses, pharmacists, community health workers, health educators, social workers, and exercise physiologists participate substantially and effectively in the care of patients with hypertension, especially the care of patients with uncomplicated hypertension. These other disciplines educate, manage treatment, and detect problems that may occur with lifelong therapies such as lack of compliance. In addition, advanced practice nonphysician providers including nurse practitioners, clinical nurse specialists, physician assistants, and clinical pharmacists are trained and licensed to diagnose, treat, and manage acute and chronic conditions, including hypertension. **Table C134.1** provides an overview of the roles and responsibilities of nonphysician health care professionals.

Patient Needs

Detection and referral. At least one-fourth of all patients initially diagnosed with hypertension remain unaware of their condition or do not return for follow-up. In the early 1970s, outreach programs were established in many high-risk communities to detect adults with hypertension. Some of these programs have continued in the United States or have been reestablished incorporating the use of nonphysician health care professionals to screen individuals; identify cases; make referrals; track and follow up, educate, and monitor referrals; and keep appointments. Organized blood pressure (BP) screenings in community sites such as churches and the workplace offer an

opportunity for staff from health care facilities to reach out into the community.

Tracking and follow-up. Once identified, many hypertensive individuals do not seek help from the medical care system. Insufficient knowledge of the consequences of uncontrolled hypertension and myths about treatment are common reasons for lack of follow-up. After screenings, nonphysician health care professionals should follow up to determine whether referrals were completed. Through phone or mailed feedback, they can learn whether individuals with elevated BP levels have sought attention from the medical care system or community-based clinics.

Follow-up care of hypertensive patients is often complicated by their not returning for office visits. Missed appointments or dropping out of care entirely relates to a limited understanding of the benefits of care, excessive costs, unforgiving work schedules, child and elder care responsibilities, and difficult logistics, such as lack of transportation, of getting to and from the health care site. Staff serve as patient advocates by facilitating keeping of appointments, obtaining resources such as transportation and free medications, and, in selected situations, making home visits, minimizing the patient's burden. Databases that are structured to allow nonphysician providers to track and follow up patients who have missed appointments have proven useful.

Education and reinforcement. Education is the first step in the process of helping individuals who are ready to make changes in their behavior to better control their hypertension. Lifestyle modification, including weight loss, sodium restriction, and exercise, requires several intervention steps: assessing baseline behaviors, education about how to make appropriate changes, counseling to set short-term goals, self-monitoring to ensure maintenance of changes, rechecking to determine whether adherence is a problem, and reinforcement of progress toward the goal of a change in behavior. Nonphysician health care providers also help patients with hypertension adhere to

Table C134.1. Role of Nonphysician Providers

	NURSES	PHARMACISTS	NURSE PRACTITIONERS/ PHYSICIAN ASSISTANTS	OFFICE ASSISTANTS	COMMUNITY HEALTH WORKERS
Screening/detection	X	X	X	X	X
Tracking/follow-up	X	X	X	X	X
Education and skill-building					
Lifestyle modification	X	X	X	X	X
Medication adherence	X	X	X	X	X
Self-measurement of blood pressure	X	X	X	X	X
Clinic/office management (preappointment reminders, educational materials, refills)	X	X		X	X
Case management	X[a]	X	X		
Coordination of community-based services				X	X

[a]Specialty-practice nurses in clinic settings may manage drug titration under protocol/supervision of a physician in some instances.

treatment recommendations (see Chapter C131). Once pharmacologic therapy has been initiated, nonphysician health care providers may be the first to note that a patient has not filled a prescription or is having difficulty with a medication or the medication schedule. Their role is to encourage discussion of side effects and to determine if the scheduling and dosing are as recommended. They encourage the use of memory enhancement devices, such as a box with the pills for each day of the week in a compartment and self-monitoring of BP and weight. A useful framework for BP control focuses on critical patient behaviors (**Table C134.2**). Home monitoring of BP is a useful adjunct to office measurement. Nonphysician health care providers ensure that patients understand their goal BP, educate them about the use of home devices and obtaining BP records, and provide feedback about control of BPs.

Roles of Clinic and Office Personnel

A team approach to hypertension management in office and community settings is highly effective in ensuring appropriate patient care and outcomes. However, little is written about how well-defined roles and responsibilities for different health professionals in practice settings (private practice, specialty, primary care, or neighborhood clinics) can improve BP control.

Office staff. The office or clinic environment is a critical factor for supporting patients. Office staff, including medical assistants and nurses, should be familiar with basic principles and should ensure that the office is supplied with appropriate health education materials (booklets, pamphlets, posters) that can be easily accessed by patients. Staff should know how to apply correct BP measurement technique to reliably identify patients with elevated BP levels. Finally, office support staff play a key role in tracking appointments by sending preappointment reminders and following up with patients who miss scheduled visits.

Office nurses. The ability of office nurses to make appropriate clinical decisions in managing patients has been well established for over 30 years. Although physicians are most often responsible for making the diagnosis of hypertension, determining secondary causes, and making initial decisions about treatment, nurses play an important role in ongoing management. In some specialty practice clinics, nurses follow protocols supervised by physicians and are responsible for a thorough history and physical,

ordering appropriate laboratory tests and contributing to the pharmacologic aspects of hypertension management.

Clinical pharmacists. Within large clinics, clinical pharmacists may play a key role in helping patients manage hypertension. They may work directly with patients to ensure that refills are obtained and that patients are educated about drug interactions and side effects. Clinical pharmacists may consult with physicians to provide their expertise on complex drug regimens or may be primarily responsible for selecting and adjusting the medication regimen in some settings.

Advanced practice nurses. Advanced practice nurses (nurse practitioners and clinical nurse specialists) practicing under protocols have been providing care management for patients with hypertension since the early 1970s. Nurses' ability to prescribe and titrate medications and help patients manage other aspects of hypertension has resulted in improved patient outcomes in clinical trials and nonresearch settings. In worksite settings, clinic office practices, and large HMOs, nurses have attained better control of BP than that achieved by physicians alone. In some studies, nurses have successfully reduced the costs of treatment.

The ongoing training by nurse care managers of other health care professionals, such as community health care workers, office support staff, including receptionists, and other health care professionals who may consult outside the office or clinic, is critical to reducing the clinical workload of the advanced practice nurses as well as the physicians.

Coordination of Community-Based Care and Services

Further progress in improving high BP control rates depend on health care providers' attitudes. Effective methods of coordinating

Table C134.2. Critical Patient Behaviors for Blood Pressure Control

Make decision to control blood pressure
Take medication as prescribed
Monitor progress toward goal
Resolve problems that block achieving blood pressure control

From Patient behavior for blood pressure control. Guidelines for professionals. *JAMA.* 1979;241(23):2534–2537, with permission.

care should optimize resources in the communities in which patients live. The ability of patients to integrate healthy BP behaviors into their daily lives improves the outcomes of treatment. This necessitates using every possible resource to provide BP monitoring, feedback on progress to goal BP, financial assistance with health care and medications, and social services to address pressing life circumstances such as unemployment or homelessness. It is most beneficial when health care providers identify and communicate with community-based resources. A neighborhood clinic, a worksite clinic, or a neighbor who can measure BP are examples of complementary sources of monitoring BP.

SUGGESTED READING

1. Burke LE, Dunbar-Jacob JM, Hill MN. Compliance with cardiovascular disease prevention strategies: a review of the research. *Ann Behav Med.* 1997;19:239–263.
2. Curzio JL, Beevers M. The role of nurses in hypertension care and research. *J Hum Hypertens.* 1997;11:541–550.
3. Hill MN. Strategies for patient education. *Clin Exp Hypertens [A].* 1989;11:1187–1201.
4. Hill MN. Interdisciplinary approach to the management of hypertension: does it work? *Cardiovasc Rev Rep.* 1998;19:49–54.
5. Hill MN, Becker DM. Roles of nurses and health workers in cardiovascular health promotion. *Am J Med Sci.* 1995;310:S123–S126.
6. Kreiger J, Collier C, Song L, Martin D. Linking community based BP measurement to clinical care: a randomized controlled trial of outreach and tracking by community health workers. *Am J Public Health.* 1999;89:856–861.
7. Miller NH, Hill MN. Nursing clinics in the management of hypertension. In: Oparil S, Weber M, eds. *A Companion to Brenner & Rector's The Kidney.* Orlando, FL: WB Saunders; 2000.
8. Miller NH, Hill M, Kottke T, Ockene IS. The multilevel compliance challenge: recommendations for a call to action. A statement for health care professionals. *Circulation.* 1997;95:1085–1090.
9. Patient behavior for blood pressure control. Guidelines for professionals. *JAMA.* 1979;241:2534–2537.
10. U.S. Department of Health and Human Services. *Churches as an Avenue to High Blood Pressure Control.* Bethesda, MD: National Institute of Health; 1992. NIH publication 92-2725.

Chapter C135

Patient Education

Daniel W. Jones, MD

KEY POINTS

- Patient education requires large amounts of provider time but is an effective adjunct to hypertension management.

- Patient education is a continuous process involving a variety of health care workers.

- Resources for patient education are abundantly available, but quality varies.

See also Chapters B102–B105, C127–C129, C131, C134, C136, and C152

Most experts and most clinicians consider patient education an integral part of hypertension patient management, but educational efforts are inconsistent.

Challenges to Effective Education

Hypertension is not obviously symptomatic and is long in duration. Treatment requires daily attention to lifestyle factors and medication for most patients. Patient education is a key element in promoting patient compliance. However, no other area of hypertension management is as challenging. Patient education requires large amounts of provider time and unfortunately is not reimbursable in most health systems. Some clinicians are unaware of the evidence for effectiveness of patient education in improving outcomes.

Benefits of Education

A number of well-conducted studies clearly document benefit. Morisky et al. evaluated 3 education interventions: exit interviews, home visits, and group classes. After 5 years of follow-up, the intervention group had significantly better blood pressure control (79% controlled vs. 50% for a comparison group). Inconsistency is another problem. Because few studies have been done to guide the approach to patient education in hypertension, methods are often haphazard. Key patient education strategies have been outlined by Hill (**Table C135.1**).

Components of Successful Programs

The best providers plan for patient education just as they plan for any other component of disease-state management. Involvement of all members of the health care team improves

Table C135.1. Patient Education Strategies in Hypertension

Identify knowledge, attitudes, beliefs, and experience
Educate about condition and treatment
Tailor the regimen to the patient
Provide reinforcement
Promote social support
Collaborate with other professionals

Table C135.2. Useful Web Sites for Hypertension Patient Education

National High Blood Pressure Education Program (NHBPEP)
  http://www.nhlbi.nih.gov/about/nhbpep/index.htm
NHBPEP patient information
  http://www.nhlbi.nih.gov/health/public/heart/index.htm#hbp
NHBPEP your guide to lowering high blood pressure
  http://www.nhlbi.nih.gov/hbp/index.html
DASH diet
  http://www.nhlbi.nih.gov/health/public/heart/hbp/dash/index.htm
American Heart Association
  http://www.americanheart.org
American Heart Association high blood pressure
  http://www.americanheart.org/presenter.jhtml?identifier=2114

effectiveness (see Chapter C134). In many settings, nurses and pharmacists provide much of the patient education. Physician involvement is a necessary component. A simple mention of a concept by a physician (such as the need to lose weight) may improve the chances that educational efforts by other members of the team will be taken more seriously.

Educational materials. A crucial element in the success of any patient education effort is the commitment of the provider to the educational process. It is impossible to draw the line between educating and motivating; good teachers are successful at both. Materials for use in patient education in blood pressure management are plentiful. There are, however, several challenges to consider. Hypertension disproportionately affects the poor and the uneducated. Attention to use of materials suitable for a patient's learning level is crucial. Another major challenge is avoiding the use of nonobjective materials. Two good sources of objective materials are the American Heart Association and the National High Blood Pressure Education Program of the National Heart, Lung, and Blood Institute. **Table C135.2** provides a list of Web sites with patient information from each of these organizations. Printed materials in multiple languages aimed at various target groups are available, as well as materials in other formats, including video.

SUGGESTED READING

1. Green LW. Educational strategies to improve compliance with therapeutic and preventative regimens: the recent evidence. In: Haynes RB, Taylor DW, Sackett DL, eds. *Compliance in Healthcare.* Baltimore, MD: Johns Hopkins University Press, 1979:157–173.
2. Grueninger UJ, Goldstein MG, Duffy FD. Patient education in hypertension: five essential steps. *J Hypertens.* 1989;7:S93–S98.
3. Hill MN. Strategies for patient education. *Clin Exp Hypertens A.* 1989;11:1187–1201.
4. Jones D, Basile J, Cushman W, et al. Managing hypertension in the southeastern United States: applying the guidelines from the Sixth Report of the Joint National Committee on Prevention, Detection, Evaluation, and Treatment of High Blood Pressure. *Am J Med Sci.* 1999;318:357–364.
5. Morisky DE, Levine DM, Green LW, et al. Five-year blood pressure control and mortality following health education for hypertension patients. *Am J Public Health.* 1983;73:153–161.

Chapter C136

Barriers to Blood Pressure Control

David J. Hyman, MD, MPH; Valory N. Pavlik, PhD, MPH

KEY POINTS

- Barriers to better blood pressure control are system related, physician related, patient related, and societal.

- Most undiagnosed and diagnosed-uncontrolled hypertension is systolic, but physicians remain unassertive in diagnosing and treating systolic hypertension.

- Most people with undiagnosed or uncontrolled hypertension see physicians regularly.

- Blood pressure measurement deficiencies in physician offices probably contribute to poor hypertension control.

See also Chapters B79, B80, B88, B93, B98, B101, B102, B104, B105, B107–C109, C127, C129, C131–C135, C137, C138, C150–C152, C167, and C173

Hypertension Control in the United States Population

Hypertension control in the United States remains limited. National survey data show that only approximately two-thirds of hypertensives are aware of their condition, and slightly more than half are on treatment, with less than 30% at goal (**Figure C136.1**). Barriers to hypertension control can be classified into 4 groups: (a) barriers to use of the health care system, such as lack of health insurance or the high cost of drugs; (b) physician-controlled decisions about the diagnosis and treatment of hypertension; (c) patient nonadherence to a prescribed drug regimen or follow-up schedule; and (d) societal barriers to a healthy lifestyle.

Barriers to System Use by Patients

Health care access. Examining the correlates of poor blood pressure (BP) control in the Third National Health and Nutri-

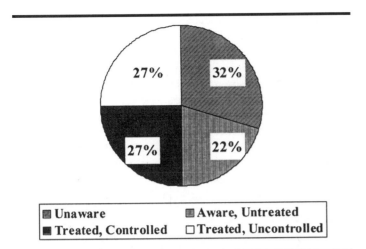

Figure C136.1. Hypertension control in the U.S. population. Third National Health and Nutrition Examination Survey Phase 2 (1991–1994).

tion Examination Survey (NHANES III) provides insight into the probable reasons for the low frequency of hypertension control. Most persons classified as having uncontrolled hypertension have health insurance and a usual source of medical care. Persons who are "unaware" of having hypertension have a mean age of 58 years; 90% of them have health insurance, approximately 80% have a usual source of health care, and 70% have seen a physician at least once within the past year with an average of more than 3 visits a year. More than 75% report having had a BP measurement within the last year. Persons who are aware of having hypertension but are untreated have demographic and health care access characteristics that are similar to those of persons who are aware of hypertension and are receiving treatment. Persons who are being treated for hypertension but whose hypertension is not at goal have an average age of 65 years; 96% of them have health insurance, 97% have a usual source of care, and 96% have seen a physician at least once within the past year with an average of 6 visits per year. Although it is important to recognize that inaccessibility to health care does not adequately explain the low levels of hypertension control in the United States, hypertensive persons without health insurance or a source of primary care are at greater risk of having their BPs uncontrolled. Any change in the health care system that leaves more people uninsured or without a usual source of care will likely lessen control or limit its improvement. For example, Hispanic Americans who have

hypertension use health care the least and have the lowest probability of being controlled. Significant problems derive from the fact that the poorest and most vulnerable segments of the population have trouble getting needed health services.

Cost. The cost of drugs is another potential barrier, but traditionally recommended "first-line" agents such as diuretics and β-blockers are generic drugs available for pennies per day. Long-acting angiotensin-converting enzyme inhibitors and calcium channel blockers are now also generic, so cost should not usually impede antihypertensive treatment. If cost is a barrier for an individual, it is likely that physician-driven drug selection is a major issue.

Physician-Controlled Barriers

Attitudes about systolic hypertension. Most of the undiagnosed, untreated, and treated-uncontrolled hypertension in the United States is isolated systolic hypertension (≥140 systolic BP and ≤90 diastolic BP). **Table C136.1** reports the mean BP for persons with uncontrolled hypertension in 3 different age strata in the NHANES III survey sample. The average diastolic pressure is above 90 mm Hg only in the stratum of persons younger than 45 years of age (<20% of all hypertensives). In an analysis of NHANES III, Franklin and colleagues estimated that approximately two-thirds of uncontrolled hypertension represents elevation in systolic BP with normal diastolic BP. The ALLHAT study has provided convincing evidence that BP control can be substantially improved. In this large community-based titration study, a final BP of 134/75 was achieved in the chlorthalidone arm, which corresponds to a control rate of 68%. Thus, physician skepticism about the feasibility of BP control in older people is not well founded.

Clinical advisory statement. In 2000, a clinical advisory was issued by the National High Blood Pressure Education Program recommending a "paradigm shift" to systolic over diastolic BP in the diagnosis and treatment of hypertension, especially in older people. There is considerable evidence that adoption of this recommendation would cause a major change in practice for United States physicians, and even more so for physicians in other countries.

Physician surveys. In a survey of self-reported physician behavior, many physicians did not start any BP treatment or adjust medications for persistently elevated systolic BP when the diastolic BP was "satisfactory." In Veterans Affairs clinics, physician inaction in the face of persistently elevated systolic

Table C136.1. Blood Pressure Levels in Uncontrolled Hypertensives by Age[a]

AGE GROUP	HYPERTENSION PRESENT BUT SUBJECT UNAWARE		ACKNOWLEDGED, UNTREATED HYPERTENSION		TREATED, UNCONTROLLED HYPERTENSION	
	MEAN BLOOD PRESSURE (MM HG)	SBP ≥140 MM HG AND DBP <90 MM HG (%)	MEAN BLOOD PRESSURE (MM HG)	SBP ≥140 MM HG AND DBP <90 MM HG (%)	MEAN BLOOD PRESSURE (MM HG)	SBP ≥140 MM HG AND DBP <90 MM HG (%)
25–44 yr	138/91	51.9 ± 7.4	141/94	25.1 ± 7.9	147/95	29.1 ± 7.9
45–64 yr	148/86	69.4 ± 3.3	152/89	53.5 ± 4.8	150/87	66.1 ± 2.8
>65 yr	153/77	91.1 ± 1.1	160/81	81.5 ± 2.7	159/78	87.6 ± 1.3
All subjects	148/83	78.8 ± 2.0	151/88	59.1 ± 2.7	155/82	76.9 ± 1.5

DBP, diastolic blood pressure; SBP, systolic blood pressure.
[a]Plus-minus (±) values are means ± standard error.
From Hyman P. Characteristics of patients with uncontrolled hypertension in the United States. *N Engl J Med.* 2001;345:479–486, with permission.

BPs has been documented by Berlowitz and colleagues. In a large sample of practice settings in a major southwestern city, 25% of persons with isolated systolic hypertension were not diagnosed as being hypertensive; in treated hypertensives, diastolic BP persistently >90 mm Hg usually triggered intensification of treatment whereas persistent systolic BP elevations did not. Oliveria and colleagues surveyed physicians about their reasoning during a specific patient encounter and reviewed the clinical records of the encounter. Physicians who responded did not act on persistently elevated systolic BPs and expressed explicit satisfaction with the values achieved. Physicians in the United States, therefore, are not following the recommendations of the current Joint National Committee on the Prevention, Evaluation, and Treatment of High Blood Pressure VI guidelines treating to reduce systolic BP to <140 mm Hg.

Reasons for physician noncompliance. The reasons for physician noncompliance are not clear. Physician adherence to many different practice guidelines is limited, so it is not surprising to find suboptimal hypertension control. Yet some strongly evidenced-based guidelines, such as using angiotensin-converting enzyme inhibitors to treat congestive heart failure, hepatic 3-methylglutaryl coenzyme A reductase inhibitors to reduce myocardial infarctions, and aspirin for secondary cardiovascular disease prevention, have become widely adopted. Thus, it is possible that the relative paucity of randomized trials demonstrating a clear benefit of treating systolic BPs in the 140 to 160 mm Hg range may contribute to the lack of physician interest in this parameter. International studies also suggest that variation in individual physician treatment thresholds, rather than health care financing issues, plays a major role. Although the United States does not have a national health insurance plan, the 27% national rate of BP control is double the Canadian rate of 13% and better than all European rates. Worldwide, physicians rarely diagnose or treat systolic BP elevations if the diastolic BP is <90 mm Hg. Because population survey data show that approximately 75% of uncontrolled hypertensives have an elevated systolic BP with a diastolic BP <90 mm Hg, physician inattention to control of systolic BP is a major barrier to overall hypertension control. Undoing physician preconceptions about tolerability problems with thiazide diuretics may be necessary before the ALLHAT results have a strong impact on clinical practice.

Age bias. Physician inaction with regard to systolic BP helps to explain why increasing age is the strongest predictor of being an unaware, aware-untreated, or treated but uncontrolled hypertensive. Systolic BP rises with age, but diastolic BP falls at older ages. The greatest lack of BP control in persons older than 65 years of age is owing to an elevation of systolic BP. Physicians are less aggressive with systolic BP elevations at all ages, but most particularly in the elderly.

Blood pressure measurement issues. Other factors that are controlled largely by physicians and are underappreciated as barriers to hypertension control are the physicians' BP measurement practices and the intervals between follow-up BP measurements. Most physicians appear to require a persistent BP elevation above a personally defined threshold before intensifying medical treatment. Little is known about how physicians use a single office-based reading, consecutive readings in a single patient visit, or readings over a series of visits.

Actual BP measurement in office practice is often imprecise (see Chapter C109). Random errors in single BP measurements could mask a persistent average elevation. In addition, there may be a systematic bias that could be very important to tighter control. Data from a large primary care clinic network showed that physicians selectively recheck BPs that they think are too high but accept BPs that are lower. Because of regression to the mean, repeat BP values are therefore lower. In addition, patients whose BP measurements are higher on repeat measurement because of random error are not titrated upward.

Visit intervals. Physicians also control the follow-up interval. Follow-up intervals are highly variable among physicians, even for similar conditions. If a physician's threshold for treating hypertension is a diastolic BP >90 mm Hg, for example, the number of persons who get treated could still be highly influenced by the follow-up strategy used. A physician who sees a patient with a diastolic BP of 92 mm Hg, reacts by advising the patient to return at weekly intervals, and then initiates or titrates BP drugs will achieve tighter hypertension control than a physician who reacts to the same patient by simply saying, "Don't worry about it. We'll look at it again in 6 months."

Patient Adherence and Compliance

Patient adherence and compliance and the strategies proposed to improve them are detailed in Chapter C131. Health professionals must be cognizant not to automatically "shift the blame" for uncontrolled hypertension by attributing it solely to patient noncompliance. Studies showing a high dropout rate for new patients with hypertension are widely cited, but studies reporting high adherence (>95% of established hypertensives remaining in treatment) are much less well known. Drug side effects are frequently proposed as the reason for lack of BP control, but the basis for this claim is questionable. Most categories of antihypertensive medications used today (including diuretics and β-blockers) have discontinuation rates in randomized double-blind trials similar to placebo.

Societal Barriers to Healthy Lifestyle

During the last several decades, many Americans have adopted healthier behaviors (see Chapters C129 and C130). Fewer Americans smoke, consume large amounts of saturated fat and cholesterol, and drive while intoxicated, and many more use seat belts while driving. With the proliferation of prepared and fast food, labor-saving devices, cars, and electronics, however, many more Americans are obese and do not exercise regularly. Although the trend toward obesity may hinder BP control overall, it does not explain why diastolic BP control is better in the United States than elsewhere or why systolic BP is so poorly controlled. Societal factors can no longer be invoked as the limiting barrier to hypertension control because the prevalence of hypertension is actually falling the United States.

SUGGESTED READING

1. Berlowitz DR, Ash AS, Hickey EC, et al. Inadequate management of blood pressure in a hypertensive population. *N Engl J Med.* 1998;339:1957–1963.
2. Franklin SS, Jacobs MJ, Wong ND, et al. Predominance of isolated systolic hypertension among middle-aged and elderly US hypertensives: analysis

based on National Health and Nutrition Examination Survey (NHANES) III. *Hypertension*. 2001;37:869–874.

3. Goff DC, Howard G, Russell GB, Labarthe DR. Birth cohort evidence of population influences on blood pressure in the United States, 1887–1994. *Ann Epidemiol*. 2001;11:271–279.

4. Hyman DJ, Pavlik VN. Self-reported hypertension treatment practices among primary care physicians: blood pressure thresholds, drug choices, and the role of guidelines and evidence-based medicine. *Arch Intern Med*. 2000;160:2281–2286.

5. Hyman D, Pavlik V, Vallbona C. Physician role in lack of awareness and control of hypertension. *J Clin Hypertens*. 2000;2:234–330.

6. Izzo JL, Levy D, Black HR. Clinical Advisory Statement: importance of systolic blood pressure in older Americans. *Hypertension*. 2000;35:1021–1024.

7. Joint National Committee on the Prevention, Evaluation, and Treatment of High Blood Pressure. The sixth report of the Joint National Committee on Prevention, Detection, Evaluation, and Treatment of High Blood Pressure. *Arch Intern Med*. 1997;157:2413–2446.

8. Oliveria SA, Lapuerta P, McCarthy BD, et al. Physician-related barriers to the effective management of uncontrolled hypertension. *Arch Intern Med*. 2002;162:387–388.

9. Pavlik VN, Hyman DJ, Vallbona C, Grim C. Selective physician blood pressure re-measurement in the office setting may contribute to poor hypertension control. *Am J Hypertens*. 2002;15:A81.

10. Spencer F, Scleparis G, Goldberg RJ, et al. Decade-long trends (1986 to 1997) in the medical treatment of patients with acute myocardial infarction: a community-wide perspective. *Am Heart J*. 2001;142:594–603.

Section 4. *Antihypertensive Drugs*

Chapter C137

Antihypertensive Drugs: Pharmacologic Principles and Dosing Effects

Joseph L. Izzo, Jr, MD; Domenic A. Sica, MD

KEY POINTS

- Underdosing and failure of adequate titration of antihypertensive drugs are major public health problems leading to poor blood pressure control. These trends can be remedied through better knowledge of dose-response relationships and pharmacodynamics.

- There are significant dose-response effects for all classes of antihypertensive drugs; a rough guide to the relative effectiveness of titration (or "steepness" of the dose-response relationships) follows: sympatholytics > calcium antagonists > diuretics > β-blockers = angiotensin-converting enzyme inhibitors = angiotensin receptor blockers.

- Different clinical end points often have different dose-response relationships to a given drug; for example, maximal reduction in proteinuria requires a higher dose of angiotensin receptor blockers than does maximal blood pressure reduction.

- Drug-host interactions that affect dose-response relationships include (a) population-related differences (e.g., lower plasma renin activity and reduced monotherapeutic effectiveness of ACE inhibitors/angiotensin receptor blockers in black hypertensives and (b) environment-related variations (e.g., salt balance or vasodilator-induced activation of the sympathetic nervous and renin-angiotensin systems).

- Drug-drug interactions can affect dose-response relationships (e.g., angiotensin-converting enzyme inhibitor effect is enhanced by diuretics or blunted by nonsteroidal antiinflammatory drugs).

- Combination drug therapy is necessary for adequate blood pressure control in *most* hypertensives.

See also Chapters B106–B108, C126–C128, C136, C138–C147, C151, and C152

Basic Principles

Pharmacodynamics versus pharmacokinetics. Pharmacokinetic properties are those related to absorption, distribution, and elimination of a drug. For most drugs and most patients, pharmacokinetic considerations are of minor importance in that they are already reflected in the approved dose ranges and dose intervals. Pharmacokinetic differences are most readily apparent in the use of certain drugs in subpopulations with impaired clearance. For example, a drug that is water soluble and principally eliminated by glomerular filtration often requires dosage adjustment in patients with renal impairment. From a practical point of view, however, it is the pharmacodynamic properties of a drug (i.e., characteristics that describe its biologic effects) that are of greatest interest in most patients.

Dosing intervals and peak:trough effects. Antihypertensive drugs are typically evaluated after a single dose to determine the time course of their effects. From such studies, an area-under-the-curve can be calculated for a drug and equated with response. Because this indicator is so cumbersome to obtain, peak and trough blood pressure (BP) effects are usually substituted for area-under-the-curve. Trough BP readings, often derived from ambulatory monitoring studies, are particularly useful in defining whether BP control has been effectively maintained throughout a dosing interval. An antihypertensive drug is approved for once-daily use if its peak effect is substantially different from placebo and its trough effect (usually BP 24 hours after the last dose) is at least 50% of its peak effect.

Dose-response relationships. A fundamental concept in therapeutics is the log-linear dose-response curve, which is critical to an accurate understanding of the effects of a given drug (**Figure C137.1**). In the case of an adrenergic receptor antagonist, for example, the range of receptor occupancy can vary from 0% to 100%. The effect of the antagonist is correlated with the logarithm of its concentration and, by extension, the logarithm of the dose. In the case of a true log-linear relationship, a 10-fold increase in dose would be needed to double the effect (point A to B in Figure C137.1); doubling the dose would then be expected to increase the effect by the logarithm of 2 (approximately 0.3, i.e., from point A to C). If the relationship were log-linear, a 4-fold dose increase would be needed to double the effect. In either case, it can be seen readily that small titration steps (increasing the existing dose by less than 100%) would be expected to have relatively little effect on a patient's BP.

A corollary to the dose-response principle is that a drug exhibits a log-dose response for its toxic effects that is typically parallel and to the right of its therapeutic effect curve. Thus, at any given clinical dose of an approved agent, the therapeutic effect is expected to be greater than the toxic effect (equivalent to moving from point B to B^1 in Figure C137.1). Decreasing the medication dose tends to decrease therapeutic and toxic effects but may allow a relatively greater decrease in toxicity (Figure C137.1, point A to A1). The difference between the therapeutic and toxic curves is sometimes called the *therapeutic window* of a drug.

Factors Affecting Dose-Response Relationships

Pharmacodynamic differences between drugs. Dose-response relationships can be visualized in a number of ways. In the case of the angiotensin receptor blockers (ARBs), the character of the curve ranges from shallow to flat when the dose is increased beyond the initial effect dose. Thiazide diuretics

typically display a moderate response at low doses, which rapidly flattens thereafter. Short-acting dihydropyridines, such as the immediate-release form of nifedipine, have an uncharacteristically steep response curve. A rough guide to the effectiveness of dose titration (or "steepness" of the dose-response relationship) for antihypertensive drug classes is sympatholytics > calcium antagonists > diuretics > β-blockers = angiotensin-converting enzyme (ACE) inhibitors = ARBs.

Pharmacodynamic differences in end point responsiveness. Different clinical end points may have different dose-response relationships to a given drug within the same individual; for example, the ARB dose required to maximally reduce proteinuria is much higher than that needed for maximal BP reduction.

Drug-drug interactions. In virtually all cases, addition of a diuretic to a preexisting drug regimen results in an enhanced response, typically reflected by (a) a leftward shift of the curve (less drug required to effect the same reduction in BP), (b) a greater peak (sometimes called *plateau*) response, or (c) a steepening of the response slope at its midpoint. In contrast, addition of a nonsteroidal antiinflammatory drug to a given regimen may have the opposite effect(s).

Drug-host interactions. A number of "host" factors are known to influence the dose-response to a particular antihypertensive medication. Some are relatively fixed and predictable (e.g., genetic predispositions), whereas some vary with the physiologic changes in the host's environment.

Population subgroups and drug responses. Black hypertensives are generally less responsive to low doses of ACE inhibitors and ARBs, yet if doses are increased, their response differs less from that of white hypertensives. Such response characteristics are shared with other low renin subgroups such as very elderly individuals and some diabetics. Another example of a genetic difference is the lower effectiveness of hydralazine in individuals who have inherited the rapid acetylator gene.

Physiologic changes. Salt balance is the most obvious physiologic factor affecting antihypertensive drug responsiveness. Salt overload blunts the effect of most antihypertensive drugs (except perhaps calcium antagonists). Conversely, sodium depletion (or concomitant diuretic therapy) enhances the effect of other antihypertensive drugs.

Pseudotolerance. Another major consideration in the pharmacodynamic dose-response relationship for an antihypertensive medication is the extent to which BP counterregulatory mechanisms are activated by BP lowering. Acute and chronic BP reduction often activates an interlinked series of mechanisms designed to restore BP. Reflex increases in cardiac output, peripheral vasoconstriction, and salt/water retention can result from baroreflex-mediated activation of the sympathetic nervous and renin-angiotensin systems. These responses are most likely to occur when arterial dilator drugs (hydralazine, minoxidil, some calcium antagonists) or high-dose diuretics are used. Clinically, it can be difficult to gauge the extent to which counterregulatory systems are activated. A relatively reliable sign is an unexplained loss of previously established BP control. A clinically relevant increase in pulse rate (>10%) should prompt consideration of lowering the dose of the provoking agent or adding a β-blocker. Sodium retention, as a means by which BP

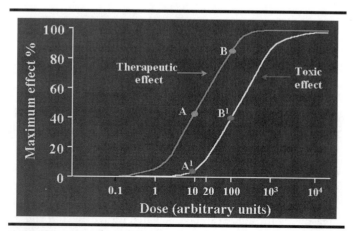

Figure C137.1. Theoretical therapeutic and toxic logarithmic-linear dose-response curves.

control is lost, is easy to recognize if peripheral edema develops. Sodium retention can still occur without peripheral edema. If this is suspected, a diuretic can be started (or if one is already in use its dose can be increased) to effect a small weight loss.

Other physiologic adaptations. Some differences in responsiveness between acute and chronic dosing may occur as a result of metabolic changes or even changes in receptor populations. True tachyphylaxis, in which enzyme induction increases drug metabolism, is generally not seen with antihypertensive drugs.

Duration of therapy. Very few long-term studies are available, but it appears that the full effects of some drugs may not be apparent until months or even years after therapy is begun. It has been speculated that favorable remodeling of the heart and blood vessels, a process that takes much longer than acute hemodynamic effects, can occur with certain agents. Thus, a dose-response relationship for an individual compound cannot be fully evaluated unless it is also considered as a function of time.

Clinical Dosing Problems Attributable to Gaps in Drug Development and Approval

The drug approval process involves a complicated series of premarketing steps in which the potential manufacturer works with the U.S. Food and Drug Administration to demonstrate safety and efficacy of an experimental drug. Unfortunately, the rules for drug development have not been carefully scrutinized until relatively recently. In the process, it has become apparent that full dose ranges of approved agents have not been adequately investigated. This a potential problem that can importantly influence the risk to benefit ratio of a drug.

Overdosing errors (lack of data on minimum therapeutic doses of older drugs). Several antihypertensive medications were introduced at doses higher than those currently recommended, including thiazide diuretics, β-blockers, alpha-methyldopa, hydralazine, and the ACE inhibitor captopril. In these cases, the failure to recognize the value of lower doses can be traced directly to a lack of data at the low end of the dose-response curve. A result of the administration of unnecessarily large doses of these medications is an impressive array of adverse effects, including proteinuria, dysgeusia, and leukopenia with captopril; sedation and depression with alpha-methyldopa; and a lupus-like syndrome associated with hydralazine. With thiazides, the use of lower doses—which are almost equally effective and are safer—was only determined by trial and error long after thiazides were approved for use.

Underdosing errors
Lack of data on maximal therapeutic doses. Failure to explore the upper ranges of the dose-response relationship occurs commonly as well. There is a powerful reluctance of drug developers to push an investigational drug to its toxic limits for fear that development will be automatically terminated. In recent years, this problem has led to a consistent trend to underdose newer agents such as ARBs, which have yet to demonstrate toxic effects different from placebo.
Inadequate titration (failure to recognize dose-response effects). Characteristic dose-response relationships for many antihypertensive drugs have been artifactually masked during drug development and approval. This is because of the scientific

inadequacy of typical end point–limited dose-titration trials. Such trials do not recognize the bias inherent to a heterogeneous response to a test agent and the impact of not testing all patients at each dose. In an end point–limited dose-titration trial, a prespecified end point (e.g., failure to achieve a nominal BP reduction ≥10 mm Hg or to reach a final BP ≤140/90 mm Hg) is used as the criterion for each titration. The (heterogeneous) response to the lowest dose can be arbitrarily subclassified into hyporesponders, normal responders, and hyperresponders, with all hyperresponders eliminated from subsequent dose titration. If a second titration step is included, the individuals ultimately receiving the highest dose are the ones who are intrinsically most resistant. The result of this systematic selection bias is the appearance of an artifactually "flat" dose-response curve (i.e., a limited maximal effect or plateau). Such bias is amplified by the degree of heterogeneity of population responses (e.g., age- and race-dependent responses to ACE inhibitors and ARBs, which are erroneously believed to have essentially flat dose-response curves). Many of the pooled dosing studies on currently available ACE inhibitors and ARBs actually demonstrate an "inexplicable" reduction in BP effect at the highest tested dose—further evidence of the impact of dose-selection bias.

Inadequate 24-hour blood pressure control (inadequate trough doses). It is sometimes mistakenly assumed that the trough to peak effect ratio for a given drug is independent of dose. This is not the case, however, for many drugs, including ACE inhibitors, which tend to reach a plateau for peak effect at lower doses than those required to achieve a maximal trough effect.

Combination Therapy

It has been recognized for decades that there is value to the use of drug combinations, not only to improve efficacy but also to reduce side effects (see Chapter C145).

Rationale. This notion was the foundation for the original triple-drug regimen of the 1980s (hydralazine, propranolol, and hydrochlorothiazide) and the stepped-care approach of the early Joint National Committee reports. Given the fact that multiple physiologic systems contribute to BP elevation and that most antihypertensive agents have a predominant (specific) mechanism of action related to one (or more) of these physiologic systems, it can be anticipated that multiple drugs will be needed to maintain BP control. Finally, it is generally recognized that "lower BP is better," yet most agents when used as monotherapy simply will not lower BP to optimal levels (ideally to 120/80 mm Hg, but at least to 140/90 mm Hg).

Fixed-dose combinations. Fixed-dose combination products were among the earliest effective oral antihypertensive agents, and many are still embraced by busy practitioners. In recent decades, fixed-dose combinations have fallen out of favor with many academic physicians and formulary groups on the grounds that they are often more expensive and are awkwardly formulated (inappropriate doses or component ratios). However, given the relatively poor overall BP control rates, the potential to deliver simultaneously greater efficacy and safety, and the improved patient acceptance that they usually bring, fixed-dose products should be reconsidered. Overall, combinations of a diuretic with an ACE inhibitor, ARB, or β-blocker or an ACE inhibitor together with a calcium antagonist offer clinically attractive 2-drug combinations.

SUGGESTED READING

1. Donnelly R, Elliott HL, Meredith PA. Concentration-effect analysis of antihypertensive drug response. Focus on calcium antagonists. *Clin Pharmacokinet.* 1994;26:472–485.
2. Johnston GD. Dose-response relationships with antihypertensive drugs. *Pharmacol Ther.* 1992;35:53–92.
3. Meredith PA, Elliot HL. Concentration-effect relationships and implications for trough-to-peak ratio. *Am J Hypertens.* 1996;9:66S–70S.
4. Meredith PA, Reid JL. The use of pharmacodynamic and pharmacokinetic profiles in drug development for planning individual therapy. In: Laragh JH, Brenner BM, eds. *Hypertension: Pathophysiology, Diagnosis, and Management.* 2nd ed. New York, NY: Raven Press Ltd; 1995:2771–2783.
5. Sica DA. Rationale for fixed-dose combinations in the treatment of hypertension: the cycle repeats. *Drugs.* 2002;62:443–462.

Chapter C138

Drug Combinations

Alan H. Gradman, MD

KEY POINTS

- More than 1 drug is required to achieve goal blood pressure in most hypertensive patients.
- Combining drugs that work by complementary pharmacologic mechanisms improves overall efficacy and tolerability.
- Fixed-drug combinations simplify treatment regimens and promote adherence.
- Most effective fixed-drug combinations include a diuretic.

See also Chapters B106–B108, C127, C128, C133, C136, C137, C139–C141, C144–C147, C151, C159, and C164

It is increasingly apparent that developing strategies for the combined use of antihypertensive drugs constitutes an essential focus of clinical therapeutics.

Multiple Drug Use in Clinical Trials

Controlled clinical trials document that to achieve diastolic blood pressures (BPs) consistent with the Sixth Report of the Joint National Committee on Prevention, Detection, Evaluation, and Treatment of High Blood Pressure (JNC VI) recommendations (<90 mm Hg), multidrug therapy is required in approximately 75% of hypertensive individuals. In patients with diabetes and renal insufficiency, an average of >3 drugs/patient are needed. The control of systolic BP also necessitates the use of combination therapy. In the Systolic Hypertension in the Elderly Program (SHEP) trial, 54% of patients with isolated systolic hypertension required >1 drug despite the fact that target BPs were generally higher than the currently recommended goal of 140 mm Hg. In the Losartan Intervention for Endpoints (LIFE) trial, treatment to goal (<140/90 mm Hg) was aggressively pursued for both systolic and diastolic BP; in more than 9,000 patients with an average baseline BP of 175/98 mm Hg, >90% required multiple agents.

Failure of Single-Drug Regimen

Although considerable variation in individual response is observed, most available drugs only reduce diastolic BP by 4 to 8 mm Hg and systolic BP by 7 to 13 mm Hg on average if corrected for placebo effects. This magnitude of effect is insufficient to achieve goal BP in most hypertensives. There are several reasons for the therapeutic inadequacy of monotherapy. It is a fundamental feature of antihypertensive drug therapy that reduction in BP by almost any pharmacologic approach results in the activation of counterregulatory mechanisms that oppose and limit the action of the primary agent (see Chapter C128).

Salt and water retention resulting from heart failure, coexistent or often unrecognized renal disease, or concurrent drug treatment (e.g., nonsteroidal antiinflammatory agents) is another common reason for the failure of monotherapy. Secondary forms of hypertension such as renal artery stenosis or primary aldosteronism play a role in some patients. The importance of partial or complete nonadherence to complicated multidose-multidrug regimens is a factor in the apparent failure of antihypertensive therapy. Thus, any means to simplify drug regimens, including once-daily dosing and the use of fixed-dose combinations, can be beneficial. Cost of medication and side effects related to drug therapy are also important reasons for patient discontinuation of drug treatment.

Goals of Combination Therapy

The goals of combination drug therapy are generally to improve efficacy and tolerability.

Efficacy. Improved BP control occurs if the agents included in a combination produce additive reductions in BP. Because hypertension is multifactorial and the exact pathophysiologic mechanisms operative in individual patients are often obscure, combining agents with different pharmacologic actions broadens the spectrum of response across a range of patient types. Efficacious 2-drug combinations include angiotensin-converting enzyme (ACE) inhibitor–thiazide, angiotensin receptor blocker (ARB)–thiazide, ACE inhibitor–calcium antagonist, β-blocker–calcium antagonist, and β-blocker–thiazide.

The results of ALLHAT confirm the necessity of combination therapy in the vast majority of hypertensive patients. In ALLHAT, target BP (< 140/90 mm Hg) was achieved in 66% of patients. Of those, a single agent was successful in 40%, indicating that only 26% of randomized patients could be controlled with monotherapy. Because target BP for diabetics (who constituted 36% of the ALLHAT cohort) is now 130/80 mm Hg, it is likely that this figure overestimates the fraction of the hypertensive population in whom monotherapy will be sufficient to reach goal BP.

Tolerability. Superior tolerability results if dose-dependent side effects (clinical or metabolic) are reduced by combining smaller doses of 2 drugs as compared to using higher doses of individual agents. This principle is the basis for low-dose combination therapy. Most drugs exhibit parallel dose-response curves for their therapeutic and toxic effects (see Figure C137.1). The degree to which these curves are separated constitutes the therapeutic index of the drug. If the curves are close together, increasing the BP response through dose titration leads to an increased frequency of side effects. Dose-dependent side effects are seen with all classes of antihypertensive agents except for ACE inhibitors and ARBs. Upward dose titration in an attempt to avoid the addition of a second agent is often a factor in the failure of monotherapy (**Figure C138.1**). Appropriate combination therapy may improve the tolerability of drugs included in the regimen because side effects associated with a particular drug are sometimes neutralized by the pharmacologic properties of a second agent. For example, the tendency for thiazides to cause hypokalemia is blunted by concomitant use of potassium-sparing diuretics, ACE inhibitors, or ARBs. The combined use of drugs with additive side effects such as verapamil with a β-blocker should be avoided.

Fixed-Drug Combinations

Rationale. Traditional teaching has stressed avoidance of fixed-drug combinations. The reason given is usually the lack of flexibility in titration of individual drug components. Pre-

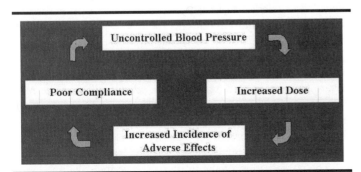

Figure C138.1. Potential consequences of monotherapy dose titration.

serving this ability may be important in selected cases, such as patients with coronary artery disease in whom the dose of β-blocker is adjusted to achieve a specific target heart rate. In the majority of hypertensives, however, this consideration is of little importance. In contrast, the advantages of fixed-drug combinations are significant. Because most patients require multiple agents to control BP, combination agents simplify the therapeutic regimen and promote adherence. Competition within the pharmaceutical industry has decreased the cost of fixed-drug combinations and many, particularly those containing low-dose diuretics, are actually less expensive to purchase than their individual components. A final advantage derives from the fact that marketed fixed-drug combinations have been carefully studied and have received FDA approval because they produce greater BP reduction than monotherapy. They thus constitute proven entities in comparison to randomly selected combinations of individual agents. A list of commonly used fixed-drug combinations is given in **Table C138.1**.

Clinical use. Fixed-drug combinations are most often used as the "second step" in patients who exhibit an inadequate response to the agent chosen initially. Low-dose combination therapy is an alternative strategy to the traditional approach of increasing the dose of the first drug until the goal is reached or side effects supervene. Although the incremental reduction in BP is often similar, dose-dependent side effects are avoided and the overall tolerability of treatment is improved.

There is also increasing use of fixed-drug combinations as initial therapy and several low-dose combinations have been approved by the U.S. Food and Drug Administration (FDA) for this purpose. Fixed-drug combinations are also being used as initial therapy in patients with severe hypertension in whom the likelihood is low that any single drug will achieve goal BP. The World Health Organization (WHO) recommends that combination drugs be used as first-line therapy in individuals with more than 7 forms of hypertension. The initial use of a combination decreases the number of office visits and shortens the time period necessary to bring the BP under control.

Importance of Diuretics in Combination Therapy

There are many reasons to consider including a diuretic whenever combination therapy is required. Low-dose diuretics constitute an excellent therapeutic selection given their safety, efficacy, low cost, and proven ability to reduce clinical events. Volume overload is a common factor in the failure of monotherapy and the routine addition of a diuretic is frequently effective in countering this tendency. Diuretics offer additive BP-lowering effects when combined with a variety of commonly used choices for initial therapy, including β-blockers, ACE inhibitors, and ARBs. In contrast, the addition of a diuretic to a calcium channel blocker is less effective, perhaps because both increase renal sodium excretion and act as vasodilators to achieve chronic BP lowering. Inclusion of a diuretic in a combination treatment regimen resulted in normalization of systolic BP in 77% compared to 46% of patients given nondiuretic-containing combinations.

Specific Combinations

Thiazides and potassium-sparing diuretics. Hypokalemia is an extremely important dose-related side effect of thiazide

Table C138.1. Combination Drugs for Hypertension

DRUG	TRADE NAME
Thiazides and potassium-sparing diuretics	
Triamterene, 37.5, 50.0, or 75.0 mg/hydrochlorothiazide, 25 or 50 mg	Dyazide, Maxzide
Spironolactone, 25 or 50 mg/hydrochlorothiazide, 25 or 50 mg	Aldactazide
Amiloride hydrochloride, 5 mg/hydrochlorothiazide, 50 mg	Moduretic
Angiotensin-converting enzyme inhibitors and diuretics	
Benazepril hydrochloride, 5, 10, or 20 mg/hydrochlorothiazide, 6.25,12.5 or 25.0 mg	Lotensin HCT
Captopril, 25 or 50 mg/hydrochlorothiazide, 15 or 25 mg	Capozide[a]
Enalapril maleate, 5 or 10 mg/hydrochlorothiazide, 12.5 or 25.0 mg	Vaseretic
Lisinopril, 10 or 20 mg/hydrochlorothiazide, 12.5 or 25.0 mg	Prinzide, Zestoretic
Angiotensin II receptor antagonists and diuretics	
Candesartan cilexetil, 16 or 32 mg/hydrochlorothiazide, 12.5 mg	Atacand HCT
Irbesartan, 150 or 300 mg/hydrochlorothiazide, 12.5 mg	Avalide
Losartan potassium, 50 or 100 mg/hydrochlorothiazide, 12.5 or 25.0 mg	Hyzaar
Telmisartan, 40 or 80 mg/hydrochlorothiazide, 12.5 mg	Micardis HCT
Valsartan, 80 or 160 mg/hydrochlorothiazide, 12.5 mg or 25.0 mg	Diovan HCT
β-Adrenergic blockers and diuretics	
Atenolol, 50 or 100 mg/chlorthalidone, 25 mg	Tenoretic
Bisoprolol fumarate, 2.5, 5.0, or 10.0 mg/hydrochlorothiazide, 6.5 mg	Ziac[a]
Metoprolol tartrate, 50 or 100 mg/hydrochlorothiazide, 25 or 50 mg	Lopressor HCT
Nadolol, 40 or 60 mg/bendroflumethiazide, 5 mg	Corzide
Propranolol hydrochloride, 40 or 80 mg/hydrochlorothiazide, 25 mg	Inderide
Propranolol hydrochloride (extended release) 80, 120, or 160 mg/ hydrochlorothiazide, 50 mg	Inderide LA
Timolol maleate, 10 mg/hydrochlorothiazide, 25 mg	Timolide
Calcium antagonists and angiotensin-converting enzyme inhibitors	
Amlodipine besylate, 2.5, 5.0, or 10.0 mg/ benazepril hydrochloride, 10 or 20 mg	Lotrel
Felodipine (extended release), 5 mg/enalapril maleate, 5 mg	Lexxel
Verapamil hydrochloride (extended release), 180 or 240 mg/trandolapril, 1, 2, or 4 mg	Tarka

[a]Approved by the U.S. Food and Drug Administration for initial therapy.
Adapted from The Sixth Report of the Joint National Committee on Prevention, Detection, Evaluation, and Treatment of High Blood Pressure. *Arch Intern Med.* 1997;157:2427.

diuretics. Combining a thiazide with a potassium-sparing diuretic such as spironolactone, triamterene, or amiloride significantly improves their safety. Because of the high incidence of hypokalemia and the resultant cardiac arrhythmias and sudden death, hydrochlorothiazide (HCTZ) should not be used at the previously recommended dose of 50 mg/day unless possibly when combined with a potassium-sparing agent.

Thiazides with angiotensin-converting enzyme inhibitors or angiotensin receptor blockers. A growing body of data supports the benefits of blocking the renin-angiotensin-aldosterone system (RAAS) on reducing clinical events, particularly in hypertensive patients with coexistent diabetes, proteinuria, renal insufficiency, left ventricular hypertrophy or established vascular or coronary artery disease. The combination of either an ACE inhibitor or an ARB with a low-dose diuretic is one of the most attractive approaches to contemporary combination therapy. The mechanisms of action of drugs included in these combinations are clearly complementary. Diuretics reduce intravascular volume, activating the RAAS. This results in vasoconstriction as well as compensatory salt and water retention, reducing the magnitude of any observed BP reduction. In the presence of an ACE inhibitor or an ARB, activation of the RAAS is prevented, and the effects of combining these agents become additive. Addition of an ACE inhibitor or ARB to a thiazide also ameliorates the hypokalemia, hyperglycemia, and hyperuremia caused by the thiazide.

ACE inhibitor–thiazide and ARB-thiazide combinations are effective in black patients who, in general, demonstrate less BP reduction compared to whites when treated with ACE inhibitors or ARBs alone.

β-Blockers and thiazides. β-blockers are effective antihypertensive agents and are a preferred therapy in patients with ischemic heart disease. Their antihypertensive effects are mediated, in part, by suppression of renin release. Therefore, like the ACE inhibitors and ARBs, β-blockers attenuate the RAAS activation that accompanies the use of thiazide diuretics. Addition of diuretics also improves the effectiveness of β-blockers in blacks and others with low renin hypertension. Combination of the cardioselective β-blocker, bisoprolol (5 mg), with very low doses of HCTZ (6.25 mg) has shown response rates equivalent to those achieved with amlodipine with a side-effect profile comparable to placebo.

Calcium antagonists and angiotensin-converting enzyme inhibitors. Calcium antagonists are among the most potent antihypertensive agents and are an essential component of therapy in patients with severe or resistant hypertension. When combined with ACE inhibitors, their BP-lowering effects are additive. Addition of an ACE inhibitor significantly improves the tolerability profile of calcium channel blockers. Through their antisympathetic effects, ACE inhibitors blunt the increases in heart rate that often accompany initiation of therapy with dihydropyridine calcium channel blockers and that may occasionally precipitate myocardial ischemia. ACE inhibitors also partially neutralize the edema of calcium antagonists, which is the most important dose-limiting side effect seen with these agents. In one study with felodipine, the incidence of edema was reduced from 10.8% to 4.1% by combining both classes of drugs. The cause for the edema produced by calcium antagonists is believed to be arteriolar dilation without matching venous dilation; the result being an increased pressure gradient across capillary membranes in dependent portions of the body. Addition of an ACE inhibitor, by producing concurrent venodilation, reduces the pressure gradient and fluid transudation.

The combination of the heart rate–lowering calcium channel blockers, verapamil and diltiazem, with ACE inhibitors may offer advantages in terms of renal protection. Unlike the dihydropyridines, diltiazem and verapamil reduce urinary albumin excretion, which appears to be a surrogate for ongoing renal damage. In a small group of patients with diabetic nephropathy, the combination of verapamil with the ACE inhibitor trandolapril reduced proteinuria to a greater extent than did either agent alone; the combination also slowed the rate of decline in renal function.

SUGGESTED READING

1. Giles TD, Sander GE. Beyond the usual strategies for blood pressure reduction: therapeutic considerations and combination therapies. *J Clin Hypertens.* 2001;3:346–353.
2. Gradman AH, Cutler NR, Davis PJ, et al. Combined enalapril and felodipine extended release (ER) for systemic hypertension. *Am J Cardiol.* 1997;79:431–435.
3. Hansson L, Zanchetti A, Carruthers SG, et al. Effects of intensive blood-pressure lowering and low-dose aspirin in patients with hypertension: principal results of the hypertension optimal treatment (HOT) randomised trial. *Lancet.* 1998;351:1755–1762.
4. Kendall MJ. Approaches to meeting the criteria for fixed dose antihypertensive combinations. Focus on metoprolol. *Drugs.* 1995;50:454–464.
5. Menard J, Bellet M. Calcium antagonists-ACE inhibitors combination therapy: objectives and methodology of clinical development. *J Cardiovasc Pharmacol.* 1993;1:S49–S54.
6. Neutel JM, Black, HR, Weber MA. Combination therapy with diuretics: an evolution of understanding. *Am J Med.* 1996;101:61S–70S.
7. Sheinfeld GR, Bakris GL. Benefits of combination angiotensin-converting enzyme inhibitor and calcium antagonist therapy for diabetic patients. *Am J Hypertens.* 1999;12:80S–85S.
8. Sica DA. Rationale for fixed-dose combinations in the treatment of hypertension: the cycle repeats. *Drugs.* 2002;62:243–262.

Chapter C139

Thiazide and Loop Diuretics

Vasilios Papademetriou, MD; Domenic A. Sica, MD; Joseph L. Izzo, Jr, MD

KEY POINTS

- Thiazide diuretics are ideal first-line agents in the treatment of hypertension because they have been proven to reduce cardiovascular mortality and morbidity in systolic and diastolic hypertension at low cost.

- Benefits of thiazide diuretics are achieved at low doses (e.g., 12.5 mg to 25.0 mg of hydrochlorothiazide or 12.5 mg of chlorthalidone daily); higher doses are rarely needed.

- In combination with any other class of antihypertensive drugs, diuretics usually provide additive blood pressure lowering effects.

- Mild biochemical abnormalities caused by low-dose diuretic therapy (hypokalemia, hyperglycemia, and hyperuricemia) are not associated with increased mortality after 6 years of follow-up in the Antihypertensive Lipid-Lowering Heart Attack Trial.

- Loop diuretics should not be used as first-line therapy in hypertension; they should be used in combination with other agents for conditions of clinically significant fluid overload (e.g., renal failure, heart failure, and fluid retention with vasodilator drugs, such as minoxidil).

See also Chapters A46, A76, B94, B106, C127, C128, C137, C138, C147, C150, C151, C159, C165, and C167

Expansion of extracellular fluid (ECF) volume plays a role in blood pressure (BP) control. Thiazide diuretics can reduce ECF volume, counteract fluid retention caused by other drugs, and dilate peripheral arterioles (**Table C139.1**). Loop diuretics are powerful natriuretic venodilator agents that reduce ECF volume and BP, particularly in conditions of reduced glomerular filtration, such as heart failure and renal failure.

THIAZIDES

Thiazide diuretics, first discovered in the early 1950s, were the first truly effective, tolerable oral antihypertensive agents. Used alone or in combination with other antihypertensives, thiazides provide a predictable and sustained antihypertensive effect in at least half of the hypertensive population, without serious side effects.

Outcome Studies in Hypertension

Early trials in diastolic hypertension. Diuretics formed the basis of a additive regimen used by the Veterans Administration (VA) Cooperative Study Group in its seminal studies begun in the 1960s that proved the benefits of BP control. Both the first (diastolic ≥105 mm Hg) and second (diastolic, 90–104 mm Hg) VA trials demonstrated reduced cardiovascular morbidity and mortality. Subsequent trials over the next 2 decades followed the lead of the VA studies. Almost all of these subsequent studies used a variant of "stepped-care" therapy (diuretic followed by adrenergic inhibitor, followed by vasodilator) that later became the basis for the several reports of the Joint Committee on the Prevention, Detection, Evaluation, and Treatment of High Blood Pressure (JNC). A metaanalysis of 18 trials and 48,220 patients has differentiated the effects of diuretics from β-blockers on

Table C139.1. Diuretics—Doses and Clinical Use

DRUG	TRADE NAME	TOTAL DAILY DOSES (FREQUENCY)	COMMENTS
Thiazide-type diuretics			
Chlorthalidone	Hygroton	12.5–50.0 (1)	More prolonged effect than hydrochlorothiazide
Hydrochlorothiazide	HydroDIURIL Microzide	12.5–50.0 (1)	
Indapamide	Lozol	1.25–5.00 (1)	
Metolazone	Zaroxolyn	2.5–10.0 (1)	Effective at glomerular filtration rate ≤10 cc, unlike other thiazide diuretics; very poor bioavailability
Metolazone	Mykrox	0.5–1.0 (1)	Improved bioavailability compared to metolazone (Zaroxolyn) results in lower dose being given
Loop diuretics			
Furosemide	Lasix	40–240 (2–3)	Shorter duration of action—multiple daily dosing to avoid rebound sodium retention
Bumetanide	Bumex	0.5–4.0 (2–3)	Same as furosemide
Torsemide	Demadex	5–100 (1–2)	Long duration of action
Ethacrynic acid	Edecrin	25–100 (2–3)	Only nonsulfonamide diuretic, ototoxicity

health outcomes. Low-dose diuretics were more effective than high-dose diuretics in the prevention of cardiovascular events. With low-dose diuretic therapy, strokes were reduced by 34%, coronary heart disease by 28%, congestive heart failure by 42%, total mortality by 10%, and cardiovascular mortality by 24%, all of which were statistically significant. High-dose diuretics reduced strokes and heart failure (see Chapter B106).

Antihypertensive Lipid-Lowering Heart Attack Trial study. The Antihypertensive Lipid-Lowering Heart Attack Trial (ALLHAT) randomized over 42,000 individuals with stage 1 or 2 hypertension to chlorthalidone, doxazosin, lisinopril, or amlodipine as initial treatment. The diuretic was proved to be superior to the α-blocker with respect to cardiovascular outcomes within 3 years. At the end of the study in year 6, the remaining 3 arms demonstrated no difference with respect to ability to prevent fatal and nonfatal cardiac events. Analysis of the secondary end points, however, demonstrated that the diuretic was superior to the angiotensin-converting enzyme (ACE) inhibitor at preventing stroke and superior to the ACE inhibitor and the calcium antagonist at preventing heart failure. The diuretic also achieved superior outcomes overall in black patients (see Chapters B106 and C167).

Isolated systolic hypertension. It is now recognized that systolic hypertension is a greater concern than diastolic hypertension for the vast majority of hypertensives (see Chapter C151). Because the most common form of hypertension is isolated systolic hypertension, specific studies have addressed the value of BP control in this group. SHEP studied the impact of chlorthalidone-based therapy compared to placebo on the incidence of stroke and other cardiovascular events over approximately 5 years. Chlorthalidone reduced the incidence of stroke by approximately 36%, myocardial infarction by approximately 27%, heart failure by approximately 55%, and overall cardiovascular morbidity by approximately 32%, all of which were statistically significant.

Mechanisms of Action of Thiazide and Thiazide-Like Diuretics

The antihypertensive effects of thiazide and thiazide-like diuretics can be separated into acute, subacute, and chronic phases, corresponding roughly to 1 to 2 weeks, 4 to 8 weeks,

and several months, respectively. Renal mechanisms are more prominent in the early phases, whereas vascular mechanisms appear to predominate in the later phases.

Renal (salt/water excretion) effects. Thiazide diuretics act by inhibiting the sodium/chloride pump in the distal convoluted tubule, which increases urinary sodium excretion. Initially, there is a variable degree of ECF contraction, but blood volume returns to normal within a few days of the onset of therapy.

Vascular (chronic hemodynamic) effects. Early on, the major hypotensive effect is due to reduction of ECF volume, cardiac preload, and cardiac output. Chronically, however, volume contraction does not persist; cardiac output returns toward baseline, whereas peripheral vascular resistance decreases. In the "subacute" or transition period between these 2 phases, a transition phase occurs in which cardiac output and systemic resistance are lower. The cellular mechanism for the relative vasodilation remains unknown but is likely to involve alterations in vascular cell ion transport.

Practical Pharmacology

Guidelines for the use of diuretics for the treatment of hypertension are provided in Table C139.1. Thiazide diuretics are among the most frequently prescribed antihypertensives. Hydrochlorothiazide (HCTZ) is the most commonly used agent, but chlorthalidone or metolazone provide similar antihypertensive effects.

Dosing. All thiazides can be given once daily, usually in the morning. It is now apparent that lower dosages of thiazides than those originally used are equally efficacious. In the elderly, a beginning dose of 12.5 mg and a maximum dose of 25.0 mg HCTZ (or its equivalent) are recommended. In the Systolic Hypertension in the Elderly Program (SHEP), 12.5 mg of chlorthalidone controlled more than 50% of patients for several years. In other groups of patients, it is rarely necessary or desirable to use ≥50 mg per day of a thiazide diuretic.

Efficacy: monotherapy versus combinations. The ability of diuretics to lower BP has been demonstrated in numerous clinical trials. As monotherapy, in low doses, diuretics can control BP in approximately 50% of patients with stage 1 or stage 2 hypertension. In combination with other drugs, diuretics can control up to 70% of patients. Diuretics can be successfully combined with β-blockers, ACE inhibitors, angiotensin receptor blockers, centrally acting agents, and even with calcium antagonists. In the VA monotherapy study, the combination of a diuretic with drugs from any other class provided the best antihypertensive effect as compared to combinations without a diuretic.

Population response patterns. Certain patient groups exhibit a high degree of salt sensitivity (see Chapters A46, A76, and B94). These same groups, particularly the so-called low-renin groups (e.g., blacks, the elderly, and diabetics) and those who manifest the metabolic syndrome (obesity, dyslipidemia, hypertension, glucose intolerance, and enhanced atherogenesis) respond well to thiazide diuretics.

Dietary modifications. A low sodium diet enhances the efficacy of diuretics and should be encouraged (see Chapter B94). It is also generally recommended that hypertensive individuals should increase their daily intake of potassium, although it is unclear that such an increase can fully overcome the kaliuretic effects of thiazides.

Drug interactions. There are beneficial and adverse interactions of thiazides with other drugs. Beneficial interactions include additive BP-lowering effects when combined with other classes of antihypertensive agents. Adverse interactions include the blunting of thiazide effects by nonsteroidal antiinflammatory drugs (see Chapter C150) and the potential to increase fatigue and lethargy when combined with β-blockers. Doses of lithium must usually be monitored closely in lithium-treated patients because thiazides can reduce lithium excretion.

Adverse Effects

When diuretics were first introduced into clinical practice, high doses (up to 200 mg daily of HCTZ) were used with potentially dangerous adverse effects. Many of these initial concerns are now less relevant with the evolved appreciation of a favorable benefit to risk ratio of low-dose diuretic therapy.

Volume depletion and hyponatremia. Severe volume depletion is very uncommon with thiazide diuretics in ambulatory patients, particularly when low doses are used. Diuretic-related volume depletion is exacerbated by excessive fluid loss from other causes (e.g., vomiting, diarrhea, and malnutrition) and is more likely with loop diuretic therapy. Hyponatremia can occur in the setting of diuretic-induced volume contraction and is typically dose-dependent and more common with thiazide than loop diuretics. Rarely, hyponatremia may occur with low-dose thiazide therapy in an idiosyncratic fashion. Reduction in the diuretic dose or discontinuation of the diuretic together with liberalization of sodium intake and, occasionally, restriction of water intake corrects this abnormality.

Hypokalemic alkalosis. Hypokalemia may develop as a result of increased delivery of sodium and chloride to the distal nephron together with the actions of sodium-retaining steroids, such as aldosterone, which accelerates the exchange of sodium for potassium and hydrogen ions. Thus, diuretics cause a form of metabolic alkalosis in a dose-dependent manner.

Potassium loss occurs mostly in the first 3 to 7 days of diuretic therapy and thereafter tends to level off or improve. Fewer than 10% of patients develop mild hypokalemia with doses of 12.5 to 25.0 mg of HCTZ daily. Hypokalemia can be further minimized by implementing a low sodium/high potassium diet. Other treatment strategies include potassium supplements or potassium-sparing diuretics. A long-standing controversy persists about the potential danger of diuretic-induced hypokalemia and the potential association with ventricular arrhythmias and sudden death. Although a few studies in the early 1980s indicated a potential arrhythmogenicity caused by diuretic-induced hypokalemia in hypertensive subjects, many other studies, including Antihypertensive Lipid-Lowering Heart Attack Trial (ALLHAT), have failed to confirm that small reductions in serum potassium (less than 0.3 mg/dL) increase the risk of sudden death. If hypokalemia does carry a cardiac risk, it is in patients with heart failure or those treated with digitalis preparations.

Lipids and glucose. Early trials suggested that thiazides increase serum lipids, but in most of these studies, long-term weight gain was a more significant cause of the lipid increases. In the ALLHAT study, minimally higher serum cholesterol was found in the chlorthalidone subgroup compared to the lisinopril or amlodipine subgroup. Overall, it seems that currently recommended doses of thiazides have a negligible effect on serum lipids. Minimal changes in fasting glucose were also found in the ALLHAT study, and the overall incidence of diabetes in the chlorthalidone group was almost 12% at the end of the study compared to approximately 8% with lisinopril. The significance of these differences has not been determined.

Other complications. Thiazide-induced hyperuricemia occurs as a result of volume contraction or because of competition of thiazides with uric acid for renal tubular secretion via the organic anion secretory pathway. In susceptible individuals, acute gouty arthritis may be precipitated, although it is uncommon. Lowering of serum magnesium with thiazides is fairly common, but the clinical significance of this finding is unclear, although magnesium loss may increase the tendency toward hypokalemia and cardiac arrhythmias in patients with heart disease. In some hypokalemic patients, it is difficult to achieve normokalemia unless magnesium depletion is first treated.

LOOP DIURETICS

Clinical Use

Loop diuretics (furosemide, ethacrynic acid, bumetanide, torsemide) should not generally be used in patients with normal renal function because they are often unable to persistently reduce ECF volume or BP. When glomerular filtration is normal, the initial diuresis with loop diuretics is often followed by rebound sodium retention, with a neutral (or sometimes positive) sodium balance. Rebound antinatriuresis is characteristic of short-acting loop diuretics, such as furosemide, especially when given once daily. Loop diuretics are generally reserved for patients with reduced glomerular filtration rates (serum creatine >2.5 mg/dL) caused by intrinsic renal disease or heart failure, in whom they are much more powerful than thiazides (see Chapter C159). They are also effective in reducing ECF volume and BP in hypertensive states that include a strong element of edema, including patients treated with potent vasodilators, such as minoxidil (see Chapter C147).

Mechanisms of Action

Loop diuretics act on transport mechanisms in the thick ascending limb of the loop of Henle to prevent chloride and sodium reabsorption from the urine. These transporters are prostaglandin-sensitive; thus, agents that interfere with prostaglandin synthesis (e.g., nonsteroidal antiinflammatory drugs) can blunt the tubular actions of loop diuretics. This class of diuretics also act as venodilators, accounting for their immediate preload-reducing effects in pulmonary edema.

Practical Pharmacology

Furosemide is relatively short-acting and may need to be used 2 to 3 times a day in some patients. Torsemide has a prolonged duration of action (up to 24 hours) and may also exert direct vasodilator effects at nondiuretic doses. In general, the adverse effects of loop diuretics are similar to those described above for thiazide diuretics. Loop diuretics increase urine calcium excretion and are not the preferred agents in female patients with osteoporosis.

SUGGESTED READING

1. Freis ED. Critique of the clinical importance of diuretic-induced hypokalemia and elevated cholesterol level. *Arch Intern Med.* 1989;149:2640–2648.
2. Freis ED. The cardiotoxicity of thiazide diuretics: review of the evidence. *J Hypertens.* 1990;8:S-23–S-32.
3. Kostis JB, Davis BR, Cutler J, et al. Prevention of heart failure by antihypertensive drug treatment in older persons with isolated systolic hypertension. *JAMA.* 1997;278:212–216.
4. Madias JE, Madias NE, Gavras HP. Nonarrhythmogenicity of diuretic-induced hypokalemia: its evidence in patients with uncomplicated hypertension. *Arch Intern Med.* 1984;144:2171–2176.
5. Major outcomes in high-risk patients randomized to angiotensin-converting enzyme inhibitor or calcium channel blocker vs diuretic. The Antihypertensive and Lipid-Lowering Treatment to Prevent Heart Attack Trial (ALLHAT). *JAMA.* 2002;288:2981–2997.
6. Medical Research Council Working Party on Mild to Moderate Hypertension. Ventricular extrasystoles during thiazide treatment: substudy of MRC mild hypertension trial. *BMJ.* 1983;287:1249–1253.
7. Moser M, Setaro JF. Antihypertensive drug therapy and regression of left ventricular hypertrophy: a review with a focus on diuretics. *Eur Heart J.* 1991;12:1034–1039.
8. Papademetriou V, Burris JF, Notargiacomo A, et al. Thiazide therapy is not a cause of arrhythmia in patients with systemic hypertension. *Arch Int Med.* 1988;148:1272–1276.
9. Papademetriou V, Price M, Notargiacomo A, et al. Effect of diuretic therapy on ventricular arrhythmias in hypertensive patients with or without left ventricular hypertrophy. *Am Heart J.* 1985;144:2171–2176.
10. Psaty MB, Smith NL, Siscovick DS, et al. Health outcomes associated with antihypertensive therapies used as first line agents. *JAMA.* 1997;277:739–745.

Chapter C140

Aldosterone Blockers and Potassium-Sparing Diuretics

Murray Epstein, MD, FACP

KEY POINTS

- Aldosterone blockers provide effective antihypertensive treatment, especially in low-renin and salt-sensitive forms of hypertension.

- Newer, more selective aldosterone blockers (e.g., eplerenone) reduce the progestational and antiandrogenic effects of spironolactone, enhancing tolerability and potentially improving adherence to therapy.

- Aldosterone blockers provide an additional benefit in the treatment of heart failure when combined with angiotensin-converting enzyme inhibitors, digoxin, and loop diuretics.

- Potassium-sparing diuretics, such as amiloride or triamterene, are generally given for essential hypertension as a fixed-dose combination with hydrochlorothiazide.

See also Chapters A9, A26, A46, A50, A77, B93, B95, C138, and C170

ALDOSTERONE BLOCKERS

Spironolactone, a nonselective aldosterone blocker, has been in clinical use for more than 2 decades. Due to resurgent interest in aldosterone as a mediator of hypertension and cardiovascular disease, a selective aldosterone blocker has been developed and recently approved.

Rationale for Aldosterone Blockade

Pathophysiology. Aldosterone exerts multiple physiologic actions that raise blood pressure, including mediation of increased extracellular fluid volume and promotion of vasoconstriction (**Table C140.1**, see Chapters A9 and A50). Pathophysiologic and outcome studies suggest another rationale for aldosterone blockade: prevention or reversal of cardiac (and perhaps vascular) target organ damage, especially fibrosis. Theoretically, there may be additional benefits achieved by aldosterone receptor blockade. Because aldosterone appears to constitute an important risk factor for cardiovascular disease, the use of aldosterone blockers, in addition to thiazides, angiotensin-converting enzyme (ACE) inhibitors, and angiotensin

Table C140.1. Pathophysiologic Actions of Aldosterone That Promote Hypertension and Increase Cardiovascular Risk

Sodium retention/volume expansion
Reduction in vascular compliance
Promotion of endothelial dysfunction
Upregulation of angiotensin II receptors
Potentiation of the pressor responses of angiotensin II
Increases in sodium influx in vascular smooth muscle cells
Fibrosis in the heart, kidneys, and vasculature
Activation of plasminogen activator inhibitor-1
Stimulation of transforming growth factor β_1
Stimulation of reactive oxygen species
Hypertrophy of vascular smooth muscle cells and myocardial cells
Increase in blood lipid levels
Hypokalemia resulting in increased potential for cardiac arrhythmias, glucose intolerance, insulin resistance
Hypomagnesemia resulting in increased potential for cardiac arrhythmias

receptor binders (ARBs) could provide additional benefit in the treatment of hypertensive end-organ damage. Thiazides increase aldosterone levels by reducing extracellular fluid volume. With drugs that block the formation or actions of angiotensin II (ACE inhibitors and ARBs), there is evidence that some patients may experience "aldosterone escape" during long-term treatment, in which aldosterone levels are initially suppressed but gradually return to baseline levels by mechanisms that remain to be fully elucidated. Spironolactone has additional renal effects decreasing urinary excretion of potassium, magnesium, and calcium.

Hypertensive end-organ damage. Aldosterone acts on renal epithelial cells in the distal tubule and collecting duct to promote sodium reabsorption and potassium excretion. In general, the endocrine or paracrine properties of aldosterone are transduced via nuclear receptors (see Chapter A9) in the epithelial cells of the kidney, colon, and salivary and sweat glands. In addition to these "genomic" effects, it has also been shown that significant "nongenomic" effects of aldosterone occur at sites including the heart, kidneys, and vasculature. In animal models, aldosterone blockade attenuates reactive fibrosis in the viable myocardium of the postinfarcted left ventricle, reduces aortic fibrosis, improves large arterial compliance, and protects normal endothelial function. Cardiac fibrosis can be reduced in these animal models with spironolactone. Clinical trials have shown that spironolactone reduces cardiac and vascular collagen turnover, improves heart rate variability, reduces ventricular arrhythmias, improves endothelial dysfunction, and dilates blood vessels. In concert, these hemodynamic and humoral actions of aldosterone have important clinical implications for the future use of aldosterone blockers in hypertension and cardiovascular and renal diseases.

Selective aldosterone blockers. Although spironolactone is an effective antialdosterone agent, its use in patients is limited by its tendency to produce undesirable sexual side effects. At standard doses, impotence and gynecomastia can be induced in men, whereas premenopausal women may experience menstrual abnormalities. These adverse effects are due to the bind-

ing of spironolactone to progesterone and androgen receptors and constitute a substantial cause of drug discontinuation. In a study involving 43 patients treated with long-term spironolactone for mineralocorticoid excess syndromes, 13 patients (30%) were switched to alternate therapy due to the occurrence of gynecomastia (6 of 20 males) and menstrual disturbances or breast pain (7 of 23 females). The Randomized Aldactone Evaluation Study (RALES) trial reported a 10% incidence of gynecomastia or breast pain in its male subjects receiving 25 to 50 mg per day of spironolactone versus 1% on placebo ($p < .001$). The recent approval of the selective aldosterone blocker eplerenone provides a treatment with improved tolerability and reduced side effects. Consequently, eplerenone should lead to an improvement in patient adherence with antialdosterone therapy.

Clinical Use

Essential hypertension. Spironolactone. Spironolactone has a proven record of success in treating hypertension, particularly when given together with a thiazide-type diuretic. Spironolactone has been shown to be effective in cases of refractory hypertension in patients whose hypertension remains poorly controlled by 3- or 4-drug therapy. Despite the general efficacy of aldosterone blockers, hypertensive patients respond heterogeneously to different types of antihypertensive drugs. Similar to other conventional thiazide-type or loop diuretics, aldosterone blockers are effective antihypertensive treatment in most patients with low-renin forms of hypertension, particularly in blacks, the elderly, and most diabetics. Aldosterone blockers are also effective in the large subgroup of individuals with metabolic syndrome (obesity, hypertension, insulin resistance, dyslipidemia, accelerated atherogenesis). Thus, the majority of hypertensive patients can be expected to respond to aldosterone blockers.
Eplerenone. In developmental studies, the selective aldosterone blocker eplerenone safely and effectively lowered blood pressure in patients with mild to moderate hypertension and diverse comorbidities, including left ventricular hypertrophy and diabetes mellitus. Eplerenone is equally effective in black and white patients, in contrast to the decreased efficacy observed with ACE inhibitors and ARBs in black patients. Eplerenone is effective and well tolerated when used alone or in combination with diverse agents, including ACE inhibitors, ARBs, calcium antagonists, and β-blockers. Eplerenone was recently approved in the United States for the treatment of hypertension.

Hyperaldosteronism. Aldosterone blockers are effective in the therapy of hyperaldosteronism, including adrenal hyperplasia, adrenal adenoma, and glucocorticoid-remediable aldosteronism (see Chapters A50, A77, and C170). Doses required in these conditions are often higher than those used in essential hypertension (**Table C140.2**).

Heart failure. In a clinical study of congestive heart failure (RALES), spironolactone was compared to placebo in its ability to reduce heart failure–related events. When given in addition to conventional therapy with ACE inhibitor, digoxin, and loop diuretic, spironolactone, 25 mg daily, reduced mortality and heart failure hospitalizations.

Table C140.2. Doses of Aldosterone Antagonists and Potassium-Sparing Diuretics in Various Clinical Conditions

DRUG	DOSING FREQUENCY	USUAL DOSE RANGES (TOTAL MG/D)		
		ESSENTIAL HYPERTENSION	HYPERALDOSTERONISM	HEART FAILURE
Spironolactone (Aldactone)	q.d.–b.i.d.	25–200	50–200[a]	25–50
Eplerenone (Inspra)	q.d.–b.i.d.	50–100	—	—

[a]Similar doses may be effective in polycystic ovary syndrome, but the drug has not been approved for that specific purpose.

Applied Pharmacology

Receptor pharmacology. Spironolactone is moderately more potent than eplerenone in competing for the mineralocorticoid receptor. Preclinical studies with eplerenone have demonstrated a 100- to 1,000-fold lower affinity for androgen and progesterone receptors than is the case for spironolactone and its active metabolite, canrenone.

Dosing. The recommended dosing range of spironolactone is 25 to 200 mg once daily in mild to moderate hypertension, and that of eplerenone is 50 to 100 mg daily. Spironolactone is not uncommonly given twice daily. Pharmacokinetic studies have disclosed no correlation between alterations in eplerenone disposition kinetics and degree of renal dysfunction.

Drug interactions. Favorable interactions include enhanced natriuresis and a potassium-sparing effect when aldosterone blockers are combined with loop or thiazide diuretics. Potentially unfavorable interactions include hyperkalemia when aldosterone antagonists are combined with ACE inhibitors or ARBs, particularly in patients who have renal insufficiency or hyporeninemic hypoaldosteronism (type IV renal tubular acidosis). Eplerenone should be used carefully with inhibitors of CYP3A4 activity (e.g., ketoconazole) because its metabolism is CYP3A4 dependent.

Adverse effects. Spironolactone may produce undesirable sexual side effects, including impotence and gynecomastia in men and menstrual abnormalities in premenopausal women. In contrast, eplerenone rarely produces these adverse effects.

POTASSIUM-SPARING DIURETICS

Other weaker diuretic compounds, such as amiloride and triamterene, can increase renal sodium excretion with relative potassium sparing. These agents tend to be relatively ineffective when used as monotherapy for hypertension but can be useful in combination with hydrochlorothiazide.

Amiloride

Mechanisms of action. Amiloride blocks epithelial sodium transport channels selectively. In the distal tubule, this action indirectly reduces aldosterone-sensitive sodium-potassium exchange and leads to increased urinary sodium excretion, with relative potassium sparing. Additional vasodilatory effects have been proposed.

Clinical use. In essential hypertension, amiloride is usually given as part of a fixed-dose combination with hydrochlorothiazide. Adverse effects are usually mild and transient and typically include gastrointestinal discomfort or, occasionally, muscle cramps.

Triamterene

Triamterene also blocks epithelial sodium transport channels, although less avidly than amiloride. Triamterene-thiazide combinations were once extremely popular on the basis of reduced potassium wasting, but their use continues to wane. In clinical practice, gastrointestinal side effects sometimes limit its use. Triamterene is a weak folic acid antagonist, but megaloblastic anemia is rare. Triamterene is incompletely absorbed and can precipitate in the urine, potentially contributing to renal stone formation. It is not indicated in patients with gout.

SUGGESTED READING

1. Delyani JA. Mineralocorticoid receptor antagonists: the evolution of utility and pharmacology. *Kidney Int*. 2000;57:1408–1411.
2. Doggrell SA, Brown L. The spironolactone renaissance. *Expert Opin Investig Drugs*. 2001;10:943–954.
3. Epstein M. Aldosterone and the hypertensive kidney: its emerging role as a mediator of progressive renal dysfunction: a paradigm shift. *J Hypertens*. 2001;19:829–842.
4. Krum H, Nolly H, Workman D, et al. Efficacy of eplerenone added to renin-angiotensin blockade in hypertensive patients. *Hypertension*. 2002;40:117–123.
5. Mantero F, Opocher G, Rocco S, et al. Long-term treatment of mineralocorticoid excess syndromes. *Steroids*. 1995;60:81–86.
6. Pitt B, Zannad F, Remme WJ, et al. The effect of spironolactone on morbidity and mortality in patients with severe heart failure. *N Engl J Med*. 1999;341:709–717.
7. Rabasseda X, Silvestre J, Castañer J. Eplerenone. *Drugs Future*. 1999;24:488–501.
8. Sica DA. Eplerenone: a new aldosterone receptor antagonist. Are the FDA's restrictions appropriate? *J Clin Hypertens (Greenwich)*. 2002;4:441–445.
9. Weber MA. Clinical implications of aldosterone blockade. *Am Heart J*. 2002;144:S12–S18.
10. Weinberger MH, Roniker B, Krause SL, Weiss RJ. Eplerenone, a selective aldosterone blocker, in mild-to-moderate hypertension. *Am J Hypertens*. 2002;15:709–716.

Chapter C141

β-Adrenergic Blockers

William H. Frishman, MD; Domenic A. Sica, MD

KEY POINTS

- β-Blockers are appropriate for initial as well as subsequent therapy of all degrees of arterial hypertension and are useful treatments for patients with hypertension who also have concomitant angina pectoris or arrhythmias.

- β-Adrenergic blockers can be differentiated from one another by presence or absence of intrinsic sympathomimetic activity, membrane stabilizing activity, β_1-receptor selectivity, α_1-adrenergic blocking activity, solubilities and routes of elimination, potencies, and duration of action.

- β-Adrenergic blockers reduce the risk of mortality and nonfatal reinfarction in survivors of acute myocardial infarction and improve clinical outcomes in patients with left ventricular dysfunction and stable symptoms who are receiving conventional heart failure therapies.

See also Chapters A1, A5, A28–A30, A 37, A38, A59, A62, B106, B107, C126–C128, C137, C138, C142, C154–C156, C164, and C165

β-Blockers are effective and safe and are widely used in the therapy of hypertension and other cardiovascular disorders.

Indications and Outcomes Studies

Hypertension. The Sixth Report of the Joint National Committee on Prevention, Detection, Evaluation, and Treatment of High Blood Pressure (JNC VI) reiterated the recommendation of previous JNC documents that β-adrenergic blockers are appropriate alternatives as first-line treatment for hypertension. These recommendations were based on reduced morbidity and mortality in large clinical trials, but most of the benefit was documented in trials of secondary cardiovascular protection rather than primary protection. In the Antihypertensive and Lipid-Lowering Treatment to Prevent Heart Attack Trial (ALLHAT) study, β-blockers were used as second-line agents in combination with diuretic, angiotensin-converting enzyme (ACE) inhibitor, or calcium antagonist. Future recommendations are likely to follow this pattern.

Angina pectoris. In the absence of contraindications, β-blockers are recommended as the initial therapy for long-term management of angina pectoris. In this regard, β-blockers provide similar clinical outcomes and are associated with fewer adverse events than calcium antagonists in randomized trials of patients who have stable angina. All β-blockers appear to be equally effective. Combined therapy with nitrates and β-blockers may be more efficacious for the treatment of angina pectoris than the use of either drug alone. Also, combined therapy with β-blockers and calcium channel blockers can provide clinical benefit for patients with angina pectoris who remain symptomatic with either agent used alone.

Antiarrhythmic effects. β-Blockers have become an important treatment modality for various cardiac arrhythmias used alone and in combination with other antiarrhythmic drugs. These agents can be quite useful in the treatment of ventricular tachyarrhythmias in the setting of myocardial ischemia and mitral valve prolapse and for other cardiovascular conditions. β-

Blockers are also useful for treating inappropriate sinus tachycardia. Although β-blockers are not potent suppressors of premature ventricular contractions, they have been shown to reduce the incidence of sudden, presumably arrhythmic, death after myocardial infarction (MI). The antiarrhythmic actions of β-blockers are considered to be a class effect because there is little evidence that indicates one β-blocker is different than another.

Myocardial infarction. The 2001 American Heart Association and American College of Cardiology guidelines for secondary prevention of MI recommend starting β-blockers in all post-MI patients and continuing therapy indefinitely. The β-Blocker Heart Attack Trial (BHAT) using propranolol and the Norwegian Multicenter Study Group trial using timolol showed significant reductions in mortality rate, reinfarction rate, or both attributable to the administered β-blocker. These early trials did not include patients with heart failure or those receiving contemporary heart failure therapies. Therein, more recent trials including the Survival and Ventricular Enlargement (SAVE) and the Acute Infarction Ramipril Efficacy (AIRE) trials showed that β-blockers provided an additional reduction in cardiovascular mortality independent of ACE inhibitors. β-Blockers without intrinsic sympathomimetic activity (ISA) are the only agents conclusively shown to decrease the rate of sudden death, overall mortality, and recurrent MI in survivors of acute MI. β-Blockers with α-blocking activity have not been broadly studied in the post-MI population. In the Carvedilol Post-Infarct Survival Control in LV Dysfunction (CAPRICORN) trial, however, mortality and nonfatal reinfarction were significantly reduced by carvedilol.

Heart failure. Two metaanalyses, each including more than 3,000 patients, have evaluated heart failure trial results for numerous β-blockers, including bisoprolol, bucindolol, carvedilol, metoprolol, and nebivolol. Both metaanalyses showed a risk reduction for mortality, hospitalization secondary to heart failure, and the combined end point of mortality and hospitalizations with β-

Table C141.1. Proposed Mechanisms to Explain the Antihypertensive Action of β-Blockers

Reduction in heart rate and cardiac output
Central nervous system effect
Inhibition of renin release
Reduction in peripheral vascular resistance (intrinsic sympathomimetic activity drugs and α,β-blockers)
Reduction in vasomotor tone
Resetting of baroreceptor function
Effects on prejunctional β-receptors; reduction in norepinephrine release
Attenuation of pressor response to catecholamines (exercise and stress)

blocker use. Several larger trials have firmly established the benefits of β-blockers in heart failure, including the U.S. Carvedilol Program and 3 large mortality trials: the Metoprolol CR/XL Randomized Intervention Trial in Congestive Heart Failure (MERIT-HF), the Cardiac Insufficiency Bisoprolol Study (CIBIS-II), and the Carvedilol Prospective Randomized Cumulative Survival (COPERNICUS) trial. There is currently not a preferred β-blocker for the treatment of heart failure.

Mechanisms of action

General mechanisms. Although there is no consensus as to the mechanisms by which β-blocking drugs lower blood pressure (BP), it is probable that some or all of the modes of action listed in **Table C141.1** are involved.

Pharmacokinetic features. β-Adrenergic blocking drugs as a group have similar therapeutic effects despite structural differences. Their varied aromatic ring structures confer many pharmacokinetic differences, including completeness of gastrointestinal absorption, degree of first-pass hepatic metabolism, lipid solubil-

ity, protein binding, volume of distribution, penetration into the central nervous system, concentration in the myocardium, rate of hepatic biotransformation, pharmacologic activity of metabolites, and renal clearance. The relevance of these variations depends on the clinical conditions present in the individual being treated.

Drug Differentiation

In contrast to other classes of antihypertensive drugs, important differences in intrinsic chemical properties of β-adrenergic blocking drugs translate into significant clinical differences in effects (**Table C141.2**).

Solubility, elimination, and duration of effects. The β-blockers can be separated into 2 broad categories by their solubilities, metabolism, and elimination routes. Lipid-soluble agents are eliminated primarily by hepatic metabolism and tend to have relatively short plasma half-lives with wider variations in plasma concentrations. Water-soluble agents that are eliminated unchanged by the kidney tend to have longer half-lives and more stable plasma concentrations. Propranolol and metoprolol are lipid-soluble, are almost completely absorbed by the small intestine, and are largely metabolized by the liver. They tend to have highly variable bioavailability and relatively short plasma half-lives. A lack of correlation between the duration of clinical pharmacologic effect and plasma half-life may explain why these drugs can be effective even when administered once or twice daily. In contrast, agents such as atenolol and nadolol are more water-soluble, are incompletely absorbed through the gut, and are eliminated unchanged by the kidney. They tend to have less variation in plasma levels and longer half-lives, allowing once-daily dosing. Differences do emerge when the duration of effect of individual β-blockers is compared (**Table C141.3**). Several β-blockers do not provide full

Table C141.2. Pharmacodynamic Properties of β-Adrenergic Blocking Drugs Used in Hypertension

DRUG	β₁-BLOCKADE POTENCY RATIO (PROPRANOLOL = 1.0)	RELATIVE β₁ SELECTIVITY	INTRINSIC SYMPATHOMIMETIC ACTIVITY	MEMBRANE-STABILIZING ACTIVITY
Acebutolol	0.3	+	+	+
Atenolol	1.0	++	0	0
Betaxolol	1.0	++	0	+
Bisoprolol[a]	10.0	++	0	0
Carteolol	10.0	0	+	0
Carvedilol[b]	10.0	0	0	++
Esmolol	0.02	++	0	0
Labetalol[c]	0.3	0	+?	0
Metoprolol	1.0	++	0	0
Nadolol	1.0	0	0	0
Nebivolol[d]	10.0	++	0	0
Oxprenolol	0.5–1.0	+	+	
Penbutolol	1.0	0	+	0
Pindolol	6.0	0	++	+
Propranolol	1.0	0	0	+
Sotalol	0.3	0	0	0
Timolol	0.6	0	0	0

+, modest effect; ++, strong effect; 0, no effect.
[a]Bisoprolol is also approved as a first-line antihypertensive therapy in combination with a very-low-dose diuretic.
[b]Carvedilol has peripheral vasodilating activity and additional α₁-adrenergic blocking activity.
[c]Labetalol has additional α₁-adrenergic blocking activity and direct vasodilatory activity (β₂-agonism); it is available for use in intravenous form for hypertensive emergencies.
[d]Nebivolol can augment vascular nitric oxide release.
From Frishman WH. *Clinical Pharmacology of the β-Adrenoceptor Blocking Drugs.* 2nd ed. Norwalk, CN: Appleton-Century-Crofts; 1984, with permission.

Table C141.3. β-Adrenergic Blocking Drugs: Doses

DRUG	TRADE NAME	USUAL RANGE (FREQUENCY/D)	COMMENT	FIXED-DOSE COMBINATION
Acebutolol	Sectral	200–800 (1)	Cardioselective, intrinsic sympathomimetic activity	
Atenolol	Tenormin	25–100 (1)	Cardioselective	Tenoretic
Betaxolol	Kerlone	10–20 (1)	Cardioselective	
Bisoprolol	Zebeta	2.5–20.0 (1)	Cardioselective, indicated as first-step therapy as combination product	Ziac
Carteolol	Cartrol	2.5–10.0 (1)		
Carvedilol	Coreg	3.125–25.000 (1–2)	Combine α- and β-blocker, postural hypotension	
Esmolol	Brevibloc		Short-acting intravenous form	
Labetalol	Normodyne, Trandate	100–400 (2)	Combined α- and β-blocker, postural hypotension	
Metoprolol	Lopressor, Toprol XL	25–200 (1,2)	Cardioselective, long-acting preparation available	
Nadolol	Corgard	40–320 (1)		Corzide
Penbutolol	Levatol	10–20 (1)		
Pindolol	Visken	5–15 (2)	Intrinsic sympathomimetic activity	
Propranolol	Inderal, Inderal-LA	10–240 (1–2)	Long-acting preparation available	Inderide
Timolol	Blocadren	20–60 (2)		Timolide

24-hour coverage and thus fail to adequately control BP during the early morning rise in BP. Dose titration is effective in some people, particularly in rate-driven forms of hypertension.

β₁-Selectivity. When used in low doses, β_1-selective blocking agents such as acebutolol, betaxolol, bisoprolol, esmolol, atenolol, and metoprolol inhibit cardiac β_1-receptors to a greater degree than β_2-receptors but have less influence on bronchial and vascular smooth muscle cells (Table C141.1). In higher doses (e.g., above approximately 50 mg/day of metoprolol), however, β_1-selective blocking agents also block β_2-receptors. β_1-Selective agents may be marginally safer than nonselective agents in patients with obstructive pulmonary disease, but selective β_1-blockers may aggravate bronchospasm in certain patients. A second theoretical advantage is that unlike nonselective β-blockers, β_1-selective blockers in low doses may not block the β_2-receptors that mediate dilatation of arterioles. It is unproven but possible that leaving the β_2-receptors unblocked and responsive to epinephrine may be functionally important in some patients with hypertension or peripheral vascular disease.

Intrinsic sympathomimetic activity or partial agonist activity. Certain β-adrenergic receptor blockers are partial agonists at β_1-adrenergic receptor sites, β_2-adrenergic receptor sites, or both. This combined action manifests itself as a neutral effect on heart rate when the sympathetic nervous system is not activated (supine rest) and a blunted increase in heart rate when the sympathetic system is activated during stress of exercise (Table C141.2). In the treatment of patients with arrhythmias, angina pectoris of effort, or hypertension, drugs with mild-to-moderate ISA appear to be as efficacious as β-blockers lacking this property. β-blocking agents with nonselective partial agonist activity can reduce peripheral vascular resistance chronically and may also cause less depression of atrioventricular conduction. It is still debated whether the presence of partial agonist activity in a β-blocker constitutes an overall advantage or disadvantage in cardiac therapy.

Combined α,β-adrenergic blocking activity. Carvedilol and labetalol are β-blockers with antagonistic properties at both α- and β-adrenergic receptors, with direct vasodilator activity. Like other β-blockers, they are useful in the treatment of hypertension and angina pectoris. However, unlike most β-blocking drugs, the additional α-adrenergic blocking actions of carvedilol and labetalol lead to a reduction in peripheral vascular resistance that acts to maintain higher levels of cardiac output.

Membrane-stabilizing activity. At concentrations well above therapeutic levels, certain β-blockers have a quinidine-like or local anesthetic membrane-stabilizing (potentially antiarrhythmic) effect on cardiomyocyte action potentials (Table C141.1). There is no evidence that membrane-stabilizing activity is responsible for any direct negative inotropic effect of the β-blockers on the usual dose range. However, membrane-stabilizing activity may be responsible for myocardial depression with massive β-blocker intoxication.

Extended-release preparations. Extended-release formulations of metoprolol and propranolol are available that allow once-daily dosing of these drugs. Studies have shown that both long-acting propranolol and metoprolol provide much smoother curves of daily plasma levels than do comparable divided doses of conventional propranolol and metoprolol. Sublingual and nasal spray formulations that can provide immediate β-blockade are being tested in clinical trials. Ultra-short-acting β-blockers are now available and may be useful when a short duration of action is desired (e.g., in patients with questionable congestive heart failure). One of these compounds, esmolol, a β_1-selective drug, has been shown to be useful in the treatment of perioperative hypertension and supraventricular tachycardias. The short half-life (<15 minutes) relates to the rapid metabolism of the drug by blood and hepatic esterases. Metabolism of β-blockers does not seem to be altered by disease states.

Clinical Usage

Blood pressure effects. Thirteen orally active β-adrenergic blockers are approved in the United States for treatment of hypertension (Tables C141.2 and C141.3). In the usual prescribed doses, β-blockers have equivalent antihypertensive efficacy. True dose equivalence among the various β-blockers has not been established, in part because few head-to-head studies have been done with individual β-blockers. β-Adrenergic blockers, alone and in combination with other antihypertensives, reduce BP in patients with combined systolic and diastolic hypertension and in most patients with isolated systolic hypertension. Uncommonly, there is a paradoxical elevation of systolic pressure during β-blockade in persons with severe aortic arteriosclerosis, presumably due to the increased stroke volume caused by rate slowing in the setting of increased impedance. Escalating doses of β-blockers and combined α,β-blockers can induce salt and water retention, making diuretics a not uncommon adjunctive therapy. Abrupt discontinuation of a β-blocker, particularly when administered in high doses, may be followed by adrenergically mediated withdrawal symptoms and the appearance of angina in patients with coronary artery disease. Therefore, a step-wise reduction in dose is advised in all high-risk patients.

Subgroups. There are few predictors of response to a β-blocker, but when hypertension is accompanied by a high pulse rate, the BP response is generally pronounced. There is a limited relationship between plasma renin activity and response to a β-blocker, and smaller studies have shown that an individual who experiences a large BP drop on a β-blocker typically responds vigorously to ACE inhibitor or angiotensin receptor blocker and less vigorously to diuretic or calcium antagonist. Certain patient subsets demonstrate lower response rates to β-blocker monotherapy, including low-renin, salt-sensitive individuals, such as the black hypertensive. Racial differences in the BP response to a β-blocker are abolished when combined with a thiazide diuretic. The elderly and diabetic respond in a fairly heterogeneous fashion to β-blocker monotherapy. β-Blockers are effective in hyperkinetic forms of hypertension as in individuals with a high cardiac awareness profile or somatic manifestations of anxiety, such as tremor, sweating, and tachycardia. Perioperative hypertension may also be treated with β-blocker therapy.

Hypertensive urgencies and emergencies. The combined α,β-blocker labetalol is the only β-blocker indicated for parenteral management of hypertensive emergencies and for treatment of intraoperative and postoperative hypertension. It can also be used in oral form to treat patients with hypertensive emergencies.

Other clinical uses. β-Blockers are indicated for angina pectoris, hypertrophic cardiomyopathy, hyperdynamic circulations, essential tremor, and headaches. Some β-adrenergic blockers are also found to reduce the risk of mortality in survivors of acute MI and to improve clinical outcomes in patients having congestive cardiomyopathy. The drugs can be used with caution in pregnancy-related hypertension. Most antihypertensive drugs, including β-blockers, reduce left ventricular mass and wall thickness, although β-blockers are generally less effective in this regard than diuretics, ACE inhibitors, calcium antagonists, and angiotensin receptor blockers. It is not known, however, whether reversal of hypertension-induced cardiac hypertrophy improves the independent risk of cardiovascular morbidity and mortality associated with left ventricular hypertrophy.

Combinations with other drugs. The antihypertensive effect of a β-blocker is fairly predictably enhanced by the simultaneous administration of a diuretic. Hydrochlorothiazide doses as low as 6.25 mg provide a substantial enough BP-lowering effect with a β-blocker to have warranted approval of the combination of bisoprolol and HCTZ as first-step therapy by the U.S. Food and Drug Administration. β-Blockers are also useful add-on therapy in the setting of vasodilator-related tachycardia, as may occur with hydralazine and minoxidil.

Adverse effects and contraindications. Most β-adrenergic blockers, at least in the usual antihypertensive dose range, should not be used in patients with asthma, chronic obstructive pulmonary disease, decompensated congestive heart failure with systolic dysfunction, heart block (greater than first degree), and sick sinus syndrome. β-Adrenergic blockers should be used with caution in insulin-dependent diabetes, because they may worsen glucose intolerance, mask the symptoms of hypoglycemia or prolong recovery from hypoglycemia, or increase the magnitude of the hypertensive response to hypoglycemia. There is probably a shorter recovery period from hypoglycemia with β_1-selective adrenergic blockers. β-Blockers should not be discontinued abruptly in patients with known ischemic heart disease. If a patient has serious contraindications to β-blockers, unacceptable side effects, or persistent angina, calcium antagonists should be administered. Long-acting dihydropyridine and nondihydropyridine agents are generally as effective as β-blockers in relieving angina. β-Blockers may increase levels of plasma triglycerides and reduce those of high-density lipoprotein cholesterol. β-Blockers with ISA α-blocking activity have little or no adverse effect on plasma lipids. There are special considerations when β-blockers are combined with other drugs. Combinations of diltiazem or verapamil with β-blockers may have additional depressant effects on the sinoatrial and atrioventricular nodes and may also promote negative inotropy. Addition of H_2-blocking agents to the combination of verapamil and β-blocker can also lead to myocardial depression. Combinations of β-blockers and reserpine may cause marked bradycardia and syncope. Combination with pseudoephedrine, ephedrine, and epinephrine can also cause elevations in blood pressure due to unopposed α-receptor–induced vasoconstriction.

SUGGESTED READING

1. Bengtsson K, Melander O, Orho-Melander M, et al. Polymorphism in the β_1 adrenergic receptor gene and hypertension. *Circulation.* 2001;104:187–190.
2. Devereux RB. Do antihypertensive drugs differ in their ability to regress left ventricular hypertrophy? *Circulation.* 1997;95:1983–1985.
3. Frishman WH. *Clinical Pharmacology of the β-Adrenoceptor Blocking Drugs.* 2nd ed. Norwalk, CN: Appleton-Century-Crofts; 1984.
4. Frishman WH. Alpha- and beta-adrenergic blocking drugs. In: Frishman WH, Sonnenblick EH, Sica D, eds. *Cardiovascular Pharmacotherapeutics.* 2nd ed. New York, NY: McGraw-Hill; 2003:67–97.
5. Frishman WH, Alwarshetty M. β-Adrenergic blockers in systemic hypertension: pharmacokinetics considerations related to JNC-VI and WHO-ISH guidelines. *Clin Pharmacokinet.* 2002;41:505–516.

6. Frishman WH, Bryzinski BS, Coulson LR, et al. A multifactorial trial design to assess combination therapy in hypertension: treatment with bisoprolol and hydrochlorothiazide. [Published correction appears in *Arch Intern Med*. 1995;155:709] *Arch Intern Med*. 1994;154:1461–1468.

7. Gress TW, Nieto J, Shahar E, et al. for the Atherosclerosis Risk in Communities Study. Hypertension and antihypertensive therapy as risk factors for type 2 diabetes mellitus. *N Engl J Med*. 2000;342:905–912.

8. Messerli FH, Grossman E, Goldbourt U. Are β blockers efficacious as first-line therapy for hypertension in the elderly? *JAMA*. 1998;279:1903–1907.

9. Opie LH. Cardiovascular drug interactions. In: Frishman WH, Sonnenblick EH, Sica D (eds). *Cardiovascular Pharmacotherapeutics*. 2nd ed. New York, NY: McGraw Hill; 2003:875–891.

10. Psaty BM, Smith NL, Siscovick DS, et al. Health outcomes associated with antihypertensive therapies used as first-line agents: a systematic review and meta-analysis. *JAMA*. 1997;277:739–745.

Chapter C142

α-Adrenoceptor Antagonists

James L. Pool, MD

KEY POINTS

- Selective α_1-adrenoceptor antagonists lower blood pressure by blocking postsynaptic vasoconstrictor effects of norepinephrine.

- Hemodynamically, selective α_1-adrenoceptor inhibitors cause balanced arterial and venous dilation, with no increase in cardiac output, but tend to cause greater blood pressure lowering in the upright compared to supine position.

- α_1-Adrenoceptor antagonists may relieve obstructive symptoms in patients with benign prostatic hypertrophy.

- α-Blockers are less effective than diuretics at reducing the incidence of heart failure.

See also Chapters A1, A27, A28, A33, A37, A38, A42, A51, B106, B107, C127, C137–C139, and C141

Rationale for α-Blockade in Hypertension

α_1-Receptors are predominantly located postsynaptically on vascular smooth muscle cells, where they are the principal sites of the vasoconstrictive action of norepinephrine (**Figure C142.1**). Five different adrenoceptor subtypes (α_{2A}, α_{2C}, β_1, β_2, and β_3) are found on vascular endothelial cells, but their roles in vasoregulation are less well understood.

Sympathetic overactivity in hypertension (see Chapter A42) and accompanying excess stimulation of postsynaptic α_1-adrenoceptors is a sound physiologic rationale for the use of selective α_1-adrenoceptor inhibitors as antihypertensive drugs. With these agents, the reduction in blood pressure (BP) is achieved with little or no change in cardiac output because of balanced venous and arterial dilation. Favorable hemodynamic effects of selective α_1-inhibitors have also been demonstrated during exercise, when cardiac performance is better preserved with α_1-blockers than β-blockers.

Clinical Effects of Selective α_1-Antagonists

Hypertension. Selective α_1-blockers (**Table C142.1**) have been shown to be effective antihypertensive agents, whether used as monotherapy or as part of a multidrug regimen. Age, race, and gender do not substantially influence BP responses to selective α_1-blockers. In general clinical practice, α_1-blockers have their widest application as a component of multiple drug regimens for the treatment of stage 2 and 3 hypertension. Their effects are additive to those of angiotensin-converting enzyme inhibitors, angiotensin receptor antagonists, β-blockers, calcium channel blockers, diuretics, and direct-acting vasodilators.

Approximately one-half of the essential hypertensives treated with monotherapy achieve diastolic BPs <90 mm Hg, providing that adequate dosages are used. In large placebo-controlled studies, doxazosin or terazosin given once daily lowered BP by approximately 10/8 mm Hg in the standing position and by approximately 9/5 mm Hg in the supine position at 24 hours post-dose.

Although less pronounced than with direct arterial vasodilators, α_1-blockers cause a degree of sodium and water retention in most patients. Concomitant use of a diuretic prevents fluid retention and markedly enhances the antihypertensive effect of α_1-blockers but also predisposes to a greater orthostatic BP decrease (lower upright than supine BP). For α_1-blockers to be effective as monotherapy, they must usually be titrated to the high end of approved dose ranges (10–20 mg daily for prazosin or terazosin, 8–16 mg daily for doxazosin).

Ventricular hypertrophy and heart failure: lack of effect.

Stimulation of the cardiac α_1-adrenoceptors causes marked trophic effects, and regression of left ventricular hypertrophy has been reported with selective α_1-adrenoceptor inhibitors. Nevertheless, in clinical trials, α_1-blockers did not provide sustained morbidity or mortality benefit to hypertensive patients, especially in primary protection against heart failure. The doxazosin arm of the Antihypertensive and Lipid-Lowering Treatment to Prevent Heart Attack Trial (ALLHAT) was discontinued prematurely because, compared with the chlor-

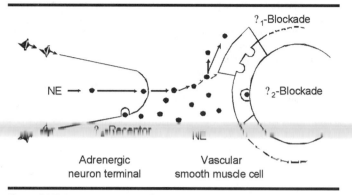

Figure C142.1. Mechanism of action of selective α_1-adrenoceptor blockade.

thalidone group, there was a 25% higher incidence of significant cardiovascular disease and a 2-fold increased incidence of congestive heart failure. Marginal positive results were found in established heart failure in the Valsartan Heart Failure Trial 2 (Val-HeFT2) study, in which α-blockers in combination with nitrates was beneficial.

Prostatism. Because of the importance of α_1-adrenoceptors in regulating the degree of constriction of urinary tract sphincters, α_1-blockers have been used for the treatment of mild obstructive uropathy in benign prostatic hypertrophy. Up to 40% of total urethral pressure is due to a-adrenergic tone, and 53% is due to static pressure from the enlarged prostate. Relaxation of this muscle tone by α_1-adrenoceptor blockade increases urinary flow and improves symptoms in patients with benign prostatic hypertrophy.

Pharmacology and Selectivity of α-Adrenoceptor Antagonists

α-Adrenoceptor blockers can be classified according to their abilities to affect specific receptor subtypes. Nonselective (α_1 + α_2) antagonists, selective presynaptic α_2-antagonists, and selective postsynaptic α_1-antagonists exist. Selective α_1-receptor antagonists (prazosin, terazosin, doxazosin) differ in their actions from nonselective α-blockers, such as phentolamine (a competitive inhibitor) and phenoxybenzamine (a noncompetitive inhibitor), primarily because the latter 2 drugs also block presynaptic α_2-adrenoceptors. Presynaptic α_2-adrenoceptors tonically inhibit neuronal norepinephrine release, so nonspecific α-blockade (i.e., α_1 + α_2 antagonism) tends to increase sympathetic nervous outflow and neuronal norepinephrine release, more than selective α_1 blockade, and includes β-adrenoceptor–mediated tachycardia, enhanced renin secretion, and attenuation of postsynaptic α_1 inhibition. Selective blockade of presynaptic α_2-adrenoceptors with yohimbine increases

BP and heart rate, and this agent is used occasionally in patients with autonomic insufficiency. These pharmacologic differences explain why nonselective α-blockers were not found to be useful in the treatment of essential hypertension.

Nonselective α_1-receptor antagonists. Phentolamine, a parenteral drug, is used almost exclusively for emergent and urgent severe hypertension with excess catecholamine release. The oral nonselective and noncompetitive α-inhibitor phenoxybenzamine remains an important agent in the preoperative management of pheochromocytomas and cases of inoperable, metastatic pheochromocytoma. These agents are generally not used in essential hypertension.

α,β-Adrenergic inhibitors. Labetalol, a nonselective β-blocker with selective α_1-adrenoreceptor antagonist effects is approximately 10% as potent as phentolamine. Although a combination α,β-antagonist, labetalol is predominately a selective postsynaptic α_1-adrenoceptor antagonist during acute intravenous or chronic oral administration. Carvedilol is another nonselective β-blocker with selective α_1-adrenoreceptor antagonist effects. Carvedilol, which is indicated for the treatment of heart failure and hypertension, acts predominantly as a β-blocker in clinical situations.

Selective α_1-receptor antagonists. Prazosin, terazosin, and doxazosin are quinazoline compounds (Table C142.1) that are postsynaptic α_1-adrenoceptor antagonists approved for the treatment of hypertension. These drugs are highly selective for α_1-adrenoceptor subtypes (α_{1A}, α_{1B}, α_{1D}) and, even when given in large doses, do not inhibit α_2-adrenoceptors, β-adrenoceptors, or the receptors for acetylcholine (muscarinic), dopamine, or 5-hydroxytryptamine.

Metabolic Effects of Selective α_1-Antagonists

Lipids. Although not specifically approved for dyslipidemia, selective α_1-adrenoceptor antagonists exert a modest beneficial effect on the serum lipid profile of hypertensive patients. Controlled studies have demonstrated that these agents lower the levels of total cholesterol (2–3%), low-density lipoprotein (LDL) cholesterol (3–4%), and triglycerides and increase the levels of high-density lipoprotein cholesterol. These modifications of the serum lipid profile are probably the result of several different mechanisms, including an increase in LDL cholesterol receptor number, a decrease in LDL cholesterol synthesis, stimulation of lipoprotein lipase activity, reduction of very-low-density lipoprotein cholesterol synthesis and secretion, and a reduction in the absorption of dietary cholesterol. In addition, the 6-hydroxy and 7-hydroxy metabolites of doxazosin inhibit the oxidation of LDL cholesterol.

Glucose tolerance. Another effect of selective α_1-inhibitors in hypertensive patients with insulin resistance, hyperglycemia, or noninsulin-dependent diabetes mellitus is an improvement in insulin sensitivity. There is usually a reduction in elevated serum insulin levels and a trend toward reduced fasting glucose. These "insulin sensitizing" effects are generally modest, however, and α_1-blockers are not specifically indicated for the treatment of hyperglycemic syndromes.

Table C142.1. Selective α_1-Antagonists

DRUG NAMES	DOSING FREQUENCY	STARTING DOSE (MG)	MAINTENANCE DOSE
Prazosin (Minipress)	b.i.d to t.i.d.	1	5–10 mg b.i.d.
Doxazosin (Cardura)	q.d. to b.i.d.	1	4–16 mg q.d.
Terazosin (Hytrin)	q.d. to b.i.d.	1	5–20 mg q.d.

Side Effects of Selective α_1-Antagonists

Selective α_1-antagonists are generally well tolerated with a short list of potential adverse effects including asthenia (2%), nasal congestion (2%), and dizziness (1%). The dizziness phenomenon with α_1-blockers is often due to the tendency of these drugs to cause greater BP reductions in the upright position, especially when used with diuretic, presumably due to reductions in cardiac preload. Some patients experience dizziness without postural hypotension. There is also a significant "first-dose phenomenon" with severe hypotension after initial exposure to the drug, but this initial effect wanes rapidly after subsequent doses, presumably as a result of subsequent salt and water retention. Syncope is uncommon, occurring in <1% of patients when small doses (1 mg or less) are used initially but is also associated with addition of α_1-blockers to a multiple drug regimen (especially if diuretic, β-blocker, or verapamil is being given). Individuals with alterations of urinary bladder function can develop incontinence with α_1-blocker–mediated relaxation of the bladder outlet. There are no clinically important adverse effects on laboratory tests and no adverse effects on renal function in hypertensive patients with normal, moderate, or severe renal impairment. In placebo-controlled trials, small decreases in hemoglobin, total protein, and albumin levels have been attributed to hemodilution secondary to mild fluid retention. Accompanying reduction of white blood cell counts is small and not progressive and remains unexplained.

SUGGESTED READING

1. Cohn JN, Archibald DG, Ziesche S, et al. Effect of vasodilator therapy on mortality in chronic congestive heart failure. Results of a Veterans Administration Cooperative Study. *N Engl J Med.* 1986;314:1547–1552.
2. Frishman WH, Kotob F. Alpha-adrenergic blocking drugs in clinical medicine. *J Clin Pharmacol.* 1999;39:7–16.
3. Guimaraes S, Moura D. Vascular adrenoceptors: an update. *Pharmacol Rev.* 2001;53:319–356.
4. Kirby RS, Pool JL. Alpha-adrenoceptor blockade in the treatment of benign prostatic hyperplasia: past, present and future. *Br J Urol.* 1997;80:521–532.
5. Kukin ML, Kalman J, Mannino M, et al. Combined alpha-beta blockade (doxazosin plus metoprolol) compared with beta blockade alone in chronic congestive heart failure. *Am J Cardiol.* 1996;77:486–491.
6. Major cardiovascular events in hypertensive patients randomized to doxazosin vs. chlorthalidone: the antihypertensive and lipid-lowering treatment to prevent heart attack trial (ALLHAT). ALLHAT Collaborative Research Group. *JAMA.* 2000;283:1967–1975.
7. Roehrborn CG, Bartsch G, Kirby R, et al. Guidelines for the diagnosis and treatment of benign prostatic hyperplasia: a comparative, international overview. *Urology.* 2001;58:642–650.
8. Sica DA, Pool JL. Current concepts of pharmacotherapy in hypertension—alpha-adrenergic blocking drugs: evolving role in clinical medicine. *J Clin Hypertens. (Greenwich)* 2000;2:138–142.

Chapter C143

Central and Peripheral Sympatholytics

Barry J. Materson, MD, MBA

KEY POINTS

- Central α_2-sympathetic agonists (methyldopa, clonidine, guanfacine) reduce blood pressure by decreasing central sympathetic outflow, peripheral vascular resistance, and heart rate. Central sympatholytics may be particularly useful in patients with concomitant anxiety, but major drawbacks include somnolence, dry mouth, rebound hypertension on withdrawal, and sensitivity reactions to transdermal-delivery systems (clonidine).

- Peripheral sympatholytics (reserpine, guanethidine) deplete nerve terminal norepinephrine, thereby decreasing reflex peripheral arterial and venous constriction, especially during upright posture, thus predisposing to orthostatic hypotension.

- Sexual dysfunction and numerous drug–drug interactions further limit clinical use of peripheral sympatholytics.

> See also Chapters A1, A2, A34, A37, A41, A42, B106, C127, C128, C137–C139, C153, and C161

Drugs that reduce sympathetic neurotransmission were some of the earliest compounds used in hypertension. Despite their overall effectiveness on blood pressure (BP), widespread clinical use remains limited by their high side-effect profile.

Central Sympatholytics

Central sympatholytics (**Table C143.1**) directly reduce sympathetic outflow to the heart and blood vessels. They are particularly useful for patients who have hypertension with associated anxiety, especially that which is manifested by sympathetic overactivity. Although central sympatholytics may be used as single-drug therapy, combination with a thiazide diuretic to block salt and water retention frequently accompanies their use. Clonidine, the prototype of this class, was shown in the Veterans Affairs Cooperative Study to be somewhat more effective in whites than in blacks and is recognized as being more effective in older than younger blacks.

Mechanism of action. Central sympatholytics stimulate α_2-receptors on the adrenergic neurons located within the rostral ventrolateral medulla, which controls sympathetic outflow.

Table C143.1. Central Sympatholytics: α_2-Agonists

Methyldopa (Aldomet)	Oral: 125-, 250-, 500-mg tablets; oral suspension and parenteral (both 50 mg/mL); usual oral dose, 500–2,000 mg/d divided into 2–4 doses
Combinations	Methyldopa + chlorothiazide (Aldoclor) Methyldopa + hydrochlorothiazide (Aldoril)
Clonidine (Catapres)	Oral: 0.1-, 0.2-, 0.3-mg tablets; usual dose, 0.2–0.6 mg in 2 doses Transdermal therapeutic system 1, 2, and 3 (containing 2.5, 5.0, and 7.5 mg, respectively); patch to be applied once weekly
Combination	Clonidine + chlorthalidone (Combipres)
Guanabenz (Wytensin)	Oral: 4- and 8-mg tablets; usual dose, 8 to 32 mg/d in 2 doses
Guanfacine (Tenex)	Oral: 1- and 2-mg tablets; usual dose, 1 to 2 mg at bedtime

This action mimics the effect of catecholamines within the central nervous system (CNS), which act to decrease sympathetic nervous system outflow. The physiologic effects of withdrawal of sympathetic nervous tone include parallel decreases in peripheral vascular resistance, heart rate, and systolic and diastolic BP in a balanced fashion. Methyldopa, the first drug in this class, requires conversion to an active agonist, α-methyl-norepinephrine, for its effect.

Drug differentiation

Methyldopa. Methyldopa is still widely used to treat pregnancy-induced hypertension. Treatment of hypertensive emergencies with intravenous methyldopa has been supplanted by more effective drugs. In this drug class, hypersensitivity reactions, including hepatitis and Coombs-positive hemolytic anemia, have been seen with methyldopa. Methyldopa and its metabolic products can interfere with some assays for catecholamines and can interfere with other therapeutic agents, such as levodopa, bromocriptine, and monoamine oxidase inhibitors.

Clonidine. Oral clonidine has a rapid onset of action (30–60 minutes) and is useful for managing hypertensive urgencies but is relatively short-acting. A transdermal patch delivery system (transdermal therapeutic system patch) provides a constant dose of drug for 7 days, but it takes 1 to 2 days to attain peak

effect, and the effect lingers from 8 to 24 hours after the patch is removed. Best absorption from the patch occurs when it is placed on the chest or upper arm. If clonidine is suddenly discontinued during treatment with high doses (usually ≥1.0 mg, although sometimes lower), rebound hypertension may occur secondary to an excessive sympathetic discharge. Rebound hypertension may be accentuated if β-blocker therapy is ongoing at the time of clonidine discontinuation. Skin hypersensitivity to the transdermal clonidine patch occurs in <15% to 20% of patients who use the transdermal therapeutic system preparation.

Guanabenz is mechanistically similar to clonidine but is somewhat longer acting, and it is slightly less prone to symptomatic hypertension with its sudden withdrawal. It is less likely to be associated with orthostatic hypotension.

Guanfacine. Guanfacine differs from the other members of this class in that its prolonged (24-hour) duration of action typically allows dosing to be once daily. Its preferable dosing time is evening to blunt the early morning surge in catecholamines and to allow for any sedative effect. As with other agents in this class, guanfacine works best when coadministered with a small dose of diuretic, which optimizes BP lowering with minimum CNS adverse effects. Adverse effects increase significantly with doses >1 mg per day.

Side and adverse effects. Somnolence and dry mouth (40%) are the most common adverse drug reactions and are the major reason central sympatholytics are discontinued. Other CNS depressants and ethanol enhance sedative effects within this drug class. Dry mouth may be quite annoying to the patient, and decreased formation of saliva may increase the risk of dental caries and periodontal disease.

Peripheral Sympatholytics

Peripheral sympatholytics have a common mechanism of action at postganglionic sympathetic nerve endings (**Table C143.2**). Reserpine has additional CNS mechanisms of action that other peripheral sympatholytics do not, so the adverse effects of all peripheral sympatholytics are not entirely comparable. Reserpine remains a widely used agent on a worldwide basis. Nevertheless, reserpine, guanethidine, and guanadrel have important and potentially dangerous interactions with other drugs that affect postganglionic catecholamine metabo-

Table C143.2. Peripheral Sympatholytics: Rauwolfia Alkaloids

Rauwolfia alkaloids	
Reserpine (Serpalan, Serpasil)	Oral: 0.1-, 0.25-mg tablets; usual dose, 0.1–0.25 mg/d
Combinations	Reserpine + chlorothiazide (Diupres, Diurigen with reserpine)
	Reserpine + chlorthalidone (Regroton, Demi-Regroton)
	Reserpine + hydrochlorothiazide (Hydropres-50)
	Reserpine + methyclothiazide (Diutensen-R)
	Reserpine + hydralazine + hydrochlorothiazide (Cam-Ap-Es, Cherapas, Ser-A-Gen, Ser-Ap-Es, Seralazide, Serpazide, Tri-Hydroserpine, Unipres)
Deserpidine (Harmonyl)	Oral: 0.25-mg tablets; usual dose, 0.25–0.50 mg/d
Combinations	Deserpidine + hydrochlorothiazide (Oreticyl, Oreticyl Forte)
	Deserpidine + methyclothiazide (Enduronyl, Enduronyl Forte)
Rauwolfia serpentina (Raudixin, Rauval, Rauverid, Wolfina)	Oral: 50-mg tablets; usual dose, 50–200 mg/d
Combination	Rauwolfia + bendroflumethiazide (Rauzide)
Postganglionic adrenergic blocking agents	
Guanethidine (Ismelin)	Oral: 10- and 25-mg tablets; usual dose, 10–50 mg/d
Guanadrel (Hylorel)	Oral: 10- and 25-mg tablets; usual dose, 10–75 mg in 2–4 doses

lism, and their use has decreased since the advent of more powerful and safer antihypertensive drugs.

Mechanism of action. Drugs of this class work by entering sympathetic neurons via catecholamine-hydrogen pump mechanism and depleting norepinephrine from storage granules in the postganglionic sympathetic nerves, thereby decreasing neurogenic vascular and cardiac tone (see Chapter A2). Because of reflex upregulation of peripheral adrenergic receptors, these agents cause exaggerated pressor responses to endogenous catecholamines. The ability to respond to upright postural change by reflex peripheral vasoconstriction is also impaired; thus, orthostatic hypotension may occur. In addition, reserpine depletes other tissue stores of catecholamines, including the heart, and it also reduces serotonin levels.

Drug differentiation. Reserpine is extremely long-acting and can be an effective and inexpensive antihypertensive agent when used in low doses (0.05 mg) with a diuretic. Most of its adverse effects occur with much higher dosage regimens. Guanethidine is difficult to titrate because of its wide therapeutic range and very long duration of action. This compound is sufficiently potent that some cases of resistant hypertension can be resolved by the addition of as little as 10 mg of guanethidine. Guanadrel is shorter-acting and easier to titrate than guanethidine and is observed to cause less diarrhea and orthostatic hypotension. Guanadrel is excreted renally and requires dosage adjustment in renally impaired patients. These drugs also typically cause salt and water retention, which attenuates their antihypertensive effect; thus, diuretic add-on therapy is almost always necessary in their long-term use.

Side and adverse effects. Reserpine causes nasal stuffiness and has been associated with significant depression. It can increase gastric acidity and risk of acid-peptic disease and intestinal motility, which may exacerbate ulcerative colitis or precipitate biliary colic. Tricyclic antidepressants interfere with the norepinephrine pump mechanism and may decrease the hypotensive effect of guanethidine and guanadrel, which also require the same pump for their biologic effects. If these drugs are added to monoamine oxidase inhibitors, a hypertensive crisis may be precipitated. This is important because monoamine oxidase inhibitors are being used increasingly in the management of Parkinson's disease. Peripheral sympatholytics may also trigger a hypertensive crisis if an occult pheochromocytoma is present. Frequent stools or diarrhea can be a problem, although less so with guanadrel. Retrograde ejaculation is another disturbing adverse reaction seen with these drugs.

SUGGESTED READING

1. Joint National Committee on Prevention, Detection, Evaluation, and Treatment of High Blood Pressure. The sixth report of the Joint National Committee on Prevention, Detection, Evaluation, and Treatment of High Blood Pressure. *Arch Intern Med.* 1997;157:2413–2446.
2. Materson BJ. Combination therapy as the initial drug treatment for hypertension: when is it appropriate? *Am J Hypertens.* 2001;14:293–295.
3. Materson BJ, Kessler WB, Alderman MH, et al. A multi-center, randomized, double-blind dose-response evaluation of step-2 guanfacine versus placebo in patients with mild-to-moderate hypertension. *Am J Cardiol.* 1986;57:32E–37E.
4. Materson BJ, Reda DJ, Cushman WC, et al. Single-drug therapy for hypertension in men: a comparison of six antihypertensive drugs with placebo. *N Engl J Med.* 1993;328:914–921.
5. Participating Veterans Administration Medical Centers. Low doses vs standard dose of reserpine: a randomized, double-blind, multiclinic trial in patients taking chlorthalidone. *JAMA.* 1982;248:2471–2477.
6. Veterans Administration Cooperative Study Group on Antihypertensive Agents. Multi-clinic controlled trial of bethanidine and guanethidine in severe hypertension. *Circulation.* 1977;55:519–525.

Angiotensin-Converting Enzyme Inhibitors

Domenic A. Sica, MD

The pivotal role for angiotensin II (Ang II) in hypertension and end-organ disease derives not only from its being a potent vasoconstrictor but also from its activation of a wide range of neural, trophic, inflammatory, and procoagulant pathways (see Chapter A3). The potential impact of angiotensin-converting enzyme (ACE) inhibition is only now becoming clear, and ACE inhibition is approved for several cardiac, renal, and vascular conditions (**Table C144.1**).

Indications and Outcomes Studies

Hypertension. ACE inhibitors are effective antihypertensive agents and are particularly useful in hypertensive diabetics (with or without proteinuria) with a neutral effect on insulin resistance and hyperlipidemia. They are also useful in patients with isolated systolic hypertension or systolic-predominant forms of hypertension because they improve vascular compliance. In patients with cerebrovascular disease, they preserve cerebral autoregulatory ability despite a reduction in blood pressure (BP). ACE inhibitors are not specific coronary vasodilators, but they do decrease myocardial oxygen consumption and thereby ischemia; thus, they can be used effectively in patients with coronary artery disease.

Heart failure. Data from several placebo-controlled or open label trials have prompted a joint American College of Cardiology and American Heart Association task group to recommend ACE inhibitors as first-line agents in all stages of heart failure (see Chapters C155 and C156). ACE inhibitors substantially

Table C144.1. U.S. Food and Drug Association Approved Indications for Angiotensin-Converting Enzyme Inhibitors

DRUG	HYPERTENSION	HEART FAILURE	DIABETIC NEPHROPATHY	HIGH-RISK CARDIOVASCULAR DISEASE
Captopril	•	• (Post-MI)[a]	•	
Benazepril	•			
Enalapril	•	•[b]		
Fosinopril	•	•		
Lisinopril	•	• (Post-MI)[a]		
Moexipril	•			
Perindopril	•			
Quinapril	•	•		
Ramipril	•	• (Post-MI)		•[c]
Trandolapril	•	• (Post-MI)		

MI, myocardial infarction.
[a]Captopril and lisinopril are indicated for heart failure treatment post–myocardial infarction and as adjunctive therapy for heart failure.
[b]Enalapril is indicated for high-risk individuals and for asymptomatic and symptomatic patients.
[c]Based on results of the Heart Outcomes Prevention Evaluation (HOPE) study.

reduce the risk of death and hospitalization for congestive heart failure, while improving its symptomatology. Statistically significant reductions in heart failure mortality have been observed with enalapril, captopril, ramipril, quinapril, trandolapril, and lisinopril. Furthermore, these agents have demonstrated improved exercise tolerance and symptomatology.

Post myocardial infarction. In post myocardial infarction patients, enalapril, captopril, lisinopril, and trandolapril have been shown to significantly reduce morbidity and mortality rates over a wide range of ventricular function, suggesting a class effect (see Chapter C154).

Nephropathy. The collaborative study group of Lewis et al. and the Ramipril Efficacy in Nephropathy (REIN) study with ramipril demonstrated in diabetics and nondiabetics with renal involvement that ACE inhibitors effectively reduce the rate of decline of renal function and urinary protein excretion in excess of that expected with BP reduction alone. ACE inhibitors have been proven useful in the setting of established type 1 insulin-dependent diabetes mellitus nephropathy, noninsulin-dependent diabetes mellitus nephropathy, normotensive type 1 insulin-dependent diabetes mellitus patients with microalbuminuria, and a variety of nondiabetic renal diseases (see Chapter C167). Also, ACE inhibitors are of proven benefit in slowing renal disease progression in blacks with hypertensive nephrosclerosis as has been shown in the African-American Study of Kidney Disease (AASK).

Stroke. The Perindopril Protection against Recurrent Stroke Study (PROGRESS) reported that a combination of perindopril and indapamide reduced the recurrence of stroke in normotensive and hypertensive patients. In this trial, stroke reduction with perindopril treatment alone was not significant, probably because of the small reduction in BP and the low dose (2–4 mg) of perindopril used. The Heart Outcomes Prevention Evaluation (HOPE) study, however, provided strong evidence that treatment with more appropriate doses of ACE inhibitor (ramipril, 10 mg daily) reduces the risk of stroke in high-risk cardiac patients. The Antihypertensive and Lipid Lowering Treatment to Prevent Heart Attack Trial (ALLHAT) found that the lisinopril treatment group had a 15% and 40% higher stroke rate in the entire study population and the black cohort, respectively. These differences favoring diuretic over ACE inhibitor therapy relative to stroke, in part related to BP differences in the treatment groups (mean follow-up systolic BP was 2 mm Hg higher for all lisinopril-treated subjects and 4-mm Hg higher in blacks). Diuretic and ACE inhibitor combination was not tested in ALLHAT. American Heart Association guidelines for the primary prevention of stroke recommend ramipril to prevent stroke in high-risk patients and in patients with diabetes and hypertension (see Chapter C160).

High-risk cardiac patients. The HOPE study compared ramipril (10 mg/day) or placebo in more than 9,500 high-risk patients against a primary composite end point (cardiovascular death, nonfatal myocardial infarction, and nonfatal stroke). The trial was stopped early (after 4.5 years of treatment) because of a 22% reduction in relative risk in the ramipril group. The benefits of ramipril were equal in those receiving or not receiving a diuretic, proving that there is additional benefit that can be achieved from combining ACE inhibitors and diuretics. The individual components of the composite end point were also significantly reduced:

32% for stroke, 26% for cardiovascular death, and 20% for myocardial infarction. In contrast, ALLHAT found no difference between lisinopril and chlorthalidone for the primary outcome (combined fatal coronary heart disease or nonfatal myocardial infarction). However, ALLHAT did not test ACE inhibitor–diuretic combinations to identify whether additional benefit could occur.

Mechanisms of Actions

Pharmacology. Ten ACE inhibitors are currently marketed in the United States (Tables C144.1 and **C144.2**). With the exception of lisinopril and captopril, ACE inhibitors are prodrugs that improve absorption but require hydrolysis. Prodrug ACE inhibitors undergo metabolic conversion to an active diacid form in the liver or intestine. ACE inhibitors are structurally heterogeneous and include sulfhydryl (captopril), phosphinyl (fosinopril), or carboxyl (all other ACE inhibitors) side groups that affect disposition and metabolism. Although ACE inhibitors can be separated by differences in absorption, protein and tissue binding, half-life, and mode of metabolic disposition, these differences rarely affect drug selection. One debated characteristic of ACE inhibitors involves their capacity to bind or penetrate into specific tissues, which may relate to lipophilicity. It has been proposed but not proven that highly lipophilic ACE inhibitors, such as quinapril and ramipril, offer superior "tissue ACE" inhibition, a characteristic of unclear clinical value.

Hormonal effects. ACE is pluripotent, catalyzing the conversion of angiotensin I (Ang I) to Ang II, the degradation of bradykinin (BK), and the metabolic breakdown of several other vasoactive peptides (see Chapters A6–A8). Reduction in Ang II is an important factor in the response to an ACE inhibitor but in an ill-defined manner. Long-term ACE inhibition is thought by some to be accompanied by "angiotensin-escape," which ostensibly results from increased generation of Ang II by non–ACE-dependent pathways. Ang II suppresses renin; when Ang II levels fall after administration of an ACE inhibitor, this inhibitory influence is removed, and plasma renin activity and Ang I increase. This excess of Ang I provides a substrate for alternative pathway enzymes, such as chymases, and is one possible explanation for the phenomenon of "Ang II escape."

ACE participates in the processing of other peptides; kininase II, which prevents BK breakdown, is identical to ACE. Increased BK stimulates the production of endothelium-derived relaxing factor (nitric oxide) and induces prostacyclin release, presumably enhancing vasodilation. Nonsteroidal antiinflammatory drugs can blunt the BP-lowering effect of ACE inhibitors (see Chapter C150). Captopril may be more susceptible to a nonsteroidal antiinflammatory drug interaction because it directly stimulates prostaglandin synthesis. A significant portion of ACE inhibitor effect can be attributed to reduced activity of the sympathetic nervous system. ACE inhibitors do not consistently reduce resting plasma catecholamine concentrations, but they tend to blunt reflex sympathetic activation seen with other vasodilating drugs.

Hemodynamic effects

Hypertension. ACE inhibitors cause a variety of interlinked hemodynamic effects. In hypertension, there is a balanced reduction of cardiac preload (through their vasodilatory effects) and

Table C144.2. Angiotensin-Converting Enzyme Inhibitors: Dosage Strengths and Treatment Guidelines

DRUG	TRADE NAME	USUAL TOTAL DAILY DOSE IN HYPERTENSION (MG) (FREQUENCY/D)[a]	USUAL TOTAL DAILY DOSE IN HEART FAILURE[a] (MG) (FREQUENCY/D)[a]	COMMENT	FIXED-DOSE COMBINATIONS[b]
Benazepril	Lotensin	20–40 (1)	Not FDA approved for heart failure		Benazepril and hydrochlorothiazide (Lotensin HCT)
Captopril	Capoten	75–300 (2–3)	18.75–150.00 (3)	Generically available	Captopril and hydrochlorothiazide (Capozide[c])
Enalapril	Vasotec	5–40 (1–2)	5–40 (2)	Generic and intravenous	Enalapril and hydrochlorothiazide (Vaseretic)
Fosinopril	Monopril	10–40 (1)	10–40 (1)	Renal and hepatic elimination	Fosinopril and hydrochlorothiazide (Monopril-HCT)
Lisinopril	Prinivil, Zestril	10–40 (1)	5–20 (1)	Generically available	Lisinopril and hydrochlorothiazide (Prinzide, Zestoretic)
Moexipril	Univasc	7.5–30.0 (1)	Not FDA approved for heart failure		Moexipril and hydrochlorothiazide (Uniretic)
Perindopril	Aceon	4–16 (1)	Not FDA approved for heart failure		
Quinapril	Accupril	20–80 (1)	10–40 (1–2)		Quinapril and hydrochlorothiazide (Accuretic)
Ramipril	Altace	5–20 (1)	10 (2)	Indicated in high-risk vascular patients	
Trandolapril	Mavik	2–8 (1)	2–4 (1)	Renal and hepatic elimination	

FDA, U.S. Food and Drug Administration.
[a]Lower doses are often recommended to initiate therapy. Higher doses are recommended for chronic therapy to provide full 24-hour coverage.
[b]Fixed-dose combinations in this class typically contain a thiazide-like diuretic.
[c]Capozide is indicated for first-step treatment of hypertension.

afterload (through direct and indirect arterial dilator effects). Because Ang II facilitates sympathetic nervous activation, ACE inhibition tends to blunt stress-induced increases in catecholamines. Heart rate effects of ACE inhibition are minimal.

Heart failure. In heart failure, ACE inhibitor use causes a marked hemodynamic improvement. Cardiac afterload is reduced because of systemic vasodilation and improved large artery compliance (see Chapter A60). Stroke volume and ejection fraction increases as a result, but myocardial oxygen consumption is not increased, in part because ACE inhibitors also reduce cardiac preload and pulmonary wedge pressures through their venodilatory effects. Finally, the antisympathetic actions of ACE inhibitors are effective to reduce tachycardia and increase ventricular filling time, another way to improve cardiac efficiency.

Class effects. Because there are few properties that separate one ACE inhibitor from another, cost has assumed added significance. *Class effect* is a phrase often invoked to legitimatize switching from one compound to another, especially when a higher-priced agent has been specifically studied in a disease state such as heart failure or diabetic nephropathy. Regarding BP responses among ACE inhibitors, class effect may apply. For other outcomes, however, differences between compounds or doses may be more important.

Clinical Usage

Blood pressure effects. BP responses to ACE inhibitors are comparable to that of most other drug classes, with response rates from 40% to 70% in stages 1 and 2 hypertension. There are a few predictors of response to an ACE inhibitor, including high plasma renin values, but there is a limited relationship between plasma renin activity and the BP response to an ACE inhibitor. On the basis of a number of trials comparing trough to peak activity ratios with 24-hour ambulatory BP monitor-

ing, fosinopril, lisinopril, perindopril, ramipril, and trandolapril can be administered once daily.

Subgroups and response patterns. Certain patient subsets demonstrate lower response rates to ACE inhibitor monotherapy, including low-renin, salt-sensitive individuals, such as diabetic and black hypertensives. The low-renin state in elderly hypertensives is an exception in that it develops not as a result of volume expansion, although these patients are salt sensitive, but because of age-related decreases in plasma renin. The elderly generally respond to ACE inhibitors, although interpretation of such a response is complicated by senescence-related renal failure having slowed the elimination of these typically renally cleared drugs, resulting in higher plasma concentrations of an ACE inhibitor. Black hypertensives are also incorrectly perceived as universally unresponsive to ACE inhibitors although wide variation exists. If adequate dose titration occurs, BP can be effectively lowered in most patients. Racial differences in BP response are abolished when an ACE inhibitor is combined with a thiazide diuretic.

Dosing

Hypertension. Information about dosing is summarized in Table C144.2. The question is often raised as to what to do if an ACE inhibitor fails to normalize BP. One approach is to increase the dose; the dose-response curve for ACE inhibitor is steep at low doses and fairly flat thereafter but not as flat as had been previously believed (see Chapter A137). Dose titration helps to improve trough effects and prolong the duration of peak effect but has less impact on the peak effect itself. This being said, the full range of ACE inhibitor doses has not been carefully studied. Also, duration of therapy matters. The final BP response to an ACE inhibitor probably requires several weeks of therapy. If a partial response to an ACE inhibitor has occurred, therapy can be continued in anticipation of an additional drop in BP over the ensuing weeks. There is no evidence to support switching from an ACE inhibitor to an ARB if the former has failed.

High-risk cardiac patients. In HOPE, low-dose ramipril (2.5 mg/day) was ineffective at preventing cardiovascular events; in general, higher doses (ramipril, 10 mg or more) are appropriate.

Heart failure. Clinical trial dosages are usually higher than those used in general practice. Initiation with low doses is recommended with titration to maximal effect. Plasma brain natriuretic peptide levels may be useful in guiding therapy (see Chapter C155). Higher doses (40 mg of enalapril or lisinopril) reduce hospitalization rates in patients with stage C heart failure (see Chapter C156). Myocardial binding, degree of change in plasma aldosterone, and changes in other neuropeptides degraded by ACE may contribute to their overall success. Because not all ACE inhibitors have been thoroughly studied in CHF, true dose equivalence can only be estimated.

Post myocardial infarction. In a hemodynamically stable patient (i.e., without hypotension) after myocardial infarction, an oral ACE inhibitor should be initiated with a low dose, generally within 24 hours of the event, particularly if the myocardial infarction is anterior and associated with depressed left ventricular function. The drug can be titrated upward rapidly if hypotension does not occur with the first dose. The hemodynamic effects and overall benefit of ACE inhibition are seen early with 40% of the 30-day increase in survival observed in days 0 to 1, 45% in days 2 to 7, and approximately 15% after day 7. The benefits of ACE inhibitor therapy in the post myocardial infarction period appear not to be the result of a substantial decline in arrhythmic mortality.

Nephropathy. ACE inhibitor regimens shown to slow the rate of CRF progression include captopril, 50 mg t.i.d.; enalapril, 20 mg per day; benazepril, 20 mg per day; and ramipril, 10 mg per day. It is presumed that renal failure increases the pharmacologic effect of these doses by reducing the renal clearance of the ACE inhibitor. Doses required to reduce proteinuria may be substantially greater than those needed to lower BP.

Combinations with other drugs. The antihypertensive effect of an ACE inhibitor is predictably enhanced by the coadministration of a diuretic. Fixed-dose combination products containing an ACE inhibitor and a diuretic capitalize on the rationale that sodium (Na^+) depletion activates renin and thereby sensitizes the individual to ACE inhibition. Low diuretic doses (6.25 mg of hydrochlorothiazide) can evoke this additive response, suggesting that even subtle alterations in Na^+ balance are sufficient to bolster the effect of ACE inhibitors. Combining an ACE inhibitor and a β-blocker was at first considered useful because the β-blocker could blunt the hyperreninemia induced by an ACE inhibitor. In practice, only a marginal additional response occurs when these drug classes are combined, however. Combination of a peripheral α-antagonist or calcium antagonist with an ACE inhibitor results in an appreciable additional response. It remains to be determined whether the combination of an ACE inhibitor and an ARB is significantly better than either given alone at maximum doses.

Adverse effects

Renal function. Functional renal insufficiency has been noted with ACE inhibitors in patients with either a solitary kidney and RAS or bilateral RAS. This phenomenon can be observed in dehydration, heart failure, and microvascular renal disease. The theme common to these conditions is reduced glomerular filtration pressure and increased intrarenal production of Ang II, which supports glomerular filtration by maximizing efferent arteriolar constriction. The abrupt removal of Ang II with an ACE inhibitor relaxes afferent and efferent arterioles and can reduce glomerular pressure to a level too low to support filtration. Discontinuation of the ACE inhibitor or careful volume repletion usually reverses the problem (see Chapter A48).

Potassium. Hyperkalemia with ACE inhibitors generally arises only in predisposed patients with reduced glomerular filtration rate or hyperaldosteronism (diabetics or CHF patients with renal failure). Use of K^+-sparing diuretics or K^+ supplements exacerbates the problem. In contrast, ACE inhibitors minimize the level of hypokalemia produced by diuretics.

Cough. A dry, nonproductive cough is seen in 10% to 20% of patients treated with ACE inhibitors. This class effect has been attributed to increased levels of BK metabolites and other vasoactive peptides. Switching among ACE inhibitors does not work, and other drugs have not proven successful in eliminating ACE inhibitor–induced cough. Angiotensin receptor blockers can be considered in ACE inhibitor–intolerant patients. Typically, the cough disappears 1 to 2 weeks after discontinuation of the ACE inhibitor.

Other. Angioneurotic edema is an unpredictable and potentially life-threatening complication of ACE inhibitor therapy occurring in <1% of treated patients and is more common in blacks than whites. It typically occurs shortly after beginning therapy with an ACE inhibitor, although it has also been seen years after beginning an ACE inhibitor. Angioneurotic edema has a distinctive pattern of involvement with severe swelling of the mouth, tongue, and upper airway. ACE inhibitors are contraindicated in pregnancy because they can also cause developmental defects if given in the second or third trimester of pregnancy but are not teratogenic per se.

SUGGESTED READING

1. ACC/AHA Guidelines for the evaluation and management of chronic heart failure in the adult: executive Summary. *Circulation.* 2001;104:2996–3007.
2. Agodoa LY, Appel L, Bakris GL, et al. Effect of ramipril vs amlodipine on renal outcomes in hypertensive nephrosclerosis: a randomized controlled trial. *JAMA.* 2001;285:2719–2728.
3. Bakris GL, Weir MR. Angiotensin-converting enzyme inhibitor-associated elevations in serum creatinine: is this a cause for concern? *Arch Intern Med.* 2000;160:685–693.
4. Dzau VJ, Bernstein K, Celermajer D, et al. The relevance of tissue angiotensin-converting enzyme: manifestations in mechanistic and endpoint data. *Am J Cardiol.* 2001;88:1L–20L.
5. Garg R, Yusuf S, for the Collaborative Group on ACE Inhibitor Trials. Overview of randomized trials of angiotensin-converting enzyme inhibitors on mortality and morbidity in patients with heart failure. *JAMA.* 1995;273:1450–1456.
6. Giatras I, Lau J, Levey SS. Effect of angiotensin-converting enzyme inhibitors on the progression of nondiabetic renal disease: a meta-analysis of randomized trials. *Ann Intern Med.* 1997;127:337–345.
7. Lewis EJ, Hunsicker LG, Bain RP, Rhode RD. The effect of angiotensin-converting enzyme inhibition on diabetic nephropathy. The Collaborative Study Group. *N Engl J Med.* 1993;329:1456–1462.
8. Schoolwerth AC, Sica DA, Ballermann BJ, Wilcox CS. Renal considerations in angiotensin converting enzyme inhibitor therapy: a statement for healthcare professionals from the Council on the Kidney in Cardiovascular Disease and the Council for High Blood Pressure Research of the American Heart Association. *Circulation.* 2001;104:1985–1991.
9. The SOLVD investigators. Effect of enalapril on survival in patients with reduced left ventricular ejection fractions and congestive heart failure. *N Engl J Med.* 1991;325:293–302.
10. Yusuf S, Sleight P, Pogue J, et al. Effects of an angiotensin-converting enzyme inhibitor, ramipril, on cardiovascular events in high-risk patients. The Heart Outcomes Prevention Evaluation Study Investigators. *N Engl J Med.* 2000;342:145–153.

Angiotensin II Receptor Blockers

Michael A. Weber, MD

Angiotensin II receptor blockers (ARBs) are used primarily for the treatment of hypertension, though recently completed clinical trials are helping to define their use for such additional indications as heart failure, post myocardial infarction, and diabetic nephropathy. Because these drugs work by blocking the effects of renin-angiotensin system activation, there was an early tendency to see them largely as well-tolerated alternatives to angiotensin-converting enzyme (ACE) inhibitors. Yet there may be meaningful pharmacologic and clinical differences between the 2 classes.

Indications and Outcome Studies

Of the 8 major clinical end point trials so far reported with ARBs, 1 has been based on hypertension, 3 have studied hypertensive patients with type 2 diabetes and nephropathy or proteinuria, and 4 have been carried out in patients with heart failure. Together, these experiences indicate that the ARBs provide clinical outcome benefits that go beyond their hemodynamic effects.

Hypertension. The Losartan Intervention for Endpoint (LIFE) study was a double-blind randomized trial that compared 4,605 patients treated with losartan-based therapy to 4,588 patients on atenolol-based therapy with respect to morbidity and mortality. The patients, aged 75 to 80 years with left ventricular hypertrophy demonstrated by electrocardiogram, were titrated from 50 mg of either losartan or atenolol to 100 mg. If blood pressure (BP) control (<140/90) was not achieved, hydrochlorothiazide and other agents could be added. Despite virtually identical BP effects on brachial BPs (**Table C145.1**), there were clear differences between the drugs on major end points (primary composite end point of cardiovascular mortality, stroke, and myocardial infarction). Losartan produced a 13% relative risk reduction ($p = .021$) compared with atenolol. There was a 25% reduction in stroke ($p = .001$), a 25% reduction in new-onset diabetes ($p = .0001$) and significantly

($p = .001$) greater regression of left ventricular hypertrophy with losartan. Those who had diabetes at baseline (Table C145.1) had outcomes that were similar to the cohort as a whole. In the subgroup with isolated systolic hypertension, a marked beneficial effect of losartan was observed on the primary end point (25% reduction) and stroke (40% reduction) relative to atenolol.

Diabetic nephropathy. The Reduction of Endpoints in NIDDM with the Angiotensin II Antagonist Losartan (RENAAL) study was a randomized double-blind placebo-controlled trial, lasting approximately 3.5 years, that compared the effects of losartan with conventional therapy (diuretics or β-blockers were primary agents and ACE inhibitors could not be used) in diabetic hypertensive patients with overt proteinuria (mean baseline albumin/creatinine ratio: 1,867 mg/g). Compared with conventional therapy, losartan reduced the primary composite end point (doubling of serum creatinine, end-stage renal disease or death) by 16% ($p = .024$). Based on similar methodology and patients (baseline urine protein: 4,016 mg/day), the Irbesartan type 2 Diabetic Nephropathy Trial (IDNT) compared irbesartan (up to 300 mg daily) with conventional therapy and also with the calcium antagonist amlodipine (up to 10 mg daily) during a 3-year period. Despite similar BP results in the 3 groups, irbesartan reduced the primary composite end point (same as in RENAAL) by 20% ($p = .02$) compared with conventional treatment, and by 23% ($p = .006$) compared with amlodipine. A third study, the Irbesartan MicroAlbuminuria (II) trial (IRMA II), demonstrated that irbesartan 300 mg daily (but not 150 mg daily) was superior to conventional antihypertensive therapy during a 2-year period in preventing progression to overt nephropathy in type 2 diabetic hypertensives with microalbuminuria. Despite their clear renal protective effects, the 3 renal studies were not designed or powered to evaluate other cardiovascular end points.

Table C145.1. Life Study[a]: Adjusted[b] Hazard Ratios (95% Confidence Interval), Losartan versus Atenolol

	WHOLE STUDY	DIABETIC PATIENTS
Primary composite end point[c]	0.87 (0.77–0.98), $p = .021$	0.76 (0.58–0.98), $p = .031$
Cardiovascular mortality	0.89 (0.73–1.07), $p = .206$	0.63 (0.41–0.95), $p = .028$
Stroke	0.75 (0.63–0.88), $p = .001$	0.79 (0.55–1.14), $p = .204$
Myocardial infarction	1.07 (0.88–1.31), $p = .491$	0.83 (0.55–1.25), $p = .373$
New-onset diabetes	0.75 (0.63–0.88), $p = .001$	Not applicable

Note: Total study: losartan (N = 4,605), atenolol (N = 4,588); diabetic patients: losartan (N = 586), atenolol (N = 609).
[a]Selected end points.
[b]For degree of left ventricular hypertrophy and Framingham risk score at baseline.
[c]Cardiovascular mortality, stroke and myocardial infarction.

Heart failure. Studies so far in heart failure have identified no meaningful differences between ARBs and ACE inhibitors on cardiovascular mortality and morbidity. In the Evaluation of Losartan in the Elderly (ELITE) studies (I and II) and in the Valsartan Heart Failure Trial (Val-HEFT) study, losartan was not found to be superior to ACE inhibition in heart failure. The latter study provided an indication for valsartan in the management of heart failure in ACE inhibitor–intolerant patients. Giving the 2 drug classes in combination may confer modest additional benefits in some studies, though these advantages may be lost if β-blockers are also given (ELITE II). It is also not clear that the effects of ARB-ACE inhibitor combinations are superior to higher doses of either class given alone. Thus, the 2 drug types probably are best regarded as alternatives to each other.

Mechanisms of Actions

Pharmacology. ARBs act by binding selectively to the AT_1 receptor (see Chapter A3). These nonpeptide oral agents can be either competitive (irbesartan, valsartan) or insurmountable (candesartan or the losartan metabolite Exp3174). Some ARBs are prodrugs that depend on conversion to an active metabolite to produce most of their clinical effects (in the case of losartan to Exp3174, the parent compound also has pharmacologic activity). There is no evidence of meaningful clinical differences between drugs that work in their parent form and those that are prodrugs. ARBs have variable bioavailability, with values as low as 13 and 15% for eprosartan and candesartan, respectively, and 60% to 80% for irbesartan. ARBs generally are administered once daily. Minor pharmacokinetic differences exist among these agents that could produce differences in their BP effects during the 24-hour treatment period. There is no evidence, though, that any of these differing pharmacologic properties materially influence the clinical effects of these drugs, especially if adequate doses are used.

Receptor subtypes. Four angiotensin II receptors have been described: AT_1, AT_2, AT_3, and AT_4 (see Chapter A3). So far, only the AT_1 and the AT_2 receptors have been well defined. The AT_1 receptor mediates most of the known physiologic actions of angiotensin II, including its hemodynamic and trophic effects. The AT_2 receptor is found primarily during fetal development and appears to mediate apoptosis and tissue remodeling/healing. Much of the time, AT_2 receptor expression is very low. It is possible that stimuli such as high BP or other cardiovascular risk factors that can injure the arterial wall also evoke the expression of AT_2 receptors, which may mediate vasodilation and inhibitory effects on cell growth. Recently, stimulation of AT_2 receptors has been shown to increase nitric oxide production and may even influence tissue kinin mechanisms. Thus, the AT_2 receptor seems to have opposing or countervailing properties to the AT_1 receptor. Tissue culture studies have confirmed that AT_1 blockade reduces cell growth and that AT_2 blockade (with nonclinical experimental agents) increases cell growth. Simultaneous blockade of the AT_1 receptor and stimulation of the AT_2 receptor (the putative situation when an ARB is used) would, therefore, result in an enhanced antiproliferative effect. These interesting possibilities, which have yet to be fully defined in the clinical setting, are summarized in **Table C145.2**.

Effects on RAAS components. ARBs cause an increase in plasma renin, angiotensin I, and angiotensin II concentrations, largely by inhibiting the negative feedback of angiotensin II on renin release. The increased angiotensin II has no direct vasoconstriction effect because the AT_1 receptor is blocked. Aldosterone levels tend to fall via AT_1 receptor blockade on adrenal zona glomerulosa cells, though this effect is minimal.

Clinical Usage

Blood pressure effects. ARBs have antihypertensive efficacy comparable to other major antihypertensive drug classes. Dose-response effects are less pronounced with ARBs and the differ-

Table C145.2. Angiotensin II Receptors and Effects of Blockade

Vascular AT_1 receptors
  Constantly expressed
  Mediate vasoconstriction
  Mediate angiotensin II arterial wall growth effects
Vascular AT_2 receptors
  Expressed only after injury (sustained hypertension might provoke expression)
  Mediate vasodilation
  Mediate antiproliferative actions
  Activate other factors (e.g., nitric oxide, tissue kinins)
Potential double action of selective AT_1 blockers
  Directly block vasoconstrictor and growth actions of angiotensin II at AT_1 receptors
  Increase circulating angiotensin II levels
  Unblocked AT_2 receptors (if expressed), stimulated by increased angiotensin II activity, mediate vasodilation and growth inhibition
  Net effect: AT_1 blockade plus AT_2 stimulation

Table C145.3. Available Drugs

GENERIC	BRAND	HALF-LIFE (H)	USUAL DOSE RANGE[a] (MG)	COMMENTS
Losartan	Cozaar; Hyzaar[b]	2	50–100	Active metabolite (E-3174), losartan is uricosuric, labeled indication in type 2 diabetic nephropathy
Valsartan	Diovan; Diovan HCT[b]	6	80–320	Labeled indication in congestive heart failure
Irbesartan	Avapro; Avalide[b]	11–15	150–300	Labeled indication in type 2 diabetic nephropathy
Eprosartan	Teveten	5–9	400–800	May have inhibitory effect on the sympathetic nervous system
Telmisartan	Micardis; Micardis HCT[b]	24	40–80	Dose dependent bioavailability of 42–58%, volume of distribution of 500 L
Candesartan cilexetil	Atacand; Atacand HCT	9–13	8–32	Active metabolite candesartan
Olmesartan medoxomil	Benicar	13	20–40	Active metabolite olmesartan

[a]Angiotensin receptor blockers are administered once daily though their effect may wane at the end of the dose interval occasionally requiring a second dose.
[b]Combination products containing hydrochlorothiazide.

ence in BP-lowering efficacy between the usual starting doses and the maximum doses is often only 4 to 8 mm Hg. As a practical matter, this property adds to the convenience of using these agents because for most of them there is only a 1-step titration regimen. The lack of dose-dependent side effects should encourage use of higher doses. Some of the principal properties of these agents, together with information about dosing, are summarized in **Table C145.3.** Some clinical trials have demonstrated differences in antihypertensive efficacy among these agents. But it is important to recognize that such differences may be influenced partly by the selection of doses, and it is also possible that other sponsored comparative studies that did not show the hoped-for differences in efficacy have not been published.

Subgroups. These drugs appear to have equal BP effects in younger and older patients as well as in men and women. As with the ACE inhibitors, ARBs appear to have less monotherapeutic efficacy in black patients than in white. It is possible that this is an issue of dosing, for some of the early data with tasosartan (an effective ARB that was withdrawn because of a possible safety concern) suggested that black patients required doses approximately 3 times as high as white patients to achieve comparable BP responses. This is an important issue, for as these drugs become used for a wider range of cardiovascular and diabetic disorders it would be critical to ensure that their potential cardiovascular and renal protective effects are made available to all population groups. Racial differences in BP response are nonexistent when ARBs are combined with thiazide diuretics.

Combination with other drugs. Because of the difference in pharmacologic properties between the ACE inhibitors and ARBs, there has been interest in the possibility that they may provide effective combination therapy. Preliminary data have shown that reduction of proteinuria with combination treatment in patients with nephropathy, for example, appears more effective than with either agent alone. Likewise, the ValHEFT also indicated that, under certain circumstances, combination therapy may be more effective than single-drug therapy. Results with BP have been mixed: Early studies with losartan suggested that minimal additional BP-lowering effects were obtained when it was combined with an ACE inhibitor. When lisinopril was combined with irbesartan, the 2 drugs in usual clinical doses had similar antihypertensive effects, but their combina-

tion had a greater effect on BP than either alone. Combinations of ARBs with such other drug classes as calcium channel blockers or β-blockers have not been well studied, though it is likely that there would be additive antihypertensive effects.

Adverse Effects

One of the principal attributes of ARBs is the absence of dose-related symptomatic and metabolic adverse events. The incidence of side effects is not different from that in placebo-treated patients; in fact, the incidence of headache is significantly higher with placebo than during treatment with the agents in this class. Cough is much less common than with ACE inhibitors, and its incidence is similar to that with other antihypertensive drugs. However, like the ACE inhibitors, ARBs are contraindicated in pregnancy.

SUGGESTED READING

1. Bakris G, Gradman A, Reif M, et al. Antihypertensive efficacy of candesartan in comparison to losartan: The CLAIM study. *J Clin Hypertens.* 2001;3:16–21.
2. Brenner BM, Cooper ME, de Zeeuw D, et al. Effects of losartan on renal and cardiovascular outcomes in patients with type 2 diabetes and nephropathy. *N Engl J Med.* 2001;345:861–869.
3. Cohn JN, Tognoni G, The Valsartan Heart Failure Trial Investigators. A randomized trial of the angiotensin-receptor blocker valsartan in chronic heart failure. *N Engl J Med.* 2001;345:1667–1675.
4. Dahlof B, Devereux RB, Kjeldsen SE, et al. for the LIFE study group. Cardiovascular morbidity and mortality in the Losartan Intervention For End point reduction in hypertension study (LIFE): a randomized trial against atenolol. *Lancet.* 2002;359:995–1003.
5. Lewis EJ, Hunsicker LG, Clarke WR, et al. Renoprotective effect of the angiotensin-receptor antagonist irbesartan in patients with nephropathy due to type 2 diabetes. *N Engl J Med.* 2001;345:51–60.
6. McKelvie RS, Yusuf S, Pericak D, et al. Comparison of candesartan, enalapril, and their combination in congestive heart failure: Randomized Evaluation of Strategies for Left Ventricular Dysfunction (RESOLVD) Pilot Study. *Circulation.* 199;100:1056–1064.
7. Parving HH, Lehnert H, Brochner-Mortensen J, et al. The effect of irbesartan on the development of diabetic nephropathy in patients with type 2 diabetes. *N Engl J Med.* 2001;345:870–878.
8. Pitt B, Poole-Wilson PA, Segal R, et al. Effect of losartan compared with captopril on mortality in patients with symptomatic heart failure: randomized trial—the Losartan Heart Failure Survival Study ELITE II. *Lancet.* 2000;355:1582–1587.
9. Russo D, Pisani A, Balletta MM, et al. Additive antiproteinuric effect of converting enzyme inhibitor and losartan in normotensive patients with IgA nephropathy. *Am J Kidney Dis.* 1999;33:851–856.
10. Weber MA, Furberg CD. Comparisons in a competitive world: when is one drug superior to another? *Am J Hypertens.* 2000;13:4, 457–459.

Chapter C146

Calcium Antagonists

Matthew R. Weir, MD; Joseph L. Izzo, Jr, MD

KEY POINTS

- Calcium antagonists (sometimes called *calcium channel blockers*) are powerful arterial dilators that are effective as antihypertensive monotherapy and in combination with other agents; they are particularly useful in reducing the incidence of stroke.

- The antihypertensive properties of calcium antagonists remain robust in all forms of hypertension, in all races, and at any age; they are effective over a wide range of dietary salt intake, which makes them useful in patients who find it difficult to reduce dietary salt consumption.

- Cardiac effects differ among calcium antagonists; they are useful in angina, but their use in arrhythmias is complex. In contrast to dihydropyridine calcium antagonists, nondihydropyridine calcium antagonists (verapamil and diltiazem) tend to slow heart rate.

- Monotherapy with dihydropyridine calcium antagonists may not provide optimal protection against heart failure or progressive renal disease, but combinations of calcium antagonists with other agents in these conditions are not contraindicated and may be useful; nondihydropyridine calcium antagonists reduce proteinuria.

- Common side effects of calcium antagonists are related to their arteriolar dilator properties, including edema, flushing, headache, and, sometimes, tachycardia.

See also Chapters A27, A33, A38, A47, A59, A60, B106–B108, C127, C128, C137, C138, C151, C153–C155, C157, C159, C164, C167, and C174

Cellular Calcium Flux

Calcium plays a critical role in cellular communication, regulation, and function, and any manipulation of transmembrane calcium flux affects a variety of cellular regulatory processes and functions (see Chapter A27). Normally, cells maintain a low resting intracellular concentration of ionized calcium in the face of large and inwardly directed concentration gradient (approximately 10,000-fold). As calcium enters the cell, it combines with calcium-binding proteins to stimulate a number of second messenger systems and cellular responses, such as nerve excitation, cardiac and vascular smooth muscle contraction, and hormone secretion. Calcium channels can be differentiated into several subtypes, but the L-type channel is the one most directly associated with blood pressure (BP) control. L-channels have activator and antagonist binding sites that can be regulated or altered experimentally and in disease states.

Calcium Antagonists Subtypes

Calcium antagonists (CAs, sometimes called *calcium channel blockers*) include a structurally and pharmacologically diverse group of compounds that fit into 3 main subclasses: phenylalkylamines, benzothiazepines, and 1,4-dihydropyridines; the prototypes of these classes are verapamil, diltiazem, and nifedipine, respectively. The pharmacologic mechanism of action common to these drugs is to decrease cellular calcium entry via the L-type calcium channel. CA subtypes are quantitatively and qualitatively distinct in that they have differential sensitivity and selectivity for binding the pharmacologic receptors along with the

calcium channel in various tissues. This differential selectivity of action has important implications for the use of these drugs in clinical medicine and explains why the CAs vary considerably in their effects on regional circulatory beds, sinus and atrioventricular nodal functions, and myocardial contractility. Thus, the CAs have quite different clinical applications, contraindications, drug-drug interactions, and side-effect profiles.

Indications and Clinical Trials

Hypertension. Both dihydropyridine (DHP) CAs and non-DHP CAs are effective alone and in combination with other agents in lowering BP. They are especially effective in isolated systolic hypertension; in the Systolic Hypertension in Europe (SYST-Eur) trial, strokes were reduced by approximately 40%, and all-cause cardiovascular morbidity and mortality were reduced by approximately 30% in isolated systolic hypertension subjects who received the DHP CA nitrendipine compared to those on placebo. The Hypertension Optimal Treatment (HOT) trial demonstrated that aggressive BP lowering to values below 140/90 mm Hg with a felodipine-based regimen was safe and effective. In the Antihypertensive and Lipid-Lowering Treatment to Prevent Heart Attack Trial (ALLHAT), the BP lowering with amlodipine was approximately 3 to 4 mm Hg greater than that seen with lisinopril and 1 to 2 mm Hg greater than chlorthalidone.

Stroke protection and cognitive function. Stroke-related morbidity and mortality in elderly patients with systolic hypertension was dramatically reduced (by approximately 40%) in

433

the SYST-Eur and Systolic Hypertension in China (SYST-China) studies. In ALLHAT, stroke protection with amlodipine was equivalent to chlorthalidone and greater than lisinopril. In SYST-Eur, a blunting of the age-related decline in cognitive function was also observed.

Angina and ischemic heart disease. Most CAs are approved for the treatment of classic, vasospastic, and unstable angina, especially in those who are unable to tolerate β blockers. A working group representing the World Health Organization and the International Society of Hypertension has recently reviewed available data and concluded that beyond their BP-lowering effects, CAs have no independent beneficial or harmful effects on coronary heart disease events, including fatal or nonfatal myocardial infarctions (MIs) and other deaths from coronary heart disease. ALLHAT demonstrated that the rates of coronary events and death were similar with amlodipine, chlorthalidone, and lisinopril. Verapamil has been demonstrated to reduce reinfarction rate and post-MI morbidity and mortality when administered 1 to 2 weeks after an MI. In this regard, verapamil is probably the CA of choice in the post-MI patient, especially in those who do not tolerate β-blockers. Diltiazem has demonstrated benefit in reducing the risk of reinfarction in patients with non–Q wave MI. As a rule, DHP CAs should not be given in the immediate post-MI period because their powerful vasodilatory effects can increase myocardial oxygen demand.

Arrhythmias. Use of CAs can be complex in the setting of arrhythmias or conduction disturbances. Non-DHPs can be useful in supraventricular tachycardias, but they are usually contraindicated in heart block.

Raynaud's phenomenon, cerebral vasospasm, and migraine headache. Peripheral vasospastic conditions can be improved by DHP CAs.

Safety Issues

Concern has been expressed in the medical and lay press about the long-term safety of CAs.

Heart failure. Amlodipine was found to be "neutral" (relatively safe but unhelpful) in patients with heart failure in the Prospective Randomized Amlodipine Survival Evaluation (PRAISE) trial. In ALLHAT, amlodipine was proven to be decidedly inferior to chlorthalidone in preventing heart failure regardless of gender, age, race, or glycemic status. Thus, CAs should not generally be used in people with significant heart failure risk or with overt heart failure.

Progressive renal disease and proteinuria

Dihydropyridine calcium antagonists. Careful review of clinical trial data in patients with renal disease indicates that monotherapy with DHP CAs may not protect as well against progression of renal disease as angiotensin-converting enzyme (ACE) inhibitors or angiotensin receptor blockers. The African American Study of Kidney disease (AASK) in nondiabetic renal disease (principally nephrosclerosis) compared combination therapy based on amlodipine to combinations based on ramipril or atenolol with respect to progression of renal disease and proteinuria. Individuals with high baseline proteinuria (>0.22 mg albumin/g creatinine) or renal impairment (baseline glomerular filtration rate

<40 mL/minute) experienced a worsening of proteinuria and an accelerated rate of decline in renal function if they were randomized to DHP CA compared to ACE inhibitor or β-blocker. In contrast, the second phase of the Appropriate Blood Pressure Control in Diabetes (ABCD) study in relatively healthy diabetics with normal renal function found that the ACE inhibitor lisinopril and the DHP CA nisoldipine conferred equivalent protection against renal deterioration or worsening of proteinuria. Thus, it would be premature to conclude that DHP CAs should not be used in patients with renal disease, especially because the combination of ACE inhibitor and CA has not been tested adequately, and lower BP itself is protective.

Nondihydropyridine calcium antagonists. Data for non-DHP CAs are somewhat different; small studies with these agents have found that they reduce proteinuria to a similar degree to that observed with ACE inhibitors. Long-term renal outcome studies with non-DHP CAs have not been completed.

Other issues. Review of available observational studies does not support any claims of an adverse effect of CAs on cancer or bleeding risk. In ALLHAT, there were no differences among chlorthalidone, amlodipine, and lisinopril with respect to bleeding episodes or cancer rates, but there was a higher rate of suicide and unintentional injury with amlodipine.

Mechanisms of Action

Vasodilatory effects. CAs uniformly reduce vascular resistance through L-channel blockade, which directly reduces intracellular calcium and indirectly blunts angiotensin II and α-adrenergic receptor–mediated vasoconstriction. Experimental maximal vasodilatory responses are inversely related to the patient's plasma renin activity or plasma angiotensin II concentration. In general, the vasodilation associated with CAs is not associated with clinically discernible reflex-mediated sympathoneural activation, although at higher doses or during periods of sympathetic excitation (stress or exercise), their sympathoexcitatory effects (increased plasma catecholamines and heart rate) are more apparent, especially with DHP CAs. CAs are more effective vasodilators in constricted than in nonconstricted vascular beds, and greater vasodepressor responses occur in patients with higher levels of BP. Although there are few head-to-head comparisons, it seems that there is little, if any, difference in BP-lowering potency between the various CAs, provided that comparable doses are given.

Renal effects. CAs facilitate natriuresis, probably principally by powerful afferent arteriolar dilatation and increased glomerular capillary pressure, with increased renal blood flow, diminished filtration fraction and renal tubular sodium reabsorption, and, possibly, by interference with aldosterone secretion. Non-DHP CAs (but not DHP CAs) diminish proteinuria, likely by improving glomerular permselectivity to proteins and by lowering systemic BP. Experimental studies have been unable to establish whether the observed reduction in proteinuria with non-DHP CAs is related to dilation of the efferent glomerular arteriole.

Cardiac effects. Cardiac function is largely unaffected by CAs, with the exception of patients who have an ejection fraction of <30%. CAs do not reduce exercise capacity, nor are they very effective in blunting stress-induced increases in systolic BP.

Dihydropyridine calcium antagonists. DHP CAs have variable effects on heart rate. Acutely, these drugs tend to induce a reflex tachycardia, but long-term studies show similar heart rates before and during therapy. Higher doses of these drugs can be expected to be associated with an increase in pulse rate. DHP CAs are less likely than non-DHP CAs to reduce cardiac output in heart failure or systolic dysfunction. Amlodipine and felodipine have been demonstrated to be relatively safe (but not necessarily beneficial) in patients with systolic dysfunction. It has been suggested that CAs may be useful for the treatment of diastolic dysfunction, perhaps through direct effects on myocardial relaxation; benefits are more likely to occur with non-DHP CAs because of their greater heart rate–lowering capacity.

Nondihydropyridine calcium antagonists. Non-DHP CA agents have more diverse cardiac effects. In the dose range used for the treatment of hypertension, non-DHP CAs usually have little effect on pulse rate. In some patients, pulse rate may be decreased by as much as 10%, but this is usually less than the pulse rate reduction observed with β-blocker therapy (−20% to −30%). Although verapamil has the greatest negative inotropic effect among the CAs, its ability to act as a coronary vasodilator, to decrease afterload, and to effectively treat diastolic dysfunction usually counterbalance any deleterious consequences of negative inotropism. Diltiazem tends to reduce sinoatrial nodal conduction, but diltiazem and verapamil block the atrioventricular node. Consequently, both can be used in the treatment of acute or chronic supraventricular arrhythmias, but verapamil is contraindicated in patients with preexcitation syndrome with rapid ventricular response because it may accentuate conduction through accessory pathways.

Clinical Use in Hypertension

CAs have been shown to be similarly effective and safe in their approved dosing range (**Table C146.1**), with monotherapy response rates in hypertension above 50%. They work equally well in younger and older patients, contrary to earlier reports that CAs were more efficacious in older patients. The drugs are also effective in black and white hypertensives, and they tend to maintain efficacy independent of salt intake or nonsteroidal antiinflammatory drug use, which makes them unique among antihypertensive drugs. CAs are also useful in cyclosporin-induced hypertension.

Pharmacokinetics and pharmacodynamics. DHP CAs are reasonably well absorbed, but they tend to undergo extensive first-pass metabolism. In general, the metabolites are inactive, with the possible exception of those of nifedipine; unlike other CAs, amlodipine does not have an extensive hepatic first-pass metabolism, which contributes to its more prolonged effect. Many of the CAs have been reformulated into sustained-release preparations, which allows for once-daily dosing. The pharmacokinetic properties of the 2 non-DHP CAs are somewhat similar (**Table C146.2**). The bioavailability of verapamil and diltiazem increases with chronic dosing, most likely secondary to saturable metabolism, which increases the pharmacodynamic duration of action such that verapamil or diltiazem (ordinarily given at least 3 times daily) can be effective when administered twice daily (Table C146.1). Verapamil and diltiazem are currently available in a variety of sustained-release formulations that allow once-daily dosing. Some of these delivery systems were specifically developed for nighttime dosing because they provide precisely timed drug delivery that coincides with circadian rhythm–related morning in blood pressure in peaks.

Alterations in pharmacodynamic effects. The pharmacokinetics of the CAs can be affected by age, intercurrent disease, and diet. In patients with renal insufficiency, the pharmacokinetics of these drugs are minimally changed. In hepatic disease states, diminished systemic clearance may necessitate dosage adjustments. Aging slows the metabolism of these drugs, presumably secondary to the accompanying decrease in hepatic blood flow, sometimes causing the need to use lower doses of

---

Table C146.1. Calcium Antagonists: Doses

DRUG	TRADE NAME	USUAL DOSE (FREQUENCY/D)	COMMENT	FIXED-DOSE COMBINATIONS
Dihydropyridines				
Amlodipine	Norvasc	2.5–10.0 (1)	Very long acting	Amlodipine and benazepril (Lotrel)
Felodipine	Plendil	2.5–20.0 (1)	Plasma levels increased with grapefruit juice intake	Felodipine and enalapril (Lexxel)
Isradipine	DynaCirc, DynaCirc SR	2.5–5.0 (1–2)	Dose dependent increase in heart rate, similar to all drugs in this class	
Nicardipine	Cardene-SR	30–60 (2)		
Nifedipine	Procardia XL, Adalat CC	30–120 (1–2)		
Nimodipine		60 (4–6)	Indicated for subarachnoid bleed	
Nisoldipine	Sular	10–40 (1)		
Nondihydropyridines				
Diltiazem	Cardizem SR, Cardizem-CD or SR, Tiazac	120–360 (1)	Inhibits cytochrome CYP3A4	Diltiazem and enalapril
Verapamil	Calan, Calan-SR, Isoptin-SR, Covera-HS, Verelan-PM	120–360 (1)	Nocturnal dosing indicated for Covera-HS and Verelan-PM	Verapamil and trandolapril (Tarka)

Table C146.2. Calcium Antagonists: Pharmacology

Available compounds
  Phenylalkylamines: verapamil
  Benzothiazepines: diltiazem
  Dihydropyridines: nifedipine, amlodipine, felodipine, isradipine
Mode of action
  Decrease cellular calcium entry via the L-type channel
  Negative inotropic effect (nondihydropyridines)
  Reduction in total peripheral resistance
  Natriuresis
  Interference with angiotensin II, α_1- and α_2-mediated vasoconstriction
Indications for use
  All forms of hypertension
  Salt-sensitive hypertension
  Diastolic dysfunction (nondihydropyridines)
  Variant angina
  Cerebral vascular disease
  Cyclosporine hypertension
Contraindications/restrictions
  Heart block and heart failure (nondihydropyridines)
  Myocardial ischemia (short-acting dihydropyridines)
  Heart failure
    Prevention properties inferior to diuretic
    Interaction of verapamil or diltiazem with β-blockers
  Renal protection inferior to angiotensin-converting enzyme inhibitor
  Proteinuria reduction inferior to angiotensin-converting enzyme inhibitor (dihydropyridines)
Common side effects
  Tachycardia (dihydropyridines)
  Edema
  Flushing
  Headache
  Constipation (verapamil)

Table C146.3. Drug-Drug Interactions with Calcium Antagonists

CALCIUM ANTAGONIST	INTERACTING DRUG	RESULT
Verapamil	Digoxin	↑ Digoxin levels by 50–90%
Diltiazem	Digoxin	↑ Digoxin level by 40%
Verapamil	β-Blockers	↑ Atrioventricular nodal blockade, hypotension, bradycardia, asystole
Verapamil, diltiazem	Cyclosporine	↑ Cyclosporine levels by 30–40%
	Cimetidine	↑ Verapamil and diltiazem levels by decreased metabolism
Verapamil	Rifampin/phenytoin	↓ Verapamil levels by enzyme induction
Dihydropyridines	α-Blockers	Excessive hypotension
	Propanolol	Increased propanolol levels
	Cimetidine	Increased area under the curve and plasma levels of calcium antagonist
Nicardipine, amlodipine	Cyclosporine	↑ Cyclosporine levels (nicardipine 40–50%, amlodipine 10%)

↓, decreased; ↑, increased.

CAs in the elderly. Several studies have demonstrated a consistent concentration-effect relationship for many of the CAs. This helps predict the effectiveness of long-term therapy from the first-dose response. In addition, the concentration-effect relationship illustrates the importance of pharmacokinetic differences between drugs and the influence of aging and disease on absolute drug effect. Withdrawal of CAs does not cause rebound hypertension, but rapid withdrawal may induce coronary artery spasm or angina pectoris, especially in patients with ischemic heart disease.

Drug combinations. The antihypertensive effect of CAs is generally additive with other antihypertensive drug classes, including thiazide diuretics. It is unclear whether addition of DHP CAs and non-DHP CAs is beneficial. If CAs are to be combined with β-blockers, it is preferable to use a DHP CA to avoid atrioventricular block or a worsening of systolic function, which may arise with the use of diltiazem or verapamil. CAs have been formulated in fixed-dose combinations with ACE inhibitors. Four fixed-dose combinations are available, 2 combining an ACE inhibitor with DHP CA (benazepril and amlodipine or enalapril and felodipine) or an ACE inhibitor with a non-DHP CA (trandolapril and verapamil or enalapril and diltiazem).

Adverse Effects

DHP CAs are generally well tolerated but do tend to have common dose-dependent side effects that are related to their potencies as arteriolar dilators, including headache, flushing, tachycardia, and edema, any of which may limit tolerability. The peripheral edema seen with CAs is not caused by net salt and water retention but rather to greater arteriolar than venous dilation and an increase in transcapillary pressure gradients. This phenomenon is dose-dependent and is linked to prolonged upright posture; pedal edema is less common with non-DHP CAs. ACE inhibitors (and perhaps angiotensin receptor blockers) are more effective than diuretics in treating the edema because of their relative abilities to lower tissue hydrostatic pressures through balanced venodilation. CAs are not associated with abnormalities in electrolyte, carbohydrate, or lipid metabolism. Drug–drug interactions are not uncommon with CAs (**Table C146.3**). For example, verapamil and diltiazem decrease cyclosporin metabolism and thereby the amount needed to maintain therapeutic drug levels.

SUGGESTED READING

1. Ad Hoc Subcommittee of the Liaison Committee of the World Health Organization and the International Society of Hypertension. Effects of calcium antagonists on the risks of coronary heart disease, cancer and bleeding. *J Hypertens.* 1997;15:105–115.
2. Agodoa LY, Appel L, Bakris GL, et al. for the African-American Study of the Kidney Disease and Hypertension (AASK) Study Group. Effect of ramipril vs amlodipine on renal outcomes in hypertensive nephrosclerosis: a randomized controlled trial. *JAMA.* 2001;6:2774–2776.
3. Elliott HL, Meredith PA. Pharmacokinetics of calcium antagonists: implications for therapy. In: Epstein M (ed). *Calcium Antagonists in Clinical Medicine.* 3rd ed. Philadelphia, PA: Hanley & Belfus; 1997:69–92.
4. Epstein M. Calcium antagonists in the management of hypertension. In: Epstein M (ed). *Calcium Antagonists in Clinical Medicine.* 3rd ed. Philadelphia, PA: Hanley & Belfus; 2002:293–314.
5. Hansen JF. Treatment with verapamil after an acute myocardial infarction: review of the Danish studies on verapamil in myocardial infarction (DAVIT I and II). *Drugs.* 191;42:43–53.
6. Lewis EJ, Hunsicker LG, Clarke WR, et al. Renoprotective effect of the angiotensin-receptor antagonist irbesartan in patients with nephropathy due to type 2 diabetes. *N Engl J Med.* 2001;345:851–860.

7. Materson BJ, Reda DJ, Cushman WC, et al. Single drug therapy for hypertension in men: a comparison of six antihypertensive agents with placebo. The Department of Veterans Affairs Cooperative Study Group on Antihypertensive Agents. *N Engl J Med.* 1993;328:914–921.

8. Piepho RW, Culbertson VL, Rhodes RS. Drug interactions with the calcium-entry blockers. *Circulation.* 1987;9:181–194.

9. Saunders E, Weir MR, Kong BW, et al. A comparison of the efficacy and safety of a β-blocker, a calcium channel blocker, and a converting enzyme inhibitor in hypertensive blacks. *Arch Intern Med.* 1990;150:1707–1713.

10. Schrier RW, Estacio RO, Esler A, Mehler P. Effects of aggressive blood pressure control in normotensive type 2 diabetic patients on albuminuria, retinopathy and strokes. *Kidney Int.* 2002;61:1086–1097.

Chapter C147

Direct Vasodilators

C. Venkata S. Ram, MD, FACC, MACP; Andrew Fenves, MD, FACP

KEY POINTS

- "Pseudotolerance" to the effects of direct arterial dilators is the result of reflex increases in sympathetic nervous activity, renin-angiotensin activation, and accompanying salt and water retention.

- Combining vasodilators with antiadrenergic drugs (β-blockers or central sympatholytics) and diuretics to form a triple-therapy regimen is necessary to limit side effects and counteract pseudotolerance mechanisms.

- Potential risk in cardiac patients and other side effects of direct arterial dilator drugs limit their use to patients with renal failure or those who are refractory to all other drugs.

- Metabolism of hydralazine, which is used to treat hypertension in pregnancy, is genetically determined.

See also Chapters A33, A37, A38, B106, B107, C118, C127, C128, C137–C139, C141, C143, C146, C148, and C165

Arterial dilator drugs act directly on vascular smooth muscle cells to cause relaxation and vasodilation. Some of these vasodilator agents, such as pinacidil, activate potassium channels. The mechanisms of action of the 2 principal arteriolar dilators used in clinical practice today, hydralazine and minoxidil, are not fully known but almost certainly involve a change in the balance between vasoconstrictive influences, such as cytosolic calcium, and vasodilatory influences, such as cyclic guanosine monophosphate. Clinical case is summarized in **Tables C147.1** and **C147.2**.

Hemodynamics and Pseudotolerance to Vasodilator Drugs

Monotherapy with arterial dilator drugs is accompanied by a fall in peripheral vascular resistance and an increase in heart rate, stroke volume, and cardiac output. Because chronic hypertension is characterized hemodynamically by increased peripheral vascular resistance, drugs that directly relax resistance arterioles would appear to be desirable in the pharmacologic management of high blood pressure (BP).

On the other hand, several physiologic mechanisms that normally act to defend BP, most notably the sympathetic nervous system, the renin-angiotensin-aldosterone system, and the accompanying renal salt and water retention, are activated by arterial dilators. As a result, the drugs such as hydralazine and minoxidil, although effective initially, tend to lose effectiveness over time because of their tendencies to activate BP defense mechanisms and cause "pseudotolerance." The first step in the pseudotolerance response is probably baroreceptor-mediated sympathetic activation, resulting in tachycardia and increased cardiac output and myocardial oxygen demand. These features make it risky to use vasodilator monotherapy in patients with known or possible coronary artery disease. Subsequent renin-angiotensin-aldosterone system activation and renal salt and water retention work in tandem to restore BP to pretreatment levels. These pseudotolerance mechanisms form the rationale for the combination of arteriolar dilators with antiadrenergic drugs (β-blockers or sympatholytic agents) and diuretics. Of note, pseudotolerance effects and some of the unpleasant vasodilatory side effects, such as flushing, headache, and palpitations, can be overcome by combining direct vasodilators with antiadrenergic agents and diuretics (**Figure C147.1**). When used in this fashion, vasodilators can be remarkably useful in the long-term management of refractory and severe hypertension.

Hydralazine

Hydralazine, a classic direct arteriolar dilator, was introduced in the early 1950s for hypertension. Although hydralazine reduces BP, pseudotolerance and other problems limit its use as monotherapy.

Clinical use. Because the efficacy of hydralazine therapy is best sustained in combination with a β-blocking drug and a diuretic, its use is restricted to patients who require multiple-drug therapy. The drug can be given twice daily, despite its short half-life. The total daily dose should be limited to 200 to 300 mg because

Table C147.1. Direct Vasodilators: Pharmacology

| DRUG (BRAND NAME) | ORAL DOSING | | | COMMENTS |
	INITIAL DOSE (MG)	DOSING FREQUENCY	TOTAL MAINTENANCE DOSE (MG/D)	
Hydralazine (Apresoline)	25	b.i.d.	100–300	Mainly used in pregnancy Usually part of triple therapy with diuretic and adrenergic inhibitor Reversible lupus-like side effects
Minoxidil (Loniten)	5	q.d.	10–40	Only for severe refractory hypertension Must be used with diuretic and adrenergic inhibitor Causes hypertrichosis

higher doses clearly pose a risk of inducing a lupus-like syndrome (see Side effects and toxicity). In fast acetylators, higher doses may be used because the risk of this reaction is less. Usually, hydralazine is added as the third agent to patients unresponsive to diuretics and β-blockers. Some authors recommend using hydralazine and β-blockers first and adding a diuretic if necessary. When a β-blocker is contraindicated, other antiadrenergic drugs, usually central α-agonists, are appropriate alternative choices to facilitate pulse rate reduction. Hydralazine, along with methyldopa, is also extensively used in pregnancy-induced hypertension because of its proven safety—maternal and fetal.

Pharmacokinetics and metabolism. After oral administration, 90% of hydralazine is absorbed from the gastrointestinal tract. Very little of the unchanged drug appears in the urine. A number of hydralazine metabolites have been identified, and the relative amounts of each may depend on the acetylation status of the individual. Acetylation of hydralazine is genetically determined by the concentration of *N*-acetyltransferase. "Slow" acetylators have a higher plasma concentration after a given dose than "fast" acetylators. The incidence of drug-induced toxicity is greater in patients who are slow acetylators, which includes approximately one-half of the U.S. population. The plasma half-life of hydralazine is only 4 hours, but its clinical action lasts from 8 to 12 hours after oral dosing. An oral dose of 75 to 100 mg is equipotent to 10 to 25 mg given parenterally.

Dosage and administration. Intramuscular or intravenous administration of hydralazine was historically used for hypertensive crises but are less popular at the present time due to the availability of other agents with more predictable BP-lowering effects and duration of action. The usual parenteral dose is 20 to 40 mg, which may be repeated as necessary. Although an effect on BP may be seen in a few minutes, the maximum effect occurs between 15 and 75 minutes. Parenteral hydralazine therapy is successfully and safely applied to the management of severe

hypertension in pregnancy and still remains a safe option in this special setting. The oral dose requirements to achieve the therapeutic goal are also unpredictable. Therapy with hydralazine can be initiated with 10 to 25 mg twice daily, which can be increased at weekly intervals to 100 to 200 mg twice daily.

Side effects and toxicity. Hydralazine causes numerous bothersome and sometimes serious side effects. In addition to the side effects described in the Clinical use section, some patients develop nausea and vomiting and, occasionally, peripheral neuropathy. Fluid retention can cause not only edema but also pseudotolerance to the vasodepressor effect of hydralazine, an effect that can be overcome by diuretic therapy, dietary restriction of salt intake, or both. Hydralazine-induced lupus usually presents with arthralgia and may be accompanied by malaise, weight loss, skin rash, splenomegaly, and pleural and pericardial effusion. Rare patients with hydralazine-induced lupus have associated glomerulonephritis. The syndrome occurs mainly in slow acetylators and is more common in women. Hydralazine-induced lupus appears between 6 and 24 months after the therapy is begun. The risk is proportional to the dosage; chronic therapy of >200 mg per day clearly enhances the risk. The syndrome is reversible after discontinuation of therapy, and full recovery occurs within weeks. In contrast to systemic lupus erythematosus, hydralazine-induced lupus is associated with antibodies directed against single-stranded DNA (surprisingly with very high titers) rather than against the native double-stranded DNA. Antibodies to histones are also frequently present.

Minoxidil

Minoxidil is a more potent vasodilator than hydralazine but is similar in its overall hemodynamic actions. Although minoxidil is extremely effective, its adverse effects limit its use in clinical practice, and its use is recommended only in hypertensive patients who are refractory to all other drugs.

Table C147.2. Direct Vasodilators: Doses

DRUG	TRADE NAME	USUAL RANGE (FREQUENCY/D)	COMMENTS
Hydralazine	Apresoline	10–100 (2–4)	Substitute for ACE inhibitors in ACE inhibitor–intolerant congestive heart failure patients, lupus syndrome
Minoxidil	Loniten	2.5–40.0 (2)	Usually requires a diuretic and β-blocker, hair growth common

ACE, angiotensin-converting enzyme.

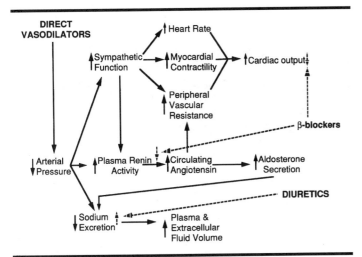

Figure C147.1. Hemodynamic consequences of direct vasodilators and the influence of concomitant therapy with a diuretic and β-blocker. Effects of concomitant therapy are shown by dashed arrows.

Clinical use. Minoxidil is frequently necessary in patients with renal insufficiency, who are often refractory to all other drugs. Some studies have shown that prolonged minoxidil therapy stabilizes or improves renal function in hypertensive patients with renal failure, and sustained BP control with minoxidil occasionally has resulted in the discontinuation of dialysis in patients with an acute or chronic component of hypertensive nephrosclerosis. The improvement in renal function is primarily due to aggressive and effective BP control, rather than a specific renoprotective effect of minoxidil. Minoxidil therapy is effective regardless of the severity or etiology of hypertension and the status of renal function. Before the availability of minoxidil, bilateral nephrectomy was the only therapeutic option in patients with uncontrolled hypertension and renal damage.

Minoxidil should always be administered with a β-blocking drug and a potent diuretic, usually of the loop-active variety, with doses adjusted as needed to prevent tachycardia and edema formation. A combination of a loop-active diuretic and a thiazide or metolazone may have to be used to treat otherwise refractory edema. In the event of contraindications to a β-blocker, a central sympatholytic drug can be used.

Pharmacokinetics. Minoxidil is completely and rapidly absorbed from the gastrointestinal tract. In patients with advanced renal failure, the absorption of the drug is delayed. It is metabolized predominantly in the liver. The elimination half-life of minoxidil varies from 3 to 4 hours, although the duration of action may be as long as 12 to 72 hours.

Dosage and administration. The usual starting dose of minoxidil is 5 mg daily. Doses are then titrated to 10 to 40 mg given once or twice daily. A few patients, particularly those with advanced renal failure, may require doses above 40 mg daily to achieve the necessary therapeutic effect.

Side effects. In addition to fluid retention and symptoms owing to the reflex activation of sympathetic tone, other specific adverse reactions occur. ST-segment depression and T-wave flattening or inversion of the electrocardiogram are sometimes seen in patients receiving minoxidil. Whether this observation represents cardiac ischemia or is a manifestation of left ventricular hypertrophy is unclear. Pericardial effusion, including tamponade, has also been reported in patients receiving minoxidil therapy. The true incidence of this side effect is not known, because many patients receiving minoxidil are already predisposed to develop fluid retention as a result of cardiac or renal dysfunction. Elevated pulmonary artery pressures have been documented in patients receiving chronic minoxidil therapy, an effect less likely to occur in patients receiving blockers concurrently. Hypertrichosis occurs in nearly all patients treated with minoxidil. This is particularly evident on the forehead and face, neck, shoulders, arms, and legs and limits it use in women. The specific mechanism for minoxidil-induced hair growth is not known, but it is probably related to increased blood flow to the hair follicles. Hypertrichosis can be treated with depilatory agents but it disappears within a few weeks after discontinuation of the drug.

SUGGESTED READING

1. Campese VM. Minoxidil: a review of its pharmacological properties and therapeutic use. *Drugs.* 1981;22:257–278.
2. Handler RP, Federman JS. Hydralazine-induced lupus. *N Y State J Med.* 1982;82:1288.
3. Koch-Weser J. Medical intelligence drug therapy. *N Engl J Med.* 1976; 295:320–323.
4. Lundeen TE, Dolan DR, Ram CV. Pericardial effusion associated with minoxidil therapy. *Postgrad Med.* 1981;70:98–100.
5. Mitchell HC, Pettinger WA. Renal function in long-term minoxidil treated patients. *J Cardiovasc Pharmacol.* 1980;2:S163–S172.
6. Ram CV. Clinical considerations in combined drug therapy of hypertension. *Prac Cardiol.* 1984;10:83–105.
7. Zacest R, Gilmore E, Koch-Weser J. Treatment of essential hypertension with combined vasodilation and beta-adrenergic blockade. *N Engl J Med.* 1972;286:617–622.

Chapter C148

Other Agents: Potassium Channel Openers, Dopamine Agonists, Serotonin-Related Agents, Renin Inhibitors, Imidazolines, and Endothelin Antagonists

Alexander M. M. Shepherd, MD, PhD

KEY POINTS

- Potassium channel openers and serotonin antagonists are already marketed in several countries, but low efficacy as monotherapy and frequent side effects limit their appeal.

- Dopamine agonists appear to have specific advantages when intravenous antihypertensive medications are warranted.

- Renin inhibitors, newer imidazolines, and endothelin-receptor antagonists are being investigated for use in human hypertension.

See also Chapters A1, A4, A12, A17, A26, A27, A33, C142, and C146

Potassium Channel Openers

Potassium channel openers increase cellular potassium conductance by opening membrane potassium channels. This results in cell membrane hyperpolarization, which causes vascular relaxation by preventing voltage-activated calcium channels from opening (see Chapter A26). Several organ systems are affected by potassium channel openers, including the cardiovascular, respiratory, reproductive, genitourinary, gastrointestinal, muscular, and central nervous systems, as well as the skin and the eye. Compounds that directly "open" adenosine triphosphate–sensitive potassium channels, including cromakalim and its negative enantiomer levcromakalim, aprikalim, pinacidil, minoxidil, diazoxide, KR-30450, BRL-34915, and nicorandil, are potent vasodilators in humans. The large number of subtypes of potassium channels is both a challenge and an opportunity, as the development of more selective agents than those currently available would minimize adverse effects.

Currently available agents cannot be used as monotherapy in hypertension because of the range of effects in multiple organ systems. Some, like nicorandil, also induce relaxation by activation of guanylate cyclase in addition to a more primary effect on potassium channels. The major hemodynamic effect preventing monotherapy with these drugs is a reactive increase in sympathetic nervous activity and cardiac output that results from the potent arterial vasodilation. Chronic therapy also produces significant fluid retention and thereby peripheral edema, a homeostatic response caused by decreased renal perfusion pressure and neurohumoral activation, especially with minoxidil. The fluid retention with minoxidil can be severe enough to warrant high-dose loop diuretic therapy or combination diuretic therapy with metolazone, or both (see Chapter C146).

Dopamine Agonists

Several decades of research have resulted in the synthesis of molecules that are more selective than dopamine, which activates dopaminergic, β-adrenergic, and α-adrenergic receptors in a dose-dependent fashion (see Chapter A1). Because the vasculature has a high density of vasodilatory dopaminergic receptors, dopamine and related agonists can lower blood pressure (BP) when used at relatively low doses.

Fenoldopam. The first of the more selective drugs to reach the market was fenoldopam mesylate, a selective peripheral dopamine$_1$ (DA$_1$) agonist. It is approved for the acute in-hospital management (for up to 48 hours) of severe hypertension. It has limited oral bioavailability and a very short elimination half-life (5–9 minutes), restricting its use to intravenous infusion for hypertensive emergencies. Fenoldopam is administered intravenously, beginning with a dose of 0.1 $\mu g/kg^{-1}/minute^{-1}$, by constant infusion. Doses are increased by 0.05 to 0.10 $\mu g/kg^{-1}/minute^{-1}$ every 10 to 20 minutes as necessary up to >1.5 $\mu g/kg^{-1}/minute^{-1}$ to reduce BP to the desired level. Fenoldopam potently dilates a number of vascular beds, including the renal circulation. Fenoldopam in a dose-dependent manner acutely improves several aspects of renal function (including creatinine clearance and urinary flow rate) as well as sodium and potassium excretion. The beneficial effects of any natriuresis with fenoldopam may be partially offset by activation of the renin-angiotensin axis. Several studies of fenoldopam have shown that it is as effective as sodium nitroprusside but that it does not produce toxic metabolites, such as thiocyanate. Fenoldopam is also useful for the intraoperative control of BP and possibly for its salutary effect on renal blood flow. The latter may be of particular importance in the at-risk renal patient receiving contrast media. BP monitoring during fenoldopam administration can be less intensive than that required for sodium nitroprusside, permitting its use in less intensive medical settings.

Fenoldopam would be expected to have interactions with other drugs that affect the dopaminergic system, including monoamine oxidase inhibitors, metoclopramide, bromocriptine, most antipsychotics, and tricyclic antidepressants. Fenoldopam increases intraocular pressure slightly, but this is unlikely to preclude its use in most patients.

Dopamine agonists in chronic hypertension. Selective peripheral DA_2 agonists could have application in the chronic therapy of hypertension because this effect would reduce plasma norepinephrine and therefore induce vasodilation. Unfortunately, currently available drugs such as bromocriptine cross the blood–brain barrier and cause unacceptable side effects resulting from central dopaminergic stimulation. Others, such as carmoxirole and ropinirole can stimulate the pituitary gland and the chemoreceptor trigger zone in the area postrema, which lie outside the blood–brain barrier, resulting in inhibition of prolactin release and nausea and vomiting. Further research may produce noncentrally acting DA_2 agonists with acceptable side-effect profiles and improved bioavailability.

Serotonin-Related Agents

Serotonin has diverse cardiophysiologic effects through its actions on the different serotonin receptor subtypes, which mediate its biologic actions (see Chapter A17). The vasoconstrictive effects of serotonin are mediated by 5-hydroxytryptamine type 2 ($5-HT_2$) serotonergic receptors, which also enhance the vasoconstrictive effects of angiotensin II and norepinephrine. Selective $5-HT_2$–blockers have been developed that are peripheral vasodilators.

Several molecules that affect peripheral or central serotonin metabolism have been studied in humans, including ketanserin, which is thought to lower BP principally by α_1-adrenergic blockade without cardiac stimulation, as well as flesinoxan, urapidil, and 5-methylurapidil. Urapidil stimulates $5-HT_{1a}$ receptors centrally and also acts as a peripheral postsynaptic α_1-receptor competitive antagonist. Beneficial effects on platelet function and fibrinolysis may account for improved outcomes in longterm trials [Prevention of Atherosclerotic Complications with Ketanserin (PACK) and Prognosis of Ischemic Risk in Atheromatous Patients under Mediatensyl (PRIHAM), with urapidil]. In addition, there may be beneficial effects on lipid profiles or insulin resistance with urapidil. Unfortunately, $5-HT_2$ serotonergic blockers may prolong the QT interval, particularly in hypokalemic patients, which may increase cardiovascular risk.

Renin Inhibitors

There have been 4 classes of renin inhibitors developed in the search for a clinically useful compound. Renin antibody use is compromised by their not being orally active. Synthetic derivatives of a renin precursor have proved to be of low potency. A modification of angiotensinogen, a pepstatin analog, binds renin but has poor specificity and binding affinity for human renin. Angiotensinogen substrate analog inhibitors are probably the most promising of these compounds.

Angiotensinogen substrate analog inhibitors that block the initial step of the renin-angiotensin-aldosterone cascade have been given the generic suffix -*kirens* (see Chapter A4). Early

work with these compounds has shown promise not only for reduction in BP in salt-depleted or diuretic-treated patients but also for the treatment of heart failure and renal disease. An impediment to the development of compounds in this class has been poor bioavailability, which relates to their peptide structure. Newer nonpeptide compounds developed to solve this problem are A-74273, zankiren, remikiren, and ciprokiren.

Imidazolines

Imidazolines are compounds with 5-member rings containing 2 nitrogens. These compounds are chemically related to clonidine and interact with a novel imidazoline-1 receptor in animals. In early clinical studies, moxonidine and rilmenidine have been shown to effectively reduce BP with a desirable hemodynamic profile (reduction in total peripheral resistance with no change in cardiac output).

Newer imidazolines have a much lower affinity for the α_2-receptor than does clonidine, a property that decreases the likelihood of nonspecific central nervous system side effects (especially sedation and dry mouth), potentially making this drug class better tolerated.

Endothelin Receptor Antagonists

Among the 3 isopeptides of endothelin (ET), ET-1, ET-2, and ET-3, ET-1 is the most potent vasoconstrictor and the main form found in blood vessels (see Chapter A12). ET-1 acts on 2 receptor subtypes, ET_A and ET_B, both of which contract vascular smooth muscle. BP is affected by several compounds designed to block ET-1 receptors of the ET_A and ET_B subclasses. At present, it is unclear whether both receptor subtypes must be blocked for sustained efficacy. The first of these agents to show efficacy in large groups of patients was bosentan, which lowers seated BP in a dose-dependent fashion without reflex sympathetic stimulation. A number of other ET-1 blockers are being developed for use in hypertension, heart failure, and the postmyocardial infarction setting.

SUGGESTED READING

1. Clozel M. Endothelin receptor antagonists: current status and perspectives. *J Cardiovasc Pharmacol.* 2000;35:S65-68.
2. Dooley M, Goa KL. Urapidil. A reappraisal of its use in the management of hypertension. *Drugs.* 1998;56:929–955.
3. Frishman WH, Hotchkiss H. Selective and nonselective dopamine receptor agonists: an innovative approach to cardiovascular disease treatment. *Am Heart J.* 1996;132:861–870.
4. Goldberg ME, Cantillo J, Nemiroff MS, et al. Fenoldopam infusion for the treatment of postoperative hypertension. *J Clin Anesth.* 1993;5:386–391.
5. Kleinert HD. Hemodynamic effects of renin inhibitors. *Am J Nephrol.* 1996;16:252–260.
6. Lawson K. Is there a therapeutic future for "potassium channel openers"? *Clin Sci (Lond).* 1996;91:651–663.
7. Messerli F. Moxonidine: a new and versatile antihypertensive. *J Cardiovasc Pharmacol.* 2000;35:S53–56.
8. Murphy MB, Murray C, Shorten GD. Fenoldopam: a selective peripheral dopamine-receptor agonist for the treatment of severe hypertension. *N Engl J Med.* 2001;345:1548–1557.
9. Ziegler D, Haxhiu MA, Kaan EC, et al. Pharmacology of moxonidine, an I1-imidazoline receptor agonist. *J Cardiovasc Pharmacol.* 1996;27:S26–37.

Antihypertensive Effects of Nonantihypertensive Drugs

Ross D. Feldman, MD

KEY POINTS

- Thiazolidinediones (glitazones) and statins have significant blood pressure–lowering effects.

- Selective phosphodiesterase-5 inhibitor (sildenafil and related compounds) can lower blood pressure or interact with nitrates or other vasoactive drugs to cause severe hypotension.

See also Chapters A22, A24, A30, A66, and C158

The history of pharmacology is replete with examples of drugs that are ultimately used for indications quite disparate from their originally approved uses. Examples include minoxidil for hair loss, β-adrenoceptor antagonists for heart failure, and acetylsalicylic acid for prevention of transient ischemic attacks or recurrent myocardial infarction. Several currently available classes of drugs approved for other indications may also lower blood pressure (BP), although none have been approved by the U.S. Food and Drug Administration for this purpose.

Thiazolidinediones

Atherosclerotic risk factors cluster with an incidence more frequent than that predicted by chance. The so-called metabolic syndrome (insulin resistance syndrome) is characterized by obesity, hypertension, dyslipidemia, and insulin resistance, the last of which may be the common basis for the vascular and lipid abnormalities evident in these patients. Thiazolidinediones [also known as *glitazones* or *insulin-sensitizers* (i.e., agents that improve hyperglycemia without increasing pancreatic insulin secretion)] have been shown to reduce BP. Troglitazone, now withdrawn because of its incidence of hepatotoxicity, lowers resting BP and also reduces the magnitude of stress-induced BP increases. Antihypertensive effects have not been seen with other hypoglycemic drug classes, including sulfonylurea drugs or with biguanide insulin sensitizers such as metformin.

The mechanism underlying the BP-lowering effect of glitazones remains unclear but may relate to improvement of abnormal endothelial function. Impaired endothelial function has been reported in diabetes and has been attributed to a range of mechanisms, including impaired fatty acid metabolism, persistent hyperinsulinemia, and chronic hyperglycemia. Troglitazone has been shown to improve flow-mediated vasodilation in subjects with insulin resistance. Troglitazone may reduce sympathetic nerve activity and has direct, nonendothelial-dependent vasodilator effects in experimental models. Whether the antihypertensive effect of troglitazone is related to its effect as an insulin-sensitizer or is more specifically related to its effect as a peroxisome proliferator-activated receptor–selective ligand (see Chapter A22) remains to be established.

Statins

Antihypertensive effects at rest and in response to stressful stimuli have been demonstrated with statins (see Chapter A43). Studies in hypertensive subjects (but not normotensive subjects) have demonstrated significant BP-lowering effects (of 5–10 mm Hg in stage 1 hypertensive patients) that may not be evident until 2 to 3 months of therapy. This delayed effect is consistent with the concept that the BP reduction is related to a change in vascular structure and is not due to reduced lipid levels themselves. The antihypertensive effect of statins also has been shown to be additive with calcium antagonists and angiotensin-converting enzyme inhibitors. It is unclear whether the antihypertensive effects of statins are class specific, or whether similar effects occur with other drugs that lower cholesterol. Pravastatin and simvastatin have been reported to reverse the endothelial dysfunction associated with hypercholesterolemia. Simvastatin also improves peripheral vascular compliance in hypercholesterolemic subjects. Statins reduce vascular free-radical release, decrease vascular smooth muscle cell migration and proliferation, and have direct antiinflammatory effects. The link between these cellular effects, reversal of endothelial dysfunction, and the antihypertensive effects of statins remains to be established.

Selective Phosphodiesterase Inhibitors

Selective inhibitors of phosphodiesterases (PDEs), especially PDE-5 and other PDEs important in the metabolism of cyclic guanosine monophosphate (cGMP) may prove to be important in the treatment of hypertension. An increase in cGMP concentrations in vascular smooth muscle has been widely recognized as an important mechanism of vasodilatation and is the predominant mechanism by which endothelial cells modulate vasodilatation via nitric oxide synthase activation. Organic nitrates that act as nitric oxide donors relax vascular smooth muscle but rapidly desensitize guanylyl cyclase, so the hypotensive effects of nitrates are rapidly attenuated during chronic therapy. However, the breakdown of cGMP is regulated by several subfamilies of PDEs, including types 3, 4, and 5 PDEs. There is increasing evidence that inhibitors of these PDEs, particularly the PDE-5 inhibitor sildenafil, have a significant antihypertensive effect. In the largest controlled study to date, sildenafil treatment was associated with a significant reduction in BP (4/4 mm Hg) in normotensive subjects, without change in heart rate at rest or with exercise. These changes have also been shown to persist in hypertensive subjects taking concomitant antihypertensive medication. Limitations in the duration of action of sildenafil as well as variability in its bioavailability make it unlikely that sildenafil will ever be shown to be a useful antihypertensive drug, although other agents that inhibit cGMP-selective PDEs may prove to be useful in treating hypertension. Marked vasodilation is also seen when sildenafil is used in combination with nitrates or α-blockers in patients in whom severe hypotension has occurred. As a result, sildenafil should not be used in individuals who require these agents.

SUGGESTED READING

1. Arima S, Kohagura K, Takeuchi K, et al. Biphasic vasodilator action of troglitazone on the renal microcirculation. *J Am Soc Nephrol*. 2002;13:342–349.
2. Arruda-Olson AM, Mahoney DW, Nehra A, et al. Cardiovascular effects of sildenafil during exercise in men with known or probable coronary artery disease: a randomized crossover trial. *JAMA*. 2002;287:719–725.
3. Bellosta S, Bernini F, Ferri N, et al. Direct vascular effects of HMG-CoA reductase inhibitors. *Atherosclerosis*. 1998;137:S101–S109.
4. Borghi C, Veronesi M, Prandin MG, et al. Statins and blood pressure regulation. *Curr Hypertens Rep*. 2001;3:281–288.
5. Egan BM, Greene EL, Goodfriend TL. Nonesterified fatty acids in blood pressure control and cardiovascular complications. *Curr Hypertens Rep*. 2001;3:107–116.
6. Glorioso N, Troffa C, Filigheddu F, et al. Effect of the HMG-CoA reductase inhibitors on blood pressure in patients with essential hypertension and primary hypercholesterolemia. *Hypertension*. 1999;34:1281–1286.
7. Nolan JJ, Ludvik B, Beerdsen P, et al. Improvement in glucose tolerance and insulin resistance in obese subjects treated with troglitazone. *N Engl J Med*. 1994;331:1188–1193.
8. Ogihara T, Rakugi H, Ikegami H, et al. Enhancement of insulin sensitivity by troglitazone lowers blood pressure in diabetic hypertensives. *Am J Hypertens*. 1995;8:316–320.
9. Sung BH, Izzo JL Jr, Dandona P, Wilson MF. Vasodilatory effects of troglitazone improve blood pressure at rest and during mental stress in type 2 diabetes mellitus. *Hypertension*. 1999;34:83–88.
10. Svensson P, de Faire U, Sleight P, et al. Comparative effects of ramipril on ambulatory and office blood pressures: a HOPE substudy. *Hypertension*. 2001;38:e28–e32.

Chapter C150

Blood Pressure Effects of Nonsteroidal Antiinflammatory Drugs and Cyclooxygenase-2 Inhibitors

Raymond R. Townsend, MD

KEY POINTS

- Nonsteroidal antiinflammatory drugs and cyclooxygenase-2 inhibitors use increases blood pressure more commonly in hypertensives than normotensives, and this effect is more pronounced on systolic blood pressure in older people.

- Alterations in sodium excretion and vascular prostaglandin metabolism are proposed mechanisms for increases in blood pressure.

- Nonsteroidal antiinflammatory drugs and cyclooxygenase-2 inhibitors use is least likely to blunt the effects of calcium antagonists compared to other classes of agents.

See also Chapters A20, A21, A33, A49, A57, A63, A66, C110, C127, C128, C139, C140–148, C151, and C173

Nonsteroidal antiinflammatory drugs (NSAIDs) and selective cyclooxygenase-2 inhibitors (COXIBs) are frequently prescribed to treat arthritis and other acute chronic pain conditions. These conditions are common in hypertensive patients, so blood pressure (BP) effects or interactions of NSAID/COXIB drugs with antihypertensive drugs are important.

Mechanisms of Blood Pressure–Raising Effects of Nonsteroidal Antiinflammatory Drugs and Cyclooxygenase-2 Inhibitors

The principal pharmacologic effect associated with either NSAID or COXIB usage is blockade of prostaglandin production (see Chapters A20 and A21). The cyclooxygenase-1 (COX-1) enzyme, largely responsible for gastric cytoprotection, is spared by COXIBs but not by NSAIDs. The COX-2 enzyme is the source of much of the circulating and renally derived prostaglandin E_2 (PGE_2) and prostacyclin (PGI_2). Although COX-2 was originally believed to be expressed mostly during inflammation, recent investigations show that it is also expressed physiologically and that its inhibition blunts certain antihypertensive medications, especially ACE inhibitors. Blockade of the COX-2 enzyme by both NSAIDs and COXIBs is thought to be the principal mechanism by which BP increases. At least 2 separate pathways have been proposed by which prostaglandins modulate BP, as diagrammed in **Figure C150.1**.

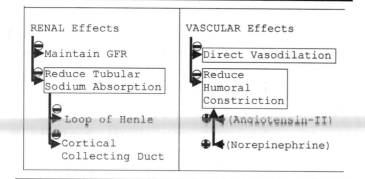

Figure C150.1. Diagram of renal and vascular mechanisms for effects of prostaglandins on blood pressure. [⊖], blood pressure–reducing effects; [⊕], blood pressure–increasing influences; GFR, glomerular filtration rate.

Blockade of prostaglandin-induced vasodilation. PGE_2 and PGI_2 are direct vasodilators that bind to prostaglandin receptors on the vascular smooth muscle cell membranes where they directly vasodilate and also counteract vasoconstriction caused by humoral factors such as angiotensin-II and catecholamines. Both NSAIDs and COXIBs decrease the production of vasodilatory prostaglandins resulting in vasoconstriction.

Renal effects. Renal actions of prostaglandins also contribute to their systemic hemodynamic effects. Prostaglandins are natriuretic. Renal prostaglandin production occurs principally in the medulla, where prostaglandins (mainly PGE_2) promote sodium loss through their actions on cells in the loop of Henle. Blockade of natriuresis with NSAIDS or COXIBs can result in sodium and water retention, weight gain, edema, and an increase in blood pressure. Additionally, renal prostaglandin production occurs in the glomerular circulation where it is important in maintaining glomerular blood flow and glomerular filtration. Because prostaglandins are vasodilatory, prostaglandin production blockade by NSAIDs or COXIBs can decrease renal blood flow and reduce glomerular filtration, thereby activating intrarenal sodium-retaining mechanisms. As with their vascular effects, these actions of prostaglandins are clinically more important in situations such as heart failure and chronic kidney disease, in which there is greater dependence on prostaglandins to maintain renal and glomerular blood flow and filtration. Infrequently, in older patients on thiazide diuretics, the combined renal effects of NSAIDs can result in disproportionate water to sodium retention with the development of hyponatremia.

Blood Pressure Modulation by Prostaglandins in Disease States

Prostaglandins act more as modulators of BP, rather than acting as primary mediators of vascular tone. As a result, the effects of prostaglandin blockade are more evident when "challenges" to BP control are present, including reduced renal function, aging, diabetes, or salt loading. In these situations, prostaglandin blockade is more likely to result in an increase in BP. In circumstances of volume depletion, impaired kidney function or heart failure that often include a degree of renal vasoconstriction, blockade of prostaglandins can further com-

promise an already diminished glomerular filtration rate and exacerbate sodium retention.

Variation in Nonsteroidal Antiinflammatory Drug and Cyclooxygenase-2 Inhibitor Effects on Blood Pressure in Hypertensives versus Normotensives

As shown in Table C150.1, NSAIDs and COXIBs have BP-increasing effects that are greater in hypertensive patients than normotensives and are in the general range of 4 to 6 mm Hg. The data shown in the table are averaged. Although the NSAID data in the table are reported as changes in "mean BP," it is principally the systolic BP that increases during NSAID or COXIB therapy and there is significant interindividual variability. Many patients have no change in BP, whereas others may have ≥20 mm Hg increases in systolic BP. The latter patients are more likely to be older, have some degree of reduced renal function, are more salt-sensitive, and generally have higher systolic BPs. The usage of NSAIDs or COXIBs in these populations therefore justifies close monitoring for BP consequences. The BP increases appear to be dose-related for both NSAIDs and COXIBs. Older patients taking NSAIDs are also more likely to initiate antihypertensive drug therapy in direct proportion to the dose of NSAID consumed. All classes of antihypertensive drug therapy, with the exception of the calcium antagonists, appear to have their antihypertensive effectiveness compromised by NSAIDs and COXIBs.

Magnitude of Blood Pressure Effects of Nonsteroidal Antiinflammatory Drugs and Cyclooxygenase-2 Inhibitors

Obtaining precise estimates of the effect on NSAID and COXIB therapy on blood pressure in humans is hampered by the heterogeneity of the agents and the conflicting results in published studies.

Nonsteroidal Antinflammatory Drugs

Metaanalyses. Two metaanalyses have evaluated the degree of blood pressure elevation associated with NSAID use and serve as the basis for the data in Table C150.1, which has certain shortcomings. Most of the subjects included in these 2

Table C150.1. Hypertensive Effects by Class and Agent

	HYPERTENSIVES	NORMALS
NSAIDs (pooled)	3.6–5.4	1.0–1.1
Indomethacin	4.8–6.0	1.0
Naproxen	3.1–6.1	ND
Piroxicam	2.9–6.2	ND
Sulindac	(–)1.6–2.2	(–)1.6
Aspirin	(–)1.8–1.0	0.6
COXIBs		
Rofecoxib	2.6–4.7	3.4
Celecoxib	(–)0.4	4.3

Note: Data for nonsteroidal antiinflammatory drugs are changes in mean arterial pressure in mm Hg; data for cyclooxygenase-2 inhibitors are systolic blood pressure changes in mm Hg.

(–), negative value; COXIBs, cyclooxygenase-2 inhibitors; ND, no data; NSAIDs, nonsteroidal antiinflammatory drugs.

metaanalyses were young, treatment periods were short (often 4–6 weeks), and an underlying disease state (arthritis or other painful condition) was not present.

Variability among different nonsteroidal antiinflammatory drugs. There appears to be variability in the hypertensive effects within the classes.

Aspirin in doses up to 1.5 g daily has no discernible effect on blood pressure. Sulindac, among the prescription NSAIDs, appears to have the least hypertensive effect. This may be related to a peculiarity in renal metabolism in which the drug is selectively metabolized within the kidney to an inactive form. Indomethacin has the most extensive documentation of effects on BP and has the greatest BP-increasing effect, followed by piroxicam.

Cyclooxygenase-2 inhibitors. COXIBs have been available only since early 1999, so their BP effects are not as well studied. Overall, their effects on renal hemodynamics appear to be similar to those of the NSAIDs. The largest source of data to date is in hypertensive patients on a large variety of antihypertensive agents treated with COXIB therapy for osteoarthritis. One study included 543 patients treated with rofecoxib and 549 treated with celecoxib; systolic BP increased by 3 mm Hg from baseline with rofecoxib with no increase seen with celecoxib. The number of patients with a combined increase of systolic BP >20 mm Hg and a final systolic BP >140 mm Hg was 14.9% in the rofecoxib group and 6.9% in the celecoxib group ($p <.01$). As with NSAIDs, treatment with calcium antagonist therapy protected against the BP increases with either COXIB.

SUGGESTED READING

1. Cannon GW, Caldwell JR, Holt P, et al. Rofecoxib, a specific inhibitor of cyclooxygenase 2, with clinical efficacy comparable with that of diclofenac sodium: results of a one-year, randomized, clinical trial in patients with osteoarthritis of the knee and hip. Rofecoxib Phase III Protocol 035 Study Group. *Arthritis Rheum.* 2000;43:978–987.

2. De Leeuw PW. Nonsteroidal anti-inflammatory drugs and hypertension. The risks in perspective. *Drugs.* 1996;51:179–187.

3. Fitzgerald GA. The choreography of cyclooxygenases in the kidney. *J Clin Invest.* 2002;110:33–34.

4. Gurwitz JH, Avorn J, Bohn RL, et al. Initiation of antihypertensive treatment during nonsteroidal anti-inflammatory drug therapy. *JAMA.* 1994; 272:781–786.

5. Johnson AG, Nguyen TV, Day RO. Do nonsteroidal anti-inflammatory drugs affect blood pressure? A metaanalysis. *Ann Intern Med.* 1994;121:289–300.

6. Pope JE, Anderson JJ, Felson DT. A metaanalysis of the effects of nonsteroidal anti-inflammatory drugs on blood pressure. *Arch Intern Med.* 1993; 153:477–484.

7. Schwartz JI, Vandormael K, Malice MP, et al. Comparison of rofecoxib, celecoxib, and naproxen on renal function in elderly subjects receiving a normal-salt diet. *Clin Pharmacol Ther.* 2002;72:50–61.

8. Whelton A, White WB, Bello AE, et al. Effects of celecoxib and rofecoxib on blood pressure and edema in patients ≥65 years of age with systemic hypertension and osteoarthritis. *Am J Cardiol.* 2002;90:959–963.

Chapter C151

Treatment of the Elderly Hypertensive: Systolic Hypertension

Jan N. Basile, MD

KEY POINTS

- Hypertension affects up to 75% of individuals 60 years of age and older, the most rapidly growing segment of our population.

- Cardiovascular risk is related to increased systolic blood pressure and pulse pressure and to decreased diastolic blood pressure, but systolic blood pressure reduction is the major target for improving outcomes in the elderly patient.

- Hypertension therapy in older individuals should include lifestyle modification, especially weight loss and sodium restriction, which may decrease the need for antihypertensive medication.

- If low initial doses are used, significant attention must be paid to adequate titration; combination therapy is usually required for optimal blood pressure control. The initial agent chosen is rarely the final agent used to achieve the recommended systolic blood pressure goal of <140 mm Hg.

See also Chapters A42, A59, A60, B82, B102, B107, C110, C119, C120, C127, C138, and C151

The *elderly*, defined as individuals ≥60 years of age, represent the most rapidly growing segment of our population. Hypertension [blood pressure (BP) ≥140/90 mm Hg] confers a 3- to 4-fold increased risk for cardiovascular disease in older compared to younger individuals. Recent recommendations emphasize that systolic BP (SBP) should be the primary target for the diagnosis and management of elderly patients with hypertension. Unfortunately, at most only approximately 20% of the elderly have their BP controlled at <140/90 mm Hg.

Age and Blood Pressure Patterns

Isolated systolic hypertension [ISH, SBP ≥140 mm Hg and diastolic BP (DBP) <90 mm Hg] represents the most common form of hypertension in the elderly. Its prevalence increases with age; two-thirds of individuals 60 years of age and older and three-fourths of those older than 75 years of age have ISH.

SBP leads to more appropriate risk stratification in the elderly. In a recent analysis of the Framingham Heart Study, knowing only the SBP correctly classified the stage of BP in 99% of adults older than 60 years of age, whereas knowing only the DBP allowed 66% to be correctly classified.

Although both an increasing DBP and SBP are directly associated with cardiovascular risk in younger populations, in those older than 60 years of age an increasing SBP and a decreasing DBP increases risk. Accordingly, the pulse pressure (SBP – DBP) is a stronger predictor of cardiovascular risk than an increased SBP or decreased DBP in the elderly. Because there has not been a clinical trial that has shown that reducing pulse pressure

reduces risk, lowering SBP continues to be the primary target for decreasing cardiovascular risk in the elderly with hypertension.

Pathophysiology

Age-related changes in aortic stiffness explain the frequent development of ISH (see Chapter A60). Whereas DBP elevation is caused by constriction of the smaller arterioles, SBP elevation is caused by the loss of distensibility of the larger arteries, especially the aorta. Age-related arterial stiffening leads to a progressive rise in SBP. The elevated systolic pressure increases left ventricular work and the risk for left ventricular hypertrophy, whereas the decreased DBP may compromise coronary blood flow.

Clinical Evaluation

All hypertensives should be evaluated, irrespective of age, using standard criteria (see Chapter C110). A few caveats apply to the elderly, however. BP is more variable in the older patient, and BP measurement can pose special problems in the elderly. Pseudohypertension should be suspected when medication causes hypotensive symptoms in elderly patients with normal BP or in those with persistently high BP without any evidence of target organ damage. In these individuals, peripheral arteries may become thickened and stiff, and the BP measurement may be an overestimation of actual intraarterial pressure. BP should be measured in the supine and standing positions because the elderly are more prone to postural hypotension, especially after a meal.

Very few elderly patients have a reversible form of hypertension (**Table C151.1**). Although renovascular hypertension is more common and often unrecognized in the elderly hyperten-

Table C151.1. Indications to Evaluate for Secondary Hypertension in the Older Patient

New onset stage 3 hypertension
Unprovoked hypokalemia or refractory hypokalemia while on thiazides, angiotensin-converting enzyme inhibitors, or angiotensin receptor blocker
Hypertension refractory to a 3-drug regimen, 1 of which is thiazide
Symptoms suggestive of pheochromocytoma
Continued creatinine rise on appropriate antihypertensive therapy
Clinical or laboratory findings suggestive of a reversible form of hypertension

sive, it is rarely cured by surgical or nonsurgical (angioplasty with stent) intervention. If BP is controlled and renal function remains normal, there is little benefit from its detection. Target organ damage is also more likely in the elderly.

Evidence-Based Benefits of Therapy in the Elderly

Lifestyle (nonpharmacologic) therapy. Reducing sodium intake and losing weight are particularly beneficial for BP control and often reduce the need for pharmacologic therapy. The Trial of Nonpharmacologic Interventions in the Elderly (TONE) showed that restricting salt to 80 mmol (2 g) per day favorably reduced SBP and DBP during the 30-month trial, and 40% of those on this low-salt diet were able to discontinue their medication. In addition, the combination of weight loss and salt restriction reduced BP more than either strategy by itself and, when used together, decreased the need for antihypertensive therapy in almost half the participants. The elderly should be encouraged to avoid excessive alcohol intake and remain as physically active as is feasible.

Treatment of isolated systolic hypertension. There is no longer any doubt that controlling BP in the older patient reduces cardiovascular and renal complications from hypertension. The minimum goals for BP lowering are SBP <140 mm Hg and DBP <90 mm Hg. Several large, prospective placebo-controlled systolic/diastolic hypertension trials conducted in the 1960s, 1970s, and 1980s found a reduction in cardiovascular morbidity and mortality when DBP was lowered to <90 mm Hg (**Table C151.2**). More recent randomized, placebo-controlled trials have shown significant benefit from drug treatment in elderly patients with ISH (**Table C151.3**). In those with stage 2 ISH (SBP of ≥160 mm Hg and a DBP <90–95 mm Hg), a reduction in stroke, heart failure, coronary events, and mortality was found. Benefit occurred when SBP was reduced by at least 20 mm Hg from baseline and to a level below the entry SBP, either 150 or 160 mm Hg. Although none of the trials achieved an average SBP of <140 mm Hg (**Table C151.4**), the Sixth Report of the Joint National Committee on Prevention, Detection, Evaluation, and Treatment of High Blood Pressure

Table C151.2. Percent Event Reduction in Clinical Trials in Older Hypertensive Patients

	STROKE	CORONARY ARTERY DISEASE	CONGESTIVE HEART FAILURE	ALL CARDIOVASCULAR DISEASE
Systolic/diastolic				
Australian	33	18	—	31
EWPHE	36	20	22	29[a]
STOP	47[a]	13[b]	51[a]	40[a]
MRC	25[a]	19	—	17[a]
HDFP	44[a]	15[a]	—	16[a]
Isolated systolic				
SHEP	33[a]	27[a]	55[a]	32[a]
Syst-EUR	42[a]	30	29	31[a]
Syst-China	38[a]	27	—	25[a]

EWPHE, European Working Party on High Blood Pressure in the Elderly; HDFP, Hypertension Detection and Follow-Up Program; MRC, Medical Research Council; SHEP, Systolic Hypertension in the Elderly Program; STOP, Swedish Trial in Old Patients; Syst-EUR, European Trial on Isolated Systolic Hypertension in the Elderly; Syst-China, Systolic Hypertension in China.
[a]Statistically significant.
[b]Myocardial infarction only.

Table C151.3. Major Clinical Trials Showing Benefit of Treating Isolated Systolic Hypertension

	SHEP (N = 4,736)	SYST-EUR (N = 4,695)	SYST-CHINA (N = 2,394)
Baseline blood pressure, SBP/DBP (mm Hg)	160–219/<90	160–219/<95	160–219/<95
Blood pressure reduction, SBP/DPB (mm Hg)	27/9	23/7	20/5
Drug therapy	Chlorthalidone	Nitrendipine	Nitrendipine
	Atenolol	Enalapril Hydrochlorothiazide	Captopril Hydrochlorothiazide
Outcomes (% ↓)			
Stroke	33	42	38
Coronary artery disease	27	30	27
Congestive heart disease	55	29	—
All cardiovascular disease	32	31	25

↓, decrease; DBP, diastolic blood pressure; SBP, systolic blood pressure; SHEP, Systolic Hypertension in the Elderly Program; Syst-EUR, European Trial on Isolated Systolic Hypertension in the Elderly; Syst-China, Systolic Hypertension in China.
From *J Clin Hypertens.* 2000;2:336, with permission.

Table C151.4. Blood Pressure in Systolic Hypertension in the Elderly Program (SHEP) and European Trial on Isolated Systolic Hypertension in the Elderly (Syst-EUR)

	SHEP (MM HG)	SYST-EUR (MM HG)
Entry	160–219/<90	160–219/<95
Goal (systolic blood pressure)	<160 + ≥21 ↓	<150 + ≥20 ↓
Baseline	170/77	174/86
Achieved: treatment	143/68	151/79
Achieved: placebo	155/72	161/84
Difference: treatment/placebo	12/4	10/5

↓, decrease.

Table C151.5. Pharmacologic Management of Hypertension in the Elderly

The primary goal of reducing blood pressure is to reduce cardiovascular events. This has been demonstrated in trials with several classes of drugs as initial therapy:
  Diuretics
  Calcium antagonists
  Angiotensin converting enzyme inhibitors
  Angiotensin receptor blocker
The evidence for β-blockers as monotherapy is less strong in the elderly.
α-Blockers should not be used as monotherapy.

(JNC VI) and a recent consensus statement recommend the minimum goal for therapy to be a SBP <140 mm Hg. In those with diabetes, renal insufficiency, or systolic heart failure, the SBP should be no more than 130 mm Hg.

Although the vascular risk of stage 1 ISH (SBP 140–159 mm Hg/DBP <90 mm Hg) is well established, no trial has been completed to test whether its treatment is beneficial. Stage 1 ISH affects 25% of the elderly population, so the results of several trials with this degree of ISH are ongoing to evaluate the treatment and prevention of this condition and will be very important.

Antihypertensive Therapy

Initial therapy. Diuretics, calcium antagonists, and angiotensin-converting enzyme inhibitors are preferred first-line drugs in older patients with systolic hypertension. Recommendations in ISH stem from several placebo-controlled outcome trials. The Systolic Hypertension in the Elderly Program (SHEP) achieved a favorable reduction in stroke and cardiovascular events using a diuretic-based strategy (with or without a β-blocker (Table C151.2). The European Trial on Isolated Systolic Hypertension in the Elderly (Syst-EUR) found a benefit using a moderately long-acting dihydropyridine calcium antagonist, nitrendipine, as initial therapy (with or without angiotensin-converting enzyme inhibitor and a diuretic). A metaanalysis of 8 placebo-controlled trials in the elderly by Staessen and colleagues (including a total of 15,693 patients followed for 4 years) found active treatment reduced coronary events by 23%, strokes by 30%, cardiovascular deaths by 18%, and total deaths by 13%, with the benefit particularly high in those older than 70 years of age. Another recent metaanalysis extends the value of therapy to those older than 80 years of age; thus, the oldest elderly seem to benefit the most from active treatment. Although all classes of antihypertensive agents effectively lower SBP and DBP in the elderly, the majority of outcome trials showing a reduction in vascular morbidity and mortality used diuretics and, when necessary, added a β-blocker. β-blocker therapy is not usually recommended as monotherapy in the elderly (unless prescribed for ischemic heart disease or heart failure) but improves outcome when used with a diuretic. Since the JNC VI report was published in 1997, several trials in the elderly (STOP-2, NORDIL, INSIGHT) have suggested that the initial agent chosen is less important than the level of BP reduction achieved (**Table C151.5**). However, there are major shortcomings of the designs of these studies, and the question of superiority of one class over another remains to be answered.

Combination therapy. Most elderly patients require 2 or more drugs to achieve the SBP goal of <140 mm Hg recommended in JNC VI. In the SHEP and the Syst-EUR trials, 40% to 50% of participants required at least 2 drugs (Table C151.3) to achieve a SBP mean of approximately 145 mm Hg, whereas DBP was <80 mm Hg (Table C151.4). In routine practice, if the SBP goal is achieved, the DBP goal is almost always reached as well.

Doses and titration. Many physicians believe that the usual dose of the initial agent in older hypertensives should be half of that used in younger hypertensives, often based on the expectation of altered pharmacokinetic renal or hepatic metabolism that often occurs in the elderly. Unfortunately, this practice often leads to underdosing and reduced control. The dose should be titrated slowly, usually every 4 to 6 weeks, until the maximum BP reduction occurs. Other agents are then added until the BP goal is attained. If not used initially, a thiazide diuretic should be included in most regimens to enhance the efficacy of other BP-lowering agents.

Potassium. The serum potassium should be kept normal. A recent retrospective analysis of SHEP found that 7% of the participants on the long-acting diuretic chlorthalidone developed hypokalemia (K <3.5 mEq/L) by the 1-year visit. Those individuals who developed hypokalemia had an event rate similar to those in the placebo group, whereas those with levels >3.5 mEq per L had significantly fewer cardiovascular events, suggesting K+ should be kept normal above 3.5 mEq per L.

Dangers of excessive blood pressure lowering. The J-curve hypothesis states that lowering DBP in those with underlying cardiovascular disease below a certain critical value increases the risk of cardiovascular death. A retrospective analysis of the SHEP trial has suggested that the few patients whose DBP was lowered to <55 mm Hg experienced no benefit in outcome when compared to the placebo group. Thus, it is prudent to exercise caution in lowering DBP to <55 mm Hg in older individuals with ISH.

SUGGESTED READING

1. Benetos A, Thomas F, Bean K, et al. Prognostic value of systolic and diastolic blood pressure in treated hypertensive men. *Arch Intern Med.* 2002;162:577–581.
2. Franklin SS, Khan SA, Wong ND, et al. Is pulse pressure useful in predicting risk for coronary heart disease? The Framingham Heart Study. *Circulation.* 1999;100:354–360.

3. Franse LV, Pahor M, Di Bari M, et al. Hypokalemia associated with diuretic use and cardiovascular events in the systolic hypertension in the elderly program. *Hypertension.* 2000;35:1025–1030.
4. Hansson L, Lindholm LH, Ekbom T, for the STOP-Hypertension-2 study group. Randomized trial of old and new antihypertensive drugs in elderly patients: cardiovascular mortality and morbidity in the Swedish Trial in Old Patients with Hypertension-2 (STOP-2) study. *Lancet.* 1999;354:1751–1756.
5. Izzo J, Levy D, Black HR. Clinical Advisory Statement. Importance of systolic blood pressure in older Americans. *Hypertension.* 2000;35:1021–1024.
6. SHEP Cooperative Research Group. Prevention of stroke by antihyperten-sive drug treatment in older persons with isolated systolic hypertension. *JAMA.* 1991;265:3255–3264.
7. Somes G, Pahor M, Shorr RI, et al. The role of diastolic blood pressure when treating isolated systolic hypertension. *Arch Intern Med.* 1999;159:2004–2009.
8. Staessen JA, Fagard R, Thijs L, et al. Morbidity and mortality in the placebo controlled European trial on isolated systolic hypertension (Syst-Eur) in the elderly. *Lancet.* 1997;350:757–764.
9. Staessen JA, Gasowski J, Wang JC, et al. Risk of untreated and treated isolated systolic hypertension in the elderly: meta-analysis of outcome trials. *Lancet.* 2000;355:865–872.

Chapter C152

Treatment of Borderline (Nonsustained) Hypertension

Stevo Julius, MD, ScD

KEY POINTS

- Patients with borderline or nonsustained hypertension have an increased likelihood of developing persistent hypertension and excess cardiovascular death.

- Approximately 30% of all young males with borderline hypertension exhibit signs of increased sympathetic activity.

- There is no consistent evidence that blood pressure responses to cold, mental stress, isometric exercise, or tilt testing predict the development of future hypertension.

- Patients with borderline hypertension but no target organ damage or diabetes should undergo a 6-month trial of nonpharmacologic management in an effort to lower self-determined blood pressure and to modify other cardiovascular risk factors; drug therapy is indicated if hypertension persists.

See also Chapters A43–A47, B98, B100, B109, C110, C112, C113, C117, C127, C129, and C130

There is a complex and distinctive pathophysiology of the syndrome of borderline or nonsustained hypertension and specific clinical measures that are indicated.

Definition

Borderline (nonsustained) hypertension occurs when blood pressure (BP) is >140/90 mm Hg at the time of measurement, but the elevation is neither permanent nor excessive. This includes (a) subjects who, out of 3 readings taken in the previous 6 months, show 1 clinic BP >140/90 mm Hg; (b) subjects with white coat hypertension (see Chapter B101), who exhibit elevated clinic BP readings but no elevated out-of-office readings; and (c) subjects with BP readings in the high-normal BP range according to The Sixth Report of the Joint National Committee on Prevention, Detection, Evaluation, and Treatment of High Blood Pressure (JNC VI) (130–139/85–89 mm Hg). According to this classification, 15% of all people 30 to 50 years old may have borderline hypertension.

Because borderline hypertensive subjects have BP that is not persistently elevated, they are occasionally diagnosed as having *labile* hypertension (as opposed to stable or sustained hypertension). This diagnosis is wrong because all evidence indicates that BP variability (lability) in these subjects is not excessive, nor is their "reactivity" to various physical stressors increased (see Chapters A43, B100, and B101). If needed, the term *labile BP* should be reserved for individuals who have "spells" of hypertension or who show wide day-to-day BP fluctuations (>30 mm Hg) irrespective of their average BP levels, such as those with baroreflex dysfunction (see Chapter C161).

Borderline Hypertension as a Precursor of Cardiovascular Diseases

Since the early 1930s, life insurance data have clearly indicated that even a single elevated office BP reading carries negative prognostic connotations. The predictive power of clinic BP readings is so strong that only a few standard treatment recommendations exist. Nevertheless, when BP measurements are repeated, <30% of subjects with borderline hypertension remain hypertensive. In addition, the cardiovascular prognosis for individuals who have just an occasional BP elevation is not normal. Over a period of 20 years, they have a 4-fold greater incidence of established hypertension and cardiovascular deaths. A study from Norway suggested that 80% of borderline hypertensives first seen in their third decade of life develop sustained hypertension after 20 years. Recently, the Framingham study reported on 6,859 subjects with high-normal BP followed for 12 years. Compared to subjects with an optimal BP at the baseline, persons with a high-normal BP had a hazard ratio of developing a major cardiovascular event of 2.5 in men and 1.6 in women. The hazard ratios were attenuated but remained significant even when the transition to hypertension was taken into account as a time-dependent covariate.

Sympathetic Overactivity and Its Consequences

Borderline hypertension is a complex pathophysiologic condition in which the elevated BP is only one of multiple cardiovascular risk factors. Approximately 30% of all young men with borderline hypertension exhibit signs of increased sympathetic activity, with increased cardiac output, stroke volume, and heart rates. Plasma norepinephrine and norepinephrine turnover rates in these patients are increased, and it has recently been shown by microneurography that the nerve traffic in sympathetic fibers is significantly elevated. Other consequences of increased sympathetic activity (see Chapters A42 and A43) include high plasma renin values (due to excessive β-adrenergic stimulation of the juxtaglomerular cells), decreased plasma volume (due to excessive α-adrenergic venular constriction), and a diminished parasympathetic inhibitory tone to the heart.

Metabolic syndrome and other linked abnormalities.
Patients with borderline hypertension tend to be overweight and have abnormalities consistent with the metabolic syndrome (see Chapters A45 and B97), including obesity, dyslipidemia, high hematocrit, and insulin resistance that put them at a higher risk for development of coronary heart disease and its complications. Acute sympathetic stimulation can cause insulin resistance by causing α-adrenergic vasoconstriction, which leads to a reduced delivery of glucose and insulin to the skeletal muscle. High insulin is predictive of the future development of atherosclerosis, most likely through the direct "trophic" effect of insulin on the blood vessel wall and the insulin-related promotion of high triglyceride and low high-density lipoprotein cholesterol values. Thus, high insulin and dyslipidemia may be directly related to excess sympathetic tone. In addition, high insulin favors increased sympathetic activity. Epidemiologic studies have shown that a higher hematocrit, which is frequently found in patients with borderline hypertension, is also a predictor of coronary mortality, most likely through the hypercoagulability of the more viscous blood. Infusion of norepinephrine causes a rapid increase in hematocrit through α-adrenergic postcapillary venoconstriction.

Therapeutic implications.
Because of a clear involvement of sympathetic overactivity in the pathogenesis of the excess coronary risk in borderline hypertension, nonpharmacologic measures such as physical conditioning and weight loss may be particularly useful. Physical training lowers both cardiac output and heart rate through a combination of decreased sympathetic and increased parasympathetic tone and improves the sensitivity of skeletal muscle to the insulin-mediated glucose incorporation. This, in turn, tends to lower plasma insulin levels.

Risk Assessment in Borderline Hypertension

Because the cardiovascular risk of a person with borderline hypertension is higher than normal, such an individual deserves

medical attention even if the absolute level of risk in borderline hypertension is too small to mandate immediate drug therapy. In a patient with borderline hypertension, the physician should assess the patient's risk status and the status of hypertension-related target organs and then individualize the approach.

Risk of sustained hypertension.
Two patients with the same average clinic BP may not have the same propensity to later development of sustained hypertension. Proven risk factors for later hypertension are average BP level, obesity and weight gain with time, tachycardia, family history of hypertension, male sex, and black race. Being overweight is a strong risk factor for future hypertension. Among risk factors for the development of hypertension, fast heart rate deserves special mention. A patient with a rapid heart rate in the physician's office and reasonably normal BP readings elsewhere is usually dismissed as having *nervous BP elevation only*. However, 10 years later, a person whose resting heart rate is >80 bpm has twice the chance of developing hypertension, even with normal BP readings. When this heart rate is combined with a transiently elevated office BP reading, the risk of hypertension quintuples. Family history is a significant predictive factor for future hypertension only if the parent required antihypertensive treatment before 50 years of age. Various "reactivity" tests (cold pressor, mental stress, isometric exercise) have been used for prediction of future hypertension among patients with borderline hypertension, but the clinical utility of such tests in regular medical practice is unclear. BP level achieved during strenuous dynamic exercise seems to be a better predictor of future BP increase than the baseline BP (see Chapter C119).

Risk of coronary heart disease.
A strong association between BP elevation and other coronary risk is seen even before the development of established hypertension. Compared with normotensive individuals, subjects with permanent or white coat borderline hypertension tend to be overweight; to have high cholesterol, triglycerides, plasma insulin, and hematocrit levels; and to have significantly decreased high-density lipoprotein cholesterol levels. It is therefore mandatory to incorporate these parameters into the evaluation of borderline hypertension testing for cardiovascular risk factors. Plasma lipids ought to be determined routinely in everyone. Fasting plasma insulin and glucose may also prove useful to gauge the effectiveness of nonpharmacologic intervention.

Target organ assessment.
Echocardiography provides reliable data to assess cardiac status in borderline hypertension, but the readings must come from a reputable laboratory (see Chapter C154). A notable proportion of patients with borderline hypertension may already show left ventricular hypertrophy or concentric remodeling (relative wall thickness, >0.45). Such subjects are at higher risk for later cardiovascular complications. Fasting blood sugar values or an oral glucose tolerance test can uncover latent glucose intolerance or diabetes (repeated fasting glucose 110–125 mg/dL = impaired glucose tolerance, fasting glucose >125 mg/dL or any glucose >200 mg/dL on an oral glucose tolerance test = diabetes). Presence of microalbuminuria (>20 mg/dL) in glucose intolerant subjects calls for particular attention and a closer follow-up. If nonpharmacologic intervention does not affect the BP or the glucose tolerance, such patients

may be considered for early BP-lowering treatment. Recent studies suggest that established hypertension treatment with ACE inhibitors and more recently the angiotensin receptor blockers reduces rate of new onset diabetes. If a decision has been made to treat a glucose intolerant, borderline hypertensive patient with drugs, ACE inhibitors and angiotensin blocking agents appear to be the preferred agents.

Out-of-Office Blood Pressure Assessment

In borderline hypertension, it is mandatory to obtain repeated BP readings outside of the physician's office (see Chapter C112). These can be obtained by patients or their relatives (usually 2 readings/day for 7 days) or by a BP-monitoring device (daytime and, when possible, nighttime readings, 2/hour). It is important to understand the context in which these measurements are taken; repeated out-of-office BPs establish a reproducible baseline against which future intervention can be evaluated and may guard against overtreatment of borderline hypertension. These readings do not decide who ought to be treated, however; a distinction that is important. Epidemiologic studies based on standard clinical BP measurements are replete with information about BP thresholds at which complication rates accelerate. Such data are not yet available for out-of-office BP readings. Out-of-office readings can also be useful in determining who should *not* be treated or who may be overtreated. If office readings alone are used to evaluate the efficacy of a regimen, some subjects will have very low out-of-office BP readings ($\leq$120/70 mm Hg) and may suffer from symptoms of hypotension.

Home BP self-determination can be used to establish a reliable BP for long-term follow-up. The standard method is to obtain 1 reading in the morning and 1 in the afternoon on 7 consecutive days. The upper limit of normality (2 standard deviations above the normal mean) is 142/92 mm Hg for men and 131/85 mm Hg for women; the upper limit for borderline hypertension (1 standard deviation above the mean) is 131/83 mm Hg for men and 121/78 mm Hg for women.

Stepwise Management of Borderline Hypertension

After home BP readings have been obtained, the following management-treatment scheme for subjects with borderline hypertension can be adopted.

Step 1. All subjects should undergo a trial of lifestyle modification (usually 6–12 months). As in patients with established hypertension, weight loss, sodium restriction, and physical exercise are preferred components of the treatment program. Almost all methods of weight loss yield an average loss of 3 to 4 kg, but there is also a strong tendency to regain the weight. However, if there is a very good correlation between weight loss and decreased BP, it becomes much easier to convince the patient to cooperate and maintain a lower weight. The Dietary Approaches to Stop Hypertension (DASH) and DASH Sodium studies suggest that such patients will benefit from a diet low in sodium and saturated fat and high in potassium, magnesium, and calories (see Chapter C129). Physical exercise is a practical way to improve the health of the patient with borderline hypertension. The training must be systematic and must include aerobic exercise (jogging, swimming, treadmill, bicycle) of suf-

ficient intensity to increase the heart rate to $\approx$130 bpm. Three 30-minute sessions per week are sufficient to achieve the maximal health benefit. Training beyond that level will not improve the BP results, but may further increase the patient's exercise capacity (see Chapter C130).

Step 2. If therapy is successful (home BP decrease of 5 mm Hg, body weight loss of 2 kg, or cholesterol reduction of 15 mg/dL), the clinician should continue with the lifestyle modifications and recheck every 6 months. If therapy is not successful, the clinician should consider pharmacologic treatment if: (a) the home average BP is >140/90 mm Hg; (b) the home BP is occasionally >140/90 mm Hg, the subject is male, and he has a positive family history of hypertension; (c) the home BP is >140/90 mm Hg, the subject is female and the home BP has increased over previous readings; or (d) the subject, regardless of gender, has home BP readings >140/90 mm Hg and abnormal levels of cholesterol or high-density lipoprotein cholesterol. Continued observation toward maximization of lifestyle modification is recommended for women who do not have additional risk factors with follow-up in 3 months. Lifestyle modification is recommended in subjects whose home BP is between 131/83 and 139/89 mm Hg. The rate of follow-up in those with additional risk factors is 3 months; in others, 6 months. Lifestyle modification is recommended in all other subjects, with 1-year follow-up.

Step 3. Excessive doses of drugs or drug combinations are not usually necessary. The choice of drug is affected by the patient's lifestyle (exercise, anxiety level, sexual dysfunction), laboratory abnormalities (glucose/lipid status), and associated conditions. Careful attention to any side effects helps minimize adherence problems. Switching classes is useful if side effects occur. The goal of treatment is to lower the home BP by 5 mm Hg of diastolic BP. If successful, treatment should be maintained for 2 years and the patient recalled on a semiannual basis. After 2 years under a physician's supervision, treatment can be discontinued with monitoring for 3 months. If the BP returns to the hypertensive range, the patient should accept lifelong treatment of the condition. If the BP does not increase, the next visit should be at 3 months, and if still not hypertensive, then each 6 months for the next 2 years. Thereafter, annual revisits may be sufficient. Patients who do not respond to small doses of drugs represent the biggest problem. Reiteration of lifestyle modification combined with treatment is in order. If this strategy does not work after 6 months, and particularly if the average BP increased (even a few mm Hg), combination treatment is in order.

SUGGESTED READING

1. Anderson EA, Sinkey CA, Lawton WJ, et al. Elevated sympathetic nerve activity in borderline hypertensive humans: evidence from direct intraneural recordings. *Hypertension.* 1989;14:177–183.
2. Joint National Committee. The sixth report of the Joint National Committee on Prevention, Detection, Evaluation, and Treatment of High Blood Pressure. *Arch Intern Med.* 1997;157:2314–2446.
3. Julius S. Coronary disease in hypertension: a new mosaic. *J Hypertens.* 1997;15(suppl 2):S3–S10.
5. Julius S, Ellis CN, Pascual AV, et al. Home blood pressure determination: value in borderline ("labile") hypertension. *JAMA.* 1974;229:663–666.
6. Julius S, Jamerson K, Mejia A, et al. The association of borderline hypertension with target organ changes and higher coronary risk. Tecumseh Blood Pressure Study. *JAMA.* 1990;264:354–358.

7. Julius S, Mejia A, Jones K, et al. "White coat" versus "sustained" borderline hypertension in Tecumseh, Michigan. *Hypertension.* 1990;16:617–623.

8. Lund-Johansen P, Omvik P. Hemodynamic patterns of untreated hypertensive disease. In: Laragh JH, Brenner BM, eds. *Hypertension: Pathophysiology, Diagnosis, and Management.* New York, NY: Raven Press Ltd; 1990:305–327.

9. Nesbitt SD, Amerena JV, Grant E, et al. Home blood pressure as a predictor of future blood pressure stability in borderline hypertension. The Tecumseh Study. *Am J Hypertens.*1997;10:1270–1280.

10. Palatini P, Julius S. Association of tachycardia with morbidity and mortality: pathophysiological considerations. *J Hum Hypertens.* 1997;11(Suppl 1):S19–S27.

11. Vasan RS, Larson MG, Leip EP, et al. Impact of high normal blood pressure on the risk of cardiovascular disease. *N Engl J Med.* 2001; 345:1291–1297.

Chapter C153

Treatment of Hypertensive Emergencies and Urgencies

Donald G. Vidt, MD

KEY POINTS

- Therapeutic decisions in a patient with accelerated hypertension depend on the severity of the associated comorbidities.

- Elevated blood pressure in the absence of symptoms of progressive target organ damage rarely requires emergency therapy and can be managed in the outpatient setting if appropriate follow-up can be provided.

- Hypertensive emergencies occur when acute or rapidly progressive target organ damage exists; these patients usually require hospitalization in an intensive care unit with blood pressure monitoring and parenteral therapy to reduce blood pressure to a safe, noncritical level, not necessarily to achieve normotension.

- Treatment of hypertensive encephalopathy (caused by abnormal autoregulation of cerebral blood flow) reverses acute neurologic abnormalities.

See also Chapters A62, A68, A69, A71, A72, C109–C111, C118, C127, C128, C133, C137, C139, C141, C143, and C146–C148

Syndromes of Severe (Stage 3) Hypertension

Therapeutic decisions in a patient with markedly elevated blood pressure (BP) (≥180 mm Hg systolic) hypertension depend on the severity of the comorbidities present in the individual patient.

Hypertensive emergencies. Hypertensive emergencies occur when severe elevations in BP are complicated by evidence of acute or rapidly progressive life-threatening target organ dysfunction. Coronary ischemia, disordered cerebral function (encephalopathy), a cerebrovascular accident, pulmonary edema, and acute arterial bleeding require immediate BP reduction (minutes to hours) to limit or prevent target organ damage and reduce risk.

Hypertensive urgencies. Hypertensive urgencies are severe elevations in BP without evidence of acute or rapidly progressive target organ dysfunction. Elevated BP alone in the absence of symptoms of progressive target organ damage rarely requires emergency therapy. BP can usually be managed by orally administered medications initiated in the emergency room (ER) with appropriate follow-up within days, depending on individual characteristics of the patient. If prompt and appropriate follow-up cannot be ensured, some hypertensive urgencies justify admission and initial management in-hospital. Examples of hypertensive emergencies and urgencies are listed in **Tables C153.1** and **C153.2**.

Table C153.1. Hypertensive Emergencies

Hypertensive encephalopathy
Malignant hypertension (some cases)
Severe hypertension in association with acute complications
    Cerebrovascular
        Intracerebral hemorrhage
        Subarachnoid hemorrhage
        Acute atherothrombotic brain infarction (with severe hypertension)
    Renal
        Rapidly progressive renal failure
    Cardiac
        Acute aortic dissection
        Acute left ventricular failure with pulmonary edema
        Acute myocardial infarction
        Unstable angina
Eclampsia or severe hypertension during pregnancy
Catecholamine excess states
    Pheochromocytoma crisis
    Food or drug interactions (tyramine) with monoamine oxidase inhibitors
    Some cases of rebound hypertension after sudden withdrawal of antihypertensive agents (i.e., clonidine, guanabenz, methyldopa)
Drug-induced hypertension (some cases)
    Overdose with sympathomimetics or drugs with similar action (e.g., phencyclidine, lysergic acid diethylamide, cocaine, phenylpropanolamine)
Head trauma
Postcoronary artery bypass hypertension
Postoperative bleeding at vascular suture lines

Table C153.2. Hypertensive Urgencies

Accelerated and malignant hypertension[a]
Extensive body burns[a]
Acute glomerulonephritis with severe hypertension[a]
Scleroderma crisis
Acute systemic vasculitis with severe hypertension[a]
Surgically related hypertension
  Severe hypertension in patients requiring immediate surgery[a]
  Postoperative hypertension[a]
  Severe hypertension after kidney transplantation
Severe epistaxis
Rebound hypertension after sudden withdrawal of antihypertensive agents
Drug-induced hypertension[a]
  Overdose with sympathomimetic agents
  Metoclopramide-induced hypertensive crisis
  Interaction between an α-adrenergic and a nonselective β-adrenergic antagonist
Episodic and severe hypertension associated with chronic spinal cord injury; autonomic hyperreflexia syndrome[a]

[a]At times may become a true hypertensive emergency.

The majority of patients presenting in the ER with stage 3 hypertension do not have a hypertensive emergency or urgency. The elevated BP is most commonly the result of inadequate treatment of hypertension or nonadherence to an antihypertensive regimen. In a few cases, a previously unrecognized form of secondary hypertension such as renovascular hypertension or primary aldosteronism may be responsible for the acute increase in BP and requires early recognition if specific therapy is to be initiated. Hypertensive patients who do not have a hypertensive emergency or urgency can safely be sent home with oral medications and arrangements made for follow-up within a few days.

Initial Assessment

Early triage is critical to assure the most timely and appropriate therapy for each patient. A thorough but expeditiously performed history and physical evaluation plus selected laboratory studies can ascertain the clinical status of the patient, provide clues to an underlying etiology of the hypertension, assess the degree of target organ involvement, and help select the most appropriate pharmacologic therapy. Initial laboratory studies should include a urinalysis with sediment examination, an electrocardiogram, a blood survey, and complete chemistry profile. A computed tomographic scan of the head should be considered in the comatose patient or when the clinical examination suggests cerebrovascular ischemia or hemorrhage. Cardiac studies are dictated by the presenting syndrome.

The algorithm in **Table C153.3** should assist the clinician in early identification of the true hypertensive emergency for immediate admission and initiation of parenteral therapy. The algorithm also helps in making the distinction between patients with a hypertensive urgency from those with high BP but no evident target organ involvement.

Treatment of Hypertensive Emergencies

Applied pathophysiology. Initial treatment is initiated to obtain a partial reduction in BP to a safer, noncritical level, although not necessarily to achieve normotension because precipitous decrease in BP may cause acute hypoperfusion of critical organs. The heart, brain, and kidneys have autoregulatory mechanisms that protect them from acute ischemia when BP is abruptly reduced within a fairly wide range of BP. The lower limit of autoregulation in hypertensive patients is shifted upward, however, and when autoregulation fails, blood flow to the cerebral, renal, and possibly coronary circulations can fall. The shift in the autoregulatory plateau is a consequence of

Table C153.3. Algorithm: Triage Evaluation

BP (MM HG)	GROUP I—HIGH BP (>180/100 MM HG)	GROUP II—URGENCY (>180/110 MM HG)	GROUP III—EMERGENCY (USUALLY >220/140 MM HG)
Symptoms	Headache Anxiety Often asymptomatic	Severe headache Shortness of breath Edema	Shortness of breath Chest pain Nocturia Dysarthria Weakness Altered consciousness
Examination	No target organ damage No clinical cardiovascular disease	Target organ damage Clinical cardiovascular disease present or stable	Encephalopathy Pulmonary edema Renal insufficiency Cerebrovascular accident Cardiac ischemia
Therapy	Observe 1–3 h Initiate/resume medication(s) Increase dosage of inadequate agent	Observe 3–6 h Lower BP with short-acting oral agents Adjust current therapy	Baseline labs Intravenous line Monitor BP May initiate parenteral therapy in the emergency room
Plan	Arrange follow-up >72 h If no prior evaluation, schedule appointment	Arrange follow-up evaluation <24 h	Immediate admission to intensive care unit Treat to initial goal BP Additional diagnostic studies

BP, blood pressure.
Adapted from Vidt DG. Emergency room management of hypertensive urgencies and emergencies. *J Clin Hypertens (Greenwich)*. 2001;3:158–164.

structural changes in the arterioles of hypertensive individuals, which do not vasodilate adequately in response to a sudden drop in BP (see Chapters A39 and A69).

Treatment goals. Aggressive treatment is appropriate, but initial therapy aimed at partial reduction in BP is probably safer for the patient with a hypertensive emergency. The initial goal of therapy is to reduce mean arterial BP by no more than 25% within minutes to 2 hours or to a BP in the range of 160/100 to 110 mm Hg. In patients with an acute aortic dissection or acute pulmonary edema, an initial reduction of pressure within minutes may be appropriate. For patients with an acute cerebrovascular accident, benefits of early reduction of BP are debatable, except for those with marked elevations (diastolic BP >130 mm Hg) in whom BP reductions should be accomplished more slowly, over a period of hours with careful attention paid to any changes in neurologic status (see Chapter C152). Therapy should be initiated before the results of all initial laboratory studies are available; additional diagnostic studies may be undertaken in situations in which the cause of the hypertension remains in doubt.

Drug therapy. Several very effective agents are available for the treatment of a hypertensive emergency. **Table C153.4** lists those agents that are readily available, together with recommended dosages, routes of administration, onset and duration of action, and selected precautions regarding usage.

Diuretics. With most parenteral agents, rapid reduction of BP is accompanied by sodium and fluid retention, which may lead to resistance to continued drug treatment. The judicious use of loop-active diuretics may be effective initially in volume-overloaded states, such as heart failure, and later in the course of therapy to maintain an adequate urine flow rate and avoid drug pseudotolerance. Loop-active diuretics are not recommended for the routine treatment of hypertensive urgencies or emergencies in the absence of fluid overload because they can cause additional reflex vasoconstriction. Furosemide (40–120 mg) or bumetanide (1–5 mg) can be given intravenously and repeated periodically to maintain an adequate urine flow rate. Alternatively, if a history of hypersensitivity to these agents is present, ethacrynic acid (50–150 mg) can be used. Fenoldopam may be useful when renal insufficiency is present.

Table C153.4. Management of Hypertensive Emergencies

AGENT	DOSE	ONSET/DURATION OF ACTION (AFTER DISCONTINUATION)	PRECAUTIONS
Parenteral vasodilators			
Sodium nitroprusside	0.25–10.00 µg/kg/min as i.v. infusion[a]; maximal dose for 10 min only	Immediate/2–3 min after infusion	Nausea, vomiting, muscle twitching; with prolonged use, may cause thiocyanate intoxication, methemoglobinemia acidosis, cyanide poisoning; bags, bottles, and delivery sets must be light resistant
Glyceryl trinitrate	5–100 µg as i.v. infusion[a]	2–5 min/5–10 min	Headache, tachycardia, vomiting, flushing, methemoglobinemia; requires special delivery systems due to the drug's binding to polyvinyl chloride tubing
Nicardipine	5–15 mg/h i.v. infusion	1–5 min/15–30 min, but may exceed 12 h after prolonged infusion	Tachycardia, nausea, vomiting, headache, increased intracranial pressure, possible protracted hypotension after prolonged infusions
Verapamil	5–10 mg i.v.; can follow with infusion of 3–25 mg/h	1–5 min/30–60 min	Heart block (first-, second-, and third-degree), especially with concomitant digitalis or β-blockers; bradycardia
Diazoxide	50–150 mg as i.v. bolus, repeated or 15–30 mg/min by i.v. infusion	2–5 min/3–12 h	Hypotension, tachycardia, aggravation of angina pectoris, nausea and vomiting, hyperglycemia with repeated injections
Fenoldopam mesylate	0.1–0.3 mg/kg/min i.v. infusion	<5 min/30 min	Headache, tachycardia, flushing, local phlebitis
Hydralazine	10–20 mg as i.v. bolus or 10–40 mg i.m.; repeat every 4–6 h	10 min i.v./ >1 h (i.v.), 20–30 min i.m./4–6 h i.m.	Tachycardia, headache, vomiting, aggravation of angina pectoris
Enalaprilat	0.625–1.250 mg every 6 h i.v.	15–60 min/12–24 h	Renal failure in patients with bilateral artery stenosis, hypotension
Parenteral adrenergic inhibitors			
Labetalol	20–80 mg as i.v. bolus every 10 min; up to 2 mg/min as i.v. infusion	5–10 min/2–6 h	Bronchoconstriction, heart block, orthostatic hypotension
Esmolol	500 µg/kg bolus injection i.v. or 25–100 µg/kg/min by infusion. May repeat bolus after 5 min or increase infusion rate to 300 µg/kg/min	1–5 min/15–30 min	First-degree heart block, congestive heart failure, asthma
Phentolamine	5–15 mg as i.v. bolus	1–2 min/10–30 min	Tachycardia, orthostatic hypotension

[a]Requires a special delivery system.

Table C153.5. **Management of Hypertensive Urgencies: Oral Agents**

AGENT	DOSE	ONSET/DURATION OF ACTION (AFTER DISCONTINUATION)	PRECAUTIONS
Captopril	25 mg p.o., repeat as needed; s.l., 25 mg	15–30 min/6–8 h; s.l. 15–30 min/2–6 h	Hypotension, renal failure in bilateral renal artery stenosis
Clonidine	0.1–0.2 mg p.o., repeat hourly as required to total dose of 0.6 mg	30–60 min/8–16 h	Hypotension, drowsiness, dry mouth
Labetalol	200–400 mg p.o., repeat every 2–3 h	30 min–2 h/2–12 h	Bronchoconstriction, heart block, orthostatic hypotension
Prazosin	1–2 mg p.o., repeat hourly, as needed	1–2 h/8–12 h	Syncope (first dose), palpitations, tachycardia, orthostatic hypotension

Follow-up therapy. Regardless of the type of hypertensive emergency or the antihypertensive agent used to control BP, an objective should be to start an oral regimen as soon as the patient can tolerate it. This allows earlier tapering and discontinuation of parenteral agents. Switching abruptly from intravenous to oral therapy may result in a precipitous rise in BP.

Hypertensive Urgencies

General management. Very high BP levels can be found in asymptomatic patients with newly diagnosed hypertension, poorly controlled BP on current regimens, or noncompliance with previous therapy. No data currently exist to show immediate benefit from acutely lowering BP in asymptomatic patients with severe hypertension, but data do suggest that an aggressive approach may be harmful, especially if arterial vasodilators are used in patients with cardiovascular risk factors. The risk of overly aggressive intervention in any hypertensive urgency must always be considered.

The caveat with hypertensive urgencies is that an elevated BP by itself rarely requires emergency therapy. An effort should be made to separate out patients with severely elevated BP and clinical evidence of target organ damage who may benefit from a period of observation in the ER after the administration of 1 or several oral medications to reduce BP over several hours (**Table C153.5**). If clinically stable, these patients can safely be discharged with oral medications with arrangements made for a follow-up visit within 24 hours in an outpatient setting.

Drug therapy. For many patients with severe hypertension, but without symptoms of target organ dysfunction, initiation of therapy with 2 agents (followed by a third if needed) is appropriate to lower BP over 24 to 48 hours. Such therapy can usually be administered in the outpatient setting, and further drug titration to optimal control can be achieved over several days to weeks as recommended in guidelines for treatment of patients with stage 2 or 3 hypertension.

Follow-up therapy. To discharge the patient from an ER or outpatient setting without a confirmed follow-up appointment is a missed opportunity to get that patient back into treatment—optimal control of BP should be a management goal.

Hypertensive Encephalopathy

General aspects. Hypertensive encephalopathy is a potentially lethal complication of severe hypertension that occurs when an increase in BP exceeds the autoregulatory ability of the brain to maintain constant cerebral perfusion. The resulting disruption of the blood–brain barrier causes diffuse cerebral edema and neurologic dysfunction. The presence of papilledema is the *sine qua non* of hypertensive encephalopathy, but it should be suspected when a severe elevation in BP is accompanied by other nonspecific neurologic signs and symptoms. This is a diagnosis of exclusion and requires that stroke, intracranial hemorrhage, seizure disorder, mental disorder, mass lesions, vasculitis, and encephalitis be ruled out. When it is suspected, however, BP should be promptly lowered as recommended in the management of a hypertensive emergency.

Drug therapy. Agents with a rapid onset of effect that can be titrated to a desirable initial BP goal are preferred. Sodium nitroprusside is an agent of choice because its rapid onset of action and short half-life allow for minute-by-minute control of BP and because it has minimal adverse effects on cerebral blood flow. Nicardipine and labetalol have also proved particularly effective in the management of hypertensive encephalopathy. Maintaining frequent neurologic assessments during the period of BP titration is imperative. BP reduction is often associated with dramatic improvement in cerebral function. Subsequent deterioration in neurologic function requires reevaluation and consideration of other possible diagnoses.

SUGGESTED READING

1. Bedoya LA, Vidt DG. Treatment of the hypertensive emergency. In: Jacobson HR, Striker GE, Klahr S, eds. *The Principles and Practice of Nephrology*, 15th ed. Philadelphia, PA: BC Decker Inc; 1991:547–557.
2. Gales MA. Oral antihypertensives for hypertensive urgencies. *Ann Pharmacother.* 1994;28:352–358.
3. Gifford RW, Jr. Management of hypertensive crises. *JAMA.* 1991;266:829–835.
4. Grossman E, Messerli FH, Grodzicki T, Kowey P. Should a moratorium be placed on sublingual nifedipine capsules given for hypertensive emergencies and pseudoemergencies? *JAMA.* 1996;276:1328–1331.
5. Kaplan NM. Management of hypertensive emergencies. *Lancet.* 1994;344:1335–1338.
6. Murphy C. Hypertensive emergencies. *Emerg Med Clin North Am.* 1995;13:973–1007.
7. Vaughan CJ, Delanty N. Hypertensive emergencies. *Lancet.* 2000;356:411–417.
8. Vidt DG. Emergency room management of hypertensive urgencies and emergencies. *J Clin Hypertens (Greenwich).* 2001;3:158–164.

Chapter C154

Treatment of Hypertension Patients with Ischemic Heart Disease

Clive Rosendorff, MD, PhD, FRCP

KEY POINTS

- In patients at high risk for the development of coronary artery disease, the antihypertensive drugs of first choice are angiotensin-converting enzyme inhibitors or long-acting calcium antagonists.

- The antihypertensive agent of first choice in patients with stable angina is a β-blocker, or if contraindicated, a long-acting calcium antagonist.

- In patients admitted to hospital with an acute coronary syndrome, hypertension should be treated with a β-blocker, or if contraindicated, verapamil or diltiazem in the absence of severe left ventricular dysfunction.

See also Chapters A65–A67, B81, B106, C110, C115–C117, C139, C141, C144, C146, and C163

Coronary artery disease limits myocardial perfusion and therefore oxygen supply (see Chapter A67). Hypertension increases myocardial oxygen demand because of the increased output impedance to left ventricular (LV) ejection, and hypertension is a common cause of LV hypertrophy. This combination of decreased oxygen supply and increased oxygen demand explains why hypertensive patients are more likely than normotensive people to have a myocardial infarction (MI) or other major coronary event and are at higher risk of dying after an acute MI.

Blood Pressure Targets in Patients with Coronary Disease

Diastolic blood pressure and the J curve. Many studies have shown that there is a continuous relationship between diastolic blood pressure (DBP) and the risk of a coronary event: the lower the DBP, the lower the risk. Some studies, however, have shown that there is a lower DBP limit of approximately 85 mm Hg below which the MI rate begins to climb, thus producing a J-shaped curve to describe the DBP-coronary risk relationship. The likely mechanism for this effect is that myocardial blood flow occurs almost entirely in diastole, and patients with occlusive coronary artery disease are less tolerant of low DBPs, especially if there is additional myocardial oxygen demand from LV hypertrophy. The Hypertension Optimal Treatment (HOT) trial was designed to answer prospectively the question whether aggressive lowering of the DBP would have a deleterious effect on cardiovascular events. In HOT, there did seem to be a small upswing in major cardiovascular events (MI and cardiovascular mortality but not stroke or renal failure) at DBP below 80 mm Hg. This apparent myocardial susceptibility to low diastolic perfusion pressures is consistent with the notion that stroke morbidity and mortality is best correlated with the level of systolic blood pressure (BP), whereas the best predictor of coronary events may be pulse pressure (see Chapter A60).

Systolic blood pressure. Pulse pressure is usually greatest in isolated systolic hypertension, in which the DBP is normal and often below 80 mm Hg, even pretreatment. However, in the elderly with isolated systolic hypertension and low DBP, no J-shaped curve has been described with antihypertensive therapy, although DBP may be reduced even further. In fact, the 3 outcome trials in the elderly with isolated systolic hypertension [Systolic Hypertension in the Elderly Program (SHEP), Systolic Hypertension in Europe (SYST-Eur), and Systolic Hypertension in China (SYST-China)] together showed decreases of 25% in MI including sudden death in the active treatment group compared with those who received placebo. Diabetic patients benefited significantly from aggressive BP lowering in the HOT trial, so that current recommendations are to lower BP in diabetic patients to below 130/85 mm Hg. Nevertheless, it may be prudent to avoid lowering the DBP below 80 mm Hg in patients with significant coronary artery disease.

Prevention of Coronary Events with Antihypertensive Drugs

See **Table C154.1.**

Diuretics and β-blockers. Early clinical trials [Hypertension Detection and Follow-Up Program (HDFP), Medical Research Council (MRC), SHEP, Swedish Trial in Old Patients with Hypertension (STOP), and MRC-elderly] used diuretics, sympathetic blocking agents, and β-blockers to investigate the value of primary prevention. These studies were based on DBP reduction and, in general, showed a significant benefit of treatment for reducing stroke morbidity and mortality in all age groups. Reduction in ischemic heart disease (IHD) was somewhat disappointing, except in older patients. In SHEP, the benefit of diuretic or β-blocker therapy on MI (25% reduction) was still not as great as it was for stroke (36% reduction). Many explanations have been advanced for the dissociation between the good stroke outcomes and the mediocre IHD ones, includ-

Table C154.1. Antihypertensive Drugs That Prevent Coronary Events

ACRONYM	REPORT	DURATION (YR)	TREATMENT	PATIENTS	MEAN AGE (YR)	TOTAL CORONARY EVENTS/1,000 PATIENTS/YR	
						ACTIVE	CONTROL/REFERENCE
Classic trials							
HDFP	1979	5	Diuretics ± reserpine/methyl-dopa ± hydralazine ± guanethidine vs. referred care	10,940	51	6	7
MRC	1985	5	Bendrofluazide or propranolol vs. placebo	17,354	51	5	4
SHEP	1991	4.5	Chlorthalidone or atenolol vs. placebo	4,736	72	15	20
STOP	1992	2	3 β-blockers + HCTZ vs. placebo	1,627	76	17	25
MRC-Elderly	1992	5.8	Atenolol or HCTZ + amiloride vs. placebo	4,396	70	7 (diuretic) 12 (β-blocker)	13
Modern trials							
Calcium channel blockers							
SYST-Eur	1997	2	Nitrendipine ± enalapril ± HCTZ vs. placebo	4,695	70	34	44
SYST-China	1998	2	Nitrendipine ± captopril or HCTZ vs. placebo	2,394	67	5	7
NORDIL	2000	5	Diltiazem (± ACEI ± diuretic or α-blocker) vs. diuretic + β-blocker (±ACEI or α-blocker)	10,881	60	6	7
INSIGHT	2000	4	Nifedipine vs. co-amilozide (HCTZ + amiloride) ± atenolol ± enalapril	6,321	65	16	17
ACE inhibitors							
UKPDS	1998	9	Captopril vs. atenolol ± furo-semide ± nifedipine ± meth-yldopa ± prazosin	758	56	26	23
CAPP	1999	6	Captopril vs. β-blockers ± diuretics	10,985	53	13	13
STOP-2	1999	6	ACE inhibitors vs. calcium antagonists or diuretic and/or β-blocker	6,614	76	13	14 (diuretics/β-blocker) 17 (calcium antago-nists)
Trials in high-risk patients							
Calcium channel blockers							
MIDAS (Multi-center Israd-ipine Diuretic Atherosclerosis Study)	1996	3	Isradipine vs. HCTZ	883	59	14	8
PREVENT (Pro-spective Ran-domized Evaluation of the Vascular Effects of Nor-vasc Trial)	2000	3	Amlodipine vs. placebo	825	57	21	25
ACE inhibitors							
HOPE	2000	5	Ramipril vs. placebo	9,297	67	93	104
PART-2	2000	4	Ramipril vs. placebo	617	61	56	61
Trials of angiotensin receptor blockers							
LIFE	2002	4.8	Losartan vs. atenolol	9,193	67	16.6	15.3

ACE, angiotensin-converting enzyme; ACEI, angiotensin I-converting enzyme; HCTZ, hydrochlorothiazide.
Note: Study names not spelled out in the table can be found in the text.

ing the potential arrhythmogenic effects of diuretic-induced hypokalemia.

Antihypertensive and Lipid-Lowering Treatment to Prevent Heart Attack Trial. The Antihypertensive and Lipid-Lowering Treatment to Prevent Heart Attack Trial (ALLHAT) in high-risk hypertensive patients showed no significant differ-ence between chlorthalidone, lisinopril, and amlodipine in nonfatal myocardial infarction plus coronary heart disease death (primary outcome of the study), combined coronary heart disease (primary outcome, coronary revascularization, hospitalized angina), or all-cause mortality. There was a superi-ority of a diuretic (chlorthalidone) over the ACE inhibitor lisin-opril in preventing stroke, and over the α-blocker doxazosin, the calcium antagonist amlodipine, and lisinopril in preventing heart failure. The results of ALLHAT were interpreted by the authors to recommend thiazide diuretics as first-line therapy for hypertensive patients who do not have compelling indication for other drugs. Diuretics probably should be part of any regimen that includes 2 or more antihypertensive drugs.

Calcium antagonists. In the last decade, trials of calcium antagonists (CAs) for the primary prevention of cardiovascular complications of hypertension [SYST-Eur, Nordic Diltiazem Study (NORDIL), SYST-China, and Intervention as a Goal in Hypertension Treatment (INSIGHT)] tended to show a significant degree of prevention of stroke, compared to placebo, diuretic, β-blocker alone, or combined therapy. The absolute risk reduction in IHD deaths and nonfatal coronary events was less impressive, with the exception of the SYST-Eur study. In SYST-Eur, however, the reference drug was placebo, and a significant number of patients in the active treatment group received 1 of the add-on agents, including enalapril, which may have influenced the results. A recent metaanalysis (Pahor et al.) of CAs as first-line antihypertensive treatment suggested that CAs were inferior to angiotensin-converting enzyme (ACE) inhibitors, with a greater risk for MI (26%), congestive heart failure (25%), and major cardiovascular events (10%), although they were as effective as ACE inhibitors in the reduction of all-cause mortality and stroke.

Angiotensin-converting enzyme inhibitors. In general, thiazide diuretics or ACE inhibitors are preferred as first-line drugs for the treatment of hypertension in patients with coronary artery disease, except of course in cases in which β-blockers are indicated for angina or arrhythmia control. Trials of ACE inhibitors [Captopril Prevention Project (CAPP) and U.K. Prospective Diabetes Study (UKPDS)] showed significant benefit of BP lowering on overall cardiovascular morbidity and mortality, especially stroke, but did not demonstrate a clearcut benefit of ACE inhibitors over conventional therapy (diuretics, β-blockers, or both) for the prevention of acute coronary events. However, STOP-2 did show that, for MI, ACE inhibitors were significantly better than CAs, and also better than conventional therapy (diuretics, β-blockers, or both), although given the low power of the study, the latter did not achieve statistical significance. In more recent trials of ACE inhibitors in patients with established coronary artery disease or high risk for coronary artery disease, the benefits of ACE inhibitors were clear. In Heart Outcomes Prevention Evaluation (HOPE), after 5 years, the relative risk for death from cardiovascular causes in the ramipril-treated group versus the placebo-treated group was 0.74; for MI, 0.80; for revascularization procedures, 0.85; for cardiac arrest, 0.63; and for heart failure, 0.77 (all highly significant). The results applied equally to hypertensive and nonhypertensive patients, and to patients with known IHD and those without coronary vascular disease. Substudies of HOPE revealed that ACE inhibition reduced progression of atherosclerosis and improved myocardial remodeling. In the smaller Prevention of Atherosclerosis with Ramipril Treatment-2 (PART-2) trial of ramipril versus placebo in high-risk patients, the treated group had a relative risk for fatal coronary artery disease of 0.43 but no difference in the MI or unstable angina rate. These relatively recent studies have served to reinforce the general idea, based on many trials, that ACE inhibition is protective in high-risk patients with and without LV dysfunction.

Angiotensin receptor blockers. The use of angiotensin receptor blockers for the treatment of hypertension in patients with coronary artery disease has a solid foundation in animal studies and surrogate end-point studies in humans. The Losartan Intervention for Endpoint (LIFE) study showed that losartan prevents more strokes and cardiovascular deaths than atenolol, but there were no significant differences in the rate of MI or hospital admissions for angina in this study.

Hypertension Treatment in Patients with Stable Angina

Nonpharmacologic and risk-factor management. The treatment of patients with symptomatic coronary artery disease is directed toward preventing MI and death and toward reducing the symptoms of angina and the occurrence of ischemia. Treatment of risk factors include, in addition to BP control, smoking cessation, management of diabetes, exercise training, lipid lowering, and weight reduction in obese patients. Less well-established are therapy with folate and vitamin B_6 in patients with elevated homocysteine levels. There is compelling evidence for the use of antiplatelet agents, aspirin if not contraindicated, otherwise clopidogrel.

β-Blockers and calcium antagonists. β-Blockers reduce angina symptoms, improve mortality, and lower BP, and should be the first drug of choice in hypertensive patients with coronary artery disease and stable angina (see Chapter C140). β-Blockers reduce cardiac output, heart rate, and slow atrioventricular conduction. The reduced inotropy and heart rate decrease myocardial oxygen demand. The slowing of heart rate prolongs the diastolic perfusion time of the coronary arteries, enhancing myocardial perfusion. The reduced cardiac output lowers BP, although there is also a significant BP-lowering effect from the blockade of β-adrenoreceptors on the cells of the renal juxtaglomerular apparatus, the major source of circulating renin. Diabetes is not a contraindication to the use of β-blockers, although the patient and doctor should be aware that the symptoms of hypoglycemia may be masked. In hypertensive LV failure, β-blockers (especially carvedilol or metoprolol) may be used as a component of the antifailure therapy, but should be started at a very low dose and titrated up very slowly (see Chapters C155 and C156). When there are contraindications to the use of β-blockers, such as obstructive airways disease, severe peripheral vascular disease, or severe bradyarrhythmias such as a high degree of atrioventricular block or the sick sinus syndrome, CAs, either long-acting dihydropyridine agents (such as amlodipine, felodipine, or a long-acting formulation of nifedipine) or nondihydropyridine drugs such as verapamil or diltiazem, are appropriate therapy for angina and hypertension. Short-acting dihydropyridine CAs have the potential to enhance the risk of adverse cardiac events and should be avoided.

One controlled study [Total Ischemic Burden European Trial (TIBET)] comparing β-blockers with CAs has reported equal efficacy in controlling stable angina, but most studies have shown β-blockers to be superior [Angina Prognosis Study in Stockholm (APSIS), Total Ischemic Burden Bisoprolol Study (TIBBS)]. Combining a β-blocker with an appropriate CA enhances antianginal efficacy. Because of the increased risk of severe bradycardia or heart block if β-blockers are used together with verapamil or diltiazem, long-acting dihydropyridine CAs are preferred for combination therapy. Other important therapies are short- or long-acting nitrates (not with sildenafil!) and lipid-lowering agents, if indicated. The role of revascularization procedures is outside the scope of this review.

Hypertension Treatment in Patients with Acute Coronary Syndromes

Unstable angina and non-ST segment elevation myocardial infarction.
Hospitalization, usually in a coronary care unit, is indicated for (a) patients with unstable angina (rest angina, new onset angina, increasing frequency and intensity of previously stable angina, or angina within 6 weeks of MI, but with normal cardiac markers of ischemia) or (b) with non-ST segment elevation MI [non-ST–elevation myocardial infarction (NSTEMI), elevated markers of myocardial injury, such as troponin I or T, or the MB isoenzyme of creatine phosphokinase, but without ST segment elevation]. Antiischemic therapy includes bed rest, continuous electrocardiogram monitoring, intravenous nitroglycerin, supplemental oxygen, morphine sulfate, β-blocker [alternatively a nondihydropyridine CA (e.g., verapamil or diltiazem) in the absence of contraindications and severe LV dysfunction]. An ACE inhibitor should be used in patients with diabetes or if hypertension persists despite treatment with nitroglycerin and a β-blocker or if there is LV systolic dysfunction or congestive heart failure.

Antiplatelet therapy with aspirin and clopidogrel and anticoagulant therapy, intravenous unfractionated heparin or subcutaneous low-molecular-weight heparin, is standard therapy. A platelet glycoprotein IIb/IIIa receptor antagonist (e.g., intravenous abciximab or oral eptifibatide or tirofiban) can be added in patients with continuing ischemia or other high-risk features and in patients in whom a percutaneous coronary intervention is planned. Because of the increased risk of hemorrhagic stroke in patients with uncontrolled hypertension who are given antiplatelet or anticoagulant therapy, hypertension should be treated aggressively. Lipid-lowering therapy is needed for patients whose low-density lipoprotein cholesterol is greater than 100 mg per dL, or whose high-density lipopro-

tein cholesterol is less than 40 mg per dL. In general, the indications for percutaneous coronary interventions and coronary artery bypass grafting are similar to those in stable angina. High-risk patients with LV systolic dysfunction, left main disease, or severe 3 vessel or 2 vessel disease with severe proximal left anterior descending coronary artery involvement should be considered for coronary artery bypass graft; lesser degrees of coronary artery disease should be evaluated for percutaneous coronary intervention on an individual basis. Follow-up BP should be controlled with a goal BP of <130/85 mm Hg.

ST-segment elevation myocardial infarction.
The management of ST-segment elevation MI (STEMI) is similar to that for unstable angina and NSTEMI, except that arrhythmia control and primary percutaneous transluminal angioplasty or thrombolytic therapy become more important. Also, in the absence of contraindications, all patients with STEMI, whether they are hypertensive or not, should receive a β-blocker and ACE inhibitor. Intravenous β-blocker therapy should be started within 12 hours of the onset of chest pain, followed by an oral β-blocker within the first 2 days. A number of large, randomized clinical trials have shown a significant morbidity and mortality benefit of ACE inhibitors started early in the course of acute STEMI. CAs do not reduce mortality rates in the setting of acute MI and should not be used except when β-blockers are contraindicated or are inadequate to control angina or supraventricular tachycardia or when adjunct therapy for BP control is necessary.

SUGGESTED READING

1. 1999 Updated ACC/AHA Guidelines for the management of patients with acute myocardial infarction. *Circulation.* 1999;100:1016–1030.
2. ACC/AHA/ACP-ASIM Guidelines for the management of patients with chronic stable angina. *Circulation.* 1999;99:2829–2848.
3. ACC/AHA Guidelines for the management of patients with unstable angina and non-ST-segment elevation myocardial infarction. *Circulation.* 2000;102:1193–1209.
4. Chrysant GS, Oparil S. Treatment of hypertension in the patient with cardiovascular disease. In: Antman EM, ed. *Cardiovascular Therapeutics.* 2nd ed. Philadelphia, PA: W.B. Saunders Company; 2002:768–795.
5. DeQuattro V, Li D, Wei H, Feng M. A review of hypertension clinical trials on morbidity/mortality. *Cardiology Special Edition.* 2001;7:57–70.
6. Pahor M, Psaty BM, Alderman MH, et al. Health outcomes associated with calcium antagonists compared with other first-line antihypertensive therapies: a meta-analysis of randomised controlled trials. *Lancet.* 2000;356:1949–1954.
7. Sleight P. Angiotensin II and trials of cardiovascular outcomes. *Am J Cardiol.* 2002;89:11A–16A.
8. Staessen JA, Wang J-G, Thijs L. Cardiovascular protection and blood pressure reduction: a meta-analysis. *Lancet.* 2001;358:1305–1315.

Management of Hypertensive Patients with Left Ventricular Hypertrophy and Diastolic Dysfunction

Richard B. Devereux, MD

KEY POINTS

- Left ventricular hypertrophy is an independent risk factor that doubles the risk of cardiovascular events and deaths.

- Patterns of left ventricular dysfunction with left ventricular hypertrophy include low midwall shortening with normal or minimally reduced ejection fraction, impaired diastolic filling with reduced late diastolic compliance (i.e., restrictive physiology), reduced ejection fraction, or combinations of impaired relaxation and compliance.

- Optimal management of left ventricular hypertrophy depends on accurately delineating the pattern of left ventricular dysfunction, relating the symptom complex to the underlying disorder, and matching the treatment to the pattern observed.

- Regression of left ventricular hypertrophy improves cardiovascular function and prognosis.

See also Chapters A59–A62, B83, C110, C115, C116, C120, C127, C139–C141, C144, C145, C154, and C156

Left ventricular hypertrophy (LVH) is a direct consequence of hypertension that functions as an independent factor for cardiovascular disease events. Effective antihypertensive therapy reduces LVH, improves cardiac function, and reduces risk.

Prognostic and Therapeutic Implications of Left Ventricular Hypertrophy and Abnormal Left Ventricular Geometry

Individuals with echocardiographic or electrocardiographic evidence of LVH are more than twice as likely to experience cardiovascular events and death (**Figure C155.1**) (see Chapter

B83) in a variety of population-based samples, including blacks, whites, women, men, and patients with or without coronary artery disease. A genetic component may also exist (see Chapter A78). The attributable risk of LVH for all-cause mortality is even greater than that of single- and multi-vessel coronary artery disease or low left ventricular (LV) ejection fraction (EF). In addition, evidence from some studies suggests that concentric LV geometry, characterized by a high relative wall thickness, is associated with a further increment in the rate of cardiovascular events. Finally, several studies using echocardiography or electrocardiography, each with design limitations, have suggested that LVH regression is associated with a lowered

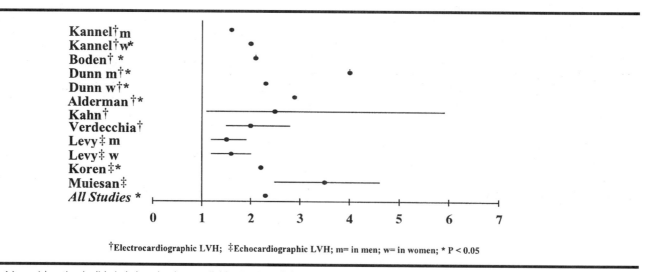

†Electrocardiographic LVH; ‡Echocardiographic LVH; m= in men; w= in women; * P < 0.05

Figure C155.1. Mean risk ratios (*solid circles*) and, when available, 95% confidence interval (*horizontal lines*) of baseline left ventricular hypertrophy (LVH) for subsequent cardiovascular morbidity in available studies. (From Vakili BA, Okin PM, Devereux RB. Prognostic significance of left ventricular hypertrophy. *Am Heart J.* 2001;141:334–341, with permission.)

event rate, suggesting that LVH regression should be a treatment goal in hypertension.

Assessment of Left Ventricular Hypertrophy

Echocardiographic definition of left ventricular hypertrophy. Echocardiography provides a sensitive and widely available tool for evaluating LV structure and function. Primary LV measurements of septal and posterior wall thickness and of LV internal dimension by the American Society of Echocardiography M-mode or 2-D methods allow calculation of LV mass by a formula validated by necropsy (r = 0.92, N = 52), with good reproducibility in a large series of hypertensive adults (intra-class correlation coefficient = 0.93). The relative wall thickness (ratio of LV wall thickness to chamber radius) provides a useful measure of LV concentricity.

High ejection fraction paradox. Echocardiograms or nuclear angiograms show high LV EF in 15% to 20% of patients with mild hypertension despite increased afterload. Part of this apparent paradox is due to a technical artifact caused by the fact that EF has been traditionally measured at the endocardium, whereas the average myocardial fiber is located at the midwall. LV wall thickening raises EF for any level of midwall shortening (MWS). Thus, myocardial contractility is assessed more accurately by expressing MWS as a percentage of the value predicted for circumferential end-systolic stress at the level of the LV midwall. Stress-corrected MWS is subnormal in approximately 20% of patients with mild to moderate hypertension and is above the upper limit of normal in only 2% or fewer of hypertensives.

Monitoring left ventricular hypertrophy as a surrogate end point. If regression of LVH is to be used as a surrogate end point in treatment of hypertensive patients, the methods of monitoring LV mass need to have good reliability with little regression to the mean. The reliability of echocardiographic LV size and wall thicknesses and LV mass and geometry, as expressed by relative wall thickness, was assessed in a sample of hypertensive patients with LVH recruited into the Prospective Randomized Enalapril Study Evaluating Regression of Ventricular Enlargement (PRESERVE) trial (N = 183). Readings by 1 blinded highly experienced reader of 2 echocardiograms performed approximately 6 weeks apart showed that there was a close relationship between LV mass determinations on the first and second echocardiograms (intraclass correlation coefficient = 0.93, $p <0.001$), with no evidence of regression to the mean except at the highest level of LV mass.

Clinical Studies of Left Ventricular Hypertrophy Regression

Metaanalyses. A metaanalysis of LVH regression considered 50 double-blind, randomized, parallel-group controlled clinical studies published through 1996 that included 13 placebo arms (N = 165) and 89 active treatment arms (N = 1,550); there were 15 studies (N = 304) with diuretics, 23 (N = 367) with β-blockers, 26 (N = 441) with calcium antagonists, and 25 (N = 438) with angiotensin-converting enzyme (ACE) inhibitors; mean duration of treatment was 29 weeks. Several factors

other than treatment were found to influence the degree of LVH regression. Predictors of LV mass reduction during treatment were higher pretreatment LV mass (r = 0.53), greater fall in systolic blood pressure (BP) (r = 0.26) or diastolic BP (r = 0.28), and longer duration of treatment (r = 0.36). After consideration of these variables, the least reduction of LV mass occurred with β-blockers and the greatest regression with ACE inhibitors ($p <.05$) and calcium antagonists ($p = .09$).

Comparator trials. Other studies have revealed a greater reduction of 24-hour pressure in diuretic-treated patients but greater LV mass reduction with ACE inhibition. The PRESERVE trial compared the effects of once daily enalapril and slow-release nifedipine. Over 70% of patients had effective BP control, and both medications reduced LV mass index substantially (by 15–17 g/m^2) at 6 and 12 months; decreased relative wall thickness suggests favorable LV remodeling. The Losartan Intervention For Endpoint Reduction in Hypertension (LIFE) trial studied composite end point reduction (stroke, myocardial infarction, cardiovascular death) in 9,193 individuals with LVH in a randomized, double-blind, parallel group design comparing the effects of losartan versus atenolol. Cornell voltage-duration product and the Sokolow-Lyon voltage combination were reduced significantly more (both $p <.001$) by losartan than atenolol therapy despite equivalent BP lowering, confirming that effective LVH regression is achieved by interruption of the renin-angiotensin system. In the large (N = 960) echocardiographic substudy of LIFE, prevention of increased stroke volume during antihypertensive therapy potentiated the LVH regression at any given degree of BP reduction. Furthermore, the degree of LVH regression was proportional to the degree of improvement in LV systolic and diastolic function.

Assessment of Left Ventricular Diastolic Function

Pathophysiology. LV diastolic function is defined by LV filling rates in relation to filling pressure. Because noninvasive methods do not provide intracardiac pressure measurements, LV diastolic filling is analyzed in 2 phases. Early diastolic filling is predominately influenced by active myocardial relaxation together with left atrium to LV pressure gradient. Late diastolic filling is reduced by increased passive stiffness of the LV due to fibrosis, higher LV relative wall thickness, or reduced left atrial to LV pressure gradient.

Mitral flow analysis. The measurements that are needed to produce a simple classification of the patterns of LV diastolic filling are based on Doppler analysis of mitral valve flow patterns. Critical measurements include (a) the peak early diastolic and atrial-phase filling velocities (E and A), (b) time required for E velocity to reach 0 ("deceleration time"), and (c) the interval between LV ejection for 1 heart beat and the beginning of transmitral blood flow for the next ("isovolumic relaxation time"). In middle-aged to elderly adults, E/A <0.8 is subnormal, whereas a ratio higher than 1.5 is supranormal, suggesting the presence of impaired relaxation or "restrictive cardiomyopathy" due to increased LV stiffness. The deceleration time is normally 150 to 250 milliseconds, with longer values suggesting impaired relaxation and shorter ones seen with restrictive physiology. Isovolumic relaxation times of 105 msec or more are prolonged in middle and older age. Impaired relaxation can be diagnosed confidently by the combination of low E/A, long isovolumic relaxation time, and long deceleration time. Restrictive filling can be diagnosed by the combination of short deceleration time and isovolumic relaxation time with E/A >1.5.

Spectrum of Left Ventricular Dysfunction in Hypertension and Left Ventricular Hypertrophy

LV dysfunction in hypertensive patients occurs as part of a complex spectrum that includes reduced contractility, LV geometric adaptation, abnormalities of LV diastolic filling, and dilated cardiomyopathy. Optimal management requires an orderly approach that delineates and relates the pattern of LV dysfunction to the symptoms and the therapy.

Left ventricular filling patterns in hypertension. In population-based samples of individuals with stage 1 or 2 hypertension, one-third to one-half have evidence of impaired LV relaxation, 3% show signs of restrictive LV filling, and 40% to 60% have normal transmitral flow patterns of LV filling (stage 3 hypertension). In more severely hypertensive patients, approximately two-thirds have abnormal relaxation, 4% have evidence of restrictive filling, one-eighth show a "pseudonormal" filling pattern (combining features of impaired relaxation and restrictive filling); only approximately one-sixth have normal filling.

Left ventricular dysfunction. In hypertension, the spectrum of LV dysfunction includes reduced EF, reduced myocardial contractility with preserved EF, impaired early diastolic LV relaxation, restrictive LV passive filling in late diastole, and various combinations of these abnormalities. Patterns of LV dysfunction are influenced by age, hypertension severity, and concomitant diseases. Reduced LV EF is relatively rare in uncomplicated asymptomatic patients with stage 1 hypertension without diabetes or renal failure (<2%). Mildly elevated EF may be seen in as many as 15% of such patients (see the section High ejection fraction paradox). In the biracial, population-based sample of hypertensive adults in the Hypertension Genetic Epidemiology Network Blood Pressure Study (HyperGEN), which did not exclude symptomatic individuals, 10% had mildly reduced EFs (40%–54%), and 3% had LV EFs <40%. Among the patients with more severe hypertension in the LIFE cohort, approximately 20% had LV EF ≤54%.

Predictors of heart failure. In echocardiographic surveys, approximately 5% of hypertensive patients have mildly decreased LV EF, and 1% have severely reduced EF (<40%) without overt heart failure. Heart failure occurs in fewer than 1% of hypertensive patients with normal EF, 5% with mild LV systolic dysfunction, and >25% with EF <40%. Similarly, heart failure occurs in approximately 2% with normal mitral E/A ratios, 5% with low E/A and in 25% with high E/A ratios. Subtle symptoms may be even more common than overt failure, including avoidance of previously routine activities and reduced performance on objective exercise tests.

Left ventricular dysfunction predicts future cardiovascular events. For instance, in a >10-year follow-up of initially asymptomatic hypertensive patients, low stress-corrected LV MWS predicted cardiovascular events and cardiovascular

death, whereas low EF occurred too uncommonly to be a significant predictor. Despite a normal EF (≤60% or ≤66%, respectively), there may be subnormal MWS when the LV wall thickness is >1.1 cm or >1.3 cm, respectively. Cardiovascular death rates are increased in individuals with extremes of low or high E/A ratios, independent of LV EF.

Management of Patients with Left Ventricular Dysfunction

Correct management of LV dysfunction depends on matching the profile of the abnormality to the treatment.

Impaired diastolic function filling with normal and increased systolic function. No available treatment directly improves LV diastolic filling as its exclusive primary action. Because of the strong associations between poorly controlled hypertension and abnormal LV geometry (concentric or eccentric hypertrophy or concentric remodeling), the goals of treatment should be to optimize BP control and to normalize LV geometry. At present, available clinical final data favor angiotensin receptor antagonists, ACE inhibitors, and long-acting calcium antagonists, in that order. A common clinical scenario is that of a patient with dyspnea or other features of heart failure in whom an echocardiogram reveals a small LV chamber size associated with high EF, poor relaxation, and the formation of systolic intracavitary gradients within the left ventricle. These patients may benefit from slowing the heart rate with β-blockers, verapamil, or diltiazem. Because they often have orthostatic hypotension due to volume depletion, diuretics or marked sodium-restriction may exacerbate the condition. Restrictive filling is usually associated with myocardial fibrosis; whether selective aldosterone antagonists ameliorate cardiac fibrosis is an experimental question that requires further study.

Hypertension with low left ventricular midwall function. Low LV MWS is strongly associated with LV hypertrophy and high relative wall thickness. Therapy should be aimed primarily at reversing LVH. ACE inhibitors, angiotensin receptor antagonists, calcium antagonists, diuretics, and β-blockers all have documented benefit, in descending order.

Hypertension with mild left ventricular systolic dysfunction. The syndrome of low LV EF is defined by an EF <55% by echo or <50% by nuclear angiogram or cardiac catheterization. LV diastolic filling pattern is then assessed by Doppler mitral inflow patterns or from nuclear angiograms. If BP is not controlled, a slightly reduced LV EF is most likely due to increased afterload. The treating physician should select an appropriate antihypertensive medication and then reevaluate LV function when BP is controlled. If arterial pressure is only minimally elevated or in the high normal range and LV EF is reduced, medications known to benefit patients with severe LV systolic dysfunction should be used, including ACE inhibitors, angiotensin receptor antagonists, β-blockers, or spironolactone. It is highly probable but as yet unproven that lower BP targets (130/80 mm Hg or lower) should be sought, as in diabetic patients.

Impaired systolic and diastolic function. Reduced systolic function is usually due to coronary artery disease or cardiomyopathy, which may occur in approximately 1% of hypertensive patients without overt heart failure. In this setting, it is appropriate to use angiotensin receptor antagonists, ACE inhibitors, β-blockers, hydralazine and nitrate in combination, or spironolactone. However, the prognosis is still poor in patients with evidence of restrictive LV filling. Investigation of agents to treat myocardial fibrosis or impaired relaxation directly is in early phases.

SUGGESTED READING

1. Bella JN, Palmieri V, Liu JE, et al. Mitral E/A ratio as a predictor of mortality in middle-aged and elderly adults: The Strong Heart Study. *Circulation.* 2002;105:1928–1933.
2. Dahlöf B, Devereux RB, Kjeldsen SE, et al. for the LIFE study group. Cardiovascular morbidity and mortality in the Losartan Intervention for Endpoint reduction in hypertension study (LIFE): a randomised trial against atenolol. *Lancet.* 2002;359:995–1003.
3. Devereux RB, Bella JN, Palmieri V, et al. Prevalence and correlates of left ventricular systolic dysfunction in a bi-racial sample of hypertensive adults: The HyperGEN Study. *Hypertension.* 2001;38:417–423.
4. Devereux RB, Palmieri V, Sharpe N, et al. Effects of once-daily angiotensin converting enzyme inhibition and calcium channel blockade-based antihypertensive treatment regimens on left ventricular hypertrophy and diastolic filling in hypertension: The PRESERVE Trial. *Circulation.* 2001;104:1248–1254.
5. Devereux RB, Roman MJ, Paranicas M, et al. A population-based assessment of left ventricular systolic dysfunction in middle-aged and older adults: The Strong Heart Study. *Am Heart J.* 2001;141:439–446.
6. Gandhi SK, Powers JC, Nomeir AM, et al. The pathogenesis of acute pulmonary edema associated with hypertension. *N Engl J Med.* 2001;344:17–22.
7. Roman MJ, Alderman MH, Pickering TG, et al. Differential effects of angiotensin converting enzyme inhibition and diuretic therapy on reductions in ambulatory blood pressure, left ventricular mass, and vascular hypertrophy. *Am J Hypertens.* 1998;11:387–396.
8. Vakili BA, Okin PM, Devereux RB. Prognostic significance of left ventricular hypertrophy. *Am Heart J.* 2001;141:334–341.
9. Wachtell K, Bella JN, Rokkedal J, et al. Change in diastolic left ventricular filling after one year of antihypertensive treatment: The LIFE trial. *Circulation.* 2002;105:1071–1076.
10. Wachtell K, Smith G, Gerdts E, et al. Left ventricular diastolic filling patterns in hypertensive patients with electrocardiographic left ventricular hypertrophy (The LIFE Study). *Am J Cardiol.* 2000;85:466–472.

Chapter C156

Treatment of Hypertensive Patients with Left Ventricular Systolic Dysfunction

John B. Kostis, MD

KEY POINTS

- Left ventricular systolic dysfunction and heart failure are common complications of aging and hypertension, in part because of increased survival after myocardial infarction.

- Heart failure can be staged according to the recommendations of the American College of Cardiology/American Heart Association Consensus Statement: stage A (at risk), stage B (asymptomatic left ventricular dysfunction), stage C (symptomatic heart failure), and stage D (end-stage disease).

- Control of hypertension especially using thiazide diuretics and fastidious management of cholesterol and other risk factors for coronary artery disease are essential for the prevention of heart failure.

- Additional therapeutic recommendations include angiotensin-converting enzyme inhibitors for stages A through D, β-blockers for stages B through D, and digitalis/diuretic for stages C through D heart failure.

See also Chapters A59–A62, A67, B81, B106, C110, C115–C117, C121, C127, C139–C142, C144–C146, C150, C154, and C155

In the last several decades, age-adjusted mortality from cardiovascular disease has decreased by approximately 50% in men and women and in different racial subsets. Fatality from acute myocardial infarction has also decreased with the advent of thrombolytic therapy, percutaneous interventions, and adjunctive pharmacologic therapy. These factors, as well as the relatively poor control of hypertension in the community and the aging of the general population, have resulted in an increased incidence of left ventricular (LV) systolic dysfunction and heart failure (HF). The prognosis of hypertensive HF patients is poor because of the high rate of morbid and mortal events imposed by systolic LV dysfunction and the frequently coexisting coronary artery disease. Better blood pressure (BP) control and use of renin-angiotensin blocking drugs markedly improve survival, however.

Pathogenesis of Left Ventricular Systolic Dysfunction

LV dysfunction and systolic HF in most people are the result of 2 overlapping but distinct pathways: hypertension and coronary artery disease.

Hypertension and aging. Uncontrolled hypertension and aging interact to exacerbate the development of HF (see Chapters A59–A62, B81, B83, C121, and C155), especially in the presence of obesity or diabetes, which further contribute to increased LV mass, LV wall thickness, and abnormal diastolic LV filling patterns. Impaired LV filling may cause the syndrome of diastolic HF with symptoms due to high pulmonary venous pressure and decreased cardiac output when the diastolic filling abnormalities are severe (see Chapter C155). In addition, LV hypertrophy due to systolic overload imposed by hypertension is associated with changes in gene expression. Impairment of systolic function is initially compensated by increased LV thickness, but ultimately, LV remodeling associated with neurohormonal activation, increased wall tension, apoptosis, myocyte loss, fibrosis, chamber dilatation, and depressed systolic function leads to HF.

Coronary artery disease. The second pathway that commonly leads to HF is LV systolic dysfunction after acute myocardial infarction, especially when dyslipidemia, diabetes, or smoking is also present. Myocardial infarction leads to reduced cardiac output, neurohormonal activation, and remodeling of the whole ventricle, resulting in LV dilatation, elevated filling pressure, systolic dysfunction, and, ultimately, systolic HF (see Chapter A62).

Other causes of heart failure. Patients with hypertension may have systolic dysfunction secondary to other causes unrelated to hypertension, such as dilated cardiomyopathy of viral, alcoholic, toxic, or other etiologies. Regardless of the cause of LV dysfunction, uncontrolled hypertension further increases the LV wall tension and LV work due to systolic overload.

Diagnosis

Overt HF is usually recognized by its congestive symptoms, but early LV systolic dysfunction may be difficult to diagnose because it can be relatively asymptomatic. Typical signs are often absent or masked in many older people. Echocardiography is useful in the majority of patients (see Chapters C117, C118, and C155).

Prevention of Heart Failure in Patients with Hypertension

Prevention of HF is a major objective of antihypertensive therapy, which should include lifestyle changes and pharmacologic treatment. Controlling hypertension prevents LV hypertrophy and acute myocardial infarction, both of which reduce the incidence of HF. Achieving the latter goal requires attention to the total risk profile of the patient and includes interventions aimed at encouraging physical activity, control of diabetes, avoidance of smoking and overweight, achieving optimum cholesterol control, and use of aspirin by high-risk patients.

Controlling BP, especially systolic BP, should be the major target of antihypertensive therapy. However, studies have shown that clinical benefits are not equal across different drug classes in spite of similar BP reductions. The calcium antagonist amlodipine was associated with a 38% higher incidence of HF, whereas angiotensin-converting enzyme (ACE) inhibition was associated with a 19% higher incidence of HF than chlorthalidone. In the Losartan Intervention for Endpoint Reduction in Hypertension Study (LIFE) in patients with hypertension

and LV hypertrophy, the angiotensin receptor blocker (ARB) losartan and the β-blocker atenolol achieved similar BP reductions, but losartan was superior in causing regression of LV hypertrophy and decreasing clinical morbid and mortal events. In the ALLHAT study, a diuretic, a calcium antagonist, an ACE inhibitor, and an α-blocker were compared to a diuretic with respect to cardiovascular outcomes. The α-blocker doxazosin was associated with a 25% higher risk for major cardiovascular events, including doubling of the risk for HF, compared to chlorthalidone.

Treatment of Hypertension and Systolic Dysfunction

Goals of therapy. The treatment of patients with hypertension and LV systolic dysfunction, with or without overt HF, should alleviate symptoms, prevent hospitalization, slow or reverse progressive LV remodeling, and decrease mortality.

Blood pressure targets. Effective treatment of HF often lowers BP to values below currently recommended targets. Very low BP is a desirable outcome for these patients because the lower the systolic BP, the lower the afterload, and the better the myocardial performance. There are no specific threshold BP levels as long as there is no functional impairment. Some patients, especially those with intervening large myocardial infarctions, develop marked LV dilatation, severe LV dysfunction, and low systolic BP (below 100 mm Hg). β-Blockers and ACE inhibitors and digitalis and diuretics should still be given to these patients, while carefully titrating diuretics. When symptomatic hypotension limits the ability to titrate β-blockers and ACE inhibitors, a lower dose of both drugs rather than a high dose of one is often necessary. In stage D HF, hypotension rather than hypertension is associated with worse prognosis.

Heart failure treatment guidelines. Current recommendations for therapy are based on the new American College of Cardiology/American Heart Association staging system (**Table C156.1**). **Stage A ("at risk").** Therapy includes control of systolic and diastolic hypertension; treatment of lipid; avoidance of behaviors that may increase the risk of HF (e.g., smoking, alcohol consumption, and illicit drug use); ACE inhibition in patients with atherosclerotic disease, diabetes mellitus, or hypertension and associated cardiovascular risk factors; control of ventricular rate in patients with supraventricular tachyarrhythmias; and treatment of thyroid disorders. **Stage B ("asymptomatic").** Therapy includes ACE inhibition and β-blockade in patients with history of myocardial infarction, regardless of ejection fraction; in those with a reduced ejection fraction, whether or not they have experienced a myocardial infarction; and in patients with a recent myocardial infarction, regardless of ejection fraction, and valve replacement or repair for patients with hemodynamically significant disease. **Stage C ("symptomatic").** Therapy includes (unless contraindicated) diuretics in patients with fluid retention, ACE inhibition in all patients, β-adrenergic blockade in all stable patients, digitalis, withdrawal of drugs known to adversely affect the clinical status of HF patients (e.g., nonsteroidal antiinflammatory drugs, most antiarrhythmic drugs, and most calcium channel blocking drugs), and probably spironolactone in patients with

Table C156.1. Stages in the Evolution of Heart Failure (HF) and Recommended Therapy by Stage

	STAGE A	STAGE B	STAGE C	STAGE D
Classification	At high risk for HF without structural heart disease or symptoms of HF	Structural heart disease without symptoms of HF	Structural heart disease with prior or current symptoms of HF	Refractory HF requiring specialized interventions
Characteristics	Patients with 　Hypertension 　Coronary artery disease 　Diabetes mellitus **or** Patients 　Using cardiotoxins 　With family history of cardiomyopathy	Patients with 　Previous myocardial infarction 　Left ventricular systolic dysfunction 　Asymptomatic valvular disease	Patients with 　Known structural heart disease 　Shortness of breath 　Fatigue or reduced exercise tolerance	Patients with marked symptoms at rest despite maximal medical therapy Patients recurrently hospitalized or those who cannot be safely discharged from the hospital without specialized interventions
Therapy	Treat hypertension Smoking cessation Treat lipid disorders Regular exercise Discourage alcohol intake and illicit drug use ACE inhibition (appropriate patients)	All measures under stage A ACE inhibitors (in appropriate patients) β-Blockers (in appropriate patients)	All measures under stage A Drugs for routine use: 　Diuretics 　ACE inhibitors 　β-Blockers 　Digitalis 　Dietary salt restriction	All measures under stages A, B, and C Mechanical assist devices Heart transplantation Continuous palliative (not intermittent) i.v. inotrope infusions Hospice care

ACE, angiotensin-converting enzyme.
Adapted from Hunt SA, Baker DW, Chin MH, et al. ACC/AHA guidelines for the evaluation and management of chronic heart failure in the adult: executive summary. A report of the American College of Cardiology/American Heart Association Task Force on Practice Guidelines (Committee to revise the 1995 Guidelines for the Evaluation and Management of Heart Failure). *J Am Coll Cardiol.* 2001;38:2101–2112.

recent or current New York Heart Association class IV symptoms, preserved renal function, and a normal potassium concentration as well as exercise training of ambulatory patients. An ARB may be used in patients who are being treated with digitalis, diuretics, and a β-blocker and who cannot be given an ACE inhibitor because of cough or angioedema, whereas a combination of hydralazine and a nitrate may be used in those who cannot be given an ACE inhibitor because of hypotension or renal insufficiency.

Stage D ("end-stage"). In addition to measures listed for patients in stages A, B, and C, the therapy of stage D ("end-stage") HF includes identification and control of fluid retention, referral for heart transplantation, referral to an HF program with expertise in the management of refractory HF, continuous intravenous infusion of a positive inotropic agent, mitral valve repair or replacement for severe secondary mitral regurgitation, mechanical assist devices, and hospice care.

Specific Drugs

Diuretics. Monotherapy with diuretics should be discouraged in patients with established HF because they may not improve survival in stages C through D HF. However, diuretic therapy is preventative and is also an essential adjunct to β-blocker and ACE inhibitor therapy to decrease congestive symptoms and signs of HF (pulmonary congestion, hepatomegaly, and edema). A particularly useful strategy is to teach the patient to adjust the amount of loop diuretic based on daily weights. In early LV dysfunction, hydrochlorothiazide can be used, but as cardiac or renal function deteriorates, loop diuretics become increasingly important. The combination of loop diuretic and thiazide can be helpful in patients with hyperkalemia.

Angiotensin-converting enzyme inhibitors and angiotensin receptor blockers. The recommendation that ACE inhibitors should be used in patients with hypertension and all stages of LV systolic dysfunction is supported by post hoc analyses of the hypertensive subsets of large controlled clinical trials, including the Studies of Left Ventricular Dysfunction (SOLVD), the Acute Infarction Ramipril Efficacy Study (AIRE) and the Trandolapril Cardiac Event Study (TRACE). All of these studies showed a significant decrease in total mortality, HF hospitalizations, ischemic end points, and cost savings because hospitalizations are costlier than medication.

ARBs can be given to patients who do not tolerate ACE inhibitors. Although the combination of ACE inhibitors and ARBs results in improved hemodynamics, the ELITE II study raised questions about the use of this combination in HF patients who also receive β-blockers, and the Valsartan Heart Failure Trial (ValHEFT) study uncovered potential adverse effects of the combination of ACE inhibitor, ARB, and β-blocker.

β-Blockers. β-Blocker therapy reduces mortality in patients with hypertension, HF, and coronary artery disease. Despite their intrinsic negative inotropic effects, β-blockers exert beneficial effects in HF by reducing heart rate, controlling BP, controlling supraventricular and ventricular arrhythmias, and exerting antiischemic effects. In a metaanalysis of controlled trials using carvedilol or bisoprolol, β-blocker use was associated with a 30% reduction in mortality and a 40% reduction in hospitalizations in patients with class II and III HF. β-Blockers (except those with partial agonist activity or intrinsic sympathomimetic activity) have been shown to reduce cardiac mortality and morbidity in patients with coronary artery disease in the majority of over 40 clinical trials.

The use of β-blockers is associated with metabolic adverse effects, including raised triglycerides, lower high-density lipoprotein cholesterol, and glucose intolerance. However, given their demonstrated benefit in hypertension, HF, and coronary artery disease, β-blockers generally should not be withheld for fear of adverse effects. In patients with mild or moderate reversible airway disease, low doses of cardioselective β-blockers do not usually produce clinically significant adverse respiratory effects, but physicians should be aware of the metabolic and bronchoconstrictive adverse effects and take appropriate measures to counteract them.

Other treatments. The addition of aldosterone antagonists, such as spironolactone, decreased mortality in HF patients already receiving ACE inhibitors or β-blockers (RALES trial). Periodic dobutamine infusions improve congestive symptoms but do not prolong life. Surgical approaches in highly selected patients may include myocardial revascularization, insertion of assist devices, or cardiac transplantation.

Aspirin and nonsteroidal antiinflammatory drugs. Aspirin is often prescribed in patients taking ACE inhibitors. ACE inhibitors reduce degradation of bradykinin, thus enhancing the production of vasodilating prostaglandins. This effect may be counteracted by aspirin, which decreases production of prostaglandins by inhibiting cyclooxygenase (see Chapter C150). Thus, nonsteroidal antiinflammatory drugs can potentially precipitate or exacerbate HF. Studies of interactions between aspirin and ACE inhibitors have yielded conflicting results, but overall, there are marked mortality benefits of both interventions. Because the gastrointestinal side effects of aspirin are more pronounced with higher doses, a dose of 80 to 160 mg of aspirin is often recommended.

Value of a Treatment Center Approach

Patients benefit from organized, multidisciplinary HF clinics offering patient education, social support, weight monitoring, and medication and dietary review. Control of hyperlipidemia, usually requiring statins, and immunization for influenza and pneumococcal pneumonia are useful. Prevention and control of diabetes and its complications are important because patients with diabetes mellitus have an increased morbidity and mortality from cardiovascular disease and account for a large percentage of morbid events.

SUGGESTED READING

1. Cohn JN. Drug therapy: the management of chronic heart failure. *N Engl J Med.* 1996;335:490–498.
2. Cohn JN. Left ventricle and arteries: structure, function, hormones, and disease. *Hypertension.* 2001;37:346–349.
3. Cook JR, Glick HA, Gerth W, et al. The cost and cardioprotective effects of enalapril in hypertensive patients with left ventricular dysfunction. *Am J Hypertens.* 1998;11:1433–1441.
4. Fortuno MA, Ravassa S, Fortuno A, et al. Cardiomyocyte apoptotic cell death in arterial hypertension: mechanisms and potential management. *Hypertension.* 2001;38:1406–1412.
5. Frohlich ED. Fibrosis and ischemia: the real risks in hypertensive heart disease. *Am J Hypertens.* 2001;14:194S–199S.
6. Furberg CD, Psaty BM, Pahor M, Alderman MH. Clinical implications of recent findings from the Antihypertensive and Lipid-Lowering Treatment to Prevent Heart Attack Trial (ALLHAT) and other studies of hypertension. *Ann Intern Med.* 2001;135:1074–1078.
7. Garg R, Yusuf S. Overview of randomized trials of angiotensin-converting enzyme inhibitors on mortality and morbidity in patients with heart failure. Collaborative Group on ACE Inhibitor Trials. *JAMA.* 1995;273:1450–1456.
8. Kostis JB. The effect of enalapril on mortal and morbid events in patients with hypertension and left ventricular dysfunction. *Am J Hypertens.* 1995;8:909–914.
9. Kostis JB, Davis BR, Cutler J, et al. SHEP Cooperative Research Group. Prevention of heart failure by antihypertensive drug treatment in older persons with isolated systolic hypertension. *JAMA.* 1997;278:212–216.
10. Salpeter S, Ormiston T, Salpeter E. Cardioselective beta-blocker use in patients with reversible airway disease. *Cochrane Database Syst Rev.* 2001;CD002992.

Treatment of Hypertensive Patients with Peripheral Arterial Disease

Jeffrey W. Olin, DO

KEY POINTS

- Patients with evidence of atherosclerotic peripheral arterial disease should be screened for the presence of coronary artery disease and should have coronary risk factors (dyslipidemia, hypertension, glucose intolerance) managed aggressively.

- Nonpharmacologic therapy (weight loss, smoking cessation, exercise) should be part of the management of peripheral arterial disease; a structured walking program has been shown to significantly increase the pain-free walking distance and maximum walking distance in patients with intermittent claudication.

- Angiotensin-converting enzyme inhibitor therapy may be the antihypertensive agent of choice in patients with peripheral arterial disease.

- β-Adrenergic blocker therapy does not worsen intermittent claudication in most subjects with peripheral arterial disease; β-blockers are also useful in patients with abdominal aortic aneurysms.

See also Chapters A65–A67, A72, B85, C110, C119, C122, C123, C129, C141, C144, C154, C163, and C164

Hypertension is clearly a risk factor for peripheral arterial disease. The Sixth Report of the Joint National Committee on Prevention, Detection, Evaluation, and Treatment of High Blood Pressure (JNC VI) identifies peripheral arterial disease (PAD) as a form of hypertensive target organ damage and assigns PAD patients to the high-risk group (group C). Treating hypertension in PAD patients reduces the risk of myocardial infarction, stroke, heart failure, and death. There are limited available data, however, whether treatment of hypertension prevents the development of claudication or alters the natural history of PAD. The Treatment of Mild Hypertension Study (TOMHS) did show, however, that drug treatment in combination with nutritional-hygienic interventions was superior to nutritional-hygienic treatment alone (placebo) in preventing the development of intermittent claudication and PAD over an average follow-up period of 4.4 years.

Recognition of Peripheral Arterial Disease

Patients with PAD may present with the symptom complex of intermittent claudication: discomfort, aching, pain, tightness, and heaviness in the buttocks, hip girdle, thighs, or calf muscles brought on by exercise and relieved by rest. There are 3 major clinical features in patients with intermittent claudication:

- The discomfort is reproducible with a consistent level of exercise from day to day.
- The discomfort completely resolves within 2 to 5 minutes after exercise has been stopped unless the patient has walked to the point of severe leg pain.
- The discomfort occurs again at approximately the same distance once walking has been resumed.

For detailed description of evaluation, see Chapter C122.

Nonpharmacologic Therapy in Peripheral Arterial Disease

JNC VI has endorsed lifestyle modifications as important adjunctive therapy in PAD patients.

Role of exercise in peripheral arterial disease. A structured walking program has been shown to significantly increase the pain-free walking distance and maximum walking distance in patients with intermittent claudication. In 26 trials of exercise conditioning summarized by Hiatt and Regensteiner, claudication pain improved an average of 134% (range, 44% to 290%), and peak walking time increased an average of 96% (range, 25% to 183%). Studies using validated disease-specific questionnaires have shown that exercise in PAD improves quality of life. In addition, a regular walking program can lower blood pressure (BP), improve survival, lower triglycerides, raise high-density lipoprotein cholesterol, and improve glucose intolerance and insulin resistance (**Table C157.1**).

The initial period of walking should be 35 minutes long, with subsequent increases of 5 minutes each session until a 50-minute session is possible. During the exercise sessions, the

Table C157.1. Beneficial Effects of Exercise in Peripheral Arterial Disease

Lowers blood pressure
Improves claudication symptoms
    Increases pain-free walking distance
    Increases maximum walking distance
Improves quality of life
Improves survival
Lowers triglycerides and raises high-density lipoprotein cholesterol
Improves glucose tolerance and insulin resistance

patient should walk on the treadmill (or outside) until a mild or moderate level of pain is reached, followed by a rest period until the pain abates. After the pain is gone, the patient resumes walking until a moderate level of claudication pain is reached, again followed by another rest period. This process is repeated until the 50-minute exercise period has elapsed. Actual treadmill exercise usually constitutes <35 minutes and rest periods <15 minutes of the 50-minute exercise period. The beneficial effects of walking dissipate quickly once the patient stops walking on a regular basis. Although exercise is clearly effective, it has several limitations. Best results are achieved in a supervised setting (similar to cardiac rehabilitation) and require a motivated patient. In addition, lack of coverage of a supervised program by most insurance companies has limited its widespread use.

Smoking cessation. Discontinuing cigarette smoking may be the single most important factor that determines whether PAD progresses. In addition, discontinuation of smoking may have a favorable effect on walking tolerance. It is important to encourage and help patients to discontinue smoking.

Special Considerations

Coronary artery disease in peripheral arterial disease patients. The mortality rate for patients with PAD is approximately 30% at 5 years, 50% at 10 years, and 75% at 15 years. More than 90% of deaths are due to myocardial infarction and stroke. The relative risk of dying of coronary heart disease in patients with PAD is 6 to 7 times that of a control population, and the relative risk of dying from any cardiovascular disease is approximately 6 times that of the control population. Several investigators have shown that the resting ankle-brachial index is an important predictor of cardiovascular mortality. There is an ~25% mortality rate at 4 years in women with an ankle-brachial index of <0.9, even in the absence of symptomatic PAD (**Figure C157.1**). All patients with evidence of PAD should therefore be screened for the presence of coronary heart disease. In addition, all patients with PAD should be on an antiplatelet agent.

Lipid abnormalities. Most patients with PAD have abnormal blood lipids, including increased serum triglycerides, increased total and low-density lipoprotein cholesterol, or decreased high-density lipoprotein cholesterol. Nonpharmacologic treat-

Table C157.2. Medical Therapy of Peripheral Arterial Disease
Stop smoking.
Achieve ideal body weight.
Structured exercise program.
Achieve goal blood pressure. [Use ACE (or angiotensin II receptor blocker) as agent of first choice.]
If hypertension is not present, consider ACE inhibitor for cardiovascular protection
Control lipids (goal low-density lipoprotein <100 mg/dL).
Prevent (ACE inhibitor or angiotensin II–blocking agent) or control diabetes.
Administer antiplatelet therapy (aspirin, clopidogrel, or both).
Consider use of cilostazol for symptoms of claudication if exercise alone is ineffective.

ACE, angiotensin-converting enzyme.

ment (weight loss, exercise) is indicated according to the Guidelines from the National Cholesterol Education Program Adult Treatment Panel III (ATPIII). The goal low-density lipoprotein cholesterol for patients with PAD should be <100 mg/dL. Statins are a very effective class of cholesterol-lowering drugs that have been shown to decrease coronary event rates, allow for regression of atherosclerosis, and help to normalize endothelial function.

Glucose intolerance and diabetes mellitus. In individuals with PAD who are also overweight [especially if the weight is distributed in the central portion of the body (i.e., "central" or "android" obesity)], coexisting glucose intolerance or insulin resistance calls for increased exercise and weight reduction. Approximately 35% to 40% of patients with PAD have diabetes mellitus. Aggressive management of diabetes is indicated. Angiotensin-converting enzyme (ACE) inhibitors or angiotensin receptor blockers are the drugs of choice in patients with PAD, diabetes, and hypertension. If hyperkalemia or worsening renal dysfunction limits the use of these drugs, other classes of antihypertensive therapy can be used. A summary of the recommended treatment of patients with peripheral arterial disease is shown in **Table C157.2**.

Treatment of Hypertension in Peripheral Arterial Disease Patients

JNC VI suggests that antihypertensive drug therapy be instituted immediately after the diagnosis of hypertension is established in patients with target organ damage (including PAD). Direct-acting vasodilators, calcium antagonists, α_1-blockers, and ACE inhibitors are all effective arteriolar vasodilators, but these agents do not acutely dilate atherosclerotic vessels and, therefore, do not tend to improve symptoms of claudication in the short term. Antihypertensive drugs have no measurable effect on walking distance or calf blood flow.

β-Blockers in peripheral arterial disease. The commonly held belief that β-blocking agents worsen intermittent claudication and shorten the amount of exercise required to bring on discomfort in the extremity now has been challenged. In a carefully performed metaanalysis of 11 randomized, controlled trials, Radack and Deck concluded that β-adrenergic blocker therapy does not worsen intermittent claudication in subjects with PAD. Ten of 11

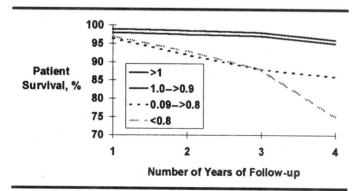

Figure C157.1. Ankle-brachial index and mortality. (From Vogt MT, Cauley JA, Newman AB, et al. Decreased ankle-arm BP index and mortality in elderly women. *JAMA.* 1993;270:465–469, with permission.)

studies in this metaanalysis showed that pain-free and maximal treadmill walking distances were not decreased by atenolol, labetalol, or pindolol. Nevertheless, some patients may experience the onset of claudication after starting β-blocker therapy. In these instances, the β-blocker should be discontinued and another agent tried. If the patient has advanced PAD with ischemic rest pain and is not a surgical candidate, β-blocker therapy should usually be discontinued (if it is safe to do so from a cardiovascular standpoint) with the hope that this may improve the peripheral circulation enough to avoid amputation. Patients with vasospastic diseases (e.g., Raynaud's phenomenon, chronic pernio) and hypertension should generally not receive β-blockers, because the extent of vasospasm may increase with the use of these drugs. Under these circumstances, calcium antagonists and α-blockers may lower the BP and decrease the severity and frequency of the vasospasm.

Angiotensin-converting enzyme inhibitors in peripheral arterial disease. Uncontrolled observations suggest that ACE inhibitors may improve walking distance in patients with intermittent claudication. Although ACE inhibitors can effectively lower BP in many patients with PAD, the overall consensus of investigators is that they do not alter walking distance significantly. Renal function should be followed closely in patients with PAD who are on ACE inhibitors because the prevalence of atherosclerotic renal artery sclerosis is high in this patient population. Anatomically significant renal artery stenosis is present in approximately 40% of patients with PAD or abdominal aortic aneurysm whereas high-grade bilateral renal artery stenosis occurs in 10% to 15% of patients. ACE inhibitors may lower cardiovascular events independent of BP lowering. In the Heart Outcomes Prevention Evaluation Study (HOPE), of the 9,297 patients entered, 4,051 patients (44%) had peripheral arterial disease (ankle-brachial index <0.9). In the entire group, the primary end point (myocardial infarction, stroke, cardiovascular death) occurred in 17.7% of patients randomized to placebo and 14.1% of patients randomized to ramipril, a relative risk reduction of 22%. The primary end point occurred in 22% of patients with PAD who received placebo compared to 14.3% of patients without PAD receiving placebo (an increase in relative risk of

approximately 50%). There was a trend toward more events in the PAD placebo group that did not reach statistical significance.

Abdominal Aortic Aneurysms

Fastidious BP control to the lowest appropriate levels is the cornerstone of nonsurgical management of abdominal aortic aneurysms. Although the data is limited and there are no large randomized trials, animal and human data suggest that β-blockers may slow the rate of aneurysmal expansion. Therefore, in the patient with an abdominal aortic aneurysm, β-blocker therapy is the antihypertensive treatment of choice if there are no contraindications to its use. Surgical resection or endovascular exclusion (aortic stent graft) of the abdominal aortic aneurysm should be considered for all symptomatic patients and in the asymptomatic patient with an aneurysm >5.0 to 5.5 cm.

SUGGESTED READING

1. Caprie Steering Committee. A randomized blinded trial of clopidogrel versus aspirin for patients at risk of ischaemic events (CAPRIE). *Lancet.* 1996;348:1329–1339.
2. Criqui MH, Langer RD, Fronek A, et al. Mortality over a period of 10 years in patients with peripheral arterial disease. *N Engl J Med.* 1992;326:381–386.
3. Gardner AW, Poehlman ET. Exercise rehabilitation programs for the treatment of claudication pain. A meta-analysis. *JAMA.* 1995;274:975–980.
4. Hiatt WR. Medical treatment of peripheral arterial disease and claudication. *New Engl J Med.* 2001;344:1608–1621.
5. Hiatt WR, Regensteiner JG, Hargarten ME, et al. Benefit of exercise conditioning for patients with peripheral arterial disease. *Circulation.* 1990;81:602–609.
6. Hirsch AT, Criqui MH, Treat-Jacobson D, et al. Peripheral arterial disease detection, awareness, and treatment in primary care. *JAMA.* 2001;286:1317–1324.
7. Radack K, Deck C. Beta-adrenergic blocker therapy does not worsen intermittent claudication in subjects with peripheral arterial disease: a meta-analysis of randomized controlled trials. *Arch Intern Med.* 1991;151:1769–1776.
8. TransAtlantic Inter-Society Consensus (TASC). Management of peripheral arterial disease (PAD). *J Vasc Surg.* 2000;31:S1–S296.
9. Vogt MT, Cauley JA, Newman AB, et al. Decreased ankle/arm BP index and mortality in elderly women. *JAMA.* 1993;270:465–469.
10. Yusuf S, Sleight P, Pogue J, et al. The Heart Outcomes Prevention Evaluation Study Investigators. Effect of angiotensin-converting-enzyme inhibitor, ramipril, on cardiovascular events in high risk patients. *N Engl J Med.* 2000;342:145–153.

Chapter C158

Sexual Dysfunction and Hypertension

L. Michael Prisant, MD

KEY POINTS

- The prevalence of sexual dysfunction increases with age and concomitant cardiac disease, hypertension, diabetes mellitus, and tobacco use.

- High-dose diuretics and drugs affecting sympathetic neurotransmission commonly cause sexual dysfunction.

- Switching antihypertensive drugs, weight reduction, and sildenafil can improve sexual function.

- Sildenafil should not be used in patients with unstable cardiac conditions; it interacts with nitrates and, perhaps, other vasoactive drugs to cause hypotension that is sometimes severe.

See also Chapters B81, B107, C110, C131, C137, and C149

Sexual dysfunction is important in the management of hypertensive patients in several ways: It is a marker of atherosclerosis, impairs quality of life, and is associated with nonadherence to treatment.

Risk Factors for Sexual Dysfunction

Epidemiologic studies. Before one can examine sexual dysfunction in men and women with hypertension, it is important to look at the population in general. The National Health and Social Life Survey recently questioned 1,749 women and 1,410 men between the ages of 18 to 59 years and found sexual dysfunction to be more common in women (43%) than men (31%). In the Massachusetts Male Aging Study (MMAS), a random survey of noninstitutionalized men between 40 to 70 years of age, the incidence of erectile dysfunction (ED) was 25.9 cases/1,000 man-years. In addition to a sexual activity survey, blood pressure (BP); height; weight; sociodemographic data; health status survey; medications; psychological tests of dominance, anger, and depression; and lipid and sex steroid hormones were measured. There was a direct relationship of ED with increasing age. Overall, 9.6% of subjects experienced complete ED, whereas 48% of men had no ED. Complete ED was more common with certain diseases, including treated heart disease (39%), treated diabetes mellitus (28%), untreated peptic ulcer (18%), treated hypertension (15%), untreated arthritis (15%), and untreated allergy (12%). Medications associated with complete ED in MMAS included vasodilators (36%), cardiac drugs (28%), hypoglycemic agents (26%), and antihypertensive drugs (14%). The use of tobacco was associated with a 2- to 3-fold increase in the rate of ED, independent of clinical condition or concomitant drug use; among subjects using antihypertensive drugs, the rate of complete impotence among nonsmokers was 7.5% compared to 21.0% among smokers.

Hypertension and antihypertensive drugs. When compared to untreated normotensives, untreated hypertensives have a higher rate of ED. It is a common belief that antihypertensive drugs cause ED, but short-term exposure to various hypertensive medicines over a 6- to 14-week period was not associated with an increased rate of self-reported ED study in a recent metaanalysis (**Figure C158.1**). One of the best prospective studies to examine sexual dysfunction in men and women was the Treatment of Mild Hypertension Study (TOMHS). In this 4-year, double-blind, randomized, controlled trial of 902 men and women with stage 1 diastolic hypertension, all subjects were treated with lifestyle changes and then randomized to treatment with placebo; acebutolol, 400 mg/day; amlodipine, 5 mg/day; chlorthalidone, 15 mg/day; doxazosin, 2 mg/day; or enalapril, 5 mg/day. If the diastolic BP was ≥95 mm Hg on 3 visits or ≥105 mm Hg on 1 visit, chlorthalidone or enalapril were added. The rate of sexual dysfunction in TOMHS was 14.4% in men and 4.9% in women. Of the 233 patients on no antihypertensive drugs at baseline, the rate of ED was 9.9%, compared to 17.6% among the 324 patients that were already receiving antihypertensive medications. The rate of ED increased progressively from 7.5% for the age group that was 45 to 49 years to 18% for the group ≥60 years. Baseline ED was significantly related to systolic BP, ranging from 8.1% in subjects whose systolic BP was less than 130 mm Hg to 20.9% in subjects whose systolic BP was ≥160 mm Hg. Through 24 months, the rate of ED was highest among subjects treated with chlorthalidone and was lowest in subjects receiving doxazosin. From 24 to 48 months, there was very little worsening of sexual frequency in subjects treated with chlorthalidone, but subjects receiving placebo had further decreases in sexual frequency. At 48 months, there was no difference among the various antihypertensive treatment groups (**Figure C158.2**).

Management

Antihypertensive drugs. It is important to gather information about sexual function before starting antihypertensive drug therapy because all antihypertensive drugs can be associated with this side effect. TOMHS is consistent with other studies that suggest that diuretics may be associated with sexual

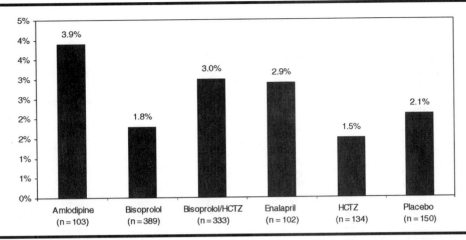

Figure C158.1.   Prevalence of short-term self-reported erectile dysfunction. There was no significant difference among the groups receiving therapy for 6 to 14 weeks in a metaanalysis of studies. HCTZ, hydrochlorothiazide. [Modified from Prisant LM, Weir MR, Frishman WH, et al. Self-reported sexual dysfunction in men and women treated with bisoprolol, hydrochlorothiazide, enalapril, amlodipine, placebo, or bisoprolol/hydrochlorothiazide. *J Clin Hypertens (Greenwich)*. 1999;1:22.]

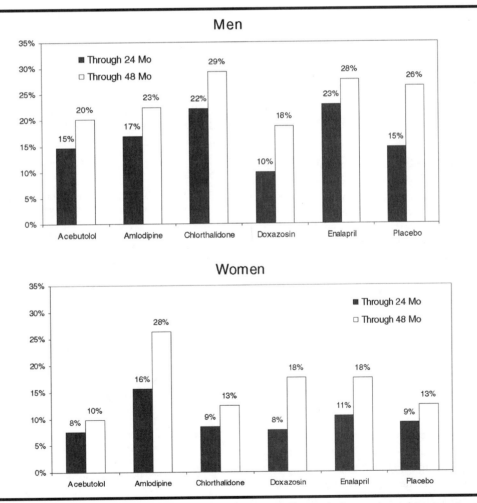

Figure C158.2.   Incidence of reported decrease in sexual frequency through 24 and 48 months by gender and treatment group. Chlorthalidone was associated with more erectile dysfunction than placebo or atenolol. Weight reduction reduced these effects of chlorthalidone. [Data from Grimm RH Jr, Grandits GA, Prineas RJ, et al. Long-term effects on sexual function of five antihypertensive drugs and nutritional hygienic treatment in hypertensive men and women. Treatment of Mild Hypertension Study (TOMHS). *Hypertension*. 1997;29:8–14.]

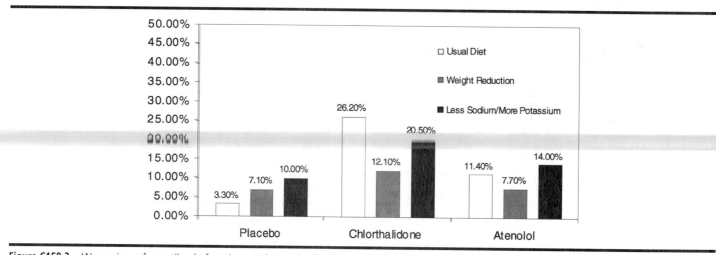

Figure C158.3. Worsening of erectile dysfunction at 6 months by drug and nonpharmacologic intervention. [Modified from Wassertheil-Smoller S, Oberman A, Blaufox MD, et al. The Trial of Antihypertensive Interventions and Management (TAIM) Study. Final results with regard to blood pressure, cardiovascular risk, and quality of life. *Am J Hypertens.* 1992;5:37–44.]

dysfunction. In contrast to common wisdom, β-blockers were not associated with a higher rate of ED than other antihypertensive drugs. Other studies show that the rate of ED is generally higher in men receiving multiple antihypertensive drugs. There are fewer data for women. As among men, there is a higher likelihood of sexual dysfunction with spironolactone, reserpine, and peripheral and central sympatholytics. Switching to alternative antihypertensive agents, such as angiotensin-converting enzyme inhibitors, angiotensin II receptor blockers, or α_1-blockers, may ameliorate the problem. Weight reduction has been shown to improve sexual function in men and women treated with chlorthalidone (**Figure C158.3**).

Phosphodiesterase type 5 inhibitors. Sildenafil is an approved alternative treatment for ED. For women, attention to foreplay, arousal, and lubrication can be helpful; data for sildenafil are not available. Sildenafil is a selective cyclic guanosine monophosphate–specific inhibitor of phosphodiesterase type 5 that releases nitric oxide, increases cyclic guanosine monophosphate in the corpus cavernosum, relaxes the helicine arteries, and allows blood to fill the lacunar spaces of the corpus cavernosum. In males with sexual dysfunction, treatment with 50 to 100 mg of sildenafil is usually effective; higher doses may be required in diabetics but are not yet approved for that purpose.

The presence of recent heart attack or stroke, significant hypertension, untreated angina, uncompensated congestive heart failure, and concomitant use of nitrates in any form precludes the use of sildenafil. There has been a general concern about the safety of sildenafil in hypertensive patients. BP-lowering effects can be significant; compared to placebo, the maximum decrease in BP from baseline 0 to 4 hours after 100 mg of sildenafil among amlodipine-treated hypertensives was 8/7 mm Hg supine and 10/8 mm Hg standing. The higher the baseline systolic or diastolic BP, the greater the decline in BP. In a *post hoc* analysis, there was no difference in the rate of adverse events associated with sildenafil in hypertensive patients on no therapy versus those taking antihypertensive drugs, but the side-effect rate caused by sildenafil was relatively high in all groups compared to placebo. The incidence of treatment-related adverse reactions in sildenafil-treated patients did not

differ greatly among subjects treated with 0 (38%), 1 (35%), 2 (31%), or ≥3 (41%) antihypertensive drugs. Side effects with sildenafil include occasional headaches, dysuria, nasal stuffiness, esophageal reflux, lightheadedness, and visual disturbances. Despite the apparent increase in adverse events, discontinuation rates were very low in placebo and sildenafil-treated patients (1%–2%), suggesting that the reported problems were relatively minor in nature. Major side effects, including symptomatic hypotension and chest pain, occurred infrequently. Recent data suggest that there is no higher incidence of fatal myocardial infarction among men taking sildenafil than in the general population.

SUGGESTED READING

1. Duncan L, Bateman DN. Sexual function in women. Do antihypertensive drugs have an impact? *Drug Saf.* 1993;8:225–234.
2. Feldman HA, Goldstein I, Hatzichristou DG, et al. Impotence and its medical and psychosocial correlates: results of the Massachusetts Male Aging Study. *J Urol.* 1994;151:54–61.
3. Grimm RH Jr, Grandits GA, Prineas RJ, et al. Long-term effects on sexual function of five antihypertensive drugs and nutritional hygienic treatment in hypertensive men and women. Treatment of Mild Hypertension Study (TOMHS). *Hypertension.* 1997;29:8–14.
4. Johannes CB, Araujo AB, Feldman HA, et al. Incidence of erectile dysfunction in men 40 to 69 years old: longitudinal results from the Massachusetts male aging study. *J Urol.* 2000;163:460–463.
5. Kloner RA, Brown M, Prisant LM, Collins M. Effect of sildenafil in patients with erectile dysfunction taking antihypertensive therapy. Sildenafil Study Group. *Am J Hypertens.* 2001;14:70–73.
6. Laumann EO, Paik A, Rosen RC. Sexual dysfunction in the United States: prevalence and predictors. *JAMA.* 1999;281:537–544.
7. Prisant LM, Carr AA, Bottini PB, et al. Sexual dysfunction with antihypertensive drugs. *Arch Intern Med.* 1994;154:730–736.
8. Prisant LM, Weir MR, Frishman WH, et al. Self-reported sexual dysfunction in men and women treated with bisoprolol, hydrochlorothiazide, enalapril, amlodipine, placebo, or bisoprolol/hydrochlorothiazide. *J Clin Hypertens (Greenwich).* 1999;1:22–26.
9. Shakir SAW, Wilton LV, Boshier A, et al. Cardiovascular events in users of sildenafil: results from first phase of prescription event monitoring in England. *BMJ.* 2001;322:651–652.
10. Wassertheil-Smoller S, Oberman A, Blaufox MD, et al. The Trial of Antihypertensive Interventions and Management (TAIM) Study. Final results with regard to blood pressure, cardiovascular risk, and quality of life. *Am J Hypertens.* 1992;5:37–44.

Treatment of Hypertension with Chronic Renal Insufficiency and Albuminuria

George L. Bakris, MD

KEY POINTS

- People younger than age 60 years with serum creatinine ≥1.5 mg/dL and those older than age 60 years with a creatinine ≥1.3 mg/dL have already lost at least 30% of their kidney function.

- The goal systolic blood pressure for people with chronic renal insufficiency of diabetic or other etiologies is ≤130 mm Hg; use of 3 to 4 different antihypertensive medications is frequently necessary to achieve goal blood pressure.

- Reduction in albumin excretion rate corresponds to a reduction in the rate of progression of renal failure.

- An angiotensin-converting enzyme inhibitor or an angiotensin receptor blocker should be included as initial blood pressure–lowering therapy and up-titrated unless contraindicated by hyperkalemia (serum [K+] ≥6 mEq/L).

- A 25% to 30% increase in serum creatinine (baseline creatinine <3 mg/dL) within the first 4 months of therapy with angiotensin-converting enzyme inhibitor or angiotensin receptor blocker in the absence of hyperkalemia (serum [K+] >6 mEq/L) correlates with long-term preservation of kidney function.

See also Chapters A38, A41, A49, A71, B84, B89, B106, C110–C113, C124, C127, C128, C137–C139, and C144–C146

Renal Insufficiency

Definition. *Chronic renal insufficiency* is defined as a glomerular filtration rate (GFR) of <90 mL/min. **Table C159.1** presents the National Kidney Foundation stages and prevalence of chronic kidney disease in the United States. It is clear from these data that approximately 27 million people have either stage 2 or 3 renal insufficiency (GFR >30 and <90 mL/min) that requires aggressive BP management. The values of serum creatinine (Cr) that correspond to these levels of GFR are noted in **Table C159.2**. The most common cause of renal insufficiency is diabetes; the second most common is hypertension associated with a variety of kidney diseases.

Renoprotective effects of antihypertensive drugs. The renoprotective effects of other classes of antihypertensive agents, such as dihydropyridine calcium antagonists (DHP-CAs), used in the absence of angiotensin-converting enzyme

(ACE) inhibitors or angiotensin receptor blockers (ARBs) are much more controversial. Only 2 prospective trials (1 in diabetic and 1 in nondiabetic kidney disease) have assessed the impact of initiating antihypertensive treatment with a DHP-CA. In both these trials of more than 700 participants, the DHP-CA, amlodipine, did not slow kidney disease progression to the same extent that was observed for ACE inhibitor or ARB in people with proteinuria and an average baseline Cr between 1.7 and 1.9 mg/dL. Conversely, in a subpopulation of blacks with hypertensive nephrosclerosis and no proteinuria [African American Study of Kidney Disease and Hypertension (AASK)], the role of renal deterioration of renal function in the amlodipine arm was not significantly different in outcome when compared to the ACE inhibitor. Moreover, in hypertension tri-

Table C159.1. Stage and Prevalence of Chronic Kidney Disease (Age ≥20 Years)

STAGE	DESCRIPTION	GLOMERULAR FILTRATION RATE (ML/MIN/1.73 M²)	PREVALENCE N (1,000s)	%
1	Normal	>90	10,259	5.8
2	Mild	60–89	21,794	12.3
3	Moderate	30–59	5,910	3.3
4	Severe	15–29	363	0.2
5	Kidney failure	<15 or dialysis	300	0.15

Table C159.2. Relationship between Glomerular Filtration Rate (GFR) Range and Serum Creatinine by Age

STAGE	GFR (ML/MIN)	ESTIMATES OF SERUM CREATININE (MG/DL) BY AGE RANGE AND AVERAGE BODY MASS[a] AGE 21 YR	AGE 75 YR
1	>90	1.0–0.8	1.0–0.7
2	60–89	2.0–1.1	1.6–1.1
3	30–59	3.5–2.1	2.7–1.7
4	15–29	7.5–3.6	4.5–2.8
5	<15 or dialysis	>7.6	>4.5

[a]Note that creatinine values will be higher if large muscle mass and lower if low muscle mass. These are approximations of GFR:creatinine ratios.

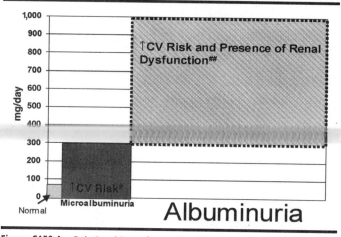

Figure C159.1. Relationship of cardiovascular and renal risk and albuminuria. In everyone who has albuminuria, proteinuria is present. Albumin makes up 40% of the protein in proteinuria. #, routine dipstick negative; ##, routine dipstick positive; ↑, increased.

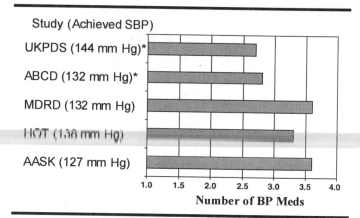

Figure C159.2. Relationship between number of antihypertensive agents and achievement of goal blood pressure (BP) in randomized clinical trials that evaluated two different levels of blood pressure. Data below are from the low BP goal. *, studies in diabetic population; SBP, systolic BP.

als that examined people without kidney disease or established heart disease, DHP-CAs reduce the risk of stroke and myocardial infarctions, which are 10 to 100 times more prevalent than end-stage renal disease (ESRD). Moreover, CAs in general should be considered as adjunctive therapy when added to an ACE inhibitor or ARB (with or without a diuretic) and are associated with a reduced risk for progression of kidney disease based on post-hoc analyses of the Reduction of End Points in NIDDM with the Angiotensin II Antagonist Losartan (RENAAL trial) in diabetic kidney disease.

Albuminuria

Definition. *Microalbuminuria* (<300 mg/day) is a major cardiovascular (CV) risk factor and is also a hallmark of renal disease (**Figure C159.1**). Microalbuminuria is clearly associated with an increased CV risk in hypertensive people but does not predict nephropathy progression in nondiabetic kidney disease. The National Kidney Foundation Proteinuria, Albuminuria, Risk Assessment, Detection, and Elimination (PARADE) task force has reviewed the evidence relating proteinuria and microalbuminuria to renal and CV risk. Screening for microalbuminuria is recommended for those at increased risk for renal or CV diseases. If proteinuria or microalbuminuria is present, further diagnostic testing may be warranted, and aggressive risk factor modification is recommended.

Benefit of therapy. Until recently, reductions in albuminuria had not been clearly associated with renal failure benefit. Now, however, numerous long-term clinical trials available in patients who have lost more than 35% of their kidney function, with or without diabetes, have demonstrated that reductions in proteinuria of 30% or more below baseline correlate with marked reduction in renal disease progression. This, in turn, led to the PARADE recommendation that therapies used to treat BP should also achieve reductions in proteinuria. The PARADE recommendation has been made on the basis of expert opinion rather than specific clinical trials, however. At present, there have been no clinical outcome studies that have established proteinuria as an independent indication for therapy.

Blood Pressure Goals

Current evidence and guidelines. No single study has prospectively assessed both CV and renal end points based on the level of BP achieved. *Post hoc* analyses of more than a dozen trials demonstrate a lower CV event rate and slower declines in kidney function in the groups with systolic BP of <140 mm Hg as compared to 10 mm Hg higher (**Figure C159.2**). All national and international recommendations including The Sixth Report of the Joint National Committee on Prevention, Detection, Evaluation, and Treatment of High Blood Pressure (JNC VI) and World Health Organization (WHO) state that the BP goal for those with nondiabetic kidney disease should be at least <130/85 mm Hg based on *post hoc* analyses of clinical trials. A recent double-blind, placebo-controlled trial in over 1,000 participants with hypertensive nephrosclerosis did not find a significant advantage in further slowing kidney disease progression by lowering BP to <130 mm Hg versus being in the range between 130 to 139 mm Hg. The evidence summarized in Figure C159.2 supports the notion of <140 mm Hg being the desired systolic BP goal to slow progression of nondiabetic kidney disease. A review of clinical studies shows that patients with renal insufficiency of any etiology with 2 different levels of BP reduction demonstrated that those randomized to the lower level of BP required an average of 3.2 different antihypertensive medications, daily (Figure C159.2). Many patients with renal disease, especially those on dialysis, take an average of 11 different medications daily. Therefore, the use of combination antihypertensive medications, such as an ACE inhibitor combined with either a diuretic or a CA, may be useful to reduce pill counts as well as co-payments at managed care pharmacies. Such long-acting combinations may also improve patient medication adherence, in addition to their expected improvement in BP control, resulting in more consistent and cost-effective control of hypertension.

A suggested approach to achieve blood pressure goals. Based on data that evaluate achievement of BP goals in the setting of an outpatient general medicine clinic, it is apparent that if an individual's SBP is greater than 15/10 mm Hg *above*

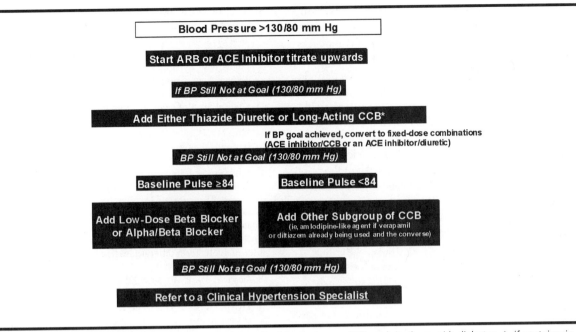

Figure C159.3. National Kidney Foundation algorithm for achieving target blood pressure (BP) goals in those with diabetes. *, if proteinuria present (>300 mg/day), non-DHP preferred; ACE, angiotensin-converting enzyme; ARB, angiotensin receptor blocker; CCB, calcium channel blocker; DHP, dihydropyridine.

the desired BP goal, then *2* different antihypertensive agents should be given simultaneously to achieve the goal. Thus, if the goal BP is 130/85 mm Hg and the patient has an office reading of >145/95 mm Hg and is not receiving treatment, the physician needs to prescribe *2* different agents. A paradigm to help achieve these goal BPs is presented in **Figure C159.3** and represents a modification of the National Kidney Foundation's Consensus report to help achieve BP goal with agents shown to slow kidney disease progression. It should be noted that the procedure of adding medications in this paradigm applies only to people with renal insufficiency or diabetes without other concomitant conditions such as angina, heart failure, or immediately following a myocardial infarction (Figure C159.3).

Blood pressure goals in dialysis. The recommended BP goals in people on dialysis must be considered. There are specific guidelines on this topic, but because the most common cause of death in such individuals is from CV events, the BP goals to reduce CV risk (i.e., 130/85 mm Hg for nondiabetic disease and <130/80 mm Hg for those with diabetes) is advised. In such patients, volume removal is the key component to achieving the BP goal, hence, patient adherence with limited volume intake between dialysis runs and aggressive fluid removal on the day of dialysis are warranted.

Specific Treatment Strategies

First-line therapy: angiotensin-converting enzyme inhibitors and angiotensin receptor blockers. A logical approach to reduce BP and proteinuria in nondiabetic renal disease is to initiate therapy with an ACE inhibitor, with the dose titrated upward to the moderate or high range (20–40 mg of lisinopril or equivalent). This recommendation is supported by a meta-analysis of clinical trials by Jafar and colleagues that showed that ACE inhibitor–based treatment reduced the risk of end-stage renal disease by 31% over other regimens in more than

1,100 people. If the ACE is not tolerated, then an ARB can be substituted. Additional therapies should be subsequently added to the ACE inhibitor or ARB after titration to the maximal dose to achieve goal BP.

Doses. The optimal dose of an ACE inhibitor or ARB needed to maximally preserve renal function remains unknown. However, the doses of these drugs used in renal outcome studies are generally higher than those observed in clinical practice. Dosing schedules for each anti–renin-angiotensin-aldosterone system drug should be familiar to clinicians, and the highest appropriate dose should be considered in all patients to comply with clinical trial evidence.

Use in renal insufficiency. Whether an ACE inhibitor or ARB should be stopped if the serum Cr increases above baseline is unclear. Based on data from clinical trials that have measured early and late changes in kidney function, a clinician should accept the following: if baseline Cr is ≤3.0 mg/dL, an increase in serum Cr of up to 30% above baseline within the first 4 months of starting treatment or reducing BP toward the goal of 130/80 to 85 mm Hg are positive prognostic signs that correlate with slower progression of renal disease. It is assumed that serum potassium is maintained <6.0 mEq/L and the rise in Cr stabilizes after this 4-month period. In the absence of heart failure, if serum Cr rises by more than 30% and continues to rise within the first 2 months of starting these agents, chronic volume depletion or bilateral renal artery stenosis needs to be ruled out.

Other drugs and combinations. ACE inhibitor–diuretic combinations are useful as initial therapy to achieve the BP goal of <130/85 mm Hg. This combination is especially efficacious in blacks and the elderly, and the use of a diuretic clearly potentiates the BP-lowering effects of ACE inhibitors. CAs are useful second-line agents that demonstrate an additive BP-reducing capability when used with either ACE inhibitors or diuretics. Moreover, ACE inhibitors, when used in concert with CAs, have resulted in a reduction of CV events. The combination of a non–DHP- and DHP-CA may allow additional BP reduction, probably in part because the non–DHP-CA tends to increase the bioavailability of the DHP-CA. Combinations of β-blockers and ACE inhibitors have failed to show any additive benefit on BP reduction, especially if the baseline pulse rate is less than 84 beats per minute. It has been observed in the Framingham study that people whose pulse rates average greater than 84 beats per minute have a higher risk of CV events as compared to those with lower heart rates.

Diuretics. In many patients with stage 2 renal insufficiency, thiazide diuretics (i.e., 12.5 to 25.0 mg/day) or CAs augment the possibility of achieving target BP goals. These agents have additive BP-reducing effects, with common side effects such as edema and hypokalemia ameliorated by the concomitant use of an ACE inhibitor. Such combinations have also been shown to reduce CV events in clinical trials of hypertension. In those with stage 3 renal insufficiency (GFR <60 mL/min) or greater, a loop diuretic is required for optimal BP-lowering effect. A thiazide such as metolazone can be added to a loop diuretic for additional BP lowering or to aid in the management of hyperkalemia but at the risk of excessive volume contraction and hypokalemia.

SUGGESTED READING

1. American Diabetes Association: clinical practice recommendations 2002. *Diabetes Care.* 2002;25:S1–S147.
2. Bakris GL, Williams M, Dworkin L, et al. Preserving renal function in adults with hypertension and diabetes: a consensus approach. National Kidney Foundation Hypertension and Diabetes Executive Committees Working Group. *Am J Kidney Dis.* 2000;36:646–661.
3. Clinical practice guidelines for chronic kidney disease: evaluation, classification and stratification. *Am J Kidney Dis.* 2002;39:S1–S231.
4. Horl MP, Horl WH. Hemodialysis-associated hypertension: pathophysiology and therapy. *Am J Kidney Dis.* 2002;39:227–244.
5. Jafar TH, Schmid CH, Landa M, et al. Angiotensin-converting enzyme inhibitors and progression of nondiabetic renal disease. A meta-analysis of patient-level data. *Ann Intern Med.* 2001;135:73–87.
6. Keane WF, Eknoyan G. Proteinuria, albuminuria, risk, assessment, detection, elimination (PARADE): a position paper of the National Kidney Foundation. *Am J Kidney Dis.* 1999;33:1004–1010.
7. Koshy S, Bakris GL. Therapeutic approaches to achieve desired blood pressure goals: focus on calcium channel blockers. *Cardiovasc Drugs Ther.* 2000;14:295–301.
8. Sica DA, Bakris GL. Type 2 diabetes: RENAAL and IDNT—the emergence of new treatment options. *J Clin Hypertens.* 2002;4:52–57.
9. Wright JT, Bakris G, Greene T, et al. Effect of blood pressure lowering and antihypertensive drug class on progression of hypertensive kidney disease: results from the AASK trial. *JAMA.* 2002;288:2421–2431.

Chapter C160

Treatment of Hypertensive Patients with Cerebrovascular Disease

Robert D. Brown, Jr, MD, MPH

KEY POINTS

- Specific blood pressure targets have not yet been identified in patients with acute cerebrovascular events, but precipitous decline in blood pressure after ischemic stroke may lead to increased infarction size.

- In acute ischemic stroke, moderate blood pressure elevation can usually be managed conservatively, but blood pressure must be more tightly controlled if thrombolytic therapy is used.

- In intracerebral and subarachnoid hemorrhage, hypertension should be treated if it is of moderate to marked severity.

- For secondary prevention, people with a transient ischemic attack or cerebral infarction benefit from reduction in blood pressure level.

See also Chapters A59, A68–A70, B81, B82, C125, C139, and C144

Hypertension is an important risk factor for transient ischemic attack, cerebral infarction, and intracerebral hemorrhage and is also commonly noted in conjunction with asymptomatic cerebrovascular occlusive disease. Optimal blood pressure (BP) treatment thresholds in people with cerebrovascular disease have not been established, but it is commonly accepted that BP treatment goals are different based on the nature of the cerebrovascular ischemic symptoms, the cause of the ischemic event, and presence of intracerebral hemorrhage or subarachnoid hemorrhage.

Cerebral Ischemia and Infarction

Hypertension after cerebral infarction is quite common. The causes of the elevated BP include pain, undiagnosed or undertreated preexisting hypertension, anxiety or agitation, reaction to artificial ventilation, hypoxia, and increased intracranial pressure. In the setting of cerebral infarction, cerebral blood flow is dependent on the systemic BP because of the impaired autoregulation in the area of the infarct. Thus, acute increases or decreases in BP may cause further damage. Management is currently based on anecdotes, animal studies, knowledge of

Table C160.1. Hypertension Management in Acute Cerebrovascular Disorders

BP LEVEL (MM HG)	MANAGEMENT
Cerebral infarction	
Diastolic BP >140	i.v. sodium nitroprusside, 0.5–1.0 µg/kg/min.
Systolic BP >220 or diastolic BP 121–140; mean BP >130	Labetalol, 10 mg i.v. over 1–2 min, repeat or double every 10–20 min, up to 300 mg. Alternate: enalaprilat, 1 mg over 5 min, then 1–5 mg every 6 h.
Systolic BP 185–220 or diastolic BP 105–120	No acute treatment, unless hemorrhagic transformation, myocardial infarction, renal failure from accelerated hypertension, or aortic dissection.
Systolic BP <185 or diastolic BP <105	No acute treatment.
Intracerebral hemorrhage	
Diastolic BP >140	i.v. sodium nitroprusside, 0.5–1.0 µg/kg/min.
Mean BP >130 mm Hg, systolic BP >180	Labetalol, 10 mg i.v. over 1–2 minutes, repeat or double every 10–20 minutes, up to 300 mg. Alternate: enalaprilat, 1.0 mg over 5 minutes, then 1–5 mg every 6 hours.
Mean BP <130, systolic BP <180	No acute treatment.
Subarachnoid hemorrhage	
Diastolic BP >140	i.v. sodium nitroprusside.
Mean BP >130 and diastolic BP <140	i.v. labetalol or enalaprilat, as noted for Cerebral infarction and Intracerebral hemorrhage.
Mean BP <130	No acute treatment.

BP, blood pressure.

intracranial vascular autoregulation, and clinical experience. There are no large trials defining optimal management after cerebral infarction and no clear guidelines to define mild hypertension. In some centers, a target systolic BP of 160 mm Hg is used, whereas in other centers, a systolic BP as high as 185 mm Hg is considered to be mild-to-moderate hypertension.

Mild-to-moderate hypertension. It is generally believed that mild-to-moderate elevations of BP after cerebral infarction should be left untreated. There is no evidence that the risk of hemorrhagic transformation or other deleterious outcomes is increased with a conservative approach to moderate hypertension in the acute ischemic stroke setting. In persons with a history of hypertension, more aggressive management of acutely elevated BP is more likely to increase infarct size, leading to poorer outcome.

Moderate-to-severe hypertension. In the acute period, there are no strict criteria as to what level of BP mandates aggressive management. In many cases, the strategy is based on the choice of whether thrombolytic agents are used.

With thrombolytic therapy. In the National Institute of Neurological Disorders and Stroke intravenous tissue plasminogen activator (t-PA) stroke study, patients were excluded from receiving intravenous t-PA for acute ischemic stroke if the BP was >185 mm Hg systolic or ≥110 mm Hg diastolic or if ongoing aggressive management was needed to meet these criteria. If intravenous t-PA is used, the goal BP should be <185 mm Hg systolic and <110 mm Hg diastolic (**Table C160.1**). In general, diastolic BP >140 mm Hg precludes candidacy for intravenous t-PA for acute ischemic stroke. In addition, persons in whom more than 2 doses of labetalol or other ongoing aggressive maneuvers are necessary to bring BP to <185 mm Hg systolic or <110 mm Hg diastolic are not considered optimal candidates for intravenous t-PA.

No thrombolytic therapy. If intravenous t-PA is not used, antihypertensive drugs may be withheld unless the estimated mean BP [(sum of systolic pressure plus double the diastolic pressure) divided by 3] is >130 mm Hg or the systolic BP is >220 mm Hg (Table C160.1). If less severe high BP (systolic BP, 185–220 mm Hg; diastolic BP, 121–130 mm Hg; mean BP >130 mm

Hg) is associated with hemorrhagic transformation, myocardial infarction, renal failure secondary to accelerated hypertension, or dissection of the thoracic aorta, then parenteral drugs must be initiated.

Choice of agents. The best agent to use in the setting of acute ischemic stroke is also not defined. Aggressive management with agents such as intravenous sodium nitroprusside is typically not needed but should be initiated if diastolic BP is >140 mm Hg (Table C160.1). Parenteral agents that are easily titrated with immediate-onset, minimal effect on cerebral blood vessels and low likelihood of causing precipitous decline in BP should be initiated (e.g., intravenous labetalol or low-dose enalapril). Sublingual use of calcium antagonists is contraindicated.

Intracerebral Hemorrhage

BP elevation is common after intracerebral hemorrhage. It is uncertain whether aggressive BP management in the setting of intracerebral hemorrhage lessens the chance of increased hemorrhage size or recurrent hemorrhage or leads to other deleterious outcomes, such as worsening diffuse cerebral ischemia or an increased zone of ischemia surrounding the hemorrhage. For persons with intracerebral hemorrhage, antihypertensive medications are typically not initiated acutely unless the mean arterial pressure is >130 mm Hg or the systolic BP is >180 mm Hg. The initial management goal should not be to rapidly achieve normotension; an appropriate initial goal would be to reduce mean arterial pressure to 110 to 130 mm Hg or systolic pressure to 140 to 160 mm Hg. Patients with a history of hypertension should be managed with particular care, and the goal levels may not be as strict. Increased intracranial pressure is also more common in intracerebral hemorrhage than in cerebral infarction, and a higher BP may be necessary to maintain a stable cerebral perfusion pressure. The antihypertensive agents recommended are similar to those used for cerebral infarction (Table C160.1).

Subarachnoid Hemorrhage

The management of hypertension after subarachnoid hemorrhage is controversial. Studies have not consistently defined a higher rate of rebleeding or death from rebleeding in persons with increased systolic BP. Among those with persistently elevated BP (mean arterial pressure >130 mm Hg), very careful reduction in BP by use of agents such as labetalol is reasonable (Table C160.1). Should any evidence of clinical deterioration or vasospasm occur, emergent reconsideration of the antihypertensive medications and fluid resuscitation must be undertaken.

Chronic Management of Hypertensive Patients after Cerebral Infarction

After a cerebral infarction has occurred, appropriate management of hypertension is a key factor for secondary prevention. It is apparent that systolic and diastolic hypertension (i.e., over 140 mm Hg systolic or over 90 mm Hg diastolic) are important, and isolated systolic hypertension should not be ignored, even if mild to moderate in severity. The beneficial effects of BP reduction in this setting include reduced risk of cerebral infarction and all stroke, and BP reduction may also reduce the risk of myocardial infarction and cardiovascular mortality. After the initial 24 hours after a cerebral infarction, an appropriate long-term hypertension management approach can be implemented.

History of treated hypertension. Patients with a history of previously treated hypertension can be restarted based on the current BP level. For patients with initial BP >220/120 mm Hg (or mean pressure >130 mm Hg), usual dosing of all antihypertensive medications may be resumed during the first day after ischemic stroke. For those with BP <220/120 mm Hg (or mean pressure <130 mm Hg), half of their usual antihypertensive medication dosages may be started at 24 hours after stroke, and if the BP decline is not marked, then the full dose of those medications may be commenced. The decision is then made regarding higher medication dosages or additional medications, based on the BP levels with the goal being <140/90 mm Hg.

History of untreated hypertension. If there is a history of hypertension and the patient is on no antihypertensive medications, chronic antihypertensive medications may be initiated 12 hours after the ischemic stroke if the initial BP is >220/120 mm Hg, or 24 hours after the ischemic stroke if the initial BP is <220/120 mm Hg.

No history of hypertension. For those without a hypertension history, if the BP is >140/90 but <220/120 mm Hg (or mean pressure <130 mm Hg), the decision regarding antihypertensive management should be made within the first several days after the ischemic stroke. If the BP is higher, chronic antihypertensive medications may be initiated at approximately 12

to 24 hours after ischemic stroke. Patients who have had a transient ischemic attack or cerebral infarction may benefit from a slight reduction in BP levels even if their in-hospital blood pressures are <140/90 mm Hg and they do not have a history of hypertension.

Choice of agents. Prevention of recurrent stroke was the principal study variable in the Perindopril Protection against Recurrent Stroke Study trial which showed a positive effect of a diuretic and angiotensin-converting enzyme inhibitor combination. Primary protection against stroke is conferred by aggressive management of systolic BP. The ability to prevent stroke has been demonstrated for several classes of drugs with diuretic [Systolic Hypertension in the Elderly Program (SHEP)], calcium antagonists (Systolic Hypertension in Europe, Hypertension Optimal Treatment), angiotensin-converting enzyme inhibitors [Heart Outcomes Prevention Evaluation (HOPE)] and angiotensin receptor blockers [Losartan Intervention for Endpoint (LIFE)]. The value of β-blockers in stroke protection is not clearly demonstrated.

SUGGESTED READING

1. Adams HP, Brott TG, Crowell RM, et al. Guidelines for the management of patients with acute ischemic stroke: a statement for healthcare professionals from a special writing group of the Stroke Council, American Heart Association. *Stroke.* 1994;25:1901–1914.
2. Blood Pressure Lowering Treatment Trialists' Collaboration. Effects of ACE inhibitors, calcium antagonists, and other blood-pressure-lowering drugs: results of prospectively designed overviews of randomised trials. *Lancet.* 2000;356:1955–1964.
3. Bosch J, Yusuf S, Pogue J, et al. on behalf of the HOPE Investigators. Use of ramipril in preventing stroke: double blind randomised trial. *BMJ.* 2002;324:1–5.
4. Broderick J, Brott T, Zucarelb M. Management of intracerebral hemorrhage. In: Batjer H, ed. *Cerebrovascular Disease.* Philadelphia, PA: Lippincott–Raven; 1996:1–17.
5. Brott T, Reed RL. Intensive care for acute stroke in the community hospital setting: the first 24 hours. *Stroke.* 1989;20:694–697.
6. Mayberg MR, Batjer HH, Dacey R, et al. Guidelines for the management of aneurysmal subarachnoid hemorrhage: a statement for healthcare professionals from a special writing group of the Stroke Council, American Heart Association. *Circulation.* 1994;90:2592–2605.
7. The National Institute of Neurological Disorders and Stroke rt-PA Stroke Study Group. Tissue plasminogen activator for acute ischemic stroke. *N Engl J Med.* 1995;333:1581–1587.
8. Powers WJ. Acute hypertension after stroke: the scientific basis for treatment decisions. *Neurology.* 1994;43:461–467.
9. Progress Collaborative Group. Randomised trial of a perindopril-based blood-pressure-lowering regimen among 6105 individuals with previous stroke or transient ischaemic attack. *Lancet.* 2001;358:1033–1041.
10. Wijdicks EF, Vermeulen M, Murray GD, et al. The effects of treating hypertension following aneurysmal subarachnoid hemorrhage. *Clin Neurol Neurosurg.* 1990;92:111–117.

Treatment of Orthostatic Disorders and Baroreflex Failure

David Robertson, MD

KEY POINTS

- Orthostatic intolerance (also called *postural tachycardia syndrome*) is characterized by a large increase in heart rate with little change in blood pressure on standing; there are many causes and multiple treatment strategies.

- Autonomic failure is characterized by severe supine hypertension and marked upright hypotension or syncope often accentuated by hypovolemia or exercise. Treatment is directed toward symptom relief and restoring functional capacities for daily life.

- Acute baroreflex failure is characterized by severe hypertension, tachycardia, headache, and sweating followed by a chronic phase that may include hypotension. Hypertensive crises are brought on by even minor emotional or physical stimuli; treatment is directed toward reducing blood pressure and excess sympathetic or vagal activity.

See also Chapters A2, A34–A37, A41–A43, C110, C113, C120, C128, and C153

Disorders of autonomic cardiovascular regulation commonly present with very high or very low blood pressures (BPs) or heart rates and patterns of extreme BP fluctuation, especially when the patient assumes the upright posture. Autonomic disorders may be considered in 3 categories: (a) mild dysautonomias, in which tachycardia may be present but orthostatic hypotension is usually absent; (b) severe dysautonomias (autonomic failure), rare conditions in which there is always orthostatic hypotension often with other neurologic problems; and (c) baroreflex failure, in which exaggerated BP and heart rate variation is exacerbated by emotional or physical stress rather than gravity.

ORTHOSTATIC INTOLERANCE SYNDROMES

The mild dysautonomias include neurally mediated syncope, in which there are episodic decreases in BP or heart rate, associated with faintness or loss of consciousness, almost always in the upright posture. The other major mild dysautonomia is orthostatic intolerance [also known as *postural tachycardia syndrome* (POTS)]. Orthostatic intolerance (OI, POTS) has the clinical hallmark of rapid heart rate on standing without orthostatic hypotension. Defined in this way, OI is not a disease but rather a syndrome.

Causes of Orthostatic Intolerance

Pathophysiologies of OI encompass structural, endocrinologic, renal, immune, toxic, and neuropathic entities (**Figure C161.1**). Among the structural entities, examples include absent venous valves and varicose veins. Volume deficits may be of 2 types: persistent hypovolemia (Bartter's syndrome and Gitelman's syndrome) or postural hypovolemia resulting from excessive transudation of fluid from the vascular compartment into the interstitial fluid compartment during upright posture. Autoimmune mechanisms may be important in many cases of OI. Neuropathic postural tachycardia syndrome appears to be due to a

partial dysautonomia. Recently, an antibody against the α_3-subunit of the N_N-nicotinic receptor on autonomic ganglia has been detected in approximately 15% of a subgroup of patients with autonomic disorders, including OI. Another rare group has a

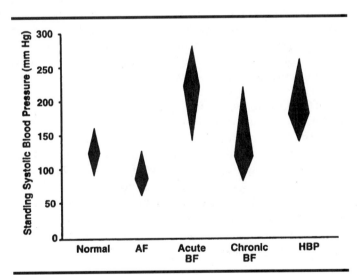

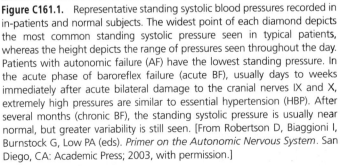

Figure C161.1. Representative standing systolic blood pressures recorded in in-patients and normal subjects. The widest point of each diamond depicts the most common standing systolic pressure seen in typical patients, whereas the height depicts the range of pressures seen throughout the day. Patients with autonomic failure (AF) have the lowest standing pressure. In the acute phase of baroreflex failure (acute BF), usually days to weeks immediately after acute bilateral damage to the cranial nerves IX and X, extremely high pressures are similar to essential hypertension (HBP). After several months (chronic BF), the standing systolic pressure is usually near normal, but greater variability is still seen. [From Robertson D, Biaggioni I, Burnstock G, Low PA (eds). *Primer on the Autonomic Nervous System*. San Diego, CA: Academic Press; 2003, with permission.]

genetic syndrome of norepinephrine transporter (NET) dysfunction. Patients with NET dysfunction complain of palpitations and orthostatic tachycardia, dizziness and lightheadedness on standing, occasional fainting, reduced exercise capacity, and fatigue. The NET is a unique gene product that subserves "reuptake" functions at the level of noradrenergic synapse (Uptake-1, see Chapter A2). In some sites, the NET is likely to be of particular importance in terminating adrenoreceptor activation. For example, in the heart where synapses are narrow, the NET is responsible for removal of 90% of the norepinephrine in the synapse.

Diagnostic Criteria

Chronic OI is characterized by the following 4 criteria: (a) symptoms of sympathetic activation on upright posture, (b) orthostatic increase in heart rate ≥ 30 beats per minute, (c) change in BP on standing $\leq 20/10$ mm Hg, (d) plasma norepinephrine during standing ≥ 600 pg per mL. OI represents the "final common pathway" for dozens of genetic and acquired autonomic and cardiovascular entities (**Table 161.1**).

Therapy of Orthostatic Intolerance

There remain many uncertainties about the consequences of OI. We do not know how many OI patients there are, nor do we understand where normal ends and where OI begins. OI and deconditioning share many clinical features, and their separation can prove challenging. Most patients with OI reduce their physical activity and therefore present with both OI and deconditioning. Finally, we know very little about the long-term outcomes of OI.

Fortunately, we are acquiring an armamentarium of treatment strategies, which in individual patients may result in improvement in symptoms. These strategies include (a) orthostatic "exercise," (b) water ingestion, (c) increased dietary salt or fludrocortisone, (d) low-dose β-blockade, (e) low-dose α_2-agonist (clonidine), and (f) low-dose α_1-agonist (midodrine). Responses to these agents are quite variable, and management is often best directed by a specialist familiar with autonomic disorders.

AUTONOMIC FAILURE

Causes

Examples of severe dysautonomias include multiple system atrophy (Shy-Drager syndrome) in which central control of autonomic function is impaired. This neurodegenerative disorder includes cerebellar and extrapyramidal abnormalities. Other examples are autonomic neuropathy due to diabetes mellitus or amyloidosis. In the latter disorders, the primary problem is damage to the peripheral autonomic nerves. Finally, there are neuro-

degenerative disorders such as "pure autonomic failure" of Bradbury-Eggleston syndrome or genetic disorders such as dopamine β-hydroxylase deficiency, in which congenital absence of norepinephrine causes profound orthostatic hypotension (**Figure C161.2**). Usually a supine and upright BP, heart rate, and plasma catecholamines suffice to diagnose severe dysautonomias. A fat pad biopsy can confirm amyloidosis.

The purpose of therapeutic interventions in patients with autonomic failure is to increase functional capacity rather than to achieve any particular level of BP. Factors such as prior ingestion of food and drugs as well as the rate of ventilation should be taken into account when assessing the patient's standing time or BP.

Importance of Volume Maintenance

Maximizing circulating blood volume is extremely important in treating orthostatic hypotension in autonomic failure. There is often a reduction in central blood volume, and many patients have a reduced total blood volume, low-normal values of central venous pressure, right atrial pressure, and pulmonary wedge pressure, even in the supine position. Liver blood flow is reduced considerably by upright posture, and blood-flow dependent drug metabolism may thus be altered. Patients with autonomic failure cannot conserve sodium during low-salt intake. This may be due to decreased renal nerve activity and perhaps to enhanced dopamine actions. In addition, renin responses to a low-salt diet and upright posture are reduced or absent during autonomic failure. This elevated supine pressure probably also contributes to the failure of the kidney to conserve salt and water, especially overnight; relative hypovolemia and orthostatic hypotension may be worse in the morning and improve during the day. Salt intake should be liberalized in all patients except those few with coexisting heart failure. Slight pedal edema is well tolerated and implies higher intravascular volume as well as increased interstitial

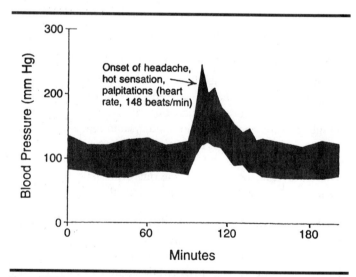

Figure C161.2. Blood pressure monitoring in a 43-year-old man approximately 2 weeks after surgical removal of a carotid body tumor. While blood pressure was being monitored, the patient's right hand was immersed in ice water for 60 seconds. The blood pressure immediately rose and continued to rise for several minutes after discontinuation of the cold stimulus. Symptoms appeared during this time and then resolved as blood pressure and heart rate returned to normal during the following 30 minutes. On some occasions, the patient had spontaneous paroxysms of similar magnitude. (From Robertson D, Hollister AS, Biaggioni I, et al. The diagnosis and treatment of baroreflex failure. *N Engl J Med* 1993;329:1449–1455, with permission.)

Table C161.1. Orthostatic Intolerance: Many Names

Effort syndrome
Hyperdynamic β-adrenergic state
Idiopathic hypovolemia
Irritable heart
Mitral valve prolapse syndrome
Neurocirculatory asthenia
Orthostatic tachycardia syndrome
Postural tachycardia syndrome
Soldier's heart
Vasoregulatory asthenia

hydrostatic pressure in the legs. Fludrocortisone is also commonly required (see the section Fludrocortisone).

Other Measures

Elastic support garments. Waist-high, custom-fitted elastic support garments (leotards) exert graded pressure on the lower body and increase interstitial hydrostatic pressure. Support stockings are not of much use unless they go at least to the waist. An abdominal binder in association with elastic stockings is even more useful and often better tolerated. Abdominal binders augment venous return from the splanchnic bed, a major source of venous pooling. Patients must be cautioned not to wear these stockings at night or when supine because the stockings increase central blood volume and supine BP, which may lead to compensatory reduction in extracellular fluid. Antigravity suits and shock suits have been used in the past with some success but are awkward and bring attention to the patient's problems.

Activities. Patients should avoid activities that involve straining or lifting heavy objects because acute increases in abdominal or intrathoracic pressure compromise venous return and can precipitate hypotension. Coughing and straining at stool or with voiding may particularly bring on hypotension. Working with one's arms above shoulder level (e.g., shaving) can lower pressure dramatically. Ambulation or shifting weight from leg to leg as opposed to standing motionless takes advantage of muscular pumping on the veins. A slightly stooped walking posture may be helpful. Squatting and standing with the legs in a "scissor" position are valuable emergency mechanisms of increasing venous return, particularly when presyncopal symptoms occur. Patients may sit with their legs over the side of the bed before standing. This minimizes hemodynamic stress, because assumption of the upright posture is broken down into 2 movements: (a) assumption of the seated posture and (b) standing from the seated posture.

Food intake. The effect of food and water on BP in chronic orthostatic hypotension can be important. In normal subjects, there is a slight tachycardia with little or no fall in BP after eating. However, patients with autonomic failure, the elderly, and those taking sympatholytic agents may exhibit large postprandial falls in BP. Even a modest amount of food may cause problems.

Exercise. A graded program of isotonic exercise such as walking is sometimes beneficial. More vigorous exercise such as jogging is rarely tolerated because postexercise decreases in BP can be severe. Swimming is usually well tolerated because in water, orthostatic hypotension is attenuated. Climbing stairs is a common hypotensive stimulus.

Drug Therapy

Drug treatment of orthostatic hypotension can be beneficial for selected patients. On the whole, however, severely affected patients are often extremely difficult to manage. The aim is for patients to have a 3-minute standing time, which usually enables patients to go about daily activities.

Fludrocortisone. Fludrocortisone (Florinef) has been the pharmacologic cornerstone in the treatment of autonomic failure. Although some patients respond to 0.1 mg daily, 0.1 mg twice daily is usually more effective, with some patients needing 0.1 mg 3 times a day. An average dose in patients with severe autonomic impairment is probably 0.1 mg twice daily given orally. Weight gain commonly occurs with fludrocortisone therapy and should be targeted at 5 to 10 lb. Fludrocortisone should generally be avoided in patients who by physical examination or history are on the verge of heart failure. The drug is begun at a dose of 0.1 mg once daily and titrated higher at 1- to 2-week intervals depending on the therapeutic response. Standing time, weight, supine BP, the presence or absence of rales and gallop rhythm, and plasma potassium and magnesium concentrations should be monitored. Most patients develop a reduction in potassium or magnesium concentration in plasma after 2 to 4 weeks of adequate dosage of fludrocortisone that may range from mild to severe, ultimately requiring replacement of potassium. Only a minority of patients require replacement of magnesium with slow-release preparations of magnesium chloride. A twice-daily dosage regimen minimizes diarrhea.

Midodrine. Midodrine is an α_1-agonist prodrug that raises BP through vasoconstriction. The dosage ranges from 2.5 mg on awakening and at noon to dosages as high as 10 mg 3 times a day. The most common limitation in the treatment of orthostatic hypotension is development of unacceptable levels of supine hypertension, which is present in most patients even in the absence of any treatment. Avoiding late day dose reduces nocturnal (supine) hypertension.

Management of Supine Hypertension

It is often necessary to accept relatively high levels of supine BP to keep the individual functionally mobile, although one must always try to avoid supine BP above 200 systolic. Most patients can maintain supine BPs in the 140 to 180/90 to 100 mm Hg range. There are a number of drugs that can be considered in treating autonomic failure and orthostatic hypotension of diverse causes, but the most important are fludrocortisone and midodrine.

Supine hypertension can be minimized by placing the head of the bed on blocks to approximately 5 to 20 degrees. In addition to attenuating nocturnal diuresis, this reduces the notable worsening of symptoms in the morning. Head-up tilt at night also may minimize nocturnal shifts of interstitial fluid from the legs into the circulation. Small meals and short-acting antihypertensive drugs (e.g., hydralazine, nifedipine) at bedtime can attenuate nocturnal hypertension.

BAROREFLEX FAILURE

Clinical Presentation

Baroreflex failure is the most dramatic of autonomic disorders (Figures C161.1 and C161.2). It presents in several ways. Sudden loss of baroreflex innervation causes acute baroreflex failure with severe hypertension and tachycardia in supine and upright postures. BPs as high as 300/160 mm Hg occur, and are usually accompanied by subjective sensations of warmth, flushing, palpitations, severe headache, and diaphoresis, similar to pheochromocytoma. After a few days, the sustained hypertensive phase gives rise to the more chronic labile BP phase. The hallmark of this phase is hypertension and tachycardia alternating with periods of hypotension, with or without bradycardia. The pressor crises usually last less than an hour and include hot flushing with pallor rather than redness. The crises tend to be brought on by even minor emotional or physical perturbations. Patients sometimes exhibit emotional volatility, but it is not always clear whether the emotional volatility is the result of the pressor crisis or the cause of it. Late in the disorder, the hypotensive phase may gradually become more pronounced and the hypertensive crises more attenuated.

Causes. Etiologies of baroreflex failure include trauma, neck irradiation, familial paraganglioma syndrome, and bilateral cell loss in the nuclei of the solitary tract due to a degenerative neurologic disease.

Diagnosis. Diagnosis of baroreflex failure is described in detail in Chapter C122. There are supranormal pressor responses to handgrip, cold pressor, and especially mental arithmetic testing. Perhaps the most helpful agent in diagnosing baroreflex failure is a small dose of clonidine; for example, 0.1 to 0.2 mg p.o. of clonidine often lowers BP precipitously in a patient with baroreflex failure. Between crises, plasma norepinephrine levels are usually normal but during attacks are dramatically elevated, often to 1,000 to 3,000 pg per mL. Over time, the pressor crises in baroreflex failure tend to become attenuated, whereas worsening more commonly occurs in pheochromocytoma, an important long-term differential point. Urinary norepinephrine levels in baroreflex failure are usually at the upper border or slightly above normal range.

Therapy

The treatment of baroreflex failure is difficult. The initial sustained hypertension phase requires hospitalization in an intensive care unit and control with nitroprusside and sympatholytic agents. In the first 2 or 3 days, apneic spells can occur if narcotics are employed, so monitoring is necessary. Once the chronic labile phase is reached, clonidine, orally or transdermally, is extremely effective, but quite high doses (0.6–2.5 mg daily in divided doses) are sometimes required but may

exacerbate hypotension. Recognition of the relationship between emotional upset and pressor crises is important. In some cases, spontaneous biofeedback treatment may result in a reduction in the number and severity of attacks. Over long periods of time, most patients may be graduated from clonidine to benzodiazepine with continued adequate control. In the rare patient with preservation of parasympathetic efferent control of heart rate (Jordan syndrome), the additional problem of episodic malignant vagotonia may require placement of a pacemaker to prevent cardiac arrest, after which long-term management of hypertension by guanadrel and attenuation of hypotension by fludrocortisone may be required.

SUGGESTED READING

1. Jacob G, Shannon JR, Costa F, et al. Neuropathic postural tachycardia syndrome. *N Engl J Med.* 2000;343:1008–1014.
2. Jordan J, Shannon JR, Black B, et al. Malignant vagotonia due to selective baroreflex failure. *Hypertension.* 1997;30:1072–1077.
3. Ketch T, Biaggioni I, Robertson RM, Robertson D. Four faces of baroreflex failure. Hypertensive crisis, volatile hypertension, orthostatic tachycardia, and malignant vagotonia. *Circulation.* 2002;105:2517–2522.
4. Low PA. *Clinical Autonomic Disorders. Evaluation and Management.* New York, NY: Little Brown and Co.; 1997.
5. Onrot J, Goldberg MR, Hollister AS, et al. Management of chronic orthostatic hypotension. *Am J Med.* 1986;80:454–464.
6. Robertson D, Biaggioni I, Burnstock G, Low PA (eds). *Primer on the Autonomic Nervous System.* San Diego, CA: Academic Press; 2003.
7. Robertson D, Hollister AS, Biaggioni I, et al. The diagnosis and therapy of baroreflex failure. *N Engl J Med.* 1993;329:1449–1455.
8. Shannon JR, Flattem NL, Jordan J, et al. Orthostatic intolerance and tachycardia associated with norepinephrine-transporter deficiency. *N Engl J Med.* 2000;342:541–549.
9. Vernino S, Low PA, Fealey RD, et al. Autoantibodies to ganglionic acetylcholine receptors in autoimmune autonomic neuropathies. *N Engl J Med.* 2001;343:847–855.

Chapter C162

Treatment of the Obese Hypertensive Patient

Xavier Pi-Sunyer, MD, MPH

KEY POINTS

- Increased fatness (body mass index) and central fat distribution (waist measurement) are associated with high blood pressure.

- Lifestyle behavioral changes of diet and activity can improve and help to control the elevated blood pressure.

- Pharmacotherapy in obese hypertensives may include weight loss drugs (sibutramine) that increase blood pressure and orlistat (Xenical), which causes steatorrhea.

- Higher doses of antihypertensive medications and drug combinations may be needed in obese hypertensive patients.

See also Chapters A11, A41, A44–A47, A53, A55, A76, B81, B87–B93, B97, B98, B103, C127–C130, C134–C136, C152, C163, C164, C166, and C167

Uncontrolled hypertension can lead to severe clinical consequences, including myocardial infarction, heart failure, stroke, and end-stage renal disease. This is even more true for obese than for lean individuals. It is therefore disquieting that so

many obese patients are not aggressively treated for hypertension. The relationship between obesity and high blood pressure has been reported in a large number of cross-sectional and longitudinal population-based studies. The effect of weight gain on blood pressure has been calculated from the Framingham study, showing that for every 10% increase in relative weight, systolic pressure increases by 6.5 mm Hg.

Blood Pressure Measurement

The measurement of blood pressure in an obese patient can be difficult. To obtain accurate readings, the compression cuff must be of an adequate size, because a cuff that is too small gives a falsely high pressure. The bladder should be wide enough to cover at least 80% of the circumference and approximately 75% of the length of the upper arm between the top of the shoulder and the olecranon. The patient should sit in a quiet room for 5 minutes before the measurement. An average of 2 or more readings should be taken, and this should be verified in the contralateral arm.

Assessment of Fat Burden

Total fat burden and fat distribution are important in blood pressure elevation.

Body mass index. The total fat burden is best assessed in a simple and economical manner by calculating the body mass index (BMI) of an individual. This is done as follows: [weight in kg/(height in m)^2] or [weight in lb/(height in in.)^2 × 703]. The BMI correlates well with the total body fat except in very muscular individuals. Central or upper body obesity has also been associated with increased blood pressure in many population-based studies.

Waist to hip ratio. Central obesity is best documented by measuring waist circumference, with >102 cm in males and >88 cm in women being considered abnormal by the NIH and WHO. A waist to hip ratio has also been used, with a ratio of >1.0 in males and >0.85 in women being considered abnormal.

Therapeutic Goals

The initial goal of weight loss therapy is to reduce body weight by approximately 10% to 15% from baseline. Such losses have been shown to be associated with significant improvements in comorbid conditions, including hypertension. Also, this amount of weight loss has been found to be achievable and maintainable with behavioral treatment and with pharmacotherapy. Weight loss tends to occur over a time frame of 6 months, with a reasonable and sustainable rate of loss of 1 to 2 lb per week.

Weight Loss Therapy

Weight loss therapy is recommended for every overweight and obese patient with hypertension.

General evaluation. When beginning to work with an obese patient, a careful preliminary assessment needs to be made. This includes discussing a patient's usual diet, food preferences, and eating habits (time, place, and person). Also, a careful history of previous weight loss attempts and why the attempts may have failed or partially succeeded needs to be taken. Habitual activity should be reviewed.

Psychosocial evaluation. Patient motivation needs to be addressed. Losing weight is a difficult procedure, and a patient needs to be appropriately motivated. It is important not to try

to embark on such an arduous program unless the patient wants to lose weight and is motivated to do so. In addition, a readiness assessment needs to be made, dealing with psychological attitudes toward weight loss, ability to increase physical activity, ability to understand nutritional guidelines, and self-control skills. Also, the environmental ambiance and social support structure of the patient should be investigated to see how that may help or hinder the weight loss attempt.

Behavior modification. Behavior modification is important in the treatment of obesity. Changing behavior is the only way to change weight permanently. Behavior modification is not an arcane art. It is a methodology for changing lifestyle habits that can be used by any primary care provider interested in identifying simple ways to break old habits and develop new ones. Behavior modification focuses on gradual, permanent changes in eating and exercise habits. There are 5 major areas in which altering behavior helps weight loss: (a) changing eating habits, (b) increasing physical activity, (c) altering attitudes, (d) developing support systems, and (e) education about nutrition. The primary focus is on self-control to achieve a gradual change in habits via incorporation of an individual's food preferences into dietary planning. The provider must be supportive and not demand perfection because there will be slips and slides along the way. The program for weight loss and weight maintenance must be adaptable to meet the needs of diverse patients. There is therefore no standardized set of rules to optimize weight reduction with a given patient.

Dietary changes. The strategies for weight loss include a hypocaloric diet, increased physical activity, and behavior modification strategies to maintain these lifestyle changes over the long term. The hypocaloric diet may be a low-fat diet, but what is most important is an overall decrease in calories. The nutritional plan must be individualized. It should take into consideration food preferences, availability, and taste, as well as cultural preferences and socioeconomic factors. In addition, attention needs to be paid to other concurrent dietary requirements of any comorbid conditions, such as the hypertension, diabetes, and dyslipidemia.

The nutritional plan must be a long-term one. It should emphasize healthy eating and stress the need to reduce calories for weight loss and then weight maintenance. The typical American diet consists of 14% protein, 40% fat, and 46% carbohydrate, of which 28% is complex carbohydrates and 18% sugar. The best plan is to educate the patient with regard to high- and low-calorie-dense foods. High-fat foods should be reduced, and heavy intake of sugar should be discouraged. Portion sizes should be reduced. Fiber should be increased. The DASH (Dietary Approaches to Stop Hypertension) diet, in conjunction with a decrease in sodium, has been reported to be successful in hypertensive patients. This diet is rich in fruits and vegetables, low in saturated and total fat, and rich in low-fat dairy food. Alcohol should be eliminated or drastically curtailed. The aim is for a 500 to 1,000 kcal deficit for the weight loss phase and then a decreased calorie intake of approximately 30 kcal per kg for weight maintenance. All of these suggestions fit in well with the Recommended Dietary Guidelines and the food pyramid promulgated by the U. S. Departments of Agriculture and of Health and Human Services. In some individuals, it may be more helpful to use a lower calorie diet of approximately 800 kcal for a time (12–24 weeks), and this is often done with liquid formulas.

Physical activity. Obese persons are extraordinarily sedentary. Physical activity is a crucial component for a weight loss and maintenance program (see Chapter C130). Exercise is important in obese hypertensive patients because it can have a direct effect in improving blood pressure control and insulin sensitivity as well as on weight loss and maintenance. Exercise increases energy expenditure, and what an obese patient needs is not only a decrease in caloric intake but also an increase in energy expenditure. Physical activity may take many forms, depending on the interests and capabilities of the patient. The important parts of an exercise program are intensity, duration, and frequency. A patient should be advised to start slowly and for short periods, but to exercise at least 5 times a week from the beginning. The plan should be to begin with low-intensity aerobic exercise (walking is probably best) and gradually work toward more intensive activity (e.g., jogging, swimming, biking, tennis). Activity should be done 5 to 7 days per week for approximately 30 minutes per day overall but may be divided into shorter segments if necessary. The exercise prescription should be individualized to the lifestyle of the individual. If social interaction and spousal or family support can be built into the exercise, the exercise program is more likely to be sustained. Enlisting outside resources such as public pools, health clubs, and gyms can be very helpful.

Maintenance of weight loss. After successful weight loss, the likelihood of weight loss maintenance is enhanced by a program consisting of dietary counseling and physical activity that should be continued indefinitely. This needs to include continued contact with the physician to ensure a persistence of the new lifestyle changes that have been instrumental in the loss of weight.

Anorectic drugs. In patients with a BMI over 27, if a 6-month trial of diet, exercise, and behavior therapy has not proven successful, pharmacotherapy can be tried. At present, there are only 2 drugs that are U.S. Food and Drug Administration approved. Sibutramine (Meridia) is a serotonin and norepinephrine reuptake inhibitor that reduces food intake by enhancing satiety. In randomized clinical trials for up to 2 years, a loss of approximately 10 to 15 lb was seen. Sibutramine can increase blood pressure and heart rate, and it may require withdrawal. The drug is contraindicated in patients with coronary artery disease. Milder side effects include dry mouth, constipation, insomnia, dizziness, and nausea. Data on safety and efficacy are only available for 2 years.

The other drug approved for weight loss is orlistat (Xenical), an inhibitor of intestinal lipase that impairs fat absorption by the gut. The net effect is to decrease absorption of dietary fat calories. This drug has undergone 2-year clinical trials with no significant adverse side effects except for a small reduction of fat-soluble vitamins. This drug causes steatorrhea as part of its action, with soft and more frequent stools. It has approximately the same effectiveness as sibutramine over a 1-year period, with 55% of orlistat-treated patients losing more than 5% of their body weight and 25% losing more than 10% of their body weight (compared to 33% and 15%, respectively, achieving the same mean weight loss in the placebo-treated group).

Surgery. For the very obese, those with BMIs above 40 or BMIs over 35 with very adverse health conditions, obesity surgery may be an appropriate option. This should be done by an interested and experienced surgical and medical team that will commit to following the patient long-term.

Public health issues. Although culturally sensitive programs need to be initiated for specific population groups, it is important to state that all geographic racial and cultural subgroups in America manifest increasing cardiovascular risk with increasing weight. There is no reason to believe that all groups do not profit from weight loss and risk factor reduction. With regard to older individuals, in general, they take on similar or greater risks for morbidity with increasing weight than do younger subjects.

Blood Pressure Management

Not all patients are able to lose weight, and even if they do lose weight, not all patients experience a return to normal blood pressures. For these obese hypertensive patients, effective antihypertensive drug therapy needs to be instituted. The general principles of pharmacotherapy for obese patients are not different from nonobese patients, but there are a few caveats. Diuretics such as hydrochlorothiazide may be required in higher doses to have an adequate effect, but they also tend to increase blood glucose and lower potassium at these higher doses. Because of these problems, it is often preferable to use diuretics in combination with other agents such as angiotensin-converting enzyme (ACE) inhibitors. β-Blockers may be effective at high doses in obese patients, but they may induce a worsening of insulin resistance and glucose intolerance. α-Adrenergic receptor blocking agents may reduce the early insulin response and increase insulin sensitivity and are theoretically attractive in obese hypertensives, but these agents do not protect against heart failure, which is relatively common in obese hypertensives. ACE inhibitors can be helpful in obese patients, reducing total peripheral vascular resistance, improving insulin sensitivity, reversing increased left ventricular mass, and protecting the kidneys. Calcium antagonists seem to help reduce peripheral vascular resistance and may promote natriuresis but often cause edema which is ameliorated by combining the calcium antagonist with an ACE inhibitor.

SUGGESTED READING

1. DeFronzo RA, Cooke CR, Andres R, et al. The effect of insulin on renal handling of sodium, potassium, calcium and phosphate in man. *J Clin Invest.* 1975;55:845–855.
2. Ferrannini E, Haffner SM, Stern MP. Essential hypertension: an insulin-resistance state. *J Cardiovasc Pharmacol.* 1990;15:S18–S25.
3. National Heart, Lung, and Blood Institute. Clinical guidelines on the identification, evaluation, and treatment of overweight and obesity in adults—the evidence report. *Obes Res.* 1998;6:51S–209S.
4. Pi-Sunyer FX. A review of long-term studies evaluating the efficacy of weight loss in ameliorating disorders associated with obesity. *Clin Ther.* 1996;18:1006–1035.
5. Pi-Sunyer FX. Obesity. In: *Conn's Current Therapy.* Philadelphia, PA: WB Saunders Co.; 1998:574–579.
6. Reisen E, Frolich ED, Messerli FH, et al. Cardiovascular changes after weight reduction in obesity hypertension. *Ann Intern Med.* 1983;98:315–319.

7. Rocchini AP. Insulin resistance, obesity, and hypertension. *J Nutr.* 1995;126:1718S–1724S.

8. Sacks FM, Svetkey LP, Vollmer WM, et al. Effects on blood pressure of reduced dietary sodium and the Dietary Approaches to Stop Hypertension (DASH) diet. *N Engl J Med.* 2001;344:3–10.

9. Schotte DE, Stunkard AJ. The effects of weight reduction on blood pressure in 301 obese patients. *Arch Intern Med.* 1990;150:1701–1704.

10. The sixth report of the Joint National Committee on prevention, detection, evaluation, and treatment of high blood pressure. *Arch Intern Med.* 1997;157:2413–2446.

Chapter C163

Treatment of the Hypertensive Patient with Lipid and Lipoprotein Abnormalities

Michael D. Cressman, DO

KEY POINTS

- Coronary heart disease risk increases progressively as total cholesterol and low-density lipoprotein cholesterol levels increase.

- Total cholesterol, triglyceride, high-density lipoprotein cholesterol, and low-density lipoprotein cholesterol levels should be determined during the basic laboratory evaluation of all hypertensive patients.

- Low-density lipoprotein cholesterol levels <100 mg/dL and non–high-density lipoprotein cholesterol (total cholesterol minus high-density lipoprotein cholesterol) levels <130 mg/dL should be achieved in high-risk hypertensive patients (hypertensive patients with coronary heart disease or with a coronary heart disease risk equivalent).

- Cholesterol-lowering drug treatment, especially with hepatic 3-methylglutaryl coenzyme A reductase inhibitors (statins), has been shown to reduce the risk of stroke and myocardial infarction in normotensive and hypertensive patients.

See also Chapters A65–A67, B81, B85, B97, B98, B103, B104, C110, C127, C129, C130, C149, C154, C157, and C164

Hypertension and hypercholesterolemia frequently coexist and can markedly increase coronary heart disease (CHD) risk. The association of systolic blood pressure (BP) and total cholesterol (TC) levels with CHD death rates in 316,000 middle-aged men free of preexisting CHD who were screened for the Multiple Risk Factor Intervention Trial (MRFIT) is summarized in **Table C163.1**. Additional prognostic information can be obtained through analysis of a blood lipid profile that includes TC, low-density lipoprotein cholesterol (LDL-C), triglyceride (TG), and high-density lipoprotein cholesterol (HDL-C) measurements.

Measurement and Classification of Blood Lipid Levels and Risk

The standard screening test is a fasting lipid profile (including TC, LDL-C, HDL-C, and TG levels), which should be obtained after a 9- to 12-hour fast during the evaluation of all hypertensive patients. Classifications of TC, LDL-C, TG, and HDL-C levels based on criteria defined in the third Adult Treatment Panel (ATP-III) of the National Cholesterol Education Program report are summarized in **Table C163.2**. An additional parameter used in hypertriglyceridemic patients is "non–HDL-C" (non–HDL-C = TC − HDL-C).

Table C163.1. Age-Adjusted Coronary Heart Disease Death Rates (per 10,000 Person-Years) by Systolic Blood Pressure and Total Cholesterol Levels in Nonsmoking Multiple Risk Factor Intervention Trial Screened Subjects (12-Year Follow-Up)

SYSTOLIC BLOOD PRESSURE, MM HG	TOTAL CHOLESTEROL LEVELS, MG/DL				
	<182	182–202	203–220	221–244	>245
<118	3.1	4.3	5.5	5.9	12.2
118–124	3.4	6.0	6.3	9.6	12.7
125–131	5.6	7.9	8.6	8.3	17.1
132–141	5.0	7.9	10.7	12.3	21.0
≥142	13.7	16.7	17.7	22.6	33.7

From Marin MJ, Hulley SB, Browner WS, et al. Serum cholesterol, blood pressure, and mortality: implications from a cohort of 361,662 men. *Lancet.* 1986;2:933–936, with permission.

Table C163.2. Classification of Blood Lipid Levels

Classification of total cholesterol levels	
Desirable	<200 mg/dL
Borderline	200–239 mg/dL
High	≥240 mg/dL
Classification of low-density lipoprotein cholesterol levels	
Optimal	<100 mg/dL
Near optimal/above optimal	100–129 mg/dL
Borderline high	130–159 mg/dL
High	160–189 mg/dL
Very high	≥190 mg/dL
Classification of serum triglyceride levels	
Normal	<150 mg/dL
Borderline-high	150–199 mg/dL
High	200–499 mg/dL
Very high	≥500 mg/dL
Classification of high-density lipoprotein cholesterol levels	
Low	<40 mg/dL
High	≥60 mg/dL

Adapted from Expert Panel on Detection, Evaluation, and Treatment of High Blood Cholesterol in Adults. Executive Summary of the third report of the National Cholesterol Education Program (NCEP) Expert Panel on Detection, Evaluation, and Treatment of High Blood Cholesterol in Adults (Adult Treatment Panel III). *JAMA.* 2001;285: 2486–2497.

Total cholesterol and low-density lipoprotein cholesterol.
Risk is influenced by the distribution of cholesterol contained in high-density lipoproteins, which do not contain apoprotein B, and non–high-density lipoproteins, which contain apoprotein B. Approximately two-thirds of cholesterol is contained in low-density lipoprotein particles that contain apoprotein B and are the principal atherogenic lipoproteins in the circulation. A TC <200 mg/dL is considered to be "desirable," whereas an LDL-C <100 mg/dL is considered to be "optimal." Although the TC level generally provides a reasonable estimate of lipid-associated CHD risk, CHD risk can vary considerably within a population.

Triglycerides, very-low-density lipoprotein, and non–high-density lipoprotein cholesterol. Fasting TG levels, which are frequently used to calculate LDL-C levels, are also useful in distinguishing higher risk individuals. When TG levels are lower than 400 mg/dL, very-low-density lipoprotein cholesterol (VLDL-C) levels can be estimated using the formula VLDL-C = TG/5. In general, individuals with elevated TG levels have an increased CHD risk, although this risk may not be explainable based on TGs per se. In the ATP-III classification scheme, a fasting TG level lower than 150 mg/dL is considered to be *normal*, TG levels of 150 to 199 mg/dL are classified as *borderline-high*, TG levels ranging from 200–499 mg/dL are considered to be *high*, and levels of 500 mg/dL or greater are classified as *very high*, respectively.

Individuals with TG levels above approximately 200 mg/dL may have an increased risk of atherosclerosis if there are elevated levels of atherogenic apoprotein B–containing particles. It has been recommended that non–HDL-C be used as a risk indicator in hypertriglyceridemic patients because it includes the cholesterol contained in all lipoproteins containing apoprotein B.

A normal TG level is considered to be <150 mg/dL and a normal VLDL-C concentration can be considered to be <30 mg/dL (VLDL-C = TG/5 when TG levels are less than 400 mg/

dL). Thus, a reasonable goal for non–HDL-C is approximately 30 mg/dL higher than LDL-C.

High-density lipoprotein cholesterol. An HDL-C <40 mg/dL is defined as *low* in the ATP-III report. Epidemiologic evidence suggests that a 1% decrease in HDL-C is associated with a 2% to 3% increase in CHD risk. However, individuals with low HDL-C levels are frequently hypertriglyceridemic and have small, dense low-density lipoprotein particles, which seem to be particularly atherogenic. These atherogenic particles and other factors that coexist in individuals with low HDL-C levels may contribute to the observed epidemiologic associations. An HDL-C ≥60 mg/dL is classified as a *high HDL-C* in ATP-III and is considered to be a negative risk factor in the recommended approach to CHD risk assessment. The presence of a high HDL-C removes or cancels 1 risk factor from the risk factor count that is used in the overall assessment of CHD risk among nondiabetic subjects with no clinical evidence of atherosclerosis.

Risk Stratification in Hypertensive Patients

Lipid profiles should be used in conjunction with clinical information (the presence or absence of clinical evidence of atherosclerosis, diabetes mellitus, and other conventional CHD risk factors) to obtain an overall or "global" assessment of CHD risk. A general principle that guides subsequent lipid management in hypertensive normotensive individuals is that the intensity of lipid altering therapy should vary directly with the level of cardiovascular risk.

The ATP-III report provides Framingham risk scoring tables that use age, gender, TC levels, HDL-C levels, systolic BP levels, the presence or absence of a history of hypertension, and current smoking status to obtain a 10-year CHD risk estimate. Hypertensive patients who have CHD, other clinical evidence of atherosclerosis (carotid artery disease, abdominal aortic aneurysm, peripheral arterial disease) or diabetes mellitus constitute a high-risk group. An additional group of high-risk patients are those with 2 or more of the major CHD risk factors (identified in **Table C163.3**) who have an estimated CHD risk

Table C163.3. Risk Status Based on Presence of Coronary Heart Disease Risk Factors Other Than Low-Density Lipoprotein Cholesterol

Positive risk factors
Age
Male ≥45 yr
Female ≥55 yr
Family history of premature coronary heart disease (definite myocardial infarction or sudden death before 55 yr of age in father or other male first-degree relative or before 65 yr of age in mother or other female first-degree relative)
Current cigarette smoking
Hypertension (blood pressure ≥140/90 mm Hg or taking antihypertensive medication)
Low high-density lipoprotein cholesterol level (<40 mg/dL)
Negative (protective) risk factor
High high-density lipoprotein cholesterol level (≥60 mg/dL)

Adapted from Expert Panel on Detection, Evaluation, and Treatment of High Blood Cholesterol in Adults. Executive Summary of the third report of the National Cholesterol Education Program (NCEP) Expert Panel on Detection, Evaluation, and Treatment of High Blood Cholesterol in Adults (Adult Treatment Panel III). *JAMA.* 2001; 285:2486–2487.

Table C163.4. Treatment Decisions Based on Low-Density Lipoprotein Levels and Coronary Heart Disease (CHD) Risk Status

PATIENT CATEGORY	LDL-C INITIATION LEVEL (MG/DL)	LOW-DENSITY LIPOPROTEIN GOAL (MG/DL)
Dietary therapy		
CHD or CHD risk equivalent[a]	≥100	<100
≥2 Risk factors (10-yr risk ≤20%)	≥130	<130
0–1 Risk factor	≥100	<100
Drug treatment		
CHD or CHD risk equivalent	≥130[b]	<100
≥2 Risk factors (10-yr risk ≤20%)	≥130 (10-yr risk 10%–20%)	<130
	≥160 (10-yr risk <10%)	<130
0–1 Risk factor	≥190[c]	≤160

LDL-C, low-density lipoprotein cholesterol.
[a]Diabetics are included in this category.
[b]Drug treatment optional with LDL-C 100–129 mg/dL.
[c]Drug treatment optional with LDL-C 160–189 mg/dL.
Adapted from Expert Panel on Detection, Evaluation, and Treatment of High Blood Cholesterol in Adults. Executive Summary of the third report of the National Cholesterol Education Program (NCEP) Expert Panel on Detection, Evaluation, and Treatment of High Blood Cholesterol in Adults (Adult Treatment Panel III). *JAMA.* 2001;285:2486–2487.

exceeding 20% over 10 years. An example of such an individual would be an elderly man with systolic hypertension who smokes and has a low HDL-C level.

Nonpharmacologic Therapy for Hypertensive Patients with Hypercholesterolemia

See **Table C163.4** for a listing of nonpharmacologic therapies for hypertensive patients with hypercholesterolemia. The principal nutritional goals for hypercholesterolemic hypertensive patients are shown in **Table C163.5**. Alcohol intake should be restricted to <2 oz per day of ethanol, and sodium intake should be <2 g per day. These measures, when combined with achievement and maintenance of desirable body weight and reduction of saturated fat and cholesterol intake, may be particularly beneficial and should be especially encouraged in hypertensive patients who have hypercholesterolemia or features of the metabolic syndrome. Clinical identification of this syndrome, according to ATP-III criteria, is based on the presence of 3 or more of the following abnormalities: increased waist circumference (>102 cm in men, >88 cm in women), TG ≥150 mg/dL, low HDL-C (<40 mg/dL in men or <50 mg/dL in women), BP

Table C163.5. Nutritional Guidelines for Management of Hypertensive Patients with Hypercholesterolemia

Nutritional goals
  Body weight within 15% of desirable level
  Alcohol, <2 oz/d ethanol
  Sodium, <2 g/d
  Saturated fat, <7% of total calories
  Cholesterol, <200 mg/d
  Viscous (soluble) fiber, 5–10 g/d
  Plant sterol/stanols, 2 g/d

130/85 mm Hg or greater, and fasting blood glucose level 110 mg/dL or greater. The metabolic syndrome is present in over 40% of individuals older than 60 years of age in the United States. Although many patients find it difficult to make dietary and other lifestyle changes, the clinician should provide appropriate counseling or referral to sources of information related to lifestyle changes. Nonpharmacologic therapy is particularly important in patients with multiple abnormalities that are responsive to dietary or other nonpharmacologic measures.

Pharmacologic Treatment of Hypercholesterolemia in the Hypertensive Patient

See Table C163.4.

Statins. Hepatic 3-methylglutaryl coenzyme A reductase inhibitors (lovastatin, pravastatin, simvastatin, fluvastatin, atorvastatin) have become the cornerstones of cholesterol-lowering drug therapy because of their favorable tolerability profile and unparalleled efficacy in lowering LDL-C levels. Convincing evidence of the benefits of statins in reducing the risk of stroke and CHD events has been obtained during the last decade, particularly in hypercholesterolemic patients with preexisting coronary artery disease. Beneficial effects have also been demonstrated in primary and secondary prevention trials among subjects with a wide range of cholesterol levels. In the Antihypertensive and Lipid-Lowering Treatment to Prevent Heart Attack Trial (ALLHAT), which was designed to determine whether treatment with an alpha-blocker, calcium antagonist, or ACE inhibitor lowered the incidence of CHD or other cardiovascular events compared to a thiazide diuretic, also had a second step that added a lipid-lowering agent (pravastatin). Total cholesterol levels were slightly higher during treatment with the thiazide diuretic when compared to the calcium antagonist ACE inhibitor groups. However, no difference in CHD incidence was observed after a mean follow-up of 4.9 years. Among moderately hypercholesterolemic participants, treatment with pravastatin reduced total cholesterol by approximately 17% compared to 8% for usual care. Although a small decrease in cardiovascular event rates was noted in the pravastatin group, differences were not statistically significant. Reduced lipid levels were accompanied by the expected differences in cardiovascular event rates, which supports the goal of aggressive modification of blood lipid levels in high-risk hypertensive patients. Comparisons of the lipid-lowering effects and cost of the currently marketed statins through their typically prescribed dose range are given in **Table C163.6**. The most feared complication of statin treatment is rhabdomyolysis, which is increased by coadministration of drugs such as cyclosporine, erythromycin, gemfibrozil, and niacin. Statins may also cause elevations in hepatic transaminase levels, which occur in approximately 0.5% to 2.0% of patients, depending on the dose administered.

Other lipid-lowering agents. Other drugs have a more limited role in the management of patients with dyslipidemia. Bile acid sequestrants (cholestyramine, colestipol, colesevelam) are primarily LDL-C–lowering agents that may increase TG levels, particularly in hypertriglyceridemic patients. Gastrointestinal side effects, including nausea, epigastric discomfort, and constipation, commonly occur with these agents, particularly early in the course of treatment. Nicotinic acid continues to be the most effective HDL-C–raising agent and tends to lower serum TG levels, LDL-C, and levels of the atherogenic lipoprotein(a). Flushing and

Table C163.6. Comparison of Low-Density Lipoprotein Cholesterol–Lowering Effects of Hepatic 3-Methylglutaryl Coenzyme A Reductase Inhibitors with Usual Starting and Maximum Doses

DRUG	DOSE (MG/D)	DECREASE IN LOW-DENSITY LIPOPROTEIN CHOLESTEROL (%)
Lovastatin	20–00	24–40
Pravastatin	20–80	24–37
Simvastatin	20–80	35–46
Fluvastatin	20–80	18–31
Atorvastatin	10–80	37–57

pruritus frequently limit tolerability to nicotinic acid treatment, although use of aspirin, slow upward dose titration, and extended-release formulations of niacin are helpful in limiting these cutaneous side effects. Fibric acid derivatives, such as fenofi-brate and gemfibrozil, are particularly effective TG-lowering agents that raise HDL-C levels but have variable effects on LDL-C concentrations. They have been shown to be effective in reducing CHD risk particularly among individuals with low HDL-C levels.

SUGGESTED READING

1. Expert Panel on Detection, Evaluation, and Treatment of High Blood Cholesterol in Adults. Executive Summary of the third report of the National Cholesterol Education Program (NCEP) Export Panel on Detection, Evaluation, and Treatment of High Blood Cholesterol in Adults (Adult Treatment Panel III). *JAMA*. 2001;285:2486–2497.
2. Ford ES, Giles WH, Dietz WH. Prevalence of the metabolic syndrome in US adults: findings from the third National Health and Nutrition Examination Survey. *JAMA*. 2002;287:356–359.
3. Gotto AM. Statin therapy and reduced incidence of stroke: implications of cholesterol-lowering therapy for cerebrovascular disease. *Arch Intern Med*. 1997;157:1283–1284.
4. Gould AL, Rossouw JE, Santanello NC, et al. Cholesterol reduction yields clinical benefit. Impact of Statin Trials. *Circulation*. 1998;97:946–952.
5. Grundy SM. Non-high-density lipoprotein cholesterol level as potential risk predictor and therapy target. *Arch Intern Med*. 2001;161:1379–1380.

Chapter C164

Treatment of Diabetes and Hypertension

Samy I. McFarlane, MD; James R. Sowers, MD

KEY POINTS

- Hypertension is twice as common in people with diabetes than in those without and accounts for up to 85% of excess cardiovascular disease risk; patients with hypertension are more prone to have diabetes than are normotensive patients.

- In type 2 diabetes, hypertension usually clusters with the other components of the cardiometabolic syndrome (microalbuminuria, central obesity, insulin resistance, dyslipidemia, hypercoagulation, increased inflammation, left ventricular hypertrophy, and hyperuricemia).

- Hypertension in people with diabetes is also associated with salt sensitivity, volume expansion, isolated systolic hypertension, loss of the nocturnal dipping of blood pressure and heart rate, increased propensity toward orthostatic hypotension, and albuminuria; hypertension and nephropathy exacerbate each other.

- Cardiovascular disease risk reduction in this high-risk population mandates aspirin, low-density lipoprotein cholesterol lowering to <100 mg/dL, and blood pressure lowering to <130/80 mm Hg with agents that also have renal and cardiovascular disease protective effects (angiotensin-converting enzyme inhibitors or angiotensin receptor blockers).

See also Chapters A22, A44–A46, A53, A60, A66, B93, B97, B98, C127, C129, C130, C136–C139, C141, C144–C146, C152, C159, C161, and C162

Hypertension is a major risk factor for cardiovascular disease (CVD) in people with diabetes, increasing the risk for coronary heart disease, stroke, retinopathy, and nephropathy. When hypertension coexists with diabetes, risk of stroke or CVD is doubled, and the risk for developing end-stage renal disease increases to 5 to 6 times compared to hypertensive patients without diabetes. Other risk factors for CVD that cluster with diabetes are central obesity, dyslipidemia, microalbuminuria, and coagulation and inflammation abnormalities.

Hypertension is approximately twice as common in patients with diabetes compared to those without the disease and accounts for up to 85% of excess CVD risk. Conversely, patients with hypertension are more prone to develop diabetes than are normotensive persons.

Specific Treatment Targets

Hypertension in patients with diabetes demonstrates other features, most of which are considered risk factors for CVD

Table C164.1. Cardiovascular Disease Risk Factors Associated with Diabetes

Hypertension
Obesity
Hyperinsulinemia/insulin resistance
Endothelial dysfunction
Microalbuminuria
Low high-density lipoprotein cholesterol levels
High triglyceride levels
Small, dense low-density lipoprotein cholesterol particles
Increased apolipoprotein B levels
Increased fibrinogen levels
Increased plasminogen activator inhibitor-1 and decreased plasminogen activator levels
Increased C-reactive protein and other inflammatory markers
Absent nocturnal dipping of blood pressure and heart rate
Salt sensitivity
Left ventricular hypertrophy
Premature/excess coronary artery disease, stroke, and peripheral vascular disease

(Table C164.1). These features can be important in selecting the optimal antihypertensive medications.

Salt sensitivity and volume expansion. Increased sensitivity to dietary salt is greatest in hypertensive patients with diabetes, obesity, renal insufficiency, or low-renin status and in blacks and the elderly. Weight reduction and moderate salt restriction have been shown in clinical trials to reduce blood pressure (BP) in diabetic patients with hypertension.

Isolated systolic hypertension. Age-related stiffening of the aorta and central arteries is accelerated in diabetes. Systolic BP increases, leading to isolated systolic hypertension, which is more common and occurs at a relatively younger age in patients with diabetes.

Loss of nocturnal decline of blood pressure. In patients with diabetes, there is a loss of the normal nocturnal drop of BP and heart rate by 24-hour ambulatory monitoring ("nondipping"), which conveys excessive risk for stroke and myocardial infarction. Microalbuminuria and increased left ventricular mass are associated with nondipping in diabetic patients. Nondipping in diabetic patients is an important factor in deciding the optimal dosing strategies of antihypertensive medications in cases in which drugs that provide consistent and sustained 24-hour BP control are advantageous.

Microalbuminuria and nephropathy. Thiazide diuretics, calcium antagonists, and, perhaps, angiotensin-converting enzyme (ACE) inhibitors are useful in isolated systolic hypertension. There is considerable evidence that hypertension in type 1 diabetes is a consequence, rather than a cause, of renal disease because nephropathy often precedes the rise in BP. Yet hypertension and nephropathy also exacerbate each other. Elevated systolic BP is a significant determining factor in the progression of microalbuminuria, which is an integral component of the metabolic syndrome. This concept is important to consider in selecting the pharmacologic therapy for hypertension in patients with diabetes in cases in which antihypertensive medications that decrease both proteinuria and BP (ACE inhibitors and angiotensin receptor blockers) are important

tools in reducing the progression of nephropathy and associated CVD risk.

Orthostatic hypotension. In patients with diabetes and autonomic dysfunction, excessive venous pooling can cause immediate or delayed orthostatic hypotension, potentially compromising cerebral blood flow and leading to intermittent lightheadedness, fatigue, unsteady gait, or syncope. Orthostatic hypotension is itself a risk factor and a diagnostic confounder. All diabetic patients should have their BP measured in the sitting and standing positions at each visit; a supine BP should also be measured at regular intervals. Increased propensity for orthostatic hypertension in patients with diabetes renders α-adrenergic receptor blockers less desirable agents for these patients. In addition, doses of all antihypertensive agents must be titrated more carefully in patients with diabetes who have greater propensity for orthostatic hypertension.

Management of Cholesterol and Other Cardiovascular Risk Factors

The goal of therapy of hypertension in people with diabetes is the reduction of CVD morbidity and mortality; therefore, all CVD risk factors (e.g., smoking, alcohol intake, inactivity, and dyslipidemia) must be controlled concomitantly. Statin therapy is especially important in reducing the incidence of myocardial infarction. The American Diabetes Association recommends lifestyle modifications, such as smoking cessation, weight loss, exercise, reduction of dietary sodium intake, and limitation of alcohol consumption, as an integral part of management.

Blood Pressure Control

Based on the results of several major randomized controlled trials, including the Hypertension Optimal Treatment (HOT) trial, the United Kingdom Prospective Diabetes Study (UKPDS), the Appropriate Blood Pressure Control in Diabetes (ABCD) trial, and the Modification of Diet in Renal Disease (MDRD) trial, the Hypertension and Diabetes Executive Working Group of the National Kidney Foundation recommends lowering the BP goal level to 130/80 mm Hg or less in patients with diabetes or renal impairment. This treatment goal was also adopted by the Canadian Hypertension Society and by the American Diabetes Association. However, despite the compelling evidence from these trials that lowering the BP significantly reduces CVD in people with diabetes, the BP goal of 130/80 mm Hg is achieved only in one-fourth of patients. Optimal control of all CVD risk factors was achieved in <10% of these patients.

Angiotensin-converting enzyme inhibitors. ACE inhibitors lower BP, attenuate albuminuria and renal disease progression, and reduce cardiovascular risk as shown in randomized controlled trials such as the Captopril Prevention Project (CAPP) and the Microalbuminuria, Cardiovascular, and Renal Outcome-Heart Outcomes Prevention Evaluation (MICRO-HOPE) study. ACE inhibitors also improved insulin resistance and prevented the development of diabetes in the HOPE study. In patients with type 1 diabetes and proteinuria, ACE inhibitor treatment was associated with a significant reduction in the risk of the combined CVD and microvascular end points in MICRO-HOPE. Furthermore, ACE inhibitors reduced heart failure incidence. With these clearly proven benefits, ACE

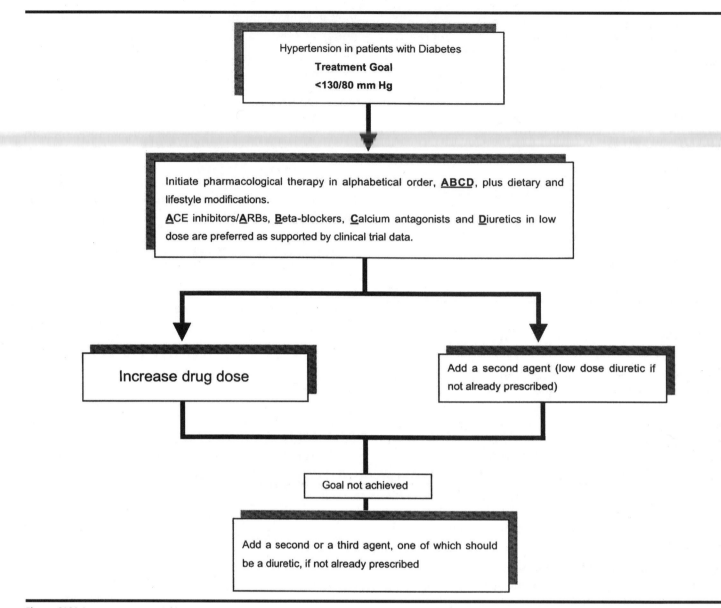

Figure C164.1.   Management of hypertension in patients with diabetes. ACE, angiotensin-converting enzyme; ARBs, angiotensin receptor blockers.

inhibitors are currently recommended as a first-line treatment and are the most prescribed antihypertensive medication for patients with diabetes and hypertension.

Angiotensin receptor blockers. Angiotensin receptor blockers (ARBs) are recommended as an initial therapy for those who do not tolerate ACE inhibitors (usually because of cough) and are an alternative to ACE inhibitors in patients with diabetes and proteinuria, heart failure, systolic dysfunction, postmyocardial infarction, and mild renal insufficiency. Three major studies—the Reduction of Endpoints in NIDDM with the Angiotensin II Antagonist Losartan (RENAAL) Study, the Irbesartan Microalbuminuria Type 2 Diabetes in Hypertensive Patients (IRMA II) Study, and the Irbesartan in Diabetic Nephropathy Trial (IDNT)—have showed that ARBs are effective in reducing the progression of renal disease in patients with type 2 diabetes and hypertension. BP control was similar in the placebo and ARB-treated groups in these studies, indicating that ARBs protect the kidney independent of BP reduction. The RENAAL study docu-

mented reduction in the initial hospitalization for heart failure. In the Losartan Intervention for Endpoint (LIFE) trial, losartan was statistically significantly superior to atenolol in reducing CVD morbidity and mortality in diabetic patients with hypertension and left ventricular hypertrophy, reducing fatal and nonfatal strokes by 25%, and new onset of diabetes by 25% compared to atenolol. These benefits were above and beyond those attributable to BP reduction alone. ARBs have been recommended as a first-line therapy for patients with diabetes and hypertension along with ACE-inhibitors (**Figure C164.1**).

β-Blockers. β-Blockers are also useful antihypertensive agents in patients with diabetes. In the UKPDS study, atenolol or ACE inhibitor reduced microvascular complications of diabetes by 37%, strokes by 44%, and death related to diabetes by 32%. Hypertensive patients receiving β-blockers have a higher risk of new diabetes than those on no medication or on other antihypertensive medications, but they have proved to have significant long-term favorable effects on CVD in hypertensive patients with diabetes and therefore should be used routinely, particularly those with underlying ischemic heart disease.

Calcium antagonists. Nondihydropyridine calcium antagonists (CAs), such as verapamil or diltiazem, may have more beneficial effects on proteinuria than dihydropyridine CAs, such as nifedipine or amlodipine. However, with the use of ACE inhibitors (or ARBs) as a first-line treatment, especially when diuretic is also present, the addition of a long-acting dihydropyridine, such as amlodipine, substantially improves BP control rates. CAs are especially useful in patients with isolated systolic hypertension or nephropathy.

Diuretics. Low-dose diuretics are effective antihypertensive agents in patients with diabetes. Adverse metabolic effects shown with large doses (e.g., 50–200 mg of hydrochlorothiazide) have not been substantiated with low-dose diuretics. In addition, diuretics are often a necessary component of combination antihypertensive therapy in people with diabetes who usually require multiple drug therapy to achieve target BP.

Combination antihypertensive therapy. To achieve a BP goal of 130/80 mm Hg or less in people with diabetes and hypertension, 2 or more antihypertensive medications are usually necessary. Indeed, in a report by our group, among 1,372 patients with hypertension and diabetes, the average number of medications required to achieve a target BP of 130/85 mm Hg was 3.1, consistent with results from other analyses from UKPDS, MDRD, HOT, and ABCD, in which more than 2 medications were often required for optimal control of BP.

SUGGESTED READING

1. Bakris GL, Williams M, Dworkin L, et al. Preserving renal function in adults with hypertension and diabetes: a consensus approach. National Kidney Foundation Hypertension and Diabetes Executive Committees Working Group. *Am J Kidney Dis.* 2000;36:646–661.
2. Brenner BM, Cooper ME, de Zeeuw D, et al. Effects of losartan on renal and cardiovascular outcomes in patients with type 2 diabetes and nephropathy. *N Engl J Med.* 2001;345:861–869.
3. Dahlof B, Devereux RB, Kjeldsen SE, et al. Cardiovascular morbidity and mortality in the Losartan Intervention For End point reduction in hypertension study (LIFE): a randomized trial against atenolol. *Lancet.* 2002;359:995–1003.
4. Gress TW, Nieto FJ, Shahar E, et al. Hypertension and antihypertensive therapy as risk factors for type 2 diabetes mellitus. Atherosclerosis Risk in Communities Study. *N Engl J Med.* 2000;342:905–912.
5. Lindholm LH, Isben H, Dahlof B, et al. Cardiovascular morbidity and mortality in patients with diabetes in the Losartan Intervention For Endpoint reduction in hypertension study (LIFE): a randomized trial against atenolol. *Lancet.* 2002;359:1004–1010.
6. McFarlane SI, Banerji M, Sowers JR. Insulin resistance and cardiovascular disease. *J Clin Endocrinol Metab.* 2001;86:713–718.
7. McFarlane SI, Jacober SJ, Winer N, et al. Control of cardiovascular risk factors in patients with diabetes and hypertension at urban academic medical centers. *Diabetes Care.* 2002;25:718–723.
8. Parving HH, Lehnert H, Brochner-Mortensen J, et al. Effect of irbesartan on the development of diabetic nephropathy in patients with type 2 diabetes. *Ugeskr Laeger.* 2001;163:5519–5524.
9. Sowers JR, Epstein M, Frohlich ED. Diabetes, hypertension, and cardiovascular disease: an update. *Hypertension.* 2001;37:1053–1059.
10. Yusuf S, Sleight P, Pogue J, et al. Effects of an angiotensin-converting-enzyme inhibitor, ramipril, on cardiovascular events in high-risk patients. The Heart Outcomes Prevention Evaluation Study Investigators. *N Engl J Med.* 2000;342:145–153.

Chapter C165

Treatment of Pregnant Hypertensive Patients

Sandra J. Taler, MD

KEY POINTS

- Most women with chronic hypertension in pregnancy have stage 1 to 2 hypertension and are candidates for nondrug therapy.

- There is no evidence that pharmacologic treatment leads to improved neonatal outcomes.

- Preeclampsia occurs in 25% of women with chronic hypertension.

- Hypertensive disorders have a high rate of recurrence (20–50%) in subsequent pregnancies.

See also Chapters A38, A57, B86, C137, C139, C141, C143, C146, C147, and C153

The key to management of hypertension in pregnancy is to differentiate preeclampsia, a pregnancy-specific syndrome of exaggerated vasoconstriction and reduced organ perfusion, from preexisting chronic hypertension. Hypertension during pregnancy is classified into 1 of 5 categories (**Table C165.1**).

Prepregnancy Assessment and Counseling

Ideally, women with hypertension should be evaluated before conception to define the severity of their hypertension and plan for potential lifestyle changes. If systolic blood pressure (SBP) is ≥180 mm Hg or diastolic blood pressure (DBP) is ≥110 mm Hg, or if treatment requires multiple antihypertensive agents, the

Table C165.1. Classification of Hypertension in Pregnancy

Chronic hypertension	BP ≥140 mm Hg systolic or 90 mm Hg diastolic before pregnancy or before 20 wk gestation Persists >12 wk postpartum
Preeclampsia	BP ≥140 mm Hg systolic or 90 mm Hg diastolic with proteinuria (>300 mg/24 h) after 20 wk gestation Can progress to eclampsia (seizures) More common in nulliparous women, multiple gestation, women with hypertension for ≥4 yr, family history of preeclampsia, hypertension in previous pregnancy, renal disease
Chronic hypertension with superimposed preeclampsia	New onset proteinuria after 20 wk in a woman with hypertension In a woman with hypertension and proteinuria before 20 wk gestation: Sudden 2- to 3-fold increase in proteinuria Sudden increase in BP Thrombocytopenia Elevated aspartate aminotransferase or alanine aminotransferase
Gestational hypertension	Hypertension without proteinuria occurring after 20 wk gestation Temporary diagnosis May represent preproteinuric phase of preeclampsia or recurrence of chronic hypertension abated in midpregnancy May evolve to preeclampsia If severe, may result in higher rates of premature delivery and growth retardation than mild preeclampsia
Transient hypertension	Retrospective diagnosis BP normal by 12 wk postpartum May recur in subsequent pregnancies Predictive of future essential hypertension

BP, blood pressure.

woman should be evaluated for potentially reversible causes. In hypertensive women planning to become pregnant, some practitioners change to antihypertensive medications known to be safe during pregnancy, such as β-blockers or methyldopa even before conception. Angiotensin-converting enzyme inhibitors and angiotensin receptor blockers should be discontinued before conception or as soon as pregnancy is confirmed.

Target organ damage. Women with a history of hypertension over several years should be evaluated for target organ damage, including left ventricular hypertrophy, retinopathy, and renal disease. If these conditions are present, women should be advised that pregnancy may worsen these conditions. Women with chronic hypertension may be at higher risk for adverse neonatal outcomes independent of the development of preeclampsia if proteinuria is present early in pregnancy. The risks of fetal loss and acceleration of maternal renal disease increase at serum creatinine levels higher than 1.4 mg per dL at conception, although it may be difficult to separate the effects of pregnancy from progression of the underlying renal disease. Preeclampsia is significantly more common in women with chronic hypertension, with an incidence of approximately 25%. Risk factors for superimposed preeclampsia include renal insufficiency, a history of hypertension for 4 years or longer, and hypertension in a previous pregnancy.

Lifestyle changes. Chronic hypertension before pregnancy requires planning for lifestyle changes. Hypertensive women are advised to restrict aerobic exercise during pregnancy based on theoretic concerns that inadequate placental blood flow may increase the risk of preeclampsia. Weight reduction is not recommended during pregnancy, even in obese women. Sodium restriction is recommended only for those women who have been successfully treated by this approach before pregnancy. As in all pregnancies, the use of alcohol and tobacco is strongly discouraged.

Treatment of Chronic Hypertension during Pregnancy

Most women with chronic hypertension in pregnancy have stage 1 to 2 hypertension (SBP of 140–179, DBP of 90–109 mm Hg, or both) and are at low risk for cardiovascular complications during pregnancy. These women are candidates for nondrug therapy because there is no evidence that pharmacologic treatment leads to improved neonatal outcomes. As blood pressure (BP) usually falls during the first half of pregnancy, hypertension may be easier to control with reduced or no medications. Home BP monitoring is a useful adjunct to close medical supervision. Although evaluation for secondary causes can usually be deferred until after delivery, all hypertensive women should be screened for pheochromocytoma at the time of discovery of the hypertension owing to the high associated morbidity and mortality of this condition if not diagnosed antepartum. The benefit of continued administration of antihypertensive drugs to pregnant women with chronic hypertension continues to be an area of debate. Some centers manage chronic hypertensives by stopping antihypertensive medications while maintaining close observation. For women with evidence for target organ damage and for those on multiple agents, medications may be tapered based on BP readings but should be continued if needed to control BP. There is evidence from several studies that antihypertensive medications prevent increase of BP to very high levels during pregnancy. Treatment should be reinstituted once BP reaches levels of 150 to 160 mm Hg systolic or 100 to 110 mm Hg diastolic.

Antihypertensive drug selection. The primary goal of treating chronic hypertension is to reduce maternal risk, but the agents selected must be safe for the fetus. Methyldopa is preferred by many as first-line therapy, based on reports of stable uteroplacental blood flow and fetal hemodynamics and follow-up studies out to 7.5 years showing no long-term adverse effects on development of children exposed to methyldopa *in utero*. Other treatment options are listed in **Table C165.2.** Based on a recent metaanalysis of 45 randomized controlled trials of treatment of stage 1 and 2 hypertension in pregnancy, there are still concerns regarding the safety of any drug treatment. In this analysis of trials using methyldopa, β-blockers, thiazide diuretics, hydralazine, calcium antagonists, and clonidine, there was a direct linear relationship between treatment-induced fall in mean arterial pressure and the proportion of small-for-gestational-age infants. The type of hypertension, type of antihypertensive agent, and duration of therapy do not explain this relationship.

There are no placebo-controlled trials evaluating the treatment of stage 3 hypertension in pregnancy, and none are likely

Table C165.2. Treatment of Chronic Hypertension in Pregnancy

AGENT	COMMENTS
Methyldopa	Preferred based on long-term follow-up studies supporting safety
β-Blockers	Reports of intrauterine growth retardation (atenolol), generally safe
Labetalol	Increasingly preferred to methyldopa owing to reduced side effects
Clonidine	Limited data
Calcium antagonists	Limited data, no increase in major teratogenicity with exposure
Diuretics	Not first-line agents, probably safe
Angiotensin-converting enzyme inhibitors, angiotensin II receptor antagonists	Contraindicated, reported fetal toxicity and death

to ever be performed owing to ethical concerns. Early reports of experience with severe chronic hypertension in the first trimester described fetal loss rates of 50% and significant maternal mortality, with most of the poor outcomes occurring in those pregnancies complicated by superimposed preeclampsia.

Influence of renal diseases on management. Women with progressive renal diseases should be encouraged to complete their childbearing while their renal function is relatively well preserved. Among women with mild renal disease (serum creatinine below 1.4 mg/dL), fetal survival is only moderately reduced and the underlying disease does not generally worsen. Moderate or severe renal insufficiency in pregnancy may accelerate hypertension and the underlying disease and markedly reduce fetal survival. A decrease in birth weight correlates directly with rising maternal serum creatinine concentration. As renal failure progresses, the hypertension has a component of volume overload and may require sodium restriction, use of diuretics, or dialysis. Chronic dialysis during pregnancy is associated with significant maternal morbidity and fetal loss and conception should be discouraged. Renal transplant recipients are advised to wait 1.5 to 2.0 years after successful transplantation and undertake pregnancy only if renal function is stable with creatinine of 2.0 mg per dL or less. Rates of prematurity are high, thus all pregnancies in transplant recipients are considered to be high risk.

Treating hypertension during lactation. Breast-feeding can usually be done safely with certain limits on antihypertensive drug choices. In mildly hypertensive mothers who wish to breast-feed for a few months, medication may be withheld with close monitoring of BP. After discontinuation of nursing, antihypertensive therapy can be reinstituted. For patients with more severe BP elevation on a single antihypertensive agent, the clinician may consider reducing the dosage while closely monitoring mother and infant. The available data regarding excretion of antihypertensive agents in human breast milk suggest that all studied agents are excreted into human breast milk, although there are differences in the milk to plasma ratio related to lipid solubility and extent of ionization of the drug at physiologic pH. No short-term adverse effects have been reported from exposure to methyldopa or hydralazine. Propanolol and labetalol are preferred if a β-blocker is indicated. Diuretics may reduce milk volume and thereby suppress lactation. Angiotensin-converting enzyme inhibitors and angiotensin receptor antagonists should be avoided based on reports of adverse fetal and neonatal renal effects. Given the scarcity of data, breast-fed infants of mothers taking antihypertensive agents should be closely monitored for potential adverse effects.

Preeclampsia

Prevention. The ability to prevent preeclampsia is limited by lack of knowledge of its underlying cause. Prevention has focused on identification of women at higher risk, followed by close clinical and laboratory monitoring aimed at early recognition of the disease and institution of intensive monitoring or delivery when indicated. Despite the encouraging results of early small trials, none of the large multicenter trials of aspirin demonstrated any benefit compared with placebo. The prevailing opinion is that women without risk factors do not benefit from treatment, but selective treatment for certain women at higher risk (specifically women with the antiphospholipid syndrome) may be reasonable. Randomized trials of calcium supplementation have demonstrated reductions in incidence of preeclampsia in women at high risk and with low calcium intake. For low-risk women in the United States, there is no evidence of benefit of calcium-enriched diets.

General management principles. Treatment for preeclampsia consists of hospitalization for bed rest, control of BP, seizure prophylaxis when signs of impending eclampsia are present, and timely delivery. Therapy is palliative and does not alter the underlying pathophysiology of the disease; at best, it may slow progression of the condition and provide time for fetal maturation. Delivery is always appropriate therapy for the mother but may compromise a fetus of less than 32 weeks' gestation. For a preterm fetus with no evidence of fetal compromise in a woman with mild disease, valuable time may be gained by postponing delivery. Antihypertensive therapy should be prescribed only for maternal safety; it does not improve perinatal outcomes and may adversely affect uteroplacental blood flow. As many women with preeclampsia were previously normotensive with BPs in the range of 100 to 110/70 mm Hg, acute elevations to mild levels (i.e., 150/100 mm Hg) may cause significant symptomatology and require treatment. It is unusual for preeclampsia to remit spontaneously, and, in most cases, the disease worsens. Regardless of gestational age, delivery should be strongly considered when there are signs of fetal distress or intrauterine growth retardation or signs of maternal risk including severe hypertension, hemolysis, elevated liver enzymes, and low platelet count (termed the *HELLP syndrome*), deteriorating renal function, visual disturbance, headache, or epigastric pain. Vaginal delivery is preferable to cesarean delivery to avoid the added stress of surgery.

Antihypertensive drug therapy. Selection of antihypertensive agents and route of administration depends on anticipated timing of delivery. If it is likely to be more than 48 hours until delivery, oral methyldopa is preferred owing to its safety record and extensive experience. Oral labetalol is an alternative choice, with other β-blockers and calcium antagonists acceptable alternatives based on limited data. If delivery is imminent, parenteral agents are practical and effective (**Table C165.3**).

Table C165.3. Treatment of Acute Severe Hypertension in Preeclampsia

Hydralazine	5 mg i.v. bolus, then 10 mg every 20–30 min to a maximum of 25 mg, repeat in several hours as necessary.
Labetalol (second-line)	20 mg i.v. bolus, then 40 mg 10 min later, 80 mg every 10 min for 2 additional doses to a maximum of 220 mg.
Nifedipine (controversial)	10 mg p.o. repeat every 20 min to a maximum of 30 mg. Caution when using nifedipine with magnesium sulfate, can see precipitous blood pressure drop. Short-acting nifedipine is not approved by U.S. Food and Drug Administration for managing hypertension.
Sodium nitroprusside (rarely when others fail)	0.25 µg/kg/min to a maximum of 5 µg/kg/min. Fetal cyanide poisoning may occur if used for more than 4 h.

Antihypertensives are administered before induction for persistent diastolic levels of 105 to 110 mm Hg or higher, aiming for levels of 95 to 105 mm Hg.

Recurrence of Hypertension

Hypertensive disorders have a high rate of recurrence (20%–50%) in subsequent pregnancies whether classified as gestational hypertension, preeclampsia, or preeclampsia superimposed on chronic hypertension. Risk factors for recurrence include early onset of hypertension in the first pregnancy, a history of chronic hypertension, persistent hypertension beyond 5 weeks postpartum, and high baseline BP early in pregnancy. Remote hypertension is more common after gestational hypertension, but women with preeclampsia have a greater tendency to develop hypertension than those with normotensive pregnancies.

SUGGESTED READING

1. American College of Obstetricians and Gynecologists. Chronic hypertension in pregnancy. ACOG Practice Bulletin #29. *Obstet Gynecol.* 2001;98:S177–S185.
2. Buchbinder A, Sibai B, Caritis S, et al. Adverse perinatal outcomes are significantly higher in severe gestational hypertension than in mild preeclampsia. *Am J Obstet Gynecol.* 2002;186:66–71.
3. Report of the National High Blood Pressure Education Program Working Group on High Blood Pressure in Pregnancy. *Am J Obstet Gynecol.* 2000;183:S1–S22.
4. Sibai BM. Treatment of hypertension in pregnant women. *N Engl J Med.* 1996;335:257–265.
5. Von Dadelszen P, Ornstein MP, Bull SB, et al. Fall in mean arterial pressure and fetal growth restriction in pregnancy hypertension: a meta-analysis. *Lancet.* 2000;355:87–92.
6. Zhang J, Troendle JF, Levine RJ. Risks of hypertensive disorders in the second pregnancy. *Paediatr Perinat Epidemiol.* 2001;15:226–231.

Chapter C166

Treatment of Hypertensive Children and Adolescents

Bonita E. Falkner, MD

KEY POINTS

- Children and adolescents with hypertension, as well as those with diabetes or chronic renal disease, benefit from treatment to lower blood pressure below the 90th percentile for age.

- Echocardiography, ambulatory blood pressure monitoring, and metabolic risk factor assessment provide useful information to guide blood pressure treatment decisions in children and adolescents.

- Lifestyle changes, especially weight loss, should be emphasized in children with high normal blood pressure.

- Pharmacologic treatment should be individualized in each child.

Also see Chapters B87, B97, B98, B102, C109, C110, C112, C127, C129, C130, C137–C139, C141–C147, and C152

Hypertension in childhood and adolescence is defined as systolic or diastolic blood pressure (BP) ≥ the 95th percentile for age, sex, and height. The challenge clinically is to identify, evaluate, and treat those children who will benefit from interventions to lower BP. Children who have BP levels substantially above the 95th percentile (by 10 to 15 mm Hg) require careful evaluation to detect a possible secondary cause of hypertension that could be correctable. These children also benefit from medical treatment to lower BP. Children with renal disease or diabetes should receive treatment to lower BP below the 90th percentile for renal protection. Fewer data are available on the benefit of intervention in children with BPs above the 90th to 95th percentile who do not have diabetes or renal disease. Children with high BP levels will continue to have high BP levels and will progress to clinical hypertension at an earlier age. In all cases, it is appropriate to use nonpharmacologic treatments.

Assessment of Hypertension and Target Organs

When there is a question as to whether pharmacologic therapy should be used in children, additional clinical information can be helpful. An echocardiogram can be used if the level of BP has caused increased cardiac mass. Twenty-four–hour ambulatory BP monitoring can provide adjunctive assessment of BP by repeated measurements throughout the day and night, resulting in information on levels and variability of BP. Values from both the echocardiogram and the ABPM should be reported and interpreted using the pediatric reference data. Many children with modest BP elevations for age are also overweight or obese and should be evaluated for other metabolic risk factors including glucose and lipid abnormalities.

Nonpharmacologic Therapy in Children and Adolescents

Nonpharmacologic therapies for BP control can be useful in children with modest hypertension or high normal BP. Children who have severe hypertension or those with uncorrectable conditions such as chronic renal disease will probably not respond to nonpharmacologic therapies alone but these interventions may still be helpful in maintaining the BP level within a satisfactory range with lower doses of drugs. The most commonly used nondrug therapies in the young are weight reduction, diet modification, and physical exercise. Lifestyle changes are difficult to effect in the young, but do provide risk-free health benefits that can be enduring.

Weight reduction. Childhood obesity has become a major health problem that will require substantial public health efforts. Overweight children and adolescents with high BP should be strongly encouraged to reduce excess weight and should be provided the education and support necessary to be successful. The recently developed childhood growth grids (http://www.cdc.gov/growthcharts) for body mass index are helpful in documenting the degree of excess weight and providing feedback to the child and family.

Diet modification. The contribution of sodium intake to elevations in BP in the young is unclear. Because the intake of sodium in Westernized societies is excessive, moderate sodium restriction is appropriate and is without adverse nutritional consequences. The Task Force has recommended reductions in sodium intake to 85 to 100 mEq (5–6 g of salt) per day for all hypertensive patients. This is a reasonable goal that can be achieved by reducing the intake of processed foods, eliminating foods with obvious salt added (pretzels and "chips") and limiting the intake of table salt. The Dietary Approach to Stop Hypertension (DASH) study detected a beneficial effect on BP from a diet that increased intake of a combination of dietary nutrients. A comparable study has not yet been conducted in children or adolescents with mild BP elevation. However, in view of the progressive dietary reduction in fresh fruits and vegetables with increasing intake of processed foods among the young, it is prudent and likely beneficial to encourage diet modifications that replace processed foods with fresh fruits and vegetables and low-fat dairy products. A reasonable approach is the "5 a day" method wherein a child or adolescent should strive to consume 5 servings a day of fruits or vegetables.

Exercise. Secular changes in physical activity have resulted in a more sedentary lifestyle among children and adolescents. Aerobic exercise decreases BP in hypertensive adolescents and is generally recommended for enhancing weight loss and improving cardiovascular fitness. In contrast, weight-lifting and body-building exercises that cause excessive increases in muscle mass tend to elevate BP. Thus, physical activities and sports that emphasize aerobic exercise should be encouraged for both children and adolescents and the potential deleterious effects of strenuous static exercise should also be mentioned. Sports participation does not impose a significant risk in hypertensive athletes. However, before sports participation, a hypertensive child or adolescent should be evaluated medically and for those who require pharmacologic therapy, adequate BP control should be achieved.

Other habits. In addition to the above lifestyle changes, use of tobacco, alcohol, and other street drugs should be strongly discouraged. Adolescent boys with high BP who are active in competitive athletics or body-building activities should be especially cautioned and discouraged from using anabolic steroids due to the potential adverse effects of these substances on BP.

Pharmacologic Therapy in Children and Adolescents

The goals of pharmacotherapy are (a) to restore the BP level to normal (below the 90th percentile) and (b) to prevent target organ damage. Pharmacologic therapy for hypertension in the young is challenging for pediatricians because there are limited clinical trial data on the efficacy, safety, and dose responses in children for most antihypertensive drugs, particularly the newer medications. In addition, the tablet strengths available often make precise dose adjustments for small children quite difficult.

Drug strategies. When pharmacologic therapy is used, treatment is individualized to achieve BP control with the most effective single drug or combination of drugs at the lowest effective dose, with minimal side effects. Treatment is usually initiated with a single antihypertensive agent; the dose of this agent is then increased until control is achieved or maximal dosage is reached. If BP control is not achieved, a second drug is usually added. Alternatively, if the first drug has no effect or is not tolerated, a different class of drug should replace the first.

Specific agents. Thiazide diuretics are generally not an optimal first step in antihypertensive therapy for pediatric patients, except in cases where fluid overload plays a significant role. β-Blockers have been used and are effective for BP control in children with hypertension but at higher doses, these agents can produce fatigue and compromise physical performance. Clinical experience is developing on the pediatric use of newer classes of antihypertensive drugs, including calcium antagonists, angiotensin-converting enzyme (ACE) inhibitors, and angiotensin II receptor blockers (ARBs). This experience to date indicates that these newer drugs are effective and well tolerated in children and frequently offer the advantage of once-daily dosing. ACE inhibitors and ARB drugs should be used with caution in sexually active adolescent girls because of the adverse effects of these drugs on the fetus. The needed pharmacodynamic and pharmacokinetic data for these drugs in chil-

Table C166.1. Treatment of Chronic Hypertension in Children

DRUG	DOSE	FREQUENCY	AVAILABLE PREPARATIONS
Diuretics			
Chlorothiazide	20–30 mg/kg/day Maximum: 2 g/day	q12–24h	Tablets: 250, 500 mg Solution: 250 mg/5 mL
Hydrochlorothiazide	1–4 mg/kg/day Maximum: 200 mg/day	q12–24h	Tablets: 25, 50, 100 mg
Metolazone	0.1–0.5 mg/kg/day Maximum: 20 mg/day (Zaroxolyn) 0.5–1.0 mg/day (Mykrox)	q24h q24h	Tablets: 2.5, 5.0, 10.0 mg (Zaroxolyn) Tablets: 0.5, 1.0 mg (Mykrox)
Furosemide	0.5–4.0 mg/kg/day Maximum: 80 mg/dose	q6–24h	Tablets: 20, 40, 80 mg Solution: 10 mg/mL, 40 mg/5 mL, 80 mg/10 mL
Spironolactone	1–3 mg/kg/day Maximum: 200 mg/day for hypertension	q16–24h	Tablets: 25, 50, 100 mg
β-Adrenergic antagonists			
Nonselective			
Propranolol	0.5–5.0 mg/kg/day Maximum: 480 mg/day	q6–12h	Tablets: 10, 20, 40, 60, 80 mg Long-acting capsules: 60, 80, 120, 160 mg Solution: 20, 40 mg/5 mL
Nadolol[a]	40–240 mg/day	q24h	Tablets: 20, 40, 80, 120, 160 mg
Selective			
Atenolol	1–2 mg/kg/day Maximum: 100 mg/day	q24h	Tablets: 25, 50, 100 mg
Metoprolol	1–4 mg/kg/day Maximum: 450 mg/day	q12–24h	Tablets: 50, 100 mg
α-Adrenergic antagonists			
Prazosin	0.02–0.50 mg/kg/day Maximum: 20 mg/day	q6–12h	Tablets: 1, 2, 5 mg
Phenoxybenzamine	0.2–4.0 mg/kg/day Maximum: 40 mg/dose	q8–12h	Capsules: 10 mg
Complex adrenergic antagonists			
Labetalol	1–4 mg/kg/day initially Maximum: 20 mg/kg/day	q8–12h	Tablets: 100, 200, 300 mg
Central α agonists			
Clonidine	5–25 mg/kg/day 0.1–0.6 mg/day Maximum: 2.4 mg/day (oral)	q6–12h q week	Tablets: 0.1, 0.2, 0.3 mg Patches: 0.1, 0.2, 0.3 mg
Methyldopa	10–65 mg/kg/day Maximum: 3 g/day Solution: 250 mg/5 mL	q6–12h	Tablets: 125, 250, 500 mg
Angiotensin-converting enzyme inhibitors			
Captopril	0.05–6.00 mg/kg/day Maximum: 200 mg/day	q8–12h	Tablets: 12.5, 25.0, 50.0, 100.0 mg
Enalapril	0.1–0.5 mg/kg/day Maximum: 40 mg/day	q12–24h	Tablets: 2.5, 5.0, 10.0, 20.0 mg
Lisinopril[a]	2.5–80.0 mg/day	q12–24h	Tablets: 5, 10, 20 mg
Quinapril[a]	1.25–80.00 mg/day	q24h	Tablets: 5, 10, 20 mg
Ramipril[a]	1.25–20.00 mg/day	q12–24h	Capsules: 1.25, 2.50, 5.00, 10.00 mg
Vasodilators			
Hydralazine	1–8 mg/kg/day Maximum: 200 mg/day	q12–24h	Tablets: 10, 25, 50, 100 mg
Minoxidil	0.2–2.0 mg/kg/day Maximum: 100 mg/day	q12–24h	Tablets: 2.5, 10.0 mg
Calcium antagonists			
Nifedipine	0.25–4.00 mg/kg/day Maximum: 180 mg/day	q6–24h	Capsules: 10, 20 mg Extended release: 30, 60, 90 mg
Isradipine	2.5–20.0 mg/day	q8–12h	Capsules: 2.5, 5.0, 10.0 mg
Amlodipine[a]	2.5–10.0 mg/day	q24h	Tablets: 2.5, 5.0, 10.0 mg
Felodipine ER	2.5–20.0 mg/day	q24h	Tablets: 2.5, 5.0, 10.0 mg
Combination drugs			
Bisoprolol/hydrochlorothiazide[a]	2.50/6.25–10.00/6.25/day	q24h	Tablets: 2.50/6.25; 5.00/6.25; 10.00/6.26
Angiotensin II receptor blocking agents			
Losartan[a]	25–100 mg/day	q12–24h	Tablets: 25, 50, 100 mg
Irbesartan[a]	75–300 mg/day	q24h	Tablets: 75, 150, 300 mg
Telmisartan[a]	20–80 mg/day	q24h	Tablets: 40, 80 mg
Candesartan[a]	2–32 mg/day	q12–24h	Tablets: 4, 8, 16, 32 mg

[a]The pediatric dose is under investigation.

Reprinted from Bonilla-Felix M, Portman RJ, Falkner B. Systemic hypertension. In: Burg FD, Ingelfinger JR, Polin RA, Gershon AA, eds. *Gellis and Kagan's Current Pediatric Therapy*. 17th ed. Philadelphia, PA: WB Saunders Co., 2002, with permission.

Table C166.2. Treatment of Hypertensive Emergencies in Children

DRUG	DOSE	ROUTE	COMMENTS
Furosemide	1–4 mg/kg/dose Maximum: 160 mg/dose	i.v., i.m., or p.o.	Nephrotoxic, ototoxic When administered i.v., infuse slowly to avoid ototoxicity Onset: 5–20 min
Hydralazine	0.1–0.5 mg/kg/dose Maximum: 50 mg/dose	i.v., i.m.	Tachycardia, flushing, salt retention Onset: 10–20 min
Diazoxide	1–5 mg/kg/dose q5–15 min Maximum: 150 mg/dose	i.v.	Pain at injected vein, sodium retention, use with diuretics Onset: 2 min
Sodium nitroprusside	0.3–10.0 mg/kg/min by continuous infusion	i.v.	Cyanide poisoning in patients with renal failure Onset: seconds
Minoxidil	0.2–1.0 mg/kg/dose Maximum: 50 mg/dose	p.o.	Hypertrichosis, salt retention, consider use with diuretics and β-blockers Onset: 30 min
Nifedipine	0.2–0.5 mg/kg/dose Maximum: 10 mg/dose	p.o., bite and swallow	Headaches, edema Onset: 2–3 min
Nicardipine	0.1–5.0 mg/kg/min	i.v.	Dizziness, flushing
Labetalol	0.2–1.0 mg/kg/dose by bolus over 2-min period or 0.4–3.0 mg/kg/h Maximum: 80 mg/dose or 300 mg/total dose	i.v. q10min Continuous i.v. infusion	Contraindicated in congestive heart failure, diabetes mellitus, and asthma Onset: 5–10 min
Phentolamine	0.05–0.20 mg/kg/dose Maximum: 5 mg/dose	i.v. or i.m.	Hypotension, arrhythmias Onset: 1–2 min
Enalaprilat	5–10 mg/kg/dose Maximum: 5 mg/dose	i.v.	Cough, angioedema, renal failure, hyperkalemia Onset: 15 min

Reprinted from Bonilla-Felix M, Portman RJ, Falkner B. Systemic hypertension. In: Burg FD, Ingelfinger JR, Polin RA, Gershon AA, eds. *Gellis and Kagan's Current Pediatric Therapy.* 17th ed. Philadelphia, PA: WB Saunders Co., 2002, with permission.

dren is slowly being developed. Drug doses for antihypertensive drugs in children and adolescents have been developed from clinical experience and small clinical trials; currently available information is summarized in **Table C166.1.**

Hypertensive Urgencies and Emergencies

Children with severe symptomatic hypertension should be admitted to the hospital for treatment and close monitoring of vital signs and neurologic status. The focus of treatment is to lower the BP as well as identify the cause of the severe hypertension. The BP level at which symptoms arise is highly variable but tends to be lower in very young children. Although acute severe hypertension must be treated promptly to prevent serious complications, rapid decreases in BP should be avoided. The goal should be to decrease BP to a safe level within a few hours, followed by a gradual decrease to normal levels. The treatment of hypertensive emergencies in children has traditionally relied exclusively on the use of parenteral drugs. However, oral agents including calcium antagonists are found to be

safe and efficient in children with acute hypertension. **Table C166.2** provides the doses of drugs used to treat hypertensive emergencies in children.

SUGGESTED READING

1. Bonilla-Felix M, Portman RJ, Falkner B. Systemic hypertension. In: Burg FD, Ingelfinger JR, Polin RA, Gershon AA, eds. *Gellis and Kagan's Current Pediatric Therapy.* 17th ed. Philadelphia, PA: WB Saunders Co., 2002.
2. Daniels SR, Kimball TR, Morrison JA, et al. Indexing left ventricular mass to account for differences in body size in children and adolescents without cardiovascular disease. *Am J Cardiol.* 1995;76:699–701.
3. Sacks FM, Svetkey LP, Vollmer WM, et al., for the DASH-Sodium Collaborative Research Group. Effects on blood pressure of reduced dietary sodium and the dietary approaches to stop hypertension (DASH) diet. *N Engl J Med.* 2001;344:3–10.
4. Soergel M, Kirschstein M, Busch C, et al. Oscillometric twenty-four hour ambulatory blood pressure values in healthy children and adolescents: a multicenter trial including 1141 subjects. *J Pediatr.* 1997;130:178–184.
5. Working Group. Update on the 1987 task force report on high blood pressure in children and adolescents: a working group report from the national high blood pressure education program. *Pediatrics.* 1996;98:649–658.

Chapter C167

Treatment of Hypertension in Minorities

Jyothsna Kodali, MD; Mahboob Rahman, MD, MS; Jackson T. Wright, Jr, MD, PhD

KEY POINTS

- Thiazide diuretics are preferred as initial therapy in nearly all hypertensives, especially blacks.

- Monotherapy with angiotensin-converting enzyme inhibitors, angiotensin receptor blockers, or β-blockers is somewhat less effective in lowering blood pressure than diuretic therapy in blacks than non-blacks, but addition of a diuretic to these drug classes eliminates racial response differences.

- Few data are available on response rates to different drugs in non-black minorities.

- Drug cost and social issues may need to be considered more often in low-income minority groups.

See also Chapters B79, B80, B88–B94, B100, B104, B106–B108, C127, C129–C131, and C136–C139

Hypertension and hypertensive target organ damage are more prevalent and severe in certain minority populations, especially blacks (see Chapters B88–B92). Clinicians should therefore be especially vigilant in evaluation and treatment of these populations.

Practical Epidemiology

The United States is an increasingly diverse nation of individuals from various racial and ethnic origins. In 1990, the U.S. Census Bureau reported population percentages of whites, 80.3%; blacks, 12.1%; Hispanics, 9%; Asian and Pacific Islanders, 2.9%; and Native Americans, 0.8%. In the past decade, the country has experienced a marked increase in minority populations and immigrants, and this trend is expected to continue. As immigrant populations acculturate, their risk for cardiovascular disease changes (see Chapter B100).

Because of the greater prevalence and severity of hypertension in blacks and, until recently, the much smaller size of other minority groups in the United States, data on hypertension in blacks exceeds the limited data in other minority groups (see Chapters B88–B92). Data from phase II (1992–1994) of the third National Health and Nutrition Survey (NHANES III) indicate that 32% of all persons with hypertension are unaware of their condition and are not receiving treatment, 15% are aware of it but are not receiving treatment, and 26% have treated but uncontrolled hypertension, leaving only 27% in whom hypertension is controlled. A slightly smaller percentage of non-Hispanic blacks than of non-Hispanic whites were unaware of their condition, and the percentage of non-Hispanic blacks with controlled hypertension was essentially the same as that among non-Hispanic whites. Although the overall prevalence of hypertension is lower among Mexican Americans than in the other 2 groups, Mexican Americans were markedly more likely than non-Hispanic whites or non-Hispanic blacks to be unaware that they had hypertension and less likely to have controlled hypertension if they were receiving treatment.

Blacks. The prevalence of hypertension is almost 40% higher in blacks in comparison with whites (32.4% vs. 23.3%) in NHANES III. The Hypertension Detection and Follow-up Program (HDFP) reported that severe hypertension (diastolic pressure ≥115 mm Hg) was 5 to 7 times more common in blacks than in whites in all age ranges except in men >80 years. This may in part explain the 80% higher stroke mortality rate, 50% higher heart disease mortality rate, and 320% greater rate of hypertension-related end-stage renal disease in blacks. Differences in obesity and lifestyle factors in young adults contribute to the higher baseline blood pressure (BP) and greater BP increase over time of blacks relative to whites (CARDIA study). In blacks, the added excess prevalence of diabetes mellitus, cigarette smoking, obesity, lipid disorders, and left ventricular hypertrophy exacerbate the greater severity of hypertension and make the need for aggressive BP control even more critical (see Chapter B89).

Hispanic Americans. Age-adjusted BP levels in Hispanic populations generally parallel that of the racial group to which they belong. BP is generally the same or lower than that of non-Hispanic whites, despite the high prevalence of obesity and type 2 diabetes mellitus. Mexican Americans in general have lower educational attainment and higher rates of unemployment and poverty than the general population. Low socioeconomic status compounded by language barriers may affect preventive and primary health care. BP control rates in Mexican Americans are among the lowest in the United States (see Chapter B90).

Asians and Pacific Islanders. Two-thirds of U.S. Asians and Pacific Islanders are foreign born. Native Hawaiians appear to be at greater risk for coronary artery disease, and the group as a whole has poorer health outcomes and lower life expectancy than other groups in Hawaii, due, at least in part, to their increased prevalence of obesity and diabetes. Although NHANES II reported that 27% of all U.S. adults 20 to 59 years of age were overweight in 1985, a study of residents of Hawaiian Homestead lands on the largely rural island of Molokai found that 65% of these native Hawaiians 20 to 59 years of age were overweight. South Asians have the highest rates of coronary artery disease of any ethnic group studied despite the fact that nearly half of this group are lifelong vegetarians. The age-adjusted prevalence of myocardial infarction or angina was approximately 3 times higher in South Asian men compared to the Framingham Offspring Study (7.2% vs. 2.5%) but was similar in women (0.3% vs. 1.0%). Immigrant South Asian men in the United States have high prevalence of coronary heart disease, non–insulin-dependent diabetes mellitus, low high-density lipoprotein cholesterol levels, and hypertriglyceridemia (insulin resistance). However, hypertension is less prevalent in South Asian men (14.2% vs. 19.1%) but similar in women (11.3% vs. 11.4%) (see Chapter B92).

Native Americans. Although the data are extremely limited, the prevalence of hypertension in Native Americans is probably similar to the general population. As in other populations, hypertension incidence is associated with obesity, age, and diabetes prevalence.

Clinical Trials Comparing Drug Therapies in Minorities

There are few studies specifically designed to evaluate racial and ethnic differences in antihypertensive drug response. However, blacks have consistently shown lesser BP response to angiotensin-converting enzyme (ACE) inhibitors, angiotensin receptor blockers, and β-blockers compared to thiazide diuretics and calcium antagonists. This finding was confirmed in the Antihypertensive and Lipid-Lowering Treatment to Prevent Heart Attack Trial (ALLHAT) in which the difference in BP lowering and reduction in cardiovascular events (including strokes and heart failure) between a thiazide-type diuretic versus an ACE inhibitor (and versus an α-blocker) was exaggerated in the black participants. Only a higher rate of heart failure was noted in the black participants on the calcium antagonist amlodipine compared to the diuretic in this study. ACE inhibitors were shown to be more effective than β-blockers and dihydropyridine calcium antagonists in preventing progression of renal disease in black patients with hypertensive renal disease.

General Principles of Management

In all populations, hypertension is associated with substantial excess morbidity and mortality. Subgroup differences in epidemiology, severity, and response to certain antihypertensive drug classes may be influenced by cultural, social, and economic access. True genetic differences have not been clearly established. Furthermore, racial and ethnic differences are quantitative rather than qualitative. Thus, although characteristics of hypertension differ among racial and ethnic groups, the presentation and management of hypertension in minority populations is largely similar to the general population.

Evaluation

The evaluation of hypertension in minorities is similar regardless of subgroup. In all, evaluation is directed at assessing severity and presence of other risk factors, target organ damage, and likelihood of secondary hypertension. The higher frequency of early onset, severe, resistant essential hypertension makes the identification of secondary hypertension more chal-

lenging in black hypertensives. Sleep disordered breathing also occurs more commonly in blacks and in the Asian population, and this racial difference is greatest at early ages. Thus, evaluation for sleep disordered breathing and other secondary causes of hypertension should be considered when the clinical presentation is suggestive of hypertension.

Treatment

Lowering BP has been shown to reduce cardiovascular events in multiple clinical trials in diverse populations. Although studies have suggested some racial differences in pathophysiologic characteristics and response to various antihypertension agents, there are no compelling data to suggest that the treatment of minorities should differ substantially from the population as a whole.

Lifestyle modification. Lifestyle modification deserves special attention in minority populations. The increasing problem of obesity in these populations makes it mandatory to emphasize caloric restriction and exercise as part of the treatment of hypertension. Reduction of salt intake should be also strongly emphasized in minority populations. In addition, the Diet Approaches to Stop Hypertension (DASH) trials clearly demonstrated the BP-lowering efficacy of diets high in fruits, vegetables, grains, and low-fat dairy products, even in the absence of weight reduction. Incorporating salt reduction into the DASH diet results in further BP reduction. It is noteworthy that blacks showed the greatest BP reduction with this diet.

Monotherapy. Based on the ALLHAT results, diuretics are preferred as initial therapy in nearly all hypertensive patients, especially black hypertensives. β-Blockers, ACE inhibitors, and calcium antagonists also reduce cardiovascular events and are reasonable alternatives in those unable to take diuretics or in combination with diuretics to achieve the BP goal. The ALLHAT data also suggested greater BP reduction and cardiovascular event reduction with calcium antagonists in black hypertensives than with ACE inhibitors or α-blockers.

Need for combination therapy. BP control can be enhanced with combination agents rather than monotherapy. The racial differences in BP among agents are usually eliminated if ACE inhibitors, angiotensin receptor blockers, or β-blockers are combined with thiazide-type diuretics or calcium antagonists. Although data are limited, there is no indication of differences in BP efficacy of specific drugs in other population subgroups. The fact that most hypertensives require more than 1 antihypertensive agent to reach BP goal diminishes the importance of debates regarding which of several agents should be prescribed first.

Medication side effects. The incidence of side effects with ACE inhibitors appears to be higher in blacks than in the general population. In particular, cough and angioedema occur at roughly twice the rates seen in whites. The reasons for these racial differences are not yet known, but different patterns of bradykinin breakdown are suspected.

Cost and other issues. The cost of drugs may also represent a significant hurdle. The lower income levels found in many minority populations can influence the likelihood of long-term adherence to therapy. It is fortunate that in addition to their unsurpassed BP lowering and reduction in clinical end points, thiazide-type diuretics are the most affordable. In addition, the availability of generic ACE inhibitors and calcium antagonists, as well as β-blockers and centrally acting agents, can increase the affordability for most patients. Many pharmaceutical firms offer special programs to aid economically disadvantaged patients. Use of such programs also can be exploited. Other social and cultural issues may also affect an individual's willingness to accept lifestyle changes or take medications. Health care providers should be familiar with these issues and be prepared to work with individuals to overcome such barriers to therapy.

SUGGESTED READING

1. The ALLHAT Officers and Coordinators for the ALLHAT Collaborative Research Group. Major cardiovascular events in hypertensive patients randomized to doxazosin vs chlorthalidone. *JAMA*. 2000;283:1967–1975.
2. The ALLHAT Officers and Coordinators for the ALLHAT Collaborative Research Group. Major outcomes in high risk hypertensive patients randomized to angiotensin-converting enzyme or calcium channel blocker vs diuretic. *JAMA*. 2002;288:2891–2997.
3. Burt VL, Whelton P, Roccella EJ, et al. Prevalence of hypertension in the US adult population: results from the Third National Health and Nutrition Examination Survey, 1988–1991. *Hypertension*. 1995;25:305–313.
4. Cushman WC, Ford CE, Cutler JA, et al. Success and predictors of blood pressure control in diverse North American settings: the Antihypertensive and Lipid-Lowering Treatment to Prevent Heart Attack Trial (ALLHAT). *J Clin Hypertens*. 2002;4:1–12.
5. Enas EA, Garg A, Davidson MA, et al. Coronary heart disease and its risk factors in the first generation immigrant Asian Indians to the USA. *Indian Heart J*. 1996;48:343–353.
6. Hyman DJ, Pavlik VN. Characteristics of patients with uncontrolled hypertension in the United States. *N Engl J Med*. 2001;345:479–486.
7. Liu K, Ruth KJ, Flack JM, et al. Blood pressure in young blacks and whites: relevance of obesity and lifestyle factors in determining differences. CARDIA Study. *Circulation*. 1996;93:60–66.
8. Rahman M, Douglas JG, Wright JT. Pathophysiology and treatment implications of hypertension in the African American population. *Endocrinol Metab Clin North Am*. 1997;26:125–144.
9. Sixth Report of the Joint National Committee on Prevention, Detection, Evaluation and Treatment of High Blood Pressure. *Arch Intern Med*. 1997;157:2413–2446.
10. Wright JT Jr, Agodoa L, Contreras G, et al. Successful blood pressure control in the African American study of kidney disease and hypertension. *Arch Intern Med*. 2002;162:1636–1643.
11. Wright JT Jr, Bakris G, Greene T, et al. for the AASK Study Group. Effect of blood pressure lowering and antihypertensive drug class on progression of hypertensive kidney disease: results from the AASK trial. *JAMA*. 2002;288:2421–2467.

Section 6. *Management of Secondary Hypertension*

Chapter C168

Management of Renovascular Hypertension

Joseph V. Nally, Jr, MD

KEY POINTS

- The goals of therapy for renovascular disease are effective control of hypertension and preservation of renal function; medical therapy, percutaneous transluminal renal angioplasty (with or without stenting), and surgery are the 3 therapeutic options.

- Medical therapy with an angiotensin-converting enzyme inhibitor (± diuretic or calcium antagonist) is appropriate for older patients who are at a higher risk for an intervention and for those who refuse an invasive procedure.

- Percutaneous transluminal renal angioplasty is the treatment of choice for fibromuscular dysplasia, but in unilateral atherosclerotic renal artery stenosis, clinical trials have not demonstrated a clear-cut benefit of intervention; intolerable side effects from antihypertensive medications or nonadherence also favor intervention.

- Angiotensin-converting enzyme inhibitors and angiotensin receptor blockers can reduce glomerular filtration rate in patients with a solitary kidney or with bilateral renal artery stenosis, but any class of antihypertensive therapy is capable of causing renal failure if systemic pressure is lowered excessively in the setting of "critical" high-grade renal artery stenosis; any adverse effect of blood pressure medications on renal function is usually reversible.

See also Chapters A37, A38, A41, A48, C110, C111, C123, C128, C144, C146, and C153

The goals of therapy for renovascular hypertension (RVHT) are effective control of blood pressure (BP) and preservation of renal function. Optimal treatment for RVHT is uncertain, as there have been no prospective randomized clinical trials comparing medical therapy, percutaneous transluminal renal angioplasty (PTRA), and surgery. PTRA (with or without renal artery stenting) or renovascular surgery usually reestablishes blood flow to an ischemic kidney but may or may not cause a

Table C168.1. Indications for Surgery or Angioplasty

Inability to control blood pressure on an appropriate antihypertensive regimen
Preservation of renal function
Intolerable side effects of medical therapy
Noncompliance with a medical regimen

significant lowering of BP. Until definitive information is available, the clinician must base decisions on a variety of factors, including the underlying risk profile of the patient and the intended goals of therapy (see Chapter C123). The type of lesion (arteriosclerosis obliterans vs. fibromuscular hyperplasia) and site of the lesion (unilateral vs. bilateral) are important considerations in deliberating the appropriate therapy. The usual indications for intervention for renal artery disease are summarized in **Table C168.1.**

General Care Issues in Older Patients

Providing optimal medical care for patients with renal artery disease secondary to atherosclerosis includes more than simply managing BP and preserving kidney function. Modification of cardiovascular risk factors is extremely important, because the majority of patient deaths are due to coronary heart disease and cerebrovascular accidents. Careful attention must be given to managing coexisting hyperlipidemia and diabetes mellitus with diet, exercise, or pharmacologic therapies. Patients must be strongly counseled to discontinue smoking.

Medical Therapy

General principles. Medical therapy is almost always required for the short term, even if patients are being prepared for interventional therapy. Chronic medical therapy may be indicated for medically unstable patients who cannot withstand intervention or for those who decline angioplasty or surgery. Medical therapy is also appropriate for older individuals with easily controlled hypertension and well-maintained renal function. For younger patients, chronic use of antihypertensive medications for 30 to 40 years seems less attractive, especially because the results of PTRA (with and without stenting) and surgery are improving.

The management of renovascular hypertension is similar to that for essential hypertension with 3 important distinctions. First, hypertension with renovascular disease may be more difficult to control and usually requires 2 or more medications of different classes. Second, vigilant attention must be given to preserving renal function during antihypertensive therapy. Finally, coexistent atherosclerotic carotid and coronary artery disease are more prevalent and often necessitate specific intervention.

Angiotensin-converting enzyme inhibitors and angiotensin receptor blockers. Before the use of angiotensin-converting enzyme (ACE) inhibitors, effective control of BP in patients with RVHT was difficult to achieve. Early reports of trials with diuretics, guanethidine, hydralazine, and β-adrenergic blockers demonstrated control of hypertension in <50% of the patients. ACE inhibitors or angiotensin receptor blockers

(ARBs) have proved to be excellent antihypertensive agents for treating RVHT, yet their potential for an adverse effect on renal function remains a concern. The initial review of captopril therapy in 269 patients demonstrated successful short-term control of BP in 74%. In a comparison of enalapril plus a diuretic with standard triple-drug therapy, control was achieved in 96% of ACE inhibitor–treated patients versus 82% of those on triple-drug therapy. The long-term efficacy of captopril combined with a β-blocker and diuretic was reported in 90% of RVHT patients.

In patients with unilateral renal artery stenosis (RAS) or other forms of moderate renal artery disease, ACE inhibitors are preferred for short-term management. ACE inhibitors may be effectively combined with other antihypertensive agents, particularly diuretics. In patients with high-grade bilateral RAS or stenosis of a solitary kidney, ACE inhibitor therapy should be used with caution.

Calcium antagonists. Calcium antagonists are quite effective in lowering BP and induce less overall acute impairment of renal function in RVHT than ACE inhibitors. Both agents demonstrate a potent antihypertensive effect, but in 2 studies, nifedipine produced a much smaller decrement in glomerular filtration rate (GFR) than captopril in patients with unilateral, bilateral, or solitary-kidney RAS. Calcium antagonists act to maintain renal blood flow and function because of their preferential preglomerular vasodilatory (afferent arteriolar) effect.

Deterioration of renal function. Any class of antihypertensive therapy is capable of reducing renal function if pressure is lowered excessively in the setting of "critical" high-grade RAS. Refractory hypertension, often associated with worsening azotemia, is a common presentation of patients with RVHT due to bilateral RAS. Failure of medical therapy in such a patient may be an indication for more aggressive interventional therapy.

Use of an ACE inhibitor or ARB may cause a reversible decrement in renal function in a kidney with hemodynamically significant stenosis, because glomerular filtration in this setting is angiotensin II–dependent. ACE inhibitor or ARB therapy removes angiotensin II–mediated vasoconstriction, particularly in the efferent arteriole, and thereby lowers glomerular pressure and GFR in the affected kidney. Acute renal insufficiency with ACE inhibition has been observed in up to 23% to 38% of patients with high-grade bilateral RAS or RAS of a solitary kidney. A mild decrease in GFR has also been noted in 20% of patients with high-grade unilateral RAS treated with enalapril and a diuretic. Fortunately, the reduction in renal function is usually reversible when the ACE inhibitor is discontinued, but complete occlusion of high-grade unilateral stenoses has been reported with the use of an ACE inhibitor and a diuretic.

Percutaneous Transluminal Renal Angioplasty

Revascularization procedures are often recommended for preservation of renal function because BP can usually be controlled with currently available antihypertensive drugs. Earlier studies had suggested that PTRA could be an effective treatment for hypertension and preservation of renal function. Factors that determine the success of PTRA include success of the initial dilatation, location of the lesion (ostial vs. nonostial), and pre-PTRA renal function.

Fibromuscular hyperplasia. PTRA should be the initial choice in younger patients with a fibromuscular lesion amenable to balloon angioplasty. Results of PTRA for fibromuscular hyperplasia have been excellent and quite comparable to surgical intervention. As many as 30% of patients with fibromuscular dysplasia have branch renal arterial involvement that may significantly increase the technical difficulty of PTRA but may not necessarily preclude this treatment modality.

Atherosclerotic disease. In patients with unilateral atherosclerotic RAS, several well-controlled studies have compared the efficacy of PTRA to either medical therapy or surgery. In a recent Dutch study of PTRA versus medical therapy that used an intention to treat analysis, BP, renal function, and daily medication doses were similar between the 2 groups at 1 year. However, at 3 months, nearly 40% of the 50 patients initially assigned to medical therapy required "rescue" PTRA because of refractory hypertension. A French randomized trial of PTRA versus medical therapy noted equivalent BPs at 6-months follow-up, but the angioplasty patients tended to require fewer medications. A randomized trial of PTRA versus surgery showed a higher primary patency rate in the surgical group, but the clinical outcome was similar because many PTRA patients with restenosis were successfully treated with a second PTRA. It was concluded that PTRA was an acceptable first-line treatment if combined with an intensive follow-up and aggressive reintervention.

Stenting. A method to improve the efficacy of PTRA (especially in ostial lesions) and to reduce the incidence of restenosis is the insertion of a balloon-expandable intravascular stent at the time of angioplasty. Several studies have documented the superior primary patency rate of PTRA with stenting for ostial atherosclerotic lesions. A prospective trial compared the outcome of PTRA alone versus PTRA plus stent in ostial atherosclerotic lesions and confirmed the higher patency rate of the PTRA plus stent group, yet the combined procedure lowered BP to a similar degree as PTRA alone. Despite the benefits of higher patency rates, it is unclear whether PTRA plus stent is superior to PTRA alone to preserve or slow deterioration of renal function.

Surgical Intervention

Surgical intervention in unilateral atherosclerotic RAS usually involves bypassing the stenotic segment or removing an atrophic kidney distal to a complete arterial occlusion. Surgery is generally more effective than PTRA in the treatment of atherosclerotic disease, with 80% to 90% of patients becoming stable or improved. Aortorenal bypass using autogenous saphenous vein or hypogastric artery is a common revascularization technique in patients with a nondiseased abdominal aorta. When an autogenous vascular graft is not available, a synthetic polytetrafluoroethylene graft can be used. Alternatively, splenorenal, hepatorenal, or ileorenal bypasses may be performed to avoid manipulation of a severely atherosclerotic aorta. In some cases, surgical revascularization is successful in preserving renal function. The mortality rate associated with surgical intervention for atherosclerotic disease varies with the degree of extrarenal vascular disease, type of surgery, and experience of the surgical team. Overall mortality rates of less than 2.5% have been reported from experienced centers for treating patients with unilateral disease and mortality rates between 3% and 6% in patients with bilateral disease. Concomitant screening for coronary or cerebrovascular disease is crucial in reducing mortality rates.

SUGGESTED READING

1. Blum U, Krumme B, Flugel P, et al. Treatment of ostial renal-artery stenoses with vascular endoprostheses after unsuccessful balloon angioplasty. *N Engl J Med*. 1997;336:459–465.
2. Franklin SS, Smith RD. Comparison of effects of enalapril plus hydrochlorothiazide versus standard triple therapy on renal function in renovascular hypertension. *Am J Med*. 1985;79:14–23.
3. Hollenberg NK. Medical therapy for renovascular hypertension: a review. *Am J Hypertens*. 1988;1:338S–343S.
4. Plouin PF, Chatellier G, Darne B, Raynaud A. Blood pressure outcome of angioplasty in atherosclerotic renal artery stenosis: a randomized trial. Essai Multicentrique Medicaments vs. Angioplastie (EMMA) Study Group. *Hypertension*. 1998;31:823–829.
5. Ribstein J, Mourad G, Mimran A. Contrasting acute effects of captopril and nifedipine on renal function in renovascular hypertension. *Am J Hypertens*. 1988;1:239–244.
6. Rimmer JM, Gennari FJ. Atherosclerotic renovascular disease and progressive renal failure. *Ann Intern Med*. 1993;118:712–719.
7. van de Ven PJ, Kaatee R, Beutler JJ, et al. Arterial stenting and balloon angioplasty in ostial atherosclerotic renovascular disease: a randomised trial. *Lancet*. 1999;353:282–286.
8. van Jaarsveld BC, Krijnen P, Pieterman H, et al. The effect of balloon angioplasty on hypertension in atherosclerotic renal-artery stenosis. Dutch Renal Artery Stenosis Intervention Cooperative Study Group. *N Engl J Med*. 2000;342:1007–1014.
9. Weibull FL, Bergqvist D, Bergentz SE, et al. Percutaneous transluminal renal angioplasty versus surgical reconstruction of atherosclerotic renal artery stenosis: a prospective randomized study. *J Vasc Surg*. 1993;18:841–850; discussion, 850–852.
10. Zierler RE, Bergelin RO, Davidson RC, et al. A prospective study of disease progression in patients with atherosclerotic renal artery stenosis. *Am J Hypertens*. 1996;9:1055–1061.

Chapter C169

Management of Pheochromocytoma

William F. Young, Jr, MD, MS; Sheldon G. Sheps, MD

KEY POINTS

- The diagnosis of a catecholamine-producing tumor is based on clinical suspicion that is confirmed biochemically (by increased urine or plasma levels of catecholamines or their metabolites) and anatomically (by computer-assisted imaging starting with the adrenals and the abdomen).

- The treatment of choice for pheochromocytomas, which are usually benign, is surgical resection after careful preoperative pharmacologic preparation.

- Hypertension is usually cured by excision of the tumor, but some individuals experience residual hypertension that requires drug therapy.

- Malignant pheochromocytoma is diagnosed when direct invasion of surrounding tissue or a metastatic lesion is found; dependent on the extent of and the location of disease, resection, radiation therapy, radiofrequency ablation, and chemotherapy should be considered.

See also Chapters A1, A2, A13, A18, A41, A42, A51, A52, C110, C127, C128, C141, C142, and C146

Catecholamine-secreting tumors are located in the adrenal medulla (pheochromocytoma) or in the extraadrenal paraganglion tissue (catecholamine-secreting paraganglioma). Prevalence estimates for pheochromocytoma vary from 0.01% to 0.10% of the hypertensive population, with an incidence of 2 to 8 cases per million people per year. These tumors occur equally in men and women, primarily in their third through fifth decades.

Clinical Presentation

Patients with catecholamine-secreting tumors may be asymptomatic, but usually symptoms are present and due to the excess circulating catecholamines. Episodic symptoms include abrupt onset of throbbing headaches, generalized diaphoresis, palpitations, anxiety, chest pain, and abdominal pain. These spells can be extremely variable in their presentation and may be spontaneous or precipitated by postural changes, anxiety, exercise, or maneuvers that increase intraabdominal pressure. The pheochromocytoma spell may last 10 to 60 minutes and may occur daily to monthly. Clinical signs include hypertension (paroxysmal in half of the patients and sustained in the other half), orthostatic hypotension, pallor, grade I to IV hypertensive retinopathy, tremor, and fever. The pathophysiology of pheochromocytoma-induced hypertension results from excess catecholamine production, but the tumors can be found in association with other endocrine abnormalities in the multiple endocrine neoplasia syndromes (see Chapter A51).

Diagnosis

The diagnostic approach to catecholamine-producing tumors is divided into 2 series of studies (**Figure C169.1**), both of which are triggered by the clinical presentation.

Biochemical tests. The diagnosis of a catecholamine-producing tumor must be confirmed biochemically by the presence of increased urine or plasma levels of catecholamines or their metabolites. Fractionated plasma metanephrines, although highly sensitive, lack sensitivity for routine screening of low-risk, nonfamilial patients. Plasma or urinary catecholamines also can be used, but urinary vanillylmandelic acid is no longer recommended because of relatively poor sensitivity and specificity.

Imaging studies. The next step is to localize the catecholamine-producing tumor to guide the surgical approach. Computer-assisted adrenal and abdominal imaging (magnetic resonance imaging or computed tomography) is the first localization test. Approximately 90% of catecholamine-producing tumors are found in the adrenals, and 98% are in the abdomen. If the abdominal imaging is negative, then scintigraphic localization with iodine-123 metaiodobenzylguanidine is indicated. This radiopharmaceutical accumulates preferentially in catecholamine-producing tumors; however, this procedure is not as definitive as initially hoped (sensitivity, 85%; specificity, 99%). Computer-assisted pelvis, chest, and neck imaging; octreotide scintigraphy; and positron emission tomography are additional localizing procedures that can be used, although they are rarely required.

Functional tests. Suppression testing with clonidine or provocative testing with glucagon, histamine, or metoclopramide is rarely needed. These tests are not recommended by all experts due to expense and potential risks (hypertension and hypotension). In general, repeat testing of catecholamines or metabolites is preferred in the usual clinical setting. The differential diagnosis of catecholamine-secreting tumors is summarized in **Table C169.1**.

Treatment

The treatment of choice for catecholamine-secreting tumors is surgical resection. Most of these tumors are benign and can

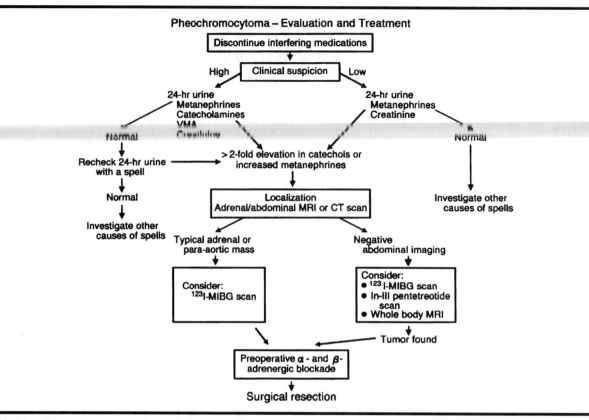

Figure C169.1. Evaluation and treatment of catecholamine-producing tumors. Clinical suspicion is triggered by the following: presence of headache, palpitations, or abnormal sweating; paroxysmal symptoms (especially hypertension); hypertension that is intermittent, unusually labile, or resistant to treatment; family history of pheochromocytoma or associated conditions; or incidentally discovered adrenal mass. For details, see text. CT, computed tomography; ^{123}I-MIBG, [^{123}I]metaiodobenzylguanidine; MRI, magnetic resonance imaging; VMA, vanillymandelic acid. (From Young WF Jr. *Pheochromocytoma: 1926–1993.* New York, NY: Elsevier Science Inc; 1993:122, with permission.)

be totally excised. Hypertension is usually cured by excision of the tumor, but some patients have residual hypertension that necessitates drug therapy. Careful preoperative pharmacologic preparation is crucial to successful treatment.

Preoperative management. Combined α- and β-adrenergic blockade is recommended before surgery to control blood pressure and to prevent intraoperative hypertensive crises. Long-acting nonselective α-adrenergic blockade (e.g., phenoxybenzamine) should be started at least 7 to 10 days before surgery to allow for expansion of the contracted blood volume. A liberal salt diet is advised during the preoperative period. Once adequate α-adrenergic blockade is achieved (e.g., resolution of spells, normal blood pressure, nasal stuffiness, mild orthostasis), β-adrenergic blockade is initiated, usually a few days before surgery. Calcium antagonists have also been used successfully at several medical centers for the preoperative preparation of pheochromocytoma patients. A few clinicians still use α-methyl-L-tyrosine (metyrosine), which inhibits the synthesis of catecholamines by blocking the enzyme tyrosine hydroxylase (see Chapter A2). Because of the significant side-effect profile of metyrosine, it is reserved primarily for those patients who, for cardiopulmonary reasons, do not tolerate combined α- and β-adrenergic blockade.

Anesthesia and surgery. Extirpation of a catecholamine-secreting tumor is a high-risk surgical procedure, and an experi-

enced surgeon and anesthesiologist team is required. The last oral doses of the antihypertensive agents can be administered early in the morning on the day of operation. Cardiovascular and hemodynamic variables must be monitored closely. Acute hypertensive crises may occur before or during operation and should be treated with nitroprusside or phentolamine administered intravenously.

In the past, an anterior midline abdominal surgical approach was usually used for adrenal pheochromocytoma. However, laparoscopic adrenalectomy is the procedure of choice in patients with solitary adrenal catecholamine-secreting tumors that are <8 cm in diameter. If the tumor is in the adrenal gland, the entire gland should be removed. Cortical-sparing procedures may be indicated in patients with bilateral adrenal tumors [e.g., von Hippel-Lindau syndrome (VHL)]. If the tumor is malignant, as much tumor as possible should be removed. Catecholamine-secreting paragangliomas of the neck, chest, and urinary bladder require specialized approaches. At major centers, the surgical mortality rate is <2%. The survival rate after removal of a benign pheochromocytoma is nearly that of age- and sex-matched controls.

Follow-up. Blood pressure usually is normal by the time of dismissal from the hospital. Approximately 2 weeks after surgery, the catecholamine secretory status should be assessed. If the levels of catecholamines and metabolites are normal, the resection of the pheochromocytoma can be considered to have been complete. Fractionated plasma metanephrines or the 24-hour urinary excretion of catecholamines or metanephrines

Table C169.1. Differential Diagnosis of Pheochromocytoma Spells

Endocrine
  Thyrotoxicosis
  Primary hypogonadism (e.g., menopausal syndrome)
  Pancreatic tumors (e.g., insulinoma)
  Medullary thyroid carcinoma
  "Hyperadrenergic" spells
Cardiovascular
  Essential hypertension, labile
  Angina and cardiovascular deconditioning
  Pulmonary edema
  Dilated cardiomyopathy
  Syncope
  Orthostatic hypotension
  Paroxysmal cardiac arrhythmia
  Aortic dissection
  Renovascular hypertension
Psychological
  Anxiety and panic attacks
  Somatization disorder
  Hyperventilation
  Factitious (e.g., drugs, Valsalva)
Pharmacologic
  Withdrawal of adrenergic-inhibiting medication (e.g., clonidine)
  Monoamine oxidase inhibitor treatment and concomitant ingestion of tyramine or a decongestant
  Sympathomimetic ingestion
  Illicit drug ingestion (e.g., cocaine, phencyclidine, lysergic acid)
  Gold myokymia syndrome
  Acrodynia (mercury poisoning)
  Vancomycin (red man syndrome)
Neurologic
  Baroreflex failure
  Postural orthostatic tachycardia syndrome (POTS)
  Autonomic neuropathy
  Migraine headache
  Diencephalic epilepsy (autonomic seizures)
  Cerebral infarction
  Cerebrovascular insufficiency
Miscellaneous
  Mastocytosis (systemic or activation disorder)
  Carcinoid syndrome
  Recurrent idiopathic anaphylaxis
  Unexplained flushing spells

should be checked annually indefinitely as surveillance for recurrence in the adrenal bed, metastatic pheochromocytoma, or delayed appearance of multiple primary tumors.

Screening for Familial Catecholamine-Secreting Tumor Syndromes

Diagnostic studies for familial disorders such as multiple endocrine neoplasia type II, VHL, neurofibromatosis type 1, familial pheochromocytoma, and familial paraganglioma should be considered during the first postoperative visit. In addition, all immediate family members should be biochemically screened for a catecholamine-secreting tumor.

Malignant Pheochromocytoma

The distinction between benign and malignant catecholamine-producing tumors cannot be made on clinical, biochemical, or histopathologic characteristics. The diagnosis of malignancy is based on finding direct local invasion or metastasis to sites that do not have chromaffin tissue, such as lymph nodes, bone, lung, and liver. Although the 5-year survival rate is <50%, many of these patients have prolonged survival and minimal morbidity. Metastatic lesions should be resected if possible. Radiofrequency ablation of hepatic and bone metastases may be very effective in selected patients. Painful skeletal metastatic lesions can be treated with external radiation therapy. Local tumor irradiation with iodine-131 metaiodobenzylguanidine has proved to be of limited therapeutic value. If the tumor is considered to be aggressive and the quality of life is affected, then combination chemotherapy may be considered. A chemotherapy program consisting of cyclophosphamide, vincristine, and dacarbazine given cyclically every 21 to 28 days has proved beneficial but not curative in these patients. Combined α- and β-adrenergic blockade is useful to control catecholamine-related symptoms.

SUGGESTED READING

1. Averbuch SD, Steakley CS, Young RC, et al. Malignant pheochromocytoma: effective treatment with a combination of cyclophosphamide, vincristine, and dacarbazine. *Ann Intern Med.* 1988;109:267–273.
2. Kinney MAO, Warner ME, vanHeerden JA, et al. Perianesthetic risks and outcomes of pheochromocytoma and paraganglioma resection. *Anesth Analg.* 2000;91:1118–1123.
3. Koch CA, Vortmeyer AO, Huang SC, et al. Genetic aspects of pheochromocytoma. *Endocr Regul.* 2001;35:43–52.
4. Kudva YC, Young WF Jr, Thompson GB, et al. Adrenal incidentaloma: an important component of the clinical presentation spectrum of benign sporadic adrenal pheochromocytoma. *Endocrinologist.* 1999;9:77–80.
5. Lenders JWM, Pacak K, McClellan MW, et al. Biochemical diagnosis of pheochromocytoma: which test is best? *JAMA.* 2002;287:1427–1434.
6. Sheps SG, Jiang N-S, Klee GG. Diagnostic evaluation of pheochromocytoma. *Endocrinol Metab Clin North Am.* 1988;17:397–414.
7. Stein PP, Black HR. A simplified diagnostic approach to pheochromocytoma: a review of the literature and report of one institution's experience. *Medicine.* 1991;70:46–66.
8. Van der Harst E, de Herder WW, Bruining HA, et al. [123I] Metaiodobenzylguanidine and [111In] octreotide uptake in benign and malignant pheochromocytomas. *J Clin Endocrinol Metab.* 2001;86:685–693.
9. Young WF Jr. Pheochromocytoma: 1926–1993. *Trends Endocrinol Metab.* 1993;4:122–127.
10. Young WF Jr, Maddox DE. Spells: in search of a cause. *Mayo Clin Proc.* 1995;70:757–765.

Chapter C170

Management of Hypercortisolism and Hyperaldosteronism

Emmanuel L. Bravo, MD

KEY POINTS

- The determination of 24-hour urinary free cortisol is the best available test for documentation of endogenous hypercortisolism.

- The preferred treatment for Cushing's syndrome is surgical resection of a pituitary or ectopic source of adrenocorticotropic hormone or removal of the cortisol-producing adrenal cortical tumor.

- The recommended initial test in suspected primary aldosteronism is the determination of urinary aldosterone excretion rate during prolonged salt loading; other mineralocorticoids may be produced by hyperplastic glands, so the coexistence of hyperkalemia, hypertension, and low plasma renin activity should prompt consideration of adrenal cortical hyperfunction.

- In primary aldosteronism, laparoscopic adenomectomy can be performed, but, because of the high prevalence of nodular hyperplasia, medical therapy with aldosterone blockers can provide effective long-term control of blood pressure.

See also Chapters A9, A10, A41, A42, A50, A77, C110, C111, and C140

Excess hormone production from the adrenal medulla or cortex can produce several curable forms of hypertension.

CUSHING'S SYNDROME

Evaluation

Clinical features. The typical clinical presentation of Cushing's syndrome includes truncal obesity, moon face, hypertension, plethora, muscle weakness and fatigue, hirsutism, emotional disturbances, and typical purple skin striae. Carbohydrate intolerance or diabetes, amenorrhea, loss of libido, easy bruising, and spontaneous fractures of ribs and vertebrae may be encountered. All patients may exhibit some of these features at the time of diagnosis. However, few, if any, have all of them.

Biochemical tests. For screening purposes, the overnight 1-mg dexamethasone-suppression test and the measurement of 24-hour urinary free cortisol have been used in most centers. With the overnight 1-mg dexamethasone-suppression test, reduction of basal plasma cortisol level to values <5 µg/dL is defined as *normal suppression*. This test is simple and has a low incidence of false normal suppression (<3%). However, it has a high incidence of false-positive results (≈20% to 30%) and does not distinguish between hypercortisolism due to Cushing's syndrome and other non-Cushing's hypercortisolemic states (stress, pregnancy, chronic strenuous exercise, psychiatric states, malnutrition, and glucocorticoid resistance). The determination of 24-hour urinary free cortisol is the best available test for documentation of endogenous hypercortisolism. A level above 100 µg per 24 hours suggests excessive production of cortisol.

Suppressive tests. The Liddle dexamethasone suppression test is regarded as one of the best methods to discriminate between Cushing's syndrome and other types of endogenous hypercortisolism. In normal subjects and patients with pseudo-Cushing's syndrome, adrenocorticotropic hormone (ACTH) release can be suppressed with low-dose administration of dexamethasone (2 mg/day divided for dosing every 6 hours, for 2 days). In patients with Cushing's syndrome, ACTH release can be inhibited only at much higher doses of dexamethasone (8 mg/day divided every 6 hours, for 2 days). In contrast, patients with the ectopic ACTH syndrome or Cushing's syndrome due to cortisol-secreting adrenal tumors usually do not respond to high-dose administration of dexamethasone. The diagnostic accuracy of the test is ≈85%.

Localization. The choice and success of treatment in Cushing's syndrome depend largely on accurate determination of the cause of the hypercortisolism. Spontaneous (endogenous) Cushing's syndrome can result from ACTH excess (ACTH-dependent) or from autonomous secretion of cortisol (ACTH-independent) (**Table C170.1**). Radioimmunoassay of plasma ACTH is the procedure of choice of pinpointing the basis for hypercortisolism. In cases in which differentiation between pituitary and ectopic sources of ACTH excess cannot be made on the basis of plasma levels alone, a computed tomography (CT) scan may be very helpful. Should these tests prove unrevealing, pharmacologic manipulation of ACTH secretion and measurement of ACTH gradients from the head and below the neck may help in differentiating pituitary from ectopic Cushing's syndrome.

Therapy

Surgical. The standard of care for the majority of cases of Cushing's syndrome is surgical resection of a pituitary or an ectopic source of ACTH or removal of a cortisol-producing

Table C170.1. Classification and Principal Diagnostic Differences in Cushing's Syndrome

TYPE	OCCURRENCE (%)	PLASMA ACTH	COMPUTED TOMOGRAPHY SCAN
ACTH-dependent	85		
Pituitary	80	Normal	Normal size adrenals
Ectopic ACTH	20	>200 pg/mL	Bilaterally enlarged adrenals
Ectopic corticotropin-releasing hormone	(rare)	>200 pg/mL	Bilaterally enlarged adrenals
ACTH-independent	15	Low/nondetectable	
Adrenal adenoma (most common)			Unilateral adrenal mass
Adrenal carcinoma			Unilateral adrenal mass
Macronodular adrenal hyperplasia			Enlarged/nodular adrenals
Primary pigmented nodular adrenal disease			Nodular adrenals

ACTH, adrenocorticotropic hormone.

adrenocortical tumor. Transsphenoidal pituitary adenomectomy is the treatment of choice in most patients, but total hypophysectomy may be required in patients with diffuse hyperplasia or in patients with a large pituitary tumor. Bilateral adrenalectomy for Cushing's disease is almost universally successful in alleviating the hypercortisolemic state. However, 10% to 38% may later develop Nelson's syndrome, with hyperpigmentation and higher risk of pituitary tumor invasion.

The potential for cure of Cushing's disease (ACTH-dependent) is related to preoperative and postoperative cortisol responses to stimulation and the basal levels of cortisol achieved after surgery. The preoperative cortisol response to corticotropin-releasing hormone stimulation is greater among those cured by surgery than among surgical failures (maximal increment in serum is 18 vs. 11 µg/dL). The 5% to 25% rate of recurrence at 3 to 5 years after initial surgical cure is associated with relatively higher basal cortisol levels after surgery (4.7 vs. 1.5 µg/dL). The cortisol response to corticotropin-releasing hormone after surgery is also significantly greater among those who later relapse than in those who remain in remission (10.9 vs. 4.3 µg/dL). Thus, cortisol levels >3.6 µg per dL after transsphenoidal adenomectomy indicate an increased risk of late recurrence.

Radiotherapy. Seeding the pituitary bed with yttrium or gold has been advocated. Among patients with Cushing's disease whose radiographic studies failed to reveal sellar changes, 65% had complete remission and 16% had partial remission at 1 year after yttrium implantation therapy.

Medical therapy. The long-acting analogue SMS 201-995 (octreotide or Sandostatin) has been used with variable success to treat ectopic ACTH syndromes, but some benefit has been reported in Cushing's disease and Nelson's syndrome. Cyproheptadine, a serotonin antagonist, has demonstrated limited success in the treatment of Cushing's disease. Cyproheptadine and bromocriptine, alone or in combination, have little effect on the elevated ACTH levels after adrenalectomy for Cushing's syndrome in patients without evidence of a pituitary tumor. Ketoconazole has been advocated as an inhibitor of adrenal (and gonadal) sterol production by inhibiting several biosynthetic steps. For rapid correction of hypercortisolism awaiting definitive intervention, ketoconazole may play a valuable role. Mitotane (*o,p'*-DDD) is an insecticide derivative that induces destruction of the zonae reticularis and fasciculata with relative sparing of the zona glomerulosa. Its use in Cushing's disease

(associated with adrenal carcinoma) is directed toward adrenal suppression, whereas the pituitary tumor itself is not treated.

APPARENT MINERALOCORTICOID EXCESS (11β-DEHYDROGENASE DEFICIENCY)

With 11β-dehydrogenase deficiency or enzyme inhibition, intrarenal levels of cortisol increase, and cortisol causes inappropriate activation of mineralocorticoid receptors (see Chapters A50 and A77). The resulting antinatriuresis and kaliuresis cause hypertension and hypokalemia. Biochemically, there are elevations in urinary-free cortisol excretion and the ratio of the urinary metabolites of cortisol to those of cortisone and prolongation of the half-life of titrated cortisol. Plasma cortisol concentrations usually are not elevated. The signs and symptoms are reversed by spironolactone or dexamethasone and are exacerbated by administration of physiologic doses of cortisol.

PRIMARY ALDOSTERONISM

Diagnosis

As in Cushing's syndrome, the appropriate therapy of patients with primary aldosteronism depends on accurately determining the cause of excessive aldosterone production. The recognizable forms of primary aldosteronism include aldosterone-producing adenoma, adrenal (glomerulosa) hyperplasia, "indeterminate hyperaldosteronism," glucocorticoid-suppressible aldosteronism, and aldosterone-producing adrenal carcinoma. Spontaneous, moderately severe hypokalemia (<3.0 mEq/L), an anomalous postural decrease in plasma aldosterone concentration, and increased plasma 18-hydroxycorticosterone values (≥100 ng/dL) distinguish an adenoma from hyperplasia. Adrenal carcinomas usually produce various adrenocorticosteroids other than aldosterone. For localization of an adenoma, an adrenal CT scan should be obtained first and is considered diagnostic if an adrenal mass is clearly identified. When the CT scan is inconclusive, adrenal venous sampling for aldosterone and cortisol levels should be done.

Hypokalemia. Hypokalemia should be considered in patients with (a) spontaneous hypokalemia (serum potassium level <3.5 mEq/L), (b) moderately severe hypokalemia (serum potassium level <3.0 mEq/L) during diuretic therapy with conventional dosages, and (3) difficulty in maintaining normal serum potassium levels during diuretic therapy despite concomitant use of oral potassium supplementation, and/or potassium-sparing agents or ACE inhibitors. Hypokalemia, whether spontaneous or provoked, provides an important clue to the presence of primary aldosteronism. However, serum potassium concentration is normal in 7% to 38% of reported cases. In addition, 10% to 12% of patients with proven cases may not have hypokalemia during short-term salt loading. Notable is the fact that in the "normokalemic" group, conventional diuretic therapy usually produces moderately severe hypokalemia, a finding previously considered unimportant in a hypertensive patient receiving a potassium-wasting diuretic agent.

Serum and urinary potassium values serve to indicate whether inappropriate kaliuresis (serum potassium ≥3.0 mEq/L, with urinary potassium excretion ≥30 mEq/L per 24 hours) occurs during salt loading. The finding of a 24-hour urinary sodium excretion rate of >250 mEq per L gives some assurance that the patient has ingested the prescribed amount of salt. Patients in whom aldosterone excretion rate is not suppressed to <14.0 μg per 24 hours with salt loading should have additional studies. Hypokalemia or suppressed plasma renin activity (PRA) provides corroborative evidence of primary aldosteronism, but absence of either or both does not exclude the diagnosis.

Plasma renin activity. Measurement of PRA under conditions of stimulation (sodium restriction, diuretic administration, and upright posture) has been used as a screening test to exclude primary aldosteronism. Suppressed activity (<1.0 ng/mL per hour) that fails to rise above 2.0 ng per mL per hour after salt and water depletion is considered a positive test. However, some patients with primary aldosteronism may have clearly unsuppressed values during normal dietary sodium intake, and a substantial number (≈35%) may have stimulated PRA (>2.0 ng/mL per hour). In addition, ≈40% of subjects with essential hypertension have suppressed PRA during normal dietary sodium intake; 15% to 20% of these patients show values <2.0 ng per mL per hour when stimulated. The large number of false-positive and false-negative results make PRA determinations of limited use in screening patients for primary aldosteronism.

Aldosterone to renin ratio. The ratio of plasma aldosterone to PRA is used to define the appropriateness of PRA for the circulating concentrations of aldosterone. It is assumed that the volume expansion associated with aldosteronism inhibits the synthesis of renin without affecting the autonomous production of aldosterone. There are 2 serious drawbacks of this test: (a) the inherent variability of PRA and of plasma levels of aldosterone, even in the presence of a tumor; and (b) the effects of drugs that suppress or prolong stimulation of PRA long after they are discontinued.

Aldosterone excretion rate during salt loading. The test with the best sensitivity and specificity for the identification of patients with primary aldosteronism is the measurement of aldosterone excretion rate during salt loading. A rate >14.0 μg per 24 hours after 3 days of salt loading (25 mL/kg of 0.9% saline over 4 hours for 3 days) distinguishes most patients with primary aldosteronism from those with essential hypertension. Only 7% of patients with primary aldosteronism have values

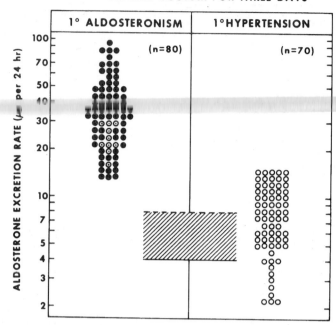

Figure C170.1. Aldosterone excretion rate after 3 days of high sodium intake. For patients with primary aldosteronism, solid circles represent adenomas (N = 70) and open circles with dotted centers represent hyperplasia (N = 10). The crosshatched area represents the mean [4.0 μg/24 hours + 2 SD (8.0 μg/24 hours)] of values obtained from 47 healthy subjects. No patient with primary aldosteronism had a value within the 95th percentile of the normal range. Two patients (14%) with primary hypertension had values that fell within the range obtained in patients with primary aldosteronism. With a reference value of >14 μg per 24 hours after a high sodium intake for 3 days, the sensitivity and specificity of the test are 96% and 93%, respectively. (From Bravo EL, Tarazi RC, Dustan HP, et al. The changing clinical spectrum of primary aldosteronism. *Am J Med.* 1983;74:641–651, with permission.)

that fall within the range for essential hypertension (**Figure C170.1**). Under the same conditions, a substantial number (39%) of patients with primary aldosteronism have plasma aldosterone values that fall within the range for essential hypertension. The recommended initial test in suspected primary aldosteronism is the determination of aldosterone excretion rate during prolonged salt loading (**Figure C170.2**). Outpatients can be evaluated by adding 10 to 12 g of sodium chloride to the normal daily sodium intake and determining the serum potassium concentration and the 24-hour urinary excretion rate of sodium, potassium, and aldosterone after 5 to 7 days. It has been suggested that adrenal hyperplasia is more common than originally thought. Hyperplastic glands may not reduce aldosterone but rather 19-nor-deoxycorticosterone or 18-hydroxydeoxycorticosterone, both of which have relatively strong mineralocorticoid activity (see Chapter A50). Neither hormone is detected by the radioimmunoassay for plasma aldosterone. Each can be determined by specialized laboratories, but such tests are not readily available to all clinicians.

Therapy

Medical. Medical management of primary aldosterone is a reasonable option for controlling blood pressure (BP) and elevating

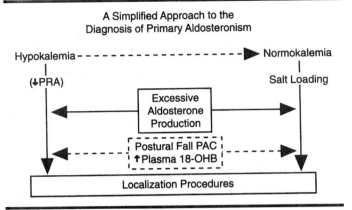

A Simplified Approach to the
Diagnosis of Primary Aldosteronism

Figure C170.2. Algorithm for the diagnosis of primary aldosteronism. ↑, increased; ↓, decreased; 18-OHB, plasma 18-hydroxycorticosterone concentration; PAC, plasma aldosterone concentration; PRA, plasma renin activity. (From Bravo EL. Primary aldosteronism. *Urol Clin North Am* 1989;16:481–486, with permission.)

serum potassium. Medical therapy is indicated in (a) patients with adrenal hyperplasia, (b) patients with adenoma who are poor surgical risks, and (c) patients with bilateral adenomas that may require bilateral adrenalectomy. Experience has been that the hypertension associated with primary aldosteronism is best treated by sustained salt and water depletion and aldosterone antagonists. Usual doses of diuretics are hydrochlorothiazide 25 to 50 mg per day or furosemide 80 to 160 mg per day in combination with either spironolactone 100 to 200 mg per day or amiloride 10 to 20 mg per day. This usually results in prompt correction of hypokalemia and normalization of BP within 2 to 4 weeks. Addition of an α-adrenergic blocker, a central sympatholytic agent, or a vasodilator may be useful to normalize arterial pressure. Other alternatives are not as effective as diuretic therapy and do not correct the metabolic abnormalities. Potential side effects of spironolactone include gynecomastia, impotence, nausea, vomiting, pigmentation, and lassitude. Hyperkalemia may occur in those patients with significant impairment of renal function. Selective aldosterone antagonists (eplerenone, see Chapter C140) with lesser side effect profiles are now being evaluated.

The efficacy of long-term medical management has been demonstrated in 24 patients with documented aldosterone-producing adenomas who were treated medically (with either spironolactone or amiloride with hydrochlorothiazide) for at least 5 years (range, 5–17 years). Systolic BP fell from 175 mm Hg to 129 mm Hg and diastolic BP from 106 mm Hg to 79 mm Hg. Serum potassium increased from 3.0 mEq per L to 4.3 mEq per L with treatment. During follow-up, no patient had a cardiovascular event or renal failure, and no tumors became malignant.

Surgical. Adrenal adenomas may now be resected through a laparoscopic approach. Operating time is similar to the conventional approach, but there is minimal blood loss, hospital stay is short (average, 2.7 days), recovery is rapid (≈2–3 weeks), and cosmetic results are excellent. In the majority of cases, surgical excision of aldosterone-producing adenomas leads to normotension as well as reversal of the biochemical defects. At the very least, surgery renders arterial pressure easier to control

with medications in those who have residual hypertension. Duration, severity of hypertension, and the degree of end-organ involvement do not predict the arterial pressure response after surgery.

Before undergoing surgery, patients should receive drug treatment for at least 3 to 6 months to decrease BP and to correct the significant potassium deficit that increases risk of cardiac arrhythmias during anesthesia. Prolonged reduction of arterial BP permits the use of intravenous fluids during surgery without producing hypertension and decreases morbidity. Administration of medications is usually continued until surgery, and glucocorticoid administration is not needed before surgery. During the immediate postoperative period, antihypertensive agents are generally not required if the patient had been normotensive for at least 3 months before surgery while receiving diuretic therapy. If hypertension becomes a problem, diuretics should be tried first and other types of antihypertensive agents later.

After the removal of an aldosterone-producing adenoma, selective hypoaldosteronism usually occurs, even in patients in whom PRA had been stimulated with chronic diuretic therapy. One likely explanation for this effect is that spironolactone may inhibit aldosterone biosynthesis by the adrenal cortex. Therefore, if indicated, potassium supplementation should be given cautiously, and serum potassium values should be monitored closely. However, sufficient residual mineralocorticoid activity usually prevents excessive renal retention of potassium, provided that sodium intake is adequate. If hyperkalemia does occur, all forms of potassium chloride supplementation should be discontinued and salt intake increased. In addition, furosemide in doses of 80 to 160 mg per day should be started. Treatment with fludrocortisone is not often necessary, but, if it is needed, 0.1 mg per day may be used as the initial dose. Abnormalities in aldosterone production can persist for as long as 3 months.

GLUCOCORTICOID-REMEDIABLE ALDOSTERONISM

Evaluation

Glucocorticoid-remediable aldosteronism is an inherited autosomal-dominant disorder that mimics an aldosterone-producing adenoma. It is caused by a genetic mutation that results in a hybrid or chimeric gene product fusing nucleotide sequences of the 11β-hydroxylase and aldosterone synthase genes.

Glucocorticoid-remediable aldosteronism should be suspected in a patient with primary aldosteronism who presents with the following clinical history: a family history of primary aldosteronism, early age of onset of hypertension, and severe hypertension with early death of affected family members resulting from cerebrovascular accident.

Treatment

The suppression of ACTH with dexamethasone usually corrects the cardiovascular and metabolic abnormalities. However, this therapy is potentially limited by untoward complications resulting from glucocorticoid excess. Alternative treatment modalities aimed at mineralocorticoid receptor blockade with spironolactone or inhibition of the mineralocorticoid-sensitive distal tubule sodium channel with amiloride may be preferable.

SUGGESTED READING

1. Arriza JL, Weinberger C, Cerelli G, et al. Cloning of human mineralocorticoid receptor complementary DNA: structural and functional kinship with the glucocorticoid receptor. *Science.* 1987;237:268–275.

2. Bravo EL. Primary aldosteronism. Issues in diagnosis and management. *Endocrinol Metab Clin North Am.* 1994;23:387–404.

3. Edwards CRW, Stewart PM, Burt D, et al. Localisation of 11 beta-hydroxysteroid dehydrogenase—tissue specific protector of the mineralocorticoid receptor. *Lancet* 1988;2:986–989.

4. Farese RV Jr, Biglieri EG, Shackleton CH, et al. Licorice-induced hypermineralocorticoidism. *N Engl J Med.* 1991;325:1223–1227.

5. Ghose RP, Hall PM, Bravo EL. Medical management of aldosterone-producing adenomas. *Ann Intern Med.* 1999;131:105–108.

6. Kaye TB, Crapo L. The Cushing syndrome: an update on diagnostic tests. *Ann Intern Med.* 1990;112:434–444.

7. Lifton RP, Dluhy RG, Powers M, et al. Hereditary hypertension caused by chimeric genes duplications and ectopic expression of aldosterone synthase. *Nat Genet.* 1992;2:66–74.

8. Miller JW, Crapo L. The medical treatment of Cushing's syndrome. *Endocr Rev.* 1993;14:443–458.

9. Walker BR, Edwards ERW. Licorice-induced hypertension and syndromes of apparent mineralocorticoid excess. *Endocrinol Metab Clin North Am.* 1994;23:359–377.

10. Winfield HN, Hamilton BD, Bravo EL. Technique of laparoscopic adrenalectomy: *Urol Clin North Am.* 1997;24:459–465.

Chapter C171

Management of Thyroid and Parathyroid Disorders

William F. Young, Jr, MD, MS

KEY POINTS

- The types of thyroid disease associated with hypertension include hyperthyroidism, hypothyroidism, and medullary thyroid carcinoma (associated with pheochromocytoma in the multiple endocrine neoplasia syndromes types IIA and IIB).

- The hypercalcemia of hyperparathyroidism is associated with an increased incidence of hypertension.

- Thyroid- and parathyroid-directed treatment in the hypertensive patient may normalize hypertension or facilitate its treatment.

See also Chapters A51, A52, C110, and C169

Dysfunction of the thyroid and parathyroid glands may be the sole cause of hypertension or may contribute significantly to underlying primary hypertension (see Chapter A52).

THYROID DYSFUNCTION

The types of thyroid disease associated with hypertension include hyperthyroidism, hypothyroidism, and medullary thyroid carcinoma (MTC) [associated with pheochromocytoma in the multiple endocrine neoplasia (MEN) type IIA and IIB syndromes].

Clinical Presentation

Hyperthyroidism. *Hyperthyroidism* is the clinical syndrome that occurs when excessive amounts of circulating thyroid hormones interact with thyroid hormone receptors on peripheral tissues. This results in increased metabolic activity and increased sensitivity to circulating catecholamines. Thyrotoxic patients usually have a high cardiac output and an increased systolic blood pressure.

Hypothyroidism. *Hypothyroidism* is the syndrome resulting from deficiency of thyroid hormones, which causes many metabolic processes to slow down. Hypothyroid patients have a 3-fold increased prevalence of hypertension, usually diastolic.

Laboratory diagnosis. The clinical suspicion of thyroid gland dysfunction may be confirmed with laboratory tests. Increased levels of blood thyroid hormones (thyroxine and triiodothyronine) and low serum levels of thyroid-stimulating hormone (TSH) are the hallmarks of hyperthyroidism. Increased sensitivity of TSH assays allows detection of low TSH levels, which are also diagnostic of hyperthyroidism. Low TSH occurs in thyrotoxicosis caused by excess thyroxine or triiodothyronine. The diagnosis of hypothyroidism is based on low serum levels of thyroid hormone and increased serum levels of TSH.

Treatment

Hyperthyroidism. The initial management of the hypertensive patient with hyperthyroidism includes the use of a β-adrenergic blocker (e.g., atenolol or propranolol) to treat the hypertension, tachycardia, and tremor. The definitive treatment of hyperthyroidism is cause-specific. Patients with autoimmune hyperthyroidism (Graves' disease) should be treated with thyroid gland ablation with radioiodine 131 (^{131}I). In the patient with hyperthyroidism caused by a multinodular goiter (Plummer's disease), ^{131}I is usually not curative, and subtotal thyroidectomy is the treatment of choice. If the hyperthyroidism is associated with acute thyroid inflammation (e.g., subacute thyroiditis), the temporary (e.g., 3 months) use of a β-adrenergic inhibitor may be the only treatment indicated.

Hypothyroidism. Treatment of thyroid hormone deficiency lowers blood pressure in most hypertensive patients. Synthetic levothyroxine (Synthroid) is the treatment of choice for hypothyroidism. The initial dosage of levothyroxine is based on body weight (1.6 µg/kg/day). The daily dosage requirement may be lower in older patients (e.g., <1.0 µg/kg/day). In patients >50 years of age or patients with cardiac disease, the initial dosage of levothyroxine should be lower (e.g., 25 to 50 µg/day) and increased every 2 weeks by 25 µg until the target dosage is achieved. Clinical and biochemical reevaluations should be completed at 2-month intervals until the serum TSH concentration is normalized.

MEDULLARY THYROID CARCINOMA

The occurrence of MTC may be sporadic or familial (familial MTC or MEN II). Although MTC does not cause hypertension, the close association with pheochromocytoma is recognized: MEN IIA (MTC, pheochromocytoma, and hyperparathyroidism) and MEN IIB (MTC, pheochromocytoma, mucosal neuromas, and marfanoid body habitus) (see Chapters A51 and C169). The MEN II syndromes are inherited as autosomal dominant traits with complete penetrance and variable expressivity.

Clinical Presentation

The usual presentation of MTC is with a thyroid nodule, a thyroid mass, or cervical lymphadenopathy. Although serum calcitonin concentrations are increased, most patients are asymptomatic. Up to 30% of patients with MTC develop watery diarrhea, presumably secondary to high circulating calcitonin levels. Serum levels of calcium and phosphorus are normal.

Laboratory Diagnosis

When the presentation is limited to a solitary thyroid nodule, the diagnosis of MTC may be made on cytologic findings from a fine-needle aspirate. In other patients, MTC may be suspected and found with genetic or biochemical testing because of a family history of MEN II. All first-degree relatives of patients with MEN II should be screened with the gene test for mutation in the *RET* protooncogene.

Treatment

The treatment of choice for MTC is surgical resection. Most centers advocate total thyroidectomy and ^{131}I ablation of the thyroid gland remnant. After this initial treatment, patients are placed on levothyroxine replacement therapy and should be followed up on an annual basis with physical examination and serum calcitonin concentration tests. If recurrent disease is suspected on the basis of increasing serum calcitonin levels, it can usually be localized with ultrasound or computerized imaging of the neck.

Screening for Other Multiple Endocrine Neoplasia Abnormalities

Clinicians should be aware of the high prevalence of other endocrine neoplasias in patients with MCT. In particular, screening for pheochromocytoma should probably be per-formed in all MCT patients because of the high cardiovascular risk (see Chapters A51 and C169). Screening of first-degree relatives should also be considered.

PRIMARY HYPERPARATHYROIDISM

Primary hyperparathyroidism is the most frequent cause of hypercalcemia, which is also associated with hypertension.

Clinical Presentation

Hypercalcemia is associated with an increased incidence of hypertension, and primary hyperparathyroidism is the most common cause of hypercalcemia. The prevalence of hypertension in patients with primary hyperparathyroidism varies from 10% to 60%. In the majority of cases, the disease is caused by a benign solitary parathyroid adenoma. However, when associated with the MEN syndromes, the hyperparathyroidism is usually due to hyperplasia of all 4 parathyroid glands. Most patients with primary hyperparathyroidism are asymptomatic. The side effects of chronic hypercalcemia may be the focus of the presentation: polyuria and polydipsia, constipation, osteoporosis, renal lithiasis, peptic ulcer disease, and hypertension.

Laboratory Diagnosis

The hallmarks of primary hyperparathyroidism are hypercalcemia, hypophosphatemia, and increased serum concentrations of parathyroid hormone. In the patient with hypercalcemia, the measurement of serum parathyroid hormone is the most specific way of making the diagnosis of primary hyperparathyroidism. If the serum concentration of parathyroid hormone is not increased, the clinical data should be reviewed and nonparathyroid causes of hypercalcemia investigated (e.g., pheochromocytoma, hyperthyroidism, cancer, multiple myeloma, vitamin D intoxication, and sarcoidosis).

Treatment

The treatment of hyperparathyroidism is surgical. Preoperative localization with sestamibi scintigraphy or neck ultrasound may facilitate minimal access parathyroidectomy in sporadic cases. In the setting of MEN, subtotal parathyroid resection (3.5 glands) of the hyperplastic glands is usually indicated.

SUGGESTED READING

1. Evans DB, Burgess MA, Goepfert H, Gagel RF. Medullary thyroid carcinoma. *Curr Ther Endocrinol Metab.* 1997;6:127–132.
2. Marzanol A, Porcelli A, Biondi B, et al. Surgical management and follow-up of medullary thyroid carcinoma. *J Surg Oncol.* 1995;59:162–168.
3. Pommier RF, Brennan MF. Medullary thyroid carcinoma. *Endocrinologist.* 1992;2:393–405.
4. Richards AM, Espiner EA, Nicholls MG, et al. Hormone, calcium and blood pressure relationships in primary hyperparathyroidism. *J Hypertens.* 1988;6:747–752.
5. Saito I, Saruta T. Hypertension in thyroid disorders. *Endocrinol Metab Clin North Am.* 1994;23:379–386.
6. Streeten DHP, Anderson GH Jr, Howland T, et al. Effects of thyroid function on blood pressure: recognition of hypothyroid hypertension. *Hypertension.* 1988;11:78–83.

Chapter C172

Management of Sleep Apnea

Virend K. Somers, MD, PhD

KEY POINTS

- Obstructive sleep apnea is widely prevalent in the general population and is especially frequent in patients who are obese, who have hypertension, or who have both conditions.

- The repetitive nocturnal hypoxemia results in acute neurohumoral activation and increased blood pressure, which carry over into daytime wakefulness.

- Effective treatment of obstructive sleep apnea reduces not only the acute neurohumoral and pressor responses, but may also result in sustained reduction in daytime sympathetic activity and lower daytime blood pressures in hypertensive patients.

See also Chapters A34, A40, A42, A44, A46, A55, B97, C110, C112, C113, C127–C129, and C162

Patients with obstructive sleep apnea (OSA) are usually, but not always, obese. The disease process is characterized by repetitive nocturnal obstructive events secondary to upper airway collapse during inspiration. The exact pathophysiology underlying the predisposition to airway collapse is not well understood but may relate to a number of factors including accumulation of adipose tissue, craniofacial characteristics, abnormal upper airway tone, and dysfunctional neural mechanisms regulating airway patency.

Hypertension in Obstructive Sleep Apnea

The repetitive nocturnal desaturations can be quite profound, reaching levels of oxygen saturation lower than 50%. Hypoxemia, together with CO_2 retention, excites the peripheral and central chemoreflexes. This elicits sympathetic activation with consequent vasoconstriction and marked increases in blood pressure (BP) (see Chapter A55). The hypoxemic and other metabolic stresses secondary to repetitive nocturnal OSA may also induce production of other humoral substances, with significant pressor and trophic consequences. For example, patients with sleep apnea manifest acute increases in catecholamines, endothelin, and markers of inflammation. The pressor effects of endothelin, for example, may persist for a number of hours. Over the long term, the arousals from sleep and the neural, humoral, and metabolic responses to repetitive nocturnal hypoxemia may result in severe daytime somnolence, cognitive impairment, increased daytime BPs and predisposition to structural and functional cardiovascular disease. There are no rigid criteria for institution of evaluation and treatment for OSA.

Diagnosis and Quantitation

The diagnosis of OSA is based on polysomnographic (PSG) monitoring of the electroencephalogram, eye movements, muscle tone, abdominal and chest movement, airflow, oxygen saturation, and, occasionally, intrathoracic pressure monitoring.

The quantification of apneas and hypopneas detected during an overnight polysomnogram is referred to as the *apnea-hypopnea index* (AHI). An AHI of up to 5 events per hour is seen in normal adults. *Mild OSA* is defined as an AHI from 5 to 20, *moderate* from 20 to 40, and *severe* as >40. Although significant OSA may be found in 2% to 4% of the adult population, the prevalence of the disorder is increased in patients with hypertension, of whom 30% to 40% may have OSA. The prevalence of OSA may be even higher in patients with resistant hypertension, particularly if they are obese.

The decision to undertake a diagnostic evaluation is based on evidence of clinical impairment (daytime somnolence, impaired driving) in the setting of a compatible history (loud snoring, witnessed apneas) or physical examination (tonsillar enlargement, retrognathia), or both. The presence of coexistent cardiovascular disease or an associated risk factor often heightens clinical suspicion. Formal diagnostic testing is not always necessary to institute innocuous therapy (i.e., positional manipulations) or behavioral modifications that may improve nighttime sleep. On the other hand, patients with some degree of risk based on this evaluation should undergo further workup. Simple overnight oximetry does have a role, particularly when interpreted by an experienced clinician. However, a "normal" appearing overnight oximetry does not rule out clinically significant OSA and should not preclude full PSG study in a patient at risk.

Obesity and sleep apnea. OSA is frequently associated with obesity, and a large percentage of patients with the syndrome are overweight. The impact of weight gain on OSA severity may be related to cervical fat deposition, intrapharyngeal adipose tissue accumulation, and effects of truncal obesity on lung volumes. Weight loss, whether from medical or dietary intervention or from bariatric surgery, has consistently been shown to improve disordered breathing during sleep. The response of OSA to weight loss varies from person to person, but even modest reductions (10% of body weight) have been shown to be of benefit. Moreover, weight loss is beneficial for overall health, particularly in those patients who have associated hypertension and other cardiovascular disease.

Treatment of obstructive sleep apnea. Mild OSA may be treated with conservative measures with the option of more aggressive, and potentially invasive, therapies later if initial treatment fails. On the other hand, moderate to severe OSA requires more aggressive therapy up front, with behavioral modifications as an adjunct therapy.

CPAP. Continuous positive airway pressure (CPAP) is the established treatment for obstructive sleep apnea hypopnea syndrome, and the gold standard therapy for patients with moderate to severe disease. CPAP involves delivery of positive pressure via a nasal mask, thereby acting as a pneumatic splint to prevent collapse of the pharyngeal airway during sleep. It is often titrated with the guidance of PSG monitoring during the second half of the study night, thereby often eliminating the need for repeat testing. CPAP provides a number of advantages as the primary form of treatment: It is noninvasive, safe, effective, and rapidly and easily applied. Indications for institution of CPAP therapy are evolving and include an abnormal AHI, with or without coexistent daytime sleepiness or increased cardiovascular risk.

Adverse effects of CPAP are few but often relate to nasal congestion or mask interface problems, both of which are often readily addressed. As with any medical therapy, patient compliance is variable and ranges from 40% to 80%. Recent advances in positive pressure airway therapy include autotitrating units that adjust the pressure applied from minute to minute, based on measurement of dynamic obstruction throughout the night. Bilevel positive airway pressure may be useful in patients with abnormal daytime ventilation who also have nocturnal sleep apnea, such as those with neuromuscular disease.

Positioning during sleep. Many patients have worsening of sleep apnea in the supine position as compared to other positions. Gravity causes the tongue and other soft tissue to fall back against the posterior pharyngeal wall when supine, thus predisposing to airway collapse. Manipulation of body position has been shown to improve the rate of disordered breathing events during sleep. This may involve sleeping on one's side and, occasionally, head and trunk elevation to 30 degrees from horizontal, which affords the airway greater stability against early closure. Other maneuvers aimed at avoiding the supine position, and, therefore, maintaining the lateral recumbent position, may be used. This may involve the use of body-length pillows along the dorsal surface of the body. Placement of tennis balls within a pocket sewn into the back of a T-shirt worn at night provides a deterrent to the supine position. Over time, the patient should become conditioned to sleeping in the lateral recumbent position. Positional therapy alone may effectively treat some patients who have purely positional sleep apnea, although it may also be used as part of a multifaceted approach to nonpositional disordered breathing.

Oral appliances. The use of oral appliances in OSA, derived primarily from case series, is based on their ability to hold the tongue forward or primarily reposition the mandible and tongue anteriorly. These appliances are molded to the shape of

the mouth and teeth and, because they have the potential to worsen airway obstruction, are fitted by dentists specialized in this field. These devices have been known to aggravate temporomandibular joint dysfunction, although newer "adjustable" appliances allow titration of the mandibular position over time. They may be useful as an adjunct to weight loss and positional therapy in patients with mild OSA. Patients should undergo a CPAP trial before use of an intraoral device given the proven efficacy of CPAP. Moreover, in patients with moderate or severe disease, intraoral devices should be reserved for those who do not tolerate or who refuse CPAP or surgical therapy.

Surgical procedures. A number of surgical procedures have been developed in an attempt to alleviate upper airway obstruction and improve airflow in patients with OSA. Tracheostomy was the first successful therapy for sleep apnea and is the only reliably effective sole surgical procedure to successfully treat OSA. However, because of the associated morbidity, it should be reserved for those cases that are refractory to other measures or for patients with clinical urgency, such as severe hypoxemia or cardiac arrhythmias. Surgery may be the preferable treatment option for patients with a specific underlying identifiable anatomic abnormality that is causing mild to moderate obstructive apnea. Examples include persistent tonsillar enlargement, nasal turbinate hypertrophy unresponsive to medical management, and nasal septal deviation. This may be especially attractive in young patients as well as older patients with few comorbidities.

Surgery is sometimes performed on patients without these strictly defined anatomic lesions. A common technique is the uvulopalatopharyngoplasty, aimed at reducing obstruction at the oropharyngeal or retropalatal region. This entails excision of the uvula, tonsillar tissue, and portions of the soft palate. However, preoperative assessment is not highly sensitive at detecting all areas of airway obstruction, and, as a consequence, only a minority of patients have long-term correction of OSA with uvulopalatopharyngoplasty. It is important to obtain follow-up PSGs to assess for response and the potential need for adjunctive CPAP therapy.

Drug therapy. Drugs that promote healthy weight loss would clearly be beneficial for OSA patients. Other pharmacologic approaches have been less rewarding and have included sex hormone supplementation, respiratory stimulants, and agents that act on neurotransmitter physiology at the level of the brain stem motor nuclei controlling the upper airway dilator muscles. Serotonin agonists and antagonists have been tried. In general, the results of pharmacologic intervention to treat the obstructive apnea per se have been mixed.

Sleep apnea in hemodialysis patients. Interest in sleep-related clinical syndromes is accelerating and novel approaches to treatment of OSA are being described. In patients with OSA and end-stage renal failure, marked improvement in AHI occurred in patients who underwent intensive nightly hemodialysis (**Figure C172.1**). Another study recently demonstrated the value of nocturnal atrial overpacing in patients with OSA. The development of pharmacologic approaches has been hindered by the complex pathophysiology underlying OSA and the mechanical nature of airway collapse.

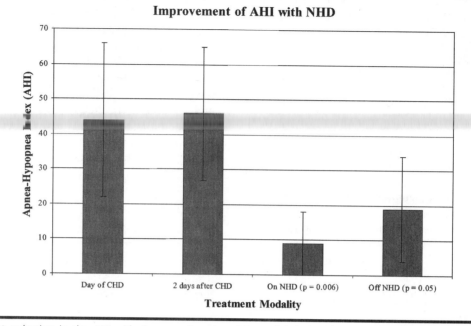

Figure C172.1. Significant reduction in the AHI with the use of nocturnal hemodialysis (NHD), as compared to limited benefits from conventional hemodialysis (CHD). Study participants underwent 6 to 15 months of daily nocturnal hemodialysis, which caused a significant reduction in their AHI ($p =$ .006). Also, on a night without NHD, participants still demonstrated a significant decrease in their AHI ($p = .05$). (Adapted from Hanly PJ, Pierratos A. Improvement of sleep apnea in patients with chronic renal failure who undergo nocturnal hemodialysis. *N Engl J Med.* 2001;344:102–107.)

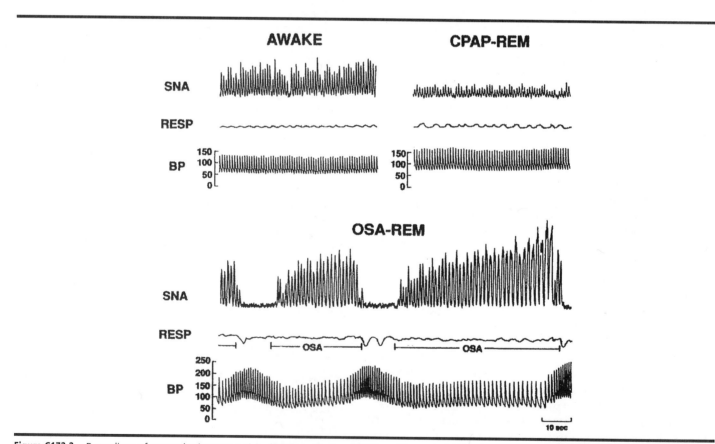

Figure C172.2. Recordings of sympathetic nerve activity (SNA), respiration (RESP), and intraarterial blood pressure (BP) in the same subject when awake (*top left*), with obstructive sleep apnea (OSA) during rapid eye movement (REM) sleep (*bottom*), and with elimination of OSA by continuous positive airway pressure (CPAP) therapy during REM sleep (*top right*). SNA is high during wakefulness, and increases further with OSA during REM. BP increases from 130/65 mm Hg when awake to 240/110 mm Hg at the end of apnea. Overall, nocturnal blood pressure is increased. Elimination of apnea by CPAP (*top right*) results in decreased sympathetic traffic and prevents BP surges during REM sleep. (From Somers VK, Dyken ME, Clary MP, Abboud FM. Sympathetic neural mechanisms in obstructive sleep apnea. *J Clin Invest.* 1995;96:1897–1904, with permission.)

Effects of Treatment on Blood Pressure and Sympathetic Activity

Acute effects. Effective treatment and prevention of the repetitive nocturnal desaturation have immediate effects on the humoral and reflex responses to hypoxemia and hypercapnia (**Figure C172.2**). Specifically, administration of CPAP results in a marked reduction in sympathetic traffic and prevents the repetitive surges in BP that are evident at the end of the apneic events. Furthermore, several hours of treatment with CPAP induces a fall in other pressor and trophic substances such as endothelin and erythropoietin. It is interesting that the change in endothelin after acute treatment with CPAP is significantly related to the reduction in BP. The consequences of acute treatment of sleep apnea may be especially important in hypertensive patients. Hypertension is associated with a potentiated chemoreflex response to hypoxemia. Thus, the adrenergic and pressor responses to equivalent levels of hypoxemia would be more marked in hypertensive individuals who already have high BPs even when awake. In a normotensive individual, severe sleep apnea can result in elevation of nocturnal BPs to levels as high as 240/110 mm Hg. These BP responses would be enhanced in hypertensive individuals with severe nocturnal apneas.

Chronic effects. It is not clear why recurrent nocturnal apneas should elicit responses that carry over into daytime wakefulness. High levels of sympathetic activity are evident in sleep apnea patients even when awake and in the absence of apneas. Effective treatment of the nocturnal desaturations may also have carryover effects into daytime wakefulness. In normotensive otherwise-healthy patients with OSA who are on no medications, treatment of sleep apnea results in a gradual decrease in tonic resting daytime sympathetic drive. This reduction in sympathetic activity becomes evident only after 1 month of treatment and is not accompanied by any substantial reduction in BP or heart rate. The absence of a significant BP reduction after chronic treatment of normotensive patients with sleep apnea has been consistent across a number of studies. Thus, although CPAP treatment lowers nocturnal BP, daytime BPs in the longer term are less affected in normotensive individuals.

Effects on BP appear to be more clear in hypertensive patients. As with normotensives, treatment with CPAP in a hypertensive patient acutely decreases the nighttime BP. Available data consistently show that treatment of sleep apnea in hypertension also results in a significant reduction in daytime BP measurements (**Figure C172.3**). There are emerging data suggesting that patients with hypertension resistant to combination therapy should be evaluated for OSA, especially if they are obese. If the apnea can be treated successfully, there is some evidence suggesting that not only do BPs decrease, but the number and dosages of medications can be substantially reduced. In patients with hypertensive heart failure who also have OSA, treatment of sleep apnea may significantly ameliorate the hypertension and the heart failure. Even sleep apneic patients with hypertension and diastolic dysfunction may experience benefit from effective treatment of their OSA.

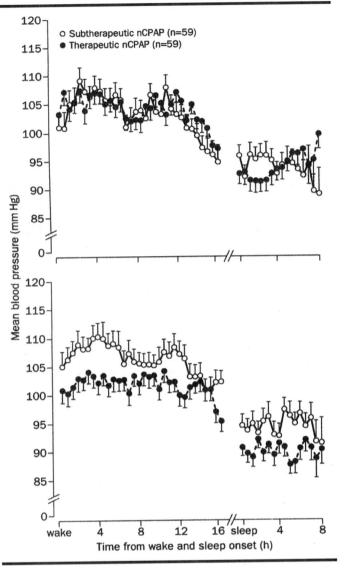

Figure C172.3. Randomized trial comparing men with sleep apnea who were treated with therapeutic versus subtherapeutic CPAP (1 cm H_2O) over a 1-month period. Mean ambulatory blood pressure profile before (*top*) and after (*bottom*) treatment. Benefit was seen during sleep and wakefulness. Severe apneics showed a better response, as did those on antihypertensive medications. nCPAP, nasal continuous positive airway pressure. (From Pepperell JC, Ramdassingh-Dow S, Crosthwaite N, et al. Ambulatory blood pressure after therapeutic and subtherapeutic nasal continuous positive airway pressure for obstructive sleep apnea: a randomized parallel trial. *Lancet.* 2002;359(9302):204–210, with permission.)

SUGGESTED READING

1. Faccenda JF, Mackay TW, Boon NA, Douglas NJ. Randomized placebo-controlled trial of continuous positive airway pressure on blood pressure in the sleep apnea-hypopnea syndrome. *Am J Respir Crit Care Med.* 2001;163:344–348.
2. Garrigue S, Bordier P, Jaïs P, et al. Benefit of atrial pacing in sleep apnea syndrome. *N Engl J Med.* 2002;346:404–412.
3. Hanly PJ, Pierratos A. Improvement of sleep apnea in patients with chronic renal failure who undergo nocturnal hemodialysis. *N Engl J Med.* 2001;344:102–107.
4. Narkiewicz K, Kato M, Phillips BG, et al. Nocturnal continuous positive airway pressure decreases daytime sympathetic traffic in obstructive sleep apnea. *Circulation.* 1999;100:2332–2335.
5. Peppard PE, Young T, Palta M, Skatrud J. Prospective study of the associa-

tion between sleep-disordered breathing and hypertension. *N Engl J Med.* 2000;342:1378–1384.

6. Pepperell JCT, Ramdassingh-Dow S, Crosthwaite N, et al. Ambulatory blood pressure after therapeutic and subtherapeutic nasal continuous positive airway pressure for obstructive sleep apnea, a randomised parallel trial. *Lancet.* 2002;359:204–210.

7. Somers VK, Dyken ME, Clary MP, Abboud FM. Sympathetic neural mechanisms in obstructive sleep apnea. *J Clin Invest.* 1995;96:1897–1904.

8. Suzuki M, Otsuka K, Guilleminault C. Long-term nasal continuous positive airway pressure administration can normalize hypertension in obstructive sleep apnea patients. *Sleep.* 1993;16:545–549.

9. Wilcox I, Grunstein RR, Hedner JA, et al. Effect of nasal continuous positive airway pressure during sleep on 24-hour blood pressure in obstructive sleep apnea. *Sleep.* 1993;16:539–544.

10. Young T, Palta M, Dempsey J, et al. The occurrence of sleep-disordered breathing among middle-aged adults. *N Engl J Med.* 1993;328:1230–1235.

Chapter C173

Management of Drug-Induced and Iatrogenic Hypertension

Ehud Grossman, MD; Franz H. Messerli, MD, FACC

KEY POINTS

- A variety of therapeutic agents and chemical substances can induce transient or sustained hypertension, exacerbate well-controlled hypertension, or antagonize the effects of antihypertensive therapy.

- Careful evaluation of a patient's drug regimen may identify chemically induced hypertension and prevent the need for lifelong antihypertensive therapy.

- When drug- or chemically induced hypertension is identified, discontinuation of the causative agent should be recommended.

- When it is not possible to avoid chemical agents that cause hypertension, institution of appropriate antihypertensive treatment is indicated.

See also Chapters A1, A41, A50, A56, A58, B96, B99, C110, C127, C137, and C150

Hypertension related to drugs and other chemical substances represents an important modifiable source of secondary hypertension. Identification of the intake of these substances is important because their elimination can obviate the need for unnecessary, costly, and potentially dangerous evaluations, treatments, or both. When drug- or chemically induced hypertension is identified, discontinuation of the causative agent should be recommended. When it is not possible to discontinue agents that cause hypertension, institution of appropriate antihypertensive treatment is indicated. In the absence of specific treatment guidelines for drug-induced hypertension, the recommended initial antihypertensive therapy should be directed to neutralize the specific mechanism causing hypertension (**Table C173.1**).

Steroids

Corticosteroids. Hypertension occurs in at least 20% of patients treated with high doses of synthetic corticosteroids. Oral cortisol increases blood pressure (BP) in a dose-dependent fashion; at a dose of 80 to 200 mg per day, systolic pressure increases by approximately 15 mm Hg, which can be apparent within 24 hours. Glucocorticoid-induced hypertension occurs more often in elderly patients and in patients with positive family history of essential hypertension. Certain exogenous compounds such as natural licorice, phenylbutazone, carbenoxolone, 9α-fluoroprednisolone, and 9α-fluorocortisol have mineralocorticoid activity. When ingested in moderate quantities, they may produce arterial hypertension characterized by the clinical picture of "pseudohyperaldosteronism" (increased exchangeable sodium and blood volume, hypokalemia with metabolic alkalosis, and suppressed plasma renin and aldosterone levels). Prolonged use of high-dose ketoconazole may alter enzymatic degradation of steroids leading to mineralocorticoid-related hypertension. Skin ointments, antihemorrhoidal preparations, ophthalmic drops, asthma inhalers, and nasal allergy sprays may contain substances with significant mineralocorticoid activity (particularly 9α-fluoroprednisolone). Some preparations also contain sympathetic amines. Discontinuation of these substances is recommended to lower BP. However, when steroid treatment is mandatory, a diuretic is often effective. Careful monitoring of potassium is necessary, however, because of the tendency for diuretics to exacerbate hypokalemia in steroid-dependent hypertension.

Sex hormones. Oral contraceptives induce hypertension in approximately 5% of users of high-dose compounds that contain at least 50 µg estrogen and 1 to 4 mg progestin. Small increases in BP have been reported even among users of modern low-dose formulations. Women with a history of high BP during pregnancy, those with a family history of hypertension, cigarette smokers, obese women, blacks, diabetics, and those

Table C173.1. Management of Drug-Induced Hypertension

INGREDIENT	MANAGEMENT	NOTES
Steroids		
Glucocorticoids	Discontinue; if not possible, start diuretics.	Monitor potassium.
Mineralocorticoids	Discontinue; if not possible, start diuretics.	Monitor potassium.
Sex hormones		
Anesthetics and narcotics		
Ketamine hydrochloride	Initial therapy, clonidine or α-blockers.	
Desflurane	Initial therapy, α-blockers or α,β-blockers.	
Naloxone	Initial therapy, α-blockers.	
Sevoflurane	Clonidine, or combination of diltiazem and nicardipine.	
Drugs affecting the sympathetic nervous system		
Ophthalmic solutions	Initial therapy, α-blockers or α,β-blockers.	Avoid β-blockers.
Antiemetic agents		Transient increase in BP.
Yohimbine hydrochloride	Discontinue.	Avoid in hypertensive patients and in those treated with tricyclic antidepressants.
Glucagon (only in patients with pheochromocytoma)	Initial therapy, intravenous phentolamine, oral phenoxybenzamine, or α_1-blockers.	
Cocaine	Initial therapy, α-blockers, nitroglycerin, and verapamil.	Most patients do not require treatment.
Anorexics	Discontinue treatment.	
Nasal decongestant	Initial therapy, α,β-blockers.	
Cough medications	Discontinue treatment.	
Sibutramine	Discontinue sibutramine or modify antihypertensive therapy.	In obese hypertensive patients, the BP reduction achieved by weight loss negates the potential increase related to the drug.
Clozapine	Discontinue; if not possible, start α-blockers or nifedipine.	
Antidepressant agents		
Monoamine oxidase inhibitors	Initial therapy, α-blockers.	
Tricyclic antidepressants	Initial therapy, α-blockers.	
Serotonin agonist	Initial therapy, α-blockers.	
Miscellaneous		
Cyclosporine	Discontinue or switch to tacrolimus; if not possible, start calcium antagonists. Other drugs are also effective.	Calcium antagonists may increase cyclosporine blood levels. Multidrug therapy may be necessary.
Tacrolimus	Discontinue; if not possible, start calcium antagonists. Other drugs are also effective.	
Recombinant human erythropoietin	Lower the dose; if unsuccessful, start calcium antagonists or α-blockers. Diuretics and angiotensin-converting enzyme inhibitors may be less effective.	Dialysis with conventional antihypertensive treatment may be effective. Phlebotomy may rapidly lower BP.
Bromocriptine disulfiram		Avoid use for suppression of lactation.
Alcohol	Moderate alcohol intake.	
Nonsteroidal antiinflammatory drugs	Calcium antagonists.	Assess the risk of an increase in BP against the expected benefit. Among cyclooxygenase-2 inhibitors, celecoxib affects BP less than rofecoxib.

BP, blood pressure.

with renal diseases may experience significant increases in BP. The usual increase in BP is minimal, but severe hypertensive episodes, including malignant hypertension, have been reported. Postmenopausal estrogen replacement therapy decreases BP slightly but is no longer recommended for cardiovascular protection. Men receiving estrogen for the treatment of prostatic cancer may also exhibit an increase in BP. Danazol, a semisynthetic androgen that is used in the treatment of endometriosis and hereditary angioedema, has been reported to induce hypertension owing to fluid retention.

Anesthetics and Narcotics

Ketamine hydrochloride, desflurane, and sevoflurane have been reported to severely increase BP owing to stimulation of the sympatholytic nervous system. Treatment with sympatholytic agents such as α-blockers, α,β-blockers, or clonidine usually lowers BP. The simultaneous use of vasoconstrictors (felypressin) with topical cocaine can result in severe hypertension. Hypertensive responses to naloxone (opiate antagonist), especially during attempted reversal of narcotic-induced anesthesia in hypertensive patients, have also been reported. Naloxone seems to acutely reverse the antihypertensive effects of clonidine and can thereby cause an acute hypertensive emergency.

Drugs Affecting Sympathetic Nervous Transmission

Phenylephrine (Neo-Synephrine) has been reported in isolated cases to severely increase BP after its administration in an ophthalmic solution. Dipivalyl adrenaline, an adrenaline prodrug used topically in the management of chronic simple glaucoma, can also increase BP. The addition of sympathomimetic agents to β-blockers can also increase BP, presumably because of unopposed α-adrenergic vasoconstriction. Use of α-blockers or agents such as labetalol or carvedilol that block both α- and β-adrenergic receptors should counteract this detrimental reaction.

Antiemetic agents such as metoclopramide, alizapride, and prochlorperazine have been reported to increase BP transiently in patients treated with cisplatin.

Yohimbine hydrochloride should be avoided or used intermittently only in hypertensive patients and in those undergoing concurrent treatment with tricyclic antidepressants.

Glucagon may induce severe hypertension in patients with pheochromocytoma. Blocking the α-adrenoceptors by intravenous phentolamine or oral agents such as phenoxybenzamine or doxazosin may prevent catastrophic cardiovascular events.

Cocaine intoxication is characterized by α-adrenergic overactivity, often associated with markedly increased BP and acute, but not chronic, hypertension. Most patients with cocaine-related hypertension do not require antihypertensive drug therapy, but if treatment is necessary, α-adrenergic receptor antagonists and combined α,β-blockers are logical choices. Nitroglycerin and verapamil reverse cocaine-induced hypertension and coronary arterial vasoconstriction and, therefore, are the agents of choice in treating patients with cocaine-associated chest pain.

Sibutramine is a novel serotonin and noradrenaline reuptake inhibitor antiobesity drug that activates the sympathetic nervous system, increasing heart rate and BP in obese normotensive subjects. Patients treated with sibutramine should be monitored for changes in BP, and the drug should be withdrawn if BP becomes elevated.

Clozapine may also raise BP by sympathetic activation, and α-adrenergic receptor antagonists are the treatment of choice.

Immunosuppressive Agents

Calcineurin inhibitor immunosuppressives (cyclosporin and tacrolimus) may induce arterial hypertension in patients undergoing organ transplantation and in those with autoimmune disease and dermatologic disorders (see Chapter A58). The risk of hypertension with these agents is unrelated to sex or race, but it is dose-related, and it increases with age of the patient and with preexisting hypertension or high serum creatinine levels. BP usually falls after the withdrawal or substitution of cyclosporine immunosuppression but may not remit completely. Calcium antagonists are the most successful agent, but other drugs are also helpful. Usually multidrug therapy is necessary. Rapamycin, a novel immunosuppressive agent that does not inhibit calcineurin, has not been reported to produce nephrotoxicity or hypertension.

Over-the-Counter Drugs

Most nonprescription anorexics contain combinations of an antihistamine and an adrenergic agonist (usually phenylpropanolamine, ephedrine, pseudoephedrine, or caffeine). α-Adrenergic intoxication induced by nasal decongestant and cough medications containing massive doses of oxymetazoline hydrochloride, phenylephrine hydrochloride, and ephedrine hydrochloride has been reported to result in severe hypertension. α-Blockers and α,β-blockers are logical choices in these cases.

Antidepressant Agents

Monoamine oxidase inhibitors can induce severe hypertension when patients consume foods containing tyramine. Tranylcypromine is the most hazardous, whereas moclobemide

and brofaromine seem to be the least likely to raise BP. α-Adrenergic receptor blockers and α,β-blockers seem appropriate for initial treatment. Tricyclic antidepressants increase BP, mainly in patients with panic disorders. Buspirone and other serotonin receptor type 1α agonists have also been reported to increase BP, especially in those also on monoamine oxidase inhibitors. Venlafaxine has a dose-dependent effect on BP that may become clinically significant at high doses. Episodes of severe hypertension have been described in patients treated with other antidepressant agents such as fluoxetine, fluoxetine plus selegiline, and thioridazine.

Antineoplastic Agents

Hypertensive reactions associated with paclitaxel treatment have been reported.

Recombinant Human Erythropoietin

Recombinant human erythropoietin (r-HuEPO) has dramatically improved the care of patients with renal failure, but this drug can increase BP in a dose-related fashion and lead to hypertension in 20% to 30% of patients treated who receive it. Hypertension may develop in some patients as early as 2 weeks and in others as late as 4 months after the start of r-HuEPO treatment. Treatment involves optimizing dialysis treatment, paying close attention to volume regulation, giving r-HuEPO subcutaneously, and careful attention to dose and frequency of administration. Hematocrit should be increased gradually so that the occurrence of hypertension can be minimized. Generally, hypertension associated with r-HuEPO has not been too difficult to control. In 1 study 42% of patients with r-HuEPO-induced hypertension were controlled with a single agent. BP can also be managed with a combination of fluid removal with dialysis and conventional antihypertensive therapy. If these measures are unsuccessful, the dose of r-HuEPO should be lowered or therapy should be held for several weeks. Phlebotomy of 500 mL of blood may rapidly lower BP in refractory patients.

Alcohol

Excessive chronic alcohol use has clearly been shown to raise BP and can also increase resistance to antihypertensive therapy. There is a dose-response relationship for the hypertensive effects of alcohol. Abstinence or at least moderation of alcohol intake to no more than approximately 1 to 2 oz of alcohol is the appropriate treatment. In some cases, BP control is extremely difficult unless abstinence from alcohol is achieved.

Nonsteroidal Antiinflammatory Drugs

Nonsteroidal antiinflammatory drugs (NSAIDs) can induce an increase in BP perhaps as much as 5 mm Hg (mean BP) and interfere with antihypertensive treatment (see Chapter C150). NSAID users also had a 40% increased risk of receiving a diagnosis of hypertension compared with nonusers. NSAIDs may interact with some antihypertensive agents such as diuretics, β-blockers, and ACE inhibitors but do not interact with calcium antagonists and central-acting drugs, the antihypertensive efficacy of which is apparently unrelated to production of prostaglandins. Indomethacin, piroxicam, and naproxen have been associated with the largest increases in BP whereas sulindac and full-dose aspirin have little BP effect. Low-dose aspirin has no effect on BP control in hypertensive patients, but newer orally effective specific cyclooxygenase-2 inhibitors (rofecoxib and celecoxib) increase BP in a dose-dependent manner. In patients who take NSAIDs, diuretics and calcium antagonists are useful.

Heavy Metals

Several studies show that cumulative exposure to lead, even at low levels sustained by the general population, may increase the risk of hypertension. Some reports suggest that arsenic or cadmium exposure also may induce hypertension in humans.

Scorpions and Black Widows

Venoms of scorpions, especially certain South American species, and black widows commonly produce a clinical picture of profuse perspiration, lacrimation, vomiting, convulsion, and cardiovascular collapse. However, occasionally hypertension and bradycardia occur. Hypertension is mediated by a massive discharge of catecholamines into the circulation produced by the venom. Therefore, α- or β-blockers are appropriate treatment in this condition.

SUGGESTED READING

1. Brem AS. Insights into glucocorticoid-associated hypertension. *Am J Kidney Dis.* 2001;37:1–10.
2. Bursztyn M, Zelig O, Or R, Nagler A. Isradipine for the prevention of cyclosporine-induced hypertension in allogeneic bone marrow transplant recipients: a randomized, double-blind study. *Transplantation.* 1997;63:1034–1036.
3. Chasan-Taber L, Willett WC, Manson JE, et al. Prospective study of oral contraceptives and hypertension among women in the United States. *Circulation.* 1996;94:483–489.
4. Clyburn EB, DiPette DJ. Hypertension induced by drugs and other substances. *Semin Nephrol.* 1995;15:72–86.
5. Frishman WH. Effects of nonsteroidal anti-inflammatory drug therapy on blood pressure and peripheral edema. *Am J Cardiol.* 2002;89:18D–25D.
6. Grossman E, Messerli FH. High blood pressure. A side effect of drugs, poisons, and food. *Arch Intern Med.* 1995;155:450–460.
7. MacMahon S. Alcohol consumption and hypertension. *Hypertension.* 1987;9:111–121.
8. McMahon FG, Weinstein SP, Rowe E, et al. Sibutramine is safe and effective for weight loss in obese patients whose hypertension is well controlled with angiotensin-converting enzyme inhibitors. *J Hum Hypertens.* 2002;16:5–11.
9. Sramek JJ, Leibowitz MT, Weinstein SP, et al. Efficacy and safety of sibutramine for weight loss in obese patients with hypertension well controlled by β-adrenergic blocking agents: a placebo-controlled, double-blind, randomised trial. *J Hum Hypertens.* 2002;16:13–19.
10. White WB, Faich G, Whelton A, et al. Comparison of thromboembolic events in patients treated with celecoxib, a cyclooxygenase-2 specific inhibitor, versus ibuprofen or diclofenac. *Am J Cardiol.* 2002;89:425–430.

Chapter C174

Management of Posttransplant Hypertension

Vincent J. Canzanello, MD

KEY POINTS

- Posttransplant hypertension is common and is associated with increased cardiovascular morbidity and mortality and an increased risk of subsequent graft dysfunction.
- Posttransplant hypertension is usually related to the use of corticosteroids and calcineurin inhibitors or to renal insufficiency.
- Many transplant recipients have additional cardiovascular comorbidities such that aggressive blood pressure lowering with combination therapy is indicated, usually to less than 130/80 mm Hg.
- Many drugs, including angiotensin-converting enzyme inhibitors, angiotensin receptor blockers, calcium antagonists, and diuretics, are safe and effective in the treatment of posttransplant hypertension.

See also Chapters A48, A49, A58, A71, C123, C124, C128, C139, C141, C144, C146, C159, C168, and C173

The long-term goal in patients with posttransplant hypertension is similar to nontransplant patients: reduced morbidity and mortality by control of blood pressure (BP), hyperglycemia, dyslipidemia, and cigarette smoking. Goal BPs should be those similar in the nontransplant setting as outlined by the Sixth Report of the Joint National Committee on the Prevention, Detection, Evaluation, and Treatment of High Blood Pressure. Many hypertensive transplant recipients have coexisting conditions, such as cardiac or renal disease, diabetes mellitus, or dyslipidemia, that require BP control to less than 130/80 mm Hg. Several goal BPs in different clinical settings are shown in **Table C174.1.** Instruction in self-measurement of BP is an integral part of many transplant programs and, in some instances, 24-hour ambulatory BP monitoring is helpful.

Exacerbating Factors

Posttransplant hypertension is usually associated with the use of immunosuppressive drugs such as calcineurin inhibitors (cyclosporine and tacrolimus) or corticosteroids. Varying degrees of renal insufficiency are important, although similar

Table C174.1. Blood Pressure Goals in Posttransplant Patients

CLINICAL SETTING	BLOOD PRESSURE GOAL (MM HG)
Office	<140/90
Out of office (home)	<135/85
Diabetes mellitus, clinical cardiovascular disease, renal insufficiency	<130/80
Proteinuric renal disease	<125/75

factors that raise BP in the nontransplant hypertensive population may be present. Corticosteroid-associated weight gain is a common occurrence after organ transplantation and is a contributing factor to the development of hypertension, diabetes mellitus, and dyslipidemia, particularly hypertriglyceridemia. Additional causes of posttransplant hypertension, particularly after renal transplantation, are shown in **Table C174.2** and should be considered in the appropriate clinical setting (see Chapter A58).

Modification of Immunosuppression Regimens

Calcineurin inhibitors such as cyclosporine and tacrolimus are well-documented causes of hypertension. Several studies in liver and renal transplantation have demonstrated a lower prevalence of hypertension with tacrolimus compared to cyclosporine. Lower doses of corticosteroids used in tacrolimus-treated patients may account, in part, for this difference. In addition, the trend toward earlier discontinuation of corticosteroids has been associated with a lower incidence of posttransplant hypertension, particularly in the setting of liver transplantation. Use of the new macrolide antibiotic sirolimus in organ transplantation is increasing. Early reports suggest this drug is less likely to be associated with hypertension compared to cyclosporine and tacrolimus. Sirolimus can have nephrotoxicity, which can cause or exacerbate hypertension.

Lifestyle Modification

Nutritional counseling is important and should focus on healthy eating habits (including total calories, protein and fat

Table C174.2. Causes of Posttransplant Hypertension

Immunosuppressive drugs
  Cyclosporine
  Tacrolimus
  Corticosteroids
Renal dysfunction
  Perioperative ischemic damage[a]
  Drug-induced nephrotoxicity
  Chronic allograft rejection[a]
  Recurrence of original renal disease[a]
Native kidneys[a]
Transplant renal artery stenosis[a]
Donor-kidney associated hypertension[a]
Miscellaneous
  Nonsteroidal antiinflammatory drugs
  Obesity
  Alcohol
  Obstructive sleep apnea

[a]Refers to renal transplant recipients.

content, sodium chloride intake, etc.). The need for regular aerobic exercise should also be emphasized.

Antihypertensive Drug Therapy Considerations

Deciding on the most appropriate drug therapy in the setting of transplant-associated hypertension has become more complex in recent years, in part due to the need to achieve multiple therapeutic goals, including (a) lowering the systemic BP to reduce cardiovascular risk, (b) maintaining optimal renal blood flow by attenuating calcineurin inhibitor-associated renal vasoconstriction, and (c) preventing long-term renal dysfunction associated with glomerular hypertension or other adverse vascular effects of calcineurin inhibitors.

In general, a single antihypertensive drug cannot achieve all of the desired goals and, as a result, many hypertensive transplant recipients require the use of 2 or more medications (**Table C174.3**). These comments generally apply to the patient who is several months posttransplantation and with stable graft function because this is the population in which the vast majority of antihypertensive drug studies have been performed. Yet, goal BPs have not been formally established for transplant recipients, and there are no clinical studies that demonstrate better outcomes at target BP below 140/90 mm Hg (Table C174.1). Nevertheless, coexisting conditions such as diabetes or heart failure may mandate lower goals. In the acute posttransplant setting (days to weeks), it may be reasonable to aim for BPs less than 160/90 mm Hg because BP may improve spontaneously with increased physical activity, mobilization of retained fluid, reduction in immunosuppressive drug doses, and improvement or stabilization of graft function.

Specific Antihypertensive Drugs

Calcium antagonists. There are several features of calcium antagonists (CAs) that make them attractive in the treatment of posttransplant hypertension. These drugs antagonize calcineurin inhibitor-induced systemic and renal vasoconstriction and thus lead to a reduction in systemic BP and an increase in renal blood flow. Whether this latter effect has long-term benefit is not yet clear. Some CAs (verapamil, diltiazem, and nicardipine) interfere with the degradation of calcineurin inhibitors, and some transplant clinicians have capitalized on this interaction to lower doses of cyclosporine or tacrolimus, reducing expense and toxicity. Long-acting dihydropyridine CAs (nifedipine, isradipine, and amlodipine) are most commonly used. Lower-extremity edema owing to local vasodilatation and other adverse events owing to systemic vasodilatation (flushing, headache, palpitations) are the most commonly reported adverse effects from these drugs. As a general rule, it is prudent to monitor the cyclosporine or tacrolimus blood levels closely during the initiation of CA therapy.

β-Blockers. β-Blockers are also effective in posttransplant hypertension, and BP effects are equivalent to CAs and angiotensin-converting enzyme (ACE) inhibitors. β-Blockers have no significant effect on renal function. Bradyarrhythmias may be a concern in the heart transplant recipient as is masking hypoglycemic symptoms in transplant recipients with diabetes mellitus. Adverse effects on lipid metabolism (increased triglyceride and reduced high-density lipoprotein cholesterol levels)

Table C174.3. Drugs Used for the Treatment of Posttransplant Hypertension

DRUG CLASS	EFFECT ON BLOOD CYCLOSPORINE LEVELS[a]	ADVERSE EFFECTS	COMMENTS
Calcium channel blockers			Should use extended-release preparations only; dihydropyridine class most extensively used
Nifedipine	None	Edema, flushing, headache, palpitations	
Amlodipine	None or minimal	Same	
Isradipine	None	Same	
Nicardipine	Increase	Same	
Diltiazem	Increase	Negative inotropic and chronotropic effects, edema, constipation	
Verapamil	Increase	Similar to diltiazem, more constipation	
β-Blockers	None	Negative inotropic and chronotropic effects, bronchospasm	Useful in patients with coronary artery disease; may attenuate vasodilatory side effects of dihydropyridine calcium channel blockers
Atenolol			
Metoprolol			
Others			
Angiotensin-converting enzyme inhibitors	None	Cough, angioedema, hyperkalemia, azotemia[b]	Requires careful monitoring of renal function and serum potassium level; demonstrated to reduce proteinuria, prevent diabetes, and reduce complications of atherosclerosis in nontransplant settings
Enalapril			
Lisinopril			
Captopril			
Others			
Angiotensin receptor blockers	None	Hyperkalemia, azotemia,[b] cough and angioedema very rare	Same as angiotensin-converting enzyme inhibitors
Losartan			
Irbesartan			
Candesartan			
Others			
Thiazide diuretics	None	Prerenal azotemia, hyponatremia, hypokalemia, hypomagnesemia, hypercalcemia, hyperglycemia, hypertriglyceridemia, hyperuricemia	Potentiate most other antihypertensive drugs; require close monitoring of clinical and laboratory status until stabilized; significantly reduced effect if glomerular filtration rate <30 mL/min
Loop diuretics	None	Prerenal azotemia, hypokalemia, hypomagnesemia, hyperuricemia	Potentiate most other antihypertensive drugs; require close monitoring of clinical and laboratory status until stabilized; effective in azotemic patients; can be used as a replacement in patients with thiazide-associated hyponatremia or hypercalcemia

[a]Limited data are available regarding interactions with tacrolimus; therefore, tacrolimus blood levels should be followed closely after starting antihypertensive drug therapy.
[b]In patients with transplant renal artery stenosis.

are of more theoretic than practical concern given the important cardiovascular benefits that these drugs have demonstrated in the general hypertensive population with or without diabetes mellitus.

Angiotensin-converting enzyme inhibitors and angiotensin receptor blockers. Plasma renin activity is generally low or suppressed up to 12 months after renal or liver transplantation using calcineurin inhibitors. As a result, ACE inhibitors and angiotensin receptor blockers (ARBs) demonstrate limited monotherapeutic effectiveness during this time interval. Their efficacy is markedly enhanced by the addition of a diuretic. In those hypertensive patients who have stable graft function for 1 year or more, ACE inhibitors and ARBs have been shown to have efficacy equivalent to CAs and β-blockers. Several studies in renal transplant recipients have shown that ACE inhibitors and ARBs reduce proteinuria to a greater extent than other drugs, despite equivalent systemic BP reduction. Although unproven, there is no reason to believe that the benefits of renal preservation demonstrated for these drugs in nontransplant patients with diabetic and nondiabetic renal disease will not be seen in transplant recipients, particularly those with chronic nephropathy owing to calcineurin inhibitors or renal graft rejection.

Many experimental studies have demonstrated the ability of these 2 drug classes to ameliorate calcineurin inhibitor–associated disturbances of endothelial and renal dysfunction. Additionally, unequivocal cardiovascular benefits of ACE inhibitors as demonstrated in the treatment with these drugs considered in the Heart Outcomes Prevention Evaluation (HOPE) study raise the question of whether organ transplant recipients should be treated with these drugs early in their course. The majority of transplant patients have as many or more cardiovascular risk factors as did the HOPE study population. Treatment might be indicated regardless of BP status given that 40% of patients in the HOPE study did not have overt hypertension.

ACE inhibitors and ARBs can exacerbate hyperkalemia associated with renal insufficiency and calcineurin inhibitor use and can also precipitate reversible acute renal failure in patients with transplant renal artery stenosis. Anemia may occur with ACE inhibitor use posttransplantation and is reversible on discontinuation of the drug. Anemia appears to be less common with ARBs, although this may reflect less clinical experience with this drug class in the transplant setting.

Diuretics

Thiazide and loop diuretics play an important role in the management of posttransplant hypertension but require careful monitoring of serum electrolytes, renal function, immunosuppressive drug levels (which can vary with renal function) and other metabolic parameters such as serum calcium, uric acid, lipid, and glucose levels. Early after transplantation, hypertension may be precipitated or exacerbated by extracellular fluid volume expansion and renal dysfunction. In patients with hyperkalemia, thiazide or loop diuretics (or a combination of both) can help in the management of serum potassium. Several studies have demonstrated the sodium sensitivity of calcineurin inhibitor–associated hypertension. In general, potassium-sparing diuretics should be avoided because patients may already have high or high-normal serum potassium levels related to renal insufficiency, use of calcineurin inhibitors, or both. Thiazide diuretics are rarely effective when the glomerular filtration rate is below 30 mL per minute (or the serum creatinine above 1.5 mg/dL). In this circumstance, use of a loop diuretic such as furosemide, bumetanide, or torsemide should be considered.

SUGGESTED READING

1. Fellstrom B. Risk factors for and management of post-transplantation cardiovascular disease. *BioDrugs.* 2001;15:261–278.
2. Hausberg M, Barenbrock M, Hohage H, et al. ACE inhibitor versus β-blocker for the treatment of hypertension in renal allograft recipients. *Hypertension.* 1999;33:862–868.
3. Mange KC, Cizman B, Joffe M, Feldman HI. Arterial hypertension and renal allograft survival. *JAMA.* 2000;283:633–638.
4. Midtvedt K, Ihlen H, Hartmann A, et al. Reduction of left ventricular mass by lisinopril and nifedipine in hypertensive renal transplant recipients: a prospective randomized double-blind study. *Transplantation.* 2001;72:107–111.
5. Midtvedt K, Neumayer H-H. Management strategies for posttransplant hypertension. *Transplantation.* 2001;70:SS64–SS69.
6. Olyaei AJ, deMattos AM, Bennett WM. A practical guide to the management of hypertension in renal transplant recipients. *Drugs.* 1999;58:1011–1027.
7. Schwenger V, Zeier M, Eberhard R. Hypertension after renal transplantation. *Curr Hypertens Rep.* 2000;2:473–477.
8. Sennesael J, Lamote J, Violet I, et al. Comparison of perindopril and amlodipine in cyclosporine-treated renal allograft recipients. *Hypertension.* 1995;26:436–444.
9. Stigant CE, Cohen J, Vivera M, Zaltzman JS. ACE inhibitors and angiotensin II antagonists in renal transplantation. *Am J Kidney Dis.* 2000;35:58–63.
10. Textor SC, Taler SJ, Canzanello VJ, et al. Posttransplantion hypertension related to calcineurin inhibitors. *Liver Transpl.* 2000;6:521–530.

Index

Note: Page numbers followed by *f* refer to figures; page numbers followed by *t* refer to tables.

diagnosis of, 464
pathogenesis of, 463–464
prevention of heart failure in, 464
treatment of hypertension and, 464–465
Leptin, 30–32
hypertension and, 31–32
insulin resistance and, 132
nonsympathetic actions of, 31
obesity and, 32
receptors, 30–31
regulation of, 30
sympathetic nervous system and, 31, 32f
Liddle's syndrome, 226
Lifestyle modifications, 379, 385–387. *See also*
Antihypertensive therapy
cost-effectiveness of, 318
for hypertension in blacks, 264–265
impact of on cardiovascular risk factors,
385–386, 386t
for posttransplant hypertension, 520
prevention and implementation strategies for,
387
risk factor clustering and, 385
in weight loss therapy for obesity, 483
Lipid-lowering agents, in hypercholesterolemia,
487–488
Lipids
abnormalities of
peripheral arterial disease and, 468
treatment of hypertension and, 485–488
α-adrenoreceptor antagonist effect on, 422
and coronary heart disease risk, 485–486, 486t
Lipooxygenase products, 58–59
activity of and atherosclerosis, 59
cellular and inflammatory effects of, 58, 59t
cyclooxygenase inhibition and, 58
inhibition of, 59
Lipoxins, 59
Loop diuretics
clinical use of, 413–414
dosing of, 412t
mechanism of action of, 414
pharmacology of, 414
for posttransplant hypertension, 522
Low birth weight, 235
Low-density lipoproteins
in atherogenesis, 193
coronary heart disease risk and, 486
Lower-extremity pressure-flow evaluation, in
peripheral arterial disease, 250
Lung sounds, in heart failure evaluation, 360

Macula densa, 16
Magnesium, dietary, blood pressure and, 284–285
Magnetic resonance imaging, 344–345
gadolinium-contrast, in renovascular imaging,
367
Medulla
arterial pressure regulation by, 100–101, 101t
caudal ventrolateral, 101
rostroventrolateral, 101
Medullary thyroid carcinoma, 511
Meiosis, 213–214, 213f
Menopause, and blood pressure, 254–255
Metabolic syndrome, 130
Metabolic syndrome X, 130
Methoxyhydroxyphenylglycol, 7
Methyldopa, 424
Microalbuminuria, 474
in diabetes, 489
in renal parenchymal disease evaluation, 369
Midodrine, in autonomic dysfunction, 481
Mineralocorticoids
cardiovascular effects of, 145–146
central nervous system effects of, 146
congenital adrenal hyperplasia and, 146
molecular pathogenesis of, 146
primary hyperaldosteronism and, 147
receptors, 24–26
antagonists, treatment of hypertension
with, 26
cardiac fibrosis and, 26
hypertension and, 26

modulation of, 24
specificity of, 24
regulation of, 144
renal effects of, 144–145
Minoxidil, 438–439
Mitogen activated protein kinase, 93–94, 94f
Multiple endocrine neoplasia syndrome, pathophysiology of, 148
Myocardial infarction
ACE inhibitors after, 426
acute, plasminogen activator inhibitor-1 in,
64–65
β-blockers for, 417
non-ST segment elevation, 459
ST-segment elevation, 459

Narcotics, hypertension associated with, 517
Natriuresis
blood flow regulation and, 112
dopamine-induced, 4
Natriuretic peptides, 42–43
actions of, 42, 43t
atrial, 42–43
brain, 42–43
clinical significance of, 43
control of secretion of, 42
C-type, 42–43
metabolism of, 43
physiologic significance of, 43
synthesis of, 42
Neck, peripheral circulation and, 362
Nedd4-2, 24, 25f
Nephritis, interstitial, 372, 372t
Nephropathy
ACE inhibitors for, 426, 428
diabetic, 489
angiotensin II receptor blockers for, 430
hypertensive, diagnosis of, 208, 208t
Nephrosclerosis, in renal parenchymal disease evaluation, 372
Nephrotic syndrome, 371
Nephrotoxicity, calcineurin, 164
Neprilysin, 18–19
actions of, 18
distribution of, 19
structure of, 18–19
Neurofibromatosis, 148
Neuropeptide Y, 38–39
actions of, 38–39
blood pressure effects, 38–39
renal effects, 39
hypertension and, 39
neurohumoral effects of, 38
receptors, 38
Neutral endopeptidase. *See* Neprilysin
Nicotinamide adenine dinucleotide phosphate,
activity of, 53–54
Nitric oxide
cellular effects of, 44–46, 45f
endothelial, release of, 44, 45f
neural, 46
nonendothelial, 46
normal endothelial function and, 189
oxidative stress and, 187
vascular physiologic effects of, 46
in vascular remodeling, 181, 182
Nitric oxide synthase, 44
endothelial, modulation of, 46
neuronal, 46
Nonantihypertensive drugs, antihypertensive
effects of, 442–443
Nonsteroidal antiinflammatory drugs (NSAIDs)
blood pressure effects of, 443–445, 444f, 444t
hypertension associated with, 518–519
for left ventricular systolic dysfunction, 466
Non-ST segment elevation myocardial infarction,
antihypertensive therapy in, 459
Noradrenaline. *See* Norepinephrine
19-Noraldosterone, 28
19-Nordeoxycorticosterone, 28
Norepinephrine, 1
metabolism of, 6–7
synthesis of, 5

Normotensive syndromes, 226, 226t
N-20 terminal peptide. *See* Proadrenomedullin N-
20 terminal peptide
Nucleus tractus solitarius, 100–101

Obesity, 219
adipose tissue angiotensinogen and, 13
antihypertensive agents and, 287–288
assessment of fat burden in, 483
blood pressure management in, 484
blood pressure measurement in, 483
body fat distribution patterns and, 129–130,
130f, 286
epidemiology and clinical importance of, 129,
130f
glucose intolerance and, 287–288
hemodynamics in, 350
hypertension and, 129–131, 130f
in Southeastern United States, 234
treatment of, 482–485
insulin resistance and, 286–287
leptin resistance and, 32
lifestyle modification for, 386
pathophysiology of obesity-related hypertension and, 130–131
in polycystic ovary syndrome, 153
public health issues and, 484
risk factor clustering in, 130, 287
salt-sensitivity and, 130–131
sleep apnea and, 512–513
therapeutic goals for, 483
weight loss therapy for, 483–484
Obstructive sleep apnea syndrome. *See* Sleep apnea,
obstructive
Occlusive coronary disease, 197
Optic nerve
circulation in, 210
retinal ischemia in, 373
Oral contraceptives, blood pressure and, 256
Organ hypertrophy, angiotensin receptor regulation of, 10
Orthostatic intolerance syndromes
causes of, 479–480, 479f
diagnostic criteria for, 480, 480t
therapy of, 480
Osteopontin, 68
Ouabain, endogenous, 48–49, 49f
synthesis of, 49
Ouabain-binding sites, 220
Ovaries, angiotensin II production in, 23
Oxidative stress, 185–188
of angiotensin II, 11
oxidation of lipoproteins in, 187
reactive oxygen species and, 185–186, 186f
regulation of gene expression and, 187
in renal parenchymal hypertension, 143
in vascular remodeling, 181, 182f
Oxygen radicals, 193–194

Paracrine factors, in baroreflex modulation, 105
Parathryoidectomy, 152
Parathyroid hormone, hypertension and, 151–152
Patient education
benefits of, 401, 401t
challenges of, 401
successful programs for, 401–402, 402t
Peripheral arterial disease, 361
diagnosis of, 250–251, 363, 364f, 365f, 467
angiography in, 251
ankle-brachial index in, 250, 363, 364f, 365f
combined assessment in, 250–251, 251t
intermittent claudication in, 250
segmental pressures and waveforms in,
364
incidence of, 251
nonpharmacologic therapy in, 467–468
progression of, 251–252
randomized controlled trials of, 252
role of exercise in, 467–468, 467t
smoking cessation in, 468
treatment of hypertension in, 468–469, 468t
Perivascular fibrosis, plasminogen activator
inhibitor-1 in, 64